D1714212

Handbook of Experimental Pharmacology

Volume 170

Editor-in-Chief

K. Starke, Freiburg i. Br.

Atherosclerosis: Diet and Drugs

Contributors

J. Ahrens, M. Anthony, T. Asahara, M. Aviram, S. Bellosta,
F. Bernini, C. Bode, C. Bolego, C. Bouchard, G. Chinetti,
A. Cignarella, R.St. Clair, P. Cullen, A. Dendorfer, P. Dominiak,
C. Fontaine, J.-C. Fruchart, B. Fuhrmann, G. Gabbiani,
J. Greeve, A.K. Groen, S. Grundy, H. Hendriks, M. Hersberger,
O.M. Hess, M. Kaplan, A. Kosters, K.M. Kostner, G.M. Kostner,
P. Kovanen, M. Kratz, F. Kuipers, T. Lakka, T. Lüscher, F. Mach,
R. Mensink, D. Müller-Wieland, R. Paoletti, K. Peters,
T. Plösch, R. Robillard, M. Rosenblatt, W. Schmitz,
H. Schunkert, B. Staels, R. Stocker, P. Suter, M.A.M.A. Thijssen,
M. Tikkanen, A. van Tol, E. Vähäkangas, A. von Eckardstein,
Q. Xu, S. Ylä-Herttuala

Editor
Arnold von Eckardstein

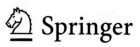 Springer

Professor
Dr. med. Arnold von Eckardstein
Institute of Clinical Chemistry
University Hospital of Zurich
Rämistrasse 100
8091 Zürich
Switzerland
e-mail: arnold.voneckardstein@usz.ch

With 78 Figures and 36 Tables

ISSN 0171-2004

ISBN-10 3-540-22569-2 Springer Berlin Heidelberg New York

ISBN-13 978-3-540-22569-0 Springer Berlin Heidelberg New York

Library of Congress Control Number: 2004113650

Springer is a part of Springer Science + Business Media
springeronline.com

© Springer-Verlag Berlin Heidelberg 2005
Printed in Germany

Editor: Dr. P. Roos
Desk Editor: S. Dathe
Cover design: *design&production* GmbH, Heidelberg, Germany
Typesetting and production: LE-TEX Jelonek, Schmidt & Vöckler GbR, Leipzig, Germany
Printed on acid-free paper   27/3150-YL - 5 4 3 2 1 0

Preface

Cardiovascular diseases continue to be the leading cause of death in the majority of industrialized countries. The most frequent underlying pathology, namely atherosclerosis, and its clinical sequelae, namely coronary heart disease, cerebrovascular disease and peripheral artery disease, remain common although for a long time we have been made aware of avoidable or modifiable etiological factors such as smoking, fat-rich diet or lack of exercise, and although these adverse lifestyle factors have been extensively addressed by population-wide primary prevention programs. Cardiovascular morbidity and mortality also remain high despite successful anti-hypertensive and lipid lowering drug therapies which help to reduce cardiovascular morbidity and mortality by about 30% in both secondary and tertiary prevention settings. This can partly be explained by the increasing life expectancy and growing proportion of elderly people, especially in Europe and North America. In addition, the World Health Organization makes the alarming prediction that probably in response to the spreading of western dietary behavior and lack of exercise resulting in an increasing prevalence of diabetes, dyslipidemia and hypertension, cardiovascular diseases rather than infectious diseases will become the most frequent cause of death worldwide.

This volume of the Handbook of Experimental Pharmacology entitled "Atherosclerosis" is divided into four parts and intends to give an overview on the pathogenesis of atherosclerosis, established treatment and prevention regimen, and of perspectives for the development of new treatment modalities.

The three chapters of part I review the state-of-the-art knowledge on the pathogenesis of atherosclerosis and its underlying risk factors. Because of its increasing prevalence and corresponding public health relevance, special attention is given to the metabolic syndrome, i.e. to the clustering of risk factors within a given individual. Although the expression of single risk factors in this situation may be moderate, affected individuals are at high risk for coronary heart disease events. In addition, due to the important etiological contribution of obesity and overweight, the metabolic syndrome is an important reason why atherosclerosis continues to be a significant public health burden.

The nine chapters of part II are devoted to the role of the various major and minor components of diet in the pathogenesis of cardiovascular risk factors and atherosclerosis. This field is currently experiencing a renaissance for two reasons: First, after fat and notably cholesterol had been accused of being "the bad guys" for a long time, novel research findings and the epidemic of obesity and diabetes produced a more differentiated view of the pathogenetic relevance of the various dietary compounds. Second, both drug and food industry have discovered diet as a therapeutic target and are currently developing drugs for the treatment and prevention of overweight and functional foods enriched by putatively cardioprotective nutrients.

The four chapters of part III give an overview of groups of drugs which in controlled intervention trials effectively prevented atherosclerotic cardiovascular disease, i.e. statins, fibrates, inhibitors of the renin-angiotensin system and antiplatelet agents. Unfortunately, beta-blockers are not covered, because the author in charge of this subject finally withdrew his commitment.

The 14 chapters of part IV present several targets and perspectives for novel pharmacological interventions. Some of these strategies led to the re-evaluation and optimization of drugs already on the market, for example nicotinic acid or agonists of peroxisome proliferating agent receptors. Other strategies helped to develop drugs which are in phase III trials and will probably be introduced into the market soon, for example inhibitors of cholesteryl ester transfer protein. Finally, some developments are still in the initial stage and must overcome methodological limitations, such as gene therapy. Especially for this part IV it is important to recall that atherosclerosis is a multifactorial disease which consequently offers many targets for treatment. Therefore, I hope that we did not leave out important developments. Some authors unfortunately withdrew their original commitment to write a chapter for this book so that, for example, important controversially discussed strategies, like hormone replacement and antibiotic therapies, are missing.

Last but not least, I wish to thank Springer Verlag and the Editorial Board for giving me the honour and chance to edit a "Handbook of Experimental Pharmacology" on atherosclerosis. I am very grateful to all authors for their excellent contributions. I also thank Mrs. Bernadette Hand (Zurich) for careful language editing and Mrs. Susanne Dathe (Springer Verlag) for her patience and help while accompanying me through this project.

Zurich, February 2005   Arnold von Eckardstein

List of Contents

List of Contributors

(Addresses stated at the beginning of respective chapters)

Ahrens, I.   443
Anthony, M.   301
Asahara, T.   777
Aviram, M.   263

Bellosta, S.   665
Bernini, F.   665
Bochaton-Piallat, M.-L.   645
Bode, C.   443
Bolego, C.   365
Bouchard, C.   137

Chinetti, G.   389
Cignarella, A.   365
Clair, R. St.   301
Cook, S.   325
Cullen, P.   3
Cynshi, O.   563

Dendorfer, A.   407
Dominiak, P.   407

Fontaine, C.   389
Fruchart, J.-C.   389
Fuhrman, B.   263

Gabbiani, G.   645
Greeve, J.   483
Groen, A.K.   465
Grundy, S.M.   107

Hendriks, H.F.J.   339
Hersberger, M.   537
Hess, O.M.   325

Jahangiri, M.   723

Kaplan, M.   263
Kosters, A.   465
Kostner, G.M.   519
Kostner, K.M.   519
Kotzka, J.   591
Kovanen, P.T.   745
Kratz, M.   195
Kuipers, F.   465

Lakka, T.A.   137
Lindstedt, K.A.   745
Lorkowski, S.   3
Lüscher, T.F.   619

Mäyränpää, M.   745
Müller-Wieland, D.   591
Mach, F.   697
Mandal, K.   723
Mensink, R.P.   165
Murayama, T.   777

Paoletti, R.   365
Peter, K.   443
Plösch, T.   465

Rauterberg, J.   3
Robillard, R.   389
Rosenblat, M.   263

Schunkert, H.   407
Spieker, L.E.   619
Staels, B.   389
Stocker, R.   563

Part I
Background

HEP (2005) 170:3–70

The Pathogenesis of Atherosclerosis

P. Cullen[1] (✉) · J. Rauterberg[1] · S. Lorkowski[1,2]

[1]Institute of Arteriosclerosis Research, Domagkstraße 3, 48149 Münster, Germany
cullen@uni-muenster.de
[2]Institute of Biochemistry, University of Münster, Münster, Germany

Abstract Worldwide, more people die of the complications of atherosclerosis than of any other cause. It is not surprising, therefore, that enormous resources have been devoted to studying the pathogenesis of this condition. This article attempts to summarize present knowledge on the events that take place within the arterial wall during atherogenesis. Classical risk factors are not dealt with as they are the subjects of other parts of this book. First, we deal with the role of endothelial dysfunction and infection in initiating the atherosclerotic lesion. Then we describe the development of the lesion itself, with particular emphasis on the cell types involved and the interactions between them. The next section of the chapter deals with the events leading to thrombotic occlusion of the atherosclerotic vessel, the cause of heart attack and stroke. Finally, we describe the advantages—and limitations—of current animal models as they contribute to our understanding of atherosclerosis and its complications.

Keywords Atherogenesis · Endothelial dysfunction · Infection · Atherosclerotic lesion · Thrombotic occlusion

1
Introduction and History

Atherosclerosis has been a companion of mankind since antiquity. Mummies from Egypt (Cockburn 1975, 1980; Magee 1998; Sandison 1962, 1981; Shattock 1909), North America (Zimmermann 1993) and China (Cockburn 1980), and dating from around 3000 B.C. to 400 A.D. showed extensive macroscopic and microscopic evidence of atherosclerosis of the aorta and of the carotid, coronary and femoral arteries (Ruffer 1911, 1920). Life expectancy even of the wealthier classes in Egypt who were subjected to mummification was in general only 25–30 years, as documented in vivid Egyptian/Roman mummy portraits dating from the first to the fourth century A.D., although some portraits of the deceased persons appear to show older individuals with wrinkles and grey hair (Egyptian Museum Cairo 1999). Even though they consumed some meat, the diet of these people was mainly vegetable and, judging from dental wear, rather coarse (Magee 1998; Ruffer 1991). Tobacco consumption was unknown although alcohol was available. It is clear therefore that atherosclerosis is an ancient process and that its pattern has always been the same regardless of race, diet and lifestyle.

It was probably Leonardo da Vinci (1452–1519) who first recognized the macroscopic changes of atherosclerosis. When he illustrated the arterial lesions in an elderly man at autopsy, he suggested that the thickening of the vessel wall was due to 'excessive nourishment' from the blood (Keele 1952; Quiney and Watts 1989). Around 1860, Félix J. Marchand (1846–1928) coined the term 'atherosclerosis' to emphasize the pathological findings of atheroma (Greek, gruel) and sclerosis (Greek, hard) seen in the intimal layer of the arteries (cited in Aschoff 1908).

From the very start, the theories concerning the pathogenesis of atherosclerosis could be divided into two broad schools, the 'cellular' and the 'humoral'. The 'cellular' school proposes that the atherosclerotic lesion mainly has its origin in changes within the artery itself. This is most commonly expressed as the 'response-to-injury' hypothesis, originally proposed in 1856 by the father of cellular pathology Rudolf Virchow (1821–1902) (Virchow 1856) and more recently championed by the late Russell Ross (1929–1999) (Ross 1993).

The 'humoral' school, by contrast, emphasizes that atherosclerosis is due to changes in the milieu within which the artery finds itself. An early proponent of such a theory was the Viennese pathologist Karl von Rokitansky (1804–1878) who in 1852 reported that fibrin plays a pivotal role in the atheromatous process (von Rokitansky 1852), a tradition that was continued by J. B. Duguid 100 years later, who also emphasized the importance of thrombosis as a factor in the pathogenesis of coronary atherosclerosis (the 'thrombogenic' hypothesis) (Duguid 1946).

Today, it is clear that aspects of both the 'cellular' and 'humoral' schools of atherogenesis are correct, in the sense that processes both outside and within the arterial wall have a profound influence on the initiation and progression of the atherosclerotic lesion. Many of the other chapters in this book deal with risk factors for atherosclerosis, with particular emphasis on diet. The present chapter will therefore confine itself to events that occur within the arterial wall during atherogenesis. Classical risk factors such as dyslipidaemia, diabetes mellitus and the metabolic syndrome, hyperhomocysteinaemia, and hypertension will not be dealt with here and we refer the reader to the relevant sections of this book for a discussion of these issues.

2
The Response-To-Injury Hypothesis of Atherosclerosis

Atherosclerosis mainly affects large and medium-sized arteries, including the aorta, the carotid arteries, the coronary arteries and the arteries of the lower extremities. The earliest lesion of atherosclerosis is called the fatty streak, which is common even in infants and young children (Napoli et al. 1997). The fatty streak is a pure inflammatory lesion, consisting only of monocyte-derived macrophages and T lymphocytes (Stary et al. 1994). In patients with hyper-cholesterolaemia, this influx of cells is preceded by lipid deposition (Napoli et al. 1997; Simionescu et al. 1986).

2.1
Endothelial Dysfunction

The response-to-injury hypothesis of atherosclerosis suggests that even before development of the fatty streak, damage to the endothelium lining the blood vessel sets the stage for lesion development. Originally, denudation of the endothelium was thought to be required (Ross and Glomset 1973), but more recent work emphasizes the importance of endothelial dysfunction (Bonetti et al. 2003; Widlansky et al. 2003). In fact, some workers have gone so far as to suggest that the endothelial status may be regarded as 'an integrated index of all atherogenic and atheroprotective factors present in an individual', a sort of 'threshold switch' that only when activated translates an unfavourable risk factor profile into actual atherosclerotic disease (Bonetti et al. 2003).

The endothelium is a continuous layer of cells that separates blood from the vessel wall. An active, dynamic tissue, endothelium controls many important functions such as maintenance of blood circulation and fluidity as well as regulation of vascular tone, coagulation and inflammatory responses (Gonzalez and Selwyn 2003). Under homeostatic conditions, the endothelium maintains normal vascular tone and blood fluidity and there is little or no expression of pro-inflammatory factors. The arterial endothelium responds to flow and to shear forces in the blood via a pathway that leads to phosphorylation of endothelial nitric oxide synthase (eNOS), which in turn produces the potent vasodilator nitric oxide (NO), thus leading to vasodilatation (Dimmler et al. 1999; Scotland et al. 2002). This response allows arteries to accommodate increases in flow and control changes in shear stress (Brouet et al. 2001). Regulation of eNOS occurs through its attachment to proteins such as caveolin (Fontana et al. 2002) and by means of phosphorylation reactions (Harrison 1997). In addition, the endothelium limits local thrombosis by producing tissue plasminogen activator, maintaining a negatively charged surface, and by secreting anticoagulant heparans and thrombomodulin (Behrendt and Ganz 2002).

Endothelial dysfunction is characterized first by a reduction in the bioavailability of vasodilators, in particular NO, whereas endothelium-derived vasoconstrictors such as endothelin 1 are increased (Bonetti et al. 2003; Yang et al. 1990). This leads to impairment of endothelium-derived vasodilatation, the functional hallmark of endothelial dysfunction. Second, endothelial dysfunction is characterized by a specific state of endothelial activation, which is characterized by a pro-inflammatory, proliferative and procoagulatory state that favours all stages of atherogenesis (Anderson 1999). Dysfunctional endothelium promotes the adhesion of leukocytes to the arterial wall and their migration into the subintimal space and also fails to inhibit the proliferation and migration of smooth muscle cells (Bonetti et al. 2003).

Many of the classical and 'newer' risk factors associated with atherosclerosis such as smoking, hyperlipidaemia, diabetes mellitus, hypertension (Celermajer et al. 1992; Libby et al. 2002), obesity (Steinberg et al. 1996), elevated C-reactive protein (Fichtlscherer et al. 2000), and chronic systemic infection (Prasad et al. 2002) have been found to be associated with endothelial dysfunction. The exact nature of the link is unknown, but may also involve reactive oxygen species. Thus, it has been postulated that at an early stage in the atherosclerotic process, oxidatively modified low-density lipoprotein (LDL) may activate protein kinase C and thus nuclear factor-κB (NFκB), a transcription factor that increases the transcription of genes encoding angiotensin converting enzyme, endothelial cell surface adhesion molecules and enzymes that further promote oxidative stress (Cai and Harrison 2000; Libby et al. 2002; Murohara et al. 1994). Reactive oxygen species may also react directly with NO, reducing its bioavailability and promoting cellular damage (Tomasian et al. 2000; Yura et al. 1999). In addition, binding of oxygen free radicals to NO may produce a toxic product, peroxynitrite, which destabilizes the production of eNOS and causes uncoupling of the enzyme, leading to production of free radicals rather than NO. Increased membrane concentrations of cholesterol lead to up-regulation of caveolin, which binds eNOS and limits NO production. Cofactors in the release of NO from arginine become oxidized and may impair eNOS function (Vasquez-Vivar et al. 1998). In addition, abnormal substrates such as asymmetric dimethylarginine may compete to block the enzyme and thus also limit NO production (Cooke 2000). It is unclear which of these mechanisms predominates in human atherosclerosis, but the end result is a failure to produce sufficient amounts of NO (Murohara et al. 1994; Ohgushi et al. 1993).

However, established cardiovascular risk factors are not the only determinants of endothelial function, as evidenced by a number of studies that showed no difference in the risk factor profile between persons with normal endothelium and persons with various stages of endothelial dysfunction (Al Suwaidi et al. 2000; Gokce et al. 2002; Halcox et al. 2002; Ohgushi et al. 1993). Although local factors, in particular haemodynamic forces such as shear stress, have been recognized as important modulators of endothelial function (Gokce et al. 2002), these findings indicate a variable endothelial susceptibility to cardiovascular risk factors and indicate the presence of other, as-yet unknown factors—including genetic predisposition—both for the prevention and the promotion of endothelial dysfunction.

Finally, it is important to note that dysfunction of the arterial endothelium is important not only at the inception of the atherosclerotic lesion, but at every stage in the life of the plaque, including in particular the events surrounding plaque rupture. This will be referred to in detail below.

2.2
The Role of Infection in Atherogenesis

The suggestion that infectious agents might be involved in the causation of atherosclerosis was first proposed by Sir William Osler (1849–1919) and others at the start of the twentieth century (Frontingham 1911; Osler 1980). In more recent times, interest has focused on four organisms: the intracellular parasite *Chlamydia pneumoniae*, the herpes viruses cytomegalovirus (CMV) and herpes simplex virus (HSV) types 1 and 2, and *Helicobacter pylori*. In addition, it has been postulated that chronic low-grade infection or recurrent infections at other sites of the body—in particular of the teeth and gums in the form of periodontitis—may also increase the risk of developing atherosclerotic disease. However, the link between infection and atherosclerosis need not be limited to these organisms. In one study of 18 atherosclerotic lesions of the carotid artery, for example, three lesions were found to contain HSV type 1 DNA, and eight contained a wide range of bacterial DNA from species that belonged either to the oral, genital or faecal commensal flora or that are present in the environment (Watt et al. 2003).

Two hypotheses have been presented to explain the presence of microorganisms in the atherosclerotic plaque: (a) a microorganism may specifically cause atherosclerosis in the same way as *H. pylori* causes gastric ulcers; (b) viruses and/or bacteria may be randomly trapped by atherosclerotic tissue during viraemia or bacteraemia.

2.2.1
Chlamydia pneumoniae

Most attention in recent years has been devoted to the link between *C. pneumoniae* and atherosclerosis. The high motivation in relation to this organism stems mainly from the fact that is amenable to treatment with antibiotics and thus might provide a rare opportunity to causally treat atherosclerosis (Kalayoglu et al. 2002). *C. pneumoniae* was first isolated in 1965, but was not properly speciated until 1989 (Grayston et al. 1990). *C. pneumoniae* has the capacity to multiply within a wide range of host cells, including macrophages and endothelial cells (Gaydos et al. 1996; Godzik et al. 1995; Kaukoranta-Tolvanen et al. 1994). Most humans encounter *C. pneumoniae* during their lives, with seropositivity rates for anti-*C. pneumoniae* antibodies achieving about 50% at 20 years and over 70% by the age of 65 years (Grayston 1992).

Four pieces of evidence suggest a role for *C. pneumoniae* in atherosclerosis: (a) some seroepidemiological studies indicate that patients with cardiovascular disease have higher titres of anti-*C. pneumoniae* antibody than controls (Danesh et al. 1997, 2000, 2002); (b) about half of all atherosclerotic lesions contain the organism or its proteins and nucleic acids. Furthermore, the pathogen has been isolated from atheroma and propagated in vitro (Kalayoglu et al. 2002); (c) in vitro studies suggest that *C. pneumoniae* can modulate the function of atheroma-associated cell types in ways that are consistent with a contribution to atherogenesis; (d) in animal studies, *C. pneumoniae* has been found to promote lesion initiation and progression, and antibiotic treatment in animals has been shown to prevent the development of atherosclerotic lesions.

Despite the strong circumstantial evidence linking *Chlamydia* to atherogenesis, however, the results of trials investigating the anti-atherosclerotic effects of antibiotic treatment in humans have been disappointing. While an early study of azithromycin treatment in male survivors of myocardial infarction with high titres of anti-*C. pneumoniae* antibody appeared to show promising results (Gupta et al. 1997), these results were not confirmed in later larger studies (Anderson et al. 1999; Dunne 2000; Muhlestein et al. 2000). At the time of writing, results are awaited from the Azithromycin and Coronary Events study of 4,000 patients with stable coronary artery disease (Jackson 2000), and from the Pravastatin or Atorvastatin Evaluation and Infection Therapy trial, which will include 4,200 patients treated with the quinolone antibiotic gatifloxacin. It is hoped that these large trials will provide a definitive answer to the question of clinical usefulness of antibiotics in treating atherosclerosis.

At present, therefore, a causal role of *C. pneumoniae* in atherogenesis must be seen as speculative. Part of this lack of clarity is due to deficiencies in available diagnostic methods to detect and monitor acute, chronic or persistent *C. pneumoniae* infection. Seroepidemiological studies have used different criteria for the diagnosis of infection. Detection of the pathogen by polymerase chain reaction and immunohistochemistry also shows excessive variation between laboratories (Apfalter et al. 2001). It is also possible that *C. pneumoniae* interacts with classical risk factors such as an atherogenic lipid profile to modulate atheroma biology, further complicating the matter (Khovidhunkit et al. 2000).

On the balance of evidence, however, it is highly unlikely that *C. pneumoniae* is required for the initiation of atherosclerosis or alone can cause this complex disease. Hyperlipidaemic animals develop atherosclerosis in germ-free conditions, cardiovascular morbidity and mortality can be reduced by lipid-lowering treatment without antibiotics, and *C. pneumoniae* is not present in all atherosclerotic lesions. For the last reason alone, *C. pneumoniae* is unable to fulfil Robert Koch's postulates with regard to its atherogenic potential. Current clinical data therefore do not warrant the use of antibiotics for the prevention or treatment of atherosclerosis in humans (Kalayoglu et al. 2002).

2.2.2
Other Infectious Agents

2.2.2.1
Cytomegalovirus

Some workers have suggested that cytomegalovirus (CMV) may be a cofactor in atherogenesis (Bruggeman et al. 1999; Epstein et al. 1996; Levi 2001). Its mode of action has been thought to be either by local invasion of the arterial wall, by effects on the host inflammatory response, by interfering with endothelial function (Grahame-Clarke et al. 2003), or by perturbation of lipid metabolism (de Boer et al. 2000a; Fong 2000; Libby et al. 1997). CMV DNA has been detected in the walls of atherosclerotic arteries, but very little is known about its ability to replicate at this location. CMV has been shown to replicate in endothelial cells and smooth muscle cells that have been isolated from human arteries. The viral replicative process disrupts control of the cell cycle and increases the amounts or activities of procoagulant proteins, reactive oxygen species, leukocyte adhesion molecules, cholesterol uptake and esterification, cell motility, and pro-inflammatory cytokines (Nerheim et al. 2004). Thus, these in vitro findings suggest ways in which CMV might promote atherogenesis and its complications. In a recent study in human coronary artery, internal mammary artery grafts and saphenous vein grafts, infection with CMV was seen only in subpopulations of intimal and adventitial cells, and was enhanced in vessels that were affected by atherosclerosis (Nerheim et al. 2004). Smooth muscle cells were completely resistant to infection with CMV.

Overall, the evidence for a causative role of CMV in atherogenesis is less strong than that for *C. pneumoniae*. The presence of viral nucleic acid within the plaque is no proof of causality, and in vitro effects cannot be extrapolated to the in vivo situation.

2.2.2.2
Herpes simplex virus, *Helicobacter pylori*

As with *C. pneumoniae* and CMV, HSV and *H. pylori* have been found in atheromatous lesions, and increased titres of antibodies to both pathogens have been used as a predictor of adverse cardiovascular events (Espinola-Klein et al. 2000). However, there is no direct evidence that they can cause the lesions of atherosclerosis.

2.2.3
Chronic Infection and Atherogenesis

2.2.3.1
Periodontitis

Multiple cross-sectional studies have demonstrated a higher incidence of atherosclerotic complications in patients with periodontal disease (Arbes et al. 1999; Grau et al. 1997; Mattila et al. 1989, 1995; Nieminen et al. 1993; Syrja-nen et al. 1989). However, a problem with cross-sectional studies is that they cannot distinguish between cause and effect. For example, it is possible that atherosclerosis might exacerbate periodontal disease by causing a systemic inflammatory response or even through subclinical ischaemia (Haynes and Stanford 2003). Prospective studies of the link between periodontal disease and atherosclerosis have been inconsistent, with some showing an increase in risk (Beck et al. 1996; Morrison et al. 1999; Wu et al. 2000), while other large studies do not (Hujoel et al. 2000; Joshipura et al. 1996). There are sev-eral possible explanations for the association between periodontal disease and atherosclerosis. First, it may reflect confounding by common risk factors that cause both conditions, such as smoking, obesity and diabetes mellitus. Second, it may reflect an individual propensity to develop an exuberant in-flammatory response to intrinsic or extrinsic stimuli. Third, the presence of an inflammatory focus in the oral cavity may exacerbate atherosclerosis by stimulating humoral or cell-mediated inflammation. Fourth, the presence of periodontal infection may lead to brief episodes of bacteraemia and inocula-tion of the atherosclerotic plaques with such periodontal pathogens as *Por-phyromonas gingivalis*, *Actinobacillus actinomycetemcomitans*, or *Bacteroides forsythus*. In one recent study, the presence of antibodies to *Porphyromonas gingivalis* was specifically linked to coronary heart disease, especially in eden-tulous individuals (Pussinen et al. 2003), while in another study, severe peri-odontal disease was associated with perturbed flow-mediated dilation of the brachial artery, presumably as a result of endothelial dysfunction (Amar et al. 2003). Severe periodontal disease has also been linked to ischaemic stroke (Grau et al. 2004).

Overall, therefore, there is suggestive evidence of a modest link between severe periodontal disease and atherosclerosis (Scannapieco et al. 2003). To test the hypothesis of causality, it will now be necessary to show that reversal of periodontal disease will reverse or at least lessen the progression or complications of atherosclerosis. This question is currently being addressed in the Periodontitis and Vascular Events trial (PAVE) that is currently being run by the United States National Institutes of Health (http://www.cscc.unc.edu/pave); however, the results of which are not expected until 2008. Until the results of PAVE and similar trials are available, a causal role of periodontal disease in atherosclerosis must remain speculative.

2.2.3.2
Infectious Burden and Atherosclerosis

It has been suggested that the risk of developing atherosclerosis is not due to infection with a single agent but rather to the number of pathogens to which a person is exposed over his or her lifetime (Epstein et al. 2000; Zhu et al. 2000, 2001). Thus, in a number of studies, risk of atherosclerosis was associated with seropositivity to *C. pneumoniae*, CMV, Epstein–Barr virus, and HSV type 2 (Espinola-Klein et al. 2000; 2002a, 2002b; Rupprecht et al. 2001), the risk of atherosclerosis increasing with an increase in the number of agents to which the patients were seropositive. It has been suggested that this effect is due to a local or systemic inflammatory response generated by the infectious agents and/or an infection-induced autoimmune response involving molecular mimicry.

The idea that infectious burden contributes to the pathogenesis of atherosclerosis must at the present time also be regarded as speculative. It is possible, for example, that individuals with greater infectious burden may appear to be at increased vascular risk only because they have less access to care or a lower socioeconomic status.

3
Development of the Atherosclerotic Lesion
3.1
Different Cell Types in Atherosclerosis: Villains or Heroes?
3.1.1
Smooth Muscle Cells

There is no doubt that proliferation of smooth muscle cells plays a role in the development of the atherosclerotic lesion, especially during its initial phases. Intimal thickening caused by proliferation of smooth muscle cells stands at the beginning of plaque development, although not all areas of intimal thickening will develop into full-blown atherosclerotic plaques. Adaptive thickening is a normal development at sites of high mechanical load, starting already at the time of birth or even earlier (Ikari et al. 1999).

Proliferation of smooth muscle cells was first suspected to play a role in development of atherosclerosis based on studies of experimental injury to the vascular wall, such as removal of the endothelium by balloon angioplasty (Ross and Glomset 1973). In this case, the vessel wall reacts by induction of proliferation of medial smooth muscle cells, migration of smooth muscle cells through the elastica interna and formation of a neointima. In the course of this process the smooth muscle cells change from a contractile to a synthetic, fibroblast-like phenotype showing higher proliferation rate and active synthesis of extracellular matrix components.

Several growth factors have been shown to be involved in this process. The role of platelet derived growth factor (PDGF) was demonstrated in early studies of balloon-induced injury by Ross et al. and Stephen M. Schwartz and coworkers (Murry et al. 1997; Bayes-Genis et al. 2000) showed that insulin-like growth factors are also involved. The animal model of endothelial injury may have a clinical correlate in the development of restenosis after coronary angioplasty in humans. In both cases, proliferation of intimal smooth muscle cells is decisive for the development of a neointima. On the other hand, narrowing of the lumen after injury results only partly from the growth of a neointima, since such narrowing also results from 'remodelling', a thickening of the media by contraction without enhancement of the tissue mass (Newby 1997).

In contrast to intimal thickening after injury, which occurs fairly rapidly, the formation of the atherosclerotic plaque is very slow. Replication of smooth muscle cells within the atherosclerotic plaque is also very sluggish with replication rates of less than 1% (Taylor et al. 1995). At present it is unknown if all intimal smooth muscle cells show uniformly slow rates of proliferation, if episodic bursts of proliferation occur, or if a small number of cells show high proliferation rates within a non-proliferating surrounding. In the early 1970s Earl P. Benditt produced a strong argument in favour of the latter possibility when he reported that atherosclerotic plaques contain large monoclonal cell populations (Benditt and Benditt 1973). This remarkable result was based on findings in women, each of whose X-chromosomes encoded a different electrophoretically discernible isoform of glucose-6-phosphate-dehydrogenase. Early in embryonic development one X-chromosome is inactivated so that each tissue normally contains a mosaic pattern of paternal and maternal X-chromosomes. However, if a single cell undergoes rapid proliferation, the newly formed tissue contains only cells producing a single isoform. The finding has been confirmed by other authors, and it is now clear that fairly large patches of the normal arterial media are also formed by cells of monoclonal origin (Chung et al. 1998).

3.1.2
Macrophages

In evolutionary terms, macrophages represent an ancient part of the immune system. Closely related cells are already found in the haemolymph of primitive multicellular organisms. The principal role of macrophages is the ingestion by phagocytosis, and hence neutralization, of non-self material, ranging from aged, necrotic, apoptotic or malignant cells to microbial invaders. They also have a central role in the regulation of the immune response and secrete a wide range of cytokines, chemokines (chemotactic cytokines) and other soluble mediators. Finally, they have a very important function in the presentation of foreign peptide antigens to T cells and thus in the initiation of the T cell-mediated immune response. Macrophages develop from circulating blood monocytes and only become fully developed at their final destination. Thus, in bone, macrophages are called osteoclasts, in the central nervous system microglia, in connective tissue histiocytes, in the kidney mesangial cells, and in the liver Kupffer cells. In order to become fully activated, tissue macrophages require exogenous signals and interaction with T cells. Once the danger has passed, macrophages may also be switched off, or deactivated, by cross-linking of inhibitory receptors, by anti-inflammatory cytokines and by certain compounds such as reactive oxygen intermediates (Bogdan 2001).

One of the principal characteristics of the atherosclerotic plaque is the presence of macrophages and macrophage-derived foam cells. These cells have been studied in detail for many years in humans, in various animal models and in cell culture. Huge amounts of information on their regulation and on their effects on other cells have been generated. Nevertheless, the central question remains as to whether macrophages fundamentally inhibit or promote the atherosclerotic process. The aim of the following section is to sketch out the main functions of the macrophage in atherosclerosis and to try to come to a provisional answer to this question.

3.1.2.1
Entry of Monocytes into the Subintimal Space

In addition to the endothelial dysfunction referred to above, an early event in atherogenesis is the activation of endothelial cells. The cause of this is not known, but it may be mediated by atherogenic lipoprotein remnants or by modified LDL. Activated endothelial cells express adhesion molecules on their surfaces. First, the glycoproteins P-selectin and E-selectin on the surface of endothelial cells bind P-selectin glycoprotein ligand-1 on the surface of monocytes in the circulation, causing these to adhere loosely in rolling fashion to the endothelium. Then, a firmer interaction of the monocyte with the endothelium is mediated by the integrins vascular cell-adhesion molecule 1 (VCAM-1) and intracellular cell-adhesion molecule 1, which bind to lymphocyte function antigen-1 and very late antigen-4, respectively, on the monocyte surface. VCAM-1 may be the pivotal molecule involved in monocyte recruitment into the atherosclerotic plaque: it is up-regulated in cultured endothelial cells in the presence of oxidized LDL, it is expressed at lesion-prone sites before the appearance of grossly visible lesions and it is fairly selective for monocytes. Moreover, atherosclerosis is reduced in mice lacking VCAM-1 (Li and Glass 2002).

Finally, adherent monocytes migrate into the subendothelial space by a process known as diapedesis under the influence of chemoattractant molecules, in particular the chemokine macrophage chemoattractant protein-1 (MCP-1), which is recognized by the chemokine CC motif receptor 2 (CCR2) on the monocyte. Monocytes isolated from persons with hypercholesterolaemia are more responsive to MCP-1 because they show increased expression of the CCR2. Oxidized LDL is itself a chemoattractant, and its oxidized phospholipid components induce expression of MCP-1 by endothelial cells (Cushing et al. 1990; Subbanagounder et al. 2002). In humans, other chemoattracts that may play a role in monocyte recruitment include interleukin (IL) 8 and its cognate chemokine receptor CXCR2 together with the macrophage inflammatory proteins 1α and 1β, and the protein RANTES (regulated upon activation, normal T cell expressed and secreted), all of which bind to the CC motif receptor 5 (CCR5) on the monocyte surface. In contrast to CCR2, the main function of CCRS is to recruit monocytes from the circulating blood, CCR5 and its ligands appear to act mainly on macrophages within the plaque (Østerud and Bjørklid 2003).

3.1.2.2
Proliferation of Macrophages in the Atherosclerotic Plaque

Accumulation of macrophages is an essential step in all phases of atherosclerotic plaque development. For a long time there was general agreement that this accumulation is caused by recruitment of monocytes from the blood, which then differentiate to macrophages within the tissue. This assumption was called into question by reports of histological markers of cell proliferation on plaque macrophages. In fact, Katsuda et al. reported that in early human lesions most proliferating cell nuclear antigen-positive cells were either monocytes/macrophages or lymphocytes (Katsuda et al. 1993). More recent reports describe the induction of macrophage proliferation by oxidized LDL. According to Hamilton et al. the proliferative effect of oxidized LDL is additive to that of a macrophage growth factor, colony stimulating factor 1 (Hamilton et al. 1999), which is required for cell survival.

Proliferation of macrophages in the presence of oxidized LDL is induced by cytokines secreted by antigen-activated T lymphocytes. Göran K. Hansson and coworkers (Paulsson et al. 2000) recently showed that a substantial portion of CD4+ cells [which are generally thought to be T helper (Th) lymphocytes] isolated from atherosclerotic plaques recognize oxidized LDL as an antigen which induces them to proliferate and to secrete cytokines. This group also demonstrated oligoclonal T cell proliferation in plaques of cholesterol-fed apolipoprotein E (apoE)-deficient mice.

Thus, despite the fact that rates of cell division in the atherosclerotic plaque are very low, accumulation of cells within the lesion is caused not only by cell immigration, but also by local that local proliferation of all cell types involved.

3.1.2.3
Formation of Foam Cells: The Macrophage Dilemma—How Does the Macrophage Deal with Excess Lipid?

To be recognized by macrophage scavenger receptors, native lipoproteins must be modified to atherogenic forms. Retention of LDL within the subendothelial extracellular matrix appears to be necessary for such modifications to occur (Skalen et al. 2002). Several lines of evidence support the hypothesis that oxidation of LDL is an essential step in its conversion to an atherogenic particle (Steinberg et al. 1989). Although macrophages, endothelial cells and smooth muscle cells can all promote oxidation of LDL in vitro, we still do not know how this process occurs in vivo. Macrophages produce lipoxygenases, myeloperoxidase, inducible nitric oxide synthase (iNOS) and NADPH oxidases, all enzymes that can oxidize LDL in vitro and that are expressed within the human atherosclerotic plaque. These enzymes – in particular myeloperoxidase, iNOS and NADPH oxidase – are the means by which macrophages generate the reactive oxygen species that are essential for microbial killing and native immunity.

Unlike other cell types, macrophages express a number of scavenger receptors that are capable of taking up oxidized LDL, including scavenger receptor A, scavenger receptor B1 (SRB1), cluster of differentiation (CD) 36, CD68, and scavenger receptor for phosphatidylserine and oxidized lipoprotein (Li and Glass 2002). As a class, these proteins tend to recognize polyanionic macromolecules and may have physiological functions in the recognition and clearance of pathogens and apoptotic cells. Of the receptors present, scavenger receptor A and CD36 appear to be the most important from a quantitative point of view in terms of uptake of modified lipoprotein. In mouse models, these two receptors accounted for between 70% and 90% of degradation of LDL modified by acetylation or oxidation. This facility may also correlate directly with atherogenesis—in atherosclerosis-prone apoE knockout mice the extent of atherosclerosis is reduced when the mice also lack either scavenger receptor A or CD36. Nevertheless, the specific role that these receptors play in the development of human atheroma remains to be determined (Nicholson 2004). Uptake of oxidized LDL is mediated primarily by CD36, which recognizes the oxidized phospholipids within the particle. By contrast, scavenger receptor A recognizes the protein components of the particle.

Exposure to oxidized LDL strongly induces expression of CD36 mRNA and protein via activation of the transcription factor peroxisome proliferator-activated receptor γ (PPARγ) (Nagy et al. 1998; Tontonoz et al. 1998). PPARγ is part of the nuclear receptor superfamily that heterodimerizes with the retinoid X receptor (RXR) in order to control the transcription of genes encoding proteins involved in adipogenesis and lipid metabolism. Two oxidized metabolites of linoleic acid present within oxidized LDL, 9-hydroxyoctadecadienoic acid (9-HODE) and 13-HODE may be responsible for this activity. Thus, macrophage expression of CD36 and foam cell formation may be driven by a cycle in which oxidized LDL drives its own uptake. Moreover, expression of CD36 increases as monocytes differentiate into macrophages. Although PPARγ is not required for macrophage differentiation, it is necessary for basal expression of CD36.

In contrast to the LDL receptor that is responsible for the physiological uptake of cholesterol-rich lipoproteins, the type A scavenger receptor and CD36 are not subject to negative feedback regulation by the intracellular cholesterol content. Thus, a central problem facing macrophages within the subintimal space is how to deal with the excess cholesterol that they ingest. Since the mammalian cell possesses no mechanisms for breaking down the sterol backbone of the cholesterol molecule, the macrophage is faced with the dilemma of how to deal with the cholesterol taken up via receptor-mediated endocytosis, a problem compounded by the fact that macrophages also ingest substantial amounts of cholesterol in the form of necrotic and apoptotic cells and cellular debris. This is not a trivial issue: as will be discussed below in more detail, excess cholesterol within the cell is toxic and can rapidly lead to cell death.

So how does the macrophage deal with the excess cholesterol? First, such cholesterol is stored in the form of cholesteryl ester droplets leading to the development of the eponymous foam cells. The cholesteryl esters present within internalized lipoproteins are first hydrolysed in lysosomes and the resulting free cholesterol is transported to other cellular sites, usually the plasma membrane. This process is disturbed in the cholesterol storage disease Niemann–Pick Type C (NPC), which is caused by mutations in the NPC1 and NPC2 proteins (Blanchette-Mackie 2000). NPC1 is a membrane spanning protein with a sterol sensing domain while NPC2 is a small cholesterol-binding protein (Carstea et al. 1997; Naureckiene 2000). On arriving at the plasma membrane, lysosome-derived free cholesterol is accessible to efflux acceptors and to the endoplasmatic reticulum where it can be re-esterified (Maxfield and Wustner 2002). The enzyme responsible for re-esterification of cholesterol is acyl-CoA:cholesterol acyltransferase (ACAT) and resides predominantly in the endoplasmatic reticulum (Chang et al. 1997). Substrate availability regulates ACAT, possibly coupled with allosteric regulation, and when a threshold level of free cholesterol is reached, ACAT activity increases dramatically (Xu and Tabas 1991). As described by us, human foam cells in vitro contain a wide variety of cholesteryl esters, principally cholesteryl eicosapentaenoate, cholesteryl docosahexaenoate, cholesteryl arachidonate, cholesteryl linoleate and cholesteryl oleate (Cullen et al. 1997). Esterification of free cholesterol serves as a detoxification mechanism, but only free cholesterol is available for efflux to cholesterol acceptors (Rothblatt et al. 1999). The cholesteryl esters present in the foam cell must therefore first be hydrolysed before they can be removed from the cells. This process is accomplished by a neutral cholesterol ester hydrolase, which is present in the cell cytosol but which has yet to be completely characterized (Vainio and Ikonen 2003).

Macrophages are able to store about twice their content of free cholesterol in the form of cholesteryl esters. However, within the atherosclerotic plaque this capacity is soon exhausted. Thus, the second means in which the plaque macrophage deals with excess cholesterol is by exporting it via a number of pathways that include transfer to high-density lipoprotein (HDL) via SRB1, transfer to apoA1- and apoE-containing lipoprotein particles via at least one adenosine triphosphate-binding cassette (ABC) transporter, and direct transfer from the cell membrane either to apoE-containing lipoproteins or to other cholesterol acceptors (Nicholson 2004).

The regulation of cholesterol efflux in the macrophage is complex and incompletely understood. A central role is played by nuclear receptors that regulate the transcription of important genes in the process. Of particular importance are the dimer RXR/PPARγ, which regulates transcription of the CD36 scavenger receptor and the liver X receptor α (LXRα) transcription factor; and RXR/LXRα, which regulates the transcription of apoE and ABCA1 (Fig. 1). We have recently found that the RXR/LXR dimer is also responsible for controlling the transcription of other proteins that may well play a role in cholesterol efflux from macrophages, notably the ABC transporter G1 and adenosine diphosphate-ribosylation factor-like protein 7 (ARL7) (Engel et al. 2004) Lorkowski et al. 2001a, 2001b). Of the components of oxidized LDL, oxysterols act as ligands for LXRα, while oxidized fatty acids act as ligands of PPARγ. Other levels of regulation of these factors also exist. For example, after binding to its receptor SRB1, HDL activates the mitogen-activated protein kinase signalling pathway, which in turn leads to phosphorylation and hence reduction of both ligand-dependent and ligand-independent transcriptional activity of PPARγ (Han et al. 2002). There is some evidence that this effect is a result of the cholesterol efflux mediated by HDL and not the addition of lipid or lipoprotein (Nicholson 2004).

In addition to transfer to HDL, either via interaction of HDL with SRB1 or to interaction of apoA1 or apoE with ABCA1 (Fig. 1), other mechanisms for cholesterol efflux exist. We, and others, have shown that apoE is capable of mediating cholesterol efflux from macrophages even in the absence of cholesterol acceptors (Cullen et al. 1996), though the physiological importance of this process in human atherosclerosis is unknown. Supporting evidence for a potentially significant role of apoE in macrophage cholesterol efflux is provided by evidence from a mouse model in which specific expression of the apoE gene in the macrophages of apoE knockout mice rescued these animals

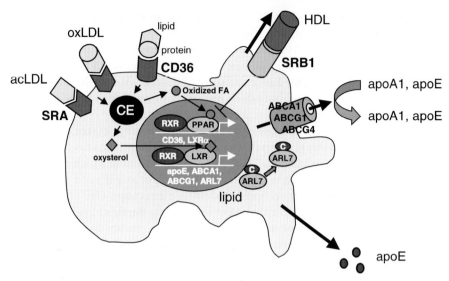

Fig. 1 Regulation of cholesterol flux in macrophages. CD36 and the ATP binding cassette transporter A1 (*ABCA1*) are regulated in response to lipid agonists derived from oxidized low-density lipoproteins (*oxLDL*), which are in turn internalized via the CD36 or the type A scavenger receptor (*SRA*). The SRA is also the principal means by which acetylated LDL is taken up into macrophages in one of the most commonly-used in vitro models of foam cell formation. CD36 and ABCA1 have major but opposite effects on macrophage lipid accumulation: increased CD36 expression increasing the intracellular content, while increased ABCA1 expression reduces cellular lipids. OxLDL increases CD36 expression because the oxidized fatty acids (*FA*) it contains act as ligands that activate the peroxisome proliferator-activated receptor γ (*PPARγ*). OxLDL also upregulates ABCA1 expression through PPARγ activation of liver X receptor α (*LXRα*). Oxysterols derived from oxLDL are ligand activators of LXRα and increase transcription of both ABCA1 and apolipoprotein (*apo*) E. The RXR/LXR dimer of transcription factors also stimulates the transcription of other genes thought to play an important role in intracellular macrophage metabolism such as the ATP binding cassette transporters G1 and G4 (*ABCG1*, *ABCG4*) and the adenosine diphosphate-ribosylation factor-like protein 7 (*ARL7*) (Engel et al. 2001, 2004; Lorkowski and Cullen 2002; Wang et al. 2004). ARL7 is induced by cholesterol loading and seems to be involved in transport of cholesterol between a perinuclear compartment and the plasma membrane, where the cholesterol is exported to high-density lipoprotein (*HDL*) via the action of ABCA1. HDL binds to its receptor scavenger receptor B1 (*SRB1*) and thus removes cholesterol from cells. Binding of HDL to SRB1 also down-regulates CD36 expression through the mitogen-activated protein kinase-mediated phosphorylation of PPARγ. The exact role of ABCG1 and of the newly-described ABC transporter ABCG4 in cholesterol efflux remains currently unknown. *CE*, Cholesteryl ester; *RXR*, retinoid X receptor. (See text for further details; adapted from Nicholson 2004)

from atherosclerosis (Bellosta et al. 1995). In the human, the relative importance of the ABCA1- and non-ABCA1-mediated pathways for apoE-dependant cholesterol efflux is unknown. A further layer of complexity is provided by the fact that both ABCA1 and ABCG1 promote the secretion of apoE in human macrophages (von Eckardstein et al. 2001).

Despite the amount of information that already exists, many components of the cholesterol balance mechanism in macrophages remain to be discovered. For example, we found that a new member of the ABC family, ABCG4 is regulated by oxysterols and retinoids in human monocyte-derived macrophages, and may also play a role in macrophage cholesterol homeostasis (Engel et al. 2001). More recently, we discovered that ARL7, a member of a family of small regulatory guanine triphosphatases (GTPases) that control vesicle budding in the secretory and endosomal pathways of cellular vesicular transport, is also regulated by LXR/RXR and is likely to mediate transport of cholesterol between a perinuclear compartment and the plasma membrane. On arriving at the plasma membrane, this cholesterol appears to be destined for ABCA1-mediated cholesterol secretion (Engel et al. 2004).

Within recent years, a further pathway of potential cholesterol efflux in the macrophage has been discovered, namely the shedding of membranes containing so-called lipid rafts (Gargalovic and Dory 2003). Lipid rafts are tightly packed, liquid-ordered plasma membrane microdomains enriched in cholesterol, sphingomyelin and glycolipids. Their unique lipid composition may serve to compartmentalize specific membrane proteins, including caveolins. Caveolae are a subset of lipid rafts that are characterized by a high caveolin content and formation of flask-shaped invaginations of the cell membrane measuring 50–100 nm in diameter (Anderson 1998). Three isoforms of caveolin exist in mammals (caveolin 1, 2 and 3), of which caveolins 1 and 2 appear to be present in human macrophages. Because of their tightly packed liquid-ordered state, lipid rafts are an unfavourable direct source of cholesterol for efflux, and the ABCA1 transporter does not associate with them, meaning that their contribution to lipid efflux is limited to the membrane shedding mentioned above (Mendez et al. 2001; Scheiffele et al. 1999; Schroeder et al. 1994). The physiological relevance of this process in humans is unknown at the present time.

3.1.2.4
The Foam Cell: Conductor in the Cellular Orchestra of the Atherosclerotic Plaque

Macrophages and foam cells are by no means passive participants in the drama of atherosclerosis. On the contrary, they play an active role at all stages of plaque development, interacting actively with each other and with other cell types, secreting a wide range of signalling molecules, modulating the inflammatory response with the plaque, and producing a range of proteins that affect the structure of the extracellular matrix. The main biological products of macrophages are listed in Table 1. The present review will focus on just a few of these products in order to illustrate the central role of the macrophage in atherogenesis. For further detail, the reader is referred to appropriate specialist reviews.

Table 1 Biological products of monocytes and macrophages

All essential components of the complement system

All factors needed to generate fibrin: all vitamin K-dependent clotting factors: FII (prothrombin), FV, FVII and FX; fibrinogen and tissue factor

Many prostaglandins (for review see Narumiya et al. 1999)

Many leukotrienes (for review see Samuelsson 2000)

Growth factors: platelet-derived growth factor (PDGF), transforming growth factor β (TGF-β), macrophage colony-stimulating factor (M-CSF), granulocyte colony-stimulating factor (GM-CSF)

Cytokines: tumour necrosis factor (TNF) α, interleukin (IL)1-β, IL-4, IL-6, IL-10, IL-12, IL-13, IL-15, IL-18, interferon γ (IFNγ)

Platelet-activating factor, lysophosphatidylcholine

Chemotactic cytokines (chemokines): macrophage chemotactic peptide (MCP) 1, MCP-2, MCP-3, IL-8, RANTES (regulated upon activation, normal T cell expressed and secreted), Epstein–Barr virus induced molecule 1 ligand chemokine (ELC), pulmonary and activation-regulated chemokine (PARC), macrophage inhibitor peptide (MIP) 1α, MIP-1β, eotaxin (CCR-3 receptor-specific, eosinophil-selective chemokine), macrophage-derived chemokines (MDC), thymus and activation-regulated chemokines (TARC), lymphocyte-directed CC chemokines (LARC) (for review, see Baggiolini 2001)

Oxygen radicals

Proteolytic enzymes

Components of extracellular matrix: type VIII collagen, type VI collagen (unpublished), other collagens (Weitkamp et al. 1999)

One of the main ways in which the macrophage affects its surroundings is by the production of potent cytokines. Chief among these is tumour necrosis factor α (TNFα), a small (17-kDa) protein that causes the release of a whole cascade of cytokines involved in the inflammatory response. TNFα exerts its principal effects by binding as a trimer to either of two membrane receptors called TNF receptor superfamily type 1A (TNFRSF1A) and TNF receptor superfamily type 1B (TNFRSF1B). This binding leads in turn to downstream activation of the transcription factor NFκB, which is translocated into the nucleus where target genes are activated. Both cytosolic and secretory phospholipase A_2 are thought to play a role in this process.

A second important cytokine is IL-x1β. During inflammation, transcription of IL-1β is stimulated by immune complexes, coagulation and complement proteins, substance P and bacterial products, most notably lipopolysaccharide. IL-1β is also induced by cytokines of lymphocyte origin such as granulocyte-macrophage colony stimulating factor (GM-CSF) and interferon γ (IFNγ). Binding of IL-1β to its receptor also activates NFκB. Together with TNFα, IL-1β is one of the main pro-inflammatory products generated by macrophages. In fact, IL-1β may mimic activation signals typically induced by TNFα (Østerud and Bjørklid 2003). IL-1β is a chemoattractant for neutrophils, induces release of neutrophils from the bone marrow to the circulation, and enhances leukocyte adherence to the endothelium. Like IL-6, IL-1β stimulates liver cells to secrete other acute phase proteins. It promotes endothelial cell proliferation and activates T cells by increasing IL-2 production and upregulating the IL-2 receptor (Østerud and Bjørklid 2003). Evidence that IL-1β is involved in atherogenesis derives from mouse models, in which blocking of IL-1β reduced plaque extent (Devlin et al. 2002; Elhage et al. 1998). IL-18 is a member of the IL-1 family and its receptor and signal transduction system are analogous to those of IL-1β (Akira 2000). IL-18 is a potent inducer of IFNγ and increased lesion development in a mouse model by provoking an IFNγ-dependent inflammatory response (Whitman et al. 2002). Moreover, IL-18 acts synergistically together with IL-12 to induce IFNγ secretion by T cells, natural killer cells and macrophages (Munder et al. 1998). In a mouse model of atherosclerosis, IL-12 was shown to promote lesion development (Lee et al. 1999a).

IFNγ plays a central role in inducing and modulating the immune response in humans. IFNγ is produced by Th1 type T lymphocytes and by activated natural killer cells. It upregulates the expression of IL-1, platelet activating factor and hydrogen peroxide by macrophages. IFNγ was shown to be atherogenic in a mouse model (Gupta et al. 1997; Nagano et al. 1997; Whitman et al. 2000).

Two further important cytokines are IL-10 and transforming growth factor β (TGF-β). IL-10 is an anti-inflammatory cytokine produced by activated macrophages and lymphocytes and has been shown to inhibit atherosclerosis formation in a mouse model (Mallat et al. 1999; Pinderski et al. 1999). TGF-β stimulates macrophage secretion of PDGF and primes macrophage chemotaxis and secretion of tissue inhibitors of matrix metalloproteinases (TIMPs). TGF-β also inhibits production of reactive oxygen and nitrogen metabolites in activated macrophages (Østerud and Bjørklid 2003).

It is important to realize that many of the cytokines produced by the macrophage have multiple and overlapping functions and that the ultimate effect also depends on the context within which the cytokine is released. The multiple and overlapping effects of some macrophage-produced cytokines are shown in Fig. 2.

A further signalling molecule that requires special mention in the context of atherogenesis is PDGF. There is much data to support the claim originally made by Russell Ross that PDGF makes a significant contribution to proliferation of smooth muscle cells in atherosclerosis (Ross et al. 1978). PDGF can be expressed by all the cells in the normal arterial wall, in particular by monocytes and macrophages. Four PDGF genes, named PDGF-A to -D exist, but only PDGF-A and PDGF-B have clearly been shown to be produced in macrophages in atherosclerosis (Evanko et al. 1998). Expression of PDGF and its receptors is increased in the atherosclerosis lesion.

3.1.2.5
Macrophage Death and Plaque Progression: Apoptosis or Necrosis?

Maintenance of a physiological ratio of free cholesterol to phospholipid in the cell membrane is essential for maintaining normal membrane fluidity (Simons and Ikonen 2000). The degree of saturation of the fatty acyl moieties of membrane phospholipids is the major determinant of lateral membrane domains, which consist of well-packed, detergent-resistant liquid-ordered rafts and more fluid, detergent-soluble liquid crystalline regions (Tabas 2002). The ability of the hydrophobic cholesterol molecule to pack tightly with the saturated fatty acyl groups of membrane phospholipids is critical for the formation of liquid-ordered rafts (Simons and Ikonen 2000), so that cholesterol depletion causes these rafts to break up. If, on the other hand, the ratio of free cholesterol to phospholipid becomes too great, then the liquid-ordered rafts become too rigid and the liquid-crystalline domains begin to lose their fluidity. These events in turn adversely affect membrane proteins that require conforma-

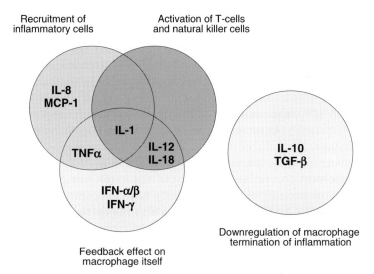

Fig. 2 Multiple and overlapping roles of macrophage-produced cytokines. Many of the cytokines produced by the macrophages within the atherosclerotic plaque have multiple and overlapping functions. Thus, interleukin 1 (*IL-1*) has functions in the recruitment of inflammatory cells and in the activation of T cells and natural killer cells, and also exerts feedback effects on the macrophage producing it. Tumour necrosis factor α (*TNFα*) helps to recruit inflammatory cells while having feedback effects on the source macrophage, while the IL-12 and IL-18 affect the source macrophage but also activate T lymphocytes and natural killer cells. By contrast, the effects of the interferons (*IFN*) α, β, and γ appears to be limited to a feedback effect on the source macrophage, while the role of IL-10 and transforming growth factor β (*TGF-β*) is limited to down-regulating the macrophage and shutting off the inflammatory response

Table 2 Potential mechanisms by which high levels of free cholesterol may kill the macrophage (from Tabas 2002)

Event	Consequence
Loss of membrane fluidity	Dysfunction of integral membrane proteins
Disruption of membrane domains	Disruption of signalling events
Induction of apoptosis	Caspase-mediated death
Intracellular cholesterol crystallization	Organelle disruption
Formation of toxic oxysterols	Oxidative damage?
Alteration of gene expression?	Change in balance of survival proteins to death proteins?

tional freedom to function properly (Yeagle 1991), such as the Na^+/K^+ ATPase, adenylate cyclase, alkaline phosphatase, rhodopsin, and transporters for glucose, organic anions, and thymidine (Tabas 2002). Thus, high free cholesterol levels may in part kill cells by inhibiting one or more vital integral membrane proteins (Table 2).

Excess membrane cholesterol may also disrupt the function of signal proteins in the membrane (Tabas 2002). Other mechanisms of toxicity include intracellular cholesterol crystallization (Kellner-Weibelo et al. 1998, 1999; Lupu et al. 1987), oxysterol formation (Brown and Jessup 1999), and triggering of apoptosis (Kellner-Weibel et al. 1998; Yao and Tabas 2000, 2001).

The response of the macrophage to excess loading with free cholesterol can be divided into two phases, an initial adaptive phase in which synthesis of phospholipids increases and a later stage when this defence is overcome and the cell dies. In the adaptive phase, an increase occurs mainly in phosphatidylcholine, synthesis of which is increased by post-translational activation of the rate-limiting enzyme in phosphatidylcholine biosynthesis, cytidine triphosphate: phosphocholine cytidylyltransferase (PCYT). How increases in free cholesterol activate PCYT is not known, but the process requires dephosphorylation of PCYT and several regulatory proteins. The up to twofold increase in cellular phosphatidylcholine leads to the appearance of whorl-like membrane structures in the cells that have been observed both in in vitro models of cholesterol loading and in lesional macrophages in a rabbit model (Shio et al. 1979).

In the face of continued exposure to rising levels of free cholesterol, the adaptive response of the macrophage will eventually fail. The basis for this adaptive failure is not known, although a decrease in PCYT activity has been seen before the onset of cellular toxicity. Morphologically, cells that are dying of free cholesterol poisoning show signs both of necrosis (e.g. disrupted cell membranes) and apoptosis (e.g. condensed nuclei) (Tabas 2002). The term apoptosis refers to the physiological process of programmed cell death that occurs in many tissues. Biochemically, apoptosis-associated caspases and their signalling pathways are activated in a portion of the cells. It is likely that a portion of the cells becomes acutely necrotic due to direct and disruptive effects of free cholesterol toxicity on membrane proteins, while others undergo a programmed apoptotic response. Some cells that first enter an apoptotic program may become necrotic later (so-called aponecrosis), perhaps as a result of chronic ATP depletion or failure of neighbouring cells to phagocytose the apoptotic bodies.

In cell culture models of macrophages loaded with free cholesterol, about 30% show such hallmarks of apoptosis as the appearance of phosphatidylserine in the outer leaflet of the cell membrane and fragmentation of the cellular DNA. These changes can be completely prevented by inhibition of a group of enzymes called caspases that are known to play a central role in apoptosis (Yao and Tabas 2001). Partial inhibition is possible by blocking the Fas receptor or the Fas signalling pathway. Activation of the Fas receptor induces apoptosis, and loading of the cell with free cholesterol causes post-translational activation of cell-surface Fas ligand, either by inducing a conformational change in the molecule or by stimulating transport of Fas ligand from intracellular stores to the plasma membrane (Yao and Tabas 2001).

Widespread mitochondrial dysfunction, indicated by a decrease in the mitochondrial transmembrane potential, is also observed in macrophages containing excessive free cholesterol (Yao and Tabas 2001). Such cells also show evidence of release of cytochrome c from the mitochondria and of activation of caspase-9. Thus, in addition to the Fas pathway, a classical mitochondrial pathway of apoptosis is activated in macrophages loaded with free cholesterol. The mechanisms by which free cholesterol triggers these events are unknown, although they appear to require the ability of free cholesterol to traffic to the cell membrane.

The presence of apoptotic and necrotic macrophages in human atherosclerotic lesions is well documented (Kockx 1998; Kockx and Herman 1998; Mitchinson et al. 1996). Among the potential causes of lesional macrophage death, toxicity due to excessive free cholesterol is a good candidate because macrophages in advanced atherosclerotic lesions are known to be loaded with free cholesterol (Tabas 1997). The functional significance of cell death is unknown. On the one hand, assuming harmless disposal of apoptotic bodies by neighbouring phagocytes, macrophage apoptosis may limit the number of intimal cells in a physiological manner that avoids inducing local inflammation. On the other hand, death of macrophages by necrosis may lead to uncontrolled proteases, inflammatory cytokines, and prothrombotic molecules, which in turn may lead to plaque rupture and acute thrombotic occlusion of the artery. Necrotic areas of advanced atherosclerotic lesions are known to be associated with death of macrophages, and ruptured plaques from human lesions have been shown to be enriched in apoptotic macrophages (Mitchinson et al. 1996).

3.1.2.6
Summary—The Macrophage in the Atherosclerotic Plaque: Friend or Foe?

Based on the above, it is unclear at the present time if the net effect of the macrophage in the atherosclerotic plaque is beneficial or harmful. Evidence exists from some mouse models that macrophages are necessary for development of the atherosclerotic plaque, and it is likely that generation of the foam cell, and in particular the overwhelming of the macrophage's capacity to deal with excess cholesterol, lie at the heart of macrophage death in the lesion. Macrophages are perhaps the central cell governing the inflammatory response within the plaque, but it is unclear if this response is physiological in that it indicates an attempt by the body to heal the atherosclerotic lesion, or if it is pathological in that it leads to growth and destabilization of the plaque. Finally, macrophages produce a very wide range of enzymes that degrade various components of the extracellular matrix. This may be one of the main mechanisms underlying plaque rupture, a complication that is compounded by macrophage expression of tissue factor and other components of the clotting cascade. On the other hand, more recent research from our own laboratory indicates that macrophages within the atherosclerotic lesion also produce a range of collagens—including several involved specifically in wound healing—and may therefore be active agents of plaque stabilization. The Janus-like nature of the macrophage within the atherosclerotic plaque is indicated in Fig. 3.

Perhaps the answer to this paradox is that net effect of the macrophage within the atherosclerotic plaque may be either beneficial or harmful depending on the stage of the lesion, its cellular composition and other compounding factors such as intercurrent illness in the host. It is in any case premature to conclude that simply because macrophage-derived foam cells are present in the advanced atherosclerotic plaque then they must be harmful, and that therefore prevention of foam cell formation must be beneficial. This is not a purely theoretical consideration. At the time of writing, ACAT inhibitors are undergoing clinical trials in humans based on just this logic (Brown 2001). Such inhibitors have been shown to prevent atherosclerosis in animal models, but the results may not apply to humans, particularly in view of the known toxic effects of raised free cholesterol levels in human macrophages (Tabas 2002). The site of action of these drugs may be the key to explaining the beneficial effects. First, even for ACAT1 inhibitors, which suppress macrophage-associated ACAT activity, the drug's ability to enter the lesion may be limited and moderate suppression of ACAT activity within the cells may be offset by increased cholesterol efflux. ACAT2 inhibitors, on the other hand, should have no direct effect on lesional macrophages and may turn out to be beneficial because of their ability to suppress production of atherogenic lipoproteins in the intestine (Buhman et al. 2000).

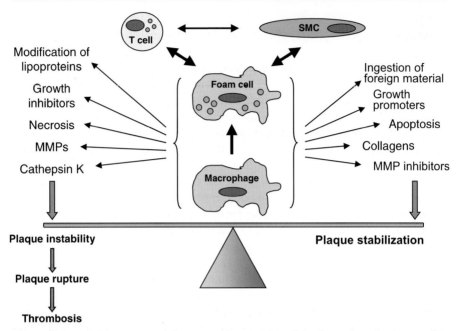

Fig. 3 The Janus-like nature of the macrophage within the atherosclerotic plaque. The macrophage of the arterial wall plays a central role in the development of the atherosclerotic plaque. The macrophage accumulates cholesterol and other lipids by uptake of modified lipoproteins and it is likely that the subsequent formation of foam cells lies at the heart of macrophage death and generation of a lipid core-containing lesion. In addition, macrophages are part of a complex network of interactions between different cell types that contribute to the pathology of the atherosclerotic artery such as smooth muscle cells (*SMCs*) and T cells. Macrophages produce an enormous range of compounds, which impact on the progression of atherosclerotic plaque formation and plaque rupture. For example, macrophages secrete several proteases such as cathepsins and matrix metalloproteinases (*MMPs*) that degrade for example collagenous components of the extracellular matrix. This may be one of the main mechanisms underlying plaque rupture. On the other hand, more recent research indicates that macrophages within the atherosclerotic lesion also produce MMP inhibitors and a range of collagens and may therefore be active agents of plaque stabilization. In addition, one of the main functions of the macrophage is to ingest—and thus to neutralize—toxic substances such as modified lipoproteins and cell detritus that would otherwise accumulate in the subintimal space. It is therefore not clear if the macrophage has a net beneficial or harmful effect on the progression of atherosclerotic plaques. The answer to this paradox may be that net effect of the macrophage within the atherosclerotic plaque may be either beneficial or harmful depending on the stage of the lesion, its cellular composition and other compounding factors such as intercurrent illness in the host

3.1.3
Mast Cells

Mast cells were first characterized in the late nineteenth century by the German physiologist Paul Ehrlich, who observed cells with metachromically staining granules in connective tissue. Ehrlich believed that the granules resulted from overfeeding of cells, and named the cells after the German word 'Mästung', to 'stuff with food' (Ehrlich 1879). His ideas regarding granule origin proved wrong, but the somewhat misleading name remained. Since then, mast cells have been shown to participate in various physiological and pathological processes, notably in allergic reactions, in the defence against parasites and bacteria, in gastric acid secretion, in lipoprotein metabolism and in autoimmune diseases (Benoist and Mathis 2002; Kovanen 1995; Metcalfe et al. 1981; Wedemeyer et al. 2000; Williams and Galli 2000).

Mast cells derive from haematopoietic stem cells in the bone marrow. The undifferentiated progenitor cells circulate in blood and in the lymphatic system before migrating to target tissues (Li and Krilis 1999; Rodewald et al. 1996), where they proliferate and differentiate into T- and TC-type mature mast cells, varying in content of tryptase, chymase and a cathepsin G-like protease as well as in immunobiology (Schechter et al. 1990; Wasserman 1990). The migration and differentiation is influenced by several cytokines such as IL-3, IL-4, and IL-9, nerve growth factor and stem cell factor (Galli et al. 1993; Madden et al. 1991; Mekori and Metcalfe 2000). The most prominent functional feature of mast cells is their ability, upon activation, to exocytose preformed mediators that are vasoactive, that regulate inflammation and cellular growth, or that have immune-modulatory effects. These mediators include the neutral proteases chymase, tryptase and carboxypeptidase A, heparin proteoglycans and histamine, prostaglandin D2, the leukotrienes B4 and C4, TNFα, TGF-β, and IL-4, IL-5, IL-6, and IL-13 (Bachert 2002; Metcalfe et al. 1997; Ra et al. 1994; Repka-Ramirez and Baraniuk 2002; Schwartz and Austen 1984; Young et al. 1987).

Mast cells are present both in normal blood vessels and in atherosclerotic lesions, where they form part of the inflammatory cell infiltrate (Kaartinen et al. 1994; Stary 1990). Increased numbers of activated mast cells are seen in the culprit lesions of patients with unstable coronary syndromes (Kaartinen et al. 1998), an observation that has led to the suggestion that mast cells participate in the pathogenesis of atherosclerosis. Indeed, there is increasing evidence that mast cells play a role in (a) recruitment of inflammatory cells; (b) foam cell formation; and (c) destabilization of atherosclerotic plaques (Kovanen 1995; Kelley et al. 2000).

3.1.3.1
Role of Mast Cells in Recruitment of Inflammatory Cells

Adhesion of circulating monocytes to the endothelium is one of the earliest steps in atherosclerosis (Li et al. 1993). Their entry into the arterial intima depends on the interaction with adhesion molecules on the surface of the endothelium. Activated mast cells secrete a variety of pro-inflammatory substances (Bradding 1996), many of which, such as TNFα, tryptase and histamine (Burns et al. 1999; Compton et al. 2000; Pober et al. 1986), cause endothelial cells to express adhesion molecules such as P-selectin and VCAM-1, which are responsible for the recruitment of monocytes and lymphocytes. Mast cells also stimulate production of macrophage chemotactic peptide 1 in fibroblasts by means of the action of TNFα and TGF-β (Gordon 2000). This in turn increases monocyte penetration into the intima. Thus, mast cells probably participate in the initiation of atherosclerosis by recruiting monocytes and lymphocytes into the vascular intima. Neutrophil infiltration has recently been shown to occur in culprit lesions in acute coronary syndromes (Naruko et al. 2002), but the triggers of this phenomenon are unknown. Both human mast cell tryptase and chymase have been shown to lead to enhanced recruitment of neutrophils into the skin of guinea pigs (He et al. 1997, 1998), but although the relevance of these findings in humans is unknown.

3.1.3.2
Role of Mast Cells in Foam Cell Formation

In atherosclerotic lesions, mast cells often reside in close association with macrophages and extracellular lipids, as well as sites of foam cell formation (Kaartinen et al. 1994b; Jeziorska et al. 1997). The 'balance theory' of atherogenesis proposes that cholesterol, carried into the arterial intima by plasma LDL, is re-circulated back to the circulation by plasma HDL. Thus, cholesterol accumulation and foam cell formation result from an imbalance between these two processes (Kovanen 1990). Increasing evidence shows that mast cells contribute to the transformation of macrophages and smooth muscle cells to foam cells in vitro by disturbing the balance between cholesterol uptake and efflux.

In order to enter the intima, LDL particles must cross the barrier of the arterial endothelium (Stender and Zilversmit 1981). Histamine from mast cells enhances vascular permeability to macromolecules (Wu and Baldwin 1992), suggesting that activated mast cells lower the endothelial barrier and increase the intimal concentration of LDL. In an animal model of passive cutaneous anaphylaxis, local activation of skin mast cells resulted in acute accumulation of LDL in areas in which mast cells were activated to secrete vasoactive components such as histamine (Ma and Kovanen 1997). Mast cells also increase the uptake of LDL by macrophages and smooth muscle cells (Kokkonen and

Kovanen 1987, 1989; Piha et al. 1995; Wang et al. 1995). The heparin proteogly-cans of mast cell granule remnants bind LDLs, facilitating chymase-mediated degradation of the apoB within the particles. This results in fusion of the LDL particles and accumulation of fused LDL on granule remnants. Granule rem-nants coated with fused LDL particles are then phagocytosed by macrophages and smooth muscle cells, thus increasing formation of foam cells. Moreover, soluble heparin proteoglycans released from activated mast cells stimulate scavenger receptor-mediated uptake of LDL (Lindstedt et al. 1992).

Efflux of cellular cholesterol is promoted by extracellular cholesterol ac-ceptors, most notably small discoidal lipid-poor preβ-migrating (preβ-) HDL (Lee et al. 1992). Mast cell chymase can proteolyse the apoA1 of preβ-HDL. This leads to reduced efflux of cholesterol from foam cells, thus increasing cholesterol deposition in the macrophages (Lee et al. 1992, 1999b; Lindstedt et al. 1996). Moreover, mast cell tryptase degrades apolipoproteins of HDL and blocks its function as an acceptor of cholesterol (Lee et al. 2002a, 2002b), although the clinical significance of this is unknown.

3.1.3.3
Role of Mast Cells in Destabilization of the Atherosclerotic Plaque

As described in detail elsewhere in this chapter, the most important mecha-nism of sudden onset of coronary syndromes such as unstable angina, acute myocardial infarction and sudden cardiac death, is erosion or rupture of an atheroma (Falk 1992; Fuster et al. 1992a, 1992b; Virmani et al. 2000). In addi-tion to macrophages, increased numbers of activated mast cells are found at sites of plaque rupture in patients who have died of acute myocardial infarction (Kovanen et al. 1995). The stability of plaques depends on the thickness and quality of the fibrous cap overlaying the lipid-rich core. The cap consists of smooth muscle cells and extracellular matrix, mostly collagen that is produced and maintained by smooth muscle cells (Lee and Libby 1997). Processes that reduce the number of smooth muscle cells, that inhibit collagen synthesis by these cells, or that increase degradation of the extracellular matrix tend to destabilize the atherosclerotic plaque.

A decrease in the number of smooth muscle cells can be caused by a lower proliferation rate or increased elimination. Mast cell-derived heparin proteo-glycans have been shown to inhibit the proliferation of smooth muscle cells in vitro (Wang and Kovanen 1999), suggesting that mast cells may participate in the regulation of smooth muscle cell growth. Since the rate of proliferation of smooth muscle cells in atherosclerotic lesions is rather low (Pickering et al. 1993), the clinical significance of such a mechanism is likely to be small. Under conditions of low proliferation, numbers of smooth muscle cells are largely controlled by cell death, either through necrosis or apoptosis. Some of the mediators released by mast cells are pro-apoptotic, such as chymase which induces cardiomyocyte apoptosis (Hara et al. 1999) and TNFα which triggers apoptosis of endothelial cells (Slowik et al. 1997). This raises the possibility that mast cells might induce apoptosis of smooth muscle cells and thus reduce plaque stability (Leskinen et al. 2001, 2003a, 2003b).

Matrix metalloproteinases (MMPs) are thought to play a prominent role in degradation of the components of the extracellular matrix of atherosclerotic plaques and to contribute to cap rupture and erosion (Galis et al. 1994; Lijnen 2002). By releasing TNFα, a potent pro-inflammatory cytokine (Kaartinen et al. 1996), mast cells induce synthesis and release of MMP9, both from adjacent macrophages (Saren et al. 1996) and from the TNFα-containing mast cells themselves (Baram et al. 2001). Moreover, TNFα has been shown to increase the expression of the MMP3, MMP8 and MMP9 in endothelial cells (Nelimarkka et al. 1998). Mast cells also synthesize and release MMP1 (Di Girolamo and Wakefield 2000), which has been found in atherosclerotic lesions (Nikkari et al. 1995).

MMPs are synthesized and secreted as zymogens, i.e. as inactive proenzymes (pro-MMPs), and must be activated after secretion (Birkedal-Hansen et al. 1993). Chymase and tryptase are both capable of activating MMPs in vitro, chymase activating pro-MMP1 and tryptase activating pro-MMP3 (Gruber et al. 1989; Saarinen et al. 1994). MMP3, in addition to being a powerful matrix-degrading enzyme, can activate other pro-MMPs, thus triggering a more extensive degradation of the surrounding extracellular matrix. In addition, chymase and tryptase can directly degrade components of the matrix such as fibronectin and vitronectin (Lohi et al. 1992; Vartio et al. 1981).

In addition to the potentially harmful effects outline above, mast cells may also have beneficial effects in atherosclerosis. Heparin proteoglycans released from activated mast cells strongly prevent collagen-induced platelet aggregation (Kauhanen et al. 2000; Lassila et al. 1997), and may thus attenuate the thrombogenicity of the exposed matrix collagen. Mast cell tryptase can interfere with coagulation by degrading fibrinogen and procoagulative kininogen (Maier et al. 1983; Schwartz et al. 1985), which could slow thrombus formation at the sites of plaque rupture. Moreover, serosal mast cells have been shown to block oxidation of LDL in vitro (Lindstedt 1993). Thus, mast cells are also anti-thrombotic and anti-oxidative cells.

3.1.4
T Lymphocytes

Atherosclerosis bears many similarities to autoimmune inflammatory diseases such as rheumatoid arthritis and multiple sclerosis (Hansson 2001; Ross 1999). As noted above, the notion that atherosclerosis has an inflammatory component was already proposed in the nineteenth century by Rudolf Virchow on the basis of light microscopic analysis of human atherosclerotic plaques. The hypothesis was later supported by electron microscopic studies and was confirmed when immunohistochemical analysis revealed that the CD14+ macrophage indeed was the major cell type in the plaque (Gown et al. 1986; Jonasson et al. 1986). More surprising was the finding that T lymphocytes were also present in substantial numbers in human atherosclerotic plaques (Jonasson et al. 1986). Recent studies demonstrated that presence of T lymphocytes has functional consequences in atherogenesis, because their complete absence reduces lesion formation during moderate hypercholesterolaemia (Dansky et al. 1997; Daugherty et al. 1997; Song et al. 2001).

T lymphocytes are cellular representatives of the specific, adaptive immune system and are designed to perform effector functions after activation by a specific antigen via the T-cell receptor. An obvious question is therefore what antigen these cells might be reactive to. In addition, is there a limited number of atherosclerosis-related antigens taking part in atherogenesis to which T cells show reactivity? The cloning of T cells specific for atherosclerosis-related antigens, such as modified LDLs (Stemme et al. 1995), heat shock proteins (Xu et al. 1993), and *C. pneumoniae* (de Boer et al. 2000b; Curry et al. 2000; Mosorin et al. 2000), from atherosclerotic lesions suggests that a cell-mediated immune reaction is taking place. Initially it was thought that atherosclerotic lesions show a monotypic or oligotypic complementarity-determining spectrum with a restricted heterogeneity of T cells (Paulsson et al. 2000). However, more recent work shows that advanced human plaques demonstrate a polyclonal T-cell composition. This does not constitute evidence that T cells are 'non-specific' (i.e. are carrying reactivities not related to atherosclerosis), but it does suggest that no single antigen reactivity dominates the T-cell population. This result in itself is not surprising, because it is known from other inflammatory conditions with known eliciting antigens that antigen-specific cells constitute a minority of infiltrating T cells. Furthermore, there is little data to support the concept of antigen-specific T-cell recruitment, suggesting instead that T-cell infiltrates arise by predominantly non-antigen specific recruitment, which may be followed by local, clonal, antigen-driven proliferation (Stemme 2001).

Many studies performed in recent years have shown pronounced effects of immunization or different approaches to immunosuppresion (Ameli et al. 1996; Fredrikson et al. 2003; Freigang et al. 1998; George et al. 1998; Maron et al. 2002; Nicoletti et al. 1998; Palinski et al. 1995; Xu et al. 1996; Zhou et al. 2001; Zhou and Hansson 2004). This is in line with the working hypothesis stating that antigen-specific T-cell activation is an important component of the atherosclerotic process. However, although interesting trials of vaccination against atherosclerosis have been performed in animals, it is unclear if a vaccination strategy would be helpful to treat or prevent atherosclerosis in humans.

The major class of T lymphocytes present in atherosclerotic lesions is CD4+. In response to the local milieu of cytokines, CD4+ cells differentiate into the Th1 or Th2 lineage (Mosmann and Sad 1996). Among the principal inducers of the Th1 and Th2 cells are IL-12 and IL-10, respectively. Activated T lymphocytes are functionally defined by the cytokines produced with IFNγ secreted from the Th1 cells and IL-4 from the Th2 cells (Daugherty and Rateri 2002). Th1 induces macrophage activation and promotes inflammation. Th1 cells accomplish this largely by secreting IFNγ, an important pro-inflammatory cytokine, which is produced in the human atherosclerotic lesion and accelerates atherosclerosis in mice (Hansson 2001). Counteracting this subset, the Th2 cell suppresses inflammation and dampens macrophage activity. Several different cytokines may be responsible for these effects, including IL-4, IL-10, and TGF-β (Hansson 2002; Hansson et al. 2002).

Thus, in summary, the presence of activated T lymphocytes in all stages of human atherosclerotic lesion implies that they are involved in the disease, although their specific role is unclear at the present time.

3.2
The Role of the Extracellular Matrix

A short look at a cross-section of a typical fibrous plaque, especially after collagen-specific staining, will immediately reveal the importance of formation of extracellular matrix in development of the atherosclerotic plaque. Large sections of the sub-intima consist of tissue that is rich in collagen but poor in cells. This exaggerated matrix deposition contributes significantly to narrowing of the arterial lumen. On the other hand, weakening of extracellular matrix in certain areas of the plaque plays a central role in plaque rupture, the most dangerous complication of atherosclerosis. 'Too much and not enough'—a description coined by Mark D. Rekhter (Rekhter 1999) aptly describes the ambivalent role of extracellular matrix formation in atherosclerosis.

Although extracellular matrix normally represents only a small part of the arterial media, its contribution to the function of the arterial wall cannot be overestimated. Extracellular matrix is the main component responsible for the elasticity and tensile strength of the arterial wall. Tensile strength is provided mainly by collagen fibres, including type I, III, and V collagens and fibril-associated components such as type XII and XIV collagens; and small proteoglycans, especially decorin and lumican. Due to their water-binding capacities, other proteoglycans, in particular the high-molecular weight versican, fill the extrafibrillar space within the extracellular matrix and contribute essentially to the regulation of water content and of the viscoelastic properties of the arterial wall. Elastic membranes providing elasticity are complex structures in which a number of microfibrillar proteins, among them fibrillin 1, are tightly associated with the rubber-like elastin.

As noted above, migration of smooth muscle cells from the media into the intima is connected with a change of phenotype from a contractile to a fibroblast-like synthetic phenotype (Owens et al. 1996). These synthetic smooth muscle cells secrete proteins of the extracellular matrix, in particular the fibril-forming collagens type I and III. This seems to be a normal physiological process at sites of high mechanical load. At some high-stress sites such as arterial bifurcations, these processes start as early as the first weeks of life and even before birth (Velican and Velican 1980). Thus, in infants, enhanced expression of type I and III collagen was localized to smooth muscle cells at a site of pressure-induced intimal thickening on the proximal site of inborn coarctation of the aorta (Jaeger et al. 1990). The formation of a neointima by recruitment of smooth muscle cells from the media is of clinical relevance in the process of restenosis after lumen widening by coronary angioplasty or atherectomy. Growth of a neointima is in this case much faster than in physiological or atherosclerotic neointma formation, leading to complete stenosis within weeks. Enhanced proliferation of smooth muscle cells stands at the beginning of this process. However, the decisive contribution to intimal thickening leading to restenosis comes from enhanced synthesis of components of the extracellular matrix (Fuster et al. 1995).

The role of enhanced formation of extracellular matrix in the development of atherosclerotic plaque is much more complicated than its role in restenosis and far from being understood. Recruitment of monocytes from the circulation and accumulation of subintimal macrophages to form a 'fatty streak' or 'xanthoma' may mark the start of atherogenesis, but most such fatty streaks/xanthomas regress and to do not develop into atherosclerotic lesions. As noted elsewhere, the distribution of fatty streaks and intimal thickenings in children differs from that in adults (Velican and Velican 1980; Virmani et al. 2000). Nevertheless, D. N. Kim observed formation of plaques in coronary arteries of pigs on a hyperlipidaemic diet preferably at locations of pre-existing intimal thickening (Kim et al. 1987). In hypercholesterolaemia in humans, lipids tend to be deposited in the intima in the vicinity of proteoglycans (Kovanen and Pentikainen 1999). Interaction with invading monocytes/macrophages leads to oxidation of LDL which provokes foam cell formation and accumulation and, via interaction with T lymphocytes, induction of an inflammatory process (Hansson 1997). Enhanced cytokine expression induces proliferation of smooth muscle cells, which in turn secrete enhanced amounts of extracellular matrix. Not only oxidized lipoproteins but also chemical modification of structural proteins of the extracellular matrix can initiate inflammation. Thus, non-enzymatic glycosylation (glycation) of collagen as it occurs in persons with diabetes mellitus increases the risk of plaque formation. Final products of glycosylation (advanced glycation end products, AGEs) activate macrophages via a specific receptor for AGEs called RAGE. They also enhance permeability of the endothelium and proliferation of smooth muscle cells and play a role in T-cell activation (for review see Vlassara 1996).

The final consequence of excessive formation of extracellular matrix is the formation of the typical atherosclerotic lesion, the fibrous cap atheroma, in which a core of accumulated and partially necrotic foam cells is surrounded and separated from the lumen by smooth muscle cell-derived fibrotic tissue. The smooth muscle cell-derived extracellular matrix plays and unclear role in this process. On the one hand accumulation of fibrotic tissue contributes to formation of the necrotic core by hindering nutrition of the deeper layers of the arterial wall; on the other hand the fibrous cap prevents the contact between the bloodstream and the thrombogenic content of the necrotic core.

The morphology of the intimal plaque extracellular matrix shows characteristic differences from the medial extracellular matrix. Extracellular matrix in the intima makes up a bigger proportion of total tissue and varies considerably in the degree of cellularity even within an atherosclerotic plaque. While in the cap region cell density is relatively high, the remainder of the intimal plaque contains very few cells. Compared to medial extracellular matrix, matrix in the intima contains more collagen and less elastin. In addition, the proportion of type III collagen is smaller and there is more type I, V and VI collagen (Barnes and Farndale 1999; Ooshima 1981; Rauterberg et al. 1993). Immunohistology shows the dominance of type I collagen in the fibrotic masses, but staining for basement membrane components reveals surprisingly strong occurrence of typical smooth muscle cell-associated basement membrane proteins such as type IV collagen, mostly in form of empty envelopes of former cells.

It is generally accepted that intimal smooth muscle cells are mainly involved in building up the fibrous cap and in synthesizing the collagenous matrix that provides its tensile strength. Invasion of macrophages is believed to weaken the cap by secretion of matrix-degrading enzymes such as MMP3 and MMP9 and cathepsins (Galis et al. 1994). Recent observations, however, suggest that macrophages may also be able to synthesize components of the extracellular matrix. Active collagen type I expression can be demonstrated by in situ hybridization only in smooth muscle cells in the vicinity of non-foamy macrophages (Jaeger et al. 1990). In the fibrous plaque atheroma is restricted to the cap and shoulders of the lesion and to the plaque base, there mostly in connection with vasa vasora. This suggests that macrophages may stimulate collagen synthesis in cells in their vicinity, probably by synthesis and secretion of TGF-β. It has been known for some time that macrophages themselves are producers of components of the extracellular matrix such as fibronectin, osteopontin, and proteoglycans. Recently, we showed that they are also able to synthesize and secrete at least one collagen (Weitkamp et al. 1999). Synthesis of type VIII collagen was found in human blood-derived macrophages at different stages of differentiation, and its expression was demonstrated by in situ hybridization in macrophages in the cap and shoulder regions of atherosclerotic plaques. The Janus-like nature of monocytes/macrophages in the atherosclerotic plaque can be understood if we bear in mind the main biologic function of this cell type as a wound healer. Beyond its main task of removing debris, the macrophage should have the ability to form a provisional matrix that allows and supports immigration of new tissue-forming cells.

3.3
The Role of Thrombus Formation

Thrombus formation plays an important role in atherogenesis (Burke et al. 2002; Libby 2000). Though there is little evidence that the formation of a blood clot is an early feature of lesion formation as was originally thought by Karl von Rokitansky (Schwartz et al. 1988; von Rokitansky 1852), thrombosis affects the growth and outcome of the pathologic process in several ways:

1. Thrombus formation at the site of an atherosclerotic lesion is the commonest cause of myocardial infarction and stroke; the thrombus may occlude the artery at the site of formation or may detach and block the blood vessel downstream.

2. In most cases, the thrombus does not occlude the artery but is organized and incorporated into the vessel wall, thus contributing to the growth of the atherosclerotic plaque.

According to Renu Virmani and her colleagues (Virmani et al. 2000), thrombus may form at the site of atherosclerosis for three reasons:

1. Rupture of the cap or shoulder of a thin fibrous cap may lead to direct contact of the highly thrombogenic core with the blood stream.

2. Erosion of the endothelial layer exposes the subendothelial collagenous matrix of the intima to the bloodstream. In autopsy studies of victims of sudden coronary death erosion was the cause of thrombus formation in about 40% of cases (Arbustini et al. 1999). Erosion is more common in women than in men.

3. Rarely, thrombus may form at the site of 'calcified nodules', small regions of mineralization that protrude from the intima into the bloodstream.

Thrombi arising due to plaque rupture often fill large areas within the plaque and may be surrounded or infiltrated by areas of haemorrhage. Haemorrhagic events occur frequently in advanced atherosclerotic lesions either by infiltration of blood from the lumen through fissures or by rupture or by degradation of vasa vasora which frequently grow at the plaque base (Kolodgie et al. 2003). Due to the high thrombogenicity of the plaque base, intra-plaque haemorrhages are usually subject to clotting and undergo essentially the same fate as lumenal thrombi.

Thrombus formation is an important part of the normal process of wound healing. In injured vessels, thrombosis is the main mechanism by which blood loss is prevented. The thrombus also serves as a provisional matrix for tissue remodelling. The thrombus initially consists of a fibrin network containing degranulated thrombocytes and other blood cells. This is followed by invasion from the blood, both by polymorphonuclear leucocytes, monocytes and lymphocytes and by mesenchymal cells of the adjacent tissue. The latter consist of endothelial cells, which lead to formation of new blood vessels, and smooth muscle cells of a migrating, proliferating and synthetic phenotype. Thrombus organization is an early phase of wound healing and tissue repair. In wound healing four distinct, overlapping phases can be defined: haemostasis, inflammation, proliferation and remodelling. The process of thrombus organization in plaques reflects these phases. The phase of thrombus formation is followed by an inflammatory phase characterized by leukocyte immigration and then by a proliferative phase, which is characterized by immigration and proliferation of smooth muscle cells and endothelium and by synthesis of extracellular matrix. In the remodelling phase, which corresponds to wound contraction, the newly formed collagenous 'scar' tissue contracts, narrowing the lumen of the vessel (Yee and Schwartz 1999). The final stage in the process is not, however, the healed wound but the enlarged plaque.

Both monocytes and polymorphonuclear leucocytes adhere to and invade thrombi, although the rate of adhesion of monocytes is greater (Kirchofer et al. 1997). Young mural thrombi often show clustering of monocytes/macrophages beneath their lumenal surface. Recently, it was shown that invading monocytes not only degrade and phagocytose tissue debris but also contribute to building of a new matrix. This is achieved not only by release of chemotactic factors that induce invasion of matrix-producing smooth muscle cells, but also by expression of matrix proteins such as type VIII collagen (Weitkamp et al. 1999).

Since the middle of the twentieth century, a debate has raged concerning the origin of the mesenchymal vascular cells contributing to thrombus organization. Some have suggested that mesenchymal endothelial or smooth muscle cells may derive from blood monocytes (Leu et al. 1988). However, no in vitro conditions have yet been described in which blood-derived monocytes differentiate into endothelial or smooth muscle cells. By contrast, monocytes in culture differentiate first into macrophages and finally into polynuclear giant cells (Zuckerman et al. 1979). The discussion recently received impetus from the detection in the circulation of stem cells, especially endothelial progenitor cells with the capacity to differentiate to mesenchymal vascular cells after invasion into thrombi (Moldovan 2003).

Another important parallel between wound repair and thrombus-driven plaque growth is that both processes are driven by almost the same panel of chemokines, cytokines and growth factors. The most important factor initiating platelet activation leading to thrombus formation in both cases is tissue factor (Tremoli et al. 1999), which is present at high concentration in plaque tissue (Asada et al. 1998; Fernandez-Ortiz et al. 1994). Invasion of monocytes is stimulated by MCP-1 and invasion and proliferation of smooth muscle cells is driven by PDGF and by thrombin. Thrombin also activates smooth muscle cells via protease-activated receptors (PARs) and stimulates synthesis of type 1 collagen by a PAR-1 mediated mechanism (Dabbagh et al. 1998). The fibrin matrix of the thrombus also supports migration of smooth muscle cells. Production of components of the extracellular matrix by smooth muscle cells is stimulated by TGF-β, which is released both by platelets and by monocyte-derived macrophages.

Finally, degradation and solubilization of thrombi is inhibited by specific anti-fibrinolytic properties of atherosclerotic vessels. Christ et al. showed that smooth muscle cells from atherosclerotic vessels produce less tissue plasminogen activator and more plasminogen activator inhibitor than smooth muscle cells from normal vessels (Christ et al. 1997).

Why did evolution allow development of an apparently self-destructive mechanism whereby thrombus formation leads to growth of the atherosclerotic plaque? Russell Ross once called atherosclerosis 'a defence mechanism gone awry' (Ross 1981). This idea fits very well to the thrombotic process in atherosclerosis. Thus, our question may be answered by another one. Why should evolution care about atherosclerosis at all? In the vast majority of cases, atherosclerosis occurs at an age that is of minor relevance for reproduction. Efficient wound healing mechanisms, however, are essential for survival at any period of life.

3.4
The Role of Calcification

Calcification is a common and early feature of atheroma. Indeed, calcification within a coronary artery is almost always an indication of the presence of an atherosclerotic plaque (Detrano et al. 2000; Sangiorgi et al. 1998; Stary 2000).

Three types of calcification are recognized in vascular tissue: cardiac valve calcification, calcification of the intimal layer associated with atherosclerosis and calcification of the tunica media (Mönckeberg calcification), which is associated with electrolyte disturbances or with metabolic disorders such as vitamin D poisoning, end-stage renal failure and diabetes mellitus. Medial calcification tends to affect arteries such as those of the abdominal viscera or the arms that are less prone to develop atherosclerosis and has never been reported in coronary arteries. It is unclear at present if medial calcification is associated with increased risk of cardiovascular events, although this may be the case in patients with diabetes mellitus (Doherty et al. 2004).

In contrast to medial calcification, calcification of the intima is seen in the distinct setting of the atherosclerotic plaque. At least two distinct patterns are seen, a punctate distribution of mineralization in the basal regions of the intima adjacent to the media, and a diffuse pattern in all areas of the intima. The latter pattern is often missed because of routine decalcification of histological specimens and is also less likely to be picked up by imaging methods (Fitzpatrick et al. 1994). The former pattern may even be accompanied by features of bone formation such as the presence of haematopoietic marrow, chondrocyte-like cells, osteoblast-like cells and osteoclast-like cells.

Several parallels exist between arterial calcification in atherosclerosis and bone formation. Three general models have been advanced. First, numerous bone-related proteins are expressed in atherosclerotic plaques at sites of calcification (Dhore et al. 2001). For this reason, it has been proposed that the mechanism of intimal arterial calcification is the same as that of bone formation (Parhami et al. 2001). Second, Cees Vermeer and colleagues have proposed a physiochemical model (Gijsbers et al. 1990; Spronk et al. 2001), whereby calcification results from a disturbance of the normal mechanism by which calcium precipitation is prevented by the presence of proteins containing γ-carboxyglutamic amino acid residues. In this model calcification occurs when matrix γ-carboxyglutamic amino acid proteins such as osteopontin and possibly other calcium chelators are no longer able to prevent the ionic calcium concentration in the extracellular fluid of the plaque from reaching sufficiently high levels to allow precipitation to occur. The third model of calcification involves the presence of osteoclast-like cells that actively inhibit calcification (Doherty et al. 2002). Many aspects of all three hypotheses are based on in vitro data and it is not known if any or all are operative in life.

Thus, overall, the role of calcification in lesion progression and in the complications of atherosclerosis is unclear at present. The main importance of calcification of the coronary arteries at the present time is therefore its usefulness as a tool to predict risk of coronary events. A range of very accurate non-invasive imaging methods exist, and many studies suggest that the coronary calcium score is a reliable and independent indicator of risk of myocardial infarction. In particular, the importance of calcification lies in the stratification of risk in asymptomatic patients at intermediate risk of coronary heart disease, in whom the calcium score appears to provide information over and above that provided by conventional risk factors.

4
From Lesion to Infarction: The Vulnerable Plaque

Until quite recently, it was assumed that the risk of myocardial infarction, stroke or sudden coronary death was related simply to the total burden of atherosclerotic disease: the greater the extent of atherosclerosis, the higher the event risk. About 10 years ago, a paradigm shift occurred when it was realized that the severe and sometimes fatal complications of atherosclerosis do not necessarily take place in those with the heaviest burden of disease. Rather, acute blockage of an artery is often caused by a clot that forms at the site of rupture of a so-called vulnerable plaque. Such vulnerable plaques consist of a lipid-rich thrombogenic core that is separated from the arterial bloodstream only by a slender and fragile layer of connective tissue, the fibrous cap. These lesions need not be large, nor need they be particularly old. No longer is the final event seen as the 'straw that breaks the camel's back', the last link in an inexorable process taking place over a very long time, but as a catastrophe resulting from an acute imbalance of stabilizing and destabilizing forces within the lesion. Such ruptures recur over many years, but do not usually cause complete occlusion of the vessel, resulting instead in mural thrombi that are incorporated into the lesion. Accordingly, rupture of the atherosclerotic plaque is often clinically silent. In addition, it is important to note that thrombosis may occur at the site of an eroded atherosclerotic plaque even without a tear in the fibrous cap of the lesion (Virmani et al. 1999, 2000).

There are therefore three main points that we need to remember:

1. The likelihood of thrombosis of an atherosclerotic vessel is not necessarily related to the volume of atherosclerotic tissue within the vessel. Rather, the likelihood of thrombosis is increased by the presence of metabolically active vulnerable plaques, which may be relatively young and small in size.

2. Thrombosis often occurs at the site of plaque rupture, but most of these thromboses are clinically silent and are incorporated into the lesion (Burke et al. 2001; Farb et al. 1996). Rupture and repair of vulnerable atherosclerotic plaques probably occur on an ongoing basis over many years.

3. Thromboses, including some leading to myocardial infarction, stroke or sudden coronary death, often occur at the site of a vulnerable atherosclerotic plaque that shows only erosion but no rupture (van der Wal et al. 1994; Virmani et al. 1999, 2000).

4.1
The Vulnerable Plaque—Rupture and Erosion

About 15 years ago, based on autopsy findings Michael J. Davies and colleagues proposed that fissuring and rupture of advanced atherosclerotic plaques are the main cause of acute myocardial infarction and sudden coronary death (Davies 1992; Davies and Thomas 1985). More recent studies, carried out in particular by Renu Virmani and colleagues at the Armed Forces Institute of Pathology in Washington DC, indicate that this picture is only partially correct (Virmani et al. 2000).

The concept of plaque rupture supposes that fracture of the fibrous cap exposes thrombogenic material, initiating platelet aggregation and coagulation in the infiltrating and overlying blood. These thrombotic changes result from activation of the clotting cascade by tissue factor, and further propagation of the thrombus through interaction of platelets with the active thrombogenic matrix. Platelet activation and thrombin formation, combined with the evulsion of thrombogenic plaque contents into the lumen of the vessel results in its sudden occlusion. This concept is based on morphological data from autopsies as well as clinical angiographic studies in which the presence of surface irregularities has been identified as evidence of plaque rupture (Ambrose et al.

1986; Giroud et al. 1992; Nobuyoshi et al. 1991). In addition, the studies by Davies and colleagues had found evidence of plaque rupture associated with thrombosis in 73% of cases (Davies 1992) This combined evidence led to the long-held and mechanistically satisfying assumption that plaque rupture is the critical event leading to coronary artery death (Ross 1999).

The major limitation of this paradigm is the lack of direct experimental test in a prospective model in humans or animals. For a variety of reasons that will be discussed in more detail below, it is unlikely that a good animal model of plaque rupture will be available in the near future (Cullen et al. 2003). Lesions in most animal models consist of masses of lipid-laden intimal macrophages without a well-developed fibrous cap, a situation that is quite atypical of human disease.

A further assumption that is unlikely to be correct in every case is that inflammation in the atherosclerotic plaque is a necessary event leading to thrombotic occlusion (Arbustini et al. 1991; Ross 1999).

Based on her findings, Renu Virmani has proposed the following classification of coronary atherosclerosis based on morphology alone as shown in Table 3 (Virmani et al. 2000). Based on this classification, the scheme for the development of the atherosclerotic plaque shown in Fig. 4 has been proposed. Examples of different stages of non-atherosclerotic arteries and atherosclerotic lesions classified according to the Virmani classification are shown in Figs. 5 and 6.

The key features defining the seven categories of lesion in the Virmani classification (initial xanthoma, intimal thickening, fibrous cap atheroma, calcified nodule, thin fibrous cap atheroma, pathological intimal thickening, fibrocalcific plaque) are the accretion of lipid in relation to the formation of the fibrous cap, changes over time in the lipid to form a necrotic core, thickening or thinning of the fibrous cap, and thrombosis. Remaining issues such as the culprit lesion associated with the thrombosis and specific plaque features representing processes critical to changes in the lesion such as angiogenesis, intraplaque haemorrhage, inflammation, calcification, cell death and proteolysis are listed as descriptive terms (Virmani et al. 2000).

Renu Virmani and colleagues propose adopting the term 'intimal xanthoma' in place of 'fatty streak', since xanthoma is a general pathological term that describes focal accumulations of fat-laden macrophages. In humans most fatty streaks/intimal xanthomas regress, as their distribution in adults is very different from that seen in children. In contrast with a widely held assumption, Renu Virmani assumes that most atherosclerotic lesions do not develop from fatty streaks/intimal xanthomas, but rather from more intimal cell masses, based mainly on the finding that the distribution of normal developmental intimal cell masses in children can be correlated with the distribution of atheroma in adults (Schwartz et al. 1995; Velican and Velican 1980).

The 'fibrous cap' of the plaque is a distinct layer of connective tissue completely covering the lipid core. It consists purely of smooth muscle cells in a collage-

Table 3 Classification of coronary atherosclerosis based on morphology according to Virmani et al. 2000

	Description	Thrombosis
Nonatherosclerotic intimal lesions		
Intimal thickening	Normal accumulation of smooth muscle cells in the intima, absence of lipid or macrophage foam cells	Thrombus absent
Intimal xanthoma, 'fatty streak'	Luminal accumulation of smooth muscle cells, no necrotic core, no fibrous cap; such lesions usually regress	Thrombus absent
Progressive atherosclerotic lesions		
Pathological intimal thickening	Smooth muscle cells in proteoglycan-rich matrix, extracellular lipid accumulation, no necrosis	Thrombus absent
Erosion	Plaque as above, luminal thrombosis	Thrombus mostly mural, occlusion rare
Fibrous cap atheroma	Well-formed necrotic core with overlying fibrous cap	Thrombus absent
Erosion	Plaque as above, luminal thrombosis, no communication of thrombus with necrotic core	Thrombus mostly mural, occlusion rare
Thin fibrous cap atheroma	Thin fibrous cap infiltrated by macrophages and lymphocytes with rare smooth muscle cells and necrotic core	Thrombus absent, may contain intraplaque haemorrhage, fibrin
Plaque rupture	Fibroatheroma with cap disruption; luminal thrombus communicates with necrotic core	Thrombus usually occlusive
Calcified nodule	Eruptive nodular calcification with underlying fibrocalcific plaque	Thrombus usually nonocclusive
Fibrocalcific plaque	Collagen-rich plaque with significant stenosis, usually contains large areas of calcification with few inflammatory cells, necrotic core may be present	Thrombus absent

nous proteoglycan matrix, with varying degrees of infiltration by macrophages and lymphocytes. Renu Virmani and colleagues define a 'thin' fibrous cap as one that is less than 65 μm thick. Fibrous caps are in fact often much thinner when they rupture—in one series of ruptured plaques they had a mean thickness of only 23 μm (Burke et al. 1997). In a series of 200 cases of sudden death, about 60% of acute thrombi resulted from rupture of a thin fibrous cap, while most of the remaining 40% of thrombi were seen at an area of plaque erosion, characterized by an area of intima denuded of endothelium where smooth muscle cells and proteoglycans are exposed to the circulating blood (Farb et al. 1995).

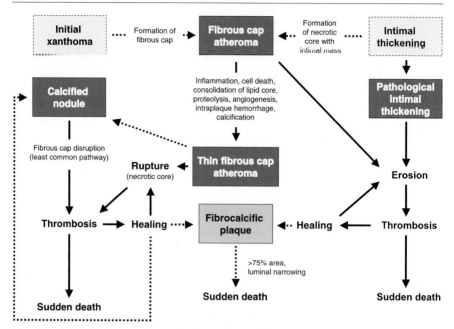

Fig. 4 Simplified scheme for classifying atherosclerotic lesions. The scheme is a modification of the current recommendations of the American Heart Association (AHA) as proposed by Renu Virmani and colleagues (Virmani et al. 2000). The boxed areas represent the seven categories of lesion. Dashed lines have been used for two categories (intimal xanthoma, intimal thickening) because there is controversy over the role that these categories play in the initial phase of lesion formation and both categories can exist without progressing to a fibrous cap atheroma (AHA type IV lesion). The processes leading to lesion progression are listed between categories. *Lines* (*solid* and *dotted*, the latter representing the least-established processes) depict current concepts of how one category may progress to another with the *thickness of the line* representing the strength of the evidence for the step depicted

A rare cause of thrombotic occlusion without rupture is the 'calcified nodule', a lesion characterized by fibrous cap disruption and thrombi in the presence of eruptive dense calcific nodules. The origin of the calcified nodule is unknown, but it may be associated with healed plaques (Virmani et al. 2000). Calcified nodules are found primarily in the right coronary artery where coronary torsion stress is maximal.

Calcified nodules should not be confused with fibrocalcific lesions that are not associated with thrombi. Fibrocalcific lesions are characterized by thick fibrous caps overlying extensive accumulations of calcium in the intima close to the media (Kragel et al. 1989). It is possible that fibrocalcific lesions are the end stage of a process of atheromatous plaque rupture and/or erosion with healing and calcification.

Despite much intensive research, we know surprisingly little about how the atherosclerotic lesion progresses and how the clinically relevant complications of stenosis, plaque erosion and plaque rupture occur.

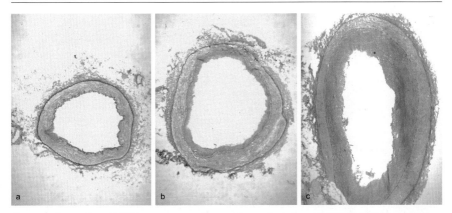

Fig. 5a–c Examples of different stages of non-atherosclerotic arteries. Samples were taken from the MAFAPS arterial tissue database and classified using the Virmani classification (Virmani et al. 2000). Human coronary arteries were obtained from hearts explanted during heart transplantation for advanced coronary heart disease as part of a tissue bank of human coronary arteries established by the MAFAPS consortium (Bellosta et al. 2002; Brinck et al. 2003). The arteries were cut into approximately 1-cm sections and snap-frozen in liquid nitrogen-cooled isopentane within minutes of explantation. Thereafter, coronary arteries were embedded and stored at −80°C until use. The grade of atherosclerosis of each sample was characterized and classified using histochemistry and immunohistology. The sections shown are stained using a van Gieson staining of the lamina elastica. **a** No intimal thickening. **b** Intimal thickening without xanthoma. **c** Intimal thickening with xanthoma

Stenosis of atherosclerotic vessels is the most common therapeutic target. However, this is the change that is least understood from a histological point of view. In an important paper published in 1987, Seymour Glagov and colleagues reported that human coronary arteries affected by atherosclerosis undergo compensatory enlargement, so that plaque mass does not correlate with the size of the lumen (Glagov et al. 1987; Virmani et al. 2000). Thus, the origin of stenosis of the lumen of atherosclerotic coronary arteries in humans is unknown, though it may be related to an attempt by the artery to heal the atherosclerotic lesion.

The origin of erosion of the coronary plaque is a complete mystery. The mechanism of fibrous cap thinning is also unknown, although we have some pointers as to how this might arise. One possibility is by means of apoptosis, yet another feature of atherosclerosis that was presciently described by Rudolf Virchow: 'thus we have here an active process which really produces new tissues but then hurries on to destruction in consequence of its own development' (Virchow 1858), cited in (Virmani et al. 2000). Many markers of apoptosis of smooth muscle cells have been found in the atherosclerotic plaque, and plaque smooth muscle cells show elevated levels of apoptosis in vitro and in vivo.

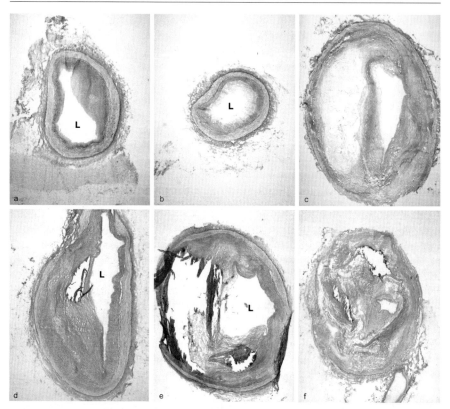

Fig. 6a–f Examples of different stages of atherosclerotic lesions. Samples were chosen from the MAFAPS arterial tissue database (Bellosta et al. 2002; Brinck et al. 2003) and classified using the Virmani classification (Virmani et al. 2000). Artery samples were obtained and processed as mentioned in the legend to Fig. 5. **a** Pathological intimal thickening. **b** Pathological intimal thickening with erosion. **c** Fibrous cap atheroma. **d** Thin fibrous cap atheroma. **e** Plaque rupture. **f** Fibrocalcific plaque. Examples for a fibrous cap atheroma with erosion and a plaque rupture by calcified nodule are not shown. *L*, Lumen

5
Animal Models of Atherosclerosis

Animals have been used for nearly a century to study atherosclerosis and have yielded very important insights into pathogenesis and therapy. However, these successes have sometimes led to uncritical transfer of results of findings in animal models to the situation in humans. In the following we will therefore focus on some of the limitations of existing models as they apply to pathology in humans. This issue has been reviewed in more detail by us elsewhere (Cullen et al. 2003).

5.1
Non-mouse Animal Models of Atherosclerosis

Rabbits develop lipid-rich arterial lesions with some of the features of atherosclerosis only if they are fed large amounts of cholesterol and fat—components that are usually lacking in their vegetarian diet. Indeed, it was in cholesterol-fed rabbits that aortic cholesterol accumulation was first noted by Nikolai Anitschkow in St. Petersburg 90 years ago (Anitschkow 1913). Such diets result in cholesterol levels many times greater than those seen in humans. The lesions that rabbits develop bear only a superficial resemblance to human atheroma, being more fatty and macrophage rich (Badimon 2001).

White Carneau pigeons develop lesions that are morphologically and ultrastructurally more similar to human atherosclerosis (Clarkson et al. 1959; Jerome and Lewis 1985, 1997; Santerre et al. 1972). However, in contrast with humans, susceptibility to atherosclerosis in these birds lies entirely at the level of the arterial wall. Cholesterol levels are normal and other risk factors are absent (Clarkson et al. 1959), the lesions in the pigeons being thought to be entirely due to an inherited (Smith et al. 2001) defect in cholesterol efflux from macrophages (Yancey and St. Clair 1992, 1994).

On a high-cholesterol diet, primates including chimpanzees, squirrel monkeys, howler monkeys, rhesus monkeys and cynomolgous monkeys develop a form of atherosclerosis that is very similar to that of humans (Malinow and Maruffo 1965, 1966; Maruffo and Malinow 1966; Stary and Malinow 1982). However, the cost of primates is prohibitive and many of these species are protected. Thus, work on atherosclerosis in primates is today generally confined to the study of complex issues such as the effects of psychological stress (Rozanski et al. 1999).

The pig is one of the most useful currently available animal models of atherosclerosis. In time, pigs develop atherosclerosis even on a normal porcine diet (Badimon et al. 1985; Fuster et al. 1985; Poeyo Palazón et al. 1998; Royo et al. 2000; Steele et al. 1985). When fed with cholesterol, they develop plasma cholesterol levels and atherosclerotic lesions that are similar to those seen in humans. The white Belgian pig variety also exhibits sudden coronary death when under stress (Badimon 2001). However, maintenance of pigs is expensive and difficult, requiring special facilities that are beyond the capabilities of most laboratories.

Dogs and rats are generally very resistant to atherosclerosis, and develop it only when their diets are very extensively modified (Badimon 2001). In recent years, however, some transgenic rat models have been produced that develop lesions resembling atherosclerosis (Herrera et al. 1999; Richardson et al. 1998; Russel et al. 1998a, 1998b).

5.2
Of Mice and Men, or Why Small Is Not Always Beautiful

Because of ease in handling, the wide knowledge base concerning mouse physiology, and the large amount of mouse genetic information available, most researchers in recent years have focused on mouse models for the study of atherosclerosis (Braun et al. 2002; Calara et al. 2001; Caligiuri et al. 1999; der Thüsen et al. 2002; Ishibashi et al. 1994; Johnson and Jackson 2001; Nakashima et al. 1994; Plump et al. 1992; Rosenfeld et al. 2000; Williams et al. 2002; Zhang et al. 1992).

Before proceeding to a description of the individual models, it is important first to recall the fundamental limitations of the mouse model. Mice do not develop atherosclerosis without genetic manipulation. They have a lipid physiology that is radically different from that of humans, most of the cholesterol being transported in HDL-like particles. Furthermore, mice weigh about 25 g, some 3,000 times less than the average human. Since mouse cells are about the same size as human cells, this means that a section of coronary artery in the mouse contains about 3,000 times fewer cells than an equivalent section of human coronary artery. This is reflected in the histology of mouse arteries, in which the endothelial layer lies directly on the internal elastic lamina and the media consists of only a few layers of smooth muscle cells. In contrast with their counterparts in humans, atherosclerotic lesions in the mouse coronary artery often extend beyond the elastic lamina (Calara et al. 2001). Remodelling of the media and aneurysms are also common in mice (Carmeliet et al. 1997; Daugherty et al. 2000; Heymans et al. 1999; Tangirala et al. 1995). Furthermore, it is difficult in mice to make a distinction between plaque erosion—as defined by endothelial denudation—and complete rupture of the fibrous cap (Calara et al. 2001). Although classical eccentric atheromas with a single fibrous cap exist in lesion-prone mouse models, multiple necrotic core areas with or without separate fibrous caps are the norm (Nakashima et al. 1994; Palinski et al. 1994; Reddick et al. 1994). As pointed out by Federico Calara and colleagues, disruption of these lesions may not mimic plaque rupture in humans, placing a fundamental limit on the applicability of mouse models for investigation of rupture mechanisms (Calara et al. 2001).

In addition to these difficulties arising from the differences between mouse and human biology, there are important issues that need to be remembered in interpreting the results obtained in mouse models that have been derived by genetic manipulation. Problems may occur, for example, when two different genetic models of a particular illness are used to investigate the effect of a third genetic manipulation. An important example in the field of atherosclerosis research concerns studies investigating knocking out the gene for the type A scavenger receptor in different genetic models of atherosclerosis. Hiroshi Suzuki and colleagues reported that deleting this scavenger receptor in apoE knockout mice reduced atherosclerotic lesion size by 60% (Suzuki et al. 1997). However, Menno de Winther and colleagues found that in the apoE3 Leiden mouse model of atherosclerosis, inactivation of the scavenger receptor actually increases lesion size (de Winther et al. 1999). A possible explanation for this difference relates to the role of apoE in the vessel wall. ApoE has been shown to mediate efflux of cholesterol from macrophages, and it is therefore possible that deficiency in apoE predisposes to macrophage foam cell formation. This process of foam cell formation might be expected to be inhibited by dele-tion of the scavenger receptor, the main route by which cholesterol-loading of macrophages occurs. By contrast, macrophages from mice bearing the *apoE3 Leiden* gene show normal apoE-mediated cholesterol efflux, so that scavenger receptor-mediated cholesterol uptake does not lead to enhanced foam cell for-mation, allowing other presumably anti-atherogenic functions of the scavenger receptor to come to the fore.

As indicated by Curt D. Sigmund, a second major problem is the genetic heterogeneity that exists among the strains used to generate transgenic and knockout mice (Sigmund 2000). This may lead to a situation where ani-mals containing exactly the same genetic manipulation exhibit profoundly different phenotypes when present on diverse genetic backgrounds. For ex-ample, the extent of atherosclerosis among apoE knockout mice on a standard atherosclerosis-prone C57BL/6 background was found to be seven times greater than apoE knockout mice with an atherosclerosis-resistant FVB genetic back-ground (Dansky et al. 1999). The ideal solution to this problem is to use inbred isogenic strains in which the experimental and control mice differ only at the target locus. The next best alternative is to develop a program of inbreed-ing to a common, congenic strain, that is, one that is genetically identical to the control strain except for the single region of the chromosome containing the target gene. This is time consuming and expensive. Six generations, or 2 years, of backcross breeding are required before the genetic backgrounds are more than 99% homogenous, with rapidly diminishing returns thereafter. For example, four more generations are needed to increase genetic homogeneity from 99.2% to 99.9% (Sigmund 2000). These problems make it imperative that a detailed description of the genetic background of all mouse models used in transgenic experiments be published, and remind us that the genetic background should always be taken into account when assessing experimental results.

5.3
Animal Models of Plaque Instability and Rupture

Despite the drawbacks mentioned above, several models have been reported recently that plausibly reproduce many of the salient features of plaque rup-tures in humans. The only non-mouse model of plaque rupture was presented by Mark D. Rekhter and colleagues in 1998 (Rekhter et al. 1998). The aim of this model was not to investigate the pathophysiological mechanisms under-lying the development of the vulnerable lesion but rather to design a model 'to evaluate plaque mechanical strength/vulnerability characteristics'. In this model, two balloon catheters were used to mechanically injure and thus pro-duce a lesion in the thoracic aorta of a cholesterol and fat-fed rabbit. A third indwelling balloon catheter was then inflated and deflated to produce rupture of the lesion. From this description, it is clear that this animal model may be suitable for measuring the mechanical strength of a plaque, and, perhaps, for investigating thrombotic sequelae, but cannot be expected to provide much information about the pathophysiology of plaque rupture in humans.

The first indirect evidence of plaque rupture in the apoE knockout mouse model of atherosclerosis appeared in 1998, when Robert L. Reddick and col-leagues reported thrombus formation in the aortas of mice that were injured by squeezing with a forceps (Reddick et al. 1998). This rather unphysiological model was followed up by a report by Michael E. Rosenfeld that elderly apoE knockout mice (60 weeks old) develop lesions in the brachiocephalic artery that are characterized by the presence of collagen-rich fibrofatty nodules and xanthomas (Rosenfeld et al. 2000). These nodules contained necrotic cores and displayed evidence of intramural bleeding. This bleeding was interpreted as possibly being due to plaque rupture. Moreover, from 42 weeks onwards, mice exhibited layered lesions, implying, the authors suggested, multiple events. In a more recent report, Rosenfeld's group reported that in 30-week-old apoE deficient mice, administration of a large dose of simvastatin (50 mg/kg/day) reduced the frequency of bleeding and calcification within lesions in the bra-chiocephalic artery, which was interpreted as evidence for 'stabilizing effects [of simvastatin] on advanced atherosclerotic lesions' (Bea et al. 2002). Fed-erico Calara and colleagues followed 82 cholesterol-fed apoE and LDL receptor knockout mice for up to 12 months and 33 chow-fed apoE knockout mice for up to 20 months (Calara et al. 2001). Of the 82 cholesterol-fed animals, three showed aortic plaque rupture and/or thrombi, while of the 33 chow-fed mice, 18 showed atherosclerosis of the coronary arteries. In 3 of these 18 animals, blood-filled channels were seen within the coronary lesions. This was taken to indicate the presence of previous plaque disruption and thrombosis, followed by recanalization. These three mice also showed deep ruptures and thrombosis of the aortic origin.

Finally, much interest was generated by two recently reported models of plaque rupture in apoE knockout mice. In the first of these, from Bristol in the United Kingdom, apoE knockout mice with an unusual mixed C57BL6/129SvJ genetic background were fed a diet containing 21% lard and 0.15% cholesterol for up to 14 months (Johnson and Jackson 2001; Williams et al. 2002). Most of these mice developed atherosclerotic plaque rupture associated with luminal thrombus at the point where the brachiocephalic artery branches into the right common carotid artery. The ruptures were characterized by fragmentation and loss of elastin and smooth muscle cells in the fibrous caps of relatively small and lipid-rich plaques overlying large complex lesions. Of 98 such mice, 51 had an acutely ruptured plaque in the brachiocephalic artery and 64 died suddenly. However, the incidence of sudden death did not differ between those with brachiocephalic rupture and those without. An undisclosed number of mice in this study also suffered myocardial infarction. In the second study, lesions were induced in apoE knockout mice by placement of a silastic collar around the carotid artery (der Thüsen et al. 2002). The resultant plaques were then incubated transluminally with adenovirus bearing a p53 transgene. Over-expression of p53, a tumour suppressor gene that promotes apoptosis, reduced the cellular and extracellular content of the cap of the lesion, with a reduced cap/intima ratio. When these mice were made hypertensive by treatment with phenylephrine, 40% developed rupture of the p53-treated plaques. Several papers have also appeared in recent years of myocardial infarction in apoE knockout mice without definite evidence of plaque rupture (Braun et al. 2002; Caligiuri et al. 1999; Kuhlencordt et al. 2001). For the sake of brevity, therefore, these models will not be discussed further here, even though some have enthused that their existence should 'finally put to rest the notion that mice cannot be models of plaque rupture' (Palinski and Napoli 2002).

5.4
Usefulness of Current Animal Models of Plaque Instability and Rupture

Of the models of plaque rupture presented thus far, none can be regarded as ideal. Both the rabbit model presented by Rekhter (Rekhter et al. 1998) and the apoE knockout mouse p53/silastic cuff model (der Thüsen et al. 2002) required such heroic measures to produce evidence of plaque rupture that they can tell us little about the pathophysiology of this condition. The usefulness of these models is thus more or less confined to studies of the mechanical process of rupture itself. More interesting from the aetiological and therapeutic points of view are the apoE mouse models in which plaque rupture was seen in elderly fat- and cholesterol-fed mice (Calara et al. 2001; Johnson and Jackson 2001; Rosenfeld et al. 2000; Williams et al. 2002). However, these models too are surrounded by caveats. In the report of Calara and colleagues (Calara et al. 2001), evidence of rupture was indirect and was seen much less frequently (about 5% of the animals) than occurs in human atherosclerosis. In the Rosenfeld model, evidence of rupture was also indirect and was seen in the brachiocephalic artery in particular (Rosenfeld et al. 2000). Finally, in the Bristol model (Johnson and Jackson 2001; Williams et al. 2002), plaque rupture was again focused on the brachiocephalic artery, and was seen only in older mice after prolonged feeding with a very-high-fat diet. The Bristol group has speculated that the predilection for plaque rupture in the brachiocephalic artery may reflect the high degree of tension in the wall of this artery in the mouse. A more general drawback of both the Rosenfeld and Bristol models is that neither shows convincing evidence of the formation of platelet- and fibrin-rich thrombus at the site of presumed rupture. This is a very important limitation, as infarction of the heart or brain in humans is not caused by rupture of the artery per se, but by the formation of an occlusive blood clot that is rich in platelets and fibrin. Perhaps as a reflection of this lack of thrombosis, death of the mice in Bristol was not related to plaque rupture. Furthermore, in the absence of thrombosis, intra-plaque haemorrhage in these models has been presumed to reflect prior plaque rupture, but this may not necessarily be the case (Majesky 2002). The Rosenfeld and Bristol models also have the disadvantages of the expense required to maintain the mice for more than a year and the variable incidence of plaque rupture.

6
Conclusions

Atherosclerosis in humans is a multi-factorial condition that develops over many years, and we are far from completely understanding its pathogenesis. Of the early lesions that form, most will regress, and some will go on to form atherosclerosis, although we do not know why a particular lesion takes one path or the other. In particular, we are in the dark about the features of atherosclerosis that lead to its clinical impact: stenosis, thrombosis and occlusion. Human coronary arteries affected by atherosclerosis undergo compensatory enlargement, and plaque mass does not correlate with the size of the lumen, so that the origin of stenosis of the lumen is unknown. Occlusive thrombosis often occurs at the site of plaque rupture, but many, perhaps even most plaque ruptures do not cause occlusive thrombosis. Equally, occlusive thrombosis may occur in the absence of plaque rupture at the site of superficial erosion of the endothelium. Perhaps the most that can be said is that occlusive thrombosis of a coronary artery requires some degree of atherosclerosis and will not occur if the vessels are normal. And although we know much of the risk factors leading to myocardial infarction, we do not know in the individual case why an occlusive clot occurs at a particular location at a particular time. Nevertheless, much knowledge of a pragmatic nature exists on how to prevent and treat atherosclerosis. This will form the subject of the remainder of this book.

References

Akira S (2000) The role of IL-18 in innate immunity. Curr Op Lipidol 12:59–63

Al Suwaidi J, Hamasaki S, Higano ST, Nishimura RA, Holmes DR Jr, Lerman A (2000) Long-term follow-up of patients with mild coronary artery disease and endothelial dysfunction. Circulation 101:948–954

Amar S, Gokce N, Morgan S, Loukideli M, Van Dyke TE, Vita JA (2003) Periodontal disease is associated with endothelial dysfunction and systemic inflammation. Arterioscler Thromb Vasc Biol 23:1245–1249

Ambrose JA, Winters SL, Arora RR, Eng A, Riccio A, Gorlin R et al. (1986) Angiographic evolution of coronary artery morphology in unstable angina. J Am Coll Cardiol 7:472–478

Ameli S, Hultgardh-Nilsson A, Regnstrom J, Calara F, Yano J, Cercek B et al. (1996) Effect of immunization with homologous LDL and oxidized LDL on early atherosclerosis in hypercholesterolemic rabbits. Arterioscler Thromb Vasc Biol 16:1074–1079

Anderson JL, Muhlestein JB, Carlquist J, Allen A, Trehan S, Nielson C et al. (1999) Randomized secondary prevention trial of azithromycin in patients with coronary artery disease and serological evidence for Chlamydia pneumoniae infection: The Azithromycin in Coronary Artery Disease: Elimination of Myocardial Infection with Chlamydia (ACADEMIC) study. Circulation 99:1540–1547

Anderson RG (1998) The caveolae membrane system. Annu Rev Biochem 67:199–225

Anderson TJ (1999) Assessment and treatment of endothelial dysfunction in coronary artery disease and implications for therapy. J Am Coll Cardiol 34:631–638

Anitschkow N (1913) Über die Veränderungen der Kaninchenaorta bei experimenteller Cholesterinsteatose. Beiträge zur pathologischen Anatomie und zur allgemeinen Pathologie 56:379–404

Apfalter P, Blasi F, Boman J, Gaydos CA, Kundi M, Maass M et al. (2001) Multicenter comparison trial of DNA extraction methods and PCR assays for detection of Chlamydia pneumoniae in endarterectomy specimens. J Clin Microbiol 39:519–524

Arbes SJ Jr., Slade GD, Beck JD (1999) Association between extent of periodontal attachment loss and self-reported history of heart attack: an analysis of NHANES III data. J Dent Res 78:1777–1782

Arbustini E, Grasso M, Diegoli M, Pucci A, Bramerio M, Ardissino D et al. (1991) Coronary atherosclerotic plaques with and without thrombus in ischemic heart syndromes: a morphologic, immunohistochemical, and biochemical study. Am J Cardiol 68:36B–50B

Arbustini E, Dal Bello B, Morbini P, Burke AP, Bocciarelli M, Specchia G et al. (1999) Plaque erosion is a major substrate for coronary thrombosis in acute myocardial infarction. Heart 82:269–272

Asada Y, Marutsuka K, Hatakeyama K, Sato Y, Hara S, Kisanuki A et al. (1998) The role of tissue factor in the pathogenesis of thrombosis and atherosclerosis. J Atheroscler Thromb 4:135–139

Aschoff KAL (1908) Über Atherosklerose und andere Sklerosen des Gafässystems. Urban and Schwarzenberg, Berlin

Bachert C (2002) The role of histamine in allergic disease: re-appraisal of its inflammatory potential. Allergy 57:287–296

Badimon L, Steele P, Badimon JJ, Bowie EJ, Fuster V (1985) Aortic atherosclerosis in pigs with heterozygous von Willebrand disease. Comparison with homozygous von Willebrand and normal pigs. Arteriosclerosis 5:366–370

Badimon L (2001) Atherosclerosis and thrombosis: lessons from animal models. Thromb Haemost 86:356–365

Baggiolini M (2001) Chemokines in pathology and medicine. J Intern Med 250:91–104

Baram D, Vaday GG, Salamon P, Drucker I, Hershkoviz R, Mekori YA (2001) Human mast cells release metalloproteinase-9 on contact with activated T cells: juxtacrine regulation by TNF-alpha. J Immunol 167:4008–4016

Barnes MJ, Farndale RW (1999) Collagens and atherosclerosis. Exp Gerontol 34:513–525

Bayes-Genis A, Conover CA, Schwartz RS (2000) The insulin-like growth factor axis: A review of atherosclerosis and restenosis. Circ Res 86:125–130

Bea F, Blessing E, Bennett B, Levitz M, Wallace EP, Rosenfeld ME (2002) Simvastatin promotes atherosclerotic plaque stability in apoE-deficient mice independently of lipid lowering. Arterioscler Thromb Vasc Biol 22:1832–1837

Beck J, Garcia R, Heiss G, Vokonas PS, Offenbacher S (1996) Periodontal disease and cardiovascular disease. J Periodontol 67:1123–1137

Behrendt D, Ganz P (2002) Endothelial function: from vascular biology to clinical applications. Am J Cardiol 90:40L–80L

Bellosta S, Mahley RW, Sanan DA, Murata J, Newland DL, Taylor JM et al. (1995) Macrophage specific expression of human apolipoprotein E reduces atherosclerosis in hypercholesterolemic apolipoprotein E-null mice. J Clin Invest 96:2170–2179

Bellosta S, Bernini F, Chinetti G, Cignarella A, Cullen P, von Eckardstein A, et al. (2002) Macrophage Function and Stability of Atherosclerotic Plaque Consortium. Macrophage function and stability of the atherosclerotic plaque: progress report of a European project. Nutr Metab Cardiovasc Dis 12:3–11

Benditt EP, Benditt JM (1973) Evidence for a monoclonal origin of human atherosclerotic plaques. Proc Natl Acad Sci USA 70:1753–1756

Benoist C, Mathis D (2002) Mast cells in autoimmune disease. Nature 420:875–878

Birkedal-Hansen H, Moore WG, Bodden MK, Windsor LJ, Birkedal-Hansen B, DeCarlo A et al. (1993) Matrix metalloproteinases: a review. Crit Rev Oral Biol Med 4:197–250

Blanchette-Mackie EJ (2000) Intracellular cholesterol trafficking: role of the NPC1 protein. Biochim Biophys Acta 1486:171–183

Bogdan C (2001) Macrophages. Nature Encyclopedia of Life Sciences; http://www.els.net/. Nature Publishing Group, London

Bonetti PO, Lerman LO, Lerman A (2003) Endothelial dysfunction—a marker of atherosclerotic risk. Arterioscler Thromb Vasc Biol 23:168–175

Bradding P (1996) Human mast cell cytokines. Clin Exp Allergy 26:13–19

Braun A, Trigatti BL, Post MJ, Sato K, Simons M, Edelberg JM et al. (2002) Loss of SR-BI expression leads to the early onset of occlusive atherosclerotic coronary artery disease, spontaneous myocardial infarctions, severe cardiac dysfunction, and premature death in apolipoprotein E-deficient mice. Circ Res 90:270–276

Brinck H, Cullen P, Exley A, Goddard MJ, Kummer S, Lorkowski S, et al. (2003) Internet-based image database for atherosclerosis research. Proceedings of the 17th International Congress and Exhibition Computer Assisted Radiology and Surgery (CARS) Elsevier, Amsterdam, p 301

Brouet A, Sonveaux P, Dessy C, Balligand JL, Feron O (2001) Hsp90 ensures the transition from the early Ca2+-dependent to the late phosphorylation-dependent activation of the endothelial nitric-oxide synthase in vascular endothelial growth factor-exposed endothelial cells. J Biol Chem 276:32663–32669

Brown AJ, Jessup W (1999) Oxysterols and atherosclerosis. Atherosclerosis 142:1–28

Brown WV (2001) Therapies on the horizon for cholesterol reduction. Clin Cardiol 24:III24–III27

Bruggeman CA, Marjorie HJ, Nelissen-Vrancken G (1999) Cytomegalovirus and atherosclerosis. Antiviral Res 43:191–200

Buhman KK, Accad M, Novak S, Choi RS, Wong JS, Hamilton RL et al. (2000) Resistance to diet-induced hypercholesterolemia and gallstone formation in ACAT2-deficient mice. Nat Med 6:1341–1347

Burke AP, Farb A, Malcolm GT, Liang YH, Smialek J, Virmani R (1997) Coronary risk factors and plaque morphology in men with coronary disease who died suddenly. N Engl J Med 336:1276–1282

Burke AP, Kolodgie FD, Farb A, Weber DK, Malcom GT, Smialek J et al. (2001) Healed plaque ruptures and sudden coronary death: evidence that subclinical rupture has a role in plaque progression. Circulation 103:934–940

Burke AP, Farb A, Kolodgie FD, Narula J, Virmani R (2002) Atherosclerotic plaque morphology and coronary thrombi. J Nucl Cardiol 9:95–103

Burns AR, Bowden RA, Abe Y, Walker DC, Simon SI, Entman ML et al. (1999) P-selectin mediates neutrophil adhesion to endothelial cell borders. J Leukoc Biol 65:299–306

Cai H, Harrison DG (2000) Endothelial dysfunction in cardiovascular diseases: the role of oxidant stress. Circ Res 87:840–844

Calara F, Silvestre M, Casanada F, Yuan N, Napoli C, Palinski W (2001) Spontaneous plaque rupture and secondary thrombosis in apolipoprotein E-deficient and LDL receptor-deficient mice. J Pathol 195:257–263

Caligiuri G, Levy B, Pernow J, Thoren P, Hansson GK (1999) Myocardial infarction mediated by endothelin receptor signaling in hypercholesterolemic mice. Proc Natl Acad Sci USA 96:6920–6924

Carmeliet P, Moons L, Lijnen R, Baes M, Lemaitre V, Tipping P et al. (1997) Urokinase-generated plasmin activates matrix metalloproteinases during aneurysm formation. Nat Genet 17:439–444

Carstea ED, Morris JA, Coleman KG, Loftus SK, Zhang D, Cummings C et al. (1997) Niemann-Pick C1 disease gene: homology to mediators of cholesterol homeostasis. Science 277:228–231

Celermajer DS, Sorensen KE, Gooch VM, Spiegelhalter DJ, Miller OI, Sullivan ID et al. (1992) Non-invasive detection of endothelial dysfunction in children and adults at risk of atherosclerosis. Lancet 340:1111–1115

Chang TY, Chang CCY, Cheng D (1997) Acyl-coenzyme A: cholesterol acyltransferase. Annu Rev Biochem 66:613–638

Christ G, Hufnagl P, Kaun C, Mundigler G, Laufer G, Huber K et al. (1997) Antifibrinolytic properties of the vascular wall. Dependence on the history of smooth muscle cell doublings in vitro and in vivo. Arterioscler Thromb Vasc Biol 17:723–730

Chung IM, Schwartz SM, Murry CE (1998) Clonal architecture of normal and atherosclerotic aorta: implications for atherogenesis and vascular development. Am J Pathol 152:913–923

Clarkson TB, Pritchard RW, Netsky MG, Lofland HB (1959) Atherosclerosis in pigeons: its spontaneous occurrence and resemblance to human atherosclerosis. AMA Arch Pathol 68:143–147

Cockburn A, Barraco RA, Reyman TA, Peck WH (1975) Autopsy of an Egyptian mummy. Science 187:1155–1160

Cockburn A (1980) Miscellaneous mummies. In: Cockburn A, Cockburn E, (eds). Mummies, disease and ancient cultures. Cambridge University Press, Cambridge

Compton SJ, Cairns JA, Holgate ST, Walls AF (2000) Human mast cell tryptase stimulates the release of an IL-8-dependent neutrophil chemotactic activity from human umbilical vein endothelial cells (HUVEC). Clin Exp Immunol 121:31–36

Cooke JP (2000) Does ADMA cause endothelial dysfunction? Arterioscler Thromb Vasc Biol 20:2032–2037

Cullen P, Fobker M, Tegelkamp K, Meyer K, Kannenberg F, Cignarella A et al. (1997) An improved method for quantification of cholesterol and cholesteryl esters in human monocyte-derived macrophages by high performance liquid chromatography with identification of unassigned cholesteryl ester species by means of secondary ion mass spectrometry. J Lipid Res 38:401–409

Cullen P, Cignarella A, von Eckardstein A, Mohr S, Assmann G (1996) Phenotype dependent differences in apolipoprotein E gene expression and protein secretion in human monocyte derived macrophages. Circulation 101:1670–1677

Cullen P, Baetta R, Bellosta S, Bernini F, Chinetti G, Cignarella A et al. (2003) Rupture of the atherosclerotic plaque. Does a good animal model exist? Arterioscler Thromb Vasc Biol 23:529–534

Curry AJ, Portig I, Goodall JC, Kirkpatrick PJ, Gaston JS (2000) T lymphocyte lines isolated from atheromatous plaque contain cells capable of responding to Chlamydia antigens. Clin Exp Immunol 121:261–269

Cushing SD, Berliner JA, Valente AJ, Territo MC, Navab M, Parhami F et al. (1990) Minimally modified low density lipoprotein induces monocyte chemotactic protein 1 in human endothelial cells and smooth muscle cells. Proc Natl Acad Sci USA 87:5134–5138

Dabbagh K, Laurent GJ, McAnulty RJ, Chambers RC (1998) Thrombin stimulates smooth muscle cell procollagen synthesis and mRNA levels via a PAR-1 mediated mechanism. Thromb Haemost 79:405–409

Danesh J, Collins R, Peto R (1997) Chronic infections and coronary heart disease: is there a link? Lancet 350:430–436

Danesh J, Whincup P, Walker M, Lennon L, Thomson A, Appleby P et al. (2000) Chlamydia pneumoniae IgG titres and coronary heart disease: prospective study and meta-analysis. BMJ 321:208–213

Danesh J, Whincup P, Lewington S, Walker M, Lennon L, Thomson A et al. (2002) Chlamydia pneumoniae IgA titres and coronary heart disease; prospective study and meta-analysis. Eur Heart J 23:371–375

Dansky HM, Charlton SA, Harper MM, Smith JD (1997) T and B lymphocytes play a minor role in atherosclerotic plaque formation in the apolipoprotein E-deficient mouse. Proc Natl Acad Sci USA 94:4642–4646

Dansky HM, Charlton SA, Sikes JL, Heath SC, Simantov R, Levin LF et al. (1999) Genetic background determines the extent of atherosclerosis in ApoE-deficient mice. Arterioscler Thromb Vasc Biol 19:1960–1968

Daugherty A, Pure E, Delfel-Butteiger D, Chen S, Leferovich J, Roselaar SE et al. (1997) The effects of total lymphocyte deficiency on the extent of atherosclerosis in apolipoprotein E-/- mice. J Clin Invest 100:1575–1580

Daugherty A, Manning MW, Cassis LA (2000) Angiotensin II promotes atherosclerotic lesions and aneurysms in apolipoprotein E-deficient mice. J Clin Invest 105:1605–1612

Daugherty A, Rateri DL (2002) T lymphocytes in atherosclerosis: the yin-yang of Th1 and Th2 influence on lesion formation. Circ Res 90:1039–1040

Davies MJ, Thomas AC (1985) Plaque fissuring: the cause of acute myocardial infarction, sudden ischaemic death, and crescendo angina. Br Heart J 53:363–373

Davies MJ (1992) Anatomic features in victims of sudden coronary death. Circulation 85:119–124

de Boer OJ, van der Wal AC, Becker AE (2000a) Atherosclerosis, inflammation, and infection. J Pathol 190:237–243

de Boer OJ, van der Wal AC, Houtkamp MA, Ossewaarde JM, Teeling P, Becker AE (2000b) Unstable atherosclerotic plaques contain T-cells that respond to Chlamydia pneumoniae. Cardiovasc Res 48:402–408

de Winther MP, Gijbels MJ, van Dijk KW, van Gorp PJ, Suzuki H, Kodama T et al. (1999) Scavenger receptor deficiency leads to more complex atherosclerotic lesions in APOE3Leiden transgenic mice. Atherosclerosis 144:315–321

der Thüsen JH, van Vlijmen BJ, Hoeben RC, Kockx MM, Havekes LM, van Berkel TJ et al. (2002) Induction of atherosclerotic plaque rupture in apolipoprotein E-/- mice after adenovirus-mediated transfer of p53. Circulation 105:2064–2070

Detrano RC, Doherty TM, Davies MJ, Stary HC (2000) Predicting coronary events with coronary calcium: pathophysiologic and clinical problems. Curr Probl Cardiol 25:374–402

Devlin CM, Kuriakose G, Hirsch E, Tabas I (2002) Genetic alterations of IL-1 receptor antagonists in mice affect plasma cholesterol level and foam cell lesion size. Proc Natl Acad Sci USA 99:6280–6285

Dhore CR, Cleutjens JP, Lutgens E, Cleutjens KB, Geusens PP, Kitslaar PJ et al. (2001) Differential expression of bone matrix regulatory proteins in human atherosclerotic plaques. Arterioscler Thromb Vasc Biol 21:1998–2003

Di Girolamo N, Wakefield D (2000) In vitro and in vivo expression of interstitial collagenase/MMP-1 by human mast cells. Dev Immunol 7:131–142

Dimmeler S, Fleming I, Fisslthaler B, Hermann C, Busse R, Zeiher AM (1999) Activation of nitric oxide synthase in endothelial cells by Akt-dependent phosphorylation. Nature 399:601–605

Doherty TM, Uzui H, Fitzpatrick LA, Tripathi PV, Dunstan CR, Asotra K et al. (2002) Rationale for the role of osteoclast-like cells in arterial calcification. FASEB J 16:577–582

Doherty TM, Fitzpatrick LA, Shaheen A, Rajavashisth TB, Detrano RC (2004) Genetic determinants of arterial calcification associated with atherosclerosis. Mayo Clin Proc 79:197–210

Duguid JB (1946) Thrombosis as a factor in the pathogenesis of coronary atherosclerosis. J Pathol Bacteriol 58:207–212

Dunne MW (2000) Rationale and design of a secondary prevention trial of antibiotic use in patients after myocardial infarction: the WIZARD (Weekly Intervention with Zithromax (azithromycin) for Atherosclerosis and its Related Disorders. J Infect Dis 181:S572–S578

Egyptian Museum Cairo. Portraits from the Desert. A temporary exhibition organised by the Kunsthistorisches Museum Vienna in conjunction with the Egyptian Museum Cairo 1999

Ehrlich P (1879) Beiträge zur Kenntniss der granulirten Bindegewebszellen und der eosinophilen Leukocythen. Arch Anat Physiol 3:166–169

Elhage R, Maret A, Pieraggi MT, Thiers JC, Arnal JF, Bayard F (1998) Differential effects of interleukin-1 receptor antagonist and tumor necrosis factor binding protein on fatty-streak formation in apolipoprotein E-deficient mice. Circulation 97:242–244

Engel T, Lorkowski S, Lueken A, Rust S, Schluter B, Berger G et al. (2001) The human ABCG4 gene is regulated by oxysterols and retinoids in monocyte-derived macrophages. Biochem Biophys Res Commun 288:483–488

Engel T, Lueken A, Bode G, Hobohm U, Lorkowski S, Schlueter B et al. (2004) ADP-ribosylation factor (ARF)-like 7 (ARL7) is induced by cholesterol loading and participates in apolipoprotein AI-dependent cholesterol export. FEBS Lett 566:241–246

Epstein SE, Speir E, Zhou YF, Guetta E, Leon M, Finkel T (1996) The role of infection in restenosis and atherosclerosois: focus on cytomegalovirus. Lancet 348:13–17

Epstein SE, Zhu J, Burnett MS, Zhou YF, Vercellotti G, Hajjar D (2000) Infection and atherosclerosis: potential roles of pathogen burden and molecular mimicry. Arterioscler Thromb Vasc Biol 20:1417–1420

Espinola-Klein C, Rupprecht HJ, Blankenberg S, Bickel C, Kopp H, Rippin G et al. (2000) Are morphological or functional changes in the carotid artery wall associated with Chlamydia pneumoniae, Helicobacter pylori, cytomegalovirus, or herpes simplex virus infection? Stroke 31:2127–2133

Espinola-Klein C, Rupprecht HJ, Blankenberg S, Bickel C, Kopp H, Rippin G et al. (2002a) Impact of infectious burden on extent and long-term prognosis of atherosclerosis. Circulation 105:15–21

Espinola-Klein C, Rupprecht HJ, Blankenberg S, Bickel C, Kopp H, Victor A et al. (2002b) Impact of infectious burden on progression of carotid atherosclerosis. Stroke 33:2581–2586

Evanko SP, Raines EW, Ross R, Gold LI, Wight TN (1998) Proteoglycan distribution in lesions of atherosclerosis depends on lesion severity, structural characteristics, and the proximity of platelet-derived growth factor and transforming growth factor-beta. Am J Pathol 152:533–546

Falk E (1992) Why do plaques rupture? Circulation 86:III30–III42

Farb A, Tang AL, Burke AP, Sessums L, Liang Y, Virmani R (1995) Sudden coronary death. Frequency of active coronary lesions, inactive coronary lesions, and myocardial infarction. Circulation 92:1701–1709

Farb A, Burke AP, Tang AL, Liang TY, Mannan P, Smialek J et al. (1996) Coronary plaque erosion without rupture into a lipid core. A frequent cause of coronary thrombosis in sudden coronary death. Circulation 93:1354–1363

Fernandez-Ortiz A, Badimon JJ, Falk E, Fuster V, Meyer B, Mailhac A et al. (1994) Characterization of the relative thrombogenicity of atherosclerotic plaque components: implications for consequences of plaque rupture. J Am Coll Cardiol 23:1562–1569

Fichtlscherer S, Rosenberger G, Walter DH, Breuer S, Dimmeler S, Zeiher AM. Elevated C-reactive protein levels and impaired endothelial vasoreactivity in patients with coronary artery disease. Circulation (2000) 102:1000–1006

Fitzpatrick LA, Severson A, Edwards WD, Ingram RT (1994) Diffuse calcification in human coronary arteries. Association of osteopontin with atherosclerosis. J Clin Invest 94:1597–1604

Fong IW (2000) Emerging relations between infectious diseases and coronary artery disease and atherosclerosis. CMAJ 163:49–56

Fontana J, Fulton D, Chen Y, Fairchild TA, McCabe TJ, Fujita N et al. (2002) Domain mapping studies reveal that the M domain of hsp90 serves as a molecular scaffold to regulate Akt-dependent phosphorylation of endothelial nitric oxide synthase and NO release. Circ Res 90:866–873

Fredrikson GN, Soderberg I, Lindholm M, Dimayuga P, Chyu KY, Shah PK et al. (2003) Inhibition of atherosclerosis in apoE-null mice by immunization with apoB-100 peptide sequences. Arterioscler Thromb Vasc Biol 23:879–884

Freigang S, Horkko S, Miller E, Witztum JL, Palinski W (1998) Immunization of LDL receptor-deficient mice with homologous malondialdehyde-modified and native LDL reduces progression of atherosclerosis by mechanisms other than induction of high titers of antibodies to oxidative neoepitopes. Arterioscler Thromb Vasc Biol 18:1972–1982

Frothingham C (1911) The relationship between acute infectious diseases and arterial lesions. Arch Intern Med 8:153–162

Fuster V, Badimon L, Badimon JJ, Chesebro JH (1992a) The pathogenesis of coronary artery disease and the acute coronary syndromes (1). N Engl J Med 326:242–250

Fuster V, Badimon L, Badimon JJ, Chesebro JH (1992b) The pathogenesis of coronary artery disease and the acute coronary syndromes (2). N Engl J Med 326:310–318

Fuster V, Lie JT, Badimon L, Rosemark JA, Badimon JJ, Bowie EJ (1985) Spontaneous and diet-induced coronary atherosclerosis in normal swine and swine with von Willebrand disease. Arteriosclerosis 5:67–73

Fuster V, Falk E, Fallon JT, Badimon L, Chesebro JH, Badimon JJ (1995) The three processes leading to post PTCA restenosis: dependence on the lesion substrate. Thromb Haemost 74:552–559

Galis ZS, Sukhova GK, Lark MW, Libby P (1994) Increased expression of matrix metalloproteinases and matrix degrading activity in vulnerable regions of human atherosclerotic plaques. J Clin Invest 94:2493–2503

Galli SJ, Iemura A, Garlick DS, Gamba-Vitalo C, Zsebo KM, Andrews RG (1993) Reversible expansion of primate mast cell populations in vivo by stem cell factor. J Clin Invest 91:148–152

Gargalovic P, Dory L (2003) Caveolins and macrophage lipid metabolism. J Lipid Res 44:11–21

Gaydos CA, Summersgill JT, Sahney NN, Ramirez JA, Quinn TC (1996) Replication of chlamydia-pneumoniae in-vitro in human macrophages, endothelial-cells, and aortic artery smooth-muscle cells. Infect Immun 64:1614–1620

George J, Afek A, Gilburd B, Levkovitz H, Shaish A, Goldberg I et al. (1998) Hyperimmunization of apo-E-deficient mice with homologous malondialdehyde low-density lipoprotein suppresses early atherogenesis. Atherosclerosis 138:147–152

Gijsbers BL, van Haarlem LJ, Soute BA, Ebberink RH, Vermeer C (1990) Characterization of a Gla-containing protein from calcified human atherosclerotic plaques. Arteriosclerosis 10:991–995

Giroud D, Li JM, Urban P, Meier B, Rutishauser W (1992) Relation of the site of acute myocardial-infarction to the most severe coronary arterial-stenosis at prior angiography. Am J Cardiol 69:729–732

Glagov S, Weisenberg E, Zarins CK, Stankunavicius R, Kolettis GJ (1987) Compensatory enlargement of human atherosclerotic coronary arteries. N Engl J Med 316:1371–1375

Godzik KL, Obrien ER, Wang SK, Kuo CC (1995) In vitro susceptibility of human vascular wall cells to infection with Chlamydia pneumoniae. J Clin Microbiol 33:2411–2414

Gokce N, Keaney JF, Hunter LM, Watkins MT, Menzoian JO, Vita JA (2002) Risk stratification for postoperative cardiovascular events via noninvasive assessment of endothelial function: a prospective study. Circulation 105:1567–1572

Gonzalez MA, Selwyn AP (2003) Endothelial function, inflammation, and prognosis in cardiovascular disease. Am J Med 115:99S–106S

Gordon JR (2000) TGFbeta1 and TNFalpha secreted by mast cells stimulated via the FcepsilonRI activate fibroblasts for high-level production of monocyte chemoattractant protein-1 (MCP-1). Cell Immunol 201:42–49

Gown AM, Tsukada T, Ross R (1986) Human atherosclerosis. II. Immunocytochemical analysis of the cellular composition of human atherosclerotic lesions. Am J Pathol 125:191–207

Grahame-Clarke C, Chan NN, Andrew D, Ridgway GL, Betteridge DJ, Emery V et al. (2003) Human cytomegalovirus seropositivity is associated with impaired vascular function. Circulation 108:678–683

Grau AJ, Buggle F, Ziegler C, Schwarz W, Meuser J, Tasman AJ et al. (1997) Association between acute cerebrovascular ischemia and chronic and recurrent infection. Stroke 28:1724–1729

Grau AJ, Becher H, Ziegler CM, Lichy C, Buggle F, Kaiser C et al. (2004) Periodontal disease as a risk factor for ischemic stroke. Stroke 35:496–501

Grayston JT, Campbell LA, Kuo CC, Mordhorst CH, Saikku P, Thom DH et al. (1990) A new respiratory tract pathogen: Chlamydia pneumoniae strain TWAR. J Infect Dis 161:618–625

Grayston JT (1992) Infections caused by Chlamydia pneumoniae strain TWAR. Clin Infect Dis 15:757–761

Gruber BL, Marchese MJ, Suzuki K, Schwartz LB, Okada Y, Nagase H et al. (1989) Synovial procollagenase activation by human mast cell tryptase dependence upon matrix metalloproteinase 3 activation. J Clin Invest 84:1657–1662

Gupta S, Leatham EW, Carrington D, Mendall MA, Kaski JC, Camm AJ. (1997a) Elevated Chlamydia pneumoniae antibodies, cardiovascular events, and azithromycin in male survivors of myocardial infarction. Circulation 96:404–407

Gupta S, Pablo AM, Jiang X, Wang N, Tall AR, Schindler C (1997b) IFN-gamma potentiates atherosclerosis in ApoE knock-out mice. J Clin Invest 99:2752–2761

Halcox JPJ, Schenke WH, Zalos G, Mincemoyer R, Prasad A, Waclawiw MA et al. (2002) Prognostic value of coronary vascular endothelial dysfunction. Circulation 106:653–658

Hamilton TA, Ohmori Y, Tebo JM, Kishore R (1999) Regulation of macrophage gene expression by pro- and anti-inflammatory cytokines. Pathobiology 67:241–244

Han J, Hajjar DP, Zhou X, Gotto AM, Jr., Nicholson AC (2002) Regulation of peroxisome proliferator-activated receptor-gamma-mediated gene expression. A new mechanism of action for high density lipoprotein. J Biol Chem 277:23582–23586

Hansson GK (1997) Cell-mediated immunity in atherosclerosis. Curr Op Lipidol 8:301–311

Hansson GK (2001) Immune mechanisms in atherosclerosis. Arterioscler Thromb Vasc Biol 21:1876–1890

Hansson GK (2002) Vaccination against atherosclerosis: science or fiction? Circulation 106:1599–1601

Hansson GK, Libby P, Schonbeck U, Yan ZQ (2002) Innate and adaptive immunity in the pathogenesis of atherosclerosis. Circ Res 91:281–291

Hara M, Matsumori A, Ono K, Kido H, Hwang MW, Miyamoto T et al. (1999) Mast cells cause apoptosis of cardiomyocytes and proliferation of other intramyocardial cells in vitro. Circulation 100:1443–1449

Harrison DG (1997) Cellular and molecular mechanisms of endothelial cell dysfunction. J Clin Invest 100:2153–2157

Haynes WG, Stanford C (2003) Periodontal disease and atherosclerosis. From dental to arterial plaque. Arterioscler Thromb Vasc Biol 23:1309–1311

He S, Peng Q, Walls AF (1997) Potent induction of a neutrophil and eosinophil-rich infiltrate in vivo by human mast cell tryptase: selective enhancement of eosinophil recruitment by histamine. J Immunol 159:6216–6225

He S, Walls AF (1998) Human mast cell chymase induces the accumulation of neutrophils, eosinophils and other inflammatory cells in vivo. Br J Pharmacol 125:1491–1500

Herrera VL, Makrides SC, Xie HX, Adari H, Krauss RM, Ryan US et al. (1999) Spontaneous combined hyperlipidemia, coronary heart disease and decreased survival in Dahl salt-sensitive hypertensive rats transgenic for human cholesteryl ester transfer protein. Nat Med 5:1383–1389.

Heymans S, Luttun A, Nuyens D, Theilmeier G, Creemers E, Moons L et al. (1999) Inhibition of plasminogen activators or matrix metalloproteinases prevents cardiac rupture but impairs therapeutic angiogenesis and causes cardiac failure. Nat Med 5:1135–1142

Hujoel PP, Drangsholt M, Spiekerman C, DeRouen TA (2000) Periodontal disease and coronary heart disease risk. JAMA 248:1406–1410

Ikari Y, Mcmanus BM, Kenyon J, Schwartz SM (1999) Neonatal intima formation in the human coronary artery. Arterioscler Thromb Vasc Biol 19:2036–2040

Ishibashi S, Goldstein JL, Brown MS, Herz J, Burns DK (1994) Massive xanthomatosis and atherosclerosis in cholesterol-fed low density lipoprotein receptor-negative mice. J Clin Invest 93:1885–1893

Jackson LA (2000) Description and status of the Azithromycin and Coronary Events Study (ACES). J Infect Dis 181:S579–S581

Jaeger E, Rust S, Scharffetter K, Roessner A, Winter J, Buchholz B et al. (1990) Localization of cytoplasmic collagen mRNA in human aortic coarctation: mRNA enhancement in high blood pressure-induced intimal and medial thickening. J Histochem Cytochem 38:1365–1375

Jerome WG, Lewis JC (1985) Early atherogenesis in White Carneau pigeons. II. Ultrastructural and cytochemical observations. Am J Pathol 1985; 119:210–222

Jerome WG, Lewis JC (1997) Cellular dynamics in early atherosclerotic lesion progression in white carneau pigeons—Spatial and temporal analysis of monocyte and smooth muscle invasion of the intima. Arterioscler Thromb Vasc Biol 17:654–664

Jeziorska M, McCollum C, Woolley DE (1997) Mast cell distribution, activation, and phenotype in atherosclerotic lesions of human carotid arteries. J Pathol 182:115–122

Johnson JL, Jackson CL (2001) Atherosclerotic plaque rupture in the apolipoprotein E knockout mouse. Atherosclerosis 154:399–406

Jonasson L, Holm J, Skalli O, Bondjers G, Hansson GK (1986) Regional accumulations of T cells, macrophages, and smooth muscle cells in the human atherosclerotic plaque. Arteriosclerosis 6:131–138

Joshipura KJ, Rimm EB, Douglass CW, Trichopoulos D, Ascherio A, Willett WC (1996) Poor oral health and coronary heart disease. J Dent Res 75:1631–1636

Kaartinen M, Penttila A, Kovanen PT (1994a) Accumulation of activated mast cells in the shoulder region of human coronary atheroma, the predilection site of atheromatous rupture. Circulation 90:1669–1678

Kaartinen M, Penttila A, Kovanen PT (1994b) Mast cells of two types differing in neutral protease composition in the human aortic intima. Demonstration of tryptase- and tryptase/chymase-containing mast cells in normal intimas, fatty streaks, and the shoulder region of atheromas. Arterioscler Thromb 14:966–972

Kaartinen M, Penttila A, Kovanen PT (1996) Mast cells in rupture-prone areas of human coronary atheromas produce and store TNF-alpha. Circulation 94:2787–2792

Kaartinen M, van der Wal AC, Van der Loos CM, Piek JJ, Koch KT, Becker AE et al. (1998) Mast cell infiltration in acute coronary syndromes: implications for plaque rupture. J Am Coll Cardiol 32:606–612

Kalayoglu MV, Libby P, Byrne GI (2002) Chlamydia pneumoniae as an emerging risk factor in cardiovascular disease. JAMA 288:2724–2731

Katsuda S, Coltrera MD, Ross R, Gown AM (1993) Human atherosclerosis. IV. Immunocytochemical analysis of cell activation and proliferation in lesions of young adults. Am J Pathol 142:1787–1793

Kauhanen P, Kovanen PT, Lassila R (2000) Coimmobilized native macromolecular heparin proteoglycans strongly inhibit platelet-collagen interactions in flowing blood. Arterioscler Thromb Vasc Biol 20:E113–E119

Kaukoranta-Tolvanen SS, Laitinen K, Saikku P, Leinonen M (1994) Chlamydia pneumoniae multiplies in human endothelial cells in vitro. Microbial Pathogenesis 16:313–319

Keele KD (1952) Leonardo da Vinci on movement of the heart and blood. Harvey and Blythe, London

Kelley JL, Chi DS, Abou-Auda W, Smith JK, Krishnaswamy G (2000) The molecular role of mast cells in atherosclerotic cardiovascular disease. Mol Med Today 6:304–308

Kellner-Weibel GL, Jerome WG, Small DM, Warner GJ, Stoltenborg JK, Kearney MA et al. (1998) Effects of intracellular free cholesterol accumulation on macrophage viability—A model for foam cell death. Arterioscler Thromb Vasc Biol 18:423–431

Kellner-Weibel G, Yancey PG, Jerome WG, Walser T, Mason RP, Phillips MC et al. (1999) Crystallization of free cholesterol in model macrophage foam cells. Arterioscler Thromb Vasc Biol 19:1891–1898

Khovidhunkit W, Memon RA, Feingold KR (2000) Infection and inflammation-induced proatherogenic changes of lipoproteins. J Infect Dis 181:S462–S472

Kim DN, Schmee J, Lee KT, Thomas WA (1987) Atherosclerotic lesions in the coronary arteries of hyperlipidemic swine. Part 1. Cell increases, divisions, losses and cells of origin in first 90 days on diet. Atherosclerosis 64:231–242

Kirchhofer D, Riederer MA, Baumgartner HR (1997) Specific accumulation of circulating monocytes and polymorphonuclear leukocytes on platelet thrombi in a vascular injury model. Blood 89:1270–1278

Kockx MM (1998) Apoptosis in the atherosclerotic plaque—Quantitative and qualitative aspects. Arterioscler Thromb Vasc Biol 18:1519–1522

Kockx MM, Herman AG (1998) Apoptosis in atherogenesis: implications for plaque destabilization. Eur Heart J 19:G23–G28

Kokkonen JO, Kovanen PT (1987) Stimulation of mast cells leads to cholesterol accumulation in macrophages in vitro by a mast cell granule-mediated uptake of low density lipoprotein. Proc Natl Acad Sci USA 84:2287–2291

Kokkonen JO, Kovanen PT (1989) Proteolytic enzymes of mast cell granules degrade low density lipoproteins and promote their granule-mediated uptake by macrophages in vitro. J Biol Chem 264:10749–10755

Kolodgie FD, Gold HK, Burke AP, Fowler DR, Kruth HS, Weber DK et al. (2003) Intraplaque hemorrhage and progression of coronary atheroma. N Engl J Med 349:2316–2325

Kovanen PT (1990) Atheroma formation: defective control in the intimal round-trip of cholesterol. Eur Heart J 11:238–246

Kovanen PT (1995) Role of mast cells in atherosclerosis. Chem Immunol 62:132–170

Kovanen PT, Kaartinen M, Paavonen T (1995) Infiltrates of activated mast cells at the site of coronary atheromatous erosion or rupture in myocardial infarction. Circulation 92:1084–1088

Kovanen PT, Pentikainen MO (1999) Decorin links low-density lipoproteins (LDL) to collagen: a novel mechanism for retention of LDL in the atherosclerotic plaque. Trends Cardiovasc Med 9:86–91

Kragel AH, Reddy SG, Wittes JT, Roberts WC (1989) Morphometric analysis of the composition of atherosclerotic plaques in the four major epicardial coronary arteries in acute myocardial infarction and in sudden coronary death. Circulation 80:1747–1756

Kuhlencordt PJ, Gyurko R, Han F, Scherrer-Crosbie M, Aretz TH, Hajjar R et al. (2001) Accelerated atherosclerosis, aortic aneurysm formation, and ischemic heart disease in apolipoprotein E/endothelial nitric oxide synthase double-knockout mice. Circulation 104:448–454

Lassila R, Lindstedt K, Kovanen PT (1997) Native macromolecular heparin proteoglycans exocytosed from stimulated rat serosal mast cells strongly inhibit platelet-collagen interactions. Arterioscler Thromb Vasc Biol 17:3578–3587

Lee M, Lindstedt LK, Kovanen PT (1992) Mast cell-mediated inhibition of reverse cholesterol transport. Arterioscler Thromb 12:1329–1335

Lee RT, Libby P (1997) The unstable atheroma. Arterioscler Thromb Vasc Biol 17:1859–1867

Lee M, von Eckardstein A, Lindstedt L, Assmann G, Kovanen PT (1999) Depletion of pre beta 1LpA1 and LpA4 particles by mast cell chymase reduces cholesterol efflux from macrophage foam cells induced by plasma. Arterioscler Thromb Vasc Biol 19:1066–1074

Lee TS, Yen HC, Pan CC, Chau LY (1999) The role of interleukin 12 in the development of atherosclerosis in ApoE-deficient mice. Arterioscler Thromb Vasc Biol 19:734–742

Lee M, Calabresi L, Chiesa G, Franceschini G, Kovanen PT (2002a) Mast cell chymase degrades apoE and apoA-II in apoA-I-knockout mouse plasma and reduces its ability to promote cellular cholesterol efflux. Arterioscler Thromb Vasc Biol 22:1475–1481

Lee M, Sommerhoff CP, von Eckardstein A, Zettl F, Fritz H, Kovanen PT (2002b) Mast cell tryptase degrades HDL and blocks its function as an acceptor of cellular cholesterol. Arterioscler Thromb Vasc Biol 22:2086–2091

Leskinen M, Wang Y, Leszczynski D, Lindstedt KA, Kovanen PT (2001) Mast cell chymase induces apoptosis of vascular smooth muscle cells. Arterioscler Thromb Vasc Biol 21:516–522

Leskinen MJ, Lindstedt KA, Wang Y, Kovanen PT (2003a) Mast cell chymase induces smooth muscle cell apoptosis by a mechanism involving fibronectin degradation and disruption of focal adhesions. Arterioscler Thromb Vasc Biol 23:238–243

Leskinen MJ, Kovanen PT, Lindstedt KA (2003b) Regulation of smooth muscle cell growth, function and death in vitro by activated mast cells—a potential mechanism for the weakening and rupture of atherosclerotic plaques. Biochem Pharmacol 66:1493–1498

Leu HJ, Feigl W, Susani M, Odermatt B (1988) Differentiation of mononuclear blood cells into macrophages, fibroblasts and endothelial cells in thrombus organization. Exp Cell Biol 56:201–210

Levi M (2001) CMV endothelitis as a factor in the pathogenesis of atherosclerosis. Cardiovasc Res 50:432–433

Li H, Cybulsky MI, Gimbrone MA, Jr., Libby P (1993) Inducible expression of vascular cell adhesion molecule-1 by vascular smooth muscle cells in vitro and within rabbit atheroma. Am J Pathol 143:1551–159

Li L, Krilis SA (1999) Mast-cell growth and differentiation. Allergy 54:306–312

Li AC, Glass CK (2002) The macrophage foam cell as a target for therapeutic intervention. Nat Med 8:1235–1242

Libby P, Egan D, Skarlatos S (1997) Roles of infectious agents in atherosclerosis and restenosis—An assessment of the evidence and need for future research. Circulation 96:4095–4103

Libby P (2000) Multiple mechanisms of thrombosis complicating atherosclerotic plaques. Clin Cardiol 23:3–7

Libby P, Ridker PM, Maseri A (2002) Inflammation and atherosclerosis. Circulation 105:1135–1143

Lijnen HR (2002) Extracellular proteolysis in the development and progression of atherosclerosis. Biochem Soc Trans 30:163–167

Lindstedt KA, Kokkonen JO, Kovanen PT (1992) Soluble heparin proteoglycans released from stimulated mast cells induce uptake of low density lipoproteins by macrophages via scavenger receptor-mediated phagocytosis. J Lipid Res 33:65–75

Lindstedt KA (1993) Inhibition of macrophage-mediated low density lipoprotein oxidation by stimulated rat serosal mast cells. J Biol Chem 268:7741–7746

Lindstedt L, Lee M, Castro GR, Fruchart JC, Kovanen PT (1996) Chymase in exocytosed rat mast cell granules effectively proteolyzes apolipoprotein AI-containing lipoproteins, so reducing the cholesterol efflux-inducing ability of serum and aortic intimal fluid. J Clin Invest 97:2174–2182

Lohi J, Harvima I, Keski-Oja J (1992) Pericellular substrates of human mast cell tryptase: 72,000 dalton gelatinase and fibronectin. J Cell Biochem 50:337–349

Lorkowski S, Kratz M, Wenner C, Schmidt R, Weitkamp B, Fobker M et al. (2001) Expression of the ATP-binding cassette transporter gene ABCG1 (ABC8) in Tangier disease. Biochem Biophys Res Commun 283:821–830

Lorkowski S, Rust S, Engel T, Jung E, Tegelkamp K, Galinski EA et al. (2001) Genomic sequence and structure of the human ABCG1 (ABC8) gene. Biochem Biophys Res Commun 280:121–131

Lorkowski S, Cullen P (2002) Subfamily G of the ATP-binding cassette transporter protein family. Pure Appl Chem 74:2057–2081

Lupu F, Danaricu I, Simionescu N (1987) Development of intracellular lipid deposits in the lipid-laden cells of atherosclerotic lesions. A cytochemical and ultrastructural study. Atherosclerosis 67:127–142

Ma H, Kovanen PT (1997) Degranulation of cutaneous mast cells induces transendothelial transport and local accumulation of plasma LDL in rat skin in vivo. J Lipid Res 38:1877–1887

Madden KB, Urban JF, Jr., Ziltener HJ, Schrader JW, Finkelman FD, Katona IM (1991) Antibodies to IL-3 and IL-4 suppress helminth-induced intestinal mastocytosis. J Immunol 147:1387–1391

Magee R (1998) Arterial disease in antiquity. Med J Australia 169:663–666

Maier M, Spragg J, Schwartz LB (1983) Inactivation of human high molecular weight kininogen by human mast cell tryptase. J Immunol 130:2352–2356

Majesky MW (2002) Mouse model for atherosclerotic plaque rupture. Circulation 105:2010–2011

Malinow MR, Maruffo CA (1965) Aortic atherosclerosis in free-ranging howler monkeys (Alouatta caraya). Nature 206:948–949

Malinow MR, Maruffo CA (1966) Naturally occurring atherosclerosis in howler monkeys (Alouatta caraya). J Atheroscler Res 6:368–380

Mallat Z, Besnard S, Duriez M, Deleuze V, Emmanuel F, Bureau MF et al. Protective role of interleukin-10 in atherosclerosis. Circ Res (1999) 85:e17–e24

Maron R, Sukhova G, Faria AM, Hoffmann E, Mach F, Libby P et al. (2002) Mucosal administration of heat shock protein-65 decreases atherosclerosis and inflammation in aortic arch of low-density lipoprotein receptor-deficient mice. Circulation 106:1708–1715

Maruffo CA, Malinow MR (1966) Dissecting aneurysm of the aorta in a howler monkey (Alouatta caraya). J Pathol Bacteriol 92:567–570

Mattila KJ, Nieminen MS, Valtonen VV, Rasi VP, Kesaniemi YA, Syrjala SL et al. (1989) Association between dental health and acute myocardial infarction. BMJ 298:779–781.

Mattila KJ, Valtonen VV, Nieminen M, Huttunen JK (1995) Dental infection and the risk of new coronary events—prospective study of patients with documented coronary-artery disease. Clin Infect Dis 20:588–592

Maxfield FR, Wustner D (2002) Intracellular cholesterol transport. J Clin Invest 110:891–898

Mekori YA, Metcalfe DD (2000) Mast cells in innate immunity. Immunol Rev 173:131–140

Mendez AJ, Lin G, Wade DP, Lawn RM, Oram JF (2001) Membrane lipid domains distinct from cholesterol/sphingomyelin-rich rafts are involved in the ABCA1-mediated lipid secretory pathway. J Biol Chem 276:3158–3166

Metcalfe DD, Kaliner M, Donlon MA (1981) The mast cell. Crit Rev Immunol 3:23–74

Metcalfe DD, Baram D, Mekori YA (1997) Mast cells. Physiol Rev 77:1033–1079

Mitchinson MJ, Hardwick SJ, Bennett MR (1996) Cell-death in atherosclerotic plaques. Curr Op Lipidol 7:324–329

Moldovan NI (2003) Current priorities in the research of circulating pre-endothelial cells. Adv Exp Med Biol 522:1–8

Morrison HI, Ellison LF, Taylor GW (1999) Periodontal disease and risk of fatal coronary heart and cerebrovascular diseases. J Cardiovasc Risk 6:7–11

Mosmann TR, Sad S (1996) The expanding universe of T-cell subsets: Th1, Th2 and more. Immunol Today 17:138–146

Mosorin M, Surcel HM, Laurila A, Lehtinen M, Karttunen R, Juvonen J et al. (2000) Detection of Chlamydia pneumoniae-reactive T lymphocytes in human atherosclerotic plaques of carotid artery. Arterioscler Thromb Vasc Biol 20:1061–1067

Muhlestein JB, Anderson JL, Carlquist JF, Salunkhe K, Horne BD, Pearson RR et al. (2000) Randomized secondary prevention trial of azithromycin in patients with coronary artery disease: primary clinical results of the ACADEMIC study. Circulation 102:1755–1760

Munder M, Mallo M, Eichmann K, Modolell M (1998) Murine macrophages secrete interferon gamma upon cobined stimulation with interleukin (IL)-12 and IL-18: a novel pathway of autocrine macrophage activation. J Exp Med 187:2103–2108

Murohara T, Kugiyama K, Ohgushi M, Sugiyama S, Ohta Y, Yasue H (1994) LPC in oxidized LDL elicits vasocontraction and inhibits endothelium-dependent relaxation. Am J Physiol 36:H2441–H2449

Murry CE, Gipaya CT, Bartosek T, Benditt EP, Schwartz SM (1997) Monoclonality of smooth muscle cells in human atherosclerosis. Am J Pathol 151:697–705

Nagano H, Mitchell RN, Taylor MK, Hasegawa S, Tilney NL, Libby P (1997) Interferon-gamma deficiency prevents coronary arteriosclerosis but not myocardial rejection in transplanted mouse hearts. J Clin Invest 100:550–557

Nagy L, Tontonoz P, Alvarez JA, Chen HW, Evans RM (1998) Oxidized LDL regulates macrophage gene expression through ligand activation of PPAR gamma. Cell 93:229–240

Nakashima Y, Plump AS, Raines EW, Breslow JL, Ross R (1994) ApoE-deficient mice develop lesions of all phases of atherosclerosis throughout the arterial tree. Arterioscler Thromb 14:133–140

Napoli C, DArmiento FP, Mancini FP, Postiglione A, Witztum JL, Palumbo G et al. (1997) Fatty streak formation occurs in human fetal aortas and is greatly enhanced by maternal hypercholesterolemia—Intimal accumulation of low density lipoprotein and its oxidation precede monocyte recruitment into early atherosclerotic lesions. J Clin Invest 100:2680–2690

Naruko T, Ueda M, Haze K, van der Wal AC, Van der Loos CM, Itoh A et al. (2002) Neutrophil infiltration of culprit lesions in acute coronary syndromes. Circulation 106:2894–2900

Narumiya S, Sugimoto Y, Ushikubi F (1999) Prostanoid receptors: structures, properties, and functions. Physiol Rev 79:1193–1226

Naureckiene S, Sleat DE, Lackland H, Fensom A, Vanier MT, Wattiaux R et al. (2000) Identification of HE1 as the second gene of Niemann-Pick C disease. Science 290:2298–2301

Nelimarkka LO, Nikkari ST, Ravanti LS, Kahari VM, Jarvelainen HT (1998) Collagenase-1, stromelysin-1 and 92 kDa gelatinase are associated with tumor necrosis factor-alpha induced morphological change of human endothelial cells in vitro. Matrix Biol 17:293–304

Nerheim PL, Meier JL, Vasef MA, Li.W.-G., Hu L, Rice JB et al. (2004) Enhanced cytomegalovirus infection in atherosclerotic human blood vessels. Am J Pathol 164:589–600

Newby AC (1997) Molecular and cell biology of native coronary and vein-graft atherosclerosis: regulation of plaque stability and vessel-wall remodelling by growth factors and cell-extracellular matrix interactions. Coron Artery Dis 8:213–224

Nicholson AC (2004) Expression of CD36 in macrophages and atherosclerosis. The role of lipid regulation and PPARg signalling. Trends Cardiovasc Med 14:8–12

Nicoletti A, Kaveri S, Caligiuri G, Bariety J, Hansson GK (1998) Immunoglobulin treatment reduces atherosclerosis in apo E knockout mice. J Clin Invest 102:910–918

Nieminen MS, Mattila K, Valtonen V (1993) Infection and inflammation as risk-factors for myocardial-infarction. Eur Heart J 14:12–16

Nikkari ST, Obrien KD, Ferguson M, Hatsukami T, Welgus HG, Alpers CE et al. (1995) Interstitial collagenase (MMP 1) expression in human carotid atherosclerosis. Circulation 92:1393–1398

Nobuyoshi M, Tanaka M, Nosaka H, Kimura T, Yokoi H, Hamasaki N et al. (1991) Progression of coronary atherosclerosis: is coronary spasm related to progression? J Am Coll Cardiol 18:904–910

Ohgushi M, Kugiyama K, Fukunaga K, Murohara T, Sugiyama S, Miyamoto E et al. (1993) Protein kinase C inhibitors prevent impairment of endothelium-dependent relaxation by oxidatively modified LDL. Arterioscler Thromb 13:1525–1532

Ooshima A (1981) Collagen alpha B chain: increased proportion in human atherosclerosis. Science 213:666–668

Osler W (1980) Modern medicine: its theory and practice. Lea and Febiger, Philadelphia

Østerud B, Bjørklid E (2003) Role of monocytes in atherogenesis. Physiol Rev 83:1069–1112

Owens GK, Vernon SM, Madsen CS (1996) Molecular regulation of smooth muscle cell differentiation. J Hypertens Suppl 14:S55–S64

Palinski W, Ord VA, Plump AS, Breslow JL, Steinberg D, Witztum JL (1994) ApoE-deficient mice are a model of lipoprotein oxidation in atherogenesis. Demonstration of oxidation-specific epitopes in lesions and high titers of autoantibodies to malondialdehyde- lysine in serum. Arterioscler Thromb 14:605–616

Palinski W, Miller E, Witztum JL (1995) Immunization of low density lipoprotein (ldl) receptor-deficient rabbits with homologous malondialdehyde-modified ldl reduces atherogenesis. Proc Natl Acad Sci USA 92:821–825

Palinski W, Napoli C (2002) Unraveling pleiotropic effects of statins on plaque rupture. Arterioscler Thromb Vasc Biol 22:1745–1750

Parhami F, Tintut Y, Patel JK, Mody N, Hemmat A, Demer LL (2001) Regulation of vascular calcification in atherosclerosis. Z Kardiol 90:27–30

Paulsson G, Zhou X, Tornquist E, Hansson GK (2000) Oligoclonal T cell expansions in atherosclerotic lesions of apolipoprotein E-deficient mice. Arterioscler Thromb Vasc Biol 20:10–17

Pickering JG, Weir L, Jekanowski J, Kearney MA, Isner JM (1993) Proliferative activity in peripheral and coronary atherosclerotic plaque among patients undergoing percutaneous revascularization. J Clin Invest 91:1469–1480

Piha M, Lindstedt L, Kovanen PT (1995) Fusion of proteolyzed low-density lipoprotein in the fluid phase: a novel mechanism generating atherogenic lipoprotein particles. Biochemistry 34:10120–10129

Pinderski Oslund LJ, Hedrick CC, Olvera T, Hagenbaugh A, Territo M, Berliner JA et al. (1999) Interleukin-10 blocks atherosclerotic events in vitro and in vivo. Arterioscler Thromb Vasc Biol 19:2847–2853

Plump AS, Smith JD, Hayek T, Aalto-Setala K, Walsh A, Verstuyft JG et al. (1992) Severe hypercholesterolemia and atherosclerosis in apolipoprotein E-deficient mice created by homologous recombination in ES cells. Cell 71:343–353

Pober JS, Gimborne MA, Jr., Lapierre DL, Mendrick W, Fiers W, Rothlein R et al. (1986) Overlapping patterns of activation of human endothelial cells by interleukin I, tumor necrosis factor, and immune interferon. J Immunol 137:1893

Prasad A, Zhu J, Halcox JP, Waclawiw MA, Epstein SE, Quyyumi AA (2002) Predisposition to atherosclerosis by infections: role of endothelial dysfunction. Circulation 106:184–190

Pueyo Palazón P, Alfón J, Gaffney P, Berrozpe M, Royo T, Badimon L (1998) Effects of reducing LDL and increasing HDL with gemfibrozil in experimental coronary lesion development and thrombotic risk. Atherosclerosis 136:333–345

Pussinen PJ, Jousilahti P, Alfthan G, Palosuo T, Asikainen S, Salomaa V (2003) Antibodies to periodontal pathogens are associated with coronary heart disease. Arterioscler Thromb Vasc Biol 24:1250–1254

Quiney JR, Watts GB. (1989) Introduction. In: Quiney JR, Watts GB (eds) Classic papers in hyperlipidemia. Science Press Limited, London

Ra C, Yasuda M, Yagita H, Okumura K. Fibronectin receptor integrins are involved in mast cell activation. J Allergy Clin Immunol 1994; 94:625–628

Rauterberg J, Jaeger E, Althaus M (1993) Collagens in atherosclerotic vessel wall lesions. Curr Top Pathol 87:163–192

Reddick RL, Zhang SH, Maeda N (1994) Atherosclerosis in mice lacking Apo E—evaluation of lesional development and progression. Arterioscler Thromb 14:141–147

Reddick RL, Zhang SH, Maeda N (1998) Aortic atherosclerotic plaque injury in apolipoprotein E deficient mice. Atherosclerosis 140:297–305

Rekhter MD, Hicks GW, Brammer DW, Work CW, Kim JS, Gordon D et al. (1998) Animal model that mimics atherosclerotic plaque rupture. Circ Res 83:705–713

Rekhter MD (1999) Collagen synthesis in atherosclerosis: too much and not enough. Cardiovasc Res 41:376–384

Repka-Ramirez MS, Baraniuk JN (2002) Histamine in health and disease. Clin Allergy Immunol 17:1–25

Richardson M, Schmidt AM, Graham SE, Achen B, DeReske M, Russell JC (1998) Vasculopathy and insulin resistance in the JCR:LA-cp rat. Atherosclerosis 138:135–146

Rodewald HR, Dessing M, Dvorak AM, Galli SJ (1996) Identification of a committed precursor for the mast cell lineage. Science 271:818–822

Rosenfeld ME, Polinsky P, Virmani R, Kauser K, Rubanyi G, Schwartz SM (2000) Advanced atherosclerotic lesions in the innominate artery of the ApoE knockout mouse. Arterioscler Thromb Vasc Biol 20:2587–2592

Ross R, Glomset JA (1973) Atherosclerosis and the arterial smooth muscle cell: proliferation of smooth muscle is a key event in the genesis of the lesions of atherosclerosis. Science 180:1332–1339

Ross R, Glomset J, Kariya B, Raines E (1978) Role of platelet factors in the growth of cells in culture. Natl Cancer Inst Monogr 48:103–108

Ross R (1981) The Gordon Wilson Lecture: atherosclerosis—a response to injury gone awry. Trans Am Clin Climatol Assoc 93:78–86

Ross R (1993) The pathogenesis of atherosclerosis: a perspective for the 1990s. Nature 362:801–809

Ross R (1999) Atherosclerosis, an inflammatory disease. N Engl J Med 340:115–126

Rothblat GH, Llera-Moya M, Atger V, Kellner-Weibel G, Williams DL, Phillips MC (1999) Cell cholesterol efflux: integration of old and new observations provides new insights. J Lipid Res 40:781–796

Royo T, Alfon J, Berrozpe M, Badimon L (2000) Effect of gemfibrozil on peripheral atherosclerosis and platelet activation in a pig model of hyperlipidemia. Eur J Clin Invest 30:843–852

Rozanski A, Blumenthal JA, Kaplan J (1999) Impact of psychological factors on the pathogenesis of cardiovascular disease and implications for therapy. Circulation 99:2192–2217

Ruffer MA (1911) On arterial lesions found in Egyptian mummies. J Pathol Bacteriol 15:453–462

Ruffer MA (1920) Remarks on the histology and pathological anatomy of Egyptian mummies. Cairo Scientific J 4:3–7

Rupprecht HJ, Blankenberg S, Bickel C, Rippin G, Hafner G, Prellwitz W et al. (2001) Impact of viral and bacterial infectious burden on long-term prognosis in patients with coronary artery disease. Circulation 104:25–31

Russell JC, Graham SE, Richardson M (1998a) Cardiovascular disease in the JCR:LA-cp rat. Mol Cell Biochem 188:113–126

Russell JC, Graham SE, Amy RM, Dolphin PJ (1998b) Cardioprotective effect of probucol in the atherosclerosis-prone JCR:LA-cp rat. Eur J Pharmacol 350:203–210

Saarinen J, Kalkkinen N, Welgus HG, Kovanen PT (1994) Activation of human interstitial procollagenase through direct cleavage of the leu(83)-thrbond by mast cell chymase. J Biol Chem 269:18134–18140

Samuelsson B (2000) The discovery of the leukotrienes. Am J Respir Crit Care Med 161:S2–S6

Sandison AT (1962) Degenerative diseases in the Egyptian mummy. Med Hist 6:77–81

Sandison AT (1981) Diseases of the ancient world. In: Anthony PP, MacSween RNM (eds) Recent advances in pathology, Vol 11. Churchill Livingstone, Edinburgh, pp 1–18

Sangiorgi G, Rumberger JA, Severson A, Edwards WD, Gregoire J, Fitzpatrick LA et al. (1998) Arterial calcification and not lumen stenosis is highly correlated with atherosclerotic plaque burden in humans: a histologic study of 723 coronary artery segments using nondecalcifying methodology. J Am Coll Cardiol 31:126–133

Santerre RF, Wight TN, Smith SC, Brannigan D (1972) Spontaneous atherosclerosis in pigeons. A model system for studying metabolic parameters associated with atherogenesis. Am J Pathol 67:1–22

Saren P, Welgus HG, Kovanen PT (1996) TNF-a and IL-1b selectively induce expression of 92-kDa gelatinase by human macrophages. J Immunol 157:4159–4165

Scannapieco FA, Bush RB, Paju S (2003) Associations between periodontal disease and riks for atherosclerosis, cardiovascular disease, and stroke. A systematic review. Ann Periodontol 8:38–53

Schechter NM, Irani AM, Sprows JL, Abernethy J, Wintroub B, Schwartz LB (1990) Identification of a cathepsin G-like proteinase in the MCTC type of human mast cell. J Immunol 145:2652–2661

Scheiffele P, Rietveld A, Wilk T, Simons K (1999) Influenza viruses select ordered lipid domains during budding from the plasma membrane. J Biol Chem 274:2038–2044

Schroeder R, London E, Brown D (1994) Interactions between saturated acyl chains confer detergent resistance on lipids and glycosylphosphatidylinositol (GPI)-anchored proteins: GPI-anchored proteins in liposomes and cells show similar behavior. Proc Natl Acad Sci USA 91:12130–12134

Schwartz LB, Austen KF (1984) Structure and function of the chemical mediators of mast cells. In: Ishizaka K (ed) Mast cell activation and mediator release. Karger, Basel, pp 271–321

Schwartz LB, Bradford TR, Littman BH, Wintroub BU (1985) The fibrinogenolytic activity of purified tryptase from human lung mast cells. J Immunol 135:2762–2767

Schwartz CJ, Valente AJ, Kelley JL, Sprague EA, Edwards EH (1988) Thrombosis and the development of atherosclerosis: Rokitansky revisited. Semin Thromb Hemost 14:189–195

Schwartz SM, de Blois D, O'Brien ER (1995) The intima: soil for atherosclerosis and restenosis. Circ Res 77:445–465

Scotland RS, Morales-Ruiz M, Chen Y, Yu J, Rudic RD, Fulton D et al. (2002) Functional reconstitution of endothelial nitric oxide synthase reveals the importance of serine 1179 in endothelium-dependent vasomotion. Circ Res 90:904–910

Shattock SG (1909) A report upon the pathological condition of the aorta of King Menephthah, traditionally regarded as the Pharoah of the Exodus. Proc Roy Soc Med Path 2:122–127

Shio H, Haley NJ, Fowler S (1979) Characterization of lipid-laden aortic cells from cholesterol-fed rabbits. III. Intracellular localization of cholesterol and cholesteryl esters. Lab Invest 41:160–167

Sigmund CD (2000) Viewpoint: are studies in genetically altered mice out of control? Arterioscler Thromb Vasc Biol 20:1425–1429

Simionescu N, Vasile E, Lupu F, Popescu G, Simionescu M (1986) Prelesional events in atherogenesis. Accumulation of extracellular cholesterol-rich liposomes in the arterial intima and cardiac valves of the hyperlipidemic rabbit. Am J Pathol 123:109–125

Simons K, Ikonen E (2000) How cell handle cholesterol. Science 290:1721–1726

Skalen K, Gustafsson M, Rydberg EK, Hulten LM, Wiklund O, Innerarity TL et al. (2002) Subendothelial retention of atherogenic lipoproteins in early atherosclerosis. Nature 417:750–754

Slowik MR, Min W, Ardito T, Karsan A, Kashgarian M, Pober JS (1997) Evidence that tumor necrosis factor triggers apoptosis in human endothelial cells by interleukin-1-converting enzyme-like protease-dependent and -independent pathways. Lab Invest 77:257–267

Smith SC, Smith EC, Taylor RL, Jr. (2001) Susceptibility to spontaneous atherosclerosis in pigeons: an autosomal recessive trait. J Hered 92:439–442

Song L, Leung C, Schindler C (2001) Lymphocytes are important in early atherosclerosis. J Clin Invest 108:251–259

Spronk HM, Soute BA, Schurgers LJ, Cleutjens JP, Thijssen HH, De Mey JG et al. (2001) Matrix Gla protein accumulates at the border of regions of calcification and normal tissue in the media of the arterial vessel wall. Biochem Biophys Res Commun 289:485–490

Stary HC, Malinow MR (1982) Ultrastructure of experimental coronary artery atherosclerosis in cynomolgus macaques. A comparison with the lesions of other primates. Atherosclerosis 43:151–175

Stary HC (1990) The sequence of cell and matrix changes in atherosclerotic lesions of coronary arteries in the first forty years of life. Eur Heart J 11:3–19

Stary HC, Chandler AB, Glagov S, Guyton JR, Insull W, Jr., Rosenfeld ME et al. (1994) A definition of initial, fatty streak, and intermediate lesions of atherosclerosis. A report from the Committee on Vascular Lesions of the Council on Arteriosclerosis, American Heart Association. Arterioscler Thromb 14:840–856

Stary HC (2000) Natural history of calcium deposits in atherosclerosis progression and regression. Z Kardiol 89:28–35

Steele PM, Chesebro JH, Stanson AW, Holmes DR, Jr., Dewanjee MK, Badimon L et al. (1985) Balloon angioplasty. Natural history of the pathophysiological response to injury in a pig model. Circ Res 57:105–112

Steinberg D, Parthasarathy S, Carew TE, Khoo JC, Witztum JL (1989) Beyond cholesterol. Modifications of low density lipoprotein that increase its atherogenicity. New Engl J Med 320:915–924

Steinberg HO, Chaker H, Leaming R, Johnson A, Brechtel G, Baron AD (1996) Obesity/insulin resistance is associated with endothelial dysfunction. Implications for the syndrome of insulin resistance. J Clin Invest 97:2601–2610

Stemme S, Faber B, Holm J, Wiklund O, Witztum JL, Hansson GK. (1995) T lymphocytes from human atherosclerotic plaques recognize oxidized low density lipoprotein. Proc Natl Acad Sci USA 92:3893–3897

Stemme S (2001) Plaque T-cell activity: not so specific? Arterioscler Thromb Vasc Biol 21:1099–1101

Stender S, Zilversmit DB (1981) Transfer of plasma lipoprotein components and of plasma proteins into aortas of cholesterol-fed rabbits. Molecular size as a determinant of plasma lipoprotein influx. Arteriosclerosis 1:38–49

Subbanagounder G, Wong JW, Lee H, Faull KF, Miller E, Witztum JL et al. (2002) Epoxy-isoprostane and epoxycyclopentenone phospholipids regulate monocyte chemotactic protein-1 and interleukin-8 synthesis. Formation of these oxidized phospholipids in response to interleukin-1beta. J Biol Chem 277:7271–7281

Suzuki H, Kurihara Y, Takeya M, Kamada N, Kataoka M, Jishage K et al. (1997) A role for macrophage scavenger receptors in atherosclerosis and susceptibility to infection. Nature 386:292–296

Syrjanen J, Peltola J, Valtonen V, Iivanainen M, Kaste M, Huttunen JK (1989) Dental infections in association with cerebral infarction in young and middle-aged men. J Intern Med 225:179–184

Tabas I (1997) Free cholesterol-induced cytotoxicity. A possible contributing factor to macrophage foam cell necrosis in advanced atherosclerotic lesions. Trends Cardiovasc Med 7:256–263

Tabas I (2002) Consequences of cellular cholesterol accumulation: basic concepts and physiological implications. J Clin Invest 110:905–911

Tangirala RK, Rubin EM, Palinski W (1995) Quantitation of atherosclerosis in murine models: correlation between lesions in the aortic origin and in the entire aorta, and differences in the extent of lesions between sexes in LDL receptor-deficient and apolipoprotein E-deficient mice. J Lipid Res 36:2320–2328

Taylor AJ, Farb AA, Angello DA, Burwell LR, Virmani R (1995) Proliferative activity in coronary atherectomy tissue. Clinical, histopathologic, and immunohistochemical correlates. Chest 108:815–820

Tomasian D, Keaney JFJr, Vita JA (2000) Antioxidants and the bioactivity of endothelium-derived nitric oxide. Cardiovasc Res 47:426–435

Tontonoz P, Nagy L, Alvarez JA, Thomazy VA, Evans RM (1998) PPAR gamma promotes monocyte/macrophage differentiation and uptake of oxidized LDL. Cell 93:241–252

Tremoli E, Camera M, Toschi V, Colli S (1999) Tissue factor in atherosclerosis. Atherosclerosis 144:273–283

Vainio S, Ikonen E (2003) Macrophage cholesterol transport: a critical player in foam cell formation. Ann Med 35:146–155

van der Wal AC, Becker AE, Vanderloos CM, Das PK (1994) Site of intimal rupture or erosion of thrombosed coronary atherosclerotic plaques Is characterized by an inflammatory process irrespective of the dominant plaque morphology. Circulation 89:36–44

Vartio T, Seppa H, Vaheri A (1981) Susceptibility of soluble and matrix fibronectins to degradation by tissue proteinases, mast cell chymase and cathepsin G. J Biol Chem 256:471–477

Vasquez-Vivar J, Kalyanaraman B, Martasek P, Hogg N, Masters BS, Karoui H et al. (1998) Superoxide generation by endothelial nitric oxide synthase: the influence of cofactors. Proc Natl Acad Sci USA 95:9220–9225

Velican D, Velican C (1980) Atherosclerotic involvement of the coronary arteries of adolescents and young adults. Atherosclerosis 36:449–460

Virchow R (1856) Phlogose und Thrombose im Gefäßsystem. Gesammelte Abhandlungen zur wissenschaftlichen Medizin. Meidinger, Frankfurt am Main, p ff

Virchow R (1858) Die Cellularpathologie in ihrer Begründung auf physiologische und pathologische Gewebelehre. Verlag von August Hirschwald, Berlin

Virmani R, Burke AP, Farb A (1999) Plaque rupture and plaque erosion. Thromb Haemost 82:1–3

Virmani R, Kolodgie FD, Burke AP, Farb A, Schwartz SM (2000) Lessons from sudden coronary death: a comprehensive morphological classification scheme for atherosclerotic lesions. Arterioscler Thromb Vasc Biol 20:1262–1275

Vlassara H (1996) Advanced glycation end-products and atherosclerosis. Ann Med 28:419–426

von Eckardstein A, Langer C, Engel T, Schaukal I, Cignarella A, Reinhardt J et al. (2001) ATP binding cassette transporter ABCA1 modulates the secretion of apolipoprotein E from human monocyte-derived macrophages. FASEB J 15:1555–1561

von Rokitansky C (1852) Über einige der wichtigsten Krankheiten der Arterien. K. K. Hof- und Staatsdruckereien Wien, Vienna

Wang Y, Lindstedt KA, Kovanen PT (1995) Mast cell granule remnants carry LDL into smooth muscle cells of the synthetic phenotype and induce their conversion into foam cells. Arterioscler Thromb Vasc Biol 1995; 15:801–810

Wang Y, Kovanen PT (1999) Heparin proteoglycans released from rat serosal mast cells inhibit proliferation of rat aortic smooth muscle cells in culture. Circ Res 84:74–83

Wang N, Lan D, Chen W, Matsuura F, Tall AR (2004) ATP-binding cassette transporters G1 and G4 mediate cellular cholesterol efflux to high-density lipoproteins. Proc Natl Acad Sci USA 101:9774–9779

Wasserman SI (1990) Mast cell biology. J Allergy Clin Immunol 86:590–593

Watt S, Aesch B, Lanotte P, Tranquart F, Quentin R (2003) Viral and bacterial DNA in carotid atherosclerotic lesions. Eur J Clin Microbiol Infect Dis 22:99–105

Wedemeyer J, Tsai M, Galli SJ (2000) Roles of mast cells and basophils in innate and acquired immunity. Curr Opin Immunol 12:624–631

Weitkamp B, Cullen P, Plenz G, Robenek H, Rauterberg J (1999) Human macrophages synthesize type VIII collagen in vitro and in the atherosclerotic plaque. FASEB J 13:1445–1457

Whitman SC, Ravisankar P, Daugherty A (2000) Exogenous interferon-gamma enhances atherosclerosis in apolipoprotein E−/−mice. Am J Pathol 157:1819–1824

Whitman SC, Ravisakar P, Daugherty A (2002) Interleukin-18 enhances atherosclerosis in apolipoprotein E(−/−) mice through release of interferon-gamma. Circ Res 90:E34–E38

Widlansky ME, Gokce N, Keaney JF, Vita JA (2003) The clinical implications of endothelial dysfunction. J Am Coll Cardiol 42:1149–1160

Williams CM, Galli SJ (2000) The diverse potential effector and immunoregulatory roles of mast cells in allergic disease. J Allergy Clin Immunol 105:847–859

Williams H, Johnson JL, Carson KG, Jackson CL (2002) Characteristics of intact and ruptured atherosclerotic plaques in brachiocephalic arteries of apolipoprotein E knockout mice. Arterioscler Thromb Vasc Biol 22:788–792

Wu NZ, Baldwin AL (1992) Transient venular permeability increase and endothelial gap formation induced by histamine. Am J Physiol 262:H1238–H1247

Wu T, Trevisan M, Genco RJ, Dorn JP, Falkner KL, Sempos CT (2000) Periodontal disease and risk of cerebrovascular disease: the first national health and nutrition examination survey and its follow-up study. Arch Intern Med 160:2749–2755

Xu Q, Kleindienst R, Waitz W, Dietrich H, Wick G (1993) Increased expression of heat shock protein 65 coincides with a population of infiltrating T lymphocytes in atherosclerotic lesions of rabbits specifically responding to heat shock protein 65. J Clin Invest 91:2693–2702

Xu QB, Kleindienst R, Schett G, Waitz W, Jindal S, Gupta RS et al. (1996) Regression of ar-teriosclerotic lesions induced by immunization with heat-shock protein 65-containing material in normocholesterolemic, but not hypercholesterolemic, rabbits. Atherosclero-sis 123:145–155

Xu XX, Tabas I (1991) Lipoproteins activate acyl-coenzyme A:cholesterol acyltransferase in macrophages only after cellular cholesterol pools are expanded to a critical threshold level. J Biol Chem 266:17040–17048

Yancey PG, St.Clair RW (1992) Cholesterol efflux is defective in macrophages from atherosclerosis-susceptible White Carneau pigeons relative to resistant show racer pigeons.
Arterioscler Thromb 12:1291–1304
Yancey PG, St.Clair RW (1994) Mechanism of the defect in cholesteryl ester clearance from
macrophages of atherosclerosis-susceptible white carneau pigeons. J Lipid Res 35:2114–
2129
Yang ZH, Richard V, von Segesser L, Bauer E, Stulz P, Turina M et al. (1990) Threshold
concentrations of endothelin-1 potentiate contractions to norepinephrine and serotonin
in human arteries: a new mechanism of vasospasm? Circulation 82:188–195
Yao PM, Tabas I (2000) Free cholesterol loading of macrophages induces apoptosis involving
the fas pathway. J Biol Chem 275:23807–23813
Yao PM, Tabas I (2001) Free cholesterol loading of macrophages is associated with widespread
mitochondrial dysfunction and activation of the mitochondrial apoptosis pathway. J Biol
Chem 276:42468–42476
Yeagle PL (1991) Modulation of membrane function by cholesterol. Biochimie 73:1303–1310
Yee KO, Schwartz SM (1999) Why atherosclerotic vessels narrow: the fibrin hypothesis.
Thromb Haemost 82:762–771
Young JD, Liu CC, Butler G, Cohn ZA, Galli SJ (1987) Identification, purification, and
characterization of a mast cell-associated cytolytic factor related to tumor necrosis
factor. Proc Natl Acad Sci USA 84:9175–9179
Yura T, Fukunaga M, Khan R, Nassar GN, Badr KF, Montero A (1999) Free readical-generated
F2-isoprostane stimulates cell proliferation and endothelin-1 expression on endothelial
cells. Kidney Int 56:471–478
Zhang SH, Reddick RL, Piedrahita JA, Maeda N (1992) Spontaneous hypercholesterolemia
and arterial lesions in mice lacking apolipoprotein E. Science 258:468–471
Zhou X, Caligiuri G, Hamsten A, Lefvert AK, Hansson GK (2001) LDL immunization in-
duces T-cell-dependent antibody formation and protection against atherosclerosis. Arterioscler Thromb Vasc Biol 21:108–114
Zhou X, Hansson GK (2004) Vaccination and atherosclerosis. Curr Atheroscler Rep 6:158–
164
Zhu J, Quyyumi AA, Norman JE, Csako G, Waclawiw MA, Shearer GM et al. (2000) Effects
of total pathogen burden on coronary artery disease risk and C-reactive protein levels.
Am J Cardiol 85:140–146
Zhu J, Nieto J, Home BD, Anderson JL, Muhlestein JB, Epstein SE (2001) Prospective study
of pathogen burden and risk of myocardial infarction or death. Circulation 103:45–51
Zimmerman MR (1993) The paleopathology of the cardiovascular system. Tex Heart I J
20:252–257
Zuckerman SH, Ackerman SK, Douglass J (1979) Long-term human peripheral blood monocyte cultures: establishment, metabolism and morphology of primary human monocyte-
macrophage cell lines. Immunology 38:401–411

HEP (2005) 170:71–105
© Springer-Verlag Berlin Heidelberg 2005

Risk Factors for Atherosclerotic Vascular Disease

A. von Eckardstein

Institute of Clinical Chemistry, University Hospital Zurich, Raemistrasse 100, 8093 Zurich, Switzerland
arnold.voneckardstein@usz.ch

Abstract Several controlled interventional trials have shown the benefit of anti-hypertensive and hypolipidaemic drugs for the prevention of coronary heart disease (CHD). International guidelines for the prevention of CHD agree in their recommendations for tertiary prevention and recommend lowering the blood pressure to below 140 mm/90 mm Hg and low density lipoprotein (LDL)-cholesterol to below 2.6 mmol/l in patients with manifest CHD.

Novel recommendations for secondary prevention are focused on the treatment of the pre-symptomatic high-risk patient with an estimated CHD morbidity risk of higher than 20% per 10 years or an estimated CHD mortality risk of higher than 5% per 10 years. For the calculation of this risk, the physician must record the following risk factors: sex, age, family history of premature myocardial infarction, smoking, diabetes, blood pressure, total cholesterol, LDL-cholesterol, high-density lipoprotein (HDL)-cholesterol, and triglyceride. This information allows the absolute risk of myocardial infarction to be computed by using scores or algorithms which have been deduced from results of epidemiological studies. To improve risk prediction and to identify new targets for intervention, novel risk factors are sought. High plasma levels of C-reactive protein has been shown to improve the prognostic value of global risk estimates obtained by the combination of conventional risk factors and may influence treatment decisions in patients with intermediate global cardiovascular risk (CHD morbidity risk of 10%–20% per 10 years or CHD mortality risk of 2%–5% per 10 years).

Keywords Risk factor · LDL cholesterol · HDL cholesterol · Triglycerides · Hypertension · Diabetes mellitus · Family history · Gene · Homocysteine · C-reactive protein · Fibrinogen · Lipoprotein(a) · Obesity · Overweight · Global risk estimation · Framingham score · PROCAM algorithm · Guidelines

1
Introduction

Atherosclerosis is a multifactorial disease whose age of onset and progression are strongly influenced by inborn and acquired risk factors. Since the pioneering work of the Framingham study, many prospective population and clinical studies have identified a series of risk factors for myocardial infarction, stroke and peripheral vascular disease, among which the pre-existence of atherosclerotic vascular disease, age, male sex, a positive family history of premature atherosclerotic disease, smoking, diabetes mellitus, hypertension, hypercholesterolaemia, hypertriglyceridaemia and low high-density lipoprotein (HDL) cholesterol are considered to be classical risk factors. Moreover, several large randomized and prospective intervention studies have demonstrated that smoking cessation as well as anti-hypertensive and lipid lowering drug therapies help to reduce cardiovascular morbidity and mortality by about 30% in both secondary and primary prevention. Therefore, the classical risk factors have become part of algorithms or scores that allow the estimation of an individual's risk to suffer a cardiovascular event or to die from it. These algorithms and scores have also become important cornerstones of international guidelines aiming at the prevention of cardiovascular disease (Anonymous 2001, 2002; de Backer et al. 2003; International Task Force for Prevention of Coronary Heart Disease 2002). They have high negative predictive values but relatively low positive predictive values (von Eckardstein et al. 2004). Therefore many patients with an estimated high or moderate risk are falsely assigned to intervention. To improve the detection of individuals at risk and also to identify novel targets for therapeutic intervention, novel genotypic and phenotypic risk factors are searched for intensively.

Usually it is required that both conventional and novel risk factors are statistically independent from other risk factors in multivariate analysis. However, dependent risk factors—such as obesity and being overweight or dietary patterns—can play an important role in the pathogenesis of atherosclerosis and represent important targets for intervention. They are classified as underlying risk factors.

In the pages that follow classical, underlying and novel risk factors are reviewed. Due to limited space and because many risk factors are covered by more specific articles in this book, each risk factor is summarized in a condensed form.

2
Classical and Independent Risk Factors

2.1
Male Sex

In industrialized countries, the average life expectancy is some 8 years less in males than in females. Before the age of 55 years, men have a threefold excess of coronary heart disease (CHD) events, a twofold excess of stroke, and a two- to threefold excess of peripheral vascular disease. The lifetime risk of CHD at the age of 40 years is one in two for men and one in three for women (Lloyd-Jones et al. 1999). The different risk persists at least until the age of 80 years and, on average, the risk of women lags by 10–15 years behind that of men. This male preponderance is remarkably consistent across 52 countries with hugely divergent rates of CHD mortality and lifestyles (Wu and von Eckardstein 2003). The universality of sex disparity makes it likely that there is an intrinsic sexual dimorphism in susceptibility to CHD that may involve genetic, hormonal, lifestyle or ageing factors.

The most popular explanation for this male preponderance in coronary arterial disease is that adult male levels of testosterone are proatherogenic and/or there is a lack of the cardioprotective effects of oestrogens in men. The lack of oestrogens and the abundance of androgens have often been regarded as the principle cause underlying this male disadvantage. Sex hormones may play a role in cardiovascular morbidity and mortality by modulating the risk factors of atherosclerosis and vascular dysfunction, by influencing the progression of subclincial coronary, cerebral and peripheral arterial vessel wall lesions to symptomatic cardiovascular disease including myocardial infarction, stroke, and claudicatio intermittens. Finally, sex hormones may influence the long-term clinical sequelae of CHD such as heart failure and arrhythmias.

The lack of an inflection point in the rate of increase in cardiovascular morbidity and mortality after menopause and the failure of controlled combined oestrogen-progestin replacement intervention trials to show prevention of coronary events in postmenopausal women (Grady et al. 2002; Writing Group for the Women's Health Initiative Investigators 2002) have shed doubts on the cardioprotective role of oestrogens. The role of testosterone in atherosclerosis is uncertain because data of clinical endpoint studies are missing, and also because data from observational studies on the associations between endogenous testosterone and CHD, as well as data from interventional studies on the effects of testosterone on cardiovascular risk factors and pre-clinical symptoms of atherosclerosis, are controversial. Likewise, data from animal and in vitro experiments do not allow any conclusion to be reached regarding the net effect of testosterone on atherosclerosis (Wu and von Eckardstein 2003).

More recent concepts suggest that non-hormonal factors play a predominant role in the sex disparity in atherosclerotic vascular disease. This could involve interactions between a multitude of genetic and environmental/lifestyle factors that are important in the pathogenesis of atherosclerosis. The sex-specific expression of candidate genes may involve diverse mechanisms ranging from sex hormone exposure in utero, imprinting on sex-specific behaviour patterns, distribution of visceral body fat to vascular and myocardial structural and functional adaptation to ageing, pressure overload and disease (Hayward et al. 2000; Liu et al. 2003; Wu and von Eckardstein 2003). For example, sex differences are detectable in vascular endothelial function, lipid loading in human monocyte-derived macrophages, and for the same amount of total body fat men accumulate a disproportionately greater volume of abdominal visceral adipose tissue than premenopausal women of the same age (Liu et al. 2003; Wu and von Eckardstein 2003).

As the clinical consequence of the higher risk in men, primary CHD prevention and hence screening and treatment of risk factors should start earlier in men (>45 years) than in women (>55 years).

2.2
Age

Autopsy data obtained from miscarried foetuses as well as from children, adolescents and young adults who died because of accidents and violence have demonstrated that atherosclerosis starts early and progresses throughout life (McGill and McMahan 2003; Tsimikakis and Witztum 2002). Already at this young age, the extent of fatty streak lesions correlates with the presence and severity of risk factors (Palinski and Napoli 2002) and vice versa, risk factors in childhood predict the occurrence of carotid atheorsclerosis in early adulthood (Li et al. 2003; Raitakari et al. 2003). In both men and women, the incidence of CHD and stroke events increases steeply with advancing age. This reflects the exposure time to risk factors and the progressively increasing burden of atherosclerotic lesions. In addition cardiovascular risk factors such as dyslipi-daemias, hypertension and diabetes mellitus become more frequent and severe with increasing age. Finally, aging is accompanied by various phenomena that are involved in the pathogenesis of atherosclerosis, for example oxidation, cell death and loss of endocrine functions.

Recent clinical trials indicate that lipid lowering and antihypertensive ther-apies reduce cardiovascular morbidity and mortality in older patients (ALL-HAT Officers and Coordinators 2002a, 2002b; Mungall et al. 2003). However, the baseline level of the therapeutic target may not necessarily identify the person with the greatest benefit from the intervention. For example, in the PROSPER study baseline levels of HDL cholesterol rather than low-density lipoprotein (LDL) cholesterol had the closest relationship with risk reduction by pravastatin treatment (Shepherd 2003; Shepherd et al. 2002).

Because of the great weight of age in algorithms and scores, which were de-duced from prospective studies in middle-aged individuals, algorithms over-estimate the absolute cardiovascular risk in individuals older than 65 years of age and underestimate the risk in young individuals. As a consequence of this Grundy et al. suggested calculating relative rather than absolute risks in elderly people (Grundy et al. 1999). Alternatively, it was suggested to define more moderate treatment goals in individuals beyond the age of 80 years.

2.3
Presence of Atherosclerotic Vessel Disease

The symptomatic presence of CHD (i.e. previous myocardial infarction, angina pectoris, angiographic demonstration of CHD, previous revascularization pro-cedure) is one of the most important risk factors for myocardial infarction, cardiac death, and stroke. In these patients, dyslipidaemia and hypertension imply a several-fold increased risk as compared with patients with similar cholesterol levels or blood pressure but without CHD. This is the basis of the aggressive treatment goals for LDL cholesterol levels and blood pressure in secondary prevention. Also, patients with clinically manifest atherosclerosis in non-coronary vessels, e.g. peripheral, cerebral and renal arteries as well as aorta are at increased risk for myocardial infarction (Anonymous 2002; International Task Force for Prevention of Coronary Heart Disease 1998).

Because the presence of atherosclerotic lesions has such a high predic-tive value for the occurrence of cardiovascular events, non-invasive methods are investigated to detect patients with pre-symptomatic arteriosclerosis. The Doppler-sonographic assessment of stenoses, plaques and intima media thick-ening in the carotid arteries identifies individuals in whom the risk of myocar-dial infarction is increased by factors of two, four and six, respectively (Bots and Groby 2002). Nowadays, electron beam computed tomography (EBCT) and multidetector-row computed tomography (MDCT) as well as magnetic resonance imaging can help to detect and quantify atherosclerotic lesions in coronary arteries. Coronary artery calcifications occur relatively early in atherosclerotic disease evolution and EBCT or MDCT have been used for diagnosis of subclinical coronary artery disease and risk assessment (Arad et al. 2000; Becker et al. 2001; Detrano et al. 1999). From the results of coronary calcium measurements by CT a future myocardial event can be predicted with sensitivities reaching as high as 89% (Arad et al. 1996; Wong et al. 2000).

2.4
Family History of Atherosclerotic Vessel Disease

Individuals who have first-degree relatives with premature CHD, have a 2- to 12-fold increased risk of myocardial infarction. The risk increases with the number and younger age of affected first-degree relatives. The highest relative risk is found in siblings of patients with premature CHD, probably due to shared genes, exposures and sociocultural environment (Anonymous 2002; Scheuner 2001). In some families, the occurrence of premature CHD is paralleled with the Mendelian inheritance of a single risk factor, for example severely elevated total and LDL cholesterol in familial hypercholesterolaemia. In the majority of cases, however, the clustering of CHD resembles diseases of polygenic origin which is only partially explained by the familial aggregation of risk factors (e.g. blood pressure, lipids, Lipoprotein(a) (Anonymous 2002; Scheuner 2001).

Consequently, global cardiovascular risk estimation should include the assessment of premature CHD in all first-degree relatives. A family history will be considered as positive for CHD if myocardial infarction or cardiac death has occurred in at least one male first-degree relative younger than 55 years or one female first-degree relative younger than 65 years. Moreover, families of patients with premature CHD should be systematically worked up to detect inherited and non-inherited risk factors and to initiate preventive measures as early as possible (Anonymous 2002; International Task Force for Prevention of Coronary Heart Disease 1998, 2002).

2.5
Smoking

Smoking is a central risk factor for coronary, cerebral and peripheral artery diseases and contributes to 30% of all coronary deaths. Duration of smoking and number of cigarettes smoked correlate with the risk of myocardial infarction and stroke. Several controlled intervention trials showed that in primary prevention cessation of smoking substantially reduces the risk of cardiac events (Anonymous 2002; International Task Force for Prevention of Coronary Heart Disease 1998). This decline in risk starts within months so that after 7 years of non-smoking the risk of an ex-smoker equals the risk of a never-smoker. Therefore smoking cessation is a prime target in both the population and the clinical strategy to reduce CHD risk (Anonymous 2001, 2002; de Backer 2003; International Task Force for Prevention of Coronary Heart Disease 1998, 2002).

2.6
Total Cholesterol, LDL Cholesterol and non-HDL Cholesterol

In many population studies including the Framingham study, the PROCAM study, or the Lipid Research Clinics Trial, the serum concentrations of total cholesterol and LDL cholesterol were found to correlate with the risk of myocardial infarction and cardiac death (Anonymous 2002; International Task Force for Prevention of Coronary Heart Disease 1998). Even in populations with low CHD incidence and low average cholesterol levels (e.g. China) this association was found. The relationship between total or LDL cholesterol and stroke or peripheral artery disease is much weaker (Anonymous 1995). For stroke it is, however, important to emphasize the impact of aetiological heterogeneity. Cholesterol levels show a positive correlation with the risk of ischaemic stroke but an inverse one with haemorrhagic stroke (Iso et al. 1989; Suh et al. 2001).

A huge body of evidence from in vitro and in vivo experiments demonstrates the causal role of cholesterol in the pathogenesis of atherosclerosis. The strongest evidence is derived from the finding of premature atherosclerosis in patients with familial hypercholesterolaemia due to defects in the LDL receptor gene as well as in animals with inborn or targeted mutations in the LDL receptor gene (Brown and Goldstein 1992; Goldstein et al. 2001).

In several controlled intervention trials, lowering of LDL cholesterol by diet and/or drugs—especially statins—was found to reduce coronary and cerebrovascular morbidity and mortality both in primary and secondary prevention and independently of the absence or presence of other risk factors (ALLHAT Officers and Coordinators 2002a; Anonymous 2002; Collins et al. 2004; Heart Protection Study Collaborative Group 2002; International Task Force for Prevention of Coronary Heart Disease 1998; Shepherd et al. 2002) (see the chapter by Paoletti et al., this volume). Both men and women benefit from LDL cholesterol lowering. Results of clinical trials suggest that a reduction of total and LDL cholesterol by 1% reduces the risk of CHD by 2% and 1% respectively. However, the benefit can be larger if LDL cholesterol levels are kept low for prolonged time. A 10% decrease in LDL cholesterol achieved at age 40 lowers relative CHD risk by 50% as opposed to 10% if begun at age 70.

Current guidelines recommend to lower LDL cholesterol below 100 mg/dl (2.6 mmol/l) in patients with manifest atherosclerosis (i.e. secondary prevention) (Anonymous 2001, 2002; de Backer 2003, International Task Force for Prevention of Coronary Heart Disease 1998, 2002). Very recent data suggest that more aggressive LDL cholesterol lowering therapy below this target value by using high dosages of atorvastatin results in even greater risk reduction (Cannon et al. 2004). In primary prevention, indications and goals of LDL lowering therapy vary depending on the presence and severity of additional risk factors (Anonymous 2001, 2002; de Backer 2003; International Task Force for Prevention of Coronary Heart Disease 1998, 2000; see Sect. 2.11).

As cholesterol is also transported in very low-density lipoprotein (VLDL) and its remnants, which also are atherogenic lipoproteins (as highlighted by premature and severe atherosclerosis in patients with type III hyperlipidaemia due to gene defects in the apolipoprotein (apo) E, as well as in apoE-deficient animals (Mahley and Rall 2001), some authors have suggested monitoring and targeting non-HDL cholesterol levels (i.e. VLDL+LDL cholesterol) rather than LDL cholesterol levels. However, only some but not all of the prospective studies proved the prognostic superiority of non-HDL cholesterol. This appears to be true especially in patients with moderate but not severe hypertriglyceridaemia (>200 mg/dl but <500 mg/dl) (Anonymous 2002). Therefore all international guidelines target LDL cholesterol rather than total or non-HDL cholesterol as primary treatment goals. Some guidelines (for example ATP III) accept non-HDL cholesterol as a secondary treatment goal in patients with moderate hypertriglyceridaemia (Anonymous 2001, 2002; de Backer 2003; International Task Force for Prevention of Coronary Heart Disease 2002).

2.7
HDL Cholesterol

Numerous clinical and epidemiological studies have demonstrated the inverse and independent association between HDL cholesterol and the risk of fatal and non-fatal CHD events (Gordon and Rifkind 1989; Hersberger and von Eckardstein 2003). Low HDL cholesterol has been found in more than 40% of patients with myocardial infarction (Genest et al. 1991). This prevalence may be even higher in some ethnic populations, e.g. Turks, Arabs or Israelis, who for unknown reasons have 10–15 mg/dl lower mean concentrations of HDL cholesterol than Caucasians and who face a dramatic increase in the incidence of cardiovascular disease (Bobak et al. 1999, Hergenc et al. 1999).

From the data of population studies, it has been calculated that every 1 mg/dl increase in HDL cholesterol lowers coronary risk by 1%. In patients with angiographically assessed CHD this association may even be stronger as the prospective and multicentric European Concerted Action on Thrombosis and Disabilities (ECAT) study, as well as the Baltimore Longitudinal Heart Study identified low HDL cholesterol as the most important biochemical risk factor for coronary events (Bolibar et al. 2000; Miller et al. 1998). However, it is not clear whether this rule can be extrapolated to the whole range of HDL cholesterol. Whereas a low HDL cholesterol level (e.g. below the 20th percentile) has been consistently found to increase cardiovascular risk, it has not been consistently shown that a high HDL cholesterol level is protective. In at least some studies, including the PROCAM study and the ECAT Angina pectoris study, individuals with the highest levels of HDL cholesterol (e.g. above the 80th percentile) did not experience fewer coronary events than individuals with HDL cholesterol in the high–normal range (e.g. 60th to 80th percentile). In certain metabolic conditions (e.g. hepatic lipase deficiency, some cases of cholesterol ester transfer protein deficiency) a high level of HDL cholesterol is rather associated with increased cardiovascular risk (Hirano et al. 1995). Hypertriglyceridaemic participants of the Copenhagen City Heart Study and the PROCAM Study with high levels of HDL cholesterol were at higher coronary risk than hypertriglyceridaemic probands with intermediate HDL cholesterol levels (Jeppesen et al. 1998; von Eckardstein et al. 1999). Interestingly, although low HDL cholesterol is also significantly associated with reduced life expectancy, in the PROCAM population and also in a Belgian population, HDL cholesterol levels in the fifth quintile were also associated with excess mortality as compared to intermediate HDL levels (Cullen et al. 1997; de Backer et al. 1998).

By convention, the risk threshold values of HDL cholesterol have been defined to be 35 mg/dl or 40 mg/dl (0.9 mmol/l or 1.05 mmol/l) in men and 45 mg/l or 50 mg/dl (1.15 mmol/l or 1.3 mmol/l) in women (Anonymous 2001, 2002; de Backer 2003; International Task Force for Prevention of Coronary Heart Disease 2002). However, as with other risk factors, the strength of the association between HDL cholesterol and cardiovascular risk depends on the presence of additional risk factors (von Eckardstein and Assmann 2000). By contrast to high LDL cholesterol, which coincides by chance with smoking and other risk factors, low HDL cholesterol is frequently confounded because of metabolic reasons with hypertriglyceridaemia, the presence of small dense LDL, impaired glucose tolerance or overt diabetes mellitus type 2, hypertension, and overweight. Actually, in many populations a low HDL cholesterol is a typical component of the metabolic syndrome or insulin resistance syndrome that precedes the manifestation of the other components including diabetes mellitus type 2 (Anonymous 2002; International Task Force for Prevention of Coronary Heart Disease 2002; Rohrer et al. 2004). Thus, although the association of HDL cholesterol with CHD is statistically independent of other risk factors, a low HDL cholesterol is frequently not the sole risk factor in a single individual (see chapters by Grund und Müller, Wieland und Kotzka).

Some controlled intervention studies demonstrated a significant benefit of patients with low HDL cholesterol from hypolipidaemic drug therapy (Gotto et al. 2000; Manninen et al. 1992; Rubins et al. 1999). Therefore, and as HDL exerts various potentially anti-atherogenic properties (reverse cholesterol transport as well as inhibition of oxidation, inflammation, coagulation and platelet aggregation), and because increasing HDL cholesterol was found to protect from atherosclerosis in several genetic animal models, HDL cholesterol has attracted a lot of interest from both clinicians and the pharmaceutical industry, not only as a marker of increased coronary risk but also as a therapeutic target (Hersberger and von Eckardstein 2003). Actually, whereas in current international guidelines a low HDL cholesterol is only an indication to start treatment of risk factors (Anonymous 2002; International Task Force for Prevention of Coronary Heart Disease 2002), it is now increasingly discussed to advocate an HDL cholesterol plasma level >1 mmol/l as a therapeutic goal (Fruchart et al. 1998). However, to date the majority of the presently available drugs does not increase HDL cholesterol levels effectively enough to reach this goal in many patients with manifest CHD or increased cardiovascular risk. Moreover, experiences of patients with inborn errors of HDL metabolism and, even more so, data from genetic animal models of HDL metabolism indicate that is it not the increase of HDL cholesterol per se but the mechanism of modifying HDL metabolism and function that is relevant for protection from atherosclerosis (Hersberger and von Eckardstein 2003) (see the chapter by Hersberger and von Eckardstein, this volume).

Several studies have investigated the question of whether HDL subpopulations or apolipoproteins have a better prognostic value than HDL cholesterol. Data are conflicting and derive mostly from small case–control studies. Prospective data have been generated in the Physicians' Health Study and the ARIC study (Sharrett et al. 2001; Stampfer et al. 1991), which did not show any superiority of HDL$_2$, HDL$_3$ or apoA-I, and most recently in the PRIME study, which found apoA-I to be a better risk indicator than HDL-C (Luc et al. 2002).

2.8
Triglycerides

The role of triglycerides as a cardiovascular risk factor is controversial. Upon univariate statistical analysis, most epidemiological studies found positive correlations between the concentration of serum triglycerides and cardiovascular event rates. However, this association did not remain stable in multivariate data analysis of many data sets. Reasons for this include the non-Gaussian frequency distribution with a preponderance of low and normal triglyceride levels (<150 mg/dl or <1.7 mmol/l) and the frequent confounding of hypertriglyceridaemia with other cardiovascular risk factors (low HDL cholesterol, hyperglycaemia, hypertension). Moreover, the risk increases only with triglycerides up to about 10 mmol/l and tends to decrease again at higher levels (Austin et al. 1998). Among others, the reason for this is the heterogeneity of triglyceride-rich lipoproteins, which also differ in atherogenicity. Cholesterol-enriched remnants of chylomicrons and VLDL (i.e. intermediate density lipoproteins) appear to be more atherogenic than their triglyceride-richer but cholesterol-poorer precursors. Nevertheless, meta-analyses of epidemiological studies revealed a statistically significant association of triglycerides with CHD which is independent of other risk factors and appears to be stronger in women than in men (Austin et al. 1998).

Because of their higher atherogenicity, tests for the measurement of remnant lipoproteins are currently being developed and evaluated. Concentrations of non-HDL cholesterol and apoB, which may reflect the number of atherogenic lipoprotein particles better than triglycerides and LDL cholesterol, were

found to correlate with CHD risk (Anonymous 2002). Also small LDL particles, which are frequently found in hypertriglyceridaemic patients, are a good
marker for the presence of atherogenic cholesterol and apoB-containing particles (Lamarche et al. 1999). However, in the clinical setting, apoB and LDL size
suffer from the lack of standardization or feasible and cheap high throughput
methods.

2.9
High Blood Pressure

The present guidelines of the World Health Organization (WHO), the International Hypertension Society and the Joint National Committee on Prevention, Detection, Evaluation and Treatment of Hypertension define hypertension as the presence of a systolic blood pressure above 140 mmHg or
diastolic blood pressure above 90 mmHg (Anonymous 1996, 1997). Hypertension has been consistently found to increase the risk of stroke, myocardial infarction and heart failure. The highest risk of myocardial infarction
is found in hypertensive patients with diabetes mellitus or dyslipidaemias,
ventricular hypertrophy, reduced renal function and proteinuria and smokers. Together with overweight, hyperglycaemia, low HDL cholesterol and
hypertriglyceridaemia hypertension is a component of the metabolic syndrome (Anonymous 2002). Several controlled, randomized and prospective
trials have demonstrated that the decrease in blood pressure achieved by beta
blockers, diuretics, angiotensin converting enzyme (ACE) inhibitors and angiotensin receptor blockers reduces cardiovascular morbidity and mortality
(ALLHAT Officers and Coordinators 2002b; Anonymous 1997a, 2002; International Task Force for Prevention of Coronary Heart Disease 1998, 2002).
Some of these drugs appear to be anti-atherogenic independently of lowering
blood pressure, e.g. ACE inhibitors (see the chapter by Dendorfer et al., this
volume).

The aggressiveness of blood pressure lowering therapy depends on the
presence of cardiovascular diseases and additional risk factors. In patients
with manifest cardiovascular disease or hypertension-induced organ damage
(ventricular hypertrophy, renal insufficiency, proteinuria) or additional risk
factors (diabetes, smoking, dyslipidaemia) or excessive hypertension (systolic
blood pressure >180 mmHg, diastolic blood pressure >100 mmHg) the therapeutic goal must be targeted aggressively by an early start of drug therapy
and frequent controls. In patients without organ damage or additional risk
factors non-pharmacological interventions (weight reduction, salt and alcohol
restriction, physical activity) can be tried for a longer time (Anonymous 1996;
1997a, 2001, 2002; de Backer 2003; International Task Force for Prevention of
Coronary Heart Disease 2002).

2.10
Diabetes

The WHO and American Diabetes Association (ADA) defined diabetes mellitus as a fasting plasma glucose level of 126 mg/dl (7 mmol/l) or higher (Alberti and Zimmet 1998; Anonymous 1997b). Both type 1 diabetes mellitus and type 2 diabetes mellitus increase the risk for coronary, cerebral and peripheral arterosclerotic vessel disease. The relative cardiovascular risk associated with diabetes mellitus is higher in women than in men so that also before menopause, women with diabetes mellitus have a substantially increased risk for myocardial infarction and stroke and both sexes are to be treated according to identical guidelines and targets (Anonymous 1997a, 2002; de Backer 2003; International Task Force for Prevention of Coronary Heart Disease 2002).

The increased risk of diabetics is associated both dependently with hyperglycaemia and independently with risk factors which accumulate in diabetic patients, for example dyslipidaemias (especially hypertriglyceridaemia and low HDL cholesterol), arterial hypertension, nephropathy, and a hypercoaguable state (for example elevated levels of fibrinogen and plasminogen activator inhibitor 1, or disturbed fibrinolysis).

In patients with type 1 diabetes mellitus but euglycaemic control, hypertension and dyslipidaemias are not more prevalent than in the non-diabetic population. However, hyperglycaemia and diabetic nephropathy frequently coincide with elevated blood pressure and dyslipidaemia so that CHD and other vascular diseases become manifest in the fourth and fifth decades of life. In patients with type 2 diabetes mellitus, risk factors are significantly more frequent than in patients with type 1 diabetes mellitus and the non-diabetic population, even if plasma glucose levels are normal. Already the pre-clinical phase of type 2 diabetes mellitus (impaired fasting glucose according to ADA, or disturbed glucose tolerance according to WHO) is frequently characterized by the presence of low HDL cholesterol, hypertriglyceridaemia and/or hypertension. The presence of these risk factors for many years before manifestation of diabetes is an important reason why at the time of clinical diagnosis many patients with diabetes mellitus type 2 are already affected with cardiovascular disease (see the chapter by Grundy, this volume).

Euglycaemic control (i.e. glycated haemoglobin <7.0%) is the most important treatment goal in patients with diabetes mellitus. However it was consistently found to reduce the risk of microvascular complications such as nephropathy and retinopathy but not the risk of macrovascular atherosclerotic events such as myocardial infarction, stroke or limb amputation (de Fronzo 1999). Therefore and because other risk factors were found to increase the risk of cardiovascular events more pronouncedly in diabetic than in non-diabetic patients, treatment of hypertension and dyslipidaemia have become cornerstones in the prevention of cardiovascular disease in patients with diabetes mellitus. Post hoc analyses of many controlled prospective intervention trials demonstrated that cardiovascular event rates are decreased by blood pressure and LDL cholesterol lowering therapies in diabetic patients as much as in non-diabetic individuals (Collins et al. 2003; Heart Protection Study Collaborative Group 2002). Therefore, many guidelines consider diabetes mellitus as a CHD equivalent and define treatment goals for blood pressure and LDL cholesterol that are identical to those defined for secondary prevention, i.e. normalization of blood pressure below 140 mmHg (systolic) and 90 mmHg (diastolic) and lowering of LDL cholesterol to below 100 mg/dl (2.6 mmol/l). Triglycerides should be less than 150 mg/dl (150 mmol/l) and HDL cholesterol above 35 mg/dl (0.9 mmol/l). Diabetic patients should not smoke (Anonymous 1997a, 2002; de Backer 2003; International Task Force for Prevention of Coronary Heart Disease 2002).

2.11
Global Cardiovascular Risk Estimation

Two recent reports on the data of more than 500,000 participants in 14 intervention trials and three observational studies showed that 80% to 90% of patients who developed clinically significant coronary heart disease had at least one of four classical risk factors, namely hypercholesterolaemia (serum cholesterol >240 mg/dl or 6.22 mmol/l), hypertension (systolic blood pressure >140 mmHg and/or diastolic blood pressure >90 mmHg), diabetes mellitus or smoking (Greenland et al. 2003; Khot et al. 2003). However, counting of risk factors has a low sensitivity and specificity because it does not take into account the graded and dose-dependent influence of risk factors and the overproportional effect of risk factor interaction. In a given individual, the presence of a single risk factor has a low positive predictive value and vice versa, the presence of several moderately expressed risk factors can produce a significant increase in cardiovascular risk. Therefore, at present the most advanced strategy for coronary risk assessment is to combine the information of several risk factors in algorithms or scores. This procedure allows calculation of an individual's absolute risk of experiencing a cardiovascular event (fatal and/or non-fatal) within the next 10 years (Assmann et al. 2002, Conroy et al. 2003, Wilson et al 1998).

Current international guidelines released by the National Cholesterol Education Program (Adult Treatment Panel III, ATP III), European Societies of Cardiology, Atherosclerosis etc. (3rd Joint European Guidelines, 3JE) or the International Task Force for the Prevention of Coronary Heart Disease/International Atherosclerosis Society (TF/IAS) base their recommendations for the indication of hypolipidaemic or anti-hypertensive drug treatment in clinically asymptomatic patients ('primary prevention') on the estimation of an individual's global risk of suffering a fatal or non-fatal cardiovascular event (ATP III and TF/IAS) (Anonymous 2002, International Task Force for Prevention of Coronary Heart Disease 2002) or of dying as a result of cardiovascular disease

(3JE) (de Backer 2003) (Tables 1 and 2). The algorithms and scores have been derived either from the US-American Framingham study (ATP III) (Anonymous 2001, 2002; Wilson et al 1998), the German PROCAM study (TF/IAS) (Assmann et al. 2002; International Task Force for Prevention of Coronary Heart Disease 2002) or pooled epidemiological data from various European cohorts (3JE) (Conroy et al. 2003; de Backer 2003). An estimated global cardiovascular morbidity plus mortality risk of more than 20% per 10 years (ATP III and TF/IAS) or an estimated cardiovascular mortality risk of greater than 5% per 10 years (3JE) in an asymptomatic patient is considered high (Anonymous 2002; de Backer 2003; International Task Force for Prevention of Coronary Heart Disease). The affected patient is advised to be treated as aggressively as a symptomatic patient with vascular disease. This implies lowering of LDL cholesterol to below 100 mg/dl (2.6 mmol/l) and systolic blood pressure below 130 mmHg. Estimated CHD risks ranging between 10% and 20% (morbidity plus mortality) or 2% and 5% (mortality) in 10 years are considered as moderate and treatment targets for LDL cholesterol and systolic blood pressure are less than 130 mg/dl (<3.4 mmol/l) and 140 mmHg, respectively. Estimated CHD risks of less than 10% (morbidity) or less than 2% (mortality) are considered low. In this case, drug treatment recommendations are not offered to the majority of individuals (Anonymous 2002; de Backer 2003; International Task Force for Prevention of Coronary Heart Disease 2003).

The three international guidelines differ in their use of various risk factors (Tables 1 and 2) and hence in their prognostic efficacy (Table 3). If validated in the German PROCAM or MONICA cohorts, the ITF/IAS guidelines have the highest specificity, positive predictive value and diagnostic efficacy, the 3JE guideline have the best sensitivity but lowest specificity, positive predictive value and diagnostic efficacy (Table 3).

Using the PROCAM algorithm as advocated by TF/IAS, 7.5% of German men aged 35–65 years have an estimated CHD risk above 20%, 15% an estimated CHD risk of 10%–20% and 72.5% an estimated CHD risk below 10%. Each group accounts for about one-third of all coronary events that occur during 10 years of follow up. Using the PROCAM algorithm, the finding of an estimated global risk above 20% in a 35–65-year-old asymptomatic German man has a positive predictive value of 32%. The finding of an estimated global risk of less than 10% has a negative predictive value of 97%. The intermediate risk of 10%–20% has positive and negative predictive values of 14% and 86%, respectively (von Eckardstein et al. 2004). The Framingham algorithm propagated by ATP III and, even more so, the SCORECARD propagated by 3JE have even lower positive predictive values and, hence, overestimate cardiovascular risk in asymptomatic German middle-aged men (Hense et al. 2003; von Eckardstein et al. 2004).

The predictive values summarized above give rise to a conceptual misunderstanding by many scientists, physicians, and patients, who believe that the assessment of classical risk factors leads to an underestimation of coronary risk

Table 1 Comparison of consensus methods for the estimation of global CHD risk according to content

	3rd Joint European Guidelines (3JE)	ITF/IAS	ATP III
Risk factors considered in the algorithm	Sex, age, smoking, systolic blood pressure, cholesterol	Age, family history, smoking, diabetes mellitus, systolic blood pressure, LDL cholesterol, HDL cholesterol, triglycerides	Age, smoking, diabetes mellitus, systolic blood pressure, cholesterol, HDL cholesterol, triglycerides
Method of risk estimation	Graphic tables (SCORECARD) in combination with hypertension (>180/110 mmHg), diabetes mellitus (yes/no), hypercholesterolaemia (total cholesterol >8 mmol/l or LDL cholesterol >6 mmol/l) as CHD equivalents	Algorithm or scoring	Scoring in combination with counting of risk factors and diabetes mellitus as CHD equivalent
Data source	SCORE: summarized CHD mortality data from 12 European studies	PROCAM (Germany)	Framingham (Massachusetts, USA)
Applicable to women	Yes	(Yes)	Yes
Age range (years)	40–65	35–65	30–75

Table 2 Comparison of consensus-methods for CHD risk estimation according to strata of risk stratification

	3JE	ITF/IAS	ATP III
High risk			
Definitions	1. Clinically manifest atherosclerosis 2. Diabetes mellitus type 2 or type 1 combined with microalbuminuria 3. Estimated CHD death risk > 5% in 10 years 4. Cholesterol > 8 mmol/l or 320 mg/dl 5. LDL cholesterol > 6 mmol/l or /240 mg/dl 6. Blood pressure > 180/110 mmHg	1. Clinically manifest atherosclerosis 2. Estimated CHD risk > 20% in 10 years	1. Clinically manifest atherosclerosis 2. Diabetes mellitus 3. Estimated CHD risk > 20% in 10 years
Treatment goals	1. LDL cholesterol < 2.6 mmol/l or 100 mg/dl blood pressure < 140/90 mmHg 2. LDL cholesterol < 2.6 mmol/l or 100 mg/dl Blood pressure < 130/80 mmHg 3.-6. LDL cholesterol < 3 mmol/l or 115 mg/dl Blood pressure < 140/90 mmHg	1.-2.: LDL cholesterol < 2.6 mmol/l or < 100 mg/dl. Blood pressure < 130/85 mmHg	1.-3.: LDL cholesterol < 2.6 mmol/l or < 100 mg/dl. Blood pressure < 130/85 mmHg
Intermediate risk			
Definitions	Estimated CHD death risk 2%–5% in 10 years	Estimated CHD risk 10%–20% in 10 years	Estimated CHD risk 10%–20% in 10 years Two or more important risk factors[a]
Treatment goals	Blood pressure < 140/90 mmHg	LDL cholesterol < 3.4 mmol/l or < 130 mg/dl Blood pressure < 140/90 mmHg	LDL cholesterol < 3.4 mmol/l or < 130 mg/dl Blood pressure < 140/90 mmHg
Moderate risk			
Definitions	Estimated CHD death risk > 2% in 10 years	Estimated CHD risk < 10% in 10 years	Estimated CHD risk < 10% in 10 years One important risk factor[a]
Treatment goals	Blood pressure < 140/90 mmHg	LDL cholesterol < 4.2 mmol/l < 160 mg/dl Blood pressure < 140/90 mmHg	LDL-C < 4.2 mmol/l < 160 mg/dl Blood pressure < 140/90 mmHg

[a] ATPIII defines the following risk factors as important: cigarette smoking, blood pressure > 140/90 mmHg or presence of anti-hypertensive medication, HDL cholesterol < 40 mg/dl (≤ 1.05 mmol/l), family history with premature CHD in first-degree relatives (women < 65 years of age, men < 55 years of age) and age (men > 45 years and women > 55 years). HDL cholesterol > 60 mg/dl (≥ 1.6 mmol/l) is considered as a negative risk factor, which should lead to subtraction of one point.

Table 3 Comparison of consensus methods for CHD risk estimation according to prognostic value in male participants of the PROCAM study

	3JE-guidelines		ITF/IAS	ATP III
	Low-risk model	High-risk model		
Prevalence of patients recommended to be treated[a]	13.5%	25%	7.5%	10.6%
Relative risk of patients recommended to be treated vs. patients not recommended to be treated[a]	4.21	5.47	6.81	4.47
Sensitivity	39.7%	64.6%	35.7%	34.5%
Specificity	88.4%	77.9%	94.5%	91.1%
Predictive value of positive test	19.8%	17.5%	32.0%	21.9%
Predictive value of negative test	95.3%	96.8%	95.3%	95.1%
Diagnostic efficacy	85.1%	77.0%	90.5%	87.3%

[a] In predicting coronary events in male participants of the PROCAM study according to risks of CHD morbidity > 20% in 10 years (ITF/IAS and ATP III) or CHD mortality > 5% in 10 years (3JE) as estimated by the various methods (325 events in 4818 men aged 35–65 years during 10 years of follow-up).

in many individuals. The opposite is the case. The detection of the relatively small percentage of individuals who will develop atherosclerotic vascular disease despite estimated low global risk would require cost-intensive screening of large populations with a low case finding probability. The more relevant problem is the high false-positive rate in individuals with a high or intermediate estimated global risk (von Eckardstein 2004).

The use of neural network statistics rather than conventional Cox-proportional hazard or multiple logistic function statistics can improve the diagnostic efficacy of global risk estimation because it can also consider dependent (i.e. underlying risk factors) and further stratify categorical risk factors (for example duration of smoking and number of cigarettes, duration and kind of treatment of diabetes mellitus). However, this strategy does not provide freely accessible algorithms and scores, but requires the communication with a central data manager for the calculation of an individual's risk (Voss et al. 2002). Moreover, even this approach does not eliminate the problem of false-positive risk assignment.

3
Underlying Risk Factors

Many epidemiological studies identified lifestyle factors as being associated with the incidence of cardiovascular diseases. However, since these risk factors at least partially affect the pathogenesis of atherosclerosis indirectly via other measurable risk factors, they frequently did not emerge as statistically independent risk factors. Nevertheless they play an important role in the pathogenesis of cardiovascular diseases and are therefore targets for prevention (Krumhout et al. 2002).

3.1
Diet and Alcohol

Prospective studies show that dietary patterns modify the baseline risk of CHD and contribute to the manifestation of overweight and obesity, elevated blood pressure, glucose intolerance and diabetes mellitus, dyslipidaemia and thrombophilia. Numerous dietary compounds modulate the pathogenetic process of atherosclerosis either negatively or positively. Details on the pro- and anti-atherogenic effects of the various dietary compounds are presented in other chapters of this book (see chapters by Lakka and Bouchard, Thijssen and Mensink, Kratz, Suter, and Tikkanen, and by Aviram and Fuhrmann, this volume). Essential goals of a healthy diet encompass (Anonymous 2002; Hu and Willett 2002; International Task Force for Prevention of Coronary Heart Disease 1998):

- Reduction of dietary fat to below 30% of calories. Dietary cholesterol should be less than 300 mg cholesterol per day. Saturated fatty acids should represent less than one-third of dietary fat and should be substituted by mono- and polyunsaturated fatty acids and complex carbohydrates.
- The diet should be enriched in whole grains as well as fresh fruits and vegetables.
- The calorie intake should be limited in order to keep or gain normal body weight.
- Patients with hypertension should limit the intake of salt (<4 g or 70 mmol of sodium chloride per day) and alcohol.
- Patients with severe dyslipidaemia, diabetes mellitus or hypertension should receive special dietary counselling.

Epidemiological studies revealed a J- or U-shaped relationship between alcohol consumption and total mortality. Teetotallers have a higher cardiovascular risk than moderate drinkers (10 g–30 g alcohol corresponding to one to three drinks per day) (Mukamal and Rimm 2001; Mukamal et al. 2003). More excessive alcohol consumption increases total mortality by increasing the incidences of accidents, suicide, liver cirrhosis, pancreatitis, various cancers, cardiomyopathy and haemorrhagic stroke. The protective effect of alcohol is frequently explained by beneficial effects on HDL cholesterol, platelet aggregation and fibrinolysis. However, drinking of alcohol does also increase blood pressure and serum levels of triglycerides (Mukamal and Rimm 2001; Mukamal et al. 2003) (see the chapter by Hendriks and van Tol, this volume). In addition it is intensively discussed whether red wine is anti-atherogenic and explains the so-called French paradox because of the additional presence of anti-oxidants (Rimm and Stampfer 2002) (see the chapter by Aviram and Fuhrmann, this volume). However, several observational studies did not find any evidence for different risk reduction by various forms of alcoholic beverages.

3.2
Physical Inactivity

Physical inactivity is an independent risk factor of myocardial infarction and predisposes for the manifestation of overweight, hypertension, diabetes mellitus, low HDL cholesterol, hypertriglyceridaemia and thrombophilia (McKechnie and Mosca 2003) (see the chapter by Lakka and Bouchard, this volume).

3.3
Obesity and Overweight

The WHO classifies obesity and overweight according to body mass index (BMI), which is calculated by division of body weight (in kg) by the square of body height (in m). The relationship between BMI and mortality is J-formed, i.e. underweight (BMI <18.5 kg/m^2) as well as overweight (BMI >25 kg/m^2) and even more so obesity (BMI >30 kg/m^2) reduce life expectancy. The excess in morbidity and mortality associated with obesity is considerably due to cardiovascular diseases. Overweight and obesity increase cardiovascular risk partially by their close association with hypertension, glucose intolerance, low HDL cholesterol and hypertriglyceridaemia. In particular, excess intra-abdominal fat predisposes to insulin resistance, which plays a pivotal role in the pathogenesis of these metabolic disorders. Simple clinical indices of central or abdominal adiposity are a waist circumference of more than 80 cm in women and more than 94 cm in men or a waist/hip ratio of over 0.85 in women and over 1 in men. Patients with a BMI of more than 30 kg/m^2 and/or a waist circumference in excess of 88 cm (women) or in excess of 102 cm (men) need special medical attention. Weight reduction increases life expectancy and reduces cardiovascular risk by lowering blood pressure and improving glucose tolerance and dyslipidaemia. In addition, weight reduction decreases the risks of accidents, certain carcinomas and chronic lung and articular diseases. Therefore ATP III has defined weight reduction in overweight and obese patients as primary goals of CHD prevention. This strategy becomes an even more important issue because the prevalence of obesity and overweight increases all over the world, most pronouncedly in children and adolescents (Anonymous 2002; Kopelman 2000, see also the chapters by Grundy, Lakka and Bouchard, and Müller-Wieland and Kotzka, this volume).

3.4
Psychosocial Factors

A low socio-economic status, lack of social support, depression and hostility are independent risk factors of CHD. They have impact on the pathogenesis of atherosclerosis both directly via neuroendocrine pathways (for example the activation of sympathetic nerves) and indirectly by the association with an unhealthy life style (e.g. smoking, lack of physical activity, atherogenic diet, overweight). In practice these factors are difficult to monitor objectively so that they are not part of models of cardiovascular risk assessment (Krantz and McCeney 2002).

4
Novel or Emerging Risk Factors

The interest in improving cardiovascular risk assessment, resulting from a better understanding of the pathogenesis of atherosclerosis and identification of new targets for anti-atherosclerotic drug therapy has always stimulated the search for novel risk factors. Thousands of cross-sectional case–control studies have identified hundreds of clinical, biochemical or genetic markers which showed statistically significant associations with coronary heart disease, stroke or peripheral vascular disease. Most of these associations were either not reproducible in other studies or not independent of classical risk factors. However, some of these emerging risk factors turned out to be robust and independent. Some of them are listed in Table 4.

Currently there is an intense discussion whether they should be introduced into routine risk assessment. To this end they must fulfil pre-defined criteria (Anonymous 2002; Hackam and Anand 2003; von Eckardstein 2004):

Table 4 Examples of emerging risk factors

Lipid risk factors
VLDL-remnants, small dense LDL, lipoprotein(a), apolipoproteins A-I, B, C-III
Prothrombotic factors
Fibrinogen, plasminogen activator inhibitor 1, tissue plasminogen activator, factor VII, von Willebrand factor, D-dimer
Inflammation markers
High sensitivity CRP, serum amyloid A, white blood cell count
Insulin resistance marker
Impaired fasting glucose, impaired glucose tolerance, insulin, indices like HOMA (homeostatic model assessment)
Others
Homocysteine

– The methods for their measurement must be precise, accurate, and internationally standardized so that the results are reliable and independent from the manufacturer and the laboratory.

– The analyte should be biologically stable so that single measurements within an individual are representative and no special pre-analytical requirements are to be fulfilled.

– Consensus must have been obtained on diagnostic cut-offs so that clinical decisions can be drawn in daily practice.

– A novel risk factor must interact with the classical risk factors so that they improve the diagnostic efficacy of global risk estimation. In addition or alternatively, they should be of special importance in subgroups of patients, e.g. in women or patients with diabetes mellitus or kidney disease, or in association with specific vascular diseases, e.g. stroke or peripheral vascular disease.

– The assessment of the risk factor should have therapeutic implications which in the ideal case are specific.

– The marker should exhibit a good cost–benefit relationship by fulfilling the criteria listed before and by being measured by easy-to-use and inexpensive tests.

In the following lipoprotein(a) (Lp(a)), C-reactive protein (CRP), fibrinogen, homocysteine and microalbuminuria are discussed in more detail as they are best documented with respect to the aforementioned criteria (Hackam and Anand 2003; von Eckardstein 2004).

4.1
Lipoprotein(a)

In several prospective clinical studies, high serum levels of Lp(a) were identified as a risk factor for CHD (Marcovina et al. 2003) (see also the chapter by Kostner and Kostner, this volume). A meta analysis of data on more than 4,000 cases revealed that patients with Lp(a) levels in the upper tertile have a 70% higher risk of CHD events as compared with patients with Lp(a) levels in the lower tertile (Danesh et al. 2000). By convention, the majority of laboratories agree on a cut-off of 30 mg/dl, above which cardiovascular risk is considered as increased (Marcovina et al. 2003). The importance of Lp(a) as a CHD risk factor will increase if elevated Lp(a) coincides with additional risk factors. In a prospective 10-year follow up of the PROCAM study, elevated Lp(a) was found to further increase coronary risk in men with elevated LDL cholesterol relative risk (RR)=2.6), low HDL cholesterol (RR=8.3) and arterial hypertension (RR=3.3). However, the effect of increased Lp(a) was much less in men with LDL cholesterol levels below 160 mg/dl (RR=1.3), HDL cholesterol above 35 mg/dl (RR=2.1), or normal blood pressure (RR=2.2). Estimation of global cardiovascular risk by multiple logistic function (MLF) analysis helped to define two high-risk quintiles of men in which 83% of all coronary events occurred. Lp(a) improved the prediction of coronary events in men with high (i.e. fifth quintile of MLF) and moderately increased (i.e. fourth quintile of MLF) global risk of coronary events (RR=2.7) but did not do so in men with low estimated global coronary risk (first to third quintiles of MLF; RR=0.01) (von Eckardstein et al. 2001).

The role of elevated Lp(a) as a risk factor of stroke is controversial (Marcovina et al. 2003). It has been identified as a risk factor for stroke in both the elderly and in the young (Ariyo et al. 2003; Strater et al. 2002). In children, adolescents and young adults it appears of special relevance for stroke risk if it occurs in association with thrombophilic risk factors such as resistance to activated protein C because of the G1691A mutation in clotting factor V (factor V Leiden) (Nowak-Gottl et al. 1999).

Because of its strong genetic determination, Lp(a) levels show little intra-individual variation. However, renal insufficiency and proteinuria cause increases in Lp(a) levels. Consequently, it is not the Lp(a) level but the size polymorphism of its protein constituent, apolipoprotein(a), which shows a significant association with coronary events in patients with renal disease (Kronenberg et al. 1999).

Lp(a) levels are influenced little by currently available drugs except sex steroids. In post hoc analyses of some intervention trials, individuals with high Lp(a) levels were found to derive an excessive benefit from statin or postmenopausal hormone replacement therapy. However, this finding has not been reproduced in the analyses of other large intervention trials (Berg et al. 1997; Shlipak et al. 2000) (see also the chapter by Kostner and Kostner, this volume).

An international Lp(a) standard has become available only recently. However, the use of this standard by different tests still gives discrepant results so that Lp(a) data from different laboratories give discrepant results (Marcovina et al. 2000).

4.2
C-Reactive Protein

Several population studies have identified mildly elevated serum levels of CRP (i.e. below the threshold level which in clinical practice is taken as the cut-off to diagnose acute bacterial infection) as a significant and independent cardiovascular risk factor. A huge observational study in the Icelandic population and a parallel meta-analysis of previously investigated populations found that CRP levels in the upper tertile increases CHD risk by 45% as compared to a 135% increase in CHD risk associated with cholesterol levels in the upper tertile (Danesh et al. 2004). The consistent finding of elevated CRP as a cardiovascular risk factor has contributed much to our current paradigm of understanding atherosclerosis as an inflammatory disease. A CRP level above 1 mg/l is considered to indicate a moderate increase in risk and a CRP level above 3 mg/l is considered to be an indicator of high risk (Pearson et al. 2003; Pepys and Hirschfield 2003; Ridker 2003). However, CRP levels are strongly influenced by acute and chronic inflammation so that levels above 10 mg/l must not be used for cardiovascular risk assessment. In this case, repeated blood samples for analysis must be taken after recovery from the acute disease (Ledue and Rifai 2003; Pearson et al. 2003). Several studies have demonstrated the interaction of CRP with global risk estimates. In three of four studies, elevated CRP levels were found to further increase the cardiovascular risk of men and women being at intermediate and high risk (i.e. >10% in 10 years as estimated with the Framingham risk score) (Albert et al. 2003; Koenig et al. 2004; Ridker et al. 2002; van der Meer et al. 2003). Post hoc analyses of intervention trials indicate that men with elevated CRP have an over-proportional benefit from aspirin and statin therapy (Ridker et al. 1997, 2001). CRP directed statin intervention studies have been initiated. As the consequence of current evidence it has been recommended that CRP measurements are used for stratification of individuals at intermediate risk. CRP measurements are not recommended for general screening and for risk stratification in low-risk individuals (because of low case-finding chance) (Pearson et al. 2003). Until recently, they were neither recommended to be used in high-risk individuals or patients with present disease (because these patients need intensive intervention regardless of CRP) (Pearson et al. 2003). However, most recently it has been suggested to introduce CRP in high-risk individuals as well for eventually defining more aggressive treatment goals, i.e. <70 mg/dl (<1.8 mmol/L) for LDL cholesterol (www.chd-taskforce.com, Grundy et al. 2004).

4.3
Fibrinogen

In several prospective studies, elevated plasma levels of fibrinogen have been identified as an independent cardiovascular risk factor (Koenig 2003). Like CRP, fibrinogen is an acute phase reactant, which is not clinically useful for cardiovascular risk assessment in patients with acute disease. There is no international consensus on a diagnostic cut-off although in the majority of studies 3.5 g/l has been used. Fibrinogen was found to further increase the risk of men with a high estimated cardiovascular risk as estimated with the Framingham score (Acevedo et al. 2002). Likewise in the PROCAM study, fibrinogen was found to increase further the risk of men with low and combined intermediate and high risk (unpublished results). Information on therapeutic interventions based on elevated fibrinogen is not available.

Plasma concentrations of the fibrinogen split product D-dimer, which is released during coagulation and therefore serves as a marker of incident thrombus formation, have evolved as an independent and perhaps even stronger risk factor of myocardial infarction and stroke than fibrinogen. However, no standardized tests and therefore internationally accepted normal ranges and cut-offs are available (Folsom 2001).

4.4
Homocysteine

Numerous case–control studies and several prospective studies have identified homocysteine as an independent cardiovascular risk factor, although it does not show the strength of association that has been found for the classical risk factors CRP, Lp(a) or fibrinogen. In a recent meta-analysis homocysteine levels in the upper quintile were associated with a 40% risk increase as compared to a relative risk of about 3 associated with systolic blood pressure or cholesterol levels in the upper quintile (Homocysteine Studies Collaboration 2002). Despite its moderate association with coronary risk, homocysteine was found to further increase the risk of high-risk individuals such as those with pre-existing coronary heart disease or those with a high estimated Framingham score risk (Homocysteine Studies Collaboration 2002). So far there is little consensus on cut-offs for homocysteine levels so that they vary from 10µmol/l to 16µmol/l. Homocysteine is the only one of the novel risk factors discussed here which is connected with a specific therapeutic intervention, namely the application of folate either alone or in combination with vitamins B6 and B12 (see the chapter by Cook and Hess, this volume). In one study, treatment of patients undergoing coronary angioplasty with this vitamin combination reduced restenosis rates and cardiovascular event rates (Schnyder et al. 2001, 2002a, 2002b). Surprisingly, however, the rates of restenosis as well as clinical events were increased upon folate/vitamins B6 and B12 treatment in another study of similar design (Lange et al. 2004). Therefore, in order to judge the clinical relevance of this marker we urgently need the outcomes of several ongoing large intervention trials that are assessing the clinical effects of homocysteine lowering vitamins.

4.5
Microalbuminuria and creatinine

Microalbuminuria is a well accepted marker for micro- and macrovascular damage in patients with diabetes mellitus or hypertension (Parving and Hovind 2002; Pontremoli et al. 2002). Therefore, and because of the proven benefit of treatment with ACE inhibitors or angiotensin II receptor antagonists in patients with microalbuminuria, consensus guidelines recommend the measurement of albuminuria in hypertensive or diabetic patients (Parving and Hovind 2002; Pontremoli et al. 2002). More and more evidence is accumulating that microalbuminuria is an important cardiovascular risk factor even in the general population (Hillege et al. 2002). It interacts with classical risk factors. It has not yet been shown, however, whether and how it further increases the risk within estimated global risk categories (Borch-Johnsen et al. 1999). Another major drawback for the wider use of microalbuminuria is the lack of agreement on the optimal specimen and the large intra-individual variation because of the great impact of fever, physical stress and menstrual bleeding on renal albumin excretion. The gold standard specimen, 24-h urine, is neither practical nor well accepted by patients. Albumin concentrations in spot urine show a good correlation with 24-h albumin excretion if taken at a defined time point (second morning urine). However, disagreement exists on whether the albumin/creatinine ratio or absolute albumin concentration should be determined. The former takes into consideration muscle mass and needs the definition of age and sex specific cut-offs; the latter is confounded by intra-individual variation in diuresis (von Eckardstein 2004).

In addition renal insufficiency is causing a dose-dependent increase in cardiovascular risk (Gupta et al. 2004; Yerkey et al. 2004). Patients with terminal renal insufficiency, i.e. requiring dialysis or hemofiltration, have an extremely elevated cardiovascular risk which is explained only partially by the clustering of both conventional (hypercholesterolaemia, hypertension, low HDL cholesterol, diabetes mellitus underlying many cases of chronic kidney disease) (Prichard 2003) and novel risk factors (elevated plasma levels of homocysteine, Lp(a), and CRP) (Muntner et al. 2004).

5
Genetic Risk Factors

The familial aggregation of cardiovascular diseases clearly demonstrates the importance of genetic predisposition to atherosclerosis. Consequently genes and genetic variants are intensively searched to understand better the pathogenesis of atherosclerosis and to develop new tests for risk assessment as well as drugs for treatment and prevention. Monogenic disorders are a rare cause of premature CHD and stroke (Table 5). Atherosclerosis is rather a polygenic and multifactorial disease in which allelic variants of various genes interact with one another as well as with environmental factors. Association studies identified a multitude of alleles which have statistically significant associations with CHD and stroke. However, in the majority of cases the associations were not reproducible and a single polymorphism had only a small impact on cardiovascular risk (Cullen and Funke 2001; Humphries et al. 2004; Sing et al. 2003). Because of this there are so far no genetic markers that could be used for screening of genetically determined cardiovascular risk. In the future, multiallelic and multiparametric tests will probably combine the information of multiple genetic markers with clinical and biochemical data to optimise the estimation of cardiovascular risk. Table 6 gives some examples for such polymorphisms (www.chd-taskforce.com).

Table 5 Examples of monogenetic diseases with increased cardiovascular risk

Phenotype	Mode of inheritance	Loci	Prevalence	Alleles
LDL cholesterol	Codominant	LDLR, APOB	1/200	1 major (ApoB3500) + >800 minor
LDL cholesterol	Recessive	LIPA, ARH,	Rare	1 major (LIPA) +
VLDL-cholesterol	Recessive	APOE, LIPC	1/5000	1 major (ApoE2/2) >10 minor
HDL cholesterol	Codominant	APOA1, LCAT, ABCA1	1/1000	>100
Triglycerides	Recessive	LIPB	1/10000	>100 minor
Sitosterol	Recessive	ABCG5, ABCG8	Rare	>50 minor
Homocysteine	Recessive	CBS, MTHFR	$1/10^6$	>10
Diabetes	Dominant	HNF1, HNF4, GK (MODY)	Rare	>100
Hypertension	Dominant	(Liddle)	rare	>10
Hypertension	Dominant	(GC-treated aldosteronism)		>10
Hypertension	Recessive	MC-Rez	rare	>10

LDLR, LDL receptor; APOB, apolipoprotein B; LIPA, acid lipase; ARH, autosomal rescessive hypercholesterolaemia gene; APOE, apolipoprotein E; LIPC hepatic lipase; APOA1, apolipoprotein A-I; LCAT, lecithin:cholesterol acyltransferase; ABCA1, ATP binding cassette transporter A1; LIPB, lipoprotein lipase; ABCG5 and ABCG8, ATP binding cassette transporters G5 and G8; CBS, cystathion beta synthase; MTHFR methlyenetetra hydrofolate reductase; HNF1 and HNF 4, hepatic nuclear factor 1 and 4; GK, glucokinase; cholesterol-C.

6
Conclusion

The classical risk factors have a high negative predictive value especially if they are combined in scores and algorithms, the use of which is currently advocated by international consensus guidelines for primary prevention of cardiovascular disease. Because costs are high relative to the small chance of finding cases, novel risk factor should not be included in unselected population-wide screening programs. However, global risk estimates have insufficient positive predictive value, and so there is a clear need to improve risk estimation in individuals at high and intermediate risk. This applies to 20% to 25% of the population. These individuals are the proper target for any novel risk factor (and non-invasive imaging method for the early detection of clinically relevant atherosclerosis). As yet, all emerging risk factors have to be investigated along these lines, before they are introduced into clinical practice. Among the novel risk factors currently under discussion, CRP has apparently been evaluated best.

Several authors advocate the use of novel risk factors in patients with existing coronary heart disease and who lack any classical risk factors. However, in this

Table 6 Examples of genetic polymorphisms affecting cardiovascular risk (from www.chd-taskforce.com)

Polymorphism and gene	Frequency of rare allele/haplo-type in general population	Odds ratio for atherosclerosis in carriers of rare allele or haplotype
G20210A polymorphisms in the factor II (prothrombin) gene	0.02	1.3
gly460trp polymorphism in the alpha adducin (*ADD1*) gene	0.19	1.3*
glu298asp (G894T) polymorphism in the endothelial nitric oxide synthase (*NOS3*) gene,	0.35	1.3*
cys112arg, arg158cys polymorphisms in the apolipoprotein E (*APOE*) gene	112cys,158cys (E2): 0.08 112cys, 158arg (E3): 0.75 112arg, 158arg (E4): 0.17 ε2/2: 0.01; ε2/3: 0.12; ε3/3: 0.59; ε3/4: 0.24; ε4/4: 0.02	ε3/3 vs. ε2/3: 1.2 ε3/4 vs. ε2/3: 1.4
leu33pro polymorphism in β3 integrin subunit (platelet glycoprotein IIIa, *ITGB3*) gene	0.15	1.2
4G/5G polymorphism in the plasminogen activator inhibitor 1 (*PAI1*) gene	0.47	1.3
val640leu polymorphism the p-selectin (*SELP*) gene	0.11	1.6
C582T polymorphism in the interleukin 4 (*IL4*) gene	0.17	1.4

secondary prevention setting, a novel risk factor is of limited use if it does not lead to specific treatment. For example, so far it is not justifiable to make decisions concerning the use of statins or aspirin in patients with manifest atherosclerosis dependent on CRP or Lp(a) levels. In this setting, parameters connected with specific treatment decisions have a great potential. However, randomized intervention studies are needed to prove the relevance of these risk factors and the benefit of the intervention based on their results.

References

Acevedo M, Pearce GL, Kottke-Marchant K, Sprecher DL (2002) Elevated fibrinogen and homocysteine levels enhance the risk of mortality in patients from a high-risk preventive cardiology clinic. Arterioscler Thromb Vasc Biol 22:1042–1045

Albert MA, Glynn RJ, Ridker PM (2003) Plasma concentration of C-reactive protein and the calculated Framingham Coronary Heart Disease Risk Score. Circulation 108:161–165

Alberti KGMM, Zimmet PZ for the WHO consultation (1998) Definition, diagnosis, and classification of diabetes mellitus and its complications. Part 1: diagnosis and classification of diabetes mellitus. Provisional report of a WHO consultation. Diabetes Med 15:539–553

ALLHAT Officers and Coordinators for the ALLHAT Collaborative Research Group. The Antihypertensive and Lipid-Lowering Treatment to Prevent Heart Attack Trial (2002a) Major outcomes in moderately hypercholesterolemic, hypertensive patients randomized to pravastatin vs usual care: The Antihypertensive and Lipid-Lowering Treatment to Prevent Heart Attack Trial (ALLHAT-LLT). JAMA 288:2998–3007

ALLHAT Officers and Coordinators for the ALLHAT Collaborative Research Group (2002b) The Antihypertensive and Lipid-Lowering Treatment to Prevent Heart Attack Trial. Major outcomes in high-risk hypertensive patients randomized to angiotensin-converting enzyme inhibitor or calcium channel blocker vs diuretic: The Antihypertensive and Lipid-Lowering Treatment to Prevent Heart Attack Trial (ALLHAT). JAMA 288:2981–2997

Anonymous (1995) Cholesterol, diastolic blood pressure, and stroke: 13,000 strokes in 450,000 people in 45 prospective cohorts. Prospective studies collaboration. Lancet 346:1647–1653

Anonymous (1996) Hypertension Control Report of a WHO Expert Committee. WHO Technical Report Series No. 862, World Health Organization, Geneva

Anonymous (1997a) The Sixth Report of the Joint National Committee on Prevention, Detection, Evaluation and Treatment of high blood pressure. Arch Intern Med 157:2413–2446

Anonymous (1997b) The Expert Committee on the Diagnosis and Classification of Diabetes mellitus: Report of the Expert Committee on the Diagnosis and Classification of Diabetes mellitus. Diabetes Care 20:1183–1197

Anonymous (2001) Executive Summary of The Third Report of The National Cholesterol Education Program (NCEP) Expert Panel on Detection, Evaluation, And Treatment of High Blood Cholesterol In Adults (Adult Treatment Panel III). JAMA 285:2486–2497

Anonymous (2002) Third Report of The National Cholesterol Education Program (NCEP) Expert Panel on Detection, Evaluation, And Treatment of High Blood Cholesterol In Adults (Adult Treatment Panel III). Final report National Cholesterol Education Program Heart, Lung and Blood Institute, National Institutes of Health NIH Publication No. 02-5215 September 2002 (http://www.nhlbi.nih.gov/guidelines/cholesterol)

Arad Y, Spadaro LA, Goodman K, Newstein D, Guerci AD (2000) Prediction of coronary events with electron beam computed tomography. J Am Coll Cardiol 36:1253–1260

Arad Y, Spadaro LA, Goodman K, Lledo-Perez A, Sherman S, Lerner G, et al. (1996) Predictive value of electron beam computed tomography of the coronary arteries. 19-month follow-up of 1173 asymptomatic subjects. Circulation 93:1951–1953

Ariyo AA, Thach C, Tracy R, Cardiovascular Health Study Investigators (2003) Lp(a) lipoprotein, vascular disease, and mortality in the elderly. N Engl J Med 349:2108–2115

Assmann G, Cullen P, Schulte H (2002) Simple scoring scheme for calculating the risk of acute coronary events based on the 10-year follow-up of the prospective cardiovascular Munster (PROCAM) study. Circulation 105:310–315

Austin MA, Hokanson JE, Edwards KL (1998) Hypertriglyceridemia as a cardiovascular risk factor. Am J Cardiol 81:7B–12B

Becker CR, Kleffel T, Crispin A, Knez A, Young J, Schoepf UJ, et al. (2001) Coronary artery calcium measurement: agreement of multirow detector and electron beam CT. Am J Roentgenol 176:1295–1298

Berg K, Dahlen G, Christophersen B, Cook T, Kjekshus J, Pedersen T (1997) Lp(a) lipoprotein level predicts survival and major coronary events in the Scandinavian Simvastatin Survival Study. Clin Genet 52:254–261

Bobak M, Hense HW, Kark J, Kuch B, Vojtisek P, Sinnreich R, Gostomzyk J, Bui M, von Eckardstein A, Junker R, Fobker M, Schulte H, Assmann G, Marmot M (1999) An ecological study of determinants of coronary heart disease rates: a comparison of Czech, Bavarian and Israeli men. Int J Epidemiol 28:437–444

Bolibar I, von Eckardstein A, Assmann G, Thompson S (2000) Short-term prognostic value of lipid measurements in patients with angina pectoris. The ECAT Angina Pectoris Study Group: European Concerted Action on Thrombosis and Disabilities. Thromb.Haemost 84:955–960

Borch-Johnsen K, Feldt-Rasmussen B, Strandgaard S, Schroll M, Jensen JS (1999) Urinary albumin excretion. An independent predictor of ischemic heart disease. Arterioscler Thromb Vasc Biol 19:1992–1997

Bots ML, Grobbee DE (2002) Intima media thickness as a surrogate marker for generalised atherosclerosis. Cardiovasc Drugs Ther 16:341–351

Brown MS, Goldstein JL (1992) Koch's postulates for cholesterol. Cell 71:187–188

Cannon CP, Braunwald E, McCabe CH, Rader DJ, Rouleau JL, Belder R, Joyal SV, Hill KA, Pfeffer MA, Skene AM (2004) Comparison of Intensive and Moderate Lipid Lowering with Statins after Acute Coronary Syndromes. N Engl J Med 350:1495–1504

Collins R, Armitage J, Parish S, Sleigh P, Peto R, Heart Protection Study Collaborative Group (2003) MRC/BHF Heart Protection Study of cholesterol-lowering with simvastatin in 5963 people with diabetes: a randomised placebo-controlled trial. Lancet 361:2005–2016

Collins R, Armitage J, Parish S, Sleight P, Peto R; Heart Protection Study Collaborative Group (2004) Effects of cholesterol-lowering with simvastatin on stroke and other major vascular events in 20536 people with cerebrovascular disease or other high-risk conditions. Lancet 363:757–767

Conroy RM, Pyorala K, Fitzgerald AP, Sans S, Menotti A, De Backer G, De Bacquer D, Ducimetiere P, Jousilahti P, Keil U, Njolstad I, Oganov RG, Thomsen T, Tunstall-Pedoe H, Tverdal A, Wedel H, Whincup P, Wilhelmsen L, Graham IM; SCORE project group (2003) Estimation of ten-year risk of fatal cardiovascular disease in Europe: the SCORE project. Eur Heart J 24:987–1003

Cullen P, Funke H (2001) Implications of the human genome project for the identification of genetic risk of coronary heart disease and its prevention in children. Nutr Metab Cardiovasc Dis 11 (Suppl 5):45–51

Cullen P, Schulte H, Assmann G (1997) The Munster Heart Study (PROCAM): total mortality in middle-aged men is increased at low total and LDL cholesterol concentrations in smokers but not in nonsmokers. Circulation 96:2128–2136

Danesh J, Collins R, Peto R (2000) Lipoprotein(a) and coronary heart disease. Meta-analysis of prospective studies. Circulation 102:1082–1085

Danesh J, Wheeler JG, Hirschfield GM, Eda S, Eiriksdottir G, Rumley A, Lowe GDO, Pepys MB, Gudnason V (2004) C-reactive protein and other circulating markers of inflammation in the prediction of coronary heart disease. N Engl J Med 350:1387–1397

De Backer G, De Bacquer D, Kornitzer M (1998) Epidemiological aspects of high density lipoprotein cholesterol. Atherosclerosis 137 (Suppl):S1–S6

De Backer G, Ambrosioni E, Borch-Johnson K, Brotons C, Cifkova R, Dallongeville J, Ebrahim S, Faergeman O, Graham I, Mancia G, Manger Cats V, Orth-Gomer K, Perk J, Pyörälä K, Rodicio JL, Sans S, Sansoy V, Sechtem U, Silber S, Thomson T, Wood D (2003) European guidelines on cardiovascular disease prevention in clinical practice: Third Joint Task Force of European and other Societies on Cardiovascular Disease Prevention in Clinical Practice (constituted by representatives of eight societies and by invited experts). Eur Heart J 24:1601–1610 (http://www.escardio.org)

DeFronzo RA (1999) Pharmacologic therapy for type 2 diabetes mellitus. Ann Intern Med 131:281–303

Detrano RC, Wong ND, Doherty TM, Shavelle RM, Tang W, Ginzton LE, et al. (1999) Coronary calcium does not accurately predict near-term future coronary events in high-risk adults. Circulation 99:2633–2638

Folsom AR (2001) Hemostatic risk factors for atherothrombotic disease: an epidemiologic view. Thromb Haemost 86:366–373

Fruchart JC, Brewer HB, Jr., Leitersdorf E (1998) Consensus for the use of fibrates in the treatment of dyslipoproteinemia and coronary heart disease. Fibrate Consensus Group. Am J Cardiol 81:912–917

Genest JJ, McNamara JR, Salem DN, Schaefer EJ (1991) Prevalence of risk factors in men with premature coronary artery disease. Am J Cardiol 67:1185–1189

Goldstein JL, Hobbs HH, Brown MS (2001) Familial Hypercholesterolemia. In: Scriver CR, Beaudet AL, Sly WS, Valle D (eds) The metabolic and molecular bases of inherited disease, 8th edn. McGraw-Hill, New York, pp 2863–2915

Gordon DJ, Rifkind BM (1989) High-density lipoprotein–the clinical implications of recent studies. N Engl J Med 321:1311–1316

Gotto AM Jr, Whitney E, Stein EA, Shapiro DR, Clearfield M, Weis S, Jou JY, Langendorfer A, Beere PA, Watson DJ, Downs JR, de Cani JS (2000) Relation between baseline and on-treatment lipid parameters and first acute major coronary events in the Air Force/Texas Coronary Atherosclerosis Prevention Study (AFCAPS/TexCAPS). Circulation 101:477–484

Grady D, Herrington D, Bittner V, Blumenthal R, Davidson M, Hlatky M, Hsia J, Hulley S, Herd A, Khan S, Newby LK, Waters D, Vittinghoff E, Wenger N, HERS Research Group (2002) Cardiovascular disease outcomes during 6.8 years of hormone therapy: Heart and Estrogen/progestin Replacement Study follow-up (HERS II). JAMA 288:49–57

Greenland P, Knoll MD, Stamler J, Neaton JD, Dyer AR, Garside DB, Wilson PW (2003) Major risk factors as antecedents of fatal and nonfatal coronary heart disease events. JAMA 290:891–897

Grundy SM, Pasternak R, Greenland P, Smith S Jr, Fuster V (1999) AHA/ACC scientific statement: Assessment of cardiovascular risk by use of multiple-risk-factor assessment equations: a statement for healthcare professionals from the American Heart Association and the American College of Cardiology. J Am Coll Cardiol 34:1348–59

Grundy SM, Cleeman JI, Merz CN, Brewer HB Jr, Clark LT, Hunninghake DB, Pasternak RC, Smith SC Jr, Stone NJ; National Heart, Lung, and Blood Institute; American College of Cardiology Foundation; American Heart Association (2004) Implications of recent clinical trials for the National Cholesterol Education Program Adult Treatment Panel III guidelines. Circulation 110:227–239

Gupta R, Birnbaum Y, Uretsky BF (2004) The renal patient with coronary artery disease: current concepts and dilemmas. J Am Coll Cardiol 44:1343–1353

Hackam DG, Anand SS (2003) Emerging risk factors for atherosclerotic vascular disease: a critical review of the evidence. JAMA 290:932–940

Hayward CS, Kelly RP, Collins P 2000 The roles of gender, the menopause and hormone replacement on cardiovascular function. Cardiovasc Res 46:28–49

Heart Protection Study Collaborative Group (2002) MRC/BHF Heart Protection Study of cholesterol lowering with simvastatin in 20,536 high-risk individuals: a randomised placebo-controlled trial. Lancet 360:7–22

Hense HW, Schulte H, Lowel H, Assmann G, Keil U (2003) Framingham risk function overestimates risk of coronary heart disease in men and women from Germany–results from the MONICA Augsburg and the PROCAM cohorts. Eur Heart J 24:937–945

Hergenc G, Schulte H, Assmann G, von Eckardstein A (1999) Associations of obesity markers, insulin, and sex hormones with HDL- cholesterol levels in Turkish and German individuals. Atherosclerosis 145:147–156

Hersberger M, von Eckardstein A (2003) Low high density lipoprotein cholesterol – physiological background, clinical importance and drug treatment. Drugs 63:1907–1945

Hillege HL, Fidler V, Diercks GF, van Gilst WH, de Zeeuw D, van Veldhuisen DJ, Gans RO, Janssen WM, Grobbee DE, de Jong PE, Prevention of Renal and Vascular End Stage Disease (PREVEND) Study Group (2002) Urinary albumin excretion predicts cardiovascular and noncardiovascular mortality in general population. Circulation 106:1777–1782

Hirano K, Yamashita S, Kuga Y, Sakai N, Nozaki S, Kihara S, Arai T, Yanagi K, Takami S, Menju M (1995) Atherosclerotic disease in marked hyperalphalipoproteinemia. Combined reduction of cholesteryl ester transfer protein and hepatic triglyceride lipase. Arterioscler Thromb Vasc Biol 15:1849–1856

Hu FB, Willett WC (2002) Optimal diets for prevention of coronary heart disease. JAMA 288:2569–2578

Humphries SE, Ridker PM, Talmud PJ (2004) Genetic testing for cardiovascular disease susceptibility: a useful clinical management tool or possible misinformation? Arterioscler Thromb Vasc Biol 24:628–636

Homocysteine Studies Collaboration (2002) Homocysteine and risk of ischemic heart disease and stroke: a meta-analysis. JAMA 288:2015–2522

International Task Force for Prevention of Coronary Heart Disease (1998) Coronary heart disease: Reducing the risk. The scientific background to primary and secondary prevention of coronary heart disease. A worldwide view. Nutr Metab Cardiovasc Dis 8:205–271

International Task Force for Prevention of Coronary Heart Disease (2002) Pocket Guide to Prevention of Coronary heart disease. http://www.chd-taskforce.de/guide.htm

Iso H, Jacobs DR Jr, Wentworth D, Neaton JD, Cohen JD (1989) Serum cholesterol levels and six-year mortality from stroke in 350,977 men screened for the multiple risk factor intervention trial. N Engl J Med 320:904–910

Jeppesen J, Hein HO, Suadicani P, Gyntelberg F (1998) Triglyceride concentration and ischemic heart disease: an eight-year follow-up in the Copenhagen Male Study. Circulation 97:1029–1036

Khot UN, Khot MB, Bajzer CT, Sapp SK, Ohman EM, Brener SJ, Ellis SG, Lincoff AM, Topol EJ (2003) Prevalence of conventional risk factors in patients with coronary heart disease. JAMA 290:898–904

Kopelman PG (2002) Obesity as a medical problem. Nature 404:635–643

Koenig W (2003) Fibrin(ogen) in cardiovascular disease: an update. Thromb Haemost 89:601–609

Koenig W, Lowel H, Baumert J, Meisinger C (2004) C-reactive protein modulates risk prediction based on the Framingham Score. Implications for future risk assessment: results from a large cohort study in southern Germany. Circulation 109:1349–1353)

Krantz DS, McCeney MK (2002) Effects of psychological and social factors on organic disease: a critical assessment of research on coronary heart disease. Annu Rev Psychol 53:341–369

Kromhout D, Menotti A, Kesteloot H, Sans S (2002) Prevention of coronary heart disease by diet and lifestyle: evidence from prospective cross-cultural, cohort, and intervention studies. Circulation 105:893–898

Kronenberg F, Neyer U, Lhotta K, Trenkwalder E, Auinger M, Pribasnig A, Meisl T, Konig P, Dieplinger H (1999) The low molecular weight apo(a) phenotype is an independent predictor for coronary artery disease in hemodialysis patients: a prospective follow-up. J Am Soc Nephrol 10:1027–1036

Lamarche B, Lemieux I, Despres JP (1999) The small, dense LDL phenotype and the risk of coronary heart disease: epidemiology, patho-physiology and therapeutic aspects. Diabetes Metab 25:199–211

Lange H, Suryapranata H, De Luca G, Borner C, Dille J, Kallmayer K, Pasalary MN, Scherer E, Dambrink JH (2004) Folate therapy and in-stent restenosis after coronary stenting. N Engl J Med 350:2673–2681

Ledue TB, Rifai N (2003) Preanalytic and analytic sources of variations in C-reactive protein measurement: implications for cardiovascular disease risk assessment. Clin Chem 49:1258–1271

Li S, Chen W, Srinivasan SR, Bond MG, Tang R, Urbina EM, Berenson GS (2003) Childhood cardiovascular risk factors and carotid vascular changes in adulthood: the Bogalusa Heart Study. JAMA 290:2271–2276

Liu PY, Death AK, Handelsman DJ (2003) Androgens and cardiovascular disease. Endocr Rev 24:313–340

Lloyd-Jones DM, Larson MG, Beiser A, Levit D (1999) Lifetime risk of developing coronary heart disease. Lancet 353:89–92

Luc G, Bard JM, Ferrieres J, Evans A, Amouyel P, Arveiler D, Fruchart JC, Ducimetiere P (2002) Value of HDL cholesterol, apolipoprotein A-I, lipoprotein A-I, and lipoprotein A-I/A-II in prediction of coronary heart disease: the PRIME Study. Prospective Epidemiological Study of Myocardial Infarction. Arterioscler Thromb Vasc Biol 22:1155–1161

Mahley RW, Rall SC (2001) Type III Hyperlipoproteinemia (Dysbetalipoproteinemia). In: Scriver CR, Beaudet AL, Sly WS, Valle D, (eds) The metabolic and molecular bases of inherited disease, 8th edn. McGraw-Hill, New York, pp 2835–2862

Manninen V, Tenkanen L, Koskinen P, Huttunen JK, Manttari M, Heinonen OP, Frick MH (1992) Joint effects of serum triglyceride and LDL cholesterol and HDL cholesterol concentrations on coronary heart disease risk in the Helsinki Heart Study. Implications for treatment. Circulation 85:37–45

Marcovina SM, Albers JJ, Scanu AM, Kennedy H, Giaculli F, Berg K, Couderc R, Dati F, Rifai N, Sakurabayashi I, Tate JR, Steinmetz A (2000) Use of a reference material proposed by the International Federation of Clinical Chemistry and Laboratory Medicine to evaluate analytical methods for the determination of plasma lipoprotein(a). Clin Chem 46:1956–1967

Marcovina SM, Koschinsky ML, Albers JJ, Skarlatos S (2003) Report of the National Heart, Lung, and Blood Institute Workshop on Lipoprotein(a) and Cardiovascular Disease: recent advances and future directions. Clin Chem 49:1785–1796

McGill HC Jr, McMahan CA (2003) Starting earlier to prevent heart disease. JAMA 290:2320–2322

McKechnie R, Mosca L (2003) Physical activity and coronary heart disease: prevention and effect on risk factors. Cardiol Rev 11:21–25

Miller M, Seidler A, Moalemi A, Pearson TA (1998) Normal triglyceride levels and coronary artery disease events: the Baltimore Coronary Observational Long-Term Study. J Am Coll Cardiol 31:1252–1257

Mukamal KJ, Rimm EB (2001) Alcohol's effects on the risk for coronary heart disease. Alcohol Res Health 25:255–261

Mukamal KJ, Conigrave KM, Mittleman MA, Camargo CA Jr, Stampfer MJ, Willett WC, Rimm EB (2003) Roles of drinking pattern and type of alcohol consumed in coronary heart disease in men. N Engl J Med 348:109–118

Mungall MM, Gaw A, Shepherd J (2003) Statin therapy in the elderly: does it make good clinical and economic sense? Drugs Aging 20:263–275

Muntner P, Hamm LL, Kusek JW, Chen J, Whelton PK, He J (2004) The prevalence of nontraditional risk factors for coronary heart disease in patients with chronic kidney disease. Ann Intern Med 140: 9–17

Nowak-Gottl U, Strater R, Heinecke A, Junker R, Koch HG, Schuierer G, von Eckardstein A (1999) Lipoprotein (a) and genetic polymorphisms of clotting factor V, prothrombin, and methylenetetrahydrofolate reductase are risk factors of spontaneous ischemic stroke in childhood. Blood 94:3678–3682

Palinski W, Napoli C (2002) The fetal origins of atherosclerosis: maternal hypercholesterolemia, and cholesterol-lowering or antioxidant treatment during pregnancy influence in utero programming and postnatal susceptibility to atherogenesis. FASEB J 16:1348–1360

Parving HH, Hovind P (2002) Microalbuminuria in type 1 and type 2 diabetes mellitus: evidence with angiotensin converting enzyme inhibitors and angiotensin II receptor blockers for treating early and preventing clinical nephropathy. Curr Hypertens Rep 4:387–393

Pearson TA, Mensah GA, Alexander RW, Anderson JL, Cannon RO 3rd, Criqui M, Fadl YY, Fortmann SP, Hong Y, Myers GL, Rifai N, Smith SC Jr, Taubert K, Tracy RP, Vinicor F (2003) Markers of inflammation and cardiovascular disease: application to clinical and public health practice: A statement for healthcare professionals from the Centers for Disease Control and Prevention and the American Heart Association. Circulation 107:499–511

Pepys MB, Hirschfield GM (2003) C-reactive protein: a critical update. J Clin Invest 111:1805–1812

Pontremoli R, Leoncini G, Ravera M, Viazzi F, Vettoretti S, Ratto E, Parodi D, Tomolillo C, Deferrari G (2002) Microalbuminuria, cardiovascular, and renal risk in primary hypertension. J Am Soc Nephrol 13 (Suppl 3):S169–S172

Prichard SS (2003) Impact of dyslipidemia in end-stage renal disease. J Am Soc Nephrol 14(9 Suppl 4):S315–S320

Raitakari OT, Juonala M, Kahonen M, Taittonen L, Laitinen T, Maki-Torkko N, Jarvisalo MJ, Uhari M, Jokinen E, Ronnemaa T, Akerblom HK, Viikari JS (2003) Cardiovascular risk factors in childhood and carotid artery intima-media thickness in adulthood: the Cardiovascular Risk in Young Finns Study. JAMA 290:2277–2283

Ridker PM (2003) Clinical application of C-reactive protein for cardiovascular disease detection and prevention. Circulation 107:363–369

Ridker PM, Cushman M, Stampfer MJ, Tracy RP, Hennekens CH (1997) Inflammation, aspirin, and the risk of cardiovascular disease in apparently healthy men. N Engl J Med 336:973–979

Ridker PM, Rifai N, Clearfield M, Downs JR, Weis SE, Miles JS, Gotto AM Jr, Air Force/Texas Coronary Atherosclerosis Prevention Study Investigators (2001) Measurement of C-reactive protein for the targeting of statin therapy in the primary prevention of acute coronary events. N Engl J Med 344:1959–1965

Ridker PM, Rifai N, Rose L, Buring JE, Cook NR (2002) Comparison of C-reactive protein and low-density lipoprotein cholesterol levels in the prediction of first cardiovascular events. N Engl J Med 347:1557–1565

Rimm EB, Stampfer MJ (2002) Wine, beer, and spirits: are they really horses of a different color? Circulation 105:2806–2807

Rohrer L, Hersberger M, von Eckardstein A (2004) High density lipoproteins in the intersection of diabetes mellitus, inflammation and cardiovascular disease. Curr Opin Lipidol 15:269–278)

Rubins HB, Robins SJ, Collins D, Fye CL, Anderson JW, Elam MB, Faas FH, Linares E, Schaefer EJ, Schectman G, Wilt TJ, Wittes J (1999): Gemfibrozil for the secondary prevention of coronary heart disease in men with low levels of high-density lipoprotein cholesterol. Veterans Affairs High-Density Lipoprotein Cholesterol Intervention Trial Study Group. N Engl J Med 341:410–418

Scheuner MT (2001) Genetic predisposition to coronary artery disease. Curr Opin Cardiol 16:251–260

Schnyder G, Roffi M, Pin R, Flammer Y, Lange H, Eberli FR, Meier B, Turi ZG, Hess OM (2001) Decreased rate of coronary restenosis after lowering of plasma homocysteine levels. N Engl J Med 345:1593–1600

Schnyder G, Roffi M, Flammer Y, Pin R, Hess OM (2002a) Effect of homocysteine-lowering therapy with folic acid, vitamin B12, and vitamin B6 on clinical outcome after percutaneous coronary intervention: the Swiss Heart study: a randomized controlled trial. JAMA 288:973–979

Schnyder G, Flammer Y, Roffi M, Pin R, Hess OM (2002b) Plasma homocysteine levels and late outcome after coronary angioplasty. J Am Coll Cardiol 40:1769–1776

Sever PS, Dahlof B, Poulter NR, Wedel H, Beevers G, Caulfield M, Collins R, Kjeldsen SE, Kristinsson A, McInnes GT, Mehlsen J, Nieminen M, O'Brien E, Ostergren J, ASCOT investigators (2003) Prevention of coronary and stroke events with atorvastatin in hypertensive patients who have average or lower-than-average cholesterol concentrations, in the Anglo-Scandinavian Cardiac Outcomes Trial–Lipid Lowering Arm (ASCOT-LLA): a multicentre randomised controlled trial. Lancet. 361:1149–1158

Sharrett AR, Ballantyne CM, Coady SA, Heiss G, Sorlie PD, Catellier D, Patsch W (2001) Coronary heart disease prediction from lipoprotein cholesterol levels, triglycerides, lipoprotein(a), apolipoproteins A-I and B, and HDL density subfractions: The Atherosclerosis Risk in Communities (ARIC) Study. Circulation 104:1108–1113

Shepherd J (2003) Preventing the next event in the elderly: the PROSPER perspective. Atheroscler Suppl 4:17–22

Shepherd J, Blauw GJ, Murphy MB, Bollen EL, Buckley BM, Cobbe SM, Ford I, Gaw A, Hyland M, Jukema JW, Kamper AM, Macfarlane PW, Meinders AE, Norrie J, Packard CJ, Perry IJ, Stott DJ, Sweeney BJ, Twomey C, Westendorp RG, PROSPER study group (2002) PROspective Study of Pravastatin in the Elderly at Risk. Pravastatin in elderly individuals at risk of vascular disease (PROSPER): a randomised controlled trial. Lancet 360:1623–1630

Shlipak MG, Simon JA, Vittinghoff E, Lin F, Barrett-Connor E, Knopp RH, Levy RI, Hulley SB (2000) Estrogen and progestin, lipoprotein(a), and the risk of recurrent coronary heart disease events after menopause. JAMA 283:1845–1852

Sing CF, Stengard JH, Kardia SL (2003) Genes, environment, and cardiovascular disease. Arterioscler Thromb Vasc Biol 23:1190–1196

Stampfer MJ, Sacks FM, Salvini S, Willett WC, Hennekens CH (1991) A prospective study of cholesterol, apolipoproteins, and the risk of myocardial infarction. N Engl J Med 325:373–381

Strater R, Becker S, von Eckardstein A, Heinecke A, Gutsche S, Junker R, Kurnik K, Schobess R, Nowak-Gottl U (2002) Prospective assessment of risk factors for recurrent stroke during childhood–a 5-year follow-up study. Lancet 360:1540–1545

Suh I, Jee SH, Kim HC, Nam CM, Kim IS, Appel LJ (2001) Low serum cholesterol and haemorrhagic stroke in men: Korea Medical Insurance Corporation Study. Lancet 357:922–925

Tsimikas S, Witztum JL (2002) Shifting the diagnosis and treatment of atherosclerosis to children and young adults: a new paradigm for the 21st century. J Am Coll Cardiol 40:2122–2124

van der Meer IM, de Maat MP, Kiliaan AJ, van der Kuip DA, Hofman A, Witteman JC (2003) The value of C-reactive protein in cardiovascular risk prediction: the Rotterdam Study. Arch Intern Med 163:1323–1328

von Eckardstein A (2004) Is there a need for novel cardiovascular risk factors? Nephrol Dial Transpl 19:761–765)

von Eckardstein A, Assmann G (2000) Prevention of coronary heart disease by raising high-density lipoprotein cholesterol? Curr Opin Lipidol 11:627–637

von Eckardstein A, Schulte H, Assmann G (1999): Increased risk of myocardial infarction in men with both hypertriglyceridemia and elevated HDL cholesterol. Circulation 99:1925

von Eckardstein A, Schulte H, Cullen P, Assmann G (2001) Lipoprotein(a) further increases the risk of coronary events in men with high global cardiovascular risk. J Am Coll Cardiol 37:434–439

von Eckardstein A, Schulte H, Assmann G (2005) Vergleich internationaler Konsensus-Empfehlungen zur Erkennung des präsymptomatischen Hochrisikopatienten für den Herzinfarkt in Deutschland. Z. Kardiologie 94:52–60

Voss R, Cullen P, Schulte H, Assmann G (2002) Prediction of risk of coronary events in middle-aged men in the Prospective Cardiovascular Munster Study (PROCAM) using neural networks. Int J Epidemiol 31:1253–1262

Wilson PW, D'Agostino RB, Levy D, Belanger AM, Silbershatz H, Kannel WB (1998) Prediction of coronary heart disease using risk factor categories. Circulation 97:1837–1847

Wong ND, Hsu JC, Detrano RC, Diamond G, Eisenberg H, Gardin JM (2000) Coronary artery calcium evaluation by electron beam computed tomography and its relation to new cardiovascular events. Am J Cardiol 86:495–498

Writing Group for the Women's Health Initiative Investigators (2002) Risks and benefits of estrogen plus progestin in healthy postmenopausal women. Principal results from the Women's Health Initiative randomised controlled trial. JAMA 288:321–333

Wu FCW, von Eckardstein A (2003) Androgens and coronary artery disease. Endocrine Rev 24:183–217

Yerkey MW, Kernis SJ, Franklin BA, Sandberg KR, McCullough PA (2004). Renal dysfunction and acceleration of coronary disease. Heart 90:961–966

HEP (2005) 170:107–133

Metabolic Syndrome: Therapeutic Considerations

S.M. Grundy

Center for Human Nutrition and Departments of Clinical Nutrition and Internal Medicine, University of Texas Southwestern Medical Center at Dallas, 5323 Harry Hines Boulevard, Y3.206, Dallas TX, 75390-9052, USA
scott.grundy@utsouthwestern.edu

Abstract The metabolic syndrome is a constellation of metabolic risk factors for atherosclerotic cardiovascular disease (ASCVD) occurring in one individual. There are five cardiovascular risk factors that accompany the metabolic syndrome: atherogenic dyslipidemia [elevated apolipoprotein B (apo B), elevated triglyceride, small low-density lipoprotein (LDL) particles, and low high-density lipoprotein (HDL)cholesterol], elevated blood pressure, elevated glucose, a prothrombotic state, and a proinflammatory state. The likelihood of an individual developing metabolic syndrome is enhance by underlying risk factors, notably, obesity, insulin resistance, lack of physical activity, advancing age, and hormonal factors (e.g., androgens and corticosteroids). Besides being at higher risk for ASCVD, persons with the metabolic syndrome are at increased risk for type 2 diabetes. Persons with the metabolic syndrome deserve management in the clinical setting to reduce the risk for both ASCVD and type 2 diabetes. The two major therapeutic strategies for treatment of affected persons are modification of the underlying risk factors and separate drug treatment of the particular metabolic risk factors when appropriate. First-line therapy for underlying risk factors is therapeutic lifestyle changes, i.e., weight loss in obese persons, increased physical activity, and anti-atherogenic diet. These changes will improve all of the metabolic risk factors. Whether use of drugs to reduce insulin resistance is effective, safe, and cost-effective before the onset of diabetes awaits the results of more clinical research. Turning to individual risk components, for atherogenic dyslipidemia, drug therapies that promote lowering of apo B and raise HDL cholesterol will be needed for higher risk patients. Treatment of categorical hypertension with drugs has become standard practice. When hyperglycemia reaches the diabetic level, glucose-lowering agents will become necessary when dietary control is no longer effective, and reduction of a prothrombotic state with low-dose aspirin may be indicated in higher-risk patients.

Keywords Metabolic syndrome · Therapeutic lifestyle changes · Pharmacology therapy · Atherogenic dyslipidemia · Insulin resistance · Hypertension · Hyperglycemia · Prothrombotic state · Proinflammatory state

1
Introduction

Clinical atherosclerotic cardiovascular disease (ASCVD) has been shown to be preceded in most people by identifiable risk factors (Kannel and Wilson 1995). These risk factors are of several types. According to the United States National Cholesterol Education Program's Adult Treatment Panel III report (US NCEP ATP III) [Third report of the National Cholesterol Education Program (NCEP) expert panel on detection, evaluation, and treatment of high blood cholesterol in adults 2002], they fall into three major categories: major, underlying, and emerging risk factors. The major risk factors are advancing age, cigarette smoking, high blood pressure, elevated serum total cholesterol [or low-density lipoprotein (LDL) cholesterol], low levels of high-density lipoprotein (HDL) cholesterol, and diabetes. The underlying risk factors are obesity (especially abdominal obesity), physical inactivity, and genetics. In addition, insulin resistance has been increasingly recognized as an underlying risk factor. The emerging risk factors include abnormalities in lipoproteins and apolipoproteins [e.g., elevated lipoprotein(a), elevated apolipoprotein B (apo B), low apolipoprotein A-I], impaired glucose tolerance (IGT)/impaired fasting glucose (IFG), a prothrombotic state, and a proinflammatory state. The latter are called emerging risk factors because they are associated with ASCVD. However, to date, they have not proved to be independent risk factors, i.e., to add substantially to the risk beyond that imparted by the major risk factors. As shown in the Framingham Heart Study (Kannel and Wilson 1995), combinations of the major risk factors are common in the population and account for much of the population burden of ASCVD.

Combinations of risk factors associated with ASCVD do not occur randomly. In fact, various patterns of combinations have been identified, among them a particular combination of risk factors of metabolic origin (metabolic risk factors). This constellation of metabolic risk factors is termed metabolic syndrome. The recent US NCEP ATP III report [Third report of the National Cholesterol Education Program (NCEP) expert panel on detection, evaluation, and treatment of high blood cholesterol in adults 2002] identified the metabolic syndrome as a multi-dimensional risk factor requiring increased attention in clinical management along with elevated LDL cholesterol (LDL-C). The inclusion of the metabolic syndrome into the cholesterol-management guidelines has generated considerable interest in the cardiovascular community. At the same time, it must be recognized that not only is the metabolic syndrome a risk factor for ASCVD, but it also frequently precedes the development of type 2 diabetes. Thus, the diabetes community has shown great interest in the metabolic syndrome as well. This interest in the metabolic syndrome is driven to no small extent by the emerging epidemic of obesity in the USA and worldwide. That obesity strongly associates with the metabolic syndrome is well established.

A fundamental issue for the medical community is how to approach the clinical management of patients who present with the metabolic syndrome. Before this issue can be addressed, questions of definition and causation must be considered. Answers will have implications for clinical management. A fundamental issue for clinical management is the question whether the medical community should give priority to therapeutic lifestyle changes or to the use of pharmacology in the treatment of the metabolic syndrome.

2
Definition of Metabolic Syndrome: Implications for Therapeutic Priority

The components that compose the metabolic syndrome are a combination of major and emerging risk factors [Third report of the National Cholesterol Education Program (NCEP) expert panel on detection, evaluation, and treatment of high blood cholesterol in adults 2002]. They can generally be divided into the following five categories:

- Atherogenic dyslipidemia: elevations of serum triglycerides, total apo B, and small LDL particles and low HDL levels
- Elevated blood pressure
- Elevated plasma glucose: IGT, IFG, or type 2 diabetes
- A prothrombotic state
- A proinflammatory state

Epidemiological studies demonstrate that persons who carry these metabolic risk factors are at increased risk for both ASCVD and type 2 diabetes (Isomaa et al. 2001; Alexander et al. 2003; Hunt et al. 2003; Lakka et al. 2002). What is not currently known is how these factors lead to an increase in risk, particularly for ASCVD. Presumably, each of the metabolic risk factors in some way affects the atherogenic process. To date, the relative contributions of each have not been worked out. A key hypothesis of the metabolic syndrome is that the metabolic risk factors are interconnected, i.e., have a common basis. This concept adds to the difficulty of determining just how each factor independently raises the risk for ASCVD. On a mechanistic basis, the relation between metabolic syndrome and type 2 diabetes is better understood. Much, but perhaps not all of this relationship is mediated through insulin resistance. The association of the metabolic syndrome with ASCVD obviously is more complex, but worthy of speculation. Such speculation can be a stimulus for research to better understand the underlying mechanisms. This research may uncover new targets for therapy. Let us therefore speculate on how each of the metabolic risk factors may be related to the risk for ASCVD.

2.1
Atherogenic Dyslipidemia

Among the risk factors for ASCVD, the relationship between elevated LDL levels and the development of atherosclerosis is best understood [Third report of the National Cholesterol Education Program (NCEP) expert panel on detection, evaluation, and treatment of high blood cholesterol in adults 2002]. In persons with elevated serum LDL, LDL enters the arterial wall and initiates an inflammatory response, building the foundation of atherogenesis. This connection between LDL and atherosclerosis is most obvious in persons with severe hypercholesterolemia. In clinical practice, the presence of excess LDL is detected by measurement of LDL-C. In persons with the metabolic syndrome, however, the LDL-C level is an incomplete description of atherogenic lipoprotein abnormalities. For example, a more important abnormality seemingly is an increase in the number of lipoprotein particles of atherogenic potential.

These particles are found in LDL, but also in triglyceride-rich very low-density lipoproteins (VLDL). Both LDL and VLDL contain apo B. When the triglyceride concentration is high, the LDL-C level is not a good indicator of the concentration (or number) of apo B-containing lipoproteins. This is true for at least two reasons. First, the LDL particles are small and partially depleted of cholesterol; hence, there are more LDL particles than shown by LDL-C. In addition, with higher triglyceride, more atherogenic particles are present in the VLDL fraction. One measure of the atherogenic lipoprotein particle number is the total apo B, which can be measured by immunological techniques. Another measure is LDL+VLDL-C (also called non-HDL-C). In most persons, the non-HDL-C level is better correlated with the total apo B level than LDL-C.

It is not known whether the measurement of total apo B captures all of the atherogenic potential of apo B-containing lipoproteins. This is because all lipoproteins carrying apo B may not have the same atherogenic potential. Increases in certain lipoprotein fractions are widely believed to be unusually atherogenic. One highly atherogenic species includes the remnants of VLDL (Krauss 1998). Another fraction of greater atherogenicity may be composed of small LDL particles (Krauss 1995). Evidence to support variable atherogenic potential among the different fractions of apo B-containing lipoproteins is mostly indirect and has not been discerned with certainty. Regardless, at present, elevations of LDL+VLDL-C (or total apo B) nevertheless appear to be a more appropriate target of lipid-lowering therapy than LDL-C in persons with the metabolic syndrome (Grundy 2002).

A low level of serum HDL is another common lipoprotein abnormality associated with the metabolic syndrome. Many studies show that low HDL levels are accompanied by an increased risk for ASCVD. The reasons, however, remain to be elucidated. Some investigators believe that HDL somehow protects against the development of atherosclerosis; if so, some of this protective effect may be lost in persons with lower HDL levels. Certainly, the mechanistic relationship between HDL levels and the development of atherosclerosis is more complicated than for LDL [Third report of the National Cholesterol Education Program (NCEP) expert panel on detection, evaluation, and treatment of high blood cholesterol in adults 2002]. HDL may be related to ASCVD in at least three ways (Vega and Grundy 1996). First, high levels of HDL may protect against the development of atherosclerosis, whereas low levels may allow for accelerated atherogenesis. Several theories are proposed to explain this protective effect. For example, HDL may prevent atherogenic modification of LDL, i.e., oxidation and precipitation. Further, it may enhance reverse cholesterol transport, i.e., the removal of excess cholesterol from the arterial wall. And finally, HDL may carry protective substances that slow down the progression of atherosclerosis. A second connection between HDL and ASCVD is that HDL is a marker for increases in atherogenic lipoproteins, i.e., increases in atherogenic VLDL and LDL. There is an inverse relationship between HDL levels and atherogenic lipoproteins in patients with atherogenic dyslipidemia. Third, low levels of HDL are associated with the non-lipid risk factors of the metabolic syndrome. Whether a low HDL level per se is a potential target for clinical intervention is uncertain at present. Several new approaches for raising HDL levels are in development. They are likely to be tested in clinical trials over the next few years. If they prove to be efficacious, they could become one new approach to the management of patients with the metabolic syndrome.

2.2
Elevated Blood Pressure

Higher levels of blood pressure have long been classified as a major risk factor for ASCVD (Chobanian et al. 2003). Hypertension undoubtedly raises the risk for ASCVD, but what are the underlying mechanisms? Does hypertension accelerate the deposition of lipid in the arterial wall? If so, by what mechanism? Does elevated blood pressure cause endothelial dysfunction allowing for more infiltration of lipoprotein into the arterial wall? Or does it change the vascular biology by otherwise damaging the arterial wall? There are no definitive answers. The available evidence suggests that higher blood pressure accelerates atherosclerosis in pre-existing, lipid-rich lesions. A simple hypothesis is that elevations of atherogenic lipoproteins initiate atherosclerosis and hypertension accelerates it. Pathological studies suggest that hypertension promotes smooth muscle cell proliferation and fibrosis. Whatever the mechanism, there is no doubt that elevated blood pressure is an attractive target for treatment in patients with the metabolic syndrome. Clinical trials amply show that blood pressure reduces the risk for stroke; but at the same time, it decreases the risk for myocardial infarction (Chobanian et al. 2003).

2.3
Elevated Plasma Glucose

Patients with type 2 diabetes are at increased risk for ASCVD. A long-standing question is whether elevated plasma glucose accelerates the development of atherosclerosis. Patients with type 1 diabetes have hyperglycemia for many years, and yet many of them do not have advanced coronary atherosclerosis. A recent study (Nathan et al. 2003), on the other hand, suggests that therapeutic lowering of glucose in patients with type 1 diabetes will slow the progression of atherosclerosis and/or reduce the frequency of major coronary events. Multiple mechanisms have been proposed by which elevated plasma glucose might promote atherosclerosis (Aronson and Rayfield 2002). They include, among others, enhancement of oxidative stress in the arterial wall, glycolyation of arterial wall proteins, deposition of advanced glycation products in the arterial wall, and activation of protein kinase C (Aronson and Rayfield 2002). There is no question that lowering of glucose levels will retard the development of microvascular disease. It is likely that glucose lowering will also reduce the progression of macrovascular disease (atherosclerosis); nonetheless, that hypoglycemic therapy will specifically reduce major ASCVD events remains to be convincingly shown in controlled clinical trials.

Because there is some uncertainty about whether the lowering of glucose levels from the diabetic range will reduce macrovascular events, it is not surprising that the evidence that glucose lowering in persons with IGT/IFG will decrease major cardiovascular events is even weaker. This is not to say that treatment of IGT/IFG with agents that lower glucose levels may fail to reduce major cardiovascular events; but if so, this has not been demonstrated. Moreover, the benefits could be due to effects of these agents other than glucose lowering per se. For example, they could reduce insulin resistance, which could modify other risk factors independently of glucose lowering.

2.4
Prothrombotic State

One of the features of the metabolic syndrome is an increase in circulating factors that shift the balance of prothrombotic to antithrombotic states towards the former (De Pergola and Pannacciulli 2002). Some of these factors are pro-coagulant, whereas others are anti-fibrinolytic. Among the latter are increases in circulating fibrinogen and Factor VII, whereas an increase in PAI-1 is anti-fibrinolytic. Although it is widely assumed that a prothrombotic state will increase the likelihood of major cardiovascular events, the evidence for this is not iron-clad, nor are the mechanisms understood. It has been suggested that a prothrombotic state causes endothelial dysfunction, which accelerates atherosclerosis (Vague et al. 1995). Another possibility, however, is that whenever a small plaque undergoes rupture or erosion, the resulting thrombosis will be larger in a person who is under the influence of a prothrombotic state. If so, this person is more likely to sustain a major life-threatening cardiovascular event. Even though the mechanisms by which a prothrombotic state predisposes to major cardiovascular events are not understood, there is strong evidence that anti-platelet therapy or anti-coagulant therapy will reduce the risk for major cardiovascular events (Pearson et al. 2002). Thus, this is indirect evidence of benefit from intervention on a prothrombotic state.

2.5
Proinflammatory State

One common feature of the metabolic syndrome is a high–normal level of C-reactive protein (CRP) (Ridker et al. 2003). This finding implies that the liver is responding to a chronic stimulation by inflammatory cytokines that promote the production of acute phase reactants, one of which is CRP. Epidemiological studies reveal that high–normal levels of CRP carry predictive power for major cardiovascular events (Ridker 2003). What is not known is the mechanistic basis for this association. One hypothesis holds that higher levels of CRP reflect the presence of unstable atherosclerotic lesions that presumably contain large quantities of macrophages; activation of these macrophages triggers the release of cytokines that cause increased synthesis of acute phase reactants by the liver. But perhaps more interesting is the question of whether the acute phase reactants made in the liver have proinflammatory properties in their own right. For example, they could deposit in existing arterial lesions to enhance the local inflammatory response. If such a mechanism pertains, then higher levels of CRP (and other acute phase reactants) possibly (a) reflect enhanced chronic inflammation in arterial lesions, and (b) contribute to atherogenesis. Even though atherogenesis represents an inflammatory response to injury, it is less than certain whether high circulating levels of CRP in individuals with the metabolic syndrome directly connect with the presence of unstable atherosclerotic plaques.

3
Pathogenesis of Metabolic Syndrome: What Does It Mean for Therapy?

The metabolic syndrome arises out of the interaction between underlying risk factors and the more distal processes that produce the metabolic risk factors. The major underlying risk factors are (a) obesity and other disorders of adipose tissue, and (b) physical inactivity and disorders of skeletal muscle. Both adipose tissue and skeletal muscle are subject to acquired and genetic disorders, and both appear to be importantly involved in the pathogenesis of the metabolic syndrome. Disorders of adipose tissue and skeletal muscle undoubtedly have adverse effects on the metabolism in other tissues, particularly but not exclusively the liver. Out of this secondary aberrant metabolism grow the metabolic risk factors. Considerations of the pathogenesis of this syndrome have important implications for therapeutic approaches. For this reason, the key features of pathogenesis deserve some review.

3.1
Underlying Risk Factors

3.1.1
Obesity and Disorders of Adipose Tissue

The majority of people expressing the metabolic syndrome are overweight or obese [Third report of the National Cholesterol Education Program (NCEP) expert panel on detection, evaluation, and treatment of high blood cholesterol in adults 2002]. In this paper, the term obesity will encompass both overweight and obese categories. Definitions for these categories vary according to national standards. The worldwide increasing frequency of the metabolic syndrome strongly correlates with an increasing prevalence of obesity. If obesity is a major underlying cause, what is its mechanistic link to the syndrome? This is one of the key questions in the pathogenesis of the metabolic syndrome. Hence we are led to ask whether systemic responses to excessive production of several factors from adipose tissue largely account for the syndrome (Lyon et al. 2003; Coppack 2001). The adipose tissue secretes a variety of factors: non-esterified fatty acids (NEFAs), inflammatory cytokines, prothrombotic factors, leptin, and adiponectin. Plasma NEFAs are the product of lipolysis of triglyceride stored in adipose tissue. Inflammatory cytokines coming out of adipose tissue include tumor necrosis factor (TNF) α and interleukin (IL)-6. A major prothrombotic factor released by adipose tissue is plasminogen activator inhibitor-1 (PAI-1). Leptin is produced in adipose tissue and suppresses the appetite, whereas another product, adiponectin, appears to reduce insulin resistance in several tissues. In the presence of obesity, the release of all of these factors is increased except for adiponectin, which is reduced. Each of the factors responds in one way or another to circulating insulin. In other words, insulin suppresses the lipolysis of triglyceride and reduces the production of inflammatory cytokines, PAI-1, and leptin; it also seemingly stimulates the production of adiponectin. As circulating insulin in obese persons fails to suppress adipose tissue products down to normal levels, we must ask whether it is not appropriate to say that adipose tissue in obese persons is insulin resistant.

If adipose tissue of obese persons is insulin resistant, what might be the reasons? Several causes have been considered (Reynisdottir et al. 1994; Engfeldt and Arner 1988; Olefsky 1977; Gruen et al. 1980; Ek et al. 2002; Ryden et al. 2002). First, adipocytes that are engorged with fat could be relatively resistant to the action of insulin. Second, in obesity, there is an increase in the number of adipocytes, each of which is engorged with triglycerides. This high number of abnormal cells could result in a greater release of bio-active substances from adipose tissue. Third, if adipose tissue in obesity produces increased amounts of inflammatory cytokines, these cytokines could down-regulate insulin signaling (Hotamisligil 2003). Insulin sensitivity of adipose tissue further appears to vary depending on the adipose tissue location. Overproduction of adipose tissue products (or underproduction of adiponectin) seems to be particularly pronounced in persons with upper body obesity (Misra and Vikram 2003). Thus, upper body adipose tissue acts as if it is more insulin resistant than lower body adipose tissue. Studies have shown that adipose tissue of women with upper body obesity is more insulin resistant than that of lower body obesity. Thus, the insulin resistance of adipose tissue in obesity is likely to be of multifactorial origin. Clearly, obesity represents a target of therapy in the management of the metabolic syndrome.

The problem of insulin resistance of obese adipose tissue is seemingly exacerbated in those who have genetic abnormalities in the insulin-signaling cascade. The transmission of the insulin signal to various metabolic control points in cells is highly complicated and, not surprisingly, subject to individual differences based on polymorphic variation in insulin-signaling proteins. Several examples have been reported in the literature. One is a polymorphism in a protein called PC-1 that interacts directly with the insulin receptor (Abate et al. 2003). Polymorphisms in other proteins in the insulin-signaling cascade, notably IRS-1 and IRS-2, could further enhance insulin resistance of adipose tissue (White 2002). A more severe disorder of adipose tissue is called lipodystrophy (Garg 2004). In this condition, there is a severe deficiency of adipose tissue. Consequently, any degree of overnutrition will lead to excessive deposition of lipids in other tissue because of a lack of storage space in adipose tissue. Patients with lipodystrophy exhibit many features of the metabolic syndrome, some of them in extreme forms (Garg 2004).

The most notable consequence of insulin resistance of obese adipose tissue is excessive release of NEFA. The result of high NEFA output is increased accumulation of lipid, particularly in muscle and liver. Lipid accumulation in muscle results in insulin resistance of this tissue (Shulman 2000). This change impairs the glucose uptake in muscle, threatening an increase in plasma glucose. The only way to avoid hyperglycemia when muscle tissue is insulin resistant is by compensatory hyperinsulinemia, i.e., a rise in plasma insulin from increased production of insulin by pancreatic beta cells. Some evidence suggests that an increase in NEFA entering beta cells is one stimulant to the overproduction of insulin (Newgard and McGarry 1995). The overload of liver with excess influx of NEFA produces a fatty liver and modifies various pathways of the hepatic metabolism of glucose and lipids. Theoretically, if NEFA release from obese adipose tissue could be dampened, this should diminish insulin resistance and might reduce other metabolic risk factors. Drugs known to inhibit adipose tissue lipolysis—acipimox (Santomauro et al. 1999) and thiazolidinediones (Boden et al. 2003)—have in fact been shown to reduce insulin resistance.

The other products released by adipose tissue—inflammatory cytokines, PAI-1, adiponectin, and leptin—may have systemic effects as well, but their role is less well defined than that of excess NEFA. A discussion of the pathogenesis of the metabolic risk factors will consider their role.

3.1.2
Physical Inactivity and Disorders of Skeletal Muscle

The major site of nutrient utilization is skeletal muscle. Physical activity enhances energy utilization in muscle and reduces insulin resistance (Perseghin et al. 1996). Conversely, physical inactivity will increase insulin resistance. In addition, regular physical activity has a prolonged beneficial effect on energy utilization by promoting muscle development. Even so, with aging, there is a gradual loss of muscle mass. This change with aging will reduce the uptake and utilization of energy by muscle. Thus, unless the nutrient intake is curtailed in parallel with the loss of muscle, excess nutrients will lead to increased obesity. Recently, it has been observed that aging muscle is accompanied by a reduction in efficiency of fatty acid oxidation in mitochondria (Petersen et al. 2003). This too will increase insulin resistance in muscle, and it will divert increased amounts of NEFA to the liver. Thus, sedentary life habits and the aging process have adverse effects on skeletal muscle metabolism and are significant contributors to the development of insulin resistance and the metabolic syndrome.

3.2
Pathogenesis of Particular Metabolic Risk Factors

3.2.1
Atherogenic Dyslipidemia

The primary driving force behind the development of atherogenic dyslipidemia is fatty liver. Excess fat in the liver derived from high plasma NEFA levels serves as a stimulus for the formation and secretion of VLDL. The result will be an increased influx of triglyceride and apo B into the circulation. Higher serum triglycerides are responsible for the reduction in size of LDL and HDL particles [Third report of the National Cholesterol Education Program (NCEP) expert panel on detection, evaluation, and treatment of high blood cholesterol in adults 2002]. When concentrations of VLDL-triglycerides are elevated, cholesterol esters in LDL and HDL are exchanged for triglycerides, reducing the size and cholesterol content of both lipoproteins. Most of the excess apo B in serum will reside in small, dense LDL particles. Another cause of low HDL-C is increased activity of hepatic lipase (Vega and Grundy 1996), which is secondary to obesity and lipid accumulation in the liver (Nie et al. 1998).

3.2.2
Elevated Blood Pressure

The causes of elevated blood pressures associated with the metabolic syndrome appear to be multifactorial. Certainly, obesity tends to be associated with higher blood pressures (Anonymous 1998); some evidence suggests that blood pressure is heightened further by physical inactivity. Multiple factors have been postulated to link the underlying risk factors to hypertension (Hall 2003). Many patients with hypertension are insulin resistant, and both compensatory hyperinsulinemia and insulin resistance itself have been implicated in raising the blood pressure. Obese persons with hypertension have been shown to retain sodium, which raises the blood volume (Hall 2003). One theory holds that mechanical compression of the kidneys with excess peri-renal fat contributes to sodium retention (Hall 2003). Finally, inflammatory factors have recently been implicated in the development of endothelial function, vasoconstriction, and higher blood pressures (Sesso et al. 2003).

3.2.3
Elevated Plasma Glucose

Insulin resistance of muscle predisposes to higher glucose levels by impairing the glucose uptake in muscle (Shulman 2000). Insulin resistance in liver secondary to fatty liver results in enhanced gluconeogenesis and increased hepatic glucose output (Haque and Sanyal 2002). Hyperinsulinemia associated with insulin resistance helps to suppress hepatic gluconeogenesis, but when the liver is insulin resistant, this suppression is partially lost. When insulin levels fall secondary to beta-cell failure, hepatic gluconeogenesis is enhanced. Thus, although compensatory overproduction of insulin by pancreatic beta-cells can prevent the onset of hyperglycemia in the presence of obesity and sedentary life habits, the insulin secretory capacity eventually declines, allowing for a rise in plasma glucose. As the insulin secretory capacity declines, the first abnormality is IGT. IFG follows, and finally, categorical hyperglycemia (type 2 diabetes) sets in. Both genetic and acquired factors may accelerate the decline in beta cell function (LeRoith 2002).

3.2.4
Prothrombotic State

In individuals with the metabolic syndrome, multiple abnormalities in coagulation and fibrinolysis the origin of which is uncertain have been reported (De Pergola and Pannacciulli 2002) . High levels of PAI-1 seemingly arise by increased PAI-1 production from excess adipose tissue. Elevated fibrinogen represents enhanced stimulation of fibrinogen in the liver, probably in response to inflammatory stimuli arising either within or outside the liver. Finally, diabetes has been implicated in the development of platelet dysfunction (Yazbek et al. 2003).

3.2.5
Proinflammatory State

A state of chronic inflammation is suggested by the presence of increased circulating cytokines and acute phase reactants (e.g., CRP). The stimulus for these changes remains to be determined. One source may be an overproduction of inflammatory cytokines by adipose tissue. Another could be cytokine overproduction by macrophages in unstable atherosclerotic plaques. Whether either source is sufficient to produce elevations of CRP is uncertain. Another possibility is that increases in CRP are secondary to the fatty liver that accompanies obesity. Hepatic responses to excess fat in the liver are variable. Occasionally, patients develop significant inflammation (nonalcoholic hepatic steotosis). Even more show low-grade increases in serum transaminases. And probably still more will have modest increases in CRP. The accumulation of lipids in tissue is presumably a stimulus for an inflammatory response of varying degrees of severity (Chitturi et al. 2002). Thus, it seems likely that lipotoxicity is the major cause of the proinflammatory state of the metabolic syndrome (Chitturi et al. 2002).

4
Clinical Management of the Metabolic Syndrome

4.1
Clinical Diagnosis of the Metabolic Syndrome

The clinical management of the metabolic syndrome of course requires the identification of subjects having the condition. In recent years, several attempts have been made to provide clinical criteria for diagnosis of the syndrome. Three different organizations have proposed clinical criteria. All of them overlap considerably, although there are significant differences, depending on the view of the fundamental pathogenesis of the condition. In the following, they are reviewed briefly.

4.1.1
World Health Organization

In 1998, a WHO consultation group (Alberti and Zimmet 1998) proposed clinical criteria that have been slightly modified, as shown in Table 1. Clinical evidence of insulin resistance is a requirement for diagnosis. Identification of insulin resistance depends on one of several criteria: type 2 diabetes, impaired

Table 1 World Health Organization clinical criteria for metabolic syndrome[a]

Insulin resistance, identified by one of the following: type 2 diabetes, impaired fasting glucose, impaired glucose tolerance, or for those with normal fasting glucose levels (<110 mg/dl) glucose uptake below the lowest quartile for background population under investigation under hyperinsulinemic, euglycemic condition

Plus any two of the following:

Antihypertensive medication and/or high blood pressure (≥ 140 mmHg systolic or ≥ 90 mmHg diastolic)

Plasma triglycerides ≥ 150 mg/dl (≥ 1.7 mmol/l)

HDL cholesterol < 35 mg/dl (< 0.9 mmol/l) in men

$\qquad$ < 39 mg/dl (1.0 mmol/l) in women

BMI > 30 kg/m^2 and/or waist:hip ratio > 0.9 in men, > 0.85 in women

Urinary albumin excretion rate

≥ 20 µg/min or albumin:creatinine ratio ≥ 30 mg/g

[a] World Health Organization: Definition, diagnosis and classification of diabetes mellitus and its complications: Report of a WHO Consultation. Part 1. Diagnosis and classification of diabetes mellitus. Geneva, World Health Organization, 1999. http://whqlibdoc.who.int/hq/1999/WHO_NCD_NCS_99.2.pdf.

fasting glucose, impaired glucose tolerance, or for those with normal fasting glucose values (<110 mg/dl), a glucose uptake below the lowest quartile for background population under hyperinsulinemic, euglycemic conditions. If a person shows evidence of insulin resistance, a diagnosis of the metabolic syndrome can be made if two or more of the following features are present: hypertension, increased body mass index (BMI) (or increased waist/hip ratio), high triglycerides, low HDL-C, and microalbuminuria. The need to carry out an oral glucose tolerance test (OGTT) in patients without elevated glucose levels seems to be a logistical disadvantage of the WHO criteria.

4.1.2
ATP III Report

In 2002, the NCEP ATP III report [Third report of the National Cholesterol Education Program (NCEP) expert panel on detection, evaluation, and treatment of high blood cholesterol in adults] suggested a somewhat different set of criteria for the diagnosis of the metabolic syndrome (Table 2). When a person has three of five characteristics listed in Table 2, the diagnosis is made. Criteria include abdominal obesity, defined by increased waist circumference, raised triglycerides, reduced HDL-C, elevated blood pressure, and raised plasma glucose. Patients with type 2 diabetes are not excluded from diagnosis if they otherwise meet the criteria of the metabolic syn-

Table 2 ATP III clinical identification of the metabolic syndrome

Risk factor	Defining level
Abdominal obesity[a]	Waist circumference[b]
Men	> 102 cm (> 40 inches)
Women	> 88 cm (> 35 inches)
Triglycerides	≥ 150 mg/dl
HDL-C	
Men	< 40 mg/dl
Women	< 50 mg/dl
Blood pressure	≥ 130 or ≥ 85 mmHg
Fasting glucose	≥ 110 mg/dl[c]

[a] Overweight and obesity are associated with insulin resistance and the metabolic syndrome. However, the presence of abdominal obesity is more highly correlated with the metabolic risk factors than is an elevated BMI. Therefore, the simple measure of waist circumference is recommended to identify the body weight component of the metabolic syndrome.

[b] Some male patients can develop multiple metabolic risk factors when the waist circumference is only marginally increased, e.g., 94–102 cm (37–39 inches). Such patients may have a strong genetic contribution to insulin resistance. They should benefit from changes in life habits, similarly to men with categorical increases in waist circumference.

[c] Recently the fasting glucose has beenlowered to ≥ 100 mg/dl (Grundy et al. 2004a, 2004b)

drome according to ATP III. However, identification of insulin resistance is not required. ATP III diagnosis does not require OGTT when patients have normoglycemia.

4.1.3
The American Association of Clinical Endocrinology

The American Association of Clinical Endocrinology (AACE) (Einhorn 2003) uses the term 'insulin resistance syndrome' instead of 'metabolic syndrome'. AACE criteria for diagnosis include many of those listed in WHO and ATP III definitions (Table 3). However, a 2-h post-prandial glucose is recommended for individuals with normoglycemia who otherwise appear to be at risk for metabolic syndrome. The diagnosis is made based on clinical judgment—no specific number of fixed criteria is required for diagnosis. A diagnosis 'insulin resistance syndrome' cannot be applied if a person already has type 2 diabetes; the two diagnoses are mutually exclusive.

Table 3 American Association of Clinical Endocrinologists' Clinical criteria for diagnosis of the insulin resistance syndrome[a]

Risk factor components	Cut-off points for abnormality
Overweight/obesity	BMI $\geq$ 25 kg/m^2
Triglycerides	$\geq$ 150 mg/dl
Low HDL cholesterol	< 40 mg/dl in men
	< 50 mg/dl in women
Elevated blood pressure	$\geq$ 130/85 mmHg
2-h Post-glucose challenge	> 140 mg/dl
Fasting glucose	Between 110 mg/dl–126 mg/dl
Other risk factors	Family history of type 2 diabetes, hypertension or CVD
	Polycystic ovary syndrome
	Sedentary lifestyle
	Advancing age
	Ethnic groups having high risk for type 2 diabetes or CVD

[a] Diagnosis depends on clinical judgment based on risk factors.

4.2
Risk Assessment for ASCVD and Type 2 Diabetes

Several prospective studies show that persons with the metabolic syndrome are at increased risk for both ASCVD and type 2 diabetes (Lakka et al. 2002; Olijhoek et al. 2004; Alexander et al. 2003). Recently, the United States National Heart Lung and Blood Institute (Grundy et al. 2004a) held a conference in which data on the risk from the metabolic syndrome was examined from the

Framingham Heart Study. The results reported by the Framingham group can be summarized as follows.

4.2.1
Metabolic Syndrome as a Predictor of ASCVD

In the Framingham Heart Study, approximately 25% of new-onset ASCVD could be attributed to the metabolic syndrome. The relative risk for ASCVD was approximately twofold higher in persons with the syndrome compared to those without. Even so, in the presence of metabolic syndrome in persons without established diabetes, the 10-year risk for coronary heart disease (CHD) did not reach the level of a CHD risk equivalent, i.e., more than 20%. In most men with the syndrome, the 10-year risk was typically in the range of 10%–20%, whereas in women, it averaged less than 10%. It is important to note that assessment of the metabolic syndrome is not a substitute for multi-factorial risk assessment for projecting the risk for ASCVD. It does not contain all of the major risk predictors such as age, cigarette smoking, and total cholesterol. Neither does it grade the severity of risk factors. The use of metabolic syndrome to assess the risk for ASCVD is a misguided effort.

4.2.2
Metabolic Syndrome as a Predictor of Diabetes

In the Framingham Heart Study, the presence of metabolic syndrome was highly predictive of new-onset type 2 diabetes. For both men and women, the presence of metabolic syndrome carried a relative risk approximately five times higher than its absence. When IFG is present, the 10-year risk for type 2 diabetes is about 40%–50%. If IGT is detected by OGTT, the 10-year risk for type 2 diabetes is approximately the same. The latter suggests the value of carrying out OGTT when metabolic syndrome by ATP III criteria is present.

4.3
Management of Underlying Risk Factors

ATP III placed increased emphasis on the metabolic syndrome for the express purpose of reducing the risk for ASCVD and type 2 diabetes through modification of the underlying risk factors with therapeutic lifestyle changes. Although some of the metabolic risk factors may require drug therapies, effective treatment of the underlying risk factors offers the best opportunity to reduce all of the metabolic risk factors simultaneously. The American Heart Association recently sponsored a conference on the management of the metabolic syndrome. The results of this conference will be highlighted in this section (Grundy et al. 2004b).

4.3.1
Overweight and Obesity

Evidence-based clinical guidelines for the management of overweight and obesity were published in 1998 by the NHLBI and National Institute of Diabetes and Digestive and Kidney Diseases (Anonymous 1998). In these guidelines, overweight and obesity were defined as BMI of 25–29.9 kg/m^2 and 30 kg/m^2 or higher, respectively. As diagnostic criteria for the metabolic syndrome, ATP III adopted obesity guidelines for abdominal obesity, which was defined as a waist circumference of 102 cm or above (>40 inches) in men and 88 cm or above (>35 inches) in women. ATP III, however, noted that some persons can develop metabolic syndrome at lesser waist circumferences [Third report of the National Cholesterol Education Program (NCEP) expert panel on detection, evaluation, and treatment of high blood cholesterol in adults 2002]. This is particularly the case in certain ethnic groups, e.g., the populations of South and Southeast Asia.

Obesity guidelines (Anonymous 1998) recommend two therapeutic approaches to weight reduction: reduced caloric intake and behavioral change. The latter should incorporate increased physical activity. The diet to be employed in weight reduction should be designed to reduce the caloric intake and be a lifetime diet, not a 'crash diet' and 'extreme diet'. The latter almost universally fail to produce long-term weight reduction. More extreme diets are popular because they promise to bring a 'quick fix' to the obesity problem. Examples include diets that are very low calorie, very low fat, or very high fat. At present, low-carbohydrate, high-fat diets are popular 'quick fix' diets in the USA. For the vast majority of overweight/obese persons, these diets ultimately fail. They are too extreme for long-term adherence. Moreover, they would not be healthy as a lifetime diet. A more realistic approach to a weight loss diet is to reduce the caloric intake by 500–1000 calories per day. A useful goal when undergoing such diets is to reduce the body weight by approximately 10% during the first 6–12 months.

A diet appropriate for long-term weight reduction is consistent with current recommendations for a healthy diet. Emphasis should be given to reducing the consumption of saturated fatty acids, trans fatty acids and cholesterol, a reduced intake of simple sugars, and ample intakes of fruits, vegetables, and whole grains. Some investigators favor a relatively high intake of unsaturated fatty acids at the expense of carbohydrates. This dietary pattern is similar to that of the 'Mediterranean diet'. Avoidance of high-carbohydrate intakes will improve atherogenic dyslipidemia and reduce a post-prandial rise in glucose and insulin (Grundy 1999). Again, as mentioned before, extremes of high-fat or low-fat intakes should be avoided.

Behavioral modification is a second major requirement for successful weight reduction (Grundy et al. 2004b). Examples of behavioral changes that will increase the chances of long-term weight reduction are:

- Setting of goals for weight reduction and physical activity
- Development of strategies to avoid situations that tempt to overeat
- Planning to prevent eating binges
- Systematic planning of meals
- Eating regular meals (avoiding eating or snacking between meals)
- Eating smaller portions (and eating slower)
- Self-monitoring of eating behavior and, if possible, keeping a diet diary
- Establishing social and group support
- Management of stressful situations
- Setting aside time for regular physical activity

Resources for patients are readily available in many places. For instance, information on dietary change and behavioral modification can be obtained on-line from the NHLBI (www.nhlbi.nih.gov) and the American Heart Association (www.americanheart.org).

Successful weight reduction will mitigate all of the risk factors of the metabolic syndrome (Anonymous 1998). It will improve atherogenic dyslipidemia, reduce blood pressure, lower plasma glucose, improve coagulation and fibrinolytic factors, and reduce the proinflammatory state. Clinical trials (Tuomilehto et al. 2001; Knowler et al. 2002) further show that even moderate weight reduction will delay the onset of type 2 diabetes in patients with prediabetes, defined as IFG or IGT (Anonymous 1998). Improvement of metabolic risk factors suggests that long-term weight reduction will reduce risk for AS-CVD (Anonymous 1998). Such a favorable outcome, although highly likely, has not been demonstrated unequivocally through controlled clinical trials.

4.3.2
Physical Inactivity

In the USA, 70% or more of the population is sedentary. The situation may be somewhat better in Europe, but social and employment forces are driving all developed and urban societies towards a sedentary existence. Physical inactivity is a major underlying risk factor for the metabolic syndrome, and regular physical activity and attaining physical fitness will correct most of the metabolic risk factors. There is growing evidence that regular activity will reduce the risk for both ASCVD and type 2 diabetes (Thompson et al. 2003).

Current recommendations for healthy physical activity (Thompson et al. 2003), which can be applied to patients with the metabolic syndrome, include 30 min of daily moderate-intensity exercise. Suggested activities that will comply with this recommendation are:

- Adding routine exercise to daily activities (e.g., brisk walking, jogging, swimming, biking, golfing, team sports)

- Using simple exercise equipment for the home (e.g., treadmills)

- Including several short (10–15-min) bouts of activity (brisk walking)

- Minimizing sedentary activities in leisure time (television watching and computer games)

4.4
Management of Metabolic Risk Factors

Although first-line therapy for the metabolic syndrome aims to improve the underlying risk factors through lifestyle changes, in higher risk patients, it may be necessary to include drug therapies directed at individual metabolic risk factors (Grundy et al. 2004b). The decision to use drug therapies heavily depends on a person's absolute risk and is determined through multi-factorial risk algorithms.

4.4.1
Atherogenic Dyslipidemia

The primary feature of atherogenic dyslipidemia is an increase in apo B-containing lipoproteins, most notably small LDL and remnant lipoproteins. In higher risk patients with the metabolic syndrome, primary therapy should therefore focus on lowering the concentrations of these atherogenic lipoproteins. Statins represent the first-line treatment for lowering apo B-containing lipoproteins. Clinical trials show that statin therapy is effective in reducing the risk for major acute coronary events in all types of patients, including those with the metabolic syndrome and type 2 diabetes [Third report of the National Cholesterol Education Program (NCEP) expert panel on detection, evaluation, and treatment of high blood cholesterol in adults 2002; Ballantyne et al. 2001; Collins et al. Heart Protection Study Collaborative Group 2003]. Most patients with the metabolic syndrome who have established ASCVD will be candidates for statin therapy [Third report of the National Cholesterol Education Program (NCEP) expert panel on detection, evaluation, and treatment of high blood cholesterol in adults 2002]. The goal of therapy is an LDL-C of <100 mg/dl (non-HDL-C <130 mg/dl or total apo B <100 mg/dl). Recent clinical trials suggest that lowering LDL-C well below 100 mg/dl will provide added risk reduction (Heart Protection Study Collaborative Group 2002; Cannon et al. 2004; Nissen et al. 2004). Many patients with type 2 diabetes are also candidates for intensive LDL-lowering therapy. The ATP III guidelines [Third report of the National Cholesterol Education Program (NCEP) expert panel on detection, evaluation, and treatment of high blood cholesterol in adults 2002] identified most patients with diabetes as being at high-risk and deserving of intensive LDL lowering. At the least, non-HDL-C should be reduced to <130 mg/dl (or total apo B to <100 mg/dl). In other countries, a more individualized approach to patients with diabetes is made, such that the intensity of therapy will depend on the estimated risk. If a patient has metabolic syndrome but not established ASCVD or diabetes, less-intensive LDL-lowering therapy is needed. In such persons, the LDL-C goal should be <130 mg/dl. A portion of these patients will require statin therapy to attain the goal of treatment.

Undoubtedly, some persons with metabolic syndrome will maintain an elevated triglyceride in spite of statin therapy. For the treatment of these patients, combining a fibrate with a statin can be considered. For example, it was shown in the VA-HIT study that fibrate therapy will reduce the risk for ASCVD events in patients who have insulin resistance and/or type 2 diabetes (Rubins et al. 1999). Although it has not been proven in controlled clinical trials that the combination of statins and fibrate will reduce the risk for cardiovascular disease (CVD) events, the finding that each type of drug independently reduces the risk provides supporting evidence for this assumption. If a fibrate is used with a statin, the drug of choice should be fenofibrate. The combination of statin and gemfibrozil carries an unacceptably high risk for severe myopathy, whereas the risk is apparently not so high with the combination of statin and fenofibrate (Vega et al. 2003). An alternative to the combination of statin and fenofibrate is the combination of statin and nicotinic acid (Bays and McGovern 2003). In terms of lowering triglycerides and raising HDL, nicotinic acid is more potent than a fibrate. On the other hand, fibrates have the advantage of having an evidence base in the VA-HIT trial and fewer side effects than nicotinic acid. Nonetheless, if patients can tolerate nicotinic acid therapy, this drug is attractive for use in combination with a statin.

Finally, a low HDL-C concentration is characteristic of the metabolic syndrome. The combinations of statin plus fibrate or statin plus nicotinic acid are useful for raising HDL levels as well as for lowering triglycerides (Vega et al. 2003; Bays and McGovern 2003). For this reason, combination drug therapy can also be considered after statin therapy if the HDL level remains low.

4.4.2
Elevated Blood Pressure

ATP III defined elevated blood pressure as a component of the metabolic syndrome as a blood pressure level of 130 mmHg or above systolic or 85 mmHg or above diastolic. The Seventh Report of the Joint National Committee (JNC7) emphasized lifestyle therapy as first-line therapy of high blood pressure (Chobanian et al. 2003). However, if lifestyle changes do not reduce the blood pressure to below 140/90 mmHg, drug therapy should be considered. An important question is whether the presence of the metabolic syndrome requires a priority in choice of anti-hypertensive medication. JNC7 does not identify a priority, but these guidelines favored first use of diuretics and beta-blockers for reasons of cost-effectiveness. It is well known that high doses of these drugs can increase insulin resistance and predispose to hyperglycemia. Consequently, if these drugs are to be used in patients with metabolic syndrome with or without type 2 diabetes, the doses of these drugs should be kept as low as practical. The use of an aldosterone receptor blocker (eplerenone or spironolactone) is an alternative to thiazides, but they have not been adequately studied in combination with other drugs in large populations. A next question is whether angiotensin converting enzyme inhibitors (ACE-I) and angiotension-receptor blockers (ARB) should be first-line therapy in patients with metabolic syndrome and/or type 2 diabetes. Their use as first-line drugs is supported by some, but not all clinical trials (Abbott and Bakris 2004). The combination of ACE-I (or ARB) plus low-dose diuretics is more attractive than higher dose diuretics (Krum et al. 2003). Other anti-hypertensive drugs (calcium channel blockers, alpha-1 blockers and central alpha-2 blockers) appear to be neutral with respect to the metabolic syndrome. In many patients, multiple drug combinations are required to achieve the goals of therapy (ALLHAT Officers and Coordinators for the ALLHAT Collaborative Research Group 2002). In those with metabolic syndrome without type 2 diabetes or CVD, the goal is to reduce the blood pressure to below 140/90 mmHg; for those with type 2 diabetes and CVD, the blood pressure is to reduce to a level of less than 130/85 mmHg (Chobanian et al. 2003).

4.4.3
Elevated Plasma Glucose

An important but unresolved question is whether drug therapy to reduce insulin resistance will reduce the risk for type 2 diabetes and CVD in persons with the metabolic syndrome. The strongest evidence to support a reduction in risk with drug therapy comes from the Diabetes Prevention Program (DPP) (Knowler et al. 2002). This clinical trial showed that metformin therapy in persons with pre-diabetes (impaired glucose tolerance and impaired fasting glucose) will reduce the risk for type 2 diabetes. The drug troglitazone was also initiated in the DPP, but withdrawn because of side effects. Nonetheless, post hoc analysis of the troglitazone data suggested a strong trend towards a reduction in risk for the development of diabetes (Grundy et al. 2004b). A similar trend for reducing the risk of developing diabetes with troglitazone was noted in another study (Buchanan et al. 2002). In spite of these trials, most authorities do not recommend that drugs reducing insulin resistance be used in patients with pre-diabetes (Grundy et al. 2004b). The benefit of reducing the risk for type 2 diabetes has not been shown to be cost effective. The currently used drugs to reduce insulin resistance are not without side effects, so that the benefit/harm ratio is not fully defined for the patient at risk for type 2 diabetes either.

Once categorical diabetes develops in a person with metabolic syndrome, clinical management turns to the control of hyperglycemia. Reducing glucose levels in patients with diabetes is known to reduce the risk for microvascular complications. Whether it will decrease the risk for macrovascular complications has not been established. This is an important question, but clinical trials yield ambiguous results. Nevertheless, according to current guidelines, the hemoglobin A1c should be reduced to less than 7%. The choice of hypoglycemic drugs beyond lifestyle changes must be individualized according to clinical judgment. Without any doubt, however, high priority should be given to the treatment of major risk factors—smoking, elevated LDL-C, and high blood pressure. Smoking cessation is imperative. LDL-C levels should be reduced to lower than 100 mg/dl [Third report of the National Cholesterol Education Program (NCEP) expert panel on detection, evaluation, and treatment of high blood cholesterol in adults 2002], and blood pressure to lower than 120/80 mmHg (Chobanian et al. 2003). A triglyceride-lowering drug (fenofibrate or nicotinic acid) can be added to statin therapy if the patient has elevated triglyceride (Rubins et al. 1999; Grundy et al. 2002).

4.4.4
Prothrombotic State

Patients with the metabolic syndrome appear to have a prothrombotic state, as suggested by elevations of fibrinogen, PAI-1, and possibly other coagulation factors. Anti-coagulant therapy in these patients is not practical; nonetheless, the risk for thrombotic events can be reduced by aspirin therapy. The American Heart Association (Pearson et al. 2002) currently recommends the use of aspirin prophylaxis when the 10-year risk for CHD is 10% or higher, as determined by the Framingham risk scoring. This recommendation can certainly be applied to patients with the metabolic syndrome who show a prothrombotic state.

4.4.5
Proinflammatory State

The possibility that the metabolic syndrome may predispose to a proinflammatory state, characterized by elevated cytokines (e.g., TNFα and IL-6) and elevations in acute phase reactants (CRP and fibrinogen), has received increased attention. There are, however, important unresolved questions: (a) what are the origins of inflammatory markers? (b) are they targets for therapy?, and (c) if so, what would be the preferred intervention? The origin is uncertain; the association between obesity and inflammatory markers suggests that excess lipids in adipose tissue or liver may elicit an inflammatory state. If so, weight reduction would be the primary intervention. Currently, there are no drugs that specifically target the proinflammatory state. Nonetheless, some investigators hold that evidence of a proinflammatory state, as suggested by elevations of CRP, justifies more intensive intervention on other risk factors of the metabolic syndrome, e.g., atherogenic dyslipidemia, hypertension, and the proinflammatory state itself. Whether CRP levels can yield information useful for decisions about the selection of risk factor intervention or the intensity of therapy nevertheless remains an open question.

References

Abate N, Carulli L, Cabo-Chan A Jr, Chandalia M, Snell PG, Grundy SM (2003) Genetic polymorphism PC-1 K121Q and ethnic susceptibility to insulin resistance. J Clin Endocrinol Metab 88:5927–5934

Abbott KC, Bakris GL (2004) What have we learned from the current trials? Med Clin North Am 88:189–207

Alberti KG, Zimmet PZ (1998) Definition, diagnosis and classification of diabetes mellitus and its complications. Part 1: diagnosis and classification of diabetes mellitus provisional report of a WHO consultation. Diabet Med 15:539–553

Alexander CM, Landsman PB, Teutsch SM, Haffner SM; Third National Health and Nutrition Examination Survey (NHANES III); National Cholesterol Education Program (NCEP) (2003) NCEP-defined metabolic syndrome, diabetes, and prevalence of coronary heart disease among NHANES III participants age 50 years and older. Diabetes 52:1210–1214

ALLHAT Officers and Coordinators for the ALLHAT Collaborative Research Group (2002) The Antihypertensive and Lipid-Lowering Treatment to Prevent Heart Attack Trial. Major outcomes in high-risk hypertensive patients randomized to angiotensin-converting enzyme inhibitor or calcium channel blocker vs diuretic: The Antihypertensive and Lipid-Lowering Treatment to Prevent Heart Attack Trial (ALLHAT). JAMA 288:2981–2997

Anonymous (1998) Executive summary of the clinical guidelines on the identification, evaluation, and treatment of overweight and obesity in adults. Arch Intern Med 158:1855–1867

Clinical Guidelines on the Identification, Evaluation, and Treatment of Overweight and Obesity in Adults–The Evidence Report. National Institutes of Health, 1998. Obes Res 6:51S–209S

Aronson D, Rayfield EJ (2002) How hyperglycemia promotes atherosclerosis: molecular mechanisms. Cardiovasc Diabetol 1:1–10

Ballantyne CM, Olsson AG, Cook TJ, Mercuri MF, Pedersen TR, Kjekshus J (2001) Influence of low high-density lipoprotein cholesterol and elevated triglyceride on coronary heart disease events and response to simvastatin therapy in 4S. Circulation 104:3046–3051

Bays HE, McGovern ME (2003) Once-daily niacin extended release/lovastatin combination tablet has more favorable effects on lipoprotein particle size and subclass distribution than atorvastatin and simvastatin. Prev Cardiol 6:179–188

Boden G, Cheung P, Mozzoli M, Fried SK (2003) Effect of thiazolidinediones on glucose and fatty acid metabolism in patients with type 2 diabetes. Metabolism 52:753–759

Buchanan TA, Xiang AH, Peters RK, Kjos SL, Marroquin A, Goico J, Ochoa C, Tan S, Berkowitz K, Hodis HN, Azen SP (2002) Preservation of pancreatic beta-cell function and prevention of type 2 diabetes by pharmacological treatment of insulin resistance in high-risk hispanic women. Diabetes 51:2796–2803

Cannon CP, Braunwald E, McCabe CH, Rader DJ, Rouleau JL, Belder R, Joyal SV, Hill KA, Pfeffer MA, Skene AM; Pravastatin or atorvastatin evaluation and infection therapy-thrombolysis in myocardial infarction 22 investigators (2004) Intensive versus moderate lipid lowering with statins after acute coronary syndromes. N Engl J Med 350:1495–1504

Chitturi S, Farrell G, Frost L, Kriketos A, Lin R, Fung C, Liddle C, Samarasinghe D, George
    J (2002) Serum leptin in NASH correlates with hepatic steatosis but not fibrosis: a man-
    ifestation of lipotoxicity? Hepatology 36:403–409
Chobanian AV, Bakris GL, Black HR, Cushman WC, Green LA, Izzo J Jr, Jones DW, Materson
    BJ, Oparil S, Wright JT Jr, Roccella EJ (2003) National Heart, Lung, and Blood Institute
    Joint National Committee on Prevention, Detection, Evaluation, National High Blood
    Pressure Education Program Coordinating Committee: The seventh report of the joint
    national committee on prevention, detection, evaluation, and treatment of high blood
    pressure: the JNC 7 report. JAMA 289:2560–2572
Collins R, Armitage J, Parish S, Sleigh P, Peto R; Heart Protection Study Collaborative Group
    (2003) MRC/BHF Heart Protection Study of cholesterol-lowering with simvastatin in
    5963 people with diabetes: a randomised placebo-controlled trial. Lancet 361:2005–2016
Coppack SW (2001) Pro-inflammatory cytokines and adipose tissue. Proc Nutr Soc 60:
    349–356
De Pergola G, Pannacciulli N (2002) Coagulation and fibrinolysis abnormalities in obesity.
    J Endocrinol Invest 25:899–904
Einhorn D (2003) ACE position statement on insulin resistance syndrome. Endocr Pract
    9:237–252
Ek I, Arner P, Ryden M, Holm C, Thorne A, Hoffstedt J, Wahrenberg H (2002) A unique
    defect in the regulation of visceral fat cell lipolysis in the polycystic ovary syndrome as
    an early link to insulin resistance. Diabetes 51:484–492
Engfeldt P, Arner P (1988) Lipolysis in human adipocytes, effects of cell size, age and of
    regional differences. Horm Metab Res Suppl 19:26–29
Garg A (2004) Acquired and inherited lipodystrophies. N Engl J Med 350:1220–1234
Gruen R, Kava R, Greenwood MR (1980) Development of basal lipolysis and fat cell size in
    the epididymal fat pad of normal rats. Metabolism 29:246–253
Grundy SM (1999) The optimal ratio of fat-to-carbohydrate in the diet. Annu Rev Nutr
    19:325–341
Grundy SM (2002) Low-density lipoprotein, non-high-density lipoprotein, and apolipopro-
    tein B as targets of lipid-lowering therapy. Circulation 106:2526–2529
Grundy SM, Vega GL, McGovern ME, Tulloch BR, Kendall DM, Fitz-Patrick D, Ganda
    OP, Rosenson RS, Buse JB, Robertson DD, Sheehan JP; Diabetes Multicenter Research
    Group (2002) Efficacy, safety, and tolerability of once-daily niacin for the treatment
    of dyslipidemia associated with type 2 diabetes: results of the assessment of diabetes
    control and evaluation of the efficacy of niaspan trial. Arch Intern Med 162:1568–1576
Grundy SM, Brewer HB Jr, Cleeman JI, Smith SC Jr, Lenfant C; American Heart Association;
    National Heart, Lung, and Blood Institute (2004a) Definition of metabolic syndrome:
    Report of the National Heart, Lung, and Blood Institute/American Heart Association
    conference on scientific issues related to definition. Circulation 109:433–438
Grundy SM, Hansen B, Smith SC Jr, Cleeman JI, Kahn RA; American Heart Association; Na-
    tional Heart, Lung, and Blood Institute; American Diabetes Association (2004b) Clinical
    management of metabolic syndrome: report of the American Heart Association/National
    Heart, Lung, and Blood Institute/American Diabetes Association conference on scientific
    issues related to management. Circulation 109:551–556
Hall JE (2003) The kidney, hypertension, and obesity. Hypertension 41:625–633
Haque M, Sanyal AJ (2002) The metabolic abnormalities associated with non-alcoholic fatty
    liver disease. Best Pract Res Clin Gastroenterol 16:709–731
Heart Protection Study Collaborative Group (2002) MRC/BHF Heart Protection Study of
    cholesterol lowering with simvastatin in 20,536 high-risk individuals: a randomised
    placebo-controlled trial. Lancet 360:7–22

Hotamisligil GS (2003) Inflammatory pathways and insulin action. Int J Obes Relat Metab Disord 27(Suppl 3):S53–S55

Hunt K, Resendez R, Williams K, Haffner S, Stern M (2003) NCEP versus WHO metabolic syndrome in relation to all cause and cardiovascular mortality in the San Antonio Heart Study (SAHS). Diabetes 52:A221

Isomaa B, Almgren P, Tuomi T, Forsen B, Lahti K, Nissen M, Taskinen MR, Group L (2001) Cardiovascular morbidity and mortality associated with the metabolic syndrome. Diabetes Care 24:683–689

Kannel WB, Wilson PW (1995) An update on coronary risk factors. Med Clin North Am 79:951–971

Knowler WC, Barrett-Connor E, Fowler SE, Hamman RF, Lachin JM, Walker EA, Nathan DM; Diabetes Prevention Program Research Group (2002) Reduction in the incidence of type 2 diabetes with lifestyle intervention or metformin. N Engl J Med 346:393–403

Krauss RM (1995) Dense low density lipoproteins and coronary artery disease. Am J Cardiol 75:53B–57B

Krauss RM (1998) Atherogenicity of triglyceride-rich lipoproteins. Am J Cardiol 81:13B–17B

Krum H, Skiba M, Gilbert RE (2003) Comparative metabolic effects of hydrochlorothiazide and indapamide in hypertensive diabetic patients receiving ACE inhibitor therapy. Diabet Med 20:708–712

Lakka HM, Laaksonen DE, Lakka TA, Niskanen LK, Kumpusalo E, Tuomilehto J, Salonen JT (2002) The metabolic syndrome and total and cardiovascular disease mortality in middle-aged men. JAMA 288:2709–2716

LeRoith D (2002) Beta-cell dysfunction and insulin resistance in type 2 diabetes: role of metabolic and genetic abnormalities. Am J Med 113(Suppl 6A):3S–11S

Lyon CJ, Law RE, Hsueh WA (2003) Minireview: adiposity, inflammation, and atherogenesis. Endocrinology 144:2195–2200

Misra A, Vikram NK (2003) Clinical and pathophysiological consequences of abdominal adiposity and abdominal adipose tissue depots. Nutrition 19:457–466

Nathan DM, Lachin J, Cleary P, Orchard T, Brillon DJ, Backlund JY, O'Leary DH, Genuth S (2003) Diabetes Control and Complications Trial; Epidemiology of Diabetes Interventions and Complications Research Group. Intensive diabetes therapy and carotid intima-media thickness in type 1 diabetes mellitus. N Engl J Med 348:2294–2303

Newgard CB, McGarry JD (1995) Metabolic coupling factors in pancreatic beta-cell signal transduction. Annu Rev Biochem 64:689–719

Nie L, Wang J, Clark LT, Tang A, Vega GL, Grundy SM, Cohen JC (1998) Body mass index and hepatic lipase gene (LIPC) polymorphism jointly influence postheparin plasma hepatic lipase activity. J Lipid Res 39:1127–1130

Nissen SE, Tuzcu EM, Schoenhagen P, Brown BG, Ganz P, Vogel RA, Crowe T, Howard G, Cooper CJ, Brodie B, Grines CL, DeMaria AN; REVERSAL Investigators (2004) Effect of intensive compared with moderate lipid-lowering therapy on progression of coronary atherosclerosis: a randomized controlled trial. JAMA 291:1071–1080

Olefsky JM (1977) Insensitivity of large rat adipocytes to the antilipolytic effects of insulin. J Lipid Res 18:459–464

Olijhoek JK, van der Graaf Y, Banga JD, Algra A, Rabelink TJ, Visseren FL; the SMART Study Group (2004) The metabolic syndrome is associated with advanced vascular damage in patients with coronary heart disease, stroke, peripheral arterial disease or abdominal aortic aneurysm. Eur Heart J 25:342–348

Pearson TA, Blair SN, Daniels SR, Eckel RH, Fair JM, Fortmann SP, Franklin BA, Goldstein LB, Greenland P, Grundy SM, Hong Y, Miller NH, Lauer RM, Ockene IS, Sacco RL, Sallis JF Jr, Smith SC Jr, Stone NJ, Taubert KA (2002) AHA Guidelines for Primary Prevention of Cardiovascular Disease and Stroke: 2002 Update: Consensus Panel Guide to Comprehensive Risk Reduction for Adult Patients Without Coronary or Other Atherosclerotic Vascular Diseases. American Heart Association Science Advisory and Coordinating Committee. Circulation 106:388–391

Perseghin G, Price TB, Petersen KF, Roden M, Cline GW, Gerow K, Rothman DL, Shulman GI (1996) Increased glucose transport-phosphorylation and muscle glycogen synthesis after exercise training in insulin-resistant subjects. N Engl J Med 335:1357–1362

Petersen KF, Befroy D, Dufour S, Dziura J, Ariyan C, Rothman DL, DiPietro L, Cline GW, Shulman GI (2003) Mitochondrial dysfunction in the elderly: possible role in insulin resistance. Science 300:1140–1142

Reynisdottir S, Ellerfeldt K, Wahrenberg H, Lithell H, Arner P (1994) Multiple lipolysis defects in the insulin resistance (metabolic) syndrome. J Clin Invest 93:2590–2599

Ridker PM (2003a) Clinical application of C-reactive protein for cardiovascular disease detection and prevention. Circulation 107:363–369

Ridker PM, Buring JE, Cook NR, Rifai N (2003b) C-reactive protein, the metabolic syndrome, and the risk of incident cardiovascular events: an 8-year follow-up of 14 719 initially healthy American women. Circulation 107:391–397

Rubins HB, Robins SJ, Collins D, Fye CL, Anderson JW, Elam MB, Faas FH, Linares E, Schaefer EJ, Schectman G, Wilt TJ, Wittes J, for the Veterans Affairs High-Density Lipoprotein Cholesterol Intervention Trial Study Group (1999) Gemfibrozil for the secondary prevention of coronary heart disease in men with low levels of high-density lipoprotein cholesterol. N Engl J Med 341:410–418

Ryden M, Dicker A, van Harmelen V, Hauner H, Brunnberg M, Perbeck L, Lonnqvist F, Arner P (2002) Mapping of early signaling events in tumor necrosis factor alpha-mediated lipolysis in human fat cells. J Biol Chem 277:1085–1091

Santomauro AT, Boden G, Silva ME, Rocha DM, Santos RF, Ursich MJ, Strassmann PG, Wajchenberg BL (1999) Overnight lowering of free fatty acids with Acipimox improves insulin resistance and glucose tolerance in obese diabetic and nondiabetic subjects. Diabetes 48:1836–1841

Sesso HD, Buring JE, Rifai N, Blake GJ, Gaziano JM, Ridker PM (2003) C-reactive protein and the risk of developing hypertension. JAMA 290:2945–2951

Shulman GI (2000) Cellular mechanisms of insulin resistance. J Clin Invest 106:171–176

Third report of the National Cholesterol Education Program (NCEP) expert panel on detection, evaluation, and treatment of high blood cholesterol in adults (Adult Treatment Panel III) (2002) Final Report. Circulation106:3143–3421

Thompson PD, Buchner D, Pina IL, Balady GJ, Williams MA, Marcus BH, Berra K, Blair SN, Costa F, Franklin B, Fletcher GF, Gordon NF, Pate RR, Rodriguez BL, Yancey AK, Wenger NK; American Heart Association Council on Clinical Cardiology Subcommittee on Exercise, Rehabilitation, and Prevention; American Heart Association Council on Nutrition, Physical Activity, and Metabolism Subcommittee on Physical Activity (2003) Exercise and physical activity in the prevention and treatment of atherosclerotic cardiovascular disease: a statement from the Council on Clinical Cardiology (Subcommittee on Exercise, Rehabilitation, and Prevention) and the Council on Nutrition, Physical Activity, and Metabolism (Subcommittee on Physical Activity). Circulation 107:3109–3116

Tuomilehto J, Lindstrom J, Eriksson JG, Valle TT, Hamalainen H, Ilanne-Parikka P, Keinanen-Kiukaanniemi S, Laakso M, Louheranta A, Rastas M, Salminen V, Uusitupa M; Finnish Diabetes Prevention Study Group (2001) Prevention of type 2 diabetes mellitus by changes in lifestyle among subjects with impaired glucose tolerance. N Engl J Med 344:1343–1350

Vague P, Raccah D, Scelles V (1995) Hypofibrinolysis and the insulin resistance syndrome. Int J Obes Relat Metab Disord 19(Suppl 1):S11–S15

Vega GL, Grundy SM (1996) Hypoalphalipoproteinemia (low high density lipoprotein) as a risk factor for coronary heart disease. Curr Opin Lipidol 7:209–216

Vega GL, Ma PT, Cater NB, Filipchuk N, Meguro S, Garcia-Garcia AB, Grundy SM (2003) Effects of adding fenofibrate (200 mg/day) to simvastatin (10 mg/day) in patients with combined hyperlipidemia and metabolic syndrome. Am J Cardiol 91:956–960

White MF (2002) IRS proteins and the common path to diabetes. Am J Physiol Endocrinol Metab 283:E413–E422

Yazbek N, Bapat A, Kleiman N (2003) Platelet abnormalities in diabetes mellitus.Coron Artery Dis 14:365–371

Part II
The Impact of Diet

HEP (2005) 170:137–163

Physical Activity, Obesity and Cardiovascular Diseases

T.A. Lakka · C. Bouchard (✉)

Pennington Biomedical Research Center, 6400 Perkins Road, Baton Rouge LA, 70808-4124, USA
bouchac@pbrc.edu

Abstract Sedentary lifestyle and overweight are major public health, clinical, and economical problems in modern societies. The worldwide epidemic of excess weight is due to imbalance between physical activity and dietary energy intake. Sedentary lifestyle, unhealthy diet, and consequent overweight and obesity markedly increase the risk of cardiovascular diseases.

Regular physical activity 45–60 min per day prevents unhealthy weight gain and obesity, whereas sedentary behaviors such as watching television promote them. Regular exercise can markedly reduce body weight and fat mass without dietary caloric restriction in overweight individuals. An increase in total energy expenditure appears to be the most important determinant of successful exercise-induced weight loss. The best long-term results may be achieved when physical activity produces an energy expenditure of at least 2,500 kcal/week. Yet, the optimal approach in weight reduction programs appears to be a combination of regular physical activity and caloric restriction. A minimum of 60 min, but most likely 80–90 min of moderate-intensity physical activity per day may be needed to avoid or limit weight regain in formerly overweight or obese individuals. Regular moderate intensity physical activity, a healthy diet, and avoiding unhealthy weight gain are effective and safe ways to prevent and treat cardiovascular diseases and to reduce premature mortality in all population groups. Although the efforts to promote cardiovascular health concern the whole population, particular attention should be paid to individuals who are physically inactive, have unhealthy diets or are prone to weight gain. They have the highest risk for worsening of the cardiovascular risk factor profile and for cardiovascular disease. To combat the epidemic of overweight and to improve cardiovascular health at a population level, it is important to develop strategies to increase habitual physical activity and to prevent overweight and obesity in collaboration with communities, families, schools, work sites, health care professionals, media and policymakers.

Keywords Physical activity · Overweight · Obesity · Cardiovascular disease ·
Health promotion

1
Introduction

Sedentary lifestyle and overweight are major public health and clinical problems. They are the most prevalent risk factors for common chronic diseases and premature mortality. More than one-half of the adults in the USA do not engage in physical activity at the level currently recommended for health promotion, e.g., 30 min or more of moderate intensity physical activity on most days of the week (Pate et al. 1995; Centers for Disease Control and Prevention 2003b; Thompson et al. 2003). What is even more alarming is that almost two-thirds of children 9–13 years of age do not participate in any organized physical activity during their leisure time and almost one in four children of this age do not engage in any leisure time physical activity (Centers for Disease Control and Prevention 2003a).

Two in three adults in the USA are currently classified as overweight [body mass index (BMI) 25.0–29.9 kg/m^2) or obese (BMI $\geq$30 kg/m^2), compared with fewer than one in four adults in the early 1960s (Kuczmarski et al. 1994; Flegal et al. 2002). This trend is similar for all age, gender and race groups (Flegal et al. 2002). More than one-half of the adults in most European and other developed countries are overweight or obese, and the prevalence of obesity is increasing rapidly in these countries (World Health Organization 2000). Overweight in childhood and adolescence has more than doubled over the past decades in the USA (Ogden et al. 2002), some European countries, and Japan (World Health Organization 2000). Adulthood and childhood overweight is increasing in many developing countries as well (World Health Organization 2000). The worldwide scenario is that the increase in childhood and adolescence over-weight will translate later into an even greater prevalence of adulthood obesity and complications such as cardiovascular diseases.

The worldwide epidemic of excess weight is a consequence of positive energy balance due to both reduced energy expenditure and increased energy intake. Urbanization and automation in recent decades has resulted in a progressive reduction in the level of habitual physical activity associated with work and chores of daily living as well as a growing amount of time spent in very sedentary activities such as watching TV, working on the computer and playing video games (World Health Organization 2000; Crespo et al. 2001). The almost unlimited availability of highly palatable, energy-dense foods and drinks and increased portion sizes are undoubtedly contributing to the current epidemic of overweight and obesity (Prentice and Jebb 1995; Grundy 1998; World Health Organization 2000; Popkin and Nielsen 2003).

The epidemic of sedentary lifestyle and overweight has serious public health and economical consequences. Physical inactivity increases the incidence of coronary heart disease, stroke, hypertension, obesity, type 2 diabetes, osteo-porosis, cancers of the breast and colon, depression and premature mortality (Pate et al. 1995; Thompson et al. 2003). Overweight and obesity increase the risk of coronary heart disease, hypertension, type 2 diabetes, dyslipidemia, gout, osteoarthritis, gallbladder disease, cancers of the breast, endometrium and colon, psychosocial problems, sleep apnea, disability and premature mor-tality (National Institutes of Health 1998; World Health Organization 2000; Fontaine et al. 2003). Physical inactivity, unhealthy diet and obesity have been estimated to account for about 14% of all deaths in the USA (McGinnis and Foege 1993; Allison et al. 1999). If current trends continue, these modifiable risk factors will overtake smoking as the primary preventable cause of death (Allison et al. 1999). According to conservative estimates, physical inactivity accounts for about 4% and obesity for about 7% of direct health care costs in the USA, figures that are comparable to those of smoking (Colditz 2000).

2
Physical Activity and Energy Balance

2.1
Fundamental Principles of Energy Balance

The most important determinants of long-term energy balance and body fat stores are energy intake and energy expenditure (Fig. 1) (Bouchard 2004). Total energy intake refers to all calories consumed as food and drink that can

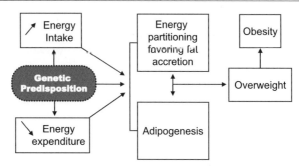

Fig. 1 Diagram of the determinants of long-term positive energy balance and fat deposition. The most important determinants of long-term energy balance and fat deposition are energy intake and energy expenditure. Nutrient partitioning is emerging as another important determinant of long-term energy balance. The amount of adipose tissue may also increase due to increased adipogenesis. (Adapted from Bouchard 2004)

be metabolized inside the body. Fat provides the most energy per unit weight (9 kcal/g), and carbohydrate (4 kcal/g) and protein (4 kcal/g) the least. Soluble fibers undergo bacterial degradation in the large intestine to produce fatty acids that are then absorbed and used as energy (1.5 kcal/g). Alcohol consumption can significantly contribute to energy balance in some individuals (7 kcal/g). In sedentary adults, basal metabolic rate accounts for 60%–70% of total energy expenditure, the thermic effect of food for about 10%, and physical activity for the remaining 20%–30%. Positive energy balance occurs when energy intake is greater than energy expenditure and promotes the storage of energy as fat (Fig. 1). Negative energy balance occurs when energy expenditure is larger than energy intake and results in the utilization of energy stores (Fig. 1). Under normal circumstances, energy balance oscillates from day to day, but the human body keeps energy stores and weight stable through multiple physiological regulatory mechanisms. Overweight and obesity develop only when positive energy balance prevails for a considerable period of time (Fig. 1).

In addition to energy intake and energy expenditure, nutrient partitioning is emerging as another important determinant of long-term energy balance (Fig. 1) (Bouchard 2004). Under positive energy balance conditions, individuals who are more likely to gain weight will partition more energy for storage in adipose tissue, which results in adipocyte hypertrophy, while those who are less likely to gain weight tend to partition relatively more for fat oxidation by skeletal muscle and other tissues (Ravussin and Smith 2002). The amount of adipose tissue may also increase due to increased adipogenesis (Fig. 1) (Bouchard 2004), which results from a complex interplay between proliferation and differentiation of preadipocytes. Mature adipocytes regulate energy balance by behaving as an endocrine and autocrine organ (Gregoire 2001). Positive energy balance may also result in storage of fat in nonadipose tissues (Ravussin and Smith 2002).

2.2
Physical Activity and Total Energy Expenditure

Regular physical activity is a major determinant of total energy expenditure. Physical activity accounts for 20%–30% of total daily energy expenditure in sedentary individuals, but it may represent up to 50% of all energy expended in persons who engage in heavy manual work or demanding exercise training (Livingstone et al. 1991). Physical activity accounts for most of the variation in total energy expenditure within and between individuals (Ravussin et al. 1986). The contribution of physical activity to total energy expenditure depends on the amount and intensity of physical activity, but also many other factors such as body mass (Ravussin et al. 1986; Livingstone et al. 1991). Total physical activity can be divided into (1) spontaneous activity such as movement of arms, legs and head, taking small steps, fidgeting, and even mastication, (2) work-related activities such as office work, (3) the activities of daily living such as climbing stairs, walking a few blocks instead of taking a car or bus, walking and cycling to and from work, household work, and yard work and (4) conditioning exercise such as walking, running, cycling, skiing, swimming, dancing, ball games, aerobics, and resistance training. Spontaneous activity can substantially increase energy cost in some individuals. In modern societies, the contribution of work-related activities to total energy expenditure is much smaller than it used to be. The activities of daily living account for most of the energy cost of physical activity in individuals who do not engage in regular exercise and who represent the majority of the populations in developed countries. In physically active individuals, however, purposeful conditioning exercise is the most important determinant of the energy expenditure of physical activity.

2.3
Physical Activity and Substrate Balance

Regular physical activity increases the capacity of the body to use lipid substrates rather than carbohydrates as a source of energy during low and moderate intensity exercise, especially when maintained over a long period of time (Hurley et al. 1986). A 20-week exercise-training program resulted in a 20% increase in fat oxidation in previously unfit individuals (Hurley et al. 1986). Regular physical activity also increased fat oxidation during the shift to a high-fat diet (Smith et al. 2000). These findings suggest that physically active individuals consume rather than store excess fat and tolerate high-fat diets better without gaining weight than sedentary persons. These observations may also partly explain why regular physical activity prevents overweight.

2.4
Physical Activity and Food Intake and Preferences

It is often said that a bout of moderate-intensity exercise stimulates appetite and leads to an increased food intake that exceeds the energy cost of the preceding activities. There is, however, little scientific evidence for this assertion. If a compensatory increase in energy intake occurs, it tends to be accurately matched to energy expenditure so that long-term energy balance is maintained (Saris 1996). Acute vigorous exercise, and possibly low-intensity exercise of long duration, can suppress appetite over the short term, but this results in a delay in the onset of eating rather than a reduction in the amount of food consumed (King et al. 1994). Although physical activity has been associated with an increased intake of carbohydrate-rich foods in some studies (Westerterp et al. 1996), whether exercise affects food and macronutrient preferences remains uncertain. However, some studies suggest that physical inactivity is associated with an increased consumption of unhealthy foods and an increased fat intake (World Health Organization 2000).

3
Physical Activity, Overweight and Obesity

3.1
Physical Activity in the Prevention of Weight Gain

Cross-sectional studies have shown that physically active adults and children are leaner and have less abdominal fat than sedentary individuals (Andersen et al. 1998; Martinez-Gonzalez et al. 1999). The difference in body adiposity between physically active and inactive individuals appears to persist from early adulthood to old age (Voorrips et al. 1992). Total energy expenditure has been inversely associated with body weight and weight gain in adults and children (Ravussin et al. 1988; Schulz and Schoeller 1994; Davies et al. 1995). Prospective epidemiological studies have observed that regular physical activity prevents unhealthy weight gain and obesity, whereas sedentary behaviors such as watching television, working at the computer or playing video games promote them (Coakley et al. 1998; Erlichman et al. 2002; Hu et al. 2003; Saris et al. 2003) (Fig. 2). It has been estimated that about 30% of new cases of obesity could be prevented by adopting a relatively active lifestyle, including more than 30 min of brisk walking and fewer than 10 h of TV watching per week (Hu et al. 2003). There is some evidence that sedentary lifestyle is a better population-level predictor of weight gain than increased caloric or fat intake (Prentice and Jebb 1995). Regular physical activity, as estimated by cardiorespiratory fitness, may play a stronger role in attenuating age-related weight gain than in promoting long-term weight loss (DiPietro et al. 1998).

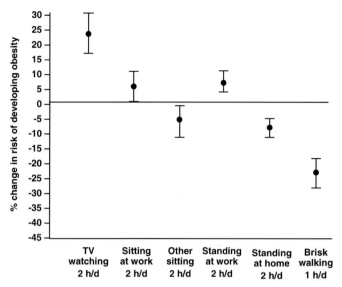

Fig. 2 Changes in the risk of developing obesity among normal-weight women associated with sedentary behaviors and regular physical activity. Regular exercise prevents unhealthy weight gain and obesity, whereas sedentary behaviors such as watching television promote them. (Adapted from Hu et al. 2003)

Epidemiological studies suggest that moderate intensity physical activity 45–60 min per day is needed to prevent unhealthy weight gain and obesity (Saris et al. 2003). Brisk walking is effective in the prevention of obesity, but low-intensity activities of daily living also appear to be beneficial (Hu et al. 2003). Vigorous exercise may provide some additional benefit beyond low-intensity and moderate-intensity physical activity in the prevention of weight gain (Coakley et al. 1998). There are no randomized controlled trials that specifically address the questions of whether regular physical activity prevents long-term weight gain and fat accumulation and what types, amount and intensity of physical activity are needed to achieve such long-term benefits. Although it is likely that physical activity is important to maintain healthy body weight and to prevent harmful weight gain, long-term energy balance will be easier to achieve if regular physical activity and a healthy diet are combined.

3.2
Physical Activity in the Promotion of Weight Loss

A number of randomized controlled trials have shown that regular physical activity can markedly reduce body weight and fat mass without dietary caloric restriction in overweight men and women (Ballor and Keesey 1991; Garrow and Summerbell 1995; Andersen et al. 1999; Ross et al. 2000; Ross and Janssen 2001; Donnelly et al. 2003; Irwin et al. 2003; Jakicic et al. 2003; Jeffery et al. 2003; Saris et al. 2003; Slentz et al. 2004). The effective exercise training programs have typically lasted for 3–12 months and have included three to five exercise sessions per week of 30–60 min each, and the total duration of physical activity has varied between 3 and 5 h per week (Ballor and Keesey 1991; Garrow and Summerbell 1995; Andersen et al. 1999; Ross et al. 2000; Ross and Janssen 2001; Donnelly et al. 2003; Irwin et al. 2003; Jakicic et al. 2003; Jeffery et al. 2003; Saris et al. 2003; Slentz et al. 2004). Regular physical activity reduces body weight and adiposity already within 3 months (Ross et al. 2000), and further reduction can be seen at least until 9 months (Kirk et al. 2003). An increase in total energy expenditure appears to be the most important determinant of successful exercise-induced weight loss. The larger the reduction in body weight and fat, the greater has been the amount of physical activity (Ross et al. 2000; Irwin et al. 2003; Jakicic et al. 2003; Jeffery et al. 2003; Slentz et al. 2004), which suggests that regular exercise decreases body adiposity in a dose-dependent manner. The best long-term results may be achieved when physical activity produces an energy expenditure of at least 2500 kcal/wk (Jeffery et al. 2003). Short-term studies have generally resulted in a greater weight and fat loss than long-term studies. The most likely explanation for this apparent discrepancy is that it is difficult to maintain high levels of energy expenditure for a long period of time (Ross and Janssen 2001; Saris et al. 2003). Indeed, adherence to the exercise-training program is a critical factor for a successful long-term weight loss. Adherence may be particularly problematic among obese subjects (Fogelholm and Kukkonen-Harjula 2000).

Most randomized controlled trials have included mainly aerobic exercise such as running, walking and cycling (Ballor and Keesey 1991; Garrow and Summerbell 1995; Andersen et al. 1999; Ross et al. 2000; Ross and Janssen 2001; Donnelly et al. 2003; Irwin et al. 2003; Jakicic et al. 2003; Jeffery et al. 2003; Saris et al. 2003; Slentz et al. 2004). However, there is some evidence that resistance training also reduces body fat (Santa-Clara et al. 2003; Schmitz et al. 2003) and that the effect is independent of other physical activities and changes in energy intake (Schmitz et al. 2003). A combination of aerobic and weight training may be more effective in producing changes in body composition than aerobic exercise alone (Santa-Clara et al. 2003). Another advantage of resistance training is that it may increase skeletal muscle mass and perhaps resting metabolic rate if the program is sufficiently intense and demanding. Resistance exercise may also improve insulin sensitivity, an important benefit for overweight and obese individuals (Ballor and Keesey 1991; Garrow and Summerbell 1995; Cuff et al. 2003). Limited evidence suggests that lifestyle activity can be effective in reducing body weight (Andersen et al. 1999). The effects of regular physical activity on cardiovascular risk factors such as insulin resistance, glucose tolerance, type 2 diabetes, dyslipidemia and elevated blood pressure are stronger if asso-

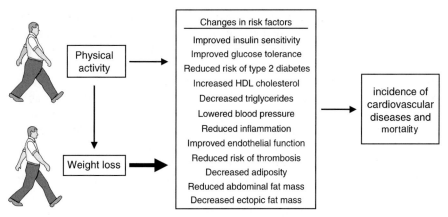

Fig. 3 Effects of regular physical activity on body weight, cardiovascular risk factors, the incidence of cardiovascular disease, and cardiovascular and total mortality. The effects of regular exercise on cardiovascular risk factors are partly mediated by weight loss and are stronger if associated with weight reduction

ciated with weight reduction (Thompson et al. 2003) (Fig. 3). Yet, the optimal approach in weight reduction programs appears to be a combination of regular physical activity and caloric restriction (Ballor and Keesey 1991; Garrow and Summerbell 1995; Ross et al. 2000; Ross and Janssen 2001; Jeffery et al. 2002; Irwin et al. 2003; Jakicic et al. 2003; Saris et al. 2003; Slentz et al. 2004). It not only results in effective weight reduction but also has the strongest effect on cardiovascular risk factors (Thompson et al. 2003). Including physical activity, especially resistance training, in weight reduction programs also helps in maintaining skeletal muscle mass (Ballor and Keesey 1991; Garrow and Summerbell 1995).

3.3
Physical Activity in the Prevention of Weight Regain After Weight Loss

Although several approaches, including dietary energy restriction and drugs, are available for weight reduction, weight maintenance after successful weight loss remains difficult. A large proportion of individuals will eventually regain weight up to their initial body weight (Jeffery et al. 2002), and new approaches to prevent weight regain are needed. Ninety percent of individuals who have been able to maintain weight after a significant weight loss report that regular physical activity is a critical component of their success (Klem et al. 1997). Randomized controlled trials have shown a modest and inconsistent effect of regular physical activity on weight maintenance (Fogelholm and Kukkonen-Harjula 2000). One explanation for the mild effect may be that the amount of physical activity has been inadequate to maintain reduced body weight in overweight and obese individuals who are prone to weight regain. Indeed, exercise programs have typically consisted of 1.5–3.0 h per week of walking or cycling, which corresponds to an energy expenditure of 500–1000 kcal per week. It is likely that much larger amounts of physical activity are required to prevent weight gain after weight loss. People who have succeeded in avoiding weight regain have reported a mean exercise energy expenditure of about 2700 kcal per week, which equals about 4 miles (6.44 km) of walking per day (Klem et al. 1997). Recent reviews have concluded that a minimum of 60 min, but most likely 80–90 min of moderate-intensity physical activity per day, corresponding to about 2000–2500 kcal per week, may be needed to avoid or limit weight regain in formerly overweight or obese individuals (Fogelholm and Kukkonen-Harjula 2000; Saris et al. 2003).

3.4
Physical Activity and Fat Distribution

There is some evidence that abdominal obesity is an independent risk factor for cardiovascular diseases and may provide additional information beyond overall adiposity (Larsson et al. 1984; Welin et al. 1987; Casassus et al. 1992; Folsom et al. 1993; Rexrode et al. 1998; Fujimoto et al. 1999; Folsom et al. 2000; Rexrode et al. 2001; Lakka et al. 2002b). Regular physical activity reduces abdominal visceral and subcutaneous fat independent of changes in dietary energy intake in healthy, overweight and obese men and women (Mourier et al. 1997; Wilmore et al. 1999; Ross et al. 2000; Donnelly et al. 2003; Irwin et al. 2003). However, regular exercise does not appear to preferentially reduce total abdominal and visceral fat beyond the changes in total adiposity (Ross et al. 2000; Irwin et al. 2003; Slentz et al. 2004). Although most studies have not been able to demonstrate a dose–response relationship between regular physical activity and reduction in abdominal adiposity (Ross and Janssen 2001), a recent study in overweight postmenopausal women showed that larger amounts of regular exercise resulted in a greater reduction in abdominal fat (Irwin et al. 2003).

As the ability of peripheral adipocytes to store fat is exceeded, the fat cells become insulin resistant, which results in increased lipolysis, release of fatty acids into the blood stream, and decreased uptake of fatty acids. This is thought to favor storage of lipids in skeletal muscle, liver, pancreas, heart, and possibly other tissues. This spillover of lipids in non-adipose tissues may contribute to the pathogenesis of lipotoxic diseases such as type 2 diabetes (Ravussin and Smith 2002; Unger 2002). There is some evidence that regular physical activity may reduce the amount of intramyocellular lipids (van Loon et al. 2003), but the issue is not entirely clear (Schrauwen-Hinderling et al. 2003). Limited evidence in rats suggests that exercise may also prevent fat accumulation in the liver (Gauthier et al. 2003).

4
Physical Activity and Cardiovascular Diseases

4.1
Physical Activity and Cardiovascular Mortality

Sedentary lifestyle is currently recognized as one of the major risk factors for atherosclerotic cardiovascular diseases, the most important cause of death in industrialized countries (Pate et al. 1995; Thompson et al. 2003). Prospective epidemiological studies have consistently shown that regular physical activity and cardiorespiratory fitness prevent cardiovascular diseases and premature cardiovascular mortality in men and women (Paffenbarger et al. 1986; Blair et al. 1989; Sandvik et al. 1993; Blair et al. 1996; Laukkanen et al. 2001) (Fig. 4). Moreover, an increase in physical activity and an improvement in cardiorespiratory fitness have been associated with reduced cardiovascular and total mortality (Paffenbarger et al. 1993; Blair et al. 1995; Erikssen et al. 1998; Wannamethee et al. 1998). The association between physical activity and cardiovascular mortality is graded with the risk being the lowest in the most active individuals and independent of conventional cardiovascular risk factors. The protective effect is strong, with the most physically active individuals generally having about half the cardiovascular mortality of the least active people. Exercise or sports in young adulthood do not prevent premature cardiovascular mortality in later years, which emphasizes the importance of lifelong engagement in physical activity (Paffenbarger et al. 1984).

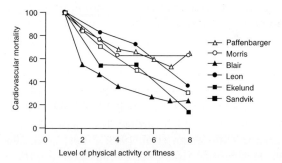

Fig. 4 Levels of physical activity (Paffenbarger, Morris, Leon) or cardiorespiratory fitness (Blair, Ekelund, Sandvik) and cardiovascular mortality. Values for more active or fit individuals are expressed as the ratio of the event rate for more active or fit divided by the event rate for least active or fit. (Adapted from Haskell 1994)

4.2
Physical Activity and Coronary Heart Disease

The epidemiological evidence on the role of regular physical activity in the prevention of atherosclerotic cardiovascular diseases is strongest for coronary heart disease (Thompson et al. 2003). Regular physical activity, an increase in the level of physical activity, and cardiorespiratory fitness prevent coronary heart disease in men and women (Lakka et al. 1994; Wannamethee et al. 1998; Manson et al. 1999; Lee et al. 2000; Sesso et al. 2000; Tanasescu et al. 2002). Moderate-intensity aerobic exercise such as walking may be as effective as more vigorous exercise in the prevention of coronary heart disease (Wannamethee et al. 1998; Manson et al. 1999). However, some studies suggest that vigorous exercise confers further protection and that the risk decreases in a dose-dependent fashion with increasing intensity of regular exercise (Tanasescu et al. 2002). Resistance training may also reduce the risk of coronary heart disease (Tanasescu et al. 2002). The accumulation of shorter daily sessions of physical activity may be as effective as longer, continuous exercise bouts (Lee et al. 2000).

Regular physical activity is also beneficial in the treatment of patients with coronary heart disease. Meta-analyses have shown that comprehensive exercise-based cardiac rehabilitation reduces total and cardiovascular mortality after myocardial infarction (Oldridge et al. 1988; O'Connor et al. 1989; Jolliffe et al. 2001). Cardiac rehabilitation programs consisting of initially supervised exercise training of 2–6 months followed by unsupervised physical activity reduced total mortality by 27% and cardiac mortality by 31% in patients who had sustained a myocardial infarction, had angina pectoris or coronary artery disease identified by angiography, or had undergone coronary artery bypass grafting or percutaneous transluminal coronary angioplasty (Jolliffe et al. 2001). However, physical activity did not reduce the risk of recurrent nonfatal myocardial infarction (Jolliffe et al. 2001).

Strenuous exercise can trigger myocardial infarction and sudden cardiac death, particularly in habitually sedentary people (Mittleman et al. 1993; Albert et al. 2000), but the absolute risk of myocardial infarction or sudden cardiac death during any particular episode of vigorous exertion is extremely low (Mittleman et al. 1993; Albert et al. 2000). Moreover, it is important to recognize that regular physical activity effectively reduces the occurrence of myocardial infarction and sudden cardiac death associated with an episode of vigorous exertion (Mittleman et al. 1993; Albert et al. 2000). Due to the potential, albeit low, cardiac risks of strenuous exercise, the current recommendations of regular moderate-intensity physical activity appear to be well justified (Pate et al. 1995; Thompson et al. 2003).

4.3
Physical Activity and Stroke

There is accumulating evidence that regular physical activity and cardiorespiratory fitness prevent ischemic stroke in men and women (Wannamethee and Shaper 1992; Lindenstrom et al. 1993; Kiely et al. 1994; Gillum et al. 1996; Sacco et al. 1998; Hu et al. 2000; Kurl et al. 2003). However, the associations are slightly weaker and less consistent than for coronary heart disease (Goldstein et al. 2001; Thompson et al. 2003). Regular exercise has been observed to protect against ischemic stroke in different ethnic groups, including Whites, Blacks and Hispanics (Sacco et al. 1998). There is some evidence that regular physical activity reduces the incidence of stroke in a dose–response manner (Wannamethee and Shaper 1992; Sacco et al. 1998; Hu et al. 2000). Whereas some studies have found that moderate-intensity physical activity such as walking is as effective as vigorous exercise in the prevention of ischemic stroke (Wannamethee and Shaper 1992), other studies suggest that more vigorous exercise confers some further protection (Sacco et al. 1998; Hu et al. 2000). The American Heart Association has recently emphasized the importance of regular physical activity for the prevention of ischemic stroke (Goldstein et al. 2001).

4.4
Physical Activity and Peripheral Artery Disease

Regular physical activity is effective in the treatment of claudication, the primary symptom of peripheral artery disease (Gardner and Poehlman 1995; Leng et al. 2000; Stewart et al. 2002). A meta-analysis of randomized controlled trials concluded that regular exercise improves maximal walking time by an average of 150 min (Leng et al. 2000), which suggests that the effect of exercise exceeds that attained with medication (Stewart et al. 2002). Clinical benefits have been observed as early as 4 weeks after the initiation of exercise and may continue to accrue after 6 months of participation (Stewart et al. 2002). Improvement in walking ability due to regular exercise results in improvement in routine daily activities (Stewart et al. 2002). Better functional capacity in turn allows for an increase in the level of physical activity, which likely improves cardiovascular risk factors and protects against future cardiovascular events in patients with peripheral artery disease (Stewart et al. 2002).

4.5
Physical Activity and Cardiovascular Risk Factors

Regular physical activity both prevents and helps in the treatment of many risk factors for atherosclerotic cardiovascular diseases (Fig. 3). Regular exercise reduces body adiposity, increases insulin sensitivity, improves glucose tolerance, reduces postprandial hyperglycemia, decreases plasma triglyceride concentrations and increases plasma high-density lipoprotein (HDL) cholesterol concentrations, decreases blood pressure, favorably affects hemostatic factors (Thompson et al. 2003), improves endothelial function (Hambrecht et al. 2000) and reduces the risk of developing metabolic syndrome (Laaksonen et al. 2002) and type 2 diabetes (Helmrich et al. 1991). The effects of regular physical activity on cardiovascular risk factors such as insulin resistance, glucose tolerance, type 2 diabetes, dyslipidemia and elevated blood pressure are stronger if associated with weight reduction (Thompson et al. 2003) (Fig. 3). Another advantage of including regular exercise in weight reduction programs is that physical activity can decrease plasma low-density lipoprotein (LDL) cholesterol and limit the reduction in plasma HDL cholesterol that often occurs with a decrease in dietary saturated fat (Stefanick et al. 1998). The favorable effects of exercise on insulin sensitivity and the lipid profile tend to dissipate a few days after the last exercise session (Thompson et al. 2001), which provides support for the recommendation that adults should participate in moderate-intensity physical activity on most days of the week (Pate et al. 1995; Thompson et al. 2003).

Most effects of regular physical activity on cardiovascular risk factors are of a lesser magnitude than those achieved by pharmacological therapies, although the impact can be significantly magnified by favorable changes in diet and weight loss (Thompson et al. 2003). For example, lifestyle intervention, including regular exercise, dietary modification and weight reduction, reduced the incidence of type 2 diabetes by 58% in persons with impaired glucose tolerance and overweight (Tuomilehto et al. 2001; Knowler et al. 2002). In fact, lifestyle intervention was found to be more effective than metformin treatment to prevent type 2 diabetes (Knowler et al. 2002). It is important to recognize that regular physical activity favorably affects many cardiovascular risk factors, and the summation of these effects results in a marked reduction in the incidence of atherosclerotic cardiovascular diseases and premature mortality (Paffenbarger et al. 1986; Blair et al. 1989; Sandvik et al. 1993; Lakka et al. 1994; Blair et al. 1996; Manson et al. 1999; Sesso et al. 2000; Lakka et al. 2001b; Tanasescu et al. 2002). There are also large individual differences in the magnitude of the effect of regular exercise on cardiovascular risk factors, and this variation in responses is influenced by age, sex, health status, body size and genetic factors (Bouchard and Rankinen 2001; Wilmore 2001).

5
Overweight, Obesity and Cardiovascular Diseases

5.1
Overweight, Obesity and Cardiovascular Mortality

Overweight and obesity are currently recognized as important risk factors for atherosclerotic cardiovascular diseases and premature mortality (National Institutes of Health 1998; National Task Force on the Prevention and Treatment of Obesity 2000; World Health Organization 2000). Prospective epidemiological studies have shown that cardiovascular and total mortality increase throughout the range of overweight and obesity (Fig. 5). Overweight and obesity predict cardiovascular mortality in both men (Lee et al. 1993; Stevens et al. 1998; Calle et al. 1999) and women (Manson et al. 1995; Stevens et al. 1998; Calle et al.

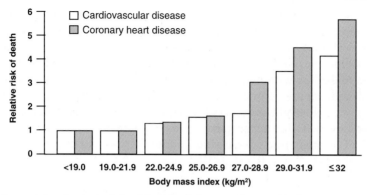

Fig. 5 Overweight, obesity and the risk of death from cardiovascular diseases and coronary heart disease. Cardiovascular and coronary mortality increase throughout the range of overweight and obesity. (Adapted from Manson et al. 1995)

1999). Obesity also markedly decreases life expectancy, particularly in young adults (Fontaine et al. 2003). The associations of overweight and obesity with cardiovascular and overall mortality may even be stronger in healthy non-smoking individuals (Manson et al. 1995; Calle et al. 1999). There is some evidence that the risk of cardiovascular diseases and cardiovascular mortality starts to increase at BMI levels as low as 22–23 kg/m^2 (Manson et al. 1990, 1995; Lee et al. 1993; Willett et al. 1995; Field et al. 2001), which suggests that the optimal BMI may be in the middle of the range of values currently considered as normal weight. Overweight and obesity increase cardiovascular and total mortality in all adult age groups, although the relative risk appears to be higher among younger individuals (Stevens et al. 1998; Calle et al. 1999). Because mortality rises dramatically with age, however, the absolute excess risk associated with overweight and obesity increases rather than decreases with age. The association of overweight and obesity with cardiovascular and total mortality was observed in both Whites and Blacks although the relative risk was greater for Whites (Calle et al. 1999).

5.2
Overweight, Obesity and Coronary Heart Disease

Prospective epidemiological studies have consistently shown that overweight and obesity are associated with an increase risk of coronary heart disease (Fig. 5). Overweight and obesity predict coronary heart disease in both men and women (Manson et al. 1990; Rimm et al. 1995; Willett et al. 1995; Rexrode et al. 1998, 2001; Folsom et al. 2000; Field et al. 2001). Abdominal obesity has been found to be a stronger risk factor for coronary heart disease than overall obesity in men and women (Larsson et al. 1984; Casassus et al. 1992; Folsom et al. 1993, 2000; Rexrode et al. 1998; Fujimoto et al. 1999; Lakka et al.

2002b) and may provide additional information beyond overall obesity in the prediction of coronary heart disease (Larsson et al. 1984; Casassus et al. 1992; Folsom et al. 1993, 2000, Rexrode et al 1998; Fujimoto et al. 1999; Lakka et al. 2002b). While the relative risk of coronary heart disease associated with obesity appears to decline with increasing age, abdominal obesity remains a strong and independent predictor of cardiovascular diseases in men of all age groups, including the elderly (Larsson et al. 1984; Rimm et al. 1995; Baik et al. 2000). However, some studies suggest that abdominal obesity is not associated with the risk of coronary heart disease independent of BMI and does not add to the predictive value of overall obesity (Rexrode et al. 2001).

5.3
Overweight, Obesity and Stroke

Prospective epidemiological studies have reported that overweight and obesity are associated with an increased risk of stroke in men and women (Walker et al. 1996; Rexrode et al. 1997; Kurth et al. 2002; Suk et al. 2003). Abdominal obesity has been more closely associated with the risk of stroke than has overall obesity, and the increased risk appears to be independent of overall obesity (Larsson et al. 1984; Welin et al. 1987; Walker et al. 1996; Suk et al. 2003). Abdominal obesity, but not overall obesity, was also associated with accelerated progression of carotid atherosclerosis in men (Lakka et al. 2001a). The association between abdominal obesity and the risk of ischemic stroke was evident in all ethnic groups, including Whites, Blacks and Hispanics (Suk et al. 2003). Obesity has been associated with an increased incidence of ischemic stroke (Rexrode et al. 1997; Suk et al. 2003), whereas the association with hemorrhagic stroke remains controversial (Rexrode et al. 1997; Kurth et al. 2002).

5.4
Overweight, Obesity and Peripheral Artery Disease

Evidence on the associations of overweight and obesity with peripheral artery disease is quite limited and is based only on cross-sectional data. One study observed an association between obesity and an increased prevalence of peripheral artery disease in elderly men (Mendelson et al. 1998). Another study found that abdominal obesity, but not overall obesity, was associated with the prevalence of peripheral artery disease in elderly men (Planas et al. 2001).

5.5
Overweight, Obesity and Cardiovascular Risk Factors

Overweight and obesity increase the risk of cardiovascular diseases partly through their effects on cardiovascular risk factors (Fig. 6). Overweight and obesity are associated with insulin resistance, impaired glucose tolerance,

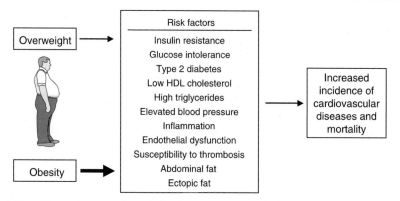

Fig. 6 The effects of overweight and obesity on cardiovascular risk factors, the incidence of cardiovascular diseases, and cardiovascular and total mortality. The effects of obesity on cardiovascular risk factors are stronger than those of overweight. The increased incidence of cardiovascular diseases and mortality associated with overweight and obesity are mediated by the effects on cardiovascular risk factors

increased incidence of type 2 diabetes, elevated blood pressure, hypertriglyceridemia, increased plasma LDL cholesterol, decreased plasma HDL cholesterol (Colditz et al. 1990; Ashton et al. 2001), as well as elevated plasma C-reactive protein, fibrinogen, plasminogen activator inhibitor-1 and other inflammatory and hemostatic factors (Visser et al. 1999; Duncan et al. 2000). Moreover, excess adiposity is a major determinant of the metabolic syndrome (Haffner and Taegtmeyer 2003), which has emerged as an important general risk factor for cardiovascular diseases (Lakka et al. 2002a). The cardiovascular risk factor profile worsens in a dose–response fashion as the BMI increases from 20 kg/m^2 to over 30 kg/m^2 (Willett et al. 1999; Ashton et al. 2001). The increase in the incidence of some risk factors such as type 2 diabetes is steep even below a BMI of 25 kg/m^2 (Willett et al. 1999). Abdominal obesity in particular is associated with unfavorable levels of risk factor, including insulin resistance, impaired glucose tolerance, elevated blood pressure, increased plasma triglycerides, LDL cholesterol and small dense LDL, and decreased plasma HDL cholesterol (Despres et al. 2001). However, the results of the association between abdominal fat and cardiovascular risk factor profile in normal weight individuals are controversial, possibly due to differences in sex and ethnic groups (Tanaka et al. 2003).

5.6
Weight Gain and Cardiovascular Diseases

Most people are not overweight when growth ends at around 20 years of age, and most excess body fat accrues in subsequent decades (Willett et al. 1999). Weight gain among men and women during early and middle adulthood has been associated with a significantly increased risk of cardiovascular diseases in a dose–response fashion (Colditz et al. 1995; Rimm et al. 1995; Willett et al. 1995, 1999; Huang et al. 1998). Men and women with even a modest weight gain of 5–10 kg during early and middle adulthood are at increased risk of coronary heart disease, type 2 diabetes and hypertension as compared with individuals who maintain their weight within 2 kg of their weight at 18–20 years of age (Colditz et al. 1995; Rimm et al. 1995; Willett et al. 1995, 1999; Huang et al. 1998). Also non-smoking women who experienced a weight gain of more than 10 kg since the age of 18 years had higher premature cardiovascular mortality than those who maintained their weight within 4 kg of their weight (Manson et al. 1995). The increased risk of coronary heart disease during adulthood associated with weight gain is evident at any level of BMI at the age of 18 years (Fig. 7).

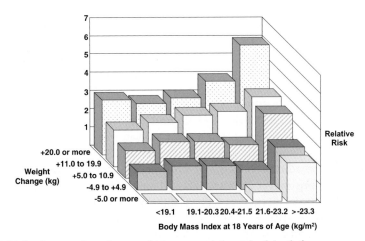

Fig. 7 Weight changes since the age of 18 years and the risk of death from coronary heart disease in women. The increased risk of coronary heart disease during adulthood associated with weight gain is evident at any level of BMI at the age of 18 years. (Adapted from Willett et al. 1995)

5.7
Weight Loss and Cardiovascular Diseases

Epidemiological prospective studies and clinical trials have shown that even modest weight reductions of 5%–10%, due to either an increase in physical activity or a decrease in energy intake or both, can substantially lower blood pressure (Lee et al. 2001); improve blood lipid profile (Lee et al. 2001), insulin sensitivity (Lee et al. 2001) and glucose tolerance (Lee et al. 2001); and decrease the incidence of type 2 diabetes (Colditz et al. 1995) and hypertension (Huang et al. 1998) among overweight individuals. In prospective epidemiological studies, intentional weight loss has been associated with a reduction or no change in cardiovascular and total mortality (Williamson et al. 1995; French et al. 1999), while unintentional weight loss, likely reflecting existing disease, has been associated with increased premature mortality (French et al. 1999). Although clinical trials have not specifically examined the effect of weight reduction on the incidence of clinical cardiovascular disease, weight loss is likely to be important in the prevention and treatment of cardiovascular diseases, because it improves many cardiovascular risk factors (Lee et al. 2001).

5.8
Weight Fluctuation and Cardiovascular Diseases

Information on the association between weight fluctuation and the risk of cardiovascular diseases is limited and inconsistent. Whereas some studies have observed that a large weight variability is associated with an increased risk of cardiovascular and total mortality, especially at the lower end of the body weight distribution (Blair et al. 1993), other studies suggest that weight variability does not predict mortality independent of weight loss or weight gain (Dyer et al. 2000).

6
Conclusions

Sedentary lifestyle and overweight are major public health, clinical, and economical problems in modern societies. The worldwide epidemic of excess weight is due to imbalance between physical activity and dietary energy intake. Sedentary lifestyle, unhealthy diet, and consequent overweight and obesity markedly increase the risk of cardiovascular diseases. Regular moderate-intensity physical activity, a healthy diet, and avoiding unhealthy weight gain are effective and safe ways to prevent and treat cardiovascular diseases and to prevent premature cardiovascular and total mortality in all population groups. Although the efforts to promote cardiovascular health concern the whole population, particular attention should be paid to individuals who are physically inactive, have unhealthy diets or are prone to weight gain. They have the highest risk for worsening of the cardiovascular risk factor profile and for cardiovascular disease. To combat the epidemic of overweight and to improve cardiovascular health at a population level, it is important to develop strategies to increase habitual physical activity and to prevent overweight and obesity in collaboration with communities, families, schools, work sites, health care professionals, media and policymakers.

References

Albert CM, Mittleman MA, Chae CU, Lee IM, Hennekens CH, Manson JE (2000) Triggering of sudden death from cardiac causes by vigorous exertion. N Engl J Med 343:1355–1361

Allison DB, Fontaine KR, Manson JE, Stevens J, VanItallie TB (1999) Annual deaths attributable to obesity in the United States. JAMA 282:1530–1538

Andersen RE, Crespo CJ, Bartlett SJ, Cheskin LJ, Pratt M (1998) Relationship of physical activity and television watching with body weight and level of fatness among children: results from the Third National Health and Nutrition Examination Survey. JAMA 279:938–942

Andersen RE, Wadden TA, Bartlett SJ, Zemel B, Verde TJ, Franckowiak SC (1999) Effects of lifestyle activity vs structured aerobic exercise in obese women: a randomized trial. JAMA 281:335–340

Ashton WD, Nanchahal K, Wood DA (2001) Body mass index and metabolic risk factors for coronary heart disease in women. Eur Heart J 22:46–55

Baik I, Ascherio A, Rimm EB, Giovannucci E, Spiegelman D, Stampfer MJ, Willett WC (2000) Adiposity and mortality in men. Am J Epidemiol 152:264–271

Ballor DL, Keesey RE (1991) A meta-analysis of the factors affecting exercise-induced changes in body mass, fat mass and fat-free mass in males and females. Int J Obes 15:717–726

Blair SN, Kampert JB, Kohl HW, 3rd, Barlow CE, Macera CA, Paffenbarger RS, Jr., Gibbons LW (1996) Influences of cardiorespiratory fitness and other precursors on cardiovascular disease and all-cause mortality in men and women. JAMA 276:205–210

Blair SN, Kohl HW, 3rd, Barlow CE, Paffenbarger RS, Jr., Gibbons LW, Macera CA (1995) Changes in physical fitness and all-cause mortality. A prospective study of healthy and unhealthy men. JAMA 273:1093–1098

Blair SN, Kohl HW, 3rd, Paffenbarger RS, Jr., Clark DG, Cooper KH, Gibbons LW (1989) Physical fitness and all-cause mortality. A prospective study of healthy men and women. JAMA 262:2395–2401

Blair SN, Shaten J, Brownell K, Collins G, Lissner L (1993) Body weight change, all-cause mortality, and cause-specific mortality in the Multiple Risk Factor Intervention Trial. Ann Intern Med 119:749–757

Bouchard C, Perusse, L., Rice, T., Rao, D.C. (2004) Genetics of Human Obesity. In: Bray GA BC (ed) Handbook of Obesity. Marcel Decker Inc., New York

Bouchard C, Rankinen T (2001) Individual differences in response to regular physical activity. Med Sci Sports Exerc 33: S446–S451; discussion S452–S443

Calle EE, Thun MJ, Petrelli JM, Rodriguez C, Heath CW, Jr. (1999) Body-mass index and mortality in a prospective cohort of U.S. adults. N Engl J Med 341:1097–1105

Casassus P, Fontbonne A, Thibult N, Ducimetiere P, Richard JL, Claude JR, Warnet JM, Rosselin G, Eschwege E (1992) Upper-body fat distribution: a hyperinsulinemia-independent predictor of coronary heart disease mortality. The Paris Prospective Study. Arterioscler Thromb 12:1387–1392

Centers for Disease Control and Prevention (2003a) Physical activity levels among children aged 9–13 years—United States, 2002. MMWR Morb Mortal Wkly Rep 52:785–788

Centers for Disease Control and Prevention (2003b) Prevalence of physical activity, including lifestyle activities among adults—United States, 2000–2001. MMWR Morb Mortal Wkly Rep 52:764–769

Coakley EH, Rimm EB, Colditz G, Kawachi I, Willett W (1998) Predictors of weight change in men: results from the Health Professionals Follow-up Study. Int J Obes Relat Metab Disord 22:89–96

Colditz G, Mariani A. (2000) The costs of obesity and sedentarism in the United States. In: Bouchard C (ed) Physical Activity and Obesity. Human Kinetics, Champaign, IL, pp 55–65

Colditz GA, Willett WC, Rotnitzky A, Manson JE (1995) Weight gain as a risk factor for clinical diabetes mellitus in women. Ann Intern Med 122:481–486

Colditz GA, Willett WC, Stampfer MJ, Manson JE, Hennekens CH, Arky RA, Speizer FE (1990) Weight as a risk factor for clinical diabetes in women. Am J Epidemiol 132:501–513

Crespo CJ, Smit E, Troiano RP, Bartlett SJ, Macera CA, Andersen RE (2001) Television watching, energy intake, and obesity in US children: results from the third National Health and Nutrition Examination Survey, 1988–1994. Arch Pediatr Adolesc Med 155:360–365

Cuff DJ, Meneilly GS, Martin A, Ignaszewski A, Tildesley HD, Frohlich JJ (2003) Effective exercise modality to reduce insulin resistance in women with type 2 diabetes. Diabetes Care 26:2977–2982

Davies PS, Gregory J, White A (1995) Physical activity and body fatness in pre-school children. Int J Obes Relat Metab Disord 19:6–10

Despres JP, Lemieux I, Prud'homme D (2001) Treatment of obesity: need to focus on high risk abdominally obese patients. BMJ 322:716–720

DiPietro L, Kohl HW, 3rd, Barlow CE, Blair SN (1998) Improvements in cardiorespiratory fitness attenuate age-related weight gain in healthy men and women: the Aerobics Center Longitudinal Study. Int J Obes Relat Metab Disord 22:55–62

Donnelly JE, Hill JO, Jacobsen DJ, Potteiger J, Sullivan DK, Johnson SL, Heelan K, Hise M, Fennessey PV, Sonko B, Sharp T, Jakicic JM, Blair SN, Tran ZV, Mayo M, Gibson C, Washburn RA (2003) Effects of a 16-month randomized controlled exercise trial on body weight and composition in young, overweight men and women: the Midwest Exercise Trial. Arch Intern Med 163:1343–1350

Duncan BB, Schmidt MI, Chambless LE, Folsom AR, Carpenter M, Heiss G (2000) Fibrinogen, other putative markers of inflammation, and weight gain in middle-aged adults—the ARIC study. Atherosclerosis Risk in Communities. Obes Res 8:279–286

Dyer AR, Stamler J, Greenland P (2000) Associations of weight change and weight variability with cardiovascular and all-cause mortality in the Chicago Western Electric Company Study. Am J Epidemiol 152:324–333

Erikssen G, Liestol K, Bjornholt J, Thaulow E, Sandvik L, Erikssen J (1998) Changes in physical fitness and changes in mortality. Lancet 352:759–762

Erlichman J, Kerbey AL, James WP (2002) Physical activity and its impact on health outcomes. Paper 2: Prevention of unhealthy weight gain and obesity by physical activity: an analysis of the evidence. Obes Rev 3:273–287

Field AE, Coakley EH, Must A, Spadano JL, Laird N, Dietz WH, Rimm E, Colditz GA (2001) Impact of overweight on the risk of developing common chronic diseases during a 10-year period. Arch Intern Med 161:1581–1586

Flegal KM, Carroll MD, Ogden CL, Johnson CL (2002) Prevalence and trends in obesity among US adults, 1999–2000. JAMA 288:1723–1727

Fogelholm M, Kukkonen-Harjula K (2000) Does physical activity prevent weight gain— a systematic review. Obes Rev 1:95–111

Folsom AR, Kaye SA, Sellers TA, Hong CP, Cerhan JR, Potter JD, Prineas RJ (1993) Body fat distribution and 5-year risk of death in older women. JAMA 269:483–487

Folsom AR, Kushi LH, Anderson KE, Mink PJ, Olson JE, Hong CP, Sellers TA, Lazovich D, Prineas RJ (2000) Associations of general and abdominal obesity with multiple health outcomes in older women: the Iowa Women's Health Study. Arch Intern Med 160:2117–2128

Fontaine KR, Redden DT, Wang C, Westfall AO, Allison DB (2003) Years of life lost due to obesity. JAMA 289:187–193

French SA, Folsom AR, Jeffery RW, Williamson DF (1999) Prospective study of intentionality of weight loss and mortality in older women: the Iowa Women's Health Study. Am J Epidemiol 149:504–514

Fujimoto WY, Bergstrom RW, Boyko EJ, Chen KW, Leonetti DL, Newell-Morris L, Shofer JB, Wahl PW (1999) Visceral adiposity and incident coronary heart disease in Japanese-American men. The 10-year follow-up results of the Seattle Japanese-American Community Diabetes Study. Diabetes Care 22:1808–1812

Gardner AW, Poehlman ET (1995) Exercise rehabilitation programs for the treatment of claudication pain. A meta-analysis. JAMA 274:975–980

Garrow JS, Summerbell CD (1995) Meta-analysis: effect of exercise, with or without dieting, on the body composition of overweight subjects. Eur J Clin Nutr 49:1–10

Gauthier MS, Couturier K, Latour JG, Lavoie JM (2003) Concurrent exercise prevents high-fat-diet-induced macrovesicular hepatic steatosis. J Appl Physiol 94:2127–2134

Gillum RF, Mussolino ME, Ingram DD (1996) Physical activity and stroke incidence in women and men. The NHANES I Epidemiologic Follow-up Study. Am J Epidemiol 143:860–869

Goldstein LB, Adams R, Becker K, Furberg CD, Gorelick PB, Hademenos G, Hill M, Howard G, Howard VJ, Jacobs B, Levine SR, Mosca L, Sacco RL, Sherman DG, Wolf PA, del Zoppo GJ (2001) Primary prevention of ischemic stroke: A statement for healthcare professionals from the Stroke Council of the American Heart Association. Circulation 103:163–182

Gregoire FM (2001) Adipocyte differentiation: from fibroblast to endocrine cell. Exp Biol Med (Maywood) 226:997–1002

Grundy SM (1998) Multifactorial causation of obesity: implications for prevention. Am J Clin Nutr 67:563S–572S

Haffner S, Taegtmeyer H (2003) Epidemic obesity and the metabolic syndrome. Circulation 108:1541–1545

Hambrecht R, Wolf A, Gielen S, Linke A, Hofer J, Erbs S, Schoene N, Schuler G (2000) Effect of exercise on coronary endothelial function in patients with coronary artery disease. N Engl J Med 342:454–460

Haskell WL (1994) J.B. Wolffe Memorial Lecture. Health consequences of physical activity: understanding and challenges regarding dose-response. Med Sci Sports Exerc 26:649–660

Helmrich SP, Ragland DR, Leung RW, Paffenbarger RS, Jr. (1991) Physical activity and reduced occurrence of non-insulin-dependent diabetes mellitus. N Engl J Med 325:147–152

Hu FB, Li TY, Colditz GA, Willett WC, Manson JE (2003) Television watching and other sedentary behaviors in relation to risk of obesity and type 2 diabetes mellitus in women. JAMA 289:1785–1791

Hu FB, Stampfer MJ, Colditz GA, Ascherio A, Rexrode KM, Willett WC, Manson JE (2000) Physical activity and risk of stroke in women. JAMA 283:2961–2967

Huang Z, Willett WC, Manson JE, Rosner B, Stampfer MJ, Speizer FE, Colditz GA (1998) Body weight, weight change, and risk for hypertension in women. Ann Intern Med 128:81–88

Hurley BF, Nemeth PM, Martin WH, 3rd, Hagberg JM, Dalsky GP, Holloszy JO (1986) Muscle triglyceride utilization during exercise: effect of training. J Appl Physiol 60:562–567

Irwin ML, Yasui Y, Ulrich CM, Bowen D, Rudolph RE, Schwartz RS, Yukawa M, Aiello E, Potter JD, McTiernan A (2003) Effect of exercise on total and intra-abdominal body fat in postmenopausal women: a randomized controlled trial. JAMA 289:323–330

Jakicic JM, Marcus BH, Gallagher KI, Napolitano M, Lang W (2003) Effect of exercise duration and intensity on weight loss in overweight, sedentary women: a randomized trial. JAMA 290:1323–1330

Jeffery RW, McGuire MT, French SA (2002) Prevalence and correlates of large weight gains and losses. Int J Obes Relat Metab Disord 26:969–972

Jeffery RW, Wing RR, Sherwood NE, Tate DF (2003) Physical activity and weight loss: does prescribing higher physical activity goals improve outcome? Am J Clin Nutr 78:684–689

Jolliffe JA, Rees K, Taylor RS, Thompson D, Oldridge N, Ebrahim S (2001) Exercise-based rehabilitation for coronary heart disease. Cochrane Database Syst Rev: CD001800

Kiely DK, Wolf PA, Cupples LA, Beiser AS, Kannel WB (1994) Physical activity and stroke risk: the Framingham Study. Am J Epidemiol 140:608–620

King NA, Burley VJ, Blundell JE (1994) Exercise-induced suppression of appetite: effects on food intake and implications for energy balance. Eur J Clin Nutr 48:715–724

Kirk EP, Jacobsen DJ, Gibson C, Hill JO, Donnelly JE (2003) Time course for changes in aerobic capacity and body composition in overweight men and women in response to long-term exercise: the Midwest Exercise Trial (MET). Int J Obes Relat Metab Disord 27:912–919

Klem ML, Wing RR, McGuire MT, Seagle HM, Hill JO (1997) A descriptive study of individuals successful at long-term maintenance of substantial weight loss. Am J Clin Nutr 66:239–246

Knowler WC, Barrett-Connor E, Fowler SE, Hamman RF, Lachin JM, Walker EA, Nathan DM (2002) Reduction in the incidence of type 2 diabetes with lifestyle intervention or metformin. N Engl J Med 346:393–403

Kuczmarski RJ, Flegal KM, Campbell SM, Johnson CL (1994) Increasing prevalence of overweight among US adults. The National Health and Nutrition Examination Surveys, 1960 to 1991. JAMA 272:205–211

Kurl S, Laukkanen JA, Rauramaa R, Lakka TA, Sivenius J, Salonen JT (2003) Cardiorespiratory fitness and the risk for stroke in men. Arch Intern Med 163:1682–1688

Kurth T, Gaziano JM, Berger K, Kase CS, Rexrode KM, Cook NR, Buring JE, Manson JE (2002) Body mass index and the risk of stroke in men. Arch Intern Med 162:2557–2562

Laaksonen DE, Lakka HM, Salonen JT, Niskanen LK, Rauramaa R, Lakka TA (2002) Low levels of leisure-time physical activity and cardiorespiratory fitness predict development of the metabolic syndrome. Diabetes Care 25:1612–1618

Lakka HM, Laaksonen DE, Lakka TA, Niskanen LK, Kumpusalo E, Tuomilehto J, Salonen JT (2002a) The metabolic syndrome and total and cardiovascular disease mortality in middle-aged men. JAMA 288:2709–2716

Lakka HM, Lakka TA, Tuomilehto J, Salonen JT (2002b) Abdominal obesity is associated with increased risk of acute coronary events in men. Eur Heart J 23:706–713

Lakka TA, Lakka HM, Salonen R, Kaplan GA, Salonen JT (2001a) Abdominal obesity is associated with accelerated progression of carotid atherosclerosis in men. Atherosclerosis 154:497–504

Lakka TA, Laukkanen JA, Rauramaa R, Salonen R, Lakka HM, Kaplan GA, Salonen JT (2001b) Cardiorespiratory fitness and the progression of carotid atherosclerosis in middle-aged men. Ann Intern Med 134:12–20

Lakka TA, Venalainen JM, Rauramaa R, Salonen R, Tuomilehto J, Salonen JT (1994) Relation of leisure-time physical activity and cardiorespiratory fitness to the risk of acute myocardial infarction. N Engl J Med 330:1549–1554

Larsson B, Svardsudd K, Welin L, Wilhelmsen L, Bjorntorp P, Tibblin G (1984) Abdominal adipose tissue distribution, obesity, and risk of cardiovascular disease and death: 13 year follow up of participants in the study of men born in 1913. Br Med J (Clin Res Ed) 288:1401–1404

Laukkanen JA, Lakka TA, Rauramaa R, Kuhanen R, Venalainen JM, Salonen R, Salonen JT (2001) Cardiovascular fitness as a predictor of mortality in men. Arch Intern Med 161:825–831

Lee IM, Blair SN, Allison DB, Folsom AR, Harris TB, Manson JE, Wing RR (2001) Epidemiologic data on the relationships of caloric intake, energy balance, and weight gain over the life span with longevity and morbidity. J Gerontol A Biol Sci Med Sci 56 Spec No 1:7–19

Lee IM, Manson JE, Hennekens CH, Paffenbarger RS, Jr. (1993) Body weight and mortality. A 27-year follow-up of middle-aged men. JAMA 270:2823–2828

Lee IM, Sesso HD, Paffenbarger RS, Jr. (2000) Physical activity and coronary heart disease risk in men: does the duration of exercise episodes predict risk? Circulation 102:981–986

Leng GC, Fowler B, Ernst E (2000) Exercise for intermittent claudication. Cochrane Database Syst Rev: CD000990

Lindenstrom E, Boysen G, Nyboe J (1993) Lifestyle factors and risk of cerebrovascular disease in women. The Copenhagen City Heart Study. Stroke 24:1468–1472

Livingstone MB, Strain JJ, Prentice AM, Coward WA, Nevin GB, Barker ME, Hickey RJ, McKenna PG, Whitehead RG (1991) Potential contribution of leisure activity to the energy expenditure patterns of sedentary populations. Br J Nutr 65:145–155

Manson JE, Colditz GA, Stampfer MJ, Willett WC, Rosner B, Monson RR, Speizer FE, Hennekens CH (1990) A prospective study of obesity and risk of coronary heart disease in women. N Engl J Med 322:882–889

Manson JE, Hu FB, Rich-Edwards JW, Colditz GA, Stampfer MJ, Willett WC, Speizer FE, Hennekens CH (1999) A prospective study of walking as compared with vigorous exercise in the prevention of coronary heart disease in women. N Engl J Med 341:650–658

Manson JE, Willett WC, Stampfer MJ, Colditz GA, Hunter DJ, Hankinson SE, Hennekens CH, Speizer FE (1995) Body weight and mortality among women. N Engl J Med 333:677–685

Martinez-Gonzalez MA, Martinez JA, Hu FB, Gibney MJ, Kearney J (1999) Physical inactivity, sedentary lifestyle and obesity in the European Union. Int J Obes Relat Metab Disord 23:1192–1201

McGinnis JM, Foege WH (1993) Actual causes of death in the United States. JAMA 270:2207–2212

Mendelson G, Aronow WS, Ahn C (1998) Prevalence of coronary artery disease, atherothrombotic brain infarction, and peripheral arterial disease: associated risk factors in older Hispanics in an academic hospital-based geriatrics practice. J Am Geriatr Soc 46:481–483

Mittleman MA, Maclure M, Tofler GH, Sherwood JB, Goldberg RJ, Muller JE (1993) Triggering of acute myocardial infarction by heavy physical exertion. Protection against triggering by regular exertion. Determinants of Myocardial Infarction Onset Study Investigators. N Engl J Med 329:1677–1683

Mourier A, Gautier JF, De Kerviler E, Bigard AX, Villette JM, Garnier JP, Duvallet A, Guezennec CY, Cathelineau G (1997) Mobilization of visceral adipose tissue related to the improvement in insulin sensitivity in response to physical training in NIDDM. Effects of branched-chain amino acid supplements. Diabetes Care 20:385–391

National Institutes of Health (1998) Clinical Guidelines on the Identification, Evaluation, and Treatment of Overweight and Obesity in Adults—The Evidence Report. National Institutes of Health. Obes Res 6 Suppl 2:51S–209S

National Task Force on the Prevention and Treatment of Obesity (2000) Overweight, obesity, and health risk. National Task Force on the Prevention and Treatment of Obesity. Arch Intern Med 160:898–904

O'Connor GT, Buring JE, Yusuf S, Goldhaber SZ, Olmstead EM, Paffenbarger RS, Jr., Hennekens CH (1989) An overview of randomized trials of rehabilitation with exercise after myocardial infarction. Circulation 80:234–244

Ogden CL, Flegal KM, Carroll MD, Johnson CL (2002) Prevalence and trends in overweight among US children and adolescents, 1999–2000. JAMA 288:1728–1732

Oldridge NB, Guyatt GH, Fischer ME, Rimm AA (1988) Cardiac rehabilitation after myocardial infarction. Combined experience of randomized clinical trials. JAMA 260:945–950

Paffenbarger RS, Jr., Hyde RT, Wing AL, Hsieh CC (1986) Physical activity, all-cause mortality, and longevity of college alumni. N Engl J Med 314:605–613

Paffenbarger RS, Jr., Hyde RT, Wing AL, Lee IM, Jung DL, Kampert JB (1993) The association of changes in physical-activity level and other lifestyle characteristics with mortality among men. N Engl J Med 328:538–545

Paffenbarger RS, Jr., Hyde RT, Wing AL, Steinmetz CH (1984) A natural history of athleticism and cardiovascular health. JAMA 252:491–495

Pate RR, Pratt M, Blair SN, Haskell WL, Macera CA, Bouchard C, Buchner D, Ettinger W, Heath GW, King AC, et al. (1995) Physical activity and public health. A recommendation from the Centers for Disease Control and Prevention and the American College of Sports Medicine. JAMA 273:402–407

Planas A, Clara A, Pou JM, Vidal-Barraquer F, Gasol A, de Moner A, Contreras C, Marrugat J (2001) Relationship of obesity distribution and peripheral arterial occlusive disease in elderly men. Int J Obes Relat Metab Disord 25:1068–1070

Popkin BM, Nielsen SJ (2003) The sweetening of the world's diet. Obes Res 11:1325–1332

Prentice AM, Jebb SA (1995) Obesity in Britain: gluttony or sloth? BMJ 311:437–439

Ravussin E, Lillioja S, Anderson TE, Christin L, Bogardus C (1986) Determinants of 24-hour energy expenditure in man. Methods and results using a respiratory chamber. J Clin Invest 78:1568–1578

Ravussin E, Lillioja S, Knowler WC, Christin L, Freymond D, Abbott WG, Boyce V, Howard BV, Bogardus C (1988) Reduced rate of energy expenditure as a risk factor for body-weight gain. N Engl J Med 318:467–472

Ravussin E, Smith SR (2002) Increased fat intake, impaired fat oxidation, and failure of fat cell proliferation result in ectopic fat storage, insulin resistance, and type 2 diabetes mellitus. Ann N Y Acad Sci 967:363–378

Rexrode KM, Buring JE, Manson JE (2001) Abdominal and total adiposity and risk of coronary heart disease in men. Int J Obes Relat Metab Disord 25:1047–1056

Rexrode KM, Carey VJ, Hennekens CH, Walters EE, Colditz GA, Stampfer MJ, Willett WC, Manson JE (1998) Abdominal adiposity and coronary heart disease in women. JAMA 280:1843–1848

Rexrode KM, Hennekens CH, Willett WC, Colditz GA, Stampfer MJ, Rich-Edwards JW, Speizer FE, Manson JE (1997) A prospective study of body mass index, weight change, and risk of stroke in women. JAMA 277:1539–1545

Rimm EB, Stampfer MJ, Giovannucci E, Ascherio A, Spiegelman D, Colditz GA, Willett WC (1995) Body size and fat distribution as predictors of coronary heart disease among middle-aged and older US men. Am J Epidemiol 141:1117–1127

Ross R, Dagnone D, Jones PJ, Smith H, Paddags A, Hudson R, Janssen I (2000) Reduction in obesity and related comorbid conditions after diet-induced weight loss or exercise-induced weight loss in men. A randomized, controlled trial. Ann Intern Med 133:92–103

Ross R, Janssen I (2001) Physical activity, total and regional obesity: dose-response considerations. Med Sci Sports Exerc 33: S521–527; discussion S528–529

Sacco RL, Gan R, Boden-Albala B, Lin IF, Kargman DE, Hauser WA, Shea S, Paik MC (1998) Leisure-time physical activity and ischemic stroke risk: the Northern Manhattan Stroke Study. Stroke 29:380–387

Sandvik L, Erikssen J, Thaulow E, Erikssen G, Mundal R, Rodahl K (1993) Physical fitness as a predictor of mortality among healthy, middle-aged Norwegian men. N Engl J Med 328:533–537

Santa-Clara H, Fernhall B, Baptista F, Mendes M, Bettencourt Sardinha L (2003) Effect of a one-year combined exercise training program on body composition in men with coronary artery disease. Metabolism 52:1413–1417

Saris WH, Blair SN, van Baak MA, Eaton SB, Davies PS, Di Pietro L, Fogelholm M, Rissanen A, Schoeller D, Swinburn B, Tremblay A, Westerterp KR, Wyatt H (2003) How much physical activity is enough to prevent unhealthy weight gain? Outcome of the IASO 1st Stock Conference and consensus statement. Obes Rev 4:101–114

Saris WHM (1996) Physical activity and body weight regulation. In: Bouchard C BG (ed) Regulation of Body Weight. Biological and Behavioural Mechanisms. Wiley, Chichester, pp 135–147

Schmitz KH, Jensen MD, Kugler KC, Jeffery RW, Leon AS (2003) Strength training for obesity prevention in midlife women. Int J Obes Relat Metab Disord 27:326–333

Schrauwen-Hinderling VB, van Loon LJ, Koopman R, Nicolay K, Saris WH, Kooi ME (2003) Intramyocellular lipid content is increased after exercise in nonexercising human skeletal muscle. J Appl Physiol 95:2328–2332

Schulz LO, Schoeller DA (1994) A compilation of total daily energy expenditures and body weights in healthy adults. Am J Clin Nutr 60:676–681

Sesso HD, Paffenbarger RS, Jr., Lee IM (2000) Physical activity and coronary heart disease in men: The Harvard Alumni Health Study. Circulation 102:975–980

Slentz CA, Duscha BD, Johnson JL, Ketchum K, Aiken LB, Samsa GP, Houmard JA, Bales CW, Kraus WE (2004) Effects of the amount of exercise on body weight, body composition, and measures of central obesity: STRRIDE—a randomized controlled study. Arch Intern Med 164:31–39

Smith SR, de Jonge L, Zachwieja JJ, Roy H, Nguyen T, Rood J, Windhauser M, Volaufova J, Bray GA (2000) Concurrent physical activity increases fat oxidation during the shift to a high-fat diet. Am J Clin Nutr 72:131–138

Stefanick ML, Mackey S, Sheehan M, Ellsworth N, Haskell WL, Wood PD (1998) Effects of diet and exercise in men and postmenopausal women with low levels of HDL cholesterol and high levels of LDL cholesterol. N Engl J Med 339:12–20

Stevens J, Cai J, Pamuk ER, Williamson DF, Thun MJ, Wood JL (1998) The effect of age on the association between body-mass index and mortality. N Engl J Med 338:1–7

Stewart KJ, Hiatt WR, Regensteiner JG, Hirsch AT (2002) Exercise training for claudication. N Engl J Med 347:1941–1951

Suk SH, Sacco RL, Boden-Albala B, Cheun JF, Pittman JG, Elkind MS, Paik MC (2003) Abdominal obesity and risk of ischemic stroke: the Northern Manhattan Stroke Study. Stroke 34:1586–1592

Tanaka S, Togashi K, Rankinen T, Perusse L, Leon AS, Rao DC, Skinner JS, Wilmore JH, Despres JP, Bouchard C (2003) Sex differences in the relationships of abdominal fat to cardiovascular disease risk among normal-weight white subjects. Int J Obes Relat Metab Disord 28:320–323

Tanasescu M, Leitzmann MF, Rimm EB, Willett WC, Stampfer MJ, Hu FB (2002) Exercise type and intensity in relation to coronary heart disease in men. JAMA 288:1994–2000

Thompson PD, Buchner D, Pina IL, Balady GJ, Williams MA, Marcus BH, Berra K, Blair SN, Costa F, Franklin B, Fletcher GF, Gordon NF, Pate RR, Rodriguez BL, Yancey AK, Wenger NK (2003) Exercise and physical activity in the prevention and treatment of atherosclerotic cardiovascular disease: a statement from the Council on Clinical Cardiology (Subcommittee on Exercise, Rehabilitation, and Prevention) and the Council on Nutrition, Physical Activity, and Metabolism (Subcommittee on Physical Activity). Circulation 107:3109–3116

Thompson PD, Crouse SF, Goodpaster B, Kelley D, Moyna N, Pescatello L (2001) The acute versus the chronic response to exercise. Med Sci Sports Exerc 33: S438–S445; discussion S452–S433

Tuomilehto J, Lindstrom J, Eriksson JG, Valle TT, Hamalainen H, Ilanne-Parikka P, Keinanen-Kiukaanniemi S, Laakso M, Louheranta A, Rastas M, Salminen V, Uusitupa M (2001) Prevention of type 2 diabetes mellitus by changes in lifestyle among subjects with impaired glucose tolerance. N Engl J Med 344:1343–1350

Unger RH (2002) Lipotoxic diseases. Annu Rev Med 53:319–336

van Loon LJ, Schrauwen-Hinderling VB, Koopman R, Wagenmakers AJ, Hesselink MK, Schaart G, Kooi ME, Saris WH (2003) Influence of prolonged endurance cycling and recovery diet on intramuscular triglyceride content in trained males. Am J Physiol Endocrinol Metab 285: E804–E811

Visser M, Bouter LM, McQuillan GM, Wener MH, Harris TB (1999) Elevated C-reactive protein levels in overweight and obese adults. JAMA 282:2131–2135

Voorrips LE, Meijers JH, Sol P, Seidell JC, van Staveren WA (1992) History of body weight and physical activity of elderly women differing in current physical activity. Int J Obes Relat Metab Disord 16:199–205

Walker SP, Rimm EB, Ascherio A, Kawachi I, Stampfer MJ, Willett WC (1996) Body size and fat distribution as predictors of stroke among US men. Am J Epidemiol 144:1143–1150

Wannamethee G, Shaper AG (1992) Physical activity and stroke in British middle aged men. BMJ 304:597–601

Wannamethee SG, Shaper AG, Walker M (1998) Changes in physical activity, mortality, and incidence of coronary heart disease in older men. Lancet 351:1603–1608

Welin L, Svardsudd K, Wilhelmsen L, Larsson B, Tibblin G (1987) Analysis of risk factors for stroke in a cohort of men born in 1913. N Engl J Med 317:521–526

Westerterp KR, Verboeket-van de Venne WP, Bouten CV, de Graaf C, van het Hof KH, Weststrate JA (1996) Energy expenditure and physical activity in subjects consuming full-or reduced-fat products as part of their normal diet. Br J Nutr 76:785–795

Willett WC, Dietz WH, Colditz GA (1999) Guidelines for healthy weight. N Engl J Med 341:427–434

Willett WC, Manson JE, Stampfer MJ, Colditz GA, Rosner B, Speizer FE, Hennekens CH (1995) Weight, weight change, and coronary heart disease in women. Risk within the 'normal' weight range. JAMA 273:461–465

Williamson DF, Pamuk E, Thun M, Flanders D, Byers T, Heath C (1995) Prospective study of intentional weight loss and mortality in never-smoking overweight US white women aged 40–64 years. Am J Epidemiol 141:1128–1141

Wilmore JH (2001) Dose-response: variation with age, sex, and health status. Med Sci Sports Exerc 33: S622–634; discussion S640–S621

Wilmore JH, Despres JP, Stanforth PR, Mandel S, Rice T, Gagnon J, Leon AS, Rao D, Skinner JS, Bouchard C (1999) Alterations in body weight and composition consequent to 20 wk of endurance training: the HERITAGE Family Study. Am J Clin Nutr 70:346–352

World Health Organization (2000) Obesity: preventing and managing the global epidemic. Report of a WHO consultation. World Health Organ Tech Rep Ser 894: i-xii, 1–253

HEP (2005) 170:165–194

Fatty Acids and Atherosclerotic Risk

M.A. Thijssen · R.P. Mensink (✉)

Department of Human Biology, Maastricht University, P.O. Box 616, 6200 MD Maastricht, The Netherlands
R.Mensink@hb.unimaas.nl

Abstract Most research concerning the effects of dietary fatty acids on atherosclerotic risk has focused on their effects on lipid and lipoprotein metabolism. However, it is known that fatty acids also influence a number of other relevant mechanisms involved in atherosclerosis such as lipid peroxidation, inflammation and haemostasis. The most favourable distribution of cholesterol over the various lipoproteins is achieved when saturated and *trans* fatty acids are replaced by a mixture of *cis*-unsaturated fatty acids. Furthermore, fatty acids from fish oil lower triacylglycerol concentrations. Effects on other atherosclerotic risk markers are less evident. Monounsaturated fatty acids may be preferable above other fatty acids with respect to low-density lipoprotein oxidation as measured by indirect in vitro assays. The relevance of these assays for the in vivo situation is, however, limited. With respect to inflammation, mainly the effects of n-3 polyunsaturated fatty acids from fish oil have been studied, but results were inconsistent. Also results from studies evaluating the effects of fatty acids on haemostatic risk markers were inconsistent, which may be partly related to the use of different analytical methods. The most consistent finding however is the potential beneficial effect of moderate intakes of fish oil on platelet aggregation. Furthermore, reducing total fat intake rather than changing the fatty acid composition of the diet may beneficially affect the coagulation system. In conclusion, while beneficial effects on atherosclerotic risk are mainly ascribed to *cis*-unsaturated fatty acids, it remains debateable whether *trans* and saturated fatty acids in the diet have to be replaced by *cis*-unsaturated fatty acids or by carbohydrates. To answer this question adequately more validated methods are needed that reflect in vivo lipid peroxidation, inflammation and haemostasis.

Keywords Fatty acids · Lipoprotein metabolism · Lipid peroxidation · Inflammation · Haemostasis

Abbreviations

CRP	C-reactive protein
DHA	Docosahexaenoic acid
EPA	Eicosapentaenoic acid
E-selectin	Selectin derived from endothelial cells
HDL	High-density lipoprotein
ICAM-1	Intercellular adhesion molecule-1
IL	Interleukin
LDL	Low-density lipoprotein
LFA-1	Leukocyte-function-associated antigen-1
MDA	Malondialdehydes
mRNA	Messenger RNA
PAI-1	Plasminogen activator inhibitor-1
PBMC	Peripheral blood mononuclear cells
PG	Prostaglandin
TBARS	Thiobarbituric acid reactive substances
TNFα	Tumour necrosis factor α

tPA   Tissue type plasminogen activator
TX   Thromboxane
VCAM-1   Vascular cell adhesion molecule-1
VLDL   Very low-density lipoprotein

1
Dietary Fatty Acids

Although dietary fats and oils always consist of a mixture of fatty acids, each fat and oil has its own characteristic fatty acid composition. Usually, one or two fatty acids are predominant (Table 1), each with its own characteristics.

Based on chain length, fatty acids can be classified as short-chain fatty acids (4–6 carbon atoms), medium-chain fatty acids (8–10 carbon atoms), long-chain fatty acids (12–18 carbon atoms) and very-long chain fatty acids (>18 carbon atoms). In addition, fatty acids may vary in the number of double bonds. Major fatty acid classes are saturated fatty acids with no double bonds, monounsaturated fatty acids with one double bond, and polyunsaturated fatty acids with two or more double bonds. Based on the position of the double bond nearest to the methyl end of the carbon chain, fatty acids are divided into families. So palmitoleic acid, a metabolite of palmitic acid, belongs to the n-7 family, oleic acid to the n-9 family, linoleic acid to the n-6 family, and α-linolenic acid to the n-3 family. Finally, the configuration of the double bond can be *cis* or *trans*.

Table 1 Major fatty acids in some edible fats ands oils

Common name	Formula	Source
Saturated fatty acids		
Medium-chain fatty acids	C4:0-C10:0	Dairy fat, coconut oil, palm kernel oil
Lauric acid	C12:0	Dairy fat, coconut oil, palm kernel oil
Myristic acid	C14:0	Dairy fat, coconut oil, palm kernel oil
Palmitic acid	C16:0	Meat, palm oil
Stearic acid	C18:0	Meat, cocoa butter
Monounsaturated fatty acids		
Oleic acid	C18:1 n-9	Olive oil, rapeseed oil, avocado, nuts
Polyunsaturated fatty acids		
Linoleic acid	C18:2 n-6	Sunflower oil, safflower oil, soybean oil
α-Linolenic acid	C18:3 n-3	Soybean oil, rapeseed oil, flaxseed
EPA	C20:5 n-3	Fish
DHA	C22:5 n-3	Fish

In most diets, about 30%–40% of total dietary energy intake is provided by fat. Palmitic and stearic acids are the most prevailing saturated fatty acids, while the most widespread monounsaturated and polyunsaturated fatty acids are oleic acid and linoleic acid, respectively.

Ultimately all fatty acids are degraded and oxidized for energy via β-oxidation in the mitochondria of cells. However, fatty acids not only provide energy, but are also important structural components of cell membranes and precursors of a wide range of eicosanoids (prostaglandins, thromboxanes and leukotrienes) involved in haemostasis and inflammation. Furthermore, fatty acids are ligands for transcription factors, thereby modulating gene expression. In this manner, dependent on their characteristics, fatty acids exert different effects on atherosclerotic risk markers. In this chapter, the effects of fatty acids on lipid and lipoprotein metabolism, lipid peroxidation, inflammation and haemostasis will be discussed (Table 2).

Table 2 Factors that are positively (↑) or negatively (↓) related to atherosclerotic risk

Risk marker	Atherosclerotic risk
Lipid and lipoprotein metabolism	
Total cholesterol	↑
LDL cholesterol	↑
HDL cholesterol	↓
Total/HDL cholesterol ratio	↑
Triacylglycerols	↑
Oxidative stress	
In vitro LDL susceptibility to oxidation	↑
Oxidized LDL	↑
F_2-isoprostanes	↑
Inflammation	
Adhesion molecules	↑
Pro-inflammatory cytokines	↑
Anti-inflammatory cytokines	↓
Haemostatic function	
Platelet aggregation	↑
Coagulation	
Factor VII	↑
Fibrinogen	↑
Prothrombin fragment 1+2	↑
Fibrinolysis	
TPA	↓
PAI-1	↑
D-dimers	↑

2
Fatty Acids and Lipoprotein Metabolism

Lipoproteins are the major transporters of lipids in the blood. While the classical risk factor for coronary heart disease is an increased concentration of serum total cholesterol, later studies have demonstrated that the various lipoprotein classes have their specific effects on cardiovascular risk.

Two major cholesterol-transporting lipoproteins are the low-density lipoproteins (LDL) and high-density lipoproteins (HDL), carrying respectively 60%–70% and 20%–30% of the total amount of cholesterol in the blood. While LDL is atherogenic, HDL may protect against atherosclerosis. Epidemiological studies now suggest that an increment of 0.1 mmol/l in LDL cholesterol results in an increase of 3.5%–4.0% in cardiovascular risk, while an increase of 0.1 mmol/l in HDL cholesterol lowers cardiovascular risk with 8%–12% (Gordon and Rifkind 1989). However, the total/HDL cholesterol ratio may be an even more specific marker to predict cardiovascular risk than total or lipoprotein cholesterol concentrations. A decrease of 0.1 unit in this ratio is associated with a 5.3% reduction in the risk of myocardial infarction (Stampfer et al. 1991). Another, less-validated, risk marker is the concentration of triacylglycerols. Triacylglycerols, which are found mainly in the very-low-density lipoproteins (VLDL), are positively related to cardiovascular risk and a 0.1 mmol/l increase in triacylglycerol is associated with a 1.4% increase in cardiovascular risk for men and a 3.7% increase for women (Hokanson and Austin 1996).

As outlined below, these cardiovascular risk markers are differently affected by the various fatty acids in the diet. However, the definition of a cholesterol-raising or cholesterol-lowering fatty acid is not straightforward. When fat is simply added to a diet, energy intake increases and as a result body weight will increase also. As body weight is an important determinant of serum total cholesterol concentrations, it will not be possible to disentangle dietary effects from those of changes in body weight. Therefore, in dietary intervention studies or meta-analyses intended to compare the effects of fatty acids on the serum lipoprotein profile, any change in the saturated, monounsaturated or polyunsaturated fatty acid, or carbohydrate composition of the diet is balanced by opposite changes in one or more of the others. Therefore, the effects of specific fatty acids are generally expressed relative to those of an iso-caloric amount of carbohydrates or of another fatty acid.

2.1
Mixtures of Saturated Fatty Acids

Well controlled dietary studies carried out in the 1950s and 1960s found that–relative to an iso-energetic amount of carbohydrate–a mixture of saturated fatty acids increased serum total cholesterol concentrations (Hegsted et al. 1965; Keys et al. 1965). These earlier studies, however, did not examine the effects of fatty acids on specific lipoproteins. From a recent meta-analysis, it can be concluded that replacement of carbohydrates with saturated fatty acids not only increased serum total cholesterol concentrations, but also those of LDL and HDL (Fig. 1). The total/HDL cholesterol ratio however was not affected. In addition, effects on the serum lipoprotein profile were dependent on the chain length of the saturated fatty acid (Mensink et al. 2003).

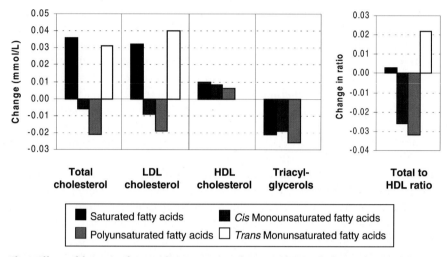

Fig. 1 Effects of the major fatty acids on serum total, LDL and HDL cholesterol, triacylglycerol concentrations and total/HDL cholesterol ratio when 1% of dietary carbohydrates is replaced by fatty acids under iso-energetic conditions

2.1.1
Medium-Chain Fatty Acids

Although medium-chain fatty acids are found in significant quantities in several natural fats and oils, the total amount in regular diets is in general low. This may explain why effects of medium-chain fatty acids on lipoprotein metabolism have not been well studied. Initially, it was suggested that medium-chain fatty acids had a neutral effect on serum total cholesterol concentrations (Hegsted et al. 1965; Keys et al. 1965). Results from two recent studies, however, suggested that relative to oleic acid, medium-chain fatty acids slightly increased serum total and LDL cholesterol, but did not affect HDL cholesterol concentrations. Triacylglycerol concentrations were slightly increased (Cater et al. 1997; Temme et al. 1997).

2.1.2
Lauric, Myristic and Palmitic Acids

Palmitic acid (C16:0) along with lauric (C12:0) and myristic (C14:0) acids, are the most potent cholesterol-raising saturated fatty acids. Their relative cholesterol elevating effects, however, are controversial. In fact, it is difficult to examine the effects of the individual saturated fatty acids, because in natural fats, high levels of one fatty acid are associated with high levels of another fatty acid. Coconut oil, for example, contains high amounts of both myristic and lauric acids, while dairy fat is rich in both myristic and palmitic acids. This makes it difficult to ascribe the observed effects to one single fatty acid. Therefore, more recent studies have used synthetic and semi-synthetic fats, specifically enriched in one of the saturated fatty acids.

Palmitic acid is the major saturated fatty acid in the diet. It is well accepted that palmitic acid raises total, LDL and HDL cholesterol and decreases triacylglycerol concentrations, relative to carbohydrates. Effects of palmitic acid relative to those of oleic acid are more controversial. In studies that compared the effects of palmolein oil (rich in palmitic acid) with olive oil (rich in oleic acid), palmitic and oleic acids had comparable effects on the serum lipoprotein profile (Choudhury et al. 1995; Ng et al. 1992). However, the majority of well-controlled studies have found that relative to oleic acid, palmitic acid increased total and LDL cholesterol concentrations (Denke and Grundy 1992; Temme et al. 1996; Zock et al. 1994).

Myristic acid has for long been suspected to be the most cholesterol-raising fatty acid (Hegsted et al. 1965). Several studies concluded that myristic acid increased total cholesterol concentrations relative to oleic acid, due to an increase in LDL as well as in HDL cholesterol (Temme et al. 1997; Zock et al. 1994). However, these effects of the semi-synthetic fats enriched in myristic acid were much less than suggested by two independent meta-analyses (Hegsted et al. 1965; Mensink et al. 2003).

Lauric acid is the fourth most common saturated fatty acid in the diet after palmitic, stearic and myristic acids. Hegsted et al. (1965) already reported that lauric acid had only a mild cholesterol-raising effect relative to carbohydrates. The effects of lauric acid on lipoprotein concentrations were compared with those of oleic acid by Denke and Grundy (1992). It was concluded that lauric acid elevated total and LDL cholesterol concentrations relative to oleic acid, but did not have any effect on HDL cholesterol and triacylglycerol concentrations. Using mixtures of natural fats, these results were confirmed by Temme et al. (1996), but in that study also an additional, significant increase in HDL cholesterol concentrations was observed.

In a recent meta-analysis the effects of the individual saturated fatty acids on the serum lipoprotein profile have been estimated (Mensink et al. 2003). Iso-energetic replacement of carbohydrates with lauric, myristic and palmitic acids all resulted in increased total, LDL and HDL cholesterol concentrations

(Fig. 2). With increasing chain length, these effects decreased. Because the cholesterol-raising effects of lauric acid were proportionally higher on HDL than on LDL cholesterol, replacement of carbohydrates by lauric acid resulted in a significantly lower total/ HDL cholesterol ratio, which suggests a decrease in atherosclerotic risk. Compared with carbohydrates, myristic and palmitic acids did not affect the ratio of total/HDL cholesterol, while lauric, myristic and palmitic acids lowered triacylglycerol concentrations to the same extent (Mensink et al. 2003).

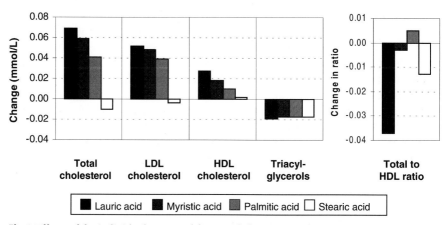

Fig. 2 Effects of the individual saturated fatty acids lauric (C12:0), myristic (C14:0), palmitic (C16:0) and stearic acid (C18:0) on serum total, LDL and HDL cholesterol, triacylglycerol concentrations and total/HDL cholesterol ratio when 1% of dietary carbohydrates is replaced by a specific fatty acid under iso-energetic conditions

2.1.3
Stearic Acid

Compared with the other long-chain saturated fatty acids, stearic acid significantly lowered total, LDL and HDL cholesterol concentrations (Tholstrup et al. 1994a, 1994b). In fact, it has been found that stearic acid and oleic acid, the major monounsaturated fatty acid, had similar effects on serum lipoproteins (Bonanome and Grundy 1988). However, other studies found an HDL cholesterol-lowering effect of stearic acid relative to unsaturated fatty acids (Kris-Etherton et al. 1993; Zock and Katan 1992). Thus, stearic and oleic acids are equivalent in their effects on LDL cholesterol and triacylglycerol, but may differ somewhat in their effects on HDL. These effects of stearic acid were confirmed by a meta-analysis, which furthermore reported that stearic acid did not change the total/HDL cholesterol ratio when compared with carbohydrates (Mensink et al. 2003).

2.2
Monounsaturated Fatty Acids

Mortality rates of coronary heart disease in traditional Mediterranean populations consuming high-fat diets rich in olive oil, a major source of monounsaturated fatty acids, are low (Keys 1970). However, previous studies concluded
that monounsaturated fatty acids had similar effects on serum total cholesterol concentrations as carbohydrates (Hegsted et al. 1965; Keys et al. 1975).
Therefore, many researchers compared the effects of monounsaturated fatty
acids, in particular of oleic acid, and carbohydrates on the distribution of
cholesterol over the different lipoproteins (Grundy 1986; Mensink and Katan
1987). From these studies it appeared that effects of oleic acid and carbohydrates on total cholesterol concentrations are indeed similar, but that oleic acid
increased HDL cholesterol and lowered very-low-density lipoprotein (VLDL)
cholesterol and triacylglycerol concentrations. As a result, a significant decrease in the total/HDL cholesterol ratio was observed. Similar conclusions
were drawn based on results of a meta-analysis (Mensink et al. 2003). Thus,
monounsaturated fatty acids have a more favourable effect on atherosclerotic
risk than carbohydrates, because of the increase in HDL and decrease in VLDL
concentrations.

2.3
Polyunsaturated Fatty Acids

Polyunsaturated fatty acids belong to either the n-6 or n-3 family. Unlike
saturated and monounsaturated fatty acids, the polyunsaturated fatty acids,
linoleic acid and α-linolenic acid, cannot be synthesized de novo by humans.
These fatty acids need to be provided by the diet and are therefore called
essential fatty acids. The most abundant essential fatty acid in the diet is
linoleic acid (C18:2n-6), while a small part of the dietary polyunsaturates is
provided by α-linolenic acid (C18:3n-3). Linoleic acid, member of the n-6
family of fatty acids, serves as the precursor of arachidonic acid (C20:4n-6),
which has important biological effects in the body. α-Linolenic acid, an n-3
fatty acid, can be converted into eicosapentaenoic acid (C20:5n-3, EPA), which
can be further elongated, desaturated and β-oxidized into docosahexaenoic
acid (C22:6n-3, DHA). However, the major part of the very-long chain fatty
acids in the human body are provided through the consumption of fatty fish,
rich in EPA and DHA.

2.3.1
n-6 Polyunsaturated Fatty Acids

Relative to carbohydrates, Keys et al. (1965) have estimated that the hypocholesterolaemic effect of linoleic acid is half as much as the hypercholesterolaemic
effect of saturated fatty acids. However, more recent meta-analyses reported

slightly lesser, but still significant, effects of linoleic acid, not only on serum total cholesterol, but also on LDL cholesterol concentrations. Moreover, linoleic acid lowered triacylglycerol and increased HDL cholesterol concentrations compared with carbohydrates. Although linoleic acid may raise HDL cholesterol less than monounsaturated and saturated fatty acids, linoleic acid still has the most favourable effect on the total/HDL cholesterol ratio (Mensink et al. 2003).

To investigate whether linoleic acid is more beneficial than oleic acid, several studies compared the effects of linoleic acid with those of oleic acid side-by-side. However, results are inconsistent, which may relate to differences in the intake of linoleic acid. When intake of linoleic acid exceeds 15% of energy, linoleic acid lowered serum total, LDL and HDL cholesterol, and serum triacylglycerol concentrations compared to oleic acid (Mattson and Grundy 1985). At more realistic intakes of linoleic acid (less than 15%), differences in effects on lipoprotein profile between linoleic and oleic acids are marginal (Hodson et al. 2001; Howard et al. 1995; Mensink and Katan 1989).

2.3.2
n-3 Polyunsaturated Fatty Acids

The principal n-3 fatty acids are EPA and DHA typically present in fatty fish and fish oils. Although dietary intake of these long-chain, highly unsaturated fatty acids is normally very low, almost 30 times lower than that of linoleic acid (Katan et al. 1994), these fatty acids lower triacylglycerol and VLDL concentrations compared to carbohydrates and other fatty acids. Furthermore, fish fatty acids may slightly raise LDL cholesterol, especially in hypertriglyceridaemic subjects, but do not affect HDL cholesterol (Harris 1997).

The metabolic precursor of the marine n-3 fatty acids is α-linolenic acid, a plant-derived fatty acid. The effects of α-linolenic acid are comparable to those of linoleic acid, an n-6 polyunsaturated fatty acid. In particular, the characteristic effects of EPA and DHA on serum triacylglycerol concentrations are not shared by α-linolenic acid (Harris 1997).

2.4
Trans Fatty Acids

Trans and *cis* isomers of unsaturated fatty acids are produced during hydrogenation of vegetable oils, either by bacteria in the first stomach (rumen) of ruminant animals or by industrial hardening of oil. The main purpose of this latter process is to convert the liquid oil into a solid or semi-solid fat, which can be used for the production of certain types of margarines or shortenings for frying or baking. More than 80% of all *trans* fatty acids in the diet are *trans* isomers of oleic acid, and more than 10% are isomers of *trans* linoleic acid.

Many studies have shown unfavourable effects of *trans* fatty acids on serum lipids. Relative to *cis*-monounsaturated fatty acids, *trans*-monounsaturated fatty acids raise total and LDL cholesterol, and lower HDL cholesterol concentrations, resulting in an increased total/HDL cholesterol ratio. Furthermore, *trans* fatty acids elevate triacylglycerol concentrations (Judd et al. 1994; Mensink and Katan 1990; Zock and Katan 1992). Effects of *trans* fatty acids and saturated fatty acids on total and LDL cholesterol concentrations are not very different. However, *trans* fatty acids lower HDL cholesterol as compared to saturated fatty acids (Judd et al. 1994; Mensink and Katan 1990). This means that the total/HDL cholesterol ratio is also unfavourably changed (Mensink et al. 2003). Therefore, *trans* fatty acids have the worst effects on blood lipids among all dietary fatty acids.

2.5
Conclusions

Dietary fatty acid composition affects the distribution of cholesterol over the various lipoproteins. Under iso-energetic metabolic conditions, the most favourable lipoprotein profile to lower atherosclerotic risk is achieved when saturated and *trans* fatty acids are replaced by a mixture of *cis*-unsaturated fatty acids. However, which unsaturated fatty acid–oleic acid, linoleic acid or fish fatty acids–is the most beneficial, is hard to conclude, because fatty acids also affect other pathways involved in the development of atherosclerosis. Furthermore, it should be noted, that not much is known about the effects of diet on the composition and particle size distribution of LDL, HDL and VLDL, which may also affect cardiovascular risk. For example, carbohydrates lower LDL cholesterol concentrations, but at the same time unfavourably change LDL particle size (Dreon et al. 1999). These effects are more difficult to translate into cardiovascular risk and are as yet not a solid basis for dietary recommendations. More information therefore is needed to elucidate how fatty acids affect lipid and lipoprotein metabolism at the molecular level.

3
Fatty Acids and Lipid Peroxidation

Reactive oxygen species, as present in vivo, induce the oxidation of lipids. This may lead to oxidative modification of LDL, which is critical in the initiation and evolution of atherosclerosis. Increased uptake of oxidized LDL by macrophages via the scavenger pathway results in the formation of foam cells and ultimately atherosclerotic plaques (Fig. 3). Oxidized LDL is cytotoxic and induces atherogenic mechanisms such as chemotaxis, and transmigration and transformation of monocytes into macrophages. In addition, oxidized LDL is a potent inducer for the production of inflammatory molecules (Berliner et al. 1995).

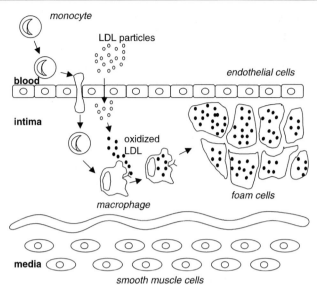

Fig. 3 Involvement of lipid peroxides and inflammation in the development of atherosclerosis. Endothelial dysfunction causes increased endothelial permeability to lipoproteins and up-regulation of leukocyte and endothelial adhesion molecules followed by the recruitment of monocytes and T lymphocytes into the arterial wall. LDL enters the intima layer of the vascular endothelium and is modified by reactive oxygen species into oxidized LDL. Oxidized LDL causes endothelial damage resulting in the release of cytokines. Monocytes recruited into the artery wall become macrophages and express scavenger receptors that bind oxidized LDL particles. Macrophages become lipid-loaded foam cells by engulfing oxidized LDL

A variety of methods has been developed to assess LDL oxidation, but no golden standard exists. In fact, there is a clear need for validated biomarkers to measure in vivo lipid peroxidation and LDL oxidation. Methods for evaluation of LDL oxidation include direct and indirect assays. Direct assays measure certain lipid peroxides, such as malondialdehydes (MDA), thiobarbituric acid reactive substances (TBARS), or conjugated dienes. However, these assays lack specificity in particular for body fluids and tissue samples. In this respect, measurement of isoprostanes is more promising. Isoprostanes are isomers of prostaglandin, which are primarily generated by free-radical mediated peroxidation of polyunsaturated fatty acids and are chemically stabile. Urinary concentrations of F_2-isoprostanes were indeed increased in patients with hypercholesterolaemia (Reilly et al. 1998). Another assay measures the concentrations of MDA-modified LDL, a lipid peroxide decomposition product, which is increased in patients with unstable atherosclerotic cardiovascular disease (Holvoet et al. 1995). Also the amount of circulating oxidized LDL can be measured and is associated with cardiovascular diseases (Holvoet et al. 1998). Furthermore, the presence of auto-antibodies against epitopes on oxidized

LDL can be quantified and is an independent predictor of the progression of atherosclerosis (Jialal and Devaraj 1996). However, all of these assays need further validation. In the past, mainly indirect assays were used, which measured the in vitro susceptibility of LDL to oxidation induced by metal ions. Usually three parameters are measured in these assays. The lag time indicates the time until oxidation of the LDL particle starts, while the rate of oxidation denotes the amount of peroxidation products formed per unit of time. Finally, the total amount of lipid peroxidation products formed can be analysed. Frequently used methods are based on the spectrophotometric measurements of the cytotoxic aldehydes, conjugated dienes, lipid hydroperoxides or apo B-100 fluorescence after induction of LDL oxidation with copper (Jialal and Devaraj 1996). Although this has been the most frequently used assay to examine effects of fatty acids on LDL oxidation, the relevance of these outcome parameters for the in vivo situation is doubtful.

Due to the presence of double bonds, the susceptibility of fatty acids to oxidative modification increases with the degree of unsaturation. Because the fatty acid composition of the diet is reflected by the fatty acid composition of the LDL particle, dietary fat therefore not only determines LDL cholesterol concentrations, but also the in vitro susceptibility of LDL to oxidative modification. Particle size may also be important, as small dense LDL is more readily modified than larger LDL (de Graaf et al. 1991), but effects of fatty acid intake on LDL particle size as related to LDL modification has not been studied indetail.

3.1
Dietary Fat and Saturated Fatty Acids

Low-fat diets and high-fat diets rich in monounsaturated fatty acids have comparable effects on the susceptibility of LDL to oxidation (Hargrove et al. 2001). Effects of saturated fatty acids on LDL oxidation have not been well examined. In theory, saturated fatty acids should beneficially affect in vitro LDL susceptibility, because they do not have any double bonds. However, some studies surprisingly found unfavourable effects on the susceptibility of LDL to oxidation, when monounsaturated fatty acids were replaced by saturated fatty acids (Kratz et al. 2002; Mata et al. 1996). In particular, the lag time was decreased. This suggests that minor dietary components from edible oils affect LDL oxidation as well.

3.2
Oleic Acid Versus Linoleic Acid

Several human studies have shown that enrichment of the diet with oleic acid at the expense of linoleic acid increased resistance of LDL to oxidative modification. When oleic acid is replaced with linoleic acid, lag time decreased, oxidation rate increased, and production of conjugated dienes was higher after copper-induced LDL oxidation (Kratz et al. 2002; Mata et al. 1996). Whether or not these results also indicate that compared with oleic acid linoleic acid elevates atherogenicity of lipoproteins in vivo has yet to be shown.

3.3
n-6 and n-3 Polyunsaturated Fatty Acids

Replacement of n-6 with n-3 polyunsaturated fatty acids in the normal diet did not affect lag time and TBARS, but conjugated diene production was significantly increased after the n-3 enriched diet (Mata et al. 1996). In another study, effects of fish oil and oils rich in n-6 polyunsaturated fatty acids were compared using indirect (LDL oxidation in vitro and TBARS) and direct (F_2-isoprostanes and MDA-modified LDL) assays, but a trend towards higher LDL susceptibility to in vitro oxidation was found only on the diet rich in n-3 fatty acids (Higdon et al. 2000). Only one study evaluated the effects of α-linolenic acid, and found a beneficial effect of α-linolenic acid above EPA and DHA on susceptibility of LDL to oxidation (Finnegan et al. 2003).

The effects of diets supplemented with n-3 polyunsaturated fatty acids, mainly EPA and DHA from fish oils, on LDL oxidation are contradictory. Using fish oil supplements for 3 or 6 weeks, some studies observed an increased susceptibility of LDL to oxidation (Leigh-Firbank et al. 2002; Oostenbrug et al. 1994), but other studies did not see any effects when supplements were given for 2 or 4 months (Bonanome et al. 1996; Higgins et al. 2001). Not only the duration of supplementation, but also differences in the doses of n-3 polyunsaturated fatty acids may explain these apparent discrepancies.

3.4
Conclusions

While polyunsaturated fatty acids have a larger hypocholesterolaemic effect, in vitro assays suggest that the effects of monounsaturated fatty acids on LDL oxidation are the most beneficial. However, the relevance of these indirect, in vitro, assays to measure LDL oxidation, for the in vivo situation is limited. Future studies should therefore use more direct measurements of lipid peroxidation products such as F_2-isoprostanes and MDA-modified LDL.

4
Fatty Acids and Inflammation

During the early phases of plaque development, inflammatory processes already play an important role, starting with the interaction between the vascular endothelium and circulating blood leukocytes. After recruitment and infiltration of mainly monocytes and T lymphocytes into the arterial intima, monocytes are transformed into macrophages, which can take up oxidized LDL rapidly. This process results in the formation of foam cells and ultimately a fatty streak (Lusis 2000). Moreover, T lymphocytes produce several pro- and anti-inflammatory cytokines, which play an important role in orchestrating the inflammatory process (Young et al. 2002). More recently, C-reactive protein (CRP), an acute phase reactant produced by the liver during systemic inflammation, has also been identified as an important risk marker for cardiovascular disease (Ridker et al. 2000).

4.1
Endothelial Cell Adhesion

Cellular adhesion molecules mediate the attachment of leukocytes to vascular endothelial cells and the subsequent *trans*-endothelial migration of monocytes and lymphocytes into the arterial wall. While selectins are involved in the initial rolling of the circulating leukocyte over the endothelium, other cellular adhesion molecules such as intercellular adhesion molecule-1 (ICAM-1) and vascular cell adhesion molecule-1 (VCAM-1), mediate the final firm attachment (Lusis 2000).

Because in vivo the accessibility of human endothelial cells is limited, effects of fatty acids on expression of adhesion molecules have been examined mainly in vitro using endothelial cell lines. From a series of experiments in which endothelial cells were incubated with various fatty acids, it was concluded that with increased degree of unsaturation of the fatty acid, VCAM-1 expression on the surface of endothelial cells decreased. These effects were observed when cells were stimulated with lipopolysaccharide or cytokines [interleukin (IL)-1α or IL-1β or tumour necrosis factor (TNF)α]. Inhibitory potencies of the fatty acids were not influenced by chain length, *cis/trans* configuration, or the position of the double bond. Results were confirmed by analysis of mRNA expression of VCAM-1. Without stimulation, however, none of the fatty acids affected VCAM-1 expression (De Caterina et al. 1998). In contrast, another study reported that addition of linoleic acid and α-linolenic acid to the medium increased mRNA expression of ICAM-1 and VCAM-1 even in unstimulated endothelial cells. On the other hand, oleic acid inhibited mRNA expression of these adhesion molecules (Toborek et al. 2002). Whether these changes in mRNA expression also resulted in changes in surface protein expression was not examined. These contrasting findings indicate that in vitro findings depend on the experimental conditions used and are difficult to extrapolate to the in vivo situation.

In contrast with endothelial cells, peripheral blood mononuclear cells (PBMC) are easily sampled which gives the opportunity to use PBMC to examine the effects of dietary fatty acids on the expression of the ligands for the endothelial adhesion molecules. Furthermore, ICAM-1 is also present on PBMC. Until now, not many studies have made use of these possibilities. In one study, effects of fish oil supplementation for 3 weeks were studied on ICAM-1 and leukocyte-function-associated antigen-1 expression, the ligand for ICAM-1. After stimulation of monocytes with interferon-γ, the expression of these adhesion molecules was lowered in the fish oil group relative to baseline values and to those of control subjects (Hughes et al. 1996). In a study with healthy volunteers, who consumed diets enriched with α-linolenic acid or fish oil for 12 weeks, no effect on ICAM-1 surface expression was found. In this latter study, PBMC were not stimulated (Wallace et al. 2003). In another study with healthy men, the effects of consumption for 2 months of a diet rich in monounsaturated fatty acids were compared with those of a regular diet. Expression of ICAM-1 on PBMC was decreased in the subjects on the monounsaturated fatty acid enriched diet (Yaqoob et al. 1998).

Alternatively, the soluble variants of the above mentioned adhesion molecules–sICAM-1, sVCAM-1 and sE-selectin–can be analysed in plasma. Increased concentrations of these soluble adhesion molecules in the blood, which may indicate increased expression of membrane-bound molecules and impaired endothelial function, are indeed associated with future cardiovascular events in apparently healthy individuals (Blankenberg et al. 2001). It should be emphasized, however, that sVCAM-1 and sE-selectin are almost exclusively derived from endothelial cells, while ICAM-1 is expressed and shed from several cell types (Gearing and Newman 1993). In patients with increased atherosclerotic risk, the effects of supplementation with relatively high doses of n-3 fatty acids (4–5 g/day) have been investigated, but results were inconsistent (Brown and Hu 2001). In healthy subjects, α-linolenic acid and fish oil, but not purified DHA, decreased sVCAM-1 expression. This suggests that possible favourable effects of fish oil should be attributed to EPA (Thies et al. 2001).

4.2
Cytokines

Inflammation is mediated by cytokines, which modulate infiltration and accumulation of immuno-competent cells (T lymphocytes and macrophages) by increasing the expression of adhesion molecules by endothelial cells. Furthermore, cytokines mediate activation and proliferation of both smooth muscle cells and macrophages. With respect to atherosclerosis, cytokines can be divided into three major classes. The pro-inflammatory cytokines typically mediate pro-atherogenic processes, whereas anti-inflammatory cytokines are involved in anti-atherogenic pathways. Major pro-inflammatory cytokines are IL-1, IL-6 and TNFα, while IL-4 and IL-10 are examples of anti-inflammatory cytokines. In addition, some cytokines, such as interferon-γ have pro- as well as anti-inflammatory effects (Young et al. 2002). TNFα, which is produced by endothelial cells, smooth muscle cells and macrophages, plays a pivotal role in the cytokine cascade as it stimulates the synthesis of other cytokines. Also IL-1 and IL-6 are versatile cytokines. IL-6, for example, is a central mediator of the acute-phase response and the primary determinant of CRP production by the liver (Yu and Rifai 2000).

In one of the earlier studies, production of the pro-inflammatory cytokines IL-1 and TNFα by in vitro stimulated PBMC was suppressed after supplementation with a high dose (18 g fish oil/day) of n-3 polyunsaturated fatty acids (Endres et al. 1989). Because these results were confirmed by some (Caughey et al. 1996), but not all studies (Thies et al. 2001; Wallace et al. 2003), it was suggested that in vitro production of pro-inflammatory cytokines is decreased only when EPA plus DHA was consumed for at least 4 weeks and daily intake exceeded 2.4 g (Kelley 2001). However, even long-term supplementation with 3.2 g fish oil/day for 6 or 12 months did not decrease in vitro production of IL-1 and TNFα after whole-blood stimulation (Blok et al. 1997). Despite these inconsistent results, fish fatty acids are considered to exert anti-inflammatory properties.

In another study, it was found that replacement of the habitual fat from the diet of Dutch volunteers by palm oil reduced TNFα production, whereas IL-6 and IL-8 (two other pro-inflammatory cytokines) concentrations were not affected (Engelberts et al. 1993). Compared to soybean oil (linoleic acid with α-linolenic acid), hydrogenated fat rich in *trans* fatty acids increased production of IL-6 and TNFα, but not of IL-1 in humans with moderately elevated LDL cholesterol levels. In this study, soybean oil and butter, the latter rich in saturated fatty acids, had similar effects (Han et al. 2002). Finally, arachidonic acid supplementation did not alter pro-inflammatory cytokine production (Kelley et al. 1998).

Though most studies investigated in vitro or ex vivo cytokine production after exposing PBMC to an inflammatory stimulant, a few studies have evaluated the effects of in particular polyunsaturated fatty acids on circulating plasma cytokine concentrations. It was found that fish oil decreased circulating concentrations of several pro- as well as anti-inflammatory cytokines in patients with a wide variety of inflammatory diseases (Kelley 2001). In healthy volunteers, fish oil did not reduce plasma cytokine concentrations (Blok et al. 1997). Compared with linoleic acid, consumption of α-linolenic acid for 3 months decreased concentrations of the pro-inflammatory IL-6 in dyslipidaemic patients (Rallidis et al. 2003).

4.3
C-reactive Protein

With the newly developed high-sensitive assays, even slightly elevated CRP concentrations can be detected in individuals with mild, non-overt inflammation that may result from the ongoing atherosclerotic process. However, effects of fatty acids on serum CRP concentrations have not been studied very well. Some studies focused on effects of n-3 fatty acids, but results are equivocal. In studies with healthy volunteers no effects of fish oil supplements on CRP concentrations were found, despite reductions of several other acute-phase proteins (Ernst et al. 1991; Madsen et al. 2003). In dyslipidaemic patients, however, replacement of linoleic acid for α-linolenic acid during 3 months reduced CRP concentrations, independently of lipid changes (Rallidis et al. 2003).

4.4
Conclusions

As atherosclerosis has a strong inflammatory component, it is important to examine the effects of fatty acids on inflammatory risk markers. Until now, many in vivo studies have focused on the effects of n-3 polyunsaturated fatty acids from fish oil. However, results are inconsistent. Effects of other fatty acids on in vivo inflammatory markers have been studied even less and this area of research clearly deserves further exploration. Furthermore, attention has to be paid to underlying mechanisms.

5
Fatty Acids and Thrombotic Tendency

Under normal physiological conditions, haemostatic balance between thrombus formation and dissolution is regulated by the endothelial wall, blood platelets, and coagulation and fibrinolytic factors. Any disturbances of this delicate balance might result in activation of the haemostatic system and in increased thrombotic tendency. In this way, the most common complications of cardiovascular disease result from thrombus formation, caused by the exposure of blood platelets to the subendothelial matrix material or disruption of an atherosclerotic plaque (Fig. 4). Thrombosis is initiated by platelet activation, adhesion and aggregation. Platelets become activated by compounds released from the endothelium, or exposed during rupture of an atherosclerotic plaque. After activation, platelets adhere on the place of injury and release their granules, which results in platelet aggregation. Activation of platelets also leads to the release of free arachidonic acid, which can be metabolized into eicosanoids. Following platelet activation, the coagulation cascade is initiated, resulting in the activation of several clotting factors. Ultimately fibrinogen is converted by activated thrombin into fibrin monomers, which polymerize into a fibrin network. In this fibrin network, blood cells and aggregated platelets are captured to form a thrombus, which can occlude the blood vessel. The dissolution of the blood thrombus is regulated by the fibrinolytic system (Kelly et al. 2001a).

Because of the findings from the 1960s showing a very low incidence of thrombosis among fish-eating Greenland Eskimos, considerable work has been carried out in the past few decades to understand how dietary fat and fatty acids, especially long-chain n-3 fatty acids, affect haemostatic risk markers.

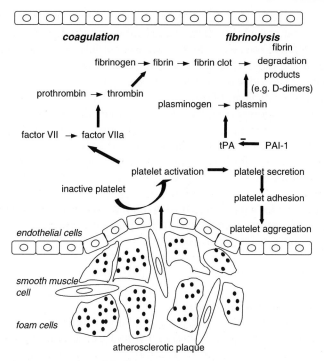

Fig. 4 Schematic representation of the haemostatic system

5.1
Platelet Aggregation

A frequently used method to assess platelet aggregability is the in vitro platelet aggregation test. However, this method measures the ability of platelets to react to a single external stimulus, a situation not comparable with platelet aggregation in vivo. Still, increased ADP-induced platelet aggregation is associated with increased atherosclerotic risk (Elwood et al. 1991). Unfortunately, however, studies are difficult to compare due to the many different methods used to measure platelet aggregation. For example, blood can be anti-coagulated with citrate, heparin or hirudin, while platelet aggregation–in either whole blood or platelet-rich plasma–can be triggered with collagen, ADP, arachidonic acid or thrombin.

Many studies have focused on the effects of n-3 polyunsaturated fatty acids. In general, collagen-induced aggregation decreased, while results of ADP-induced aggregation were very inconsistent (Mutanen 1997). Effects of other fatty acids have also been examined, but results are conflicting. When saturated fatty acids in the diet are replaced by oleic acid or linoleic acid, platelet aggregation was increased, decreased, or not changed. Comparable conflicting results have been found when oleic and linoleic acids were compared side-by-side (Lahoz et al. 1997; Mutanen et al. 1992; Turpeinen et al. 1998a). Some studies compared the effects of the different saturated fatty acids with each other. Relative to oleic acid, medium-chain fatty acids, lauric, myristic or palmitic acids did not affect collagen-induced whole blood aggregation. Furthermore, ADP-induced aggregation was not changed by medium-chain fatty acids or myristic acid (Temme et al. 1998). Thus, dietary fatty acids can modulate platelet aggregation, but the use of many different in vitro methods makes comparison and extrapolation to the in vivo situation difficult.

5.2
Eicosanoid Production

Thromboxanes (TX) and prostaglandins (PG), two eicosanoids, play an important role in the haemostatic balance. Both types of eicosanoids are synthesized from the C20 fatty acids, arachidonic acid (C20:4n-6) and eicosapentaenoic acid (C20:5n-3, EPA), after release from membrane phospholipids (Fig. 5). Eicosanoids of the n-2 series such as thromboxane A_2 (TXA$_2$) are synthesized from the n-6 fatty acid arachidonic acid in platelets, while prostaglandin I_2 (PGI$_2$) is synthesized in the vascular endothelium. TXA$_2$ is a potent vasoconstrictor and a stimulus for platelet aggregation, whereas PGI$_2$ has opposite effects. Eicosanoids of the n-3 series such as thromboxane A_3 (TXA$_3$) and prostacyclin (PGI$_3$) are principal metabolites of the n-3 fatty acid EPA. However, TXA$_3$ is biologically less active than TXA$_2$, while the anti-aggregatory effects of PGI$_3$ and PGI$_2$ are comparable. This may explain why fish oils lower platelet aggregation (Abeywardena and Head 2001).

Eicosanoids have a short half-life time and are quickly catabolized into their stable metabolites, such as TXB$_2$ and 6-keto-PGF$_{1\alpha}$. These metabolites

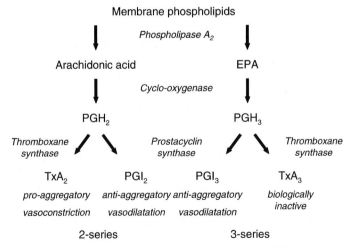

Fig. 5 Formation of eicosanoids from n-3 and n-6 polyunsaturated fatty acids

can be converted into respectively 2,3 dinor-TXB_2 or 11-dehydro-TXB_2, and 2,3 dinor-6-keto-$PGF_{1\alpha}$, which are excreted in the urine. In this way, analysis of these urinary metabolites represents a non-invasive surrogate to assess in vivo eicosanoid formation (Oates et al. 1988). In line with the anti-aggregatory effects of fish oils, several studies showed that n-3 fatty acids indeed decreased urinary excretion of TXA_2 metabolites. Prostaglandin excretion, however, was not always affected (Abeywardena and Head 2001; Lahoz et al. 1997). With respect to saturated fatty acids, lauric, myristic, palmitic and stearic acids had similar effects on urinary thromboxane and prostaglandin excretion (Blair et al. 1994; Mustad et al. 1993). Also, the effects of *trans* fatty acids were comparable with those of stearic acid (Turpeinen et al. 1998b). Furthermore, n-6 polyunsaturated fatty acids increased urinary 11-dehydro-TXB_2 excretion compared with saturated and monounsaturated fatty acids, which seemed to reflect ADP-induced platelet aggregation results (Lahoz et al. 1997).

5.3
Blood Coagulation

Important risk markers of the blood coagulation system associated with cardiovascular events are factor VII, fibrinogen and prothrombin fragment 1+2 (Miller et al. 1996). Factor VII plays a key role in the initiation of the tissue factor pathway of blood coagulation. Ultimately, the blood coagulation cascade results in the formation of an insoluble fibrin clot from fibrinogen, which can be cleaved by thrombin. Fragment 1+2, a prothrombin fragment, reflects the amount of prothrombin converted into thrombin.

5.3.1
Factor VII

Increased concentrations of coagulation factor VII, which are associated with fatal cardiovascular events (Miller et al. 1996), can be lowered by reducing total fat intake. In contrast, effects of the individual fatty acids were negligible, although some studies have indicated that stearic acid may slightly decrease factor VII (Kelly et al. 2001b; Tholstrup et al. 1994a). This, however, might be explained by the poorer digestibility and absorption of the high-stearic acid fats used in these studies. Interestingly, in one study it was reported that replacement of oleic acid for lauric or palmitic acids increased factor VII activity only in women (Temme et al. 1999). These sex-specific effects need to be confirmed in future experiments. Markedly, while n-3 fatty acids from fish oil affected platelet aggregation favourably, no effects on factor VII were observed (Agren et al. 1997).

Likewise, post-prandial studies have indicated that the total fat content of the diet, rather than the fatty acid composition, increased factor VII concentrations (Hunter et al. 1999; Sanders et al. 2000). In one study, post-prandial increases in activity of factor VII were less after consumption of meals rich in saturated fat, especially stearic acid, than after consumption of meals enriched with unsaturated fatty acids (Tholstrup et al. 2003).

5.3.2
Fibrinogen

Although fibrinogen plays a crucial role in the clotting cascade to stabilize a loose thrombus, it is doubtful whether this functional role of fibrinogen explains the association between fibrinogen and atherosclerosis (Miller et al. 1996). Because fibrinogen is also an acute phase reactant, fibrinogen concentrations might also increase, at least in part, as a consequence of inflammatory reactions that occur in atherosclerosis. However, dietary fatty acid composition does not seem to regulate fibrinogen levels (Agren et al. 1997; Hunter et al. 2000; Junker et al. 2001; Temme et al. 1999; Tholstrup et al. 1994b).

5.3.3
Prothrombin Fragment 1+2

Fasting prothrombin fragment 1+2 concentrations are not changed by the fatty acid composition of the diet (Agren et al. 1997; Hunter et al. 2000; Junker et al. 2001; Temme et al. 1999). Post-prandially, however, concentrations increased after a high-fat meal independently of the fatty acid composition, which agrees with the finding that high-fat diets increase factor VII (Hunter et al. 2001).

5.4
Fibrinolysis

Fibrinolysis is initiated by the conversion of plasminogen into plasmin through the action of tissue plasminogen activator (tPA). Plasmin catalyses the degradation of cross-linked fibrin of a thrombus. tPA activity is inhibited by plasminogen activator inhibitor-1 (PAI-1). Decreased concentrations of tPA and elevated concentrations of PAI-1 are associated with increased atherosclerotic risk. Furthermore, degradation products of cross-linked fibrin like D-dimers reflect fibrinolytic activity and increased concentrations are surprisingly associated with an increased risk for atherosclerosis (Ridker 1997).

5.4.1
Tissue Plasminogen Activator

Several studies examined the effects of fatty acid composition of the diet on tissue plasminogen activator (tPA) activity, but no different effects of specific fatty acids were found (Hunter et al. 2000; Junker et al. 2001; Mutanen and Aro 1997; Tholstrup et al. 1994a). Also reduction of dietary fat content did not affect tPA activity (Marckmann et al. 1994). Post-prandial tPA levels also did not change significantly from fasting levels after consumption of a high-fat meal (Hunter et al. 2001; Tholstrup et al. 1996). However, in one study diets rich in saturated fatty acids (stearic, palmitic or a mixture of myristic with palmitic acids) resulted in a greater rise in post-prandial tPA concentrations than unsaturated test fats rich in oleic, linoleic or *trans* fatty acids (Tholstrup et al. 2003).

5.4.2
Plasminogen Activator Inhibitor-1

While high-fat diets do not affect plasminogen activator inhibitor-1 (PAI-1) concentrations, effects of the fatty acid composition of the diet on PAI-1 are not uniform. Although some studies concluded that n-3 polyunsaturated fatty acids increased PAI-1 activity, others found no effects. A recent meta-analysis however concluded that fish oil had no specific effects on PAI-1 (Hansen et al. 2000). Effects of other fatty acids on PAI-1 are also marginal, although in one study an increase in PAI-1 activity was found when oleic acid in the diet was replaced by palmitic acid (Temme et al. 1999). Post-prandially, however, PAI-1 concentrations decreased, but these changes were not related to the fat content or fatty acid composition of the diet (Hunter et al. 2001; Salomaa et al. 1993).

5.4.3
D-dimers

No changes in D-dimers concentrations after consumption of specific fatty acids have been detected (Junker et al. 2001; Mutanen and Aro 1997; Turpeinen and Mutanen 1999).

5.5
Conclusions

Interpretation of the effects of fatty acids on haemostatic risk markers is difficult, partly due to the use of several methods and difficulties in extrapolating in vitro findings to the more complex in vivo situation. The most consistent finding is that n-3 fatty acids lower collagen-induced in vitro platelet aggregation. Furthermore, reducing total fat intake rather than changing the fatty acid composition of the diet may beneficially affect the coagulation system.

6
Concluding Remarks

To prevent the development of atherosclerosis, no doubt exists that the dietary intake of *trans* fatty acids should be as low as possible. Saturated fat intake should also decrease, although effects of the various saturated fatty acids differ. These conclusions are based mainly on effects of fats and oils on the lipoprotein profile, because effects on the other atherosclerotic risk markers discussed in this chapter are less evident. An exception, however, are the potential beneficial effects of moderate intakes of fish oil on inflammatory markers and on platelet aggregation, while total fat intake has unfavourable effects on both fasting and post-prandial factor VII concentrations. Furthermore, monounsaturated fatty acids may be preferable above polyunsaturated fatty acids with respect to oxidative processes measured by indirect in vitro assays. However, this latter conclusion has to be confirmed by direct methods measuring lipid peroxidation products.

The question can then be raised if saturated and *trans* fatty acids have to be replaced by unsaturated fatty acids or by carbohydrates. The favourable effects of unsaturated fatty acids on lipoprotein metabolism might be opposed by unfavourable effects of high-fat diets on thrombotic tendency, mainly due to effects on the coagulation system. Furthermore, high-fat diets might promote weight gain resulting in obesity. Also increased amounts of dietary fat have been related to changes in insulin sensitivity leading to diabetes and increased cancer risk. However, evidence for these latter associations are still a matter of debate. With respect to atherosclerosis, both prospective epidemiological and intervention studies have shown that high-unsaturated fat diets lower atherosclerotic risk (Sacks and Katan 2002). Therefore, fat is not necessarily bad, as long as body weight is not increased. However, when body weight is increased, it is advisable to reduce not only the intake of fat, but also of the other macronutrients.

References

Abeywardena MY, Head RJ (2001) Longchain n-3 polyunsaturated fatty acids and blood vessel function. Cardiovasc Res 52:361–371

Agren JJ, Vaisanen S, Hanninen O, Muller AD, Hornstra G (1997) Hemostatic factors and platelet aggregation after a fish-enriched diet or fish oil or docosahexaenoic acid supplementation. Prostaglandins Leukot Essent Fatty Acids 57:419–421

Berliner JA, Navab M, Fogelman AM, Frank JS, Demer LL, Edwards PA, Watson AD, Lusis AJ (1995) Atherosclerosis: basic mechanisms. Oxidation, inflammation, and genetics. Circulation 91:2488–2496

Blair IA, Dougherty RM, Iacono JM (1994) Dietary stearic acid and thromboxane-prostacyclin biosynthesis in normal human subjects. Am J Clin Nutr 60:1054S–1058S

Blankenberg S, Rupprecht HJ, Bickel C, Peetz D, Hafner G, Tiret L, Meyer J (2001) Circulating cell adhesion molecules and death in patients with coronary artery disease. Circulation 104:1336–1342

Blok WL, Deslypere JP, Demacker PN, van der Ven-Jongekrijg J, Hectors MP, van der Meer JW, Katan MB (1997) Pro- and anti-inflammatory cytokines in healthy volunteers fed various doses of fish oil for 1 year. Eur J Clin Invest 27:1003–8

Bonanome A, Biasia F, De Luca M, Munaretto G, Biffanti S, Pradella M, Pagnan A (1996) n-3 fatty acids do not enhance LDL susceptibility to oxidation in hypertriacylglycerolemic hemodialyzed subjects. Am J Clin Nutr 63:261–266

Bonanome A, Grundy SM (1988) Effect of dietary stearic acid on plasma cholesterol and lipoprotein levels. N Engl J Med 318:1244–1248

Brown AA, Hu FB (2001) Dietary modulation of endothelial function: implications for cardiovascular disease. Am J Clin Nutr 73:673–686

Cater NB, Heller HJ, Denke MA (1997) Comparison of the effects of medium-chain triacylglycerols, palm oil, and high oleic acid sunflower oil on plasma triacylglycerol fatty acids and lipid and lipoprotein concentrations in humans. Am J Clin Nutr 65:41–45

Caughey GE, Mantzioris E, Gibson RA, Cleland LG, James MJ (1996) The effect on human tumor necrosis factor alpha and interleukin 1 beta production of diets enriched in n-3 fatty acids from vegetable oil or fish oil. Am J Clin Nutr 63:116–122

Choudhury N, Tan L, Truswell AS (1995) Comparison of palmolein and olive oil: effects on plasma lipids and vitamin E in young adults. Am J Clin Nutr 61:1043–1051.

De Caterina R, Bernini W, Carluccio MA, Liao JK, Libby P (1998) Structural requirements for inhibition of cytokine-induced endothelial activation by unsaturated fatty acids. J Lipid Res 39:1062–1070

de Graaf J, Hak-Lemmers HL, Hectors MP, Demacker PN, Hendriks JC, Stalenhoef AF (1991) Enhanced susceptibility to in vitro oxidation of the dense low density lipoprotein subfraction in healthy subjects. Arterioscler Thromb 11:298–306

Denke MA, Grundy SM (1992) Comparison of effects of lauric acid and palmitic acid on plasma lipids and lipoproteins. Am J Clin Nutr 56:895–898

Dreon DM, Fernstrom HA, Williams PT, Krauss RM (1999) A very low-fat diet is not associated with improved lipoprotein profiles in men with a predominance of large, low-density lipoproteins. Am J Clin Nutr 69:411–418

Elwood PC, Renaud S, Sharp DS, Beswick AD, O'Brien JR, Yarnell JW (1991) Ischemic heart disease and platelet aggregation. The Caerphilly Collaborative Heart Disease Study. Circulation 83:38–44

Endres S, Ghorbani R, Kelley VE, Georgilis K, Lonnemann G, van der Meer JW, Cannon JG, Rogers TS, Klempner MS, Weber PC, et al. (1989) The effect of dietary supplementation with n-3 polyunsaturated fatty acids on the synthesis of interleukin-1 and tumor necrosis factor by mononuclear cells. N Engl J Med 320:265–271

Engelberts I, Sundram K, Van Houwelingen AC, Hornstra G, Kester AD, Ceska M, Francot GJ, van der Linden CJ, Buurman WA (1993) The effect of replacement of dietary fat by palm oil on in vitro cytokine release. Br J Nutr 69:159–167

Ernst E, Saradeth T, Achhammer G (1991) n-3 fatty acids and acute-phase proteins. Eur J Clin Invest 21:77–82

Finnegan YE, Howarth D, Minihane AM, Kew S, Miller GJ, Calder PC, Williams CM (2003) Plant and marine derived (n-3) polyunsaturated fatty acids do not affect blood coagulation and fibrinolytic factors in moderately hyperlipidemic humans. J Nutr 133:2210–2213

Gearing AJ, Newman W (1993) Circulating adhesion molecules in disease. Immunol Today 14:506–512

Gordon DJ, Rifkind BM (1989) High-density lipoprotein–the clinical implications of recent studies. N Engl J Med 321:1311–1316

Grundy SM (1986) Comparison of monounsaturated fatty acids and carbohydrates for lowering plasma cholesterol. N Engl J Med 314:745–748

Han SN, Leka LS, Lichtenstein AH, Ausman LM, Schaefer EJ, Meydani SN (2002) Effect of hydrogenated and saturated, relative to polyunsaturated, fat on immune and inflammatory responses of adults with moderate hypercholesterolemia. J Lipid Res 43:445–452

Hansen J, Grimsgaard S, Nordoy A, Bonaa KH (2000) Dietary supplementation with highly purified eicosapentaenoic acid and docosahexaenoic acid does not influence PAI-1 activity. Thromb Res 98:123–132

Hargrove RL, Etherton TD, Pearson TA, Harrison EH, Kris-Etherton PM (2001) Low fat and high monounsaturated fat diets decrease human low density lipoprotein oxidative susceptibility in vitro. J Nutr 131:1758–1763

Harris WS (1997) n-3 fatty acids and serum lipoproteins: human studies. Am J Clin Nutr 65:1645S–1654S

Hegsted DM, McGandy RB, Myers ML, Stare FJ (1965) Quantitative effects of dietary fat on serum cholesterol in man. Am J Clin Nutr 17:281–295

Higdon JV, Liu J, Du SH, Morrow JD, Ames BN, Wander RC (2000) Supplementation of postmenopausal women with fish oil rich in eicosapentaenoic acid and docosahexaenoic acid is not associated with greater in vivo lipid peroxidation compared with oils rich in oleate and linoleate as assessed by plasma malondialdehyde and F(2)-isoprostanes. Am J Clin Nutr 72:714–722

Higgins S, Carroll YL, McCarthy SN, Corridan BM, Roche HM, Wallace JM, O'Brien NM, Morrissey PA (2001) Susceptibility of LDL to oxidative modification in healthy volunteers supplemented with low doses of n-3 polyunsaturated fatty acids. Br J Nutr 85:23–31

Hodson L, Skeaff CM, Chisholm WA (2001) The effect of replacing dietary saturated fat with polyunsaturated or monounsaturated fat on plasma lipids in free-living young adults. Eur J Clin Nutr 55:908–915

Hokanson JE, Austin MA (1996) Plasma triglyceride level is a risk factor for cardiovascular disease independent of high-density lipoprotein cholesterol level: a meta-analysis of population-based prospective studies. J Cardiovasc Risk 3:213–219

Holvoet P, Perez G, Zhao Z, Brouwers E, Bernar H, Collen D (1995) Malondialdehyde-modified low density lipoproteins in patients with atherosclerotic disease. J Clin Invest 95:2611–2619

Holvoet P, Vanhaecke J, Janssens S, Van de Werf F, Collen D (1998) Oxidized LDL and malondialdehyde-modified LDL in patients with acute coronary syndromes and stable coronary artery disease. Circulation 98:1487–1494

Howard BV, Hannah JS, Heiser CC, Jablonski KA, Paidi MC, Alarif L, Robbins DC, Howard WJ (1995) Polyunsaturated fatty acids result in greater cholesterol lowering and less triacylglycerol elevation than do monounsaturated fatty acids in a dose-response comparison in a multiracial study group. Am J Clin Nutr 62:392–402

Hughes DA, Pinder AC, Piper Z, Johnson IT, Lund EK (1996) Fish oil supplementation inhibits the expression of major histocompatibility complex class II molecules and adhesion molecules on human monocytes. Am J Clin Nutr 63:267–272

Hunter KA, Crosbie LC, Horgan GW, Miller GJ, Dutta-Roy AK (2001) Effect of diets rich in oleic acid, stearic acid and linoleic acid on postprandial haemostatic factors in young healthy men. Br J Nutr 86:207–215

Hunter KA, Crosbie LC, Weir A, Miller GJ, Dutta-Roy AK (1999) The effects of structurally defined triglycerides of differing fatty acid composition on postprandial haemostasis in young, healthy men. Atherosclerosis 142:151–158

Hunter KA, Crosbie LC, Weir A, Miller GJ, Dutta-Roy AK (2000) A residential study comparing the effects of diets rich in stearic acid, oleic acid, and linoleic acid on fasting blood lipids, hemostatic variables and platelets in young healthy men. J Nutr Biochem 11:408–416

Jialal I, Devaraj S (1996) Low-density lipoprotein oxidation, antioxidants, and atherosclerosis: a clinical biochemistry perspective. Clin Chem 42:498–506

Judd JT, Clevidence BA, Muesing RA, Wittes J, Sunkin ME, Podczasy JJ (1994) Dietary *trans* fatty acids: effects on plasma lipids and lipoproteins of healthy men and women. Am J Clin Nutr 59:861–868

Junker R, Kratz M, Neufeld M, Erren M, Nofer JR, Schulte H, Nowak-Gottl U, Assmann G, Wahrburg U (2001) Effects of diets containing olive oil, sunflower oil, or rapeseed oil on the hemostatic system. Thromb Haemost 85:280–286

Katan MB, Zock PL, Mensink RP (1994) Effects of fats and fatty acids on blood lipids in humans: an overview. Am J Clin Nutr 60:1017S–1022S

Kelley DS (2001) Modulation of human immune and inflammatory responses by dietary fatty acids. Nutrition 17:669–673

Kelley DS, Taylor PC, Nelson GJ, Mackey BE (1998) Arachidonic acid supplementation enhances synthesis of eicosanoids without suppressing immune functions in young healthy men. Lipids 33:125–130

Kelly CM, Smith RD, Williams CM (2001a) Dietary monounsaturated fatty acids and haemostasis. Proc Nutr Soc 60:161–170

Kelly FD, Sinclair AJ, Mann NJ, Turner AH, Abedin L, Li D (2001b) A stearic acid-rich diet improves thrombogenic and atherogenic risk factor profiles in healthy males. Eur J Clin Nutr 55:88–96

Keys A (1970) Coronary heart disease in seven countries. Circulation 41: 191–198

Keys A, Anderson JT, Grande F (1965) Serum cholesterol response to changes in the diet. IV. Particular saturated fatty acids in the diet. Metabolism 14:776–787

Keys A, Anderson JT, Grande F (1975) Serum cholesterol response to changes in the diet. IV. Particular saturated fatty acids in the diet. Metabolism 14:776–787

Kratz M, Cullen P, Kannenberg F, Kassner A, Fobker M, Abuja PM, Assmann G, Wahrburg U (2002) Effects of dietary fatty acids on the composition and oxidizability of low-density lipoprotein. Eur J Clin Nutr 56:72–81

Kris-Etherton PM, Derr J, Mitchell DC, Mustad VA, Russell ME, McDonnell ET, Salabsky D, Pearson TA (1993) The role of fatty acid saturation on plasma lipids, lipoproteins, and apolipoproteins: I. Effects of whole food diets high in cocoa butter, olive oil, soybean oil, dairy butter, and milk chocolate on the plasma lipids of young men. Metabolism 42:121–129

Lahoz C, Alonso R, Ordovas JM, Lopez-Farre A, de Oya M, Mata P (1997) Effects of dietary fat saturation on eicosanoid production, platelet aggregation and blood pressure. Eur J Clin Invest 27:780–787

Leigh-Firbank EC, Minihane AM, Leake DS, Wright JW, Murphy MC, Griffin BA, Williams CM (2002) Eicosapentaenoic acid and docosahexaenoic acid from fish oils: differential associations with lipid responses. Br J Nutr 87:435–445

Lusis AJ (2000) Atherosclerosis. Nature 407:233–241

Madsen T, Christensen JH, Blom M, Schmidt EB (2003) The effect of dietary n-3 fatty acids on serum concentrations of C-reactive protein: a dose-response study. Br J Nutr 89:517–522

Marckmann P, Sandstrom B, Jespersen J (1994) Low-fat, high-fiber diet favorably affects several independent risk markers of ischemic heart disease: observations on blood lipids, coagulation, and fibrinolysis from a trial of middle-aged Danes. Am J Clin Nutr 59:935–939

Mata P, Alonso R, Lopez-Farre A, Ordovas JM, Lahoz C, Garces C, Caramelo C, Codoceo R, Blazquez E, de Oya M (1996) Effect of dietary fat saturation on LDL oxidation and monocyte adhesion to human endothelial cells in vitro. Arterioscler Thromb Vasc Biol 16:1347–1355

Mattson FH, Grundy SM (1985) Comparison of effects of dietary saturated, monounsaturated, and polyunsaturated fatty acids on plasma lipids and lipoproteins in man. J Lipid Res 26:194–202

Mensink RP, Katan MB (1987) Effect of monounsaturated fatty acids versus complex carbohydrates on high-density lipoproteins in healthy men and women. Lancet 1:122–125

Mensink RP, Katan MB (1989) Effect of a diet enriched with monounsaturated or polyunsaturated fatty acids on levels of low-density and high-density lipoprotein cholesterol in healthy women and men. N Engl J Med 321:436–441

Mensink RP, Katan MB (1990) Effect of dietary *trans* fatty acids on high-density and low-density lipoprotein cholesterol levels in healthy subjects. N Engl J Med 323:439–445

Mensink RP, Zock PL, Kester AD, Katan MB (2003) Effects of dietary fatty acids and carbohydrates on the ratio of serum total to HDL cholesterol and on serum lipids and apolipoproteins: a meta-analysis of 60 controlled trials. Am J Clin Nutr 77:1146–1155

Miller GJ, Bauer KA, Barzegar S, Cooper JA, Rosenberg RD (1996) Increased activation of the haemostatic system in men at high risk of fatal coronary heart disease. Thromb Haemost 75:767–771

Mustad VA, Kris-Etherton PM, Derr J, Reddy CC, Pearson TA (1993) Comparison of the effects of diets rich in stearic acid versus myristic acid and lauric acid on platelet fatty acids and excretion of thromboxane A2 and PGI2 metabolites in healthy young men. Metabolism 42:463–469

Mutanen M (1997) *Cis*-unsaturated fatty acids and platelet function. Prostaglandins Leukot Essent Fatty Acids 57:403–410

Mutanen M, Aro A (1997) Coagulation and fibrinolysis factors in healthy subjects consuming high stearic or *trans* fatty acid diets. Thromb Haemost 77:99–104

Mutanen M, Freese R, Valsta LM, Ahola I, Ahlstrom A (1992) Rapeseed oil and sunflower oil diets enhance platelet in vitro aggregation and thromboxane production in healthy men when compared with milk fat or habitual diets. Thromb Haemost 67:352–356

Ng TK, Hayes KC, DeWitt GF, Jegathesan M, Satgunasingam N, Ong AS, Tan D (1992) Dietary palmitic and oleic acids exert similar effects on serum cholesterol and lipoprotein profiles in normocholesterolemic men and women. J Am Coll Nutr 11:383–390

Oates JA, FitzGerald GA, Branch RA, Jackson EK, Knapp HR, Roberts LJ, 2nd (1988) Clinical implications of prostaglandin and thromboxane A2 formation (1). N Engl J Med 319:689–698

Oostenbrug GS, Mensink RP, Hornstra G (1994) Effects of fish oil and vitamin E supplementation on copper-catalysed oxidation of human low density lipoprotein in vitro. Eur J Clin Nutr 48:895–898

Rallidis LS, Paschos G, Liakos GK, Velissaridou AH, Anastasiadis G, Zampelas A (2003) Dietary alpha-linolenic acid decreases C-reactive protein, serum amyloid A and interleukin-6 in dyslipidaemic patients. Atherosclerosis 167:237–242

Reilly MP, Pratico D, Delanty N, DiMinno G, Tremoli E, Rader D, Kapoor S, Rokach J, Lawson J, FitzGerald GA (1998) Increased formation of distinct F2 isoprostanes in hypercholesterolemia. Circulation 98:2822–2828

Ridker PM (1997) Fibrinolytic and inflammatory markers for arterial occlusion: the evolving epidemiology of thrombosis and hemostasis. Thromb Haemost 78:53–59

Ridker PM, Hennekens CH, Buring JE, Rifai N (2000) C-reactive protein and other markers of inflammation in the prediction of cardiovascular disease in women. N Engl J Med 342:836–843

Sacks FM, Katan M (2002) Randomized clinical trials on the effects of dietary fat and carbohydrate on plasma lipoproteins and cardiovascular disease. Am J Med 113 Suppl 9B: 13S–24S

Salomaa V, Rasi V, Pekkanen J, Jauhiainen M, Vahtera E, Pietinen P, Korhonen H, Kuulasmaa K, Ehnholm C (1993) The effects of saturated fat and n-6 polyunsaturated fat on postprandial lipemia and hemostatic activity. Atherosclerosis 103:1–11

Sanders TA, de Grassi T, Miller GJ, Morrissey JH (2000) Influence of fatty acid chain length and *cis/trans* isomerization on postprandial lipemia and factor VII in healthy subjects (postprandial lipids and factor VII). Atherosclerosis 149:413–420

Stampfer MJ, Sacks FM, Salvini S, Willett WC, Hennekens CH (1991) A prospective study of cholesterol, apolipoproteins, and the risk of myocardial infarction. N Engl J Med 325:373–381

Temme EH, Mensink RP, Hornstra G (1996) Comparison of the effects of diets enriched in lauric, palmitic, or oleic acids on serum lipids and lipoproteins in healthy women and men. Am J Clin Nutr 63:897–903

Temme EH, Mensink RP, Hornstra G (1997) Effects of medium chain fatty acids (MCFA), myristic acid, and oleic acid on serum lipoproteins in healthy subjects. J Lipid Res 38:1746–1754

Temme EH, Mensink RP, Hornstra G (1998) Individual saturated fatty acids and effects on whole blood aggregation in vitro. Eur J Clin Nutr 52:697–702

Temme EH, Mensink RP, Hornstra G (1999) Effects of diets enriched in lauric, palmitic or oleic acids on blood coagulation and fibrinolysis. Thromb Haemost 81:259–263

Thies F, Miles EA, Nebe-von-Caron G, Powell JR, Hurst TL, Newsholme EA, Calder PC (2001) Influence of dietary supplementation with long-chain n-3 or n-6 polyunsaturated fatty acids on blood inflammatory cell populations and functions and on plasma soluble adhesion molecules in healthy adults. Lipids 36:1183–1193

Tholstrup T, Andreasen K, Sanstrom B (1996) Acute effect of high-fat meals rich in either stearic or myristic acid on hemostatic factors in healthy young men. Am J Clin Nutr 64:168–176

Tholstrup T, Marckmann P, Jespersen J, Sandstrom B (1994a) Fat high in stearic acid favorably affects blood lipids and factor VII coagulant activity in comparison with fats high in palmitic acid or high in myristic and lauric acids. Am J Clin Nutr 59:371–377

Tholstrup T, Marckmann P, Jespersen J, Vessby B, Jart A, Sandstrom B (1994b) Effect on blood lipids, coagulation, and fibrinolysis of a fat high in myristic acid and a fat high in palmitic acid. Am J Clin Nutr 60:919–925

Tholstrup T, Miller GJ, Bysted A, Sandstrom B (2003) Effect of individual dietary fatty acids on postprandial activation of blood coagulation factor VII and fibrinolysis in healthy young men. Am J Clin Nutr 77:1125–1132

Toborek M, Lee YW, Garrido R, Kaiser S, Hennig B (2002) Unsaturated fatty acids selectively induce an inflammatory environment in human endothelial cells. Am J Clin Nutr 75:119–125

Turpeinen AM, Mutanen M (1999) Similar effects of diets high in oleic or linoleic acids on coagulation and fibrinolytic factors in healthy humans. Nutr Metab Cardiovasc Dis 9:65–72

Turpeinen AM, Pajari AM, Freese R, Sauer R, Mutanen M (1998a) Replacement of dietary saturated by unsaturated fatty acids: effects of platelet protein kinase C activity, urinary content of 2,3-dinor-TXB2 and in vitro platelet aggregation in healthy man. Thromb Haemost 80:649–655

Turpeinen AM, Wubert J, Aro A, Lorenz R, Mutanen M (1998b) Similar effects of diets rich in stearic acid or *trans*-fatty acids on platelet function and endothelial prostacyclin production in humans. Arterioscler Thromb Vasc Biol 18:316–322

Wallace FA, Miles EA, Calder PC (2003) Comparison of the effects of linseed oil and different doses of fish oil on mononuclear cell function in healthy human subjects. Br J Nutr 89:679–689

Yaqoob P, Knapper JA, Webb DH, Williams CM, Newsholme EA, Calder PC (1998) Effect of olive oil on immune function in middle-aged men. Am J Clin Nutr 67:129–135

Young JL, Libby P, Schonbeck U (2002) Cytokines in the pathogenesis of atherosclerosis. Thromb Haemost 88:554–567

Yu H, Rifai N (2000) High-sensitivity C-reactive protein and atherosclerosis: from theory to therapy. Clin Biochem 33:601–610

Zock PL, de Vries JH, Katan MB (1994) Impact of myristic acid versus palmitic acid on serum lipid and lipoprotein levels in healthy women and men. Arterioscler Thromb 14:567–575

Zock PL, Katan MB (1992) Hydrogenation alternatives: effects of *trans* fatty acids and stearic acid versus linoleic acid on serum lipids and lipoproteins in humans. J Lipid Res 33:399–410

HEP (2005) 170:195–213
© Springer-Verlag Berlin Heidelberg 2005

Dietary Cholesterol, Atherosclerosis and Coronary Heart Disease

M. Kratz

Division of Metabolism, Endocrinology and Nutrition, University of Washington, School of Medicine, P.O. Box 356426, Seattle WA, 98195–6426, USA
mkratz@u.washington.edu

Abstract As early as at the beginning of the last century, animal studies have pointed to a causal role of dietary cholesterol in atherogenesis. In humans, however, most observational studies have not provided convincing evidence for an impact of cholesterol intake on coronary heart disease (CHD). Rather, these studies have consistently established a close association between a certain eating pattern and the risk of CHD. This eating pattern has usually been characterized by a high intake of total fat, saturated fatty acids (SFA) and cholesterol, and a low intake of fiber and polyunsaturated fatty acids (PUFA). In typical western diets the amounts of total fat, SFA, and cholesterol are strongly correlated with each other, while they are negatively related to the intake of fiber and PUFA. Thus, it has not been possible to determine whether the association between the above mentioned eating pattern and CHD is due to the high consumption of SFA, cholesterol, both, or an insufficient supply of one or more protective factors such as fiber or PUFA. As the consumption of eggs leads to a high intake of cholesterol without necessarily resulting in high uptake levels of SFA and total fat, several groups have tried to elucidate the effect of cholesterol by investigating the relationship between the consumption of eggs and the development of CHD. Based on these studies, the association between dietary cholesterol and CHD risk is, if anything, minor in nature. This is consistent with the finding that an increase in dietary cholesterol intake results in only a minimal increase in the total/high-density lipoprotein cholesterol ratio. Taken together these studies suggest that the association between dietary cholesterol and CHD is small, as most subjects can effectively adapt to higher levels of cholesterol intake. Nevertheless, lowering dietary cholesterol content might reduce the risk of CHD considerably in a subgroup of individuals who are highly responsive to changes in cholesterol intake.

Keywords Cholesterol · Atherosclerosis · Coronary heart disease · Diet

1
Introduction

For more than a decade now scientists have tried to elucidate whether dietary changes can beneficially affect the risk of individuals to coronary heart disease (CHD). It was noted very early that atherosclerotic lesions consist largely of cholesterol (Cowdry 1933). Thus, it was assumed as early as the beginning of the last century that the amount of cholesterol in the diet might be a major contributing factor in the development of atherosclerotic lesions. The early suggestion that dietary cholesterol induces or exacerbates atherosclerosis led to the conduction of feeding experiments in a variety of animal models. These experiments will be briefly discussed in Sect. 2.1. However, soon more and more questions arose on whether the findings yielded in these experiments were transferable to CHD in humans. This brought about a large number of observational and interventional studies in humans (Sect. 2.2). Soon it was discovered that serum concentrations of total, low-density lipoprotein (LDL)- and high-density lipoprotein (HDL)-cholesterol are closely associated with CHD risk. Numerous studies were then conducted to elucidate the impact of dietary cholesterol on the serum levels of these lipids in order to assess the qualitative and quantitative relationship between dietary cholesterol and CHD risk indirectly. Findings from these studies will be discussed in Sect. 3, along with a brief summary of the basics of cholesterol metabolism.

2
Dietary Cholesterol, Atherosclerosis and CHD

2.1
Animal Studies

At the beginning of the twentieth century, Russian scientists were the first to generate atherosclerotic lesions in rabbits by feeding them diets rich in meat, milk, and/or eggs (Weiss and Minot 1933). First, it was assumed that overconsumption of animal protein was the cause of the observed vascular changes. However, Anitschkow (1933) suspected dietary cholesterol to be causally related to atherosclerosis. This hypothesis was corroborated when he could induce atherosclerotic lesions in rabbits by feeding them vegetable oil enriched in cholesterol (Anitschkow 1933). Since those days, numerous studies using a variety of different species have provided general support for the idea that the consumption of a diet rich in cholesterol is associated with the development of atherosclerotic lesions (reviewed by Cowdry 1933 and Kritchevsky 1995). However, transferring these findings to the human situation is questionable. Recent years have provided more and more evidence of species differences in lipid and lipoprotein metabolism, atherosclerotic lesion formation, the localization of lesions, and the events leading to a clinical event such as plaque rupture or hemostasis and thrombosis (Moghadasian et al. 2001; Rosenfeld et al. 2002). Inference from the animal model to humans is most obviously aggravated by the fact that the susceptibility to dietary cholesterol varies widely even between closely related species. For example, Rudel (1997) recently compared the atherogenic response of five different primate species to dietary fat and cholesterol. From all the animals used for experiments on dietary cholesterol and atherosclerosis these nonhuman primates are most closely related to humans. The serum total and LDL-cholesterol response to dietary cholesterol differed widely between the five species. Upon enrichment of a saturated fatty acid (SFA)-rich diet with cholesterol, LDL-cholesterol increased between 361% and 1,094%, while HDL-cholesterol decreased in most species. In all species, this effect of dietary cholesterol on LDL-cholesterol was several fold more pronounced than what can be expected even in the most cholesterol-responsive human subjects (compare Sect. 3). Also, the reduction of HDL-cholesterol concentrations upon consumption of a cholesterol-enriched diet implies that lipoprotein metabolism is very differently regulated in human beings and these nonhuman primates. These studies of different animal species have undoubtedly provided much valuable insight into the biochemical and physiological processes involved in atherogenesis. Nevertheless, these experiments have not been helpful in answering the question of whether small changes in dietary cholesterol intake have an effect on the risk of CHD in humans. Thus, this article will summarize the relevant data from studies in humans that have either directly or indirectly tried to shed light on this subject.

2.2
Human Studies

2.2.1
Intervention Studies

In humans, controlled long-term primary prevention or intervention studies that investigate the impact of dietary changes on CHD risk are hard to conduct. First of all, it is difficult to ensure compliance of the subjects for a prolonged period of time. Also, ethical concerns more or less forbid the long-term administration of study diets that are hypothesized to be atherogenic. Nevertheless, some intervention studies, mostly with institutionalized subjects, have been published that investigated the effect of dietary manipulations on CHD. In these studies, however, the dietary cholesterol content was changed along with the fatty acid composition, which makes it difficult to determine the impact of dietary cholesterol alone.

Among the first intervention studies to be published was the London Medical Research Council Study. In this study, 393 male myocardial infarction survivors were randomized either into a control group or to receive dietetic advice to minimize SFA and cholesterol intake and to include a plant oil rich in ω-6-polyunsaturated fatty acids (PUFA) into their diet (Research Committee to the Medical Research Council 1968). After a period of 2–7 years there were no statistically significant differences between these groups with regard to major relapses or deaths from CHD. In the Oslo Diet-Heart Study (Leren 1970), 412 male survivors of a myocardial infarction were randomized to either the typical Norwegian diet or to the experimental group. The latter was given dietary advice to reduce their intake of SFA and cholesterol and to increase their intake of oils rich in ω-6-PUFA. The study duration was 5 years with a subsequent 6-year follow-up. Eleven years after the beginning of the study, 79 subjects had died from CHD in the experimental diet group compared to 94 in the control group ($P=0.004$).

While the dietary intervention in these two studies consisted of dietary advice to consume a more 'healthy' diet, two studies have been conducted where the participants were directly supplied with the respective diets. Dayton and colleagues (1969) published the results of their well controlled randomized dietary intervention trial conducted in 846 middle aged and elderly men, most of whom were free of CHD. These subjects, inhabitants of a U.S. veterans' domicile, were given either a diet rich in SFA and cholesterol or a low-cholesterol diet rich in ω-6-PUFA. After a study period of more than 8 years, 96 subjects in the control group had suffered from primary or secondary end points compared with 66 in the experimental group, which was a highly significant difference. In the Finnish Mental Hospital Study (Miettinen et al. 1983; Turpeinen et al. 1979), male and female patients of a mental hospital, all initially free of CHD, were included into a cross-over study of two dietary periods. The patients of one hospital received a low-cholesterol diet rich in ω-6-PUFA for the first 6 years, followed by the control diet, which was rich in cholesterol and SFA, for another 6 years. The patients in another hospital received these diets in reverse order. In men, there was a highly significant difference between the two dietary regimes with regard to the primary end points ($P=0.001$), which were major electrocardiogram changes or coronary death. In women, this difference was not significant.

Taken together, these intervention studies suggest that the risk of cardiovascular disease and coronary death in primary and possibly also secondary prevention can be reduced by decreasing the intake of cholesterol and SFA while increasing the consumption of ω-6-PUFA. Thus, these studies are in line with the proposition that a reduction in dietary cholesterol might reduce the risk of CHD. However, as the experimental diets in these studies differed in both the dietary fat composition and cholesterol content, they do not provide direct support for a causal role of dietary cholesterol in the etiology of CHD.

2.2.2
Observational Studies

Because of the above mentioned problems with long-term dietary intervention studies, the relationship between dietary cholesterol and CHD has mostly been addressed by observational studies. Epidemiological investigations on diet–disease relationships, however, face the major problem that humans do not consume isolated nutrients, but complex food items that consist of mixtures of known and unknown constituents. Within a diet study, only a limited amount of nutrients, food items or food groups can be assessed. In the available observational studies these usually comprised total energy, protein, carbohydrate, total fat, SFA, monounsaturated fatty acids, PUFA, and cholesterol intake. Because these are highly associated with each other in typical western diets (Howell et al. 1997), it is difficult to discern between their individual effects. For example, food items rich in cholesterol mostly are also rich in total fat and SFA. Another problem is that findings might be confounded by positive or negative associations with nutrients or food items that have not been assessed. For example, eating patterns that provide a high amount of cholesterol usually contain a high amount of meat, dairy or other animal products and a proportionately smaller amount of food items from plant origin such as vegetables, legumes, and fruit. A retrospective case–control study conducted in northern Italy showed that all these food groups in themselves are associated with the risk of CHD. In this study, the habitual food intake of 287 female survivors of a myocardial infarction and 649 controls were analyzed. These data demonstrated that the risk of acute myocardial infarction was directly associated with the consumption of meat, ham, salami, and butter, and inversely with the consumption of fish, carrots, green vegetables, and fresh fruit (Gramenzi et al. 1990). Basically, CHD risk was associated with food items high in total fat, SFA, and cholesterol, while it was negatively associated with food items that, with the exception of fish, contained no cholesterol and only low amounts of SFA. The higher risk associated with the consumption of the animal products might have been due to their higher SFA content, their higher cholesterol content, their lower fiber content, or another as yet unknown factor. The essential point to bear in mind is that from these kinds of studies it is difficult to determine the contributions of individual nutrients or food items to disease.

Up to now, several observational studies have shown positive associations between cholesterol intake and CHD. One of these was the Honolulu Heart Program, a prospective cohort study in more than 8,000 Japanese men (McGee et al. 1984). Main findings were that men who developed CHD had lower average intakes of calories, carbohydrates, and vegetable protein. These men also had higher average intakes from protein, fat, SFA, PUFA (all in percentage of calories), and cholesterol (per 1000 kcal) than those who remained free of CHD. In multivariate analysis including age, systolic blood pressure, serum cholesterol, cigarettes smoked per day, and physical activity, dietary cholesterol intake was still significantly associated with higher risk. This indicates that a high dietary cholesterol intake might, at least partly, increase the incidence of CHD through mechanisms that are independent from its effect on serum cholesterol levels. While this is one possibility, this finding might as well indicate that high dietary cholesterol intake is associated with one or several other dietary factors that affect CHD risk independently from serum lipid concentrations.

An association between dietary cholesterol content and cardiovascular disease has also been found in the Western Electric Study, which prospectively followed 1824 middle-aged men for a period of 25 years (Shekelle et al. 1981; Shekelle and Stamler 1989). An analysis by means of a relative hazards model, which included allowance for age, diastolic blood pressure, cigarettes smoked per day, body mass index, serum cholesterol, and intake of energy, SFA, PUFA, and alcohol showed that a higher cholesterol intake was significantly associated with increased mortality from cardiovascular diseases. Although this information was not provided, the data imply that the general eating pattern must have been different between the quintiles of cholesterol intake. Particularly, the consumption of vegetables, fruit, and legumes is likely to have been distinctly different. In the Ireland-Boston Diet-Heart Study, investigators found that those subjects who died from CHD had a higher intake of SFA and cholesterol and a lower intake of PUFA than those who did not die from CHD (Kushi et al. 1985). Furthermore, a vegetable-foods score and the intake of fiber, vegetable protein, and starch were lower among those who died from CHD. The authors noted that "it is difficult to separate the effects of increased consumption of SFA and dietary cholesterol from those of decreased consumption of vegetable protein and fiber, since these two usually go hand in hand in individual diets." Basically, the same is true for a study published by Mann and colleagues (1997). The main finding from their prospective cohort study was that an increased consumption of total fat, SFA, animal fat, and dietary cholesterol was associated with an increased risk of fatal ischemic heart disease. Taken together, these studies provide support for an association between dietary cholesterol intake and CHD. However, they do not rule out the possibility that dietary cholesterol is more an indicator of a certain 'unhealthy' eating pattern than a crucial causal trigger of the disease.

This problem is further illustrated by findings from the Zutphen Study, the EURODIAB IDDM Complications Study, the Health Professionals Follow-Up Study, and the Seven Countries Study. In the Zutphen Study, dietary cholesterol intake per 1,000 kcal was positively related to CHD (Kromhout and de Lezene Coulander 1984). However, these authors also found energy intake to be inversely related to CHD risk. Dividing the dietary content of a nutrient by another confounding nutritional factor tends to make this variable positively associated with risk of disease (Willett 1998). Accordingly, the authors of the Zutphen Study noted that this relationship was "no longer statistically significant when energy intake per kg of body weight was added to the logistic model." In the EURODIAB IDDM Study, increased intake of cholesterol was related to a higher prevalence of cardiovascular disease (Toeller et al. 1999). However, this association was no longer significant after adjustment for dietary fiber intake. A similar finding was reported by Ascherio et al. (1996) from the Health Professionals Follow-up Study. These investigators also reported that the intake of cholesterol was associated with an increased risk of CHD. In this study, the association was largely explained by confounding differences in fiber intake. In a report of findings from the Seven Countries Study, 25-year death rates from CHD were positively related to the consumption of SFA, *trans* fatty acids, and dietary cholesterol (Kromhout et al. 1995). However, the average intakes of SFA, *trans* fatty acids, and dietary cholesterol of the different cohorts were highly correlated. Therefore, the authors noted that "independent effects of the individual fatty acids and dietary cholesterol on serum cholesterol and CHD mortality could not be analyzed in multivariate analysis."

Rather than identifying a single dietary component associated with increased risk these studies provide strong evidence that a certain eating pattern increases risk. While the identified eating pattern in most studies included a high consumption of dietary cholesterol, it always also included a high intake of SFA, with concomitantly low consumption of putatively protective factors such as PUFA, fiber, vegetables, legumes, and fruit.

Investigators of the Framingham Study tried to circumvent the problem of the association between dietary cholesterol and the intake of SFA, energy, PUFA, and fiber (Dawber et al. 1982). These authors investigated whether egg consumption was associated with the risk of CHD. Eggs provide a high amount of cholesterol without a high amount of total fat and SFA. Also, the uptake of cholesterol through egg consumption does not necessarily have an impact on the whole eating pattern. For example, taking up the amount of cholesterol contained in one egg from meat or dairy products likely leads to a considerable replacement of other foods such as vegetables or fruit. In the Framingham cohort, egg consumption was estimated for a subgroup of 912 subjects, and the relationship with CHD was investigated. No association was found. Essentially the same approach was taken by Hu and colleagues (1999), who analyzed data from two large prospective cohort studies, the Health Professionals Study and the Nurses Health Study. The incidence of nonfatal and fatal CHD and stroke corresponding to the daily egg consumption was determined in 37,851 men and 80,082 women. After adjustment for age, smoking, and other potential CHD risk factors, no evidence for an overall significant association between egg consumption and risk of CHD and stroke was found. The authors found a significant association between egg consumption and CHD and stroke in only a subgroup of diabetic patients. The CHD risk of those patients in the highest quintile of egg consumption (more than one egg per day) was substantially increased compared with the patients in the lowest quintile (less than one egg per week). This latter finding might be explained by certain abnormalities in lipid metabolism that make diabetic subjects more susceptible to dietary cholesterol. The reason for this finding might also be that the impact of dietary cholesterol on CHD is in general minor in nature. Thus, the relationship became apparent only in a subgroup that is generally more prone to the development of cardiovascular disease. Besides this observation, the authors concluded that "these findings suggest that consumption of up to one egg per day is unlikely to have substantial overall impact on the risk of CHD or stroke among healthy men and women."

In addition to the studies discussed above, a large number of observational studies did not find any relationship between the intake of dietary cholesterol and the risk of CHD. Among these were the Honolulu Heart Study, the Puerto Rico Heart-Health Program, the Lipid Research Clinics Prevalence Follow-up Study, the Nurses Health Study, the Alpha-Tocopherol Beta-Carotene Cancer Prevention Study, the Hawaii Cardiovascular Study, and the Frammingham Study (Bassett et al. 1969; Esrey et al. 1996; Finegan et al. 1968; Garcia-Palmieri et al. 1980; Gordon et al. 1981; Hu et al. 1997; Khaw and Barrett-Connor 1987; Morris et al. 1977; Pietinen et al. 1997; Posner et al. 1991; Yano et al.1978).

Taken together, the observational studies conducted to date provide convincing evidence that the development of CHD is promoted by a certain eating pattern that is associated with high cholesterol intake. However, the large number of studies that has not found any association between dietary cholesterol and CHD, and the studies on the impact of egg consumption suggest that dietary cholesterol alone has a minor, if any, effect on CHD.

3
Dietary Cholesterol and Serum Lipid and Lipoprotein Concentrations

3.1
Dietary Cholesterol and Serum Concentrations of Total, LDL-, and HDL-Cholesterol

As both interventional and observational studies have not been able to fully elucidate the impact of dietary cholesterol on CHD, numerous studies have been undertaken to address this issue indirectly by measuring the effect of dietary cholesterol on serum lipid and lipoprotein concentrations. It has been well established that total and LDL-cholesterol levels are positively, and that HDL-cholesterol is negatively associated with risk of CHD. Also, reducing LDL-cholesterol concentrations by means of lipid-lowering drugs has repeatedly been shown to reduce the risk of a cardiovascular event. More details on this issue are provided in the chapter by von Eckardstein, this volume.

Howell and colleagues (1997) conducted a large meta-analysis of 224 studies published on the effect of dietary fat and cholesterol on plasma lipid and lipoprotein concentrations. Based on multivariate regression analyses the predicted serum total cholesterol response to a 100 mg/day increase in dietary cholesterol was an increase of 2.2 mg/dl. However, the authors also observed a large inter-individual variability in response to changes in dietary cholesterol content. In the majority of individuals, an increase in dietary cholesterol intake had a relatively small effect on plasma cholesterol concentrations. Howell et al. ascribe this low responsiveness to dietary cholesterol to "the existence of precise feedback mechanisms balancing the input of exogenous dietary cholesterol and endogenous synthesis of cholesterol". These mechanisms and the metabolic reasons for the distinct inter-individual variability in serum cholesterol response to dietary cholesterol will be discussed in Sect. 3.2. Dietary cholesterol showed a positive bivariate correlation with serum LDL-cholesterol levels, but in multivariate linear regression analysis including the different dietary fatty acids, dietary cholesterol was no longer significantly associated with LDL-cholesterol. Neither was the dietary cholesterol content significantly associated with HDL-cholesterol concentrations in this meta-analysis. By contrast, serum triglyceride concentrations were increased by 1.44 mg/dl for each 100 mg/day increase in dietary cholesterol content.

The findings by Howell and colleagues essentially are in agreement with those of a recent meta-analysis of studies that specifically investigated the effect of dietary cholesterol from eggs on serum lipids and lipoproteins (Weggemans et al. 2001a). In a total of 17 studies conducted on this subject, the authors found an increase in total cholesterol of 2.2 mg/dl and of HDL-cholesterol of 0.3 mg/dl per 100 mg/day increase in dietary cholesterol content. Overall, this led to an increase in the total/HDL-cholesterol ratio by 0.02 units.

Although these two meta-analyses yielded consistent results, it might well be that they underestimated the effect of increases in dietary cholesterol on serum lipids when baseline cholesterol intake is low. This is suggested by an earlier meta-analysis conducted by Paul Hopkins (1992). In contrast to other groups, this author used a nonlinear regression analysis including baseline dietary cholesterol content to evaluate the effect of additional uptake of dietary cholesterol on total serum cholesterol. A good fit to the data of 29 controlled studies was provided by the equation:

$$y = 1.22\left(e^{-0.00384x_0}\right)\left(1 - e^{-0.00136x}\right). \tag{6.1}$$

In this equation, y is the change in serum cholesterol (in mmol/l), x is added dietary cholesterol, and x_0 is baseline dietary cholesterol (both in mg/day). This equation reflects that the serum cholesterol elevating effect of a certain amount of dietary cholesterol is lower at high baseline cholesterol intake levels (Fig. 1).

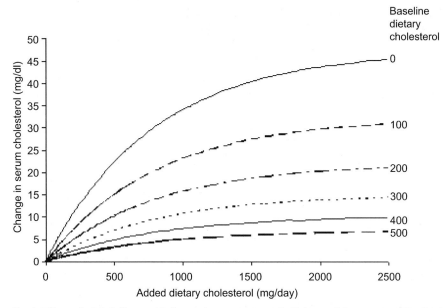

Fig. 1 Effect of added dietary cholesterol on serum total cholesterol [courtesy of Dr. Paul N. Hopkins, reproduced by permission of the American Society for Clinical Nutrition (Hopkins 1992)]. These curves are based on a nonlinear regression analysis model that included baseline dietary cholesterol content to estimate changes in serum total cholesterol concentration in response to changes in dietary cholesterol intake. The increase in serum cholesterol concentration in response to additional cholesterol intake is more pronounced at lower compared with higher baseline cholesterol intake levels

For example, the serum cholesterol concentration of an average person increases by 6.0 mg/dl when dietary cholesterol intake is increased from 0 to 100 mg per day. This figure would drop to a mere increase of 1.3 mg/dl when dietary cholesterol intake was increased from 400 to 500 mg per day. The average American consumes 256 mg cholesterol per day. According to the Hopkins model, the serum cholesterol concentration could on average be lowered by about 6 mg/dl if the intake was lowered to 100 mg per day. While a reduction in total serum cholesterol by 6 mg/dl sounds considerable, one should keep in mind that the reduction in LDL-cholesterol is only slightly more pronounced than that in HDL-cholesterol. Thus, the ratio of LDL-/HDL-cholesterol would on average be reduced only marginally by this measure. Moreover, a further reduction by 60% of the already relatively low intake would call for considerable changes in dietary habits of most Americans. However, there are many individuals who consume much more cholesterol than 256 mg per day. Also, some subjects are much more sensitive to the serum cholesterol-elevating effect of dietary cholesterol. Thus, a reduction in dietary cholesterol intake might lead to a distinctly more pronounced reduction in total and LDL-cholesterol concentrations in these subgroups of the population.

3.2
Factors Affecting Responsiveness to Dietary Cholesterol

Along with a brief summary of the basics of cholesterol metabolism, particularly cholesterol absorption and endogenous synthesis, the possible causes for the differences in responsiveness to dietary cholesterol will be discussed in this chapter.

As mentioned in the previous section, it has been known for several years that the inter-individual serum cholesterol response to dietary cholesterol intake varies widely. In 1986, Katan and colleagues (Katan et al. 1986) reported consistent differences of healthy individuals in their serum cholesterol responses to dietary cholesterol. In a follow-up study, the same group found that the responsiveness of serum cholesterol to dietary cholesterol highly correlates with the responsiveness to dietary SFA (Katan et al. 1988). Thus, it seems that the subgroup of highly responsive subjects would benefit most from a consequent change in the eating pattern to avoid food items rich in SFA and cholesterol.

These inter-individual differences in responsiveness can partly be attributed to differences in percent cholesterol absorption. Bosner and colleagues (1999) measured cholesterol absorption from dietary sources by a dual stable isotope method, and reported a mean absorption rate of 56%, with a wide range from 29% to 80%. In this study, percent cholesterol absorption was significantly higher in African–Americans than in all other racial groups, but was independent of age and sex. Similar absorption rates were found by McNamara and colleagues (1987), while other groups reported somewhat lower numbers in the range of 45% to 47% (Connor and Lin 1974; Heinemann et al. 1993; Miettinen and Kesaniemi 1989). Interestingly, Ostlund et al. (1999) observed that the relative rate of dietary cholesterol absorbed decreases with increasing intake of cholesterol.

As depicted in Fig. 2, cholesterol is incorporated into micelles, which are formed by the interaction between cholesterol, fatty acids, and bile salts. Factors that interfere with this mechanism are the dietary contents of fiber and phytosterols such as β-sitosterol or campesterol (Brown et al. 1999; Law 2000). Therefore, the effect of dietary cholesterol on serum lipid and lipoprotein concentrations is lower on a background diet rich in fiber and phytosterols. The exact mechanism by which cholesterol is then taken up into the enterocyte is not clear. Several mechanisms are feasible. The scavenger receptor class B type 1 has been implicated in the specific removal of cholesterol from mixed micelles, but this mechanism has as yet not been fully elucidated (discussed by Lu et al. 2001). A recent publication by Kramer et al. (2003) suggests that intestinal absorption of cholesterol is not regulated by a single protein, but by a complex machinery that includes an as yet unidentified cholesterol-binding protein of 80 kDa. Also, another integral membrane protein with a molecular weight of 145 kDa seems to be involved in discharging cholesterol back

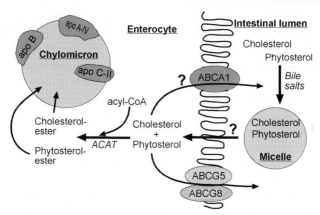

Fig. 2 Basic mechanisms of cholesterol absorption. After being incorporated into micelles, sterols are taken up by enterocytes by an as yet unidentified mechanism. Phytosterols are then discharged back into the intestinal lumen almost completely (see chapter by Tikkanen, this volume), while a portion of the cholesterol might also be discharged, possibly by means of a mechanism involving the ATP-binding cassette transporter A1. The majority of the sterols are then esterified by catalytic activity of the enzyme acyl-coenzyme A: cholesterol acyltransferase, and sterol esters are incorporated into chylomicrons together with triglycerides, phospholipids, and a number of apolipoproteins (apos) including apoB-48, apoC-II and apoA-IV

into the intestinal lumen (Kramer et al. 2003). This function has also been attributed to the ATP-binding cassette transporter A1 (Knight et al. 2003); however, this is not fully supported by all the available data (discussed in Lu et al. 2001).

After cholesterol has been taken up into the enterocyte, it is esterified with a fatty acid by means of acyl-coenzyme A: cholesterol acyltransferase (ACAT). The esterification step catalyzed by ACAT might play a major role in cholesterol absorption. In mice lacking ACAT2, which is specifically expressed in cells of the intestinal mucosa, the capacity to absorb dietary cholesterol was distinctly reduced (Buhman et al. 2000). A large number of other proteins have been implicated in the regulation of cholesterol absorption, including those affecting synthesis and secretion of bile by the liver (summarized in Lu et al. 2001).

After the esterification step, cholesterol esters, triglycerides, phospholipids, and a variety of apolipoproteins (apos) including apoA-IV, apoB-48, and apoC-II are assembled into chylomicrons. Chylomicrons then enter the circulation through the thoracic duct. These large lipoproteins contain about 98% triglycerides, which are hydrolyzed from its surface by means of lipoprotein lipase located at the capillary endothelial surface in muscle and adipose tissue. This turns the chylomicrons into so-called chylomicron remnants, which are relatively richer in cholesterol and protein. Chylomicron remnants are selectively removed from the circulation by binding of their apoE or apoB molecules to their specific receptors on the surface of liver cells. Thus, dietary and biliary cholesterol ultimately enters the liver. Cholesterol esters are hydrolyzed in lysosomes, and enter the intracellular pool of free cholesterol. In hepatocytes, the intracellular free cholesterol pool is important in regulating both endogenous cholesterol synthesis and LDL-receptor expression. If the concentration of intracellular free cholesterol is high, the activities of the key enzyme of cholesterol synthesis, 3-hydroxy-3-methylglutaryl coenzyme A reductase and of the LDL-receptor are suppressed (Dietschy et al. 1993). This results in a reduced endogenous synthesis of cholesterol, a reduced uptake of LDL particles from the circulation and thus an increase in serum LDL-cholesterol concentrations. Free cholesterol can be esterified by ACAT, which reduces the amount of intracellular free cholesterol. This esterification is to a certain degree regulated by the types of fatty acids accessible to ACAT.

Even this basic description of the biochemical and physiological mechanisms involved in cholesterol metabolism makes it clear that defects in a number of different proteins might theoretically have an impact on the serum cholesterol response to dietary cholesterol. Up to now, common polymorphisms in the genes encoding apoA-IV and apoE have most clearly been associated with changed serum lipid responses to dietary cholesterol.

The gene that has been most closely and consistently associated with responsiveness of serum cholesterol to dietary cholesterol has been the apoA-IV gene. Several groups independently found that subjects carrying a glutamine for histidine mutation at amino acid 360 in at least one allele are significantly less responsive to changes in dietary cholesterol (Clifton et al. 1997; McCombs et al. 1994; Ordovas et al. 1995; Weggemans et al. 2001c). Only Weggemans et al. (2000) found no effect of this polymorphism on responsiveness to dietary cholesterol in a group of healthy Dutch subjects.

Sarkkinen and colleagues (1998) found that the apoE genotype modified the lipid response to changes in both dietary fat and cholesterol in mildly hypercholesterolemic subjects. The response to dietary changes was greatest in subjects with apoE genotype 4/4 compared with subjects not carrying an apoE 4 allele. Ordovas et al. (1995) reported a similar finding. According to these authors the apoE genotype effects are modulated by alterations in the amount and composition of dietary fat rather than dietary cholesterol. This latter finding is consistent with a report by Weggemans and colleagues. In their study, the response to dietary cholesterol did not differ between subjects with various apoE genotypes (Weggemans et al. 2001b).

A number of other genes have also been implicated in the responsiveness to dietary fat and cholesterol, including apoA-I, apoC-III, apoB, lipoprotein lipase, cholesterol ester transfer protein, and lecithin-cholesterol acyltransferase. Possible implications of mutations in these genes have recently been summarized and discussed by Ye and Kwiterovich (Ye and Kwiterovich 2000).

The available evidence clearly suggests that most humans are able to adapt to an increase in dietary cholesterol intake to a considerable degree. Reasons for the relatively small impact of dietary cholesterol on serum lipid and lipoprotein concentrations in most subjects include that only a portion of the intestinal cholesterol is absorbed, that the relative amount absorbed decreases with increased intake, and that a reduction in endogenous cholesterol synthesis partly compensates for an increased uptake (McNamara et al. 1987). On the other hand, minor defects in genes encoding proteins involved in cholesterol or lipoprotein metabolism attenuate the adaptive capabilities and increase the responsiveness to dietary cholesterol.

4
Conclusions

Taken together, the studies presented in this chapter support the hypothesis that an eating pattern that is associated with a high intake of dietary cholesterol might increase atherogenesis and the risk of CHD. However, by the strictest scientific standards, the evidence that dietary cholesterol itself is associated with CHD risk is not ultimate. In particular, the strong correlation between dietary cholesterol content and the extent of atherosclerosis seen in animal studies could be explained by large species-differences in the response to dietary cholesterol. In contrast to most animal species including nonhuman primates, the majority of humans is able to effectively adapt to changes in dietary cholesterol intake. Consistent with these findings is the fact that observational studies have not yielded convincing and definite evidence for an effect of dietary cholesterol on CHD risk. These investigations point much more strongly to an effect of a certain eating pattern on disease risk rather than an effect of dietary cholesterol alone. In particular, this eating pattern is characterized by a high intake of food items of animal origin such as meat, cheese, butter, cream and milk, leading to a high intake of total fat, SFA and cholesterol. Also, such a diet pattern usually is associated with a simultaneously lower intake in food items such as vegetables, legumes, whole grain products, plant oils, or fruit. Thus, the increased CHD risk found in a group of individuals with a high intake of SFA and cholesterol might be due to the increased consumption of SFA, or cholesterol, or both. Alternatively, it could also be due to lower consumption of PUFA, fiber, or certain vitamins.

In addition to this frail scientific evidence from observational studies, the relationship between dietary cholesterol and serum lipid and lipoprotein concentrations is, on average, also rather weak. Meta-analyses have shown that dietary cholesterol increases the crucial total-cholesterol/HDL-cholesterol ratio only minimally.

Finally, food items don't consist of isolated nutrients, but are rather complex. For example, the consumption of eggs might slightly increase the total cholesterol/HDL-cholesterol ratio, but other components of eggs might out-weigh this adverse effect in other regards. For example, it was recently reported that the consumption of eggs distinctly reduces postprandial glycemia and in-sulinemia (Pelletier et al. 1996). Eggs have also been shown to be a good source of highly bioavailable lutein and zeaxanthin (Handelman et al. 1999). Thus, in this example, eggs might slightly increase the ratio of total/HDL-cholesterol, but compensate or even overcompensate this by other beneficial health effects. While this is to a certain degree speculative as the health benefits of these features might not be immediately clear, the point this author wants to make is that food items should not be categorized into 'good' and 'bad' foods based on only one component. Natural food is very complex, and it might be a mistake to ignore the vast majority of complex interactions that we as yet do not know enough about.

What the large amount of studies has demonstrated so far is that with regard to CHD risk dietary cholesterol is, if any, only a minor factor in the large majority of the population, especially when compared with other dietary factors such as SFA, unsaturated fats, *trans*-fatty acids, or fiber. However, the explicit recommendation to lower cholesterol intake might nevertheless be appropriate for a subgroup of individuals who respond strongly to dietary cholesterol.

Despite the lack of definitive information on the impact of dietary choles-terol, it is relatively easy to recommend a certain eating pattern for CHD risk prevention in the general population. Rather than single nutrients, the strongest positive association to the risk not only of CHD but also of type 2 di-abetes mellitus and cancer is provided by an eating pattern that is characterized by a high consumption of meat, cheese, butter and cream and a concomitantly low intake of vegetables, legumes, plant oils, whole grains, and fruit. Thus, the mostly recommended eating pattern is low in animal fats but rich in food from plant sources (Krauss et al. 2000). A diet complying with this recommended eating pattern not only is low in cholesterol, but also low in SFA and *trans*-fatty acids and high in PUFA and fiber. It is still the subject of intense discussion whether the consumption of food items that provide dietary cholesterol with-out large amounts of SFA such as eggs or seafood should be restricted in the context of such a diet. The available evidence suggests that this question, however, is of minor importance. For the time being, it should be answered in relation to a patient's overall eating pattern as well as his or her dietary preferences and global cardiovascular risk profile.

Acknowledgements The author would like to thank Rebecca Wittmann and Daniel Rutzick for critically reading the manuscript.

References

Anitschkow (1933) Experimental arteriosclerosis in animals. In: Cowdry EV (ed) Arterios-clerosis—a survey of the problem, 1st edn. The Macmillan Company, New York, pp 271–322

Ascherio A, Rimm EB, Giovannucci EL, Spiegelman D, Stampfer M, Willett WC (1996) Dietary fat and risk of coronary heart disease in men: cohort follow up study in the United States. BMJ 313:84–90

Bassett DR, Abel M, Moellering RC, Jr., Rosenblatt G, Stokes J, III (1969) Coronary heart disease in Hawaii: dietary intake, depot fat, stress, smoking, and energy balance in Hawaiian and Japanese men. Am J Clin Nutr 22:1483–1503

Bosner MS, Lange LG, Stenson WF, Ostlund RE, Jr. (1999) Percent cholesterol absorption in normal women and men quantified with dual stable isotopic tracers and negative ion mass spectrometry. J Lipid Res 40:302–308

Brown L, Rosner B, Willett WW, Sacks FM (1999) Cholesterol-lowering effects of dietary fiber: a meta-analysis. Am J Clin Nutr 69:30–42

Buhman KK, Accad M, Novak S, Choi RS, Wong JS, Hamilton RL, Turley S, Farese RV, Jr. (2000) Resistance to diet-induced hypercholesterolemia and gallstone formation in ACAT2-deficient mice. Nat Med 6:1341–1347

Clifton P, Kind K, Jones C, Noakes M (1997) Response to dietary fat and cholesterol and genetic polymorphisms. Clin Exp Pharmacol Physiol 24:A21–A25

Connor WE, Lin DS (1974) The intestinal absorption of dietary cholesterol by hypercholes-terolemic (type II) and normocholesterolemic humans. J Clin Invest 53:1062–1070

Cowdry EV (1933) Arteriosclerosis—A survey of the problem, 1st edn. The Macmillan Company, New York

Dawber TR, Nickerson RJ, Brand FN, Pool J (1982) Eggs, serum cholesterol, and coronary heart disease. Am J Clin Nutr 36:617–625

Dayton S, Pearce ML, Hashimoto S, Dixon WJ, Tomiyasu U (1969) A controlled clinical trial of a diet high in unsaturated fat in preventing complication of atherosclerosis. Circulation XL:1–63

Dietschy JM, Turley SD, Spady DK (1993) Role of liver in the maintenance of cholesterol and low density lipoprotein homeostasis in different animal species, including humans. J Lipid Res 34:1637–1659

Esrey KL, Joseph L, Grover SA (1996) Relationship between dietary intake and coronary heart disease mortality: lipid research clinics prevalence follow-up study. J Clin Epidemiol 49:211–216

Finegan A, Hickey N, Maurer B, Mulcahy R (1968) Diet and coronary heart disease: dietary analysis on 100 male patients. Am J Clin Nutr 21:143–148

Garcia-Palmieri MR, Sorlie P, Tillotson J, Costas R, Jr., Cordero E, Rodriguez M (1980) Relationship of dietary intake to subsequent coronary heart disease incidence: The Puerto Rico Heart Health Program. Am J Clin Nutr 33:1818–1827

Gordon T, Kagan A, Garcia-Palmieri M, Kannel WB, Zukel WJ, Tillotson J, Sorlie P, Hjortland M (1981) Diet and its relation to coronary heart disease and death in three populations. Circulation 63:500–515

Gramenzi A, Gentile A, Fasoli M, Negri E, Parazzini F, La Vecchia C (1990) Association be-tween certain foods and risk of acute myocardial infarction in women. BMJ 300:771–773

Handelman GJ, Nightingale ZD, Lichtenstein AH, Schaefer EJ, Blumberg JB (1999) Lutein and zeaxanthin concentrations in plasma after dietary supplementation with egg yolk. Am J Clin Nutr 70:247–251

Heinemann T, Axtmann G, von Bergmann K (1993) Comparison of intestinal absorption of cholesterol with different plant sterols in man. Eur J Clin Invest 23:827–831

Hopkins PN (1992) Effects of dietary cholesterol on serum cholesterol: a meta-analysis and review. Am J Clin Nutr 55:1060–1070

Howell WH, McNamara DJ, Tosca MA, Smith BT, Gaines JA (1997) Plasma lipid and lipoprotein responses to dietary fat and cholesterol: a meta-analysis. Am J Clin Nutr 65:1747–1764

Hu FB, Stampfer MJ, Manson JE, Rimm E, Colditz GA, Rosner BA, Hennekens CH, Willett WC (1997) Dietary fat intake and the risk of coronary heart disease in women. N Engl J Med 337:1491–1499

Hu FB, Stampfer MJ, Rimm EB, Manson JE, Ascherio A, Colditz GA, Rosner BA, Spiegelman D, Speizer FE, Sacks FM, Hennekens CH, Willett WC (1999) A prospective study of egg consumption and risk of cardiovascular disease in men and women. JAMA 281:1387–1394

Katan MB, Berns MA, Glatz JF, Knuiman JT, Nobels A, de Vries JH (1988) Congruence of individual responsiveness to dietary cholesterol and to saturated fat in humans. J Lipid Res 29:883–892

Katan MB, Beynen AC, de Vries JH, Nobels A (1986) Existence of consistent hypo- and hyperresponders to dietary cholesterol in man. Am J Epidemiol 123:221–234

Khaw KT, Barrett-Connor E (1987) Dietary fiber and reduced ischemic heart disease mortality rates in men and women: a 12-year prospective study. Am J Epidemiol 126:1093–1102

Knight BL, Patel DD, Humphreys SM, Wiggins D, Gibbons GF (2003) Inhibition of cholesterol absorption associated with a PPAR alpha-dependent increase in ABC binding cassette transporter A1 in mice. J Lipid Res 44:2049–2058

Kramer W, Girbig F, Corsiero D, Burger K, Fahrenholz F, Jung C, Muller G (2003) Intestinal cholesterol absorption: identification of different binding proteins for cholesterol and cholesterol absorption inhibitors in the enterocyte brush border membrane. Biochim Biophys Acta 1633:13–26

Krauss RM, Eckel RH, Howard B, Appel LJ, Daniels SR, Deckelbaum RJ, Erdman JW, Kris-Etherton P, Goldberg IJ, Kotchen TA, Lichtenstein AH, Mitch WE, Mullis R, Robinson K, Wylie-Rosett J, St Jeor S, Suttie J, Tribble DL, Bazzarre TL (2000) AHA Dietary Guidelines: revision 2000: A statement for healthcare professionals from the Nutrition Committee of the American Heart Association. Circulation 102:2284–2299

Kritchevsky D (1995) Dietary protein, cholesterol and atherosclerosis: a review of the early history. J Nutr 125:589S–593S

Kromhout D, de Lezene Coulander C (1984) Diet, prevalence and 10-year mortality from coronary heart disease in 871 middle-aged men. The Zutphen Study. Am J Epidemiol 119:733–741

Kromhout D, Menotti A, Bloemberg B, Aravanis C, Blackburn H, Buzina R, Dontas AS, Fidanza F, Giaipaoli S, Jansen A, Karvonen M, Katan M, Nissinen A, Nedeljkovic S, Pekkanen J, Pekkarinen M, Punsar S, Rasanen L, Simic B, Toshima H (1995) Dietary saturated and *trans*-fatty-acids and cholesterol and 25-year mortality from coronary-heart-disease—the 7 countries study. Prev Med 24:308–315

Kushi LH, Lew RA, Stare FJ, Ellison CR, el Lozy M, Bourke G, Daly L, Graham I, Hickey N, Mulcahy R (1985) Diet and 20-year mortality from coronary heart disease. The Ireland-Boston Diet-Heart Study. N Engl J Med 312:811–818

Law MR (2000) Plant sterol and stanol margarines and health. West J Med 173:43–47

Leren P (1970) The Oslo diet-heart study. Eleven-year report. Circulation 42:935–942

Lu K, Lee MH, Patel SB (2001) Dietary cholesterol absorption; more than just bile. Trends Endocrinol Metab 12:314–320

Mann JI, Appleby PN, Key TJ, Thorogood M (1997) Dietary determinants of ischaemic heart disease in health conscious individuals. Heart 78:450–455

McCombs RJ, Marcadis DE, Ellis J, Weinberg RB (1994) Attenuated hypercholesterolemic response to a high-cholesterol diet in subjects heterozygous for the apolipoprotein A-IV-2 allele. N Engl J Med 331:706–710

McGee DL, Reed DM, Yano K, Kagan A, Tillotson J (1984) Ten-year incidence of coronary heart disease in the Honolulu Heart Program. Relationship to nutrient intake. Am J Epidemiol 119:667–676

McNamara DJ, Kolb R, Parker TS, Batwin H, Samuel P, Brown CD, Ahrens EH, Jr. (1987) Heterogeneity of cholesterol homeostasis in man. Response to changes in dietary fat quality and cholesterol quantity. J Clin Invest 79:1729–1739

Miettinen M, Turpeinen O, Karvonen MJ, Pekkarinen M, Paavilainen E, Elosuo R (1983) Dietary prevention of coronary heart disease in women: the Finnish mental hospital study. Int J Epidemiol 12:17–25

Miettinen TA, Kesaniemi YA (1989) Cholesterol absorption: regulation of cholesterol synthesis and elimination and within-population variations of serum cholesterol levels. Am J Clin Nutr 49:629–635

Moghadasian MH, Frohlich JJ, McManus BM (2001) Advances in experimental dyslipidemia and atherosclerosis. Lab Invest 81:1173–1183

Morris JN, Marr JW, Clayton DG (1977) Diet and heart: a postscript. BMJ 2:1307–1314

Ordovas JM, Lopez-Miranda J, Mata P, Perez-Jimenez F, Lichtenstein AH, Schaefer EJ (1995) Gene-diet interaction in determining plasma lipid response to dietary intervention. Atheroscler 118 Suppl:S11–S27

Ostlund RE, Jr., Bosner MS, Stenson WF (1999) Cholesterol absorption efficiency declines at moderate dietary doses in normal human subjects. J Lipid Res 40:1453–1458

Pelletier X, Thouvenot P, Belbraouet S, Chayvialle JA, Hanesse B, Mayeux D, Debry G (1996) Effect of egg consumption in healthy volunteers: influence of yolk, white or whole-egg on gastric emptying and on glycemic and hormonal responses. Ann Nutr Metab 40:109–115

Pietinen P, Ascherio A, Korhonen P, Hartman AM, Willett WC, Albanes D, Virtamo J (1997) Intake of fatty acids and risk of coronary heart disease in a cohort of Finnish men. The Alpha-Tocopherol, Beta-Carotene Cancer Prevention Study. Am J Epidemiol 145:876–887

Posner BM, Cobb JL, Belanger AJ, Cupples LA, d'Agostino RB, Stokes J, III (1991) Dietary lipid predictors of coronary heart disease in men. The Framingham Study. Arch Intern Med 151:1181–1187

Research Committee to the Medical Research Council (1968) Controlled trial of soya-bean oil in myocardial infarction. Lancet 2:693–699

Rosenfeld ME, Carson KG, Johnson JL, Williams H, Jackson CL, Schwartz SM (2002) Animal models of spontaneous plaque rupture: the holy grail of experimental atherosclerosis research. Curr Atheroscler Rep 4:238–242

Rudel LL (1997) Genetic factors influence the atherogenic response of lipoproteins to dietary fat and cholesterol in nonhuman primates. J Am Coll Nutr 16:306–312

Sarkkinen E, Korhonen M, Erkkila A, Ebeling T, Uusitupa M (1998) Effect of apolipoprotein E polymorphism on serum lipid response to the separate modification of dietary fat and dietary cholesterol. Am J Clin Nutr 68:1215–1222

Shekelle RB, Shryock AM, Paul O, Lepper M, Stamler J, Liu S, Raynor WJ, Jr. (1981) Diet, serum cholesterol, and death from coronary heart disease. The Western Electric study. N Engl J Med 304:65–70

Shekelle RB, Stamler J (1989) Dietary cholesterol and ischaemic heart disease. Lancet 1:1177–1179

Toeller M, Buyken AE, Heitkamp G, Scherbaum WA, Krans HM, Fuller JH (1999) Associations of fat and cholesterol intake with serum lipid levels and cardiovascular disease: the EURODIAB IDDM Complications Study. Exp Clin Endocrinol Diabetes 107:512–521

Turpeinen O, Karvonen MJ, Pekkarinen M, Miettinen M, Elosuo R, Paavilainen E (1979) Dietary prevention of coronary heart disease: the Finnish Mental Hospital Study. Int J Epidemiol 8:99–118

Weggemans RM, Zock PL, Katan MB (2001a) Dietary cholesterol from eggs increases the ratio of total cholesterol to high-density lipoprotein cholesterol in humans: a meta-analysis. Am J Clin Nutr 73:885–891

Weggemans RM, Zock PL, Meyboom S, Funke H, Katan MB (2000) Apolipoprotein A4-1/2 polymorphism and response of serum lipids to dietary cholesterol in humans. J Lipid Res 41:1623–1628

Weggemans RM, Zock PL, Ordovas JM, Pedro-Botet J, Katan MB (2001b) Apoprotein E genotype and the response of serum cholesterol to dietary fat, cholesterol and cafestol. Atherosclerosis 154:547–555

Weggemans RM, Zock PL, Ordovas JM, Ramos-Galluzzi J, Katan MB (2001c) Genetic poly-morphisms and lipid response to dietary changes in humans. Eur J Clin Invest 31:950–957

Weiss, Minot GR (1933) Nutrition in relation to atherosclerosis. In: Cowdry EV (ed) Arteriosclerosis—A survey of the problem, 1st edn. The Macmillan Company, New York, pp 233–248

Willett W (1998) Nutritional Epidemiology, 2nd edn. Oxford University Press, New York, Oxford

Yano K, Rhoads GG, Kagan A, Tillotson J (1978) Dietary intake and the risk of coronary heart disease in Japanese men living in Hawaii. Am J Clin Nutr 31:1270–1279

Ye SQ and Kwiterovich PO, Jr. (2000) Influence of genetic polymorphisms on responsiveness to dietary fat and cholesterol. Am J Clin Nutr 72:1275S–1284S

HEP (2005) 170:215–230

Plant Sterols and Stanols

M.J. Tikkanen

Department of Medicine, Division of Cardiology, Helsinki University Central Hospital,
00290 Helsinki, Finland
matti.tikkanen@hus.fi

Abstract The expanding market of 'functional foods' containing plant sterols and stanols has focused interest on their cholesterol-lowering effects as well on possible adverse effects. Trials of cholesterol lowering demonstrate that intake of 2 g/day of plant sterols and stanols reduces serum low-density lipoprotein (LDL) cholesterol concentrations by approximately 10%. Safety concerns regarding elevations in serum plant sterol levels, or effects on fat-soluble vitamin absorption or hypothetical effects on serum sex hormone balance have received attention and been addressed in studies. Plant sterol (but not stanol) supplementation increased serum plant sterol concentrations but these levels remained much lower than those observed in homozygous sitosterolemia making an adverse health effect unlikely. Prolonged statin therapy also causes elevations in all cholesterol-adjusted plant sterol levels as well as small but significant elevations in serum unadjusted campesterol levels from baseline. This is probably caused by a statin-induced reduction in biliary cholesterol efflux resulting in a diminished intestinal cholesterol pool. The diminished competition with cholesterol molecules allows more plant sterol molecules to become incorporated in mixed micelles facilitating their uptake in enterocytes. With the exception of β-carotene, reductions in serum concentrations of fat-soluble (pro)vitamins are usually abolished by adjustment for cholesterol suggesting that they reflect reductions in carrier lipoproteins, mainly LDL. The small reductions in serum β-carotene are not regarded as a major concern, nor have any adverse effects on sex hormone metabolism been demonstrated apart from parenteral administration of large doses in experimental animals. However, as increasing consumer populations become exposed to a large variety of food products enriched with plant sterols and stanols the likelihood of rare adverse effects increases and surveillance is necessary.

Keywords Phytosterols · Phytostanols · Cholesterol absorption · Cholesterol lowering

1
Background

Introduction of 'functional foods' containing plant sterols and stanols, mainly in fat-soluble esterified form, has produced urgent interest in their proposed beneficial cholesterol-lowering effects, as well as in possible adverse effects. These substances were first incorporated in margarines and other dietary fats, and later studies were carried out using low-fat or fat-free foods fortified with plant sterols. Low-fat food products containing plant stanols and sterols are currently being introduced. Large and rapidly growing consumer populations are therefore exposed to a variety of food products containing these substances.

The usual intake of plant sterols in unsupplemented Western diets varies between 150 and 350 mg/day and plant stanol intake is around 50 mg/day (Miettinen et al. 1990). Many investigators have proposed that daily intake of significantly larger quantities of these natural substances obtained from edible vegetables might provide the basis for population strategies of cholesterol lowering, and their potential usefulness has been recognized by the National Cholesterol Education Program in the United States (Expert Panel 2001). However, while cholesterol-lowering drugs have to be tested in large-scale clinical endpoint trials, plant sterols and stanols can be marketed without any such trials. Commercially available supplemented foods generally contain 2 g plant stanol or sterol in daily portions. Simultaneous use of several such products (e.g., margarine, yogurt, cheese) may increase the daily dose several-fold. This makes it even more important to investigate the effects of various doses of different sterols and stanols and their derivatives in populations with different diets and also in combination with various drugs. In comparison to the expanding market of foods enriched with these substances, the field covered by investigations appears limited indeed.

2
Structure of Plant Sterols and Stanols

Plant sterols (phytosterols) and their saturated forms plant stanols (phytostanols) cannot be synthesized in animal organisms. They are derived exclusively from vegetables and vegetable oils and they are thought to have a role in plants similar to that of cholesterol in animals. More than 40 different plant sterols have been identified but the most abundant ones are sitosterol and campesterol. The chemical structures of plant sterols are very similar to cholesterol (Fig. 1). Sitosterol differs from cholesterol in that it has an additional ethyl group in its side chain (24-ethylcholesterol), while campesterol has a methyl group instead (24-methylcholesterol). Some natural as well as commercially produced stanols differ from sterols in that the Δ-5 double bond has been saturated to form 5α-stanols. For some reason, these very small structural differences profoundly affect the absorption efficacy from the intestine. Although 50% of the cholesterol entering the intestinal lumen is absorbed, plant sterols are absorbed to a much smaller extent and stanols only minimally: absorption ranges between 10% and 15% for campesterol and between 4% and 7% for sitosterol (Salen et al. 1992; Heinemann et al. 1993; Lütjohann et al. 1995), and only 1% of sitostanol is absorbed (Czubayko et al. 1991). Even these values may be overestimates as much smaller absorption rates have been reported in recent studies using mass spectroscopy with deuterated standards: absorption was 1.9% for campesterol, 0.5% for sitosterol and absorption of the corresponding stanols was only one-tenth of the parent sterol (Ostlund et al. 2002) Serum plant sterol levels are used as markers of cholesterol absorption effectiveness (see Sect. 3.1).

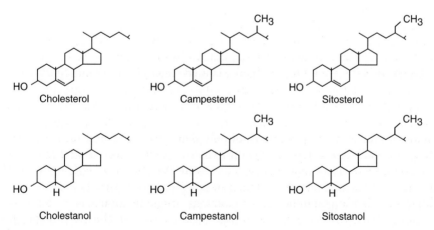

Fig. 1 Structures of major plant sterols and stanols

3
Role of Intestinal Metabolism

3.1
Plant Sterols as Markers of Cholesterol Absorption

Small amounts of noncholesterol sterols are present in serum. The concentrations of plant sterols are 500- or 1,000-fold lower than cholesterol concentrations and must be determined by high-performance liquid chromatography or gas-liquid chromatography. These water-insoluble substances are transported exclusively in lipoprotein molecules, mainly in the large low-density lipoprotein (LDL) fraction. Thus, their concentrations are altered by changes in their carrier lipoprotein concentrations, e.g., they are elevated in hypercholesterolemia and may fall when LDL levels decrease. Their levels are therefore preferably expressed as ratios to cholesterol, i.e., plant sterol:cholesterol (mmol/mol). The ratios of sitosterol, campesterol and avenasterol as well as the cholesterol metabolite cholestanol correlate positively with the fractional absorption of dietary cholesterol measured by the sterol balance technique (Miettinen et al. 1990) and they serve as markers of cholesterol absorption. These ratios are reliable markers under conditions of unchanged dietary intake of plant sterols. The cholesterol precursor sterols cholestenol, desmosterol and lathosterol correlate positively with cholesterol synthesis and their ratios (precursor sterol:cholesterol) serve as markers of cholesterol synthesis (Miettinen 1970).

3.2
Cholesterol Absorption and the Exogenous Pathway of Cholesterol Metabolism

Some 1,200–1,700 mg of cholesterol enter the lumen of the small intestine every day in people adhering to a typical Western diet. Approximately one-third of this is of dietary origin, and two-thirds is derived from the bile and to a limited extent to sloughing of the intestinal mucosa (Fig. 2). Fifty percent of this sterol is absorbed and 50% is excreted (Bosner et al. 1999; Sudhop et al. 2002).

Dietary sterols together with other lipids enter the small intestine in an emulsion which mixes with bile as well as pancreatic juice which contains cholesterol esterase. The latter enzyme hydrolyzes the proportion of cholesterol which is in esterified form. The next essential step in the sterol absorption process is to solubilize cholesterol (or other sterols) into mixed micelles consisting of bile acids, monoacyl-glycerol, phospholipids and fatty acids. The incorporation into micelles makes it possible for the cholesterol to be transferred through the unstirred water-layer separating the enterocyte brush border membrane from the bulk of the aqueous phase of intestinal contents. The mechanisms underlying the uptake of sterols by the enterocyte are not fully known. It has been recently demonstrated that Niemann–Pick C1 Like 1 (NPC1L1) protein, the expression of which is enriched in the brush border of intestinal enterocytes,

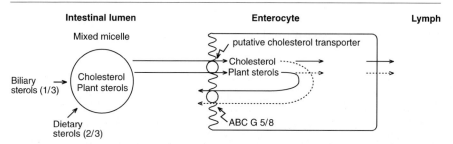

Fig. 2 Schematic representation of the absorption process of cholesterol and plant sterols. *Arrows* indicate directions of sterol transport. *Dotted arrows* indicate reduced transport. Cholesterol and plant sterols appear to share a common transporter mediating uptake into the enterocyte, which is likely to be the Niemann-Pick C1 Like 1 protein which is proposed to reside in the ezetimibe-sensitive pathway responsible for intestinal sterol absorption. The ABC G5/8-mediated transfer back into the intestinal lumen is more effective for plant sterols than for cholesterol resulting in very limited secretion of plant sterols into the lymph

plays a critical role in the cholesterol absorption process (Altmann et al. 2004). This process appears to be also regulated by the ATP-binding cassette (ABC) subfamily G, member 5 and 8 (ABCG5 and ABCG8) transporter proteins which pump plant sterols from the enterocytes into the intestinal lumen (Berge et al. 2000; Lee et al. 2001). The ABCG5/8 function selectively keeps the absorption of plant sterols low, but loss of this function by mutation of one of these transporter genes was shown to cause hyperabsorption of plant sterols resulting in sitosterolemia (phytosterolemia) (Berge et al. 2000; Lee et al. 2001). The role of ABCG5/8 in cholesterol absorption may not be crucial as sitosterolemia patients reportedly have cholesterol absorption rates in the high–normal range (Salen et al. 1989; Lütjohann et al. 1995). However, studies in experimental animals suggest that the role of ABCG5/8, although limited under conditions of low dietary intake of cholesterol, may become more significant during high cholesterol intake (Turley and Dietschy 2003).

Within the enterocyte, cholesterol is esterified by acyl CoA:cholesterol acyltransferase-2. The newly formed cholesteryl ester becomes incorporated together with apolipoprotein B48, triacylglycerols, and some free sterols in nascent chylomicrons in a process regulated by microsomal triglyceride transfer protein. The chylomicrons are transported with intestinal lymph through the thoracic duct to the circulation. This mechanism effluxes approximately 700 mg cholesterol daily into the bloodstream (Turley and Dietschy 2003). During the transport of chylomicrons in the circulation triacylglycerols are hydrolyzed by endothelial lipoprotein lipase in the capillaries which results in the formation of smaller particles called chylomicron remnants which can be taken up by receptors in the liver. Accordingly, increased influx of cholesterol via this exogenous pathway downregulates HMGCoA reductase suppressing endogenous synthesis of cholesterol, and, conversely, reduced influx upregulates the enzyme causing increased hepatic synthesis (Dietschy et al. 1993).

Thus, high cholesterol absorption rates are associated with suppressed cholesterol synthesis, and conversely, low cholesterol absorption rates correlate with increased synthesis (Miettinen et al. 2000).

3.3
Mechanism of the Cholesterol-Lowering Action of Plant Sterols and Stanols

One current theory is that plant sterols and stanols act in the intestinal lumen by displacing cholesterol from the mixed micelles which are necessary for their solubilization and transport to the brush border of enterocytes (Heinemann 1991; Nissinen et al. 2002) (Fig. 2). It appears that a daily intake of 2 g plant sterols or stanols is enough to competitively displace significant amounts of cholesterol molecules from the micelles resulting in markedly reduced absorption.

In addition, studies involving a novel specific inhibitor of cholesterol absorption, ezetimibe, have raised the possibility that cholesterol and plant sterols may share a common transporter protein which facilitates their uptake by the enterocytes. Accordingly, ezetimibe was shown to lower plasma plant sterol concentrations in sitosterolemic patients (von Bergmann et al. 2002). There is now compelling evidence that this ezetimibe-sensitive transporter protein or 'permease' is the NPC1L1 protein residing in the brush border of enterocytes (Altmann et al. 2004).

4
Cholesterol-Lowering Efficacy of Plant Sterols and Stanols

4.1
Trials of Cholesterol Lowering

Early treatments consisted of rather high doses of plant sterols, up to 18 g/day, which caused reductions in serum cholesterol of about 10% (Pollak 1953,1985; Best et al. 1994,1995; Farquhar et al. 1956). Later on, investigators observed that, depending on the physical form, smaller plant sterol quantities could achieve similar cholesterol absorption inhibition as the higher doses (Lees et al. 1977; Lees and Lees 1976; Grundy and Mok 1977). Further developments were the discovery that hydrogenation of sterols to stanols resulted in more efficient inhibition of cholesterol absorption (Ikeda and Sugano 1978; Sugano et al. 1976,1977; Heinemann et al. 1986,1993; Becker et al. 1993). It had been proposed earlier that the crystalline form of sterols might not be optimal for their action and that esterification with fatty acids would facilitate their incorporation in dietary fats enhancing inhibition of cholesterol absorption (Mattson et al. 1982). Studies in the 1990s carried out in Finland demonstrated that esterification of plant stanols indeed improved their ability to interfere with cholesterol absorption (Vanhanen and Miettinen 1992; Vanhanen et al. 1994; Gylling et al. 1995,1997; Gylling and Miettinen 1994, 1996).

A recent meta-analysis (Katan et al. 2003) of double-blind trials comparing foods with and without added plant stanols or sterols has summarized current expert opinion. In most but not all (Tikkanen et al. 2001) of the 41 trials listed, stanols or sterols were esterified, and in all trials they were solubilized in fat-containing foods. On average, the reduction in LDL cholesterol with increasing stanol or sterol dose appeared to level off at intakes of 2 g/day with little additional decrease at doses exceeding 2.5 g/day. In an analysis excluding low-dose trials (<1.1 g/day) and trials in children, stanols decreased LDL cholesterol by 10.1% (27 trials, mean dose 2.5 g/day) while sterols decreased LDL cholesterol by 9.7% (21 trials, mean dose 2.3 g/day). In general, stanols or sterols had very little effect on high-density lipoprotein (HDL) cholesterol or triglyceride levels (Katan et al. 2003).

The majority of trials have been short-term studies of 3–10 weeks. However, Miettinen et al. (1995) reported a 1-year trial of cholesterol lowering using sitostanol-ester margarine in a mildly hypercholesterolemic population. This landmark study laid the basis for the marketing of the first sitostanol-ester margarine, followed later by sitosterol-ester margarine and other fortified foods, also including low-fat products. It was shown that replacement of 24 g of dietary fat daily with a margarine containing 2.6 g of sitostanol-ester reduced LDL cholesterol by 14.1% (vs. 1.1% in the control group). In one arm of the study, 1.8 g/day of stanol lowered LDL cholesterol by 8.5% in comparison to placebo. The trial also demonstrated that serum campesterol levels were significantly decreased in the sitostanol-ester margarine group, the greatest reductions in LDL cholesterol concurring with those in campesterol (Miettinen et al. 1995). A recent 1-year trial using 1.6 g/day of plant sterol-ester reported a placebo-corrected reduction in LDL cholesterol by 6% (Hendriks et al. 2003). Because data were based on single studies and the treatment doses were not identical, it has not been possible to reach consensus regarding the issue whether the long-term efficacies of sterols and stanols are different (Katan et al. 2003). Recently, Miettinen and Gylling (2004) pointed out that plant sterols but not stanols reduced bile acid synthesis which could in the long term counteract cholesterol-lowering efficacy of sterols.

4.2
Combination of Plant Stanols with Statin Therapy

Additive efficacy has been studied mainly by using combinations of statin and stanol margarine. In a trial of 167 patients receiving statin therapy, an additional lowering of LDL cholesterol by 10% was achieved by adding stanol-ester margarine (Blair et al. 2000). Somewhat greater reductions in LDL cholesterol by 14%–20% have been reported in smaller studies in which stanol-ester margarine intake was started in statin-treated patients with coronary heart disease, familial hypercholesterolemia or type 2 diabetes (Gylling et al. 1997; Vuorio et al. 2000; Gylling and Miettinen 1996). The effects are greater than the 6% additional reduction in LDL cholesterol usually achieved by doubling the statin dose. Statin treatment apparently reduces the intestinal cholesterol pool as a consequence of reduced synthesis decreasing biliary cholesterol excretion, and therefore facilitates absorption of plant sterols leading in some situations to elevated serum concentrations (see Sect. 5.1.2)

5
Safety Aspects Concerning Plant Sterol and Stanol Supplementation of Foods

The enrichment of foods with substances that may have effects on circulating levels of plant sterols or fat-soluble vitamins and antioxidants, or on hormonal factors, poses a public health concern. Although the effects may be relatively small, large populations will be exposed and some individuals may consume a variety of sterol and stanol-containing food components raising the daily intake to high levels. Concerns have arisen regarding elevated serum plant sterol levels because they have been linked to promotion of atherosclerosis in patients with the very rare disorder sitosterolemia (phytosterolemia). Low carotenoid and fat-soluble vitamin levels could have adverse health effects, and some animal studies have raised the possibility that plant sterols could have estrogenic properties.

5.1
Serum Plant Sterol and Stanol Concentrations

5.1.1
Effects of Dietary Plant Sterol and Stanol Intake on Their Concentrations in Serum

There is some concern regarding the physiologic effects of elevations in serum plant sterol and stanol concentrations. This arises from the knowledge that in a rare autosomally inherited metabolic disorder called sitosterolemia (phytosterolemia) elevated serum plant sterol concentrations are associated with tendon xanthomas and premature atherosclerotic disease (Bhattacharyya and Connor 1974; Lee et al. 2001). Although sitosterolemia shares some clinical characteristics with homozygous familial hypercholesterolemia, sitosterolemia patients differ in that they have normal or moderately elevated serum cholesterol but markedly elevated serum plant sterol (sitosterol, campesterol, stigmasterol, avenasterol) and plant stanol levels. Sitosterol levels usually range between 10 and 30 mg/dl (Patel et al. 1998) while sitosterol and campesterol levels rarely exceed 1 mg/dl in normal individuals. Parents have normal cholesterol and sitosterol levels in their serum suggesting that one functional copy of the gene is enough to maintain normal sterol metabolism. Mutational analyses have revealed that sitosterolemia is caused by mutation in either one of two ATP binding cassette transporter genes, ABCG5 or ABCG8 (Berge et al. 2000; Lee et al. 2001) coding for two transporter proteins (sterolins 1 and 2). Sitosterolemia patients appear to hyperabsorb sterols from the intestine and, in addition, to have an inability to excrete sterols into the bile. Several different underlying mechanisms explaining the disorder are possible. One possibility is that the sterolin transporters have a bi-directional function. They mediate the entry of plant sterols and cholesterol from the intestinal lumen into the enterocytes having a higher affinity for cholesterol in this process, and they pump sterols back into the lumen, having a higher affinity for plant sterols (Fig. 2). Analogous mechanisms could apparently work for the excretion of sterols from hepatocytes into the bile. In sitosterolemia, loss of the sterolin function would result in reduced transport of plant sterols out of the entero-cytes into the intestinal lumen and out of the hepatocytes into the bile, causing increased serum and hepatic levels of these substances.

Several studies have indicated that administration of varying doses (0.63–12 g/day) of sitosterol results in increases in serum sitosterol levels by 13%–68% and in reductions of serum campesterol concentrations by 17%–27% (Jones et al. 1997; Schlierf et al. 1978; Becker et al. 1992; Vanhanen and Miettinen 1992; Becker et al. 1993; Miettinen and Vanhanen 1994). On the other hand, sitostanol administration consistently resulted in significant reductions in both serum sitosterol and serum campesterol concentrations (Vanhanen and Miettinen 1992; Becker et al. 1993; Miettinen and Vanhanen 1994; Vanhanen et al. 1993, 1994; Gylling and Miettinen 1994; Miettinen et al. 1995; Weststrate and Meijer 1998) while serum sitostanol was barely detectable (Heinemann et al. 1986).

In summary, dietary intake of 2 g/day of plant sterols usually increases serum sitosterol to some extent and results in doubling of serum campesterol concentrations (Hallikainen et al. 2000; Nguyen et al. 1999). Consumption of sterol-ester margarine produces mean serum levels of plant sterols (sitosterol and campesterol combined) of approximately 1.5 mg/dl (Weststrate and Meijer 1998; Hallikainen et al. 2000), corresponding to a 50% increase from baseline but still constituting only 5%–15% of the serum plant sterol concentrations in homozygous sitosterolemia. However, serum plant sterol levels also increase during long-term statin therapy which has caused concern in some investiga-tors. This will be discussed in Sect. 5.1.2.

5.1.2
Effects of Cholesterol-Lowering Drugs on Serum Plant Sterol and Stanol Concentrations

Miettinen et al. (2003) reported a continuous, time-dependent statin-induced increase in serum cholesterol-adjusted concentrations of sterols that are re-garded as cholesterol absorption markers. In the 1-year comparison study between atorvastatin and simvastatin, this effect was more evident in pa-tients receiving atorvastatin, and even the unadjusted serum concentrations of campesterol and sitosterol were elevated from their respective baseline levels of 0.6 mg/dl and 0.3 mg/dl by about 10%. Conversely, simvastatin caused a 10% reduction in the corresponding concentrations. However, in a previous study, the same investigators demonstrated increased serum campesterol during simvastatin treatment. They divided the Finnish subgroup of the 4S into quartiles according to the cholestanol:cholesterol ratio (the highest ratio indicating highest cholesterol absorption) (Miettinen et al. 2000). In the highest quartile (high absorption associated with low synthesis) the authors noted a slightly smaller reduction in serum cholesterol compared to the lowest quartile (low absorption associated with high synthesis), as well as an increase in serum campesterol from 0.7 mg/dl to 0.9 mg/dl after 5 years. This seemed to indicate that patients with high basal cholesterol synthesis responded to statin therapy somewhat better than those with low basal synthesis. Some other studies seem to support this (Thompson et al. 2002). Miettinen et al. (1998) also reported that although simvastatin therapy in the 4S subgroup reduced coronary events in other quartiles, it did not in the highest quartile (hyperabsorbers, low synthesizers). However, the slightly smaller decrease in serum cholesterol achieved in the highest quartile was too small to explain differences in clinical endpoints. The authors pointed out that baseline serum plant sterol levels were highest in this quartile and increased most during the 5-year study implying that an adverse effect could not be excluded during extended statin therapy (Miettinen et al. 2003). Since plant sterols are transported in lipoprotein particles, mainly in the large LDL fraction, statin-induced increases are attenuated or abolished by the LDL-lowering effect of the treatment. The finding that campesterol levels unadjusted for cholesterol nevertheless increased, deserves attention.

5.2
Effects on Serum Fat-Soluble Vitamin and Carotenoid Concentrations

Because of their mechanism of action, plant sterol- and stanol-enriched foods could potentially affect absorption of fat-soluble vitamins and other lipophilic substances. Most of these molecules are transported in the circulation by lipoprotein particles, mainly in the large LDL fraction. Accordingly, their levels should be expressed both as absolute concentrations as well as in relation to serum cholesterol. Katan et al. (2003) summarized 18 plant sterol and stanol trials that had used doses of 1.5 g/day or more and reported serum or plasma concentrations of fat-soluble vitamins. On the average, serum carotenoid (α-carotene, β-carotene and lycopene) levels decreased significantly in the treatment groups compared to controls. Following adjustment for change in serum cholesterol, only the reduction in β-carotene remained statistically significant (Katan et al. 2003), although this was not observed in all trials (Hallikainen et al. 2000). The findings indicate that the decreases in carotenoid concentrations were partly caused by decreases in carrier lipoprotein (mainly LDL) concentrations, and, at least for β-carotene, by reduced absorption. The reduction in α-tocopherol was completely abolished when corrected for the change in serum cholesterol. On the average, concentrations of vitamin D and vitamin A (retinol) did not change during plant sterol or stanol administration. Vitamin K1 (Hendriks et al. 1999) and vitamin K-dependent clotting factors (Plat and Mensink 2000) remained unaltered during stanol feeding

5.3
Effects on Hormone Metabolism

The resemblance of the ring structure of plant sterols with that of estrogens has prompted investigations concerning possible phytoestrogenic effects of plant sterols (Ling and Jones 1995). Estrogenic effects of plant sterols have been suggested in animal studies. Subcutaneous administration of large doses of sitosterol (0.5–5 mg/kg per day) to rats reduced sperm count and had other antifertility effects (Malini and Vanithakumari 1991). Weak estrogenicity has been suggested based on biological assays in fish and breast cancer cell lines (Mellanen et al. 1996; Tremblay and Van Der Kraak 1998). As summarized by Baker et al (1999), estrogenicity data have been produced in studies using subcutaneous administration of various sitosterol containing mixtures. Oral administration did not appear to have estrogenic activity as measured by uterotrophic assay in the rat. Moreover, plant sterols did not bind to estrogen receptors, nor did they stimulate transcriptional activity of the human estrogen receptor in a recombinant yeast strain (Baker et al. 1999). A study carried out in man reported no significant changes in plasma concentrations of sex hormones (Hendriks et al. 2003). Based on current knowledge, dietary intake of plant sterols or stanols is very unlikely to have effects on sex hormone concentrations or on fertility.

6
Conclusions

Cholesterol-lowering studies indicate that intake of 2 g/day of plant sterols and stanols reduces serum LDL cholesterol concentrations by approximately 10%. Based on cholesterol-lowering trials of coronary prevention this translates to a decrease of 15%–20% in coronary heart disease events over a period of 5 years. Safety concerns regarding effects on fat-soluble vitamin absorption, elevations of serum concentrations of plant sterols, and hypothetical effects on serum sex hormone concentrations have been addressed in many studies. With the exception of β-carotene, reductions in serum levels of fat-soluble (pro)vitamins are usually abolished by correction for changes in serum cholesterol suggesting that these alterations reflect decreases in serum levels of carrier lipoproteins. For reductions in serum β-carotene, also impaired absorption can contribute but the small reductions do not appear to be of major concern. Serum plant sterol concentrations became elevated during supplementation but remained much lower than the levels observed in sitosterolemia making an adverse health effect unlikely, although no safety data are available for prolonged intake exceeding 1 year. Plant stanol intake, on the other hand, does not increase but decreases serum sterol levels with negligible increases in serum plant stanol concentrations. Prolonged treatment with statins also causes small but significant mean increases in serum campesterol concentrations from baseline as well as elevations in all cholesterol-adjusted plant sterol levels. This effect is probably caused by reduction of the intestinal cholesterol pool, which facilitates incorporation of plant sterols into mixed micelles enhancing their uptake into enterocytes. While adverse health outcomes due to this effect appear unlikely in view of the established benefit of statin therapy, exploration of possible subgroups of individuals with markedly increased plant sterol absorption during long-term statin therapy are indicated. Adverse effects on steroid hormones are speculative and do not appear to exist except in experimental animals receiving large parenteral doses. Despite lack of clinical endpoint trials, sterol and stanol supplementation of foods can be regarded as a safe therapeutic alternative when moderate lowering of LDL cholesterol is aimed at. As larger consumer populations will become exposed to these substances, the likelihood of rare adverse effects will increase, necessitating safety monitoring in subsets of such populations.

References

Altmann SW, Davis HR Jr, Zhu L-J, Yao X, Hoos LM, Tetzloff G, Iyer SPN, Maguire M, Golonko A, Zeng M, Wang L, Murgolo N, Graziano MP (2004) Niemann-Pick C1 Like 1 protein is critical for intestinal cholesterol absorption. Science 303:1201–1204

Baker VA, Hepburn PA, Kennedy SJ, Jones PA, Lea LJ, Sumpter JP, Ashby J (1999) Safety evaluation of phytosterol esters. Part 1. Assessment of oestrogenicity using a combination of in vivo and in vitro assays. Food Chem Toxicol 37:13–22

Becker M, Staab D, von Bergmann K (1993) Treatment of severe familial hypercholesterolemia in childhood with sitosterol and sitostanol. J Pediatr 122:292–296

Berge KE, Tian H, Graf GA, Yu L, Grishin NV, Shultz J, Kwiterovich P, Shan B, Barnes R, Hobbs HH (2000) Accumulation of dietary cholesterol in sitosterolemia caused by mutations in adjacent ABC transporters. Science 290:1771–1775

von Bergmann K, Salen G, Lütjohann D et al. (2002) Ezetimibe effectively reduces serum plant sterols in patients with sitosterolemia. Atherosclerosis 3 (suppl):232

Best MM, Duncan CH, Van Loon EJ, Wathen JD (1954) Lowering of serum cholesterol by administration of a plant sterol. Circulation 10:201–206

Best MM, Duncan CH, Van Loon EJ, Wathen JD (1955) The effects of sitosterol on serum lipids. Am J Med 19:61–70

Bhattacharyya AK, Connor WE (1974) Beta-sitosterolemia and xanthomatosis. A newly described lipid starage disease in two sisters. J Clin Invest 53:1033–1043

Blair SN, Capuzzi DM, Gottlieb SO, Nguyen T, Morgan JM, Cater NB (2000) Incremental reduction of serum total cholesterol and low-density lipoprotein cholesterol with the addition of plant stanol ester-containing spread to statin therapy. Am J Cardiol 86:46–52

Blomqvist SM, Jauhiainen M, Van Tol A, Hyvönen M, Torstila I, Vanhanen HT (1993) Effect of sitostanol ester on composition and size distribution of LDL and HDL. Nutr Metab Cardiovasc Dis 3:158–164

Bosner MS, Lange LG, Stenson WF, Ostlund RE Jr. (1999) Percent cholesterol absorption in normal women and men quantified with dual stable isotopic tracers and negative ion mass spectrometry. J Lipid Res 40:302–308

Czubayko F, Beumers B, Lammsfuss S, Lütjohann D, von Bergmann K (1991) A simplified micro-method for quantification of fecal excretion of neutral and acidic sterols for outpatient studies in humans. J Lipid Res 32:1861–1867

Dietschy JM, Turley SD, Spady DK (1993) Role of liver in the maintenance of cholesterol and low density lipoprotein homeostasis in different animal apecies, including humans. J Lipid Res 34:1637–1659

Expert Panel on Detection, Evaluation, and Treatment of High Blood Cholesterol in Adults (Adult Treatment Panel III) (2001) Executive Summary of the Third Report of the National Cholesterol Education Program (NCEP). JAMA 285:2486–2497

Farquhar JW, Smith RE, Dempsey ME (1956) The effect of beta sitosterol on the serum lipids of young men with arteriosclerotic heart disease. Circulation 14:77–82

Grundy SM, Mok HYI (1977) Determination of cholesterol absorption in man by intestinal perfusion. J Lipid Res 18:263–271

Gylling H, Miettinen TA (1994) Serum cholesterol and cholesterol and lipoprotein metabolism in hypercholesterolaemic NIDDM patients before and during sitostanol ester-margarine treatment. Diabetologia 37:773–780

Gylling H, Miettinen TA (1996) Effects of inhibiting cholesterol absorption and synthesis on cholesterol and lipoprotein metabolism in hypercholesterolemic non-insulin-dependent diabetic men. J Lipid Res 37:1776–1785

Gylling H, Radhakrishnan R, Miettinen TA (1997) Reduction of serum cholesterol in postmenopausal women with previous myocardial infarction and cholesterol malabsorption induced by dietary sitostanol ester margarine: women and dietary sitostanol. Circulation 96:4226–4231

Gylling H, Siimes MA, Miettinen TA (1995) Sitostanol ester margarine in dietary treatment of children with familial hypercholesterolemia. J Lipid Res 36:1807–1812

Hallikainen MA, Sarkkinen ES, Gylling H, Erkkilä AT, Uusitupa MI (2000) Comparison of the effects of plant sterol ester and plant stanol ester-enriched margarines in lowering serum cholesterol concentrations in hypercholesterolaemic subjects on a low-fat diet. Eur J Clin Nutr 54:715–725

Hallikainen MA, Sarkkinen ES, Uusitupa MI (2000) Plant stanol esters affect serum cholesterol concentrations of hypercholesterolemic men and women in a dose-dependent manner. J Nutr 130:767–776

Heinemann T, Leiss O, von Bergmann K (1986) Effect of low-dose sitostanol on serum cholesterol in patients with hypercholesterolemia. Atherosclerosis 61:219–223

Heinemann T, Kullak-Ublick G-A, Pietruck B, von Bergmann K (1991) Mechanisms of action of plant sterols on inhibition of cholesterol absorption. Comparison of sitosterol and sitostanol. Eur J Clin Pharmacol 40:S59–S63

Heinemann T, Axtmann G, von Bergmann K (1993) Comparison of intestinal absorption of cholesterol with different plant sterols in man. Eur J Clin Invest 23:827–831

Hendriks HF, Brink EJ, Meijer GW, Princen HM, Ntanios FY (2003) Safety of long-term consumption of plant sterol esters-enriched spread. Eur J Clin Nutr 57:681–692

Hendriks HFJ, Weststrate JA, van Vliet T, Meijer GW (1999) Spreads enriched with three different levels of vegetable oil sterols and the degree of cholesterol lowering in normocholesterolaemic and mildly hypercholesterolaemic subjects. Eur J Clin Nutr 53:319–327

Homan R, Krause BR (1997) Established and emerging strategies for inhibition of cholesterol absorption. Curr Pharm Design 3:29–44

Ikeda I, Sugano M (1978) Comparison of absorption and metabolism of β-sitosterol and β-sitostanol in rats. Atherosclerosis 30:227–237

Jones PJH, MacDougall DE, Ntanios F, Vanstone CA (1997) Dietary phytosterols as cholesterol-lowering agents in humans. Can J Physiol Pharmacol 75:217–227

Katan MB, Grundy SM, Jones P, Law M, Miettinen T, Paoletti R, for the Stresa Workshop participants (2003) Efficacy and safety of plant stanols and sterols in the management of blood cholesterol levels. Mayo Clin Proc 78:965–978

Lee M-H, Lu K, Patel SB (2001) Genetic basis of sitosterolemia. Curr Opin Lipidol 12:141–149

Lee M-H, Lu K, Hazard S, Yu H, Shulenin S, Hidaka H, Kojima H, Allikmets R, Sakuma N, Pegoraro R, Srivasava AK, Salen G, Dean M, Patel SB (2001) Identification of a gene, ABCG5, important in the regulation of dietary cholesterol absorption. Nat Genet 27:79–83

Lees RS, Lees AM (1976) Effects of sitosterol therapy on plasma lipid and lipoprotein concentrations. In: Greten H (ed) Lipoprotein metabolism. Springer-Verlag, New York, 119–124

Lees AM, Mok HYI, Lees RS, McCluskey MA, Grundy SM (1977) Plant sterols as cholesterol-lowering agents: clinical trials in patients with hypercholesterolemia and studies of sterol balance. Atherosclerosis 28:325–338

Ling WH, Jones PJH (1995) Dietary phytosterols: a review of metabolism, benefits and side effects. Life Sci 57:195–206

Lütjohann D, Björkhem I, Beil UF, von Bergmann K (1995) Sterol absorption and sterol balance in phytosterolemia evaluated by deuterium-labeled sterols: effect of sitostanol treatment. J Lipid Res 36:1763–1773

Malini T and Vanithakumari G (1991) Antifertility effects of β-sitosterol in male albino rats. J Ethnopharmacol 35:149–153

Mattson FH, Grundy SM, Crouse JR (1982) Optimizing the effect of plant sterols on cholesterol absorption in man. Am J Clin Nutr 35:697–700

Mellanen P, Petänen T, Lehtimäki J, Mäkelä S, Gylund G, Holmbom B, Mannila E, Oikari A, Santti R (1996) Wood-derived estrogens: studies in vitro with breast cancer cell lines and in vivo in trout. Toxicol Appl Pharmacol 136:381–388

Miettinen TA (1970) Detection of changes in human cholesterol metabolism. Ann Clin Res 2:300–320

Miettinen TA, Tilvis RS, Kesäniemi YA (1990) Serum plant sterols and cholesterol precursors reflect cholesterol absorption and synthesis in volunteers of a randomly selected male population. Am J Epidemiol 131:20–31

Miettinen TA, Puska P, Gylling H, Vanhanen H, Vartiainen E (1995) Reduction of serum cholesterol with sitostanol-ester margarine in a mildly hypercholesterolemic population. New Engl J Med 333:1308–1312

Miettinen TA, Gylling H, Strandberg T, Sarna S, for the Finnish 4S investigators (1998) Baseline serum cholestanol as predictor of recurrent coronary events in subgroup of Scandinavian Simvastatin Survival Study. British Med J 316:1127–1130

Miettinen TA, Strandberg TE, Gylling H for the Finnish 4S investigators (2000) Noncholesterol sterols and cholesterol lowering by long-term simvastatin treatment in coronary patients: relation to basal serum cholestanol. Arterioscl Thromb Vasc Biol 20:1340–1346

Miettinen TA (2001) Cholesterol absorption inhibition: A strategy for cholesterol-lowering therapy. Int J Pract 55:710–716

Miettinen TA, and Gylling H (2002) Ineffective decrease of serum cholesterol by simvastatin in a subgroup of hypercholesterolemic coronary patients. Atherosclerosis 164:147–152

Miettinen TA, Gylling H (2003) Cholesterol synthesis and absorption in coronary patients with lipid triad and isolated high LDL cholesterol in a 4S subgroup. Atherosclerosis 168:343–349

Miettinen TA, Gylling H, Lindbohm N, Miettinen TE, Rajaratnam RA, Relas H (2003) Serum noncholesterol sterols during inhibition of cholesterol synthesis by statins. J Lab Clin Med 141:131–137

Miettinen TA, Gylling H (2004) Plant stanol and sterol esters in prevention of cardiovascular diseases. Ann Med 36:126–134

Nguyen TT, Dale LC, von Bergmann K, Croghan IT (1999) Cholesterol-lowering effect of stanol ester in a US population of mildly hypercholesterolemic men and women: a randomized controlled trial. Mayo Clin Proc 74:1198–1206

Nissinen M, Gylling H, Vuoristo M, and Miettinen TA (2002) Micellar distribution of cholesterol and phytosterols after duodenal plant stanol ester infusion. Am J Physiol 282:G1009–G1015

Ostlund RE Jr, McGill JB, Zeng C-M, Covey DF, Stearns J, Stenson WF, Spilburg CA (2002) Gastrointestinal absorption and plasma kinetics of soy Δ5-phytosterols and phytostanols in humans. Am J Physiol Endocrinol Metab 282: E911–E916

Patel SB, Salen G, Hikada H, Kwiterovich Jr PO, Stalenhoef AFH, Miettinen TA, Grundy SM, Lee M-H, Rubenstein JS, Polymeropoulos MH, Brownstein MJ (1998) Mapping a gene involved in regulating dietary cholesterol absorption: the sitosterolemia locus is found at chromosome 2p21. J Clin Invest 102:1041–1044

Plat J, Mensink RP (2000) Vegetable oil based versus wood based stanol ester mixtures: effects on serum lipids and hemostatic factors in non-hypercholesterolemic subjects. Atherosclerosis 148:101–112

Pollak OJ (1953) Reduction of blood cholesterol in man. Circulation 7:702–706

Pollak OJ (1985) Effect of plant sterols on serum lipids and atherosclerosis. Pharmacol Ther 31:177–208

Salen G, Shefer S, Nguyen L, Ness GC, Tint GC, Shore V (1992) Sitosterolemia. J Lipid Res 33:945–955

Salen G, Shore V, Tint GS, Forte T, Shefer S, Horak I, Horak E, Dayal B, Nguyen L, Batta AK, Lindgren FT, Kwiterovich PO Jr. (1989) Increased sitosterol absorption, decreased removal, and expanded body pools compensate for reduced cholesterol synthesis in sitosterolemia with xanthomatosis. J Lipid Res 30:1319–1330

Sudhop T, Lütjohann D, Kodal A, Igel M, Tribble DL, Shah S (2002) Inhibition of intestinal cholesterol absorption by ezetimibe in humans. Circulation 106:1943–1948

Sugano M, Kamo F, Ikeda I, Morioka H (1976) Lipid-lowering activity of phytostanols in rats. Atherosclerosis 24:301–109

Sugano M, Morioka H, Ikeda I (1977) A comparison of hypocholesterolemic activity of β-sitosterol and β-sitostanol in rats. J Nutr 107:2011–2019

Tikkanen MJ, Höqström P, Tuomilehto J, Keinänen–Kiukaannjemi S, Sundvall J, Karppanen H (2001) Effects of a diet based on low-fat foods enriched with nonesterified plant sterols and mineral nutrients on serum cholesterol. Am J Cardiol 88:1157–1162

Tremblay L, Van Der Kraak G (1998) Use of a series of homologous in vitro and in vivo assays to evaluate the endocrine modulating actions of β-sitosterol in rainbow trout. Aquatic Toxicol 43:149–162

Turley SD, Dietschy JM (2003) Sterol absorption by the small intestine Curr Opin Lipidol 14:233–240

Vanhanen HT, Kajander J, Lehtovirta H, Miettinen TA (1994) Serum levels, absorption
    efficiency, faecal elimination, and synthesis of cholesterol during increasing doses of
    dietary sitostanol esters in hypercholesterolaemic subjects. Clin Sci 87:61–67
Vanhanen HT, Miettinen TA (1992) Effects on unsaturated and saturated dietary plant sterols
    on their serum contents. Clin Chim Acta 205:97–107
Vuorio AF, Gylling H, Turtola H, Kontula K, Ketonen P, Miettinen TA (2000) Stanol ester
    margarine alone and with simvastatin lowers serum cholesterol in families with familial
    hypercholesterolemia caused by the FH-North Karelia mutation. Arterioscler Thromb
    Vasc Biol 20:500–506
Weststrate JA, Meijer GW (1998) Plant sterol-enriched margarines and reduction of plasma
    total- and LDL-cholesterol concentrations in normocholesterolaemic and mildly hyper-
    cholesterolaemic subjects. Eur J Clin Nutr 52:334–343

HEP (2005) 170:231–261

Carbohydrates and Dietary Fiber

P.M. Suter

Department of Medicine, Medical Policlinic, University Hospital Zürich, Rämistrasse 100, 8091 Zürich, Switzerland
paolo.suter@usz.ch

Abstract The most widely spread eating habit is characterized by a reduced intake of dietary fiber, an increased intake of simple sugars, a high intake of refined grain products, an altered fat composition of the diet, and a dietary pattern characterized by a high glycemic load, an increased body weight and reduced physical activity. In this chapter the effects of this eating pattern on disease risk will be outlined. There are no epidemiological studies showing that the increase of glucose, fructose or sucrose intake is directly and independently associated with an increased risk of atherosclerosis or coronary heart disease (CHD). On the other hand a large number of studies has reported a reduction of fatal and non-fatal CHD events as a function of the intake of complex carbohydrates—respectively 'dietary fiber' or selected fiber-rich food (e.g., whole grain cereals). It seems that eating too much 'fast' carbohydrate [i.e., carbohydrates with a high glycemic index (GI)] may have deleterious long-term consequences. Indeed the last decades have shown that a low fat (and consecutively high carbohydrate) diet alone is not the best strategy to combat modern diseases including atherosclerosis. Quantity and quality issues in carbohydrate nutrient content are as important as they are for fat. Multiple lines of evidence suggest that for cardiovascular disease prevention a high sugar intake should be avoided. There is growing evidence of the high impact of dietary fiber and foods with a low GI on single risk factors (e.g., lipid pattern, diabetes, inflammation, endothelial function etc.) as well as also the development of the endpoints of atherosclerosis especially CHD.

Keywords Carbohydrates · Dietary fiber · Glucose · Fructose · Glycemic index · Obesity · Metabolic syndrome · Diabetes mellitus

1
Introduction

Despite enormous advances in the elucidation of its pathogenesis, atherosclerosis, represents the major health problem in our society. In many less acculturated societies, a Westernized lifestyle increases the prevalence of atherosclerosis and the corresponding risk factors as well as endpoints. The economic development and concomitant changes in lifestyle (especially regarding our dietary habits) has led to an altered disease pattern and increased the risk for atherosclerosis (Perry 2002). The Westernization of eating habits includes a reduced intake of dietary fiber, an increased intake of simple sugars and refined grain products, altered fat composition of the diet and a dietary pattern characterized by a high glycemic load. This dietary changes correlate with increased body weight and reduced physical activity (Egusa et al. 2002). There are different single dietary components (e.g., saturated fat) that are associated with the development of atherosclerosis. However, single dietary risk factors are less important than the dietary pattern as a whole. Dietary modification represents a cornerstone in the prevention and therapy of all modern chronic diseases. Several recent studies focusing on more global changes of the diet, i.e., changes of the dietary pattern have led to a greater improvement of cardiovascular risk than strategies focusing only on changes of single components of the diet (Tucker et al. 1992; Appel et al. 1997; Schulze and Hu 2002; van-Dam et al. 2002; Jenkins et al. 2003). The current recommendations for the prevention of coronary heart disease (CHD) encourage the consumption of a low-fat diet rich in fruit and vegetables (which means rich in antioxidants, in many other non-nutritive compounds and in complex carbohydrates). However, the promotion of a low-fat diet alone leads to a compensatory increased intake of carbohydrates and especially of simple sugars and refined grain products, which is not without risk for the pathogenesis of chronic diseases.

Carbohydrates are a large group of metabolically very heterogeneous substrates. From the biochemical point of view, carbohydrates can be divided into two large groups according to their degree of polymerization: simple carbohydrates (or simple sugars) and complex carbohydrates (Cho et al. 1999). Simple carbohydrates include monosaccharides (e.g., glucose or fructose) and disaccharides [e.g., saccharose (=sucrose), maltose or lactose]. The complex carbohydrates include polysaccharides (e.g., starch and non-starch polysaccharides such as celullose or hemicellulose, and pectins). The complex carbohydrates also include the compounds generally known as 'dietary fiber'. From the medical and physiological point of view it may be better to classify carbohydrates or, more generally, their food sources based on their glycemic or insulinemic response after ingestion. This classification corresponds to the concept of the glycemic index (GI). Since the postprandial incremental area for blood glucose might change as a function of absorption kinetics, some authors also use the term 'slow carbohydrates' or 'fast carbohydrates' ('fast sugars') (Jenkins et al. 2002). The different classifications indicate that the source of carbohydrate in the diet may be as important as (or even more important than) their amount. The latter is also true for several forms and sources of dietary fatty acids. On the other hand, the different classifications also reflect the controversies surrounding the role of the physiological and pathophysiological effects of different sugars. Some of this controversy as well the insecurity for the consumer will be discussed in this chapter. Initially, the role of complex carbohydrates as a central component in the cardioprotective dietary pattern will be examined. In the second part of this short review, the focus will be directed at the role of the GI, the effect carbohydrate on the different lipoproteins, and the effects of selected carbohydrates on the risk of atherogenesis. This review focuses on the effects carbohydrates have on lipids, and less on other risk factors. Table 1 summarizes the effect of different carbohydrates sources and forms on the different lipid fractions and other risk factors.

2
Epidemiology

Due to difficulties in the assessment of the exact composition of carbohydrate intake, epidemiological studies revealed inconsistent correlations between carbohydrates and atherosclerosis and CHD. In the present context, the most important carbohydrates are the monosaccharides glucose and fructose, the disaccharide sucrose, and complex carbohydrates summarized as dietary fiber. There are no epidemiological studies showing that the increase in glucose, fructose or sucrose intake directly and independently correlates with an increased risk of atherosclerosis or CHD. Despite this lack of epidemiological evidence for selected sugars, one cannot ignore data suggesting that the amount and form of carbohydrate might play a part in the pathogenesis of atherosclerosis.

Table 1 Direct effects of the different forms of carbohydrates (CHO) and CHO food sources on selected risk factors for atherosclerosis and chronic disease risk%

CHO Class / Food	Total cholesterol	LDL	HDL	TG	Lp(a)	HT	Insulin resistance	Metabolic syndrome	CAD	Diabetes	Obesity
Dietary fiber											
Soluble	↓	↓	↑	↓	–	↓	↓	↓	↓	↓	↓
Insoluble	(↓)	(↓)	↑	↓	–	↓	↓	↓	↓	↓	↓
Sucrose	?	?	↓	↑	–	(↑)	(↑)	(↑)	?	↑	↑
Fructose	(↑)	(↑)	↓	↑	–	(↑)	(↑)	(↑)	?	↑	↑
Low GI food	↓	↓	↑	↓	–	↓	↓	↓	↓	↓	↓
High GI food	(↑)	(↑)	↓	↑	–	↑	↑	↑	↑	↑	↑
Wholegrains	↓	↓	↑	↓	–	↓	↓	↓	↓	↓	↓

Many of the described effects are a function of the amount and setting, i.e., associated risk factors, see text for details.

CHO, Carbohydrates;
HT, hypertension;
CHD, coronary heart disease;
TG, triglycerides;
HDL, HDL–cholesterol;
LDL, LDL–cholesterol;
GI, glycemic index;
↓ reduction;
↑ increase,
– no effect,
? not known,
() inconsistent controversial results.

Nearly 40 years ago, Yudkin postulated, based on epidemiological observations, that different hormonal and metabolic abnormalities leading to CHD may be caused by a high sucrose intake (Yudkin 1960, 1978). In the Scottish Heart Health Study, Bolton-Smith and Woodward (1994) studied the effects of different sugars (extrinsic, intrinsic, and lactose) and of dietary fat/sugar ratio on the CHD prevalence. In this cross-sectional study the sugar intake was assessed with a food-frequency questionnaire. More than 10,000 participants were divided into groups with newly diagnosed CHD, previously diagnosed CHD and no CHD. In these three groups, the men's sugar consumption differed, the women's did not. The odds ratios showed a trend for a U-shaped relationship between the prevalence of CHD and the intake of extrinsic sugar (Bolton-Smith and Woodward 1994). After adjustment for other CHD risk factors, the relationship between sugar intake and CHD lost its statistical significance. In addition, there was no correlation between the fat/sugar ratio and the prevalence of CHD. These results are interesting but in view of the methodological difficulties to assess sugar intake the results must be interpreted with caution.

More recently, several studies showed an increased risk for CHD, type 2 diabetes and dyslipidemia in individuals consuming a diet with a high glycemic load (see also Sect. 5) (Augustin et al. 2002).

In agreement with these observations, certain mono- and disaccharides, especially fructose and sucrose, respectively, may negatively modulate the risk of atherosclerosis through different mechanisms, as will be discussed later in this chapter.

On the other hand, a large set of studies reported a reduction of fatal and nonfatal CHD events as a function of increased intake of complex carbohydrates or 'dietary fiber', respectively, or selected fiber-rich food (e.g., wholegrain cereals). The degree of risk reduction (comparing the highest and lowest intake levels of total dietary fiber) varied from 20% (Khaw and Barrett-Connor 1987) to 50% (Humble et al. 1993) depending on various characteristics of the populations studied. In the majority of studies, including the Nurses' Health Study (Wolk et al. 1999) and the Iowa Women's Health Study (Jacobs et al. 1998), the difference between the lowest and the highest quartiles of consumption amounted to a risk reduction of 30%. In the Nurses' Health Study, the age-adjusted relative risk for major CHD events was 0.53 [95% confidence interval (CI), 0.40–0.69] for women in the highest quintile of total dietary fiber intake as compared to women in the lowest intake quintile. The median total dietary fiber intake of the two extremes was 22.9 g/day and 11.5 g/day, respectively (Wolk et al. 1999). However, the reduced CHD risk was only associated with a higher intake of cereal fibers and whole grains (Wolk et al. 1999), but not with refined grain intake (Jacobs et al. 2000). This is important, as the industrial processing of wholegrain foods changes the quality and the physiological effects of food considerably. The studies cited above investigated the whole diet and total dietary fiber intake. However, a considerable risk reduction is achievable only by increasing the ingestion of selected fiber-rich foods. A recent study using data from Norway analyzed the self reported bread intake (refined white bread, light whole grain bread, and dense whole grain bread) and the mortality risk (Jacobs et al. 2001). The study reported significant inverse hazard rate ratios (HRR) for total mortality with an increasing intake of wholegrain bread. Furthermore, the HRR were graded across all wholegrain bread score categories (category 5 versus category 1 HRR, 0.75; 95% CI, 0.63–0.89 in men, and HRR, 0.66, 95% CI, 0.44–0.98 in women) (Jacobs et al. 2001). In general, wholegrain foods have a low GI. Correspondingly, a diet with a high GI or glycemic load (GL) is associated with an increased risk of fatal and nonfatal myocardial infarction and also with type 2 diabetes (Liu et al. 2000; Augustin et al. 2002). Some studies failed to report this correlation, perhaps as a result of methodological issues (van Dam et al. 2000).

Insulin resistance, the metabolic syndrome and finally type 2 diabetes are central risk factors for the development of atherosclerosis. Again, there are no convincing epidemiological data on the relationship between the intake of total carbohydrates or certain sugars and the risk of type 2 diabetes. In view of the difficulties of assessing the intake of certain sugars in epidemiological studies, the important relationship between obesity and the risk of diabetes and finally the metabolic and pathophysiological interrelationships of the major energy substrates (i.e., fat and carbohydrate), it is not surprising that epidemiological relationships are missing or inconsistent (Castro-Cabezas et al. 2001; Frayn 2003; Mokdad et al. 2003). The role of carbohydrates in the treatment of diabetes is well established but it has to be remembered that there is currently no supportive evidence for the assumption that the percentage of calories from carbohydrates is of major pathophysiological importance in the development of type 2 diabetes as long as body weight is maintained (Franz and Bantle 1999). By contrast, because diabetes is very frequently confounded with a high carbohydrate intake, fibers even have favorable effects on the risk of diabetes due to their lower caloric content. Using the GI or GL approach, several studies observed a higher risk for the development of type 2 diabetes in subjects consuming a high GI (GL) diet. Other studies did not find any relationship (Stevens et al. 2002), which may again be the result of the methodologies used (e.g., the chance of finding a relationship increases if an increasing number of items included in the food frequency questionnaire) (Salmeron et al. 1997). In the study by Salmeron et al. (1997), the risk for diabetes was especially high in individuals consuming a combination of a diet with a high GI and a low intake of dietary fiber. In most studies, the intake of complex carbohydrates is associated with a reduction of the risk of diabetes. Through an increased dietary fiber intake, the risk of developing diabetes can be reduced by up to 40% (Fung et al. 2002), which also translates into favorable effects on the risk of atherosclerosis (Aronson and Rayfield 2002).

3
Consumption and Dietary Sources of Carbohydrates

In the last decades, food consumption has changed considerably. According to data obtained by the US Economic Research Service, the average daily calorie consumption in the USA in 2000 exceeded the intake level of 1985 by 12% (approximately 300 calories) (Economic-Research-Service 2003). Refined grains (i.e., food with a very high GI) accounted for approximately 44% of the increase, added fats for 24%, added sugars for 23%, fruit and vegetables for 8% (Economic-Research-Service 2003). These data clearly show that the increase in energy intake was not at all caused by very healthy choices! The average annual flour and cereal product consumption (again, all food items with a high GI) rose from 135 pounds (61 kg) in 1970 to 200 pounds (90 kg) in 2000 (Putnam et al. 2002). The total of daily Pyramid-Based-Servings per capita was 9.97, of which 7.69 servings consisted of white and whole-wheat flour (Putnam et al. 2002). The daily caloric sweetener supply was 31.4 teaspoons (approximately 150 g) per capita (adjusted for loss and waste) (Putnam et al. 2002). The consumption of added sugars is nearly three times as high as the recommended consumption of 12 teaspoons (approximately 56 g) per day. The intake of fruit (in pounds, fresh weight) increased by only 17% from 240 pounds (108 kg) in 1970 to 280 pounds in 2000 (Putnam et al. 2002). These data give an idea about the intake of carbohydrates and the changes during the last few years. Nevertheless, looking at these data we should remember the difficulties of assessing correctly any consumption data in general, and on sugars at the individual and the population level in particular (Sigman-Grant and Morita 2003). Despite some constraints, these consumption data show that we eat too much 'fast' carbohydrates (i.e., carbohydrates with a high GI). Some consequences of this behavior will be discussed in this chapter.

In nonprocessed food, glucose and fructose are found in similar small amounts (fruit, vegetables and berries). A higher content is found in honey and glucose syrup (e.g., corn syrup) and in so-called high-fructose corn syrup, HFCS). The latter contains large amounts of fructose and glucose. The major unprocessed dietary sources of sucrose are fruit, vegetables, berries and natural honey. The major part of consumed sucrose comes from sugar cane and sugar beet (Mann 2001).

4
The Cardioprotective Dietary Pattern: The role of Carbohydrates

The relationship between certain dietary components (e.g., cholesterol and saturated fatty acids, SFA) and atherosclerosis in general or certain atherosclerotic diseases (CHD) is well established. Therefore, the diet–heart hypothesis focusing on dietary cholesterol and saturated fatty acids has dominated research as well as clinical practice for the last 40 years. More than 30 years ago, a look at the global prevalence of diseases lead to the conclusion that the intake of highly-refined foods (including highly refined carbohydrate) increases the risk of CHD (Trowell 1972), and that an increased intake of unrefined carbohydrates (complex carbohydrate in the form of nondigestible dietary fiber) may be protective. Extraction, purification, and refinement of dietary carbohydrate sources are only a very recent phenomenon in human evolution (Spiller 2002; Walker et al. 2003), as is the pandemia of chronic diseases. Worldwide nutrition-related health patterns have changed significantly during the last decades and this has led to a change of the risk factor profile for atherosclerosis and other diseases and, in consequence, of disease patterns also (Bermudez and Tucker 2003; Ciccarone et al. 2003; Galal 2003; Newby et al. 2003). In view of the epidemiological trends of CHD, the dietary approach was only partially helpful. CHD mortality has declined during the last 20 years as a result of improved medical treatments (Capewell et al. 1999). CHD morbidity, however, has declined little. There is increasing evidence that a greater risk reduction may be achieved by multiple dietary changes rather than by a monocausal or monofactorial strategy, such as the reduction of saturated fat or cholesterol intake. A dietary pattern reducing the risk for the development of chronic diseases, including atherosclerosis and CHD, is characterized by a predominant intake of nonhydrogenated unsaturated fats as the main form of dietary fat, whole grains as the main form of carbohydrate, a high intake of fruit, vegetables and legumes as well as a higher intake of omega-3-fatty acids (Joshipura et al. 1999, 2001; Hu and Willett 2002). The increased intake of complex nonrefined carbohydrate plays an important part in the overall protective dietary pattern. The higher the intake of refined food, the worse the overall cardiovascular risk profile (e.g., regarding hypertension, hyperglycemia, hypercholesterolemia) (van Dam et al. 2003). This protective dietary pattern is further characterized by a high dietary fiber intake, a low intake of refined sugar, a high level of physical activity, abstinence from smoking and the maintenance of a healthy body weight. For clinical practice, the promotion of a healthy dietary pattern, i.e., of a whole diet approach, is useful on an individual as well as population level for the prevention of chronic diseases and the control of specific risk factors such as obesity, hypertension, physical inactivity, smoking and others (Appel et al. 1997; Walker et al. 2003; Sacks et al. 2001; Trichopoulou et al. 2003; Roberts et al. 2002). Although the beneficial effects of a healthy diet cannot be linked to a single nutrient (Wirfält et al. 2001), it has to be emphasized that a high intake of dietary fiber and of whole cereal grains is a central component of a healthy eating pattern.

4.1
Dietary Fiber

'Dietary fiber' is a term most consumers use widely and know well. However, from the scientific point of view, the term is obscure, lacking a uniformly accepted definition (Cho et al. 1999). Plant substances resisting hydrolysis during small bowel digestion are regarded as dietary fiber. The Macronutrient Report of the Institute of Medicine's Dietary Reference Intakes states that dietary fiber consists of nondigestible carbohydrates and lignin that are intrinsic and intact in plants, and further that functional fiber consists of isolated nondigestible carbohydrate eliciting beneficial physiological effects in humans (Institute of Medicine 2002). The term 'total fiber' stands for the sum of dietary fiber and functional fiber. The American Association of Cereal Chemists (De Vries 2003) defines dietary fiber as follows: "...the edible parts of plants or analogous carbohydrates that are resistant to digestion and absorption in the human small intestine with complete or partial fermentation in the large intestine. Dietary fiber includes polysaccharides, oligosaccharides, lignin, and associated plant substances. Dietary fibers promote beneficial physiological effects including laxation, and/or blood cholesterol attenuation, and/or blood glucose attenuation" (De Vries 2003). Despite this new definition of dietary fiber, the controversy will probably continue. For clinical purposes, a classification of dietary fibers according to their solubility and bacterial fermentation characteristics and thus their major clinical effects is more reasonable.

4.2
Soluble or Insoluble Dietary Fiber?

Epidemiological studies showed that an increased intake of soluble (Rimm et al. 1996; Kushi et al. 1999; Bazzano et al. 2003) and total (insoluble and soluble) (Rimm et al. 1996; Kushi et al. 1999) dietary fiber from different food sources (especially wholegrain foods) reduced the risk of CHD. Data from adults participating in the National Health and Nutrition Examination Survey I (NHANES I) during an average follow-up of 19 years revealed that the relative risk of CHD for those in the highest (median soluble fiber intake 5.9 g/day) compared with those in the lowest (0.9 g/day) quartile of soluble dietary fiber intake was 0.85 (95% CI, 0.74–0.98; $P=0.004$ for trend) for CHD events and 0.90 (95% CI, 0.82–0.99; $P=0.01$ for trend) for cardiovascular disease (CVD) events (Bazzano et al. 2003). Soluble fiber has a bigger impact on CHD risk factors (especially lipid factors) than does insoluble fiber (Spiller 1993). Nevertheless, in many epidemiological studies the cereal fiber consumption (which has a lower soluble fiber content) was inversely related to the CHD risk (Liu et al. 1999; for a review see Truswell 2002). Data from the Nurses Health Study showed an inverse relationship between wholegrain intake and CHD risk (Liu et al. 1999). In this study, the CHD risk decreased from 1.0 in the lowest quintile to 0.75 in the highest quintile of wholegrain intake (95 % CI, 0.59–0.95; P for trend=0.01) after adjustment for the classical risk factors (Liu et al. 1999). The subgroup of individuals who had never smoked was protected most effectively (R=0.49 for the extreme quintiles of whole grain intake; 95% CI, 0.30–0.79; P for trend=0.003) (Liu et al. 1999). In the same study, the risk of ischemic stroke also decreased with an increasing wholegrain intake (Liu et al. 2000). After adjustment for the classical risk factors, the relative risk for ischemic stroke from the lowest to the highest quintiles of whole grain intake declined from 1.0 to 0.68 (95% CI, 0.35–0.69), 0.69 (95% CI, 0.51–0.95), 0.49 (95% CI, 0.35–0.69), and 0.57 (95% CI, 0.42–0.78; for trend P=0.003) (Liu et al. 2000). A hospital-based case–control study reported protective effects of dietary fiber on nonfatal acute myocardial infarction (Negri et al. 2003), although the causal mechanisms of these effects remain unclear. In view of the diet–heart hypothesis that emphasizes the dietary fat intake and the known effects of soluble fibers on lipoprotein metabolism, the protective effects of dietary fiber on CHD are surprising as cereals mainly contain insoluble fibers. However, as cereal grains contain several cardioprotective compounds, such as antioxidants, unsaturated fatty acids, phytosterols and, last but not least, total dietary fiber, these findings are not astonishing (Slavin 2003). Again, the example of fiber intake and the apparently paradoxical reduction of CHD emphasizes the importance of multiple interacting mechanisms by which a diet may elicit cardioprotective effects and underlines the importance of the dietary pattern as discussed above.

In the daily diet, we usually ingest a mixture of soluble and insoluble dietary fiber. About 25% of fiber from cereal sources is water soluble (Spiller 1993). The apparently paradoxical finding that cereal grains (cereal fibers) are cardiopro-tective despite the relatively low content of soluble fiber strongly supports the theory that it is much more important to follow a cardioprotective dietary pat-tern than to focus on single food components. The American Heart Association recommends a daily fiber intake of 25–30 g/day (van Horn 1997). It is difficult to separate the effects of soluble and insoluble fibers, as a balanced diet is com-posed of a combination of the two major types of fiber. In general, wheat, rice, rye and the majority of grains contain a large portion of insoluble dietary fibers (Spiller 1993). An exception from this rule is oats, being a very good source of soluble fiber (Spiller 1993; Bell et al. 1999). Legumes are excellent sources of both types of fiber (Spiller 1993). The fiber content of fruit and vegetables is generally lower than the one of legumes and cereal grains (Spiller 1993).

There are many direct and indirect mechanisms by which dietary fiber may protect from atherosclerosis, the latter including cholesterol absorption, cholesterol synthesis as well as lipid-independent mechanisms (e.g., protection of endothelial dysfunction) (Spiller 1993). Clinical and in vitro studies showed that the direct lowering effect on cholesterol is mainly associated with the ingestion of soluble fibers (Spiller 1993; Fernandez 2001). Most studies in humans reported that wheat fiber had no significant effects on dyslipidemia.

Wheat fiber does not lower total cholesterol, low-density lipoprotein (LDL)-cholesterol and triglycerides (TG), and it does not have a significant effect on high-density lipoprotein (HDL)-cholesterol (Spiller 1993; Truswell 2002).

Cereals and cereal products (e.g., wheat grains, rye or oats) are our main sources of dietary fiber. The total dietary fiber content of cereals varies from 10% to 15 %, however, the content of soluble fiber varies from 20% (wheat) to approximately 50% (oats) (Spiller 1993). Dietary fiber consumption has been dramatically reduced during the last 50 years (Spiller 2002), mainly as a result of the increased refinement of cereal (wholegrain) products and the production of white flour (Spiller 2002). This change in the dietary pattern and an increase in the prevalence of chronic diseases including CHD, hypertension, obesity, diabetes, the metabolic syndrome and certain types of cancer appeared simultaneously. The cereals with the highest content of soluble fiber are oats, rye and barley. Their consumption results in favorable lipid effects, including the lowering of cholesterol (Davidson et al. 1991; Bourdon et al. 1999; Leinonen et al. 1999, 2000).

The fiber of oats is characterized by the high content of β-glucan (the major soluble fiber of oats) and lowers lipid levels significantly. A meta-analysis (based on 10 out of 20 studies meeting the inclusion criteria) by Ripsin et al. (1992) reported a total cholesterol lowering effect of oats amounting to -0.13 mmol/l (95% CI, -0.19 to -0.017 mmol/l). The effect was more pronounced in subjects with higher plasma cholesterol and in studies using a dose of 3 g β-glucan. There is a linear inverse relationship between the daily dose of β-glucan and the change of total cholesterol and/or LDL-cholesterol from baseline (Davidson et al. 1991). Nearly 50 studies on the effects of oats or β-glucan on plasma cholesterol and other plasma lipids have been published and showed consistent results (Bartnikowska 1999; Webster 2002). As a function of specific study characteristics (degree of dyslipidemia, body weight status and weight loss during intervention, type of oats used), plasma cholesterol declined by more than 20% (Bartnikowska 1999; Anderson et al. 1984). The effects of β-glucan are more pronounced in individuals with high total cholesterol, and in general there is no HDL-cholesterol lowering effect occurring. The content of the soluble oat fiber varies in different oat products from 4 to 5 g in rolled oats and from 6 to 7.5 g in oat bran (Webster 2002). In view of the consistent effects of oats on total and LDL-cholesterol, an authorized health claim on the relationship between the β-glucan soluble fiber from whole oat sources and a reduced risk of CHD has been formulated (Food and Drug Administration 2002). According to the Food and Drug Administration (FDA) regulation rolled oats, oat bran and whole oat flour, the soluble fraction of oat bran or whole oat flour with a β-glucan content of up to 10% on a dry weight basis (dwb) and not less than the one of the starting material (dwb), is an appropriate source of β-glucan soluble fiber for this health claim (Food and Drug Administration 2002).

Other cereal-based sources of soluble fiber are rye, barley and rice bran. An increased consumption of soluble fibers from these sources improves the lipid profile. The ingestion of a rather large amount of rye bread (20% of the daily energy intake, thus increasing the fiber intake by 15 g) for 4 weeks without any other change in the usual diet resulted in a decrease of total cholesterol by 8% (−0.53 mmol/l, P=0.002) and LDL-cholesterol (−0.36 mmol/l) (Leinonen et al. 1999). To achieve this effect, the subjects in the study by Leinonen et al. (1999) had to ingest about eight slices of rye bread per day, which is much higher than the two to three slices of bread currently consumed by the average Finnish person. Similar effects on total and LDL-cholesterol have been reported after the intake of barley or rice bran (Cicero and Gaddi 2001; Rajnarayana et al. 2001). Usually, large amounts of these fibers are needed and the effects are comparatively small even when enriched barley-derived β-glucan is used (Delaney et al. 2003; Keogh et al. 2003). To obtain a clinically relevant effect, large quantities of the corresponding food sources need to be ingested (Keogh et al. 2003), which is not necessarily easy to achieve. Further, our society consumes some of these food items in small quantities only and the acceptance of these foods is often too low to significantly reduce the risk at the population level.

A good source of soluble fiber is psyllium (psyllium seed husk) that is also associated with a considerable reduction of plasma cholesterol levels. Anderson et al. (2000) studied the effectiveness of 5.1 g psyllium twice per day in reducing plasma cholesterol as compared to a cellulose placebo. During this 26-week trial, the serum of total cholesterol and LDL-cholesterol declined by 4.7% and 6.7%, respectively (Anderson et al. 2000). The active component of psyllium seems to be a highly-branched arabinoxylan consisting of a xylose backbone and arabinose- and xylose-containing side chains (Marlett and Fischer 2003). The effects of psyllium and other dietary fiber sources are comparatively small. However, it should not be forgotten that they represent only a part of a more holistic approach, i.e. a change of the whole dietary pattern alone or even combined with drugs.

The combination of psyllium with an increased intake of MUFA (monounsaturated fatty acids) may favorably modify the lipid effects of viscous soluble fibers. A higher MUFA intake (approximately 12% of MUFA, 29% of total fat) in combination with a defined soluble fiber intake from psyllium (1.4 g/MJ) improved the triacylglycerol reduction (16.6±5.5%, P=0.006) and the ratio of LDL/HDL cholesterol (7.3±2.8%, P=0.015) compared to the psyllium phase without MUFA (Jenkins et al. 1997).

5
Glycemic Index and Atherosclerosis

During the last few years there has been increasing evidence that metabolic abnormalities surrounding glucose and insulin metabolism are key events in the pathogenesis of many chronic diseases including atherosclerosis. Overweight and obesity are often associated with the metabolic syndrome that is characterized by abdominal obesity (waist circumference in men >102 cm and in women >88 cm), elevated plasma TG concentration ($\geq$1.69 mmol/l), low HDL-cholesterol (<1.0 mol/l in men and >1.29 mmol/l in women), an increased blood pressure ($\geq$130/85 mmHg) and an elevated plasma glucose (>6.1 mmol/l) (Adult Treatment Panel III 2002). The metabolic syndrome can be observed in all age groups of our society at an increasing rate (Ford et al. 2002). A basic pathophysiological event triggering the development of the metabolic syndrome is insulin resistance (Reaven 2002, Stolar and Chilton 2003). Lifestyle factors such as body weight or physical activity are important modulators of insulin resistance (Reusch 2002). Many studies showed that low GI diets may favorably influence the pathogenesis of insulin resistance and especially several of the clinical consequences and endpoints (Liu et al. 2000; van Dam et al. 2000; Stevens et al. 2002; Liu et al. 2000; Brand-Miller et al. 2003; Ford and Liu 2001; Liu 2002, Ludwig 2003). The GI corresponds to the increase in blood glucose concentration after the ingestion of the corresponding food (standardized to obtain 50 g CHO) as compared to the increase in blood glucose after the ingestion of glucose or white bread (Jenkins et al. 1981). The glycemic response is subject to many different influences, such as the composition of starch and polysaccharides, the amount of soluble fiber, food processing and cooking, as well as interactions with other food components (e.g., protein or fat) (Augustin et al. 2002). Dietary fibers and their composition are important determinants of the GI (Bjoerck and Elmstahl 2003), however, the absolute content of glucose seems to be the major determinant (Engelyst et al. 2003). Accordingly, it is not surprising that the GIs of whole-wheat bread or white bread are very similar, although the fiber content varies considerably. As the GI is defined according to the increase of the plasma glucose, only sugars leading to a change in the plasma glucose are considered to be a determinant of the GI. Sugar (sucrose or ordinary table sugar), however, plays a very important role in nutrition and health maintenance, as a disaccharide (composed of glucose and fructose) with a relatively small GI, as long as it is not ingested in large amounts. Still, the comparatively low GI of sucrose will be significantly altered by a disproportionally high glucose intake. It is therefore recommended not to eat more than 10 teaspoons (50 g) of sugar. However, in view of the very high sugar content of many popular foods, this maximum of 10 teaspoons is frequently exceeded (e.g., a 12-oz (330 ml) soft drink contains approximately 10 teaspoons of sugar). The present sugar intake in the USA is more than 30 % higher than in the year 1983 (Center for Science in Public Interest CSPI 2003). From the pathophysiological and biochemical point of view, the high sugar content of our diet favors the development of chronic and acute diseases through pathophysiological events linked to a high GI. Epidemiological studies reported a relationship between the GI and the risk of CHD (Liu et al. 2000). This is not surprising, as the GI is associated with different cardiovascular risk factors such as insulin sensitivity, metabolic syndrome and diabetes, dyslipidemia (low HDL-cholesterol–high TG), hypertension or inflammation (Ford and Liu 2001; Sciarrone et al. 1993; Sacks and Katan 2002). HDL-cholesterol is one of the central lipid determinants for the risk of atherosclerosis. Ford and Liu (2001) examined data from the NHANES III and identified a high dietary GI to be an independent determinant of HDL-cholesterol. In obese individuals, the ingestion of a low GI/low fat/high protein diet was associated with an improved metabolic risk profile (Dumesnil et al. 2001). In addition, such a diet may have favorable long-term effects on body weight regulation, since its food components alleviate hunger and increase satiation (Dumesnil et al. 2001; Ball et al. 2003).

Again, for the treatment of patients high GI foods do not need to be avoided altogether. It is the overall composition of the diet that is important. Adding fiber-rich foods or isolated dietary fiber (e.g., β-glucan) to high GI foods reduces the GI (Jenkins et al. 2002). Moreover, foods with a high GI can easily be identified in the diet of patients by using published tables (Foster-Powell et al. 2002).

The concept of the GI is very appealing but nevertheless controversial (Raben 2002). However, in view of the deleterious effects of insulin resistance and the metabolic syndrome, the GI-hypothesis describing hyperglycemia and the overproduction of insulin fits well into the pathophysiological cascade of atherosclerosis. Further, societies with a low prevalence of chronic diseases, including atherosclerosis, do consume a low GI diet (Jenkins et al. 2003).

6
Carbohydrates and Selected Risk Factors

6.1
Obesity and Diabetes

Obesity, especially abdominal obesity, is one of the most important risk factor for atherosclerosis. There is no other single risk factor that is positively associated with most of the classical cardiovascular risk factors (Bosello and Zamboni 2000; Alexander 2001; Lakka et al. 2002). Obesity is increasing worldwide, and this development is paralleled by a rise in the prevalence of the metabolic syndrome and frank diabetes mellitus type 2 (Ford et al. 2002; Popkin and Doak 1998). Especially abdominal obesity leads to an unfavorable clustering of various risk factors that constitute the metabolic syndrome (Reaven 2002). A shift from traditional to modern diets includes a shift from staple foods with a high starch and dietary fiber content to diets characterized by the consumption of processed starch and cereal products. This shift in diet contributes to an increasing prevalence of overweight, obesity and type 2 diabetes (Fung et al. 2002). Type 2 diabetes is associated with an increased risk for atherosclerosis due to different mechanisms including dyslipidemia (Stolar and Chilton 2003; Solymoss et al. 2003). An increased intake of wholegrain foods has been associated with a reduced risk for developing diabetes and heart disease. A higher wholegrain intake is associated with higher insulin sensitivity (Liese et al. 2003) and thus a reduced risk for developing diabetes. A high fiber diet was found to exert long-term favorable effects on glucose tolerance and dyslipidemia, regardless of the composition of the dietary fiber (Bosello et al. 1980; Villaume et al. 1984). Some controversial results can be explained by the insufficient duration of the corresponding interventions. Most foods eliciting favorable effects on glucose tolerance and lipid status are characterized by a low GI. It is debatable whether a low GI diet presents an advantage for obese individuals for weight reduction purposes. Ebbeling et al. (2003) found that in obese adolescents an ad libitum, reduced-GL diet was more effective for body weight control than a conventional energy-restricted, reduced-fat diet (Ebbeling et al. 2003).

The consumption of fiber-rich foods (e.g., fiber-rich bread) was associated with a lower risk for abdominal obesity (Wirfält et al. 2001). A diet with an increased GI or GL is associated with an increased risk for fatal and nonfatal myocardial infarction (Liu et al. 2000). This is only true, however, for overweight individuals who will soon account for the largest fraction of the US population (Kuczmarski et al. 1994; McLellan 2002). In the study by Liu et al. (2000) the GL was only associated with a greater CHD risk in individuals with a body mass index (BMI) greater than 23 kg/m^2. This observation is in agreement with the pathophysiological relationship between body weight, insulin resistance, and carbohydrate intake. A recent meta-analysis confirmed that the consumption of a low-GI diet may be useful in the management of diabetes (Brand-Miller et al. 2003).

6.2
LDL-Cholesterol

LDL-cholesterol lowering remains a key strategy for the primary and secondary prevention of CHD (Expert Panel on Detection 2001). According to these guidelines, the therapeutic approach for LDL control should include dietary and pharmacological strategies. However, in view of the powerful effects of modern drug therapy, dietary strategies are often neglected. Several studies reported an additional decrease in LDL-cholesterol from 5% (Hunninghake et al. 1993) to 10% (Clifton et al. 1994) if drugs were combined with dietary fiber as compared to the drug regimen alone. These studies mainly included diets low in saturated fatty acids. Implementing a more global dietary approach in patients on cholesterol-lowering drugs in the form of the so-called Pritikin diet, i.e., a diet with a very low fat content (<10% from fat) and rich in complex carbohydrates, in combination with an exercise program, lead to an additional reduction of total cholesterol (−19%), of LDL-cholesterol (−20%), and TG (−29%) (P<0.01 for all parameters) (Barnard et al. 1997). After the completion of this intervention, 60% of the patients met the LDL goal of the National Cholesterol Education Program (NCEP) compared to only 27% at the start of the intervention (Barnard et al. 1997). In this study, the additional lipid lowering effects were much more pronounced than in most other studies, which is a result of the rather extreme and strongly supervised intervention. This intervention study lasted only 3 weeks and long-term compliance to such a program may be a problem. The dramatic effects described above are a result of the combination approach of diet, exercise and also body weight changes and are hardly achievable for the majority of patients. Ingesting 5–10 g of soluble fiber will result in a reduction of LDL-cholesterol of approximately 5%. A meta-analysis by Brown et al. (1999) concluded that each gram of soluble fiber of the diet will result in a total cholesterol change of −0.045 mmol/l (95% CI, −0.054 to −0.035) and a LDL-cholesterol change of −0.057 mmol/l (95 % CI, −0.070 to −0.044) (Brown et al. 1999). At first glance, this effect is small, but it translates into considerable risk reduction if a large enough quantity is ingested for long enough. The ingestion of 9 g/d of psyllium leads to a decrease in LDL-cholesterol of 6%–7% (Brown et al. 1999). The effects of the major soluble fiber in the form of oats, psyllium, or pectin on plasma lipids were not significantly different, as shown by the results of this meta-analysis. Other soluble fibers, such as isolated β-glucan, normal and/or defatted flaxseed (Prasad 2000; Lucas et al. 2002) or konjacmannan (Chen et al. 2003) showed a dose–response relationship to LDL-cholesterol lowering in the range of approximately 7%–20 %. It has to be remembered that the food matrix and/or the food processing (including cooking) methods can exert adverse effects on the hypocholesterolemic properties of the β-glucan of oats, but also of other dietary fibers (Kerckhoffs et al. 2003).

6.3
HDL-Cholesterol

Dietary fiber per se has no direct effect on HDL-cholesterol. In view of the effects of dietary fiber as well as the GI and/or load on TG levels, it is not surprising that HDL-cholesterol is favorably influenced as a function of the quality of the ingested carbohydrate. A low GI or GL diet may represent an ideal strategy for the maintenance of higher HDL-cholesterol levels (Ford and Liu 2001). An evaluation of the data from NHANES III (Ford and Liu 2001) showed an inverse relationship between GI and GL and HDL-cholesterol concentration across all subgroups of participants categorized by sex or BMI. After adjusting for different covariates and considering GI as a continuous variable, a change in the GI by 15 units was found to increase the HDL-cholesterol concentration by 0.06 mmol/l ($P<0.001$). The latter effect seems small, but in view of the big impact of small changes of HDL-cholesterol on the risk for CHD and the simultaneous reduction of LDL-cholesterol these effects translate into a large clinical benefit (Asztalos and Schaefer 2003). Older and newer studies reported that a high sucrose intake is associated with a lower HDL-cholesterol (Ernst et al. 1980; Archer et al. 1998). The HDL-cholesterol lowering effect of sucrose is not surprising, as a higher sucrose intake (>20% of total energy) leads to an increase in the plasma TG concentration (see Sect. 6.4). The TG enrichment of HDL leads to an increased catabolism of apolipoprotein A-1 (apoA-1) and thus to a decline in HDL-cholesterol (Lamarche et al. 1999).

6.4
Triglycerides

During the last few years evidence has accumulated that an elevated TG concentration represents an independent risk factor for CHD (Austin et al. 1998). The increase in plasma TG concentration in response to already small increases in carbohydrate intake is well known and a universal phenomenon. Neither the pathophysiological mechanisms nor the clinical consequences are well understood (Parks and Hellerstein 2000). Simple sugars and starch have the strongest effect on TG levels, which, however, is modulated by dietary fiber. As recently reviewed by Anderson (2000), several metabolic ward studies reported that a high-carbohydrate/low-fiber diet increases fasting TG levels by 53% on average (95% CI, 34–71%). In contrast, high-carbohydrate/high fiber diets lead to a decrease in fasting TG of approximately 10% (95 % CI, −1 to −17) (Anderson 2000). Only the combination of a high carbohydrate diet and weight loss avoided the increase in TG concentration (Lichtenstein et al. 1994).

In a very elegant study Hudgins et al. (1996) observed that a eucaloric low fat/high carbohydrate diet stimulates fatty acid synthesis, and that this effect is identical in lean and obese subjects (Hudgins et al. 2000). The stimulation of fatty acid synthesis is increased after the equicaloric substitution of simple carbohydrates for complex carbohydrates (Hudgins et al. 1998). The stimulatory effect was higher on a 10%-fat diet than on a 30%-fat diet (Hudgins et al. 2000). These important data prove that not only the amount but also the type of carbohydrate is an important determinant for the rate of fatty acid synthesis. Further, they support some critiques on the low-fat dietary approach to atherosclerosis. Many unfavorable effects of the diet on risk factors are more important in obese individuals. The data from Hudgins et al. (2000) showed no significant difference in the carbohydrate-induced fatty acid synthesis in lean and obese subjects, despite the increased insulin levels in the obese subjects. They also described a correlation between fasting TG levels and fatty acid synthesis on the 10%-fat carbohydrate diet. The effect of carbohydrates on TG levels occurs on all levels of intake but increases with increasing carbohydrate intake and decreasing fat intake and shows considerable individual variation (Parks and Hellerstein 2000; Retzlaff et al. 1995). Dietary fructose, consumed in larger amounts, also has a very strong effect on the plasma triglyceride concentration (see Sect. 7) (Bantle et al. 2000). The TG modulating effects of the different carbohydrates are counteracted by physical activity and exercise (Suter et al. 2001; Laaksonen et al. 2002; Gill and Hardman 2003) or other dietary components such as more complex carbohydrates (Hudgins et al. 1998).

The relationship between high carbohydrate intake and plasma TG is one of the most consistent biochemical observations in carbohydrate metabolism and nutrition. How much carbohydrate is too much carbohydrate? This question cannot be answered yet today and varies as a function of unknown genetic factors, the baseline lipoprotein pattern and especially the presence of other cardiovascular risk factors. For an individual presenting with increased body weight, physical inactivity, high fasting TG and/or hyperinsulinemia the intake of simple carbohydrate and starch should be low to moderate. In view of the present evidence, probably the lower the better.

6.5
Postprandial Lipemia

More than 20 years ago, Zilversmit and Mamo et al. postulated that atherosclerosis is to a larger extent a postprandial phenomenon (Zilversmit 1979; Zilversmit 1995; Mamo et al. 1997). Postprandial lipemia as well as hormonal changes occurring during the postprandial phase seem to represent important modulators of atherosclerosis. The postprandial clearance of TG-rich lipoproteins represents a major determinant of HDL-cholesterol concentration (Miesenböck and Patsch 1992). As a consequence of the diet–heart hypothesis low-fat, high-carbohydrate diets have been promoted. However, such a diet will also lead to an increase in the postprandial lipemia (increased peak TG concentration, increased TG area under the curve and an increased duration of the postprandial lipemia) (Leinonen et al.1999; Flatt et al. 1985; Jeppsen et al. 1995; Dubois et al. 1998; Parks 2001). Postprandial lipemia is affected by many nonmodifiable (e.g., genetic) and modifiable factors, e.g., exercise, alcohol, obesity, body composition, the baseline TG concentration and substrate composition of the diet (Suter et al. 2001; Hyson et al. 2003). A diet high in carbohydrate causes increased postprandial TG concentrations and, as a consequence, a decrease in HDL-cholesterol concentration and lipoprotein particle size as well as the occurrence of small dense LDL particles (Koutsari et al. 2000; Lemieux et al. 2000). Physical activity is a central modulator of postprandial lipemia (Hardman and Herd 1998). Present evidence suggests that carbohydrate enhances postprandial lipemia only in physically inactive individuals (Koutsari and Hardman 2001). Recently, Koutsari and Hardman (2001) reported that the increase in the postprandial TG response of more than one-third on a high-carbohydrate diet (70% of energy) could be reversed by a low degree of daily physical activity of 30 min of daily walking. The outcome of this short-term study may be extrapolated to the longer term, since many Asian and African populations do not show increased postprandial lipemia in the presence of high level physical activity, although they consume large quantities of carbohydrate as their staple food (Xie et al. 1998). However, as soon as a Western lifestyle is adapted, this favorable risk profile is lost (Bermudez and Tucker 2003; Dwyer et al. 2003). Without changing the pattern of physical activity, a low-carbohydrate diet significantly decreases the fasting and post-prandial triglyceride plasma concentration, increases HDL-cholesterol and improves the total cholesterol/HDL-cholesterol ratio in normal-weight and normolipidemic individuals (Volek et al. 2003). Especially overweight or obese individuals not pursuing regular (i.e., daily) physical activity should avoid a high intake of simple carbohydrate, particularly if they are hypertriglyceridemic.

6.6
Inflammation

An elevated C-reactive protein (CRP) value has been identified as an independent CHD risk factor (Jialal and Devaraj 2003). Pharmacological and non-pharmacological strategies can help reduce inflammation and, hence, CRP levels. Recently, Jenkins et al. (2003) evaluated the lipid-lowering effects of a dietary portfolio according to the present recommendations (i.e., low in saturated fat together with plant sterols and viscous fibers) as compared to a statin. In this study, the participants were randomized to obtain, during 1 month, a diet containing very low amounts of saturated fat, consisting of milled whole-wheat cereals and low-fat dairy products (=control group). Another group obtained the same diet plus 20 mg of lovastatin (=lovastatin group). The third group corresponded to the so-called dietary portfolio group and received a diet with a higher content of plant stanols (1 g/1000 kcal), rich in soy protein (21.4 g/1000 kcal), viscous fibers (9.8 g/1000 kcal) and almonds (14 g/1000 kcal). The mean ± SE reduction of LDL-cholesterol was significant in all three groups, but was lowest in the control group (8 ± 2.1 %) and very similar in the lovastatin and dietary portfolio group (28.6 ± 3.2% versus 30.9 ± 3.6%) (Jenkins et al. 2003). The mean reductions in CRP levels amounted to 10% in the control group (P=nonsignificant), 33% in the lovastatin group (P=0.002) and 28% in the dietary portfolio group (P=0.02) (Jenkins et al. 2003). The CRP reduction was not related to changes in LDL-cholesterol, which–if this had been the case–would have suggested direct effects of the diet or certain dietary components. Different dietary factors have been reported to lower CRP levels (Clifton 2003) such as a cholesterol-lowering diet, weight loss or a change in most of the traditional cardiovascular disease risk factors (Esposito et al. 2003; Saito et al. 2003).

7
The Role of Sucrose and Fructose

Ordinary sugar (sucrose or saccharose) is a disaccharide formed by glucose and fructose. As discussed above, the major carbohydrate-related determinant of the glycemic index is glucose. Sucrose as a disaccharide, consisting of equal parts of fructose and glucose, has a rather low GI. However, in the setting of a large sucrose intake the impact of the corresponding relatively high glucose intake may become pathophysiologically relevant (see also Sect. 5). A low intake of fructose, on the other hand, is metabolically inert and may have favorable effects (Moore et al. 2000). However, this inertness of fructose is lost if fructose is consumed in large amounts, since it bypasses the major regulatory steps of glycolysis. Glycerol-3-phosphate, which is formed from fructose-1-phosphate, is the starting point for TG synthesis. Accordingly, a high intake of fructose increases the availability of the TG backbone glycerol-3-phosphate and, thereby, TG and very-low-density lipoprotein (VLDL) synthesis (Frayn and Kingman 1995). In a randomized, balanced cross-over study during which two identical diets were fed, except that crystalline fructose was added to one diet and crystalline glucose to the other, Bantle et al. (2000) illustrated the effect of fructose on plasma lipids. Fifty-five percent of total energy in these diets was provided by carbohydrate, including 17% and 3% provided by fructose in the fructose and glucose regimens, respectively. In males participating in this study, the high fructose intake led to a significantly higher fasting, postprandial, and daylong plasma TG concentration as compared to the glucose regimen (Bantle et al. 2000). Others reported a similar effect of fructose on the plasma lipid pattern (Reiser et al. 1989).

The increase of fructose from fruit and vegetables is comparatively small in view of the large fraction of added sugar (in the form of HFCS or sucrose in numerous processed foods and beverages). From the metabolic point of view, it is conceivable that a continuously high intake of fructose may have long-term adverse effects, especially if these dietary habits are practiced for several decades, start early in life and are combined with a lifestyle characterized by a low level of physical activity. For fructose, there are no controlled long-term data available and accordingly, no final conclusion can be drawn. Nevertheless, there are rather consistent experimental data for potential adverse effects that need to be taken seriously in view of the continuous increase in sucrose intake as well as the pandemia of obesity. The potentially adverse effects are more pronounced in the setting of a low dietary fiber intake, a higher body weight status (Lichtenstein et al. 1994) and last but not least a low level of physical activity (Wood et al. 1994; Durstine et al. 2002; Petitt and Cureton 2003). Although the data are not yet conclusive and are controversial, a high intake of added sugars should be avoided, especially in the presence of increased body weight and physical inactivity. This recommendation is also in agreement with the present dietary guidelines and American Heart Association (AHA) recommendations (Howard and Wylie-Rosett 2002). The pathophysiological potential of the combination of a high-sucrose and high-fat diet in atherogenesis is supported by animal data (Yin et al. 2002), even though these data, resulting from animal testing, need to be interpreted with caution. An increased carbohydrate intake, especially an increased sucrose intake, is associated with decreased lipid oxidation and thus an increased risk for a positive fat balance and for obesity (Acheson et al. 1982; Flatt 1993). The latter is also associated with a decreased catabolism of triglyceride-rich lipoproteins TRL, resulting in prolonged lipemia (Brunzell et al. 1973). Although some experimental conditions may be rather artificial, sucrose leads to a dose-dependent increase in the triglyceride concentration (Albrink and Ullrich 1986; Raben et al. 1998; Marckmann et al. 2000). In a short-term study (11 days) by Albrink and Ullrich (1986), the sucrose effect was counteracted by the addition of dietary fiber at the lower intake levels (36% sucrose diet). However, at high intake levels (52% in this study), dietary fiber had no effect. In this study, a lower intake (<18%) of sucrose had no effect on the TG concentration, which may be due to the lower fructose intake. Most studies are only short term and some evidence suggests that the effects of increasing the TG of high-carbohydrate, high sugar diets may become less relevant over time (Saris et al. 2000), as long as certain adaptive mechanisms are working. The latter may be impaired or lost in overweight and obese subjects or in the presence of insulin resistance and/or physical inactivity, respectively. The hypertriglyceridemic effects of sucrose and other carbohydrates are modulated by the body weight status, fat distribution pattern and physical activity (Durstine et al. 2002; Petitt and Cureton 2003; Roust et al. 1994).

8
Conclusion and Recommendations

During the last decades, a low-fat (and consecutively high carbohydrate) diet has been promoted for the combat of modern diseases including atherosclerosis. We now know that low-fat diets are not very helpful in the control of the chronic diseases of the modern society. Further, we do know that not all fats are 'bad fats'. A diet high in monounsaturated and polyunsaturated fatty acids is promoted and regarded as very healthy (de Lorgeril et al. 1999; Trichopoulou et al. 2003). Besides the latter discoveries it was found that not all carbohydrates are equal regarding the metabolic response pattern as well as the pathophysiological potential. Quantity and quality issues are as important for dietary carbohydrate as for dietary fat. A recent Scientific Statement for Health professionals issued by the AHA about the role of sugar in cardiovascular disease concluded that high sugar intake should be avoided (Howard and Wylie-Rosett 2002), as there is no nutritional value in sugar other than calories. A high intake of sugar displaces nutrient-dense foods and should be controlled accordingly (Howard and Wylie-Rosett 2002).

In this chapter, we focused on a few selected aspects of carbohydrates and dietary fiber regarding the risk of atherosclerosis, especially the metabolic risk factors related to lipoprotein metabolism. There is growing evidence of the high impact of dietary fiber and foods with a low GI on single risk factors (e.g. lipid pattern, diabetes, inflammation, endothelial function etc.) as well as the development of clinical endpoints of atherosclerosis, especially of CHD. The present evidence is not yet complete, but we nevertheless do have enough evidence for action, i e., implementation. In view of the very potent drugs used for the treatment of dyslipidemia, hypertension or diabetes, the important role of dietary factors in prevention and therapy gets lost and even forgotten. We do know about the additive effects of drug combinations. However, we forget about the additive effects of the combination of dietary and pharmacological strategies (Clemmer et al. 2001; Foster et al. 2003). There are many drugs available and the right choice is important. Equally, there is no single diet that is optimal for each and every patient. Nevertheless, as reviewed in this chapter, an eating pattern for the prevention of chronic diseases including atherosclerosis should contain a large fraction of dietary fiber (whole cereal grains) and moderate amounts of disaccharides (sucrose and fructose). The ingestion of the latter should be avoided, especially in patients with overweight, physical inactivity, insulin resistance or the metabolic syndrome. Such a dietary pattern has favorable effects on the major cardiovascular risk factors and may also help control body weight (Foster et al. 2003). The promotion of healthy protective dietary strategies (such as increasing the intake of complex carbohydrates or of wholegrain diets) is more effective than forbidding single unhealthy food habits (Michels and Wolk 2002). It is important to recognize that there are different fats and carbohydates. Present evidence suggests that at least compliant individuals increase their chance of finding the 'Garden of Eden' (Jenkins et al. 2003) on Earth with the help of a plant-based diet, rich in complex (nondigestible) carbohydrates.

References

Acheson K, Flatt JP, Jéquier E (1982) Glycogen synthesis versus lipogenesis after a 500 gram carbohydrate meal in man. Metabolism 31:1234–1240

Adult-Treatment-Panel-III (2002) Third Report of the National Cholesterol Education Program (NCEP) Expert Panel on Detection, Evaluation, and Treatment of High Blood Cholesterol in Adults (Adult Treatment Panel III) final report. Circulation 106:3143–3421

Albrink MJ, Ullrich IH (1986) Interaction of dietary sucrose and fiber on serum lipids in healthy young men fed high carbohydrate diets. Am J Clin Nutr 43:419–428

Alexander JK (2001) Obesity and coronary heart disease. Am J Med Sci 321:215–224

Anderson JW (2000) Dietary Fiber prevents carbohydrate-induced hypertriglyceridemia. Curr Athero Rep 2:536–541

Anderson JW, Story L, Sieling B, Chen WJ, Petro MS, Story J (1984) Hypocholesterolemic effects of oat-bran or bean intake for hypercholesterolemic men. Am J Clin Nutr 40:1146–1155

Anderson JW, Davidson MH Blonde L, Brown WV, Howard WJ, Ginsberg H, Allgood LD, Weingand KW (2000) Long-term cholesterol-lowering effects of psyllium as an adjunct to diet therapy in the treatment of hypercholesterolemia. Am J Clin Nutr 71:1433–1438

Appel LJ, Moore TJ, Obarzanek E, Vollmer WM, Svetkey LP, Sacks FM, Bray GA, Vogt TM, Cutler JA, Windhauser MM (1997) A clinical trial of the effects of dietary patterns on blood pressure. N Engl J Med 336:1117–1124

Archer SL, Liu K, Dyer AR, Ruth KJ, Jacobs DR, Van-Horn L, Hilner JE, Savage PJ (1998) Relationship between changes in dietary sucrose and high density lipoprotein cholesterol: the CARDIA Study. Coronary Artery Risk Development in Young Adults. Ann Epidemiol 8:433–438

Aronson D, Rayfield EJ (2002) How hyperglycemia promotes atherosclerosis: molecular mechanisms. Cardiovascular Diabetology 1:1–10

Asztalos BF, Schaefer EJ (2003) HDL in atherosclerosis: actor or bystander? Atheroscler 4(Suppl):21–29

Augustin LS, Franceschi S, Jenkins DJA, Kendall CWC, La-Vecchia C (2002) Glycemic index in chronic disease: A review. Eur J Clin Nutr 56:1049–1071

Austin MA, Holkanson JE, Edwards KL (1998) Hypertriglyceridemia as a cardiovascular risk factor. Am J Cardiol 81:7B–12B

Ball SD, Keller KR, Moyer-Mileur LJ, Ding YW, Donaldsen D, Jackson DW (2003) Prolongation of Satiety After Long Versus Moderately High Glycemic Index Meals in Obese Adolescents. Pediatrics 111:488–494

Bantle JP, Raatz SK, Thomas W, Georgopoulos A (2000) Effects of dietary fructose on plasma lipids in healthy subjects. Am J Clin Nutr 72:1128–1134

Barnard RJ, DiLauro SC, Inkeles SB (1997) Effects of intensive diet and exercise intervention in patients taking cholesterol-lowering drugs. Am J Cardiol 15:1112–1114

Bartnikowska E (1999) The role of dietary fiber in the prevention of lipid metabolism disorders. In: Cho SS, Prosky L, Dreher M. Complex carbohydrates in foods. Marcel Dekker Inc., NewYork, pp 53–62

Bazzano LA, He J, Ogden LG, Loria CM, Whelton PK (2003) Dietary fiber intake and reduced risk of coronary heart disease in US men and women. Arch Intern Med 163:1897–1904

Bell S, Goldman VM, Bistrian BR, Arnold AH, Ostroff G, Forse RA (1999) Effect of beta-glucan from oats and yeast on serum lipids. Crit Rev Food Sci Nutr 39:189–202

Bermudez OI, Tucker KL (2003) Trends in dietary patterns of Latin American populations. Cad Saude Publica 19(Suppl 1):S87–S99

Bjoerck I, Elmstahl HL (2003) The glycemic index: importance of dietary fiber and other food properties. Proceeding of the Nutrition Society 62:201–206

Bolton-Smith C, Woodward M (1994) Coronary heart disease: prevalence and dietary sugars in Scotland. J Epidemiol Community Health 48:119–222

Bosello O, Zamboni M (2000) Visceral obesity and metabolic syndrome. Obes Rev 1:47–56

Bosello O, Ostuzzi R, Armellini F, Micciolo R, Scuro LA (1980) Glucose tolerance and blood lipids in bran-fed patients with impaired glucose tolerance. Diabetes Care 26:272–277

Bourdon I, Yokoyama W, Davis P, Hudson C, Backus R, Richter D, Knuckles B, Schneeman BO (1999) Postprandial lipid, glucose, insulin, and cholecystokinin responses in men fed barley pasta enriched with beta-glucan. Am J Clin Nutr 69:55–63

Brand-Miller J, Hayne S, Petocz P, Colagiuri S (2003) Low-glycemic index diets in the management of diabetes: a meta-analysis of randomized controlled trials. Diabetes Care 26:2261–2267

Brown L, Rosner B, Willett W, Sacks FM (1999) Cholesterol-lowering effects of dietary fiber: a meta-analysis. Am J Clin Nutr 69:30–42

Brunzell JD, Hazzard WR, Porte D, Bierman EL (1973) Evidence for a common, saturable, triglyceride removal mechanism for chylomicrons and very low density lipoproteins in man. J Clin Invest 52:1578–1585

Capewell S, Morrison CE, McMurray JJ (1999) Contributions of modern cardiovascular treatment and risk factor changes in the decline in coronary heart disease mortality in Scotland between 1975 and 1994. Heart 81:380–386

Castro-Cabezas M, Halkes CJ, Erkelens DW (2001) Obesity and free fatty acids: double trouble. Nutr Metab Cardiovasc Dis 11:134–142

Center for Science in Public Interest (CSPI), Website accessed October 20, 2003. http://www.cspinet.org/reports/sugar/sugarorigin.html

Chen HL, Sheu WH, Tai TS, Liaw YP, Chen YC (2003) Konjac supplement alleviated hypercholesterolemia and hyperglycemia in type 2 diabetic subjects—a randomized double-blind trial. J Am Coll Nutr 22:36–42

Cho SS, Prosky L, Dreher M (1999) Complex carbohydrates in foods. Marcel Dekker Inc., New York

Ciccarone E, Di Castelnuovo A, Salcuni M, Siani A, Giacco A, Donati MB, De Gaetano G, Capani F, Iacoviello L (2003) A high-score Mediterranean dietary pattern is associated with a reduced risk of peripheral arterial disease in Italian patients with Type 2 diabetes. J Thromb Haemostasis 1:1744–1752

Cicero AF, Gaddi A (2001) Rice bran oil and gamma-oryzanol in the treatment of hyperlipoproteinaemias and other conditions. Phytother Res 15:277–289

Clemmer KF, Binkoski AE, Coval SM, Zhao G, Kris-Etherton PM (2001) Diet and drug therapy: A dynamic duo for reducing coronary heart disease risk. Curr Athero Rep 3:507–513

Clifton PM (2003) Diet and C-reactive protein. Curr Atheroscler Rep 5:431–436

Clifton P, Noakes M, Nestel P (1994) Gender and diet interactions with simvastatin treatment. Atherosclerosis 110:25–33

Davidson MH, Dugan LD, Burns JH, Bova J, Story K, Drennan KB (1991) The hypocholesterolemic effects of beta-glucan in oatmeal and oat bran. A dose controlled study. JAMA 265:1833–1839

Delaney B, Nicolosi RJ, Wilson TA, Carlson T, Frazer S, Zheng GH, Hess R, Ostergren K, Haworth J, Knutson N (2003) Beta-glucan fractions from barley and oats are similarly antiatherogenic in hypercholesterolemic Syrian golden hamsters. J Nutr 133:468–475

de-Lorgeril M, Salen P, Martin JL, Monjaud I, Delaye J, Mamelle N (1999) Mediterranean diet, traditional risk factors, and the rate of cardiovascular complications after myocardial infarction: final report of the Lyon Diet Heart Study. Circulation 99:779–785

DeVries JW (2003) On defining dietary fibre. Proc Nutr Soc 62:37–43

Dubois C, Beaumier G et al. (1998) Effects of graded amounts (0–50 g) of dietary fat on postprandial lipemia and lipoproteins in normolipidemic adults. Am J Clin Nutr 67:31–38

Dumesnil JG, Turgeon J, Tremblay A, Poirier P, Gilbert M, Gagnon L, St-Pierre S, Garneau C, Lemieux I, Pascot A (2001) Effect of a low-glycaemic index–low-fat–high protein diet on the atherogenic metabolic risk profile of abdominally obese men. Br J Nutr 86:557–568

Durstine JL, Grandjean PW, Cox CA, Thompson PD (2002) Lipids, lipoproteins, and exercise. J Cardiopulm Rehabil 22:385–398

Dwyer T, Emmanuel SC, Janus ED, Wu Z, Hynes KL, Zhang C (2003) The emergence of coronary heart disease in populations of Chinese descent. Atherosclerosis 167:303–310

Ebbeling CB, Leidig MM, Sinclair KB, Hangen JP, Ludwig DS (2003) A reduced-glycemic load diet in the treatment of adolescent obesity. Arch Pediatr Adolesc Med 157:773–779

Economic-Research-Service (2003) U.S. Department of Agriculture. Briefing room: Food consumption. (2003) Economic-Research-Service, 3743 (Accessed October 10, 2003)

Egusa G, Watanabe H, Ohshita K, Fujikawa R, Yamane K, Okubo M, Kohno N (2002) Influence of the extent of westernization of lifestyle on the progression of preclinical atherosclerosis in Japanese subjects. J Atheroscler Thromb 9:299–304

Engelyst KN, Vinoy S, Engelyst HN, Lang V (2003) Glycemic index of cereal products explained by their content of rapidly and slowly available glucose. Br J Nutr 89:329–339

Ernst N, Fisher M, Smith W, Gordon T, Rifkind BM, Little JA, Mishkel MA, Williams OD (1980) The association of plasma high-density lipoprotein cholesterol with dietary intake and alcohol consumption. The Lipid Research Clinics Prevalence Study. Circulation 62:41–52

Esposito K, Pontillo A, Di-Palo C, Giugliano G, Masella M, Marfella R, Giugliano D (2003) Effect of weight loss and lifestyle changes on vascular inflammatory markers in obese women: a randomized trial. JAMA 289:1799–1804

Expert Panel on Detection, Evaluation, and Treatment of High Blood Cholesterol in Adults (2001) Executive summary of the third report of the National Cholesterol Education Program (NCEP) expert panel on detection, evaluation, and treatment of high blood cholesterol in adults (Adult Treatment Panel III) JAMA 285:2486–2497

Fernandez ML (2001) Soluble fiber and nondigestible carbohydrate effects on plasma lipids and cardiovascular risk. Curr Opinion Lipidol 12:35–40

Flatt JP (1993) The impact of dietary fat and carbohydrates on body weight maintenance. In: Altschul AM. Low-calorie foods handbook. Marcel Dekker Inc., New York, pp 441–477

Flatt JP (1993) The impact of dietary fat and carbohydrates on body weight maintenance. In: Altschul AM (ed.) Low-calorie foods handbook. Marcel Dekker Inc., New York,:441–477

Food and Drug Administration (2002). Food labeling: health claims; soluble dietary fiber from certain foods and coronary heart disease. Interim final rule. Fed Regist 67:61773–61783

Ford ES, Liu S (2001) Glycemic index and serum high-density lipoprotein cholesterol concentration among us adults. Arch Intern Med 161:572–576

Ford ES, Giles WH, Dietz WH (2002) Prevalence of the metabolic syndrome among US adults: findings from the third National Health and Nutrition Examination Survey. JAMA 2002 287:356–359

Foster-Powell K, Holt SHA, Brand-Miller JC (2002) International table of glycemic index and glycemic load values: 2002. Am J Clin Nutr 76:5–56

Foster GD, Wyatt HR, Hill JO, McGuckin BG, Brill C, Mohammed BS, Szapary PO, Rader DJ, Edman JS, Klein S (2003) A randomized trial of a low-carbohydrate diet for obesity. N Engl J Med 348:2082–2090

Franz MJ, Bantle JP, Wyatt HR, Hill JO, McGuckin BG, Brill C, Mohammed BS, Szapary PO, Rader Franz MJ, Bantle JP (1999) American Diabetes Association Guide to Medical Nutrition Therapy for Diabetes. American Diabetes Association, Alexandria, VA

Frayn KN (2003) Metabolic regulation. A human perspective. 2nd edn. Blackwell Science Ltd., Oxford

Frayn KN, Kingman SM (1995) Dietary sugars and lipid metabolism in humans. Am J Clin Nutr 62(Suppl):250S–261S

Fung TT, Hu FB et al. (2002) Whole-grain intake and the risk of type 2 diabetes: a prospective study in men. Am J Clin Nutr 76:535–540

Galal O (2003) Nutrition-related health patterns in the Middle East. Asia Pac J Clin Nutr 12:337–343

Gill JMR, Hardman AE (2003) Exercise and postprandial lipid metabolism: an update on potential mechanisms and interactions with high-carbohydrate diets. J Nutr Biochem 14:122–132

Hardman AE, Herd SL (1998) Exercise and postprandial lipid metabolism. Proc Nutr Soc 57:63–72

Howard BV, Wylie-Rosett J (2002) Sugar and cardiovascular disease (AHA Scientific Statement). Circulation 106:523–527

Hu FB, Willett WC (2002) Optimal diets for prevention of coronary heart disease. JAMA 288:2569–2578

Hudgins LC, Hellerstein MK, Seidman C, Neese J, Diakun J, Hirsch J (1996) Human fatty acid synthesis is stimulated by a eucaloric low fat, high carbohydrate diet. J Clin Invest 97:2081–2091

Hudgins LC, Seidman CE, Diakun J, Hirsch J (1998) Human fatty acid synthesis is reduced after the substitution of dietary starch for sugar. Am J Clin Nutr 67:631–639

Hudgins LC, Hellerstein MK, Seidman CE, Neese RA, Tremaroli JD, Hirsch J (2000) Relationship between carbohydrate-induced hypertriglyceridemia and fatty acid synthesis in lean and obese subjects. J Lipid Res 41:595–604

Humble CG, Malarcher AM, Tyroler HA (1993) Dietary fiber and coronary heart disease in middle-aged hypercholesterolemic men. Am J Prev Med 9:197–202

Hunninghake DB, Stein EA, Dujovne CA, Harris WS, Feldman EB, Miller VT, Tobert JA, Laskarzewski PM, Quiter E, Held J (1993) The efficacy of intensive dietary therapy alone or combined with lovastatin in outpatients with hypercholesterolemia. N Engl J Med 238:1213–1219

Hyson D, Rutledge JC et al. (2003) Postprandial Lipemia and Cardiovascular Disease. Curr Athero Rep 5:437–444

Institute of Medicine (2002) Dietary reference intakes for energy, carbohydrates, fiber, fat, fatty acids, cholesterol, protein, and amino acids. National Academy Press, Washington, DC

Jacobs DR, Meyer KA, Kushi LH, Folsom AR (1998) Whole-grain intake may reduce the risk of ischemic heart disease death in postmenopausal women: The Iowa Women's Health Study. Am J Clin Nutr 68:248–257

Jacobs DR, Pereira MA, Meyer KA, Kushi LH (2000) Fiber from whole grain, but not refined grains, is inversely associated with all-cause mortality in older women: The Iowa women's health study. J Am Coll Nutr 19(Suppl 3):236S–330S

Jacobs DR, Meyer HE, Solvoll K (2001) Reduced mortality among whole grain bread eaters in men and women in the Norwegian County Study. Eur J Clin Nutr 55:137–143

Jenkins DJ, Wolever, Vidgen E, Kendall CW, Ransom TP, Mehling CC, Mueller S, Cunnane SC, O'Connell NC, Setchell KD (1997) Effect of psyllium in hypercholesterolemia at two monounsaturated fatty acid intakes. Am J Clin Nutr 65:1524–1533

Jenkins DJ, Wolever TM, Taylor RH, Barker H, Fielden H, Baldwin JM, Bowling AC, Newman HC, Jenkins AL, Goff DV (1981) Glycemic index of foods: a physiological basis for carbohydrate exchange. Am J Clin Nutr 4:362–366

Jenkins AL, Jenkins DJ, Zdravkovic U, Wursch P, Vuksan V (2002) Depression of the glycemic index by high levels of beta-glucan fiber in two functional foods tested in type 2 diabetes. Eur J Clin Nutr 56:622–628

Jenkins DJ, Kendall CW, Augustin LS, Vuksan V (2002) High-complex carbohydrate or lente carbohydrate foods? Am J Med 30(Suppl 9B):30S–37S

Jenkins DJ, Kendall CW, Marchie A, Faulkner DA, Wong JM, de-Souza R, Emam A, Parker TL, Vidgen E, Lapsley KG (2003) Effects of a dietary portfolio of cholesterol-lowering foods vs lovastatin on serum lipids and C-reactive protein. JAMA 290:502–510

Jenkins DJA, Kendall CWC, Marchie A, ., Jenkins AL, Connelly PW, Jones PJH, Vuksan V (2003) The Garden of Eden—plant based diets, the genetic drive to conserve cholesterol and its implication for heart disease in the 21st century. Compar Biochem Physiol (Part A) 136:141–151

Jeppesen J, Chen YI, Zhou MY, Schaaf P, Coulston A, Reaven GM (1995) Postprandial triglyceride and retinyl ester responses to oral fat: effects of fructose. Am J Clin Nutr. 61:787–791

Jialal I, Devaraj S (2003) Role of C-reactive protein in the assessment of cardiovascular risk. Am J Cardiol 91:200–202

Joshipura KJ, Ascherio A, Manson JE, Stampfer MJ, Rimm EB, Speizer FE, Hennekens CH, Spiegelman D, Willett WC (1999) Fruit and vegetable intake in relation to risk of ischemic stroke. JAMA 282:1233–1239

Joshipura KJ, Hu FB, Manson J, E, , Stampfer M, J, , Rimm EB, Speizer FE, Colditz G, Ascherio A, Rosner B, Spiegelman D et al. (2001) The effect of fruit and vegetable intake on risk for coronary heart disease. Ann Intern Med 134:1106–1114

Keogh GF, Cooper GJ, Mulvey TB, McArdle BH, Coles GD, Monro JA, Poppitt SD (2003) Randomized controlled crossover study of the effect of a highly beta-glucan-enriched barley on cardiovascular disease risk factors in mildly hypercholesterolemic men. Am J Clin Nutr 78:711–718

Kerckhoffs DA, Hornstra G, Mensink RP (2003) Cholesterol-lowering effect of beta-glucan from oat bran in mildly hypercholesterolemic subjects may decrease when beta-glucan is incorporated into bread and cookies. Am J Clin Nutr 78:221–227

Khaw KT, Barrett-Connor E (1987) Dietary fiber and reduced ischemic heart disease mortality rates in men and women: a 12 year prospective study. Am J Epidemiol 126:1093–1102

Koutsari C, Hardman AE (2001) Exercise prevents the augmentation of postprandial lipemia attributable to a low-fat high-carbohydrate diet. Br J Nutr 86:197–205

Koutsari C, Malkova D et al. (2000) Postprandial lipemia after short-term variation in dietary fat and carbohydrates. Metabolism 49:1150–1155

Kuczmarski RJ, Flegal KM et al. (1994) Increasing prevalence of overweight among US adults: the National Health and Nutrition Examination Survey, 1960–1991. JAMA 272:205–211

Kushi LH, Meyer KA, Jacobs DR (1999) Cereals, legumes, and chronic disease risk reduction: Evidence from epidemiological studies. Am J Clin Nutr 70:451S–458S

Laaksonen DE, Lakka HM, Salonen JT, Niskanen LK, Rauramaa R, Lakka TA (2002) Low levels of leisure-time physical activity and cardiorespiratory fitness predict development of the metabolic syndrome. Diabetes care 25:1612–1618

Lakka HM, Salonen JT et al. (2002) Obesity and weight gain are associated with increased incidence of hyperinsulinemia in non-diabetic men. Horm Metab Res 34:492–498

Lamarche B, Uffelman KD, Carpentier A, Cohn JS, Steiner G, Barrett PH, Lewis GF (1999) Triglyceride enrichment of HDL enhances in vivo metabolic clearance of HDL apo A-I in healthy men. J Clin Invest 103:1191–1199

Leinonen K, Liukkonen K, Poutanen K, Uusitupa M, Mykkanen H (1999) Rye bread decreases postprandial insulin response but does not alter glucose response in healthy Finnish subjects. Eur J Clin Nutr 53:262–267

Leinonen KS, Poutanen KS, Mykkanen HM (2000) Rye bread decreases serum total and LDL cholesterol in men with moderately elevated serum cholesterol. J Nutr 130:164–170

Lemieux I, Couillard C et al. (2000) The small, dense LDL phenotype as a correlate of postprandial lipemia in men. Atherosclerosis 153:423–432

Lichtenstein AH, Ausman LM, Carrasco W, Jenner JL, Ordovas JM, Schaefer EJ (1994) Short-term consumption of a low-fat diet beneficially affects plasma lipid concentrations only when accompanied by weight loss. Hypercholesterolemia, low-fat diet, and plasma lipids. Arterioscler Thromb 14:1751–1760

Liese AD, Roach AK, Sparks KC, Marquart L, D'Agostino RB, Mayer-Davis EJ (2003) Whole-grain intake and insulin sensitivity: the Insulin Resistance Atherosclerosis Study. Am J Clin Nutr 78:965–971

Liu S (2002) Intake of refined carbohydrates and whole grain foods in relation to risk of type 2 diabetes mellitus and coronary heart disease. J Am Coll Nutr 21:298–306

Liu S, Stampfer MJ, Hu FB, Giovannuci E, Rimm E, Manson JAE, Hennekens CH, Willett WC (1999) Whole-grain consumption and risk of coronary heart disease: results from the Nurses Health Study. Am J Clin Nutr 70:412–419

Liu S, Manson JE, Stampfer MJ, Rexrode KM, Hu FB, Rimm EB, Willett WC (2000) Whole grain consumption and risk of ischemic stroke in women: A prospective study. JAMA 284:1534–1540

Liu S, Willett WC, Stampfer MJ, Hu FB, Franz M, Sampson L, Hennekens CH, Manson JE (2000) A prospective study of dietary glycemic load, carbohydrate intake, and risk of coronary heart disease in US women. Am J Clin Nutr 71:1455–1461

Lucas EA, Wild RD, Hammond LJ, Khalil DA, Juma S, Daggy BP, Stoecker BJ, Arjmandi BH (2002) Flaxseed improves lipid profile without altering biomarkers of bone metabolism in postmenopausal women. J Clin Endocrinol Metab 87:1527–1532

Ludwig DS (2003) Dietary glycemic index and the regulation of body weight. Lipids 38: 117–121

Mamo JCL, Yu KCW et al. (1997) Is atherosclerosis exclusively a postprandial phenomenon? Clin Exper Pharmacol Physiol 24:288–293

Mann J (2001) Carbohydrates. In: Bowman BA, Russell RM (eds) Present knowledge in nutrition, 8th edn. ILSI Press, Washington, D.C., pp 59–82

Marckmann P, Raben A, Astrup A (2000) Ad libidum intake of low-fat diets rich in either starch foods or sucrose: effects on blood lipids, factor VII coagulant activity, and fibrinogen. Metabolism 49:731–735

Marlett JA, Fischer MH (2003) The active fraction of psyllium seed husk. Proceedings of the Nutrition Society 62:207–209

McLellan F (2002) Obesity rising to alarming levels around the world. Lancet 359:1412

Michels KB, Wolk A (2002) A prospective study of variety of healthy foods and mortality in women. Int J Epidemiol 31:847–854

Miesenböck G, Patsch JR (1992) Postprandial hyperlipidemia: the search for the atherogenic lipoprotein. Curr Opin Lipidol 3:196–201

Mokdad AH, Ford ES, Bowman BA, Dietz WH, Vinicor F, Bales VS, Marks JS (2003) Prevalence of obesity, diabetes, and obesity-related health risk factors, 2001. JAMA 289:76–79

Moore MC, Charrington AD, Mann SL, Davis SN (2000) Acute fructose administration decreases the glycemic response to an oral glucose tolerance test in normal adults. J Clin Endocrinol Metab 85:4515–1519

Negri E, La-Vecchia C, Pelucchi C, Bertuzzi M, Tavani A (2003) Fiber intake and the risk of nonfatal acute myocardial infarction. Eur J Clin Nutr 57:464–470

Newby PK, Muller D, Hallfrisch J, Qiao N, Andres R, Tucker KL (2003) Dietary patterns and changes in body mass index and waist circumference in adults. Am J Clin Nutr 77:1417–1425

Parks EJ (2001) Recent findings in the study of postprandial lipemia. Curr Athersoscler Rep 3:462–470

Parks EJ, Hellerstein MK (2000) Carbohydrate-induced hypertriacylglycerolemia: historical perspectives and review of the biological mechanisms. Am J Clin Nutr 71:412–433

Perry IJ (2002) Healthy diet and lifestyle clustering and glucose intolerance. Proceedings of the Nutrition Society 61:543–551

Petitt DS, Cureton KJ (2003) Effects of prior exercise on postprandial lipemia: a quantitative review. Metabolism 52:418–424

Popkin BM, Doak CM (1998) The obesity epidemic is a worldwide phenomenon. Nutr Rev 56:106–114

Prasad K (2000) Flaxseed: A source of hypocholesterolemic and antiatherogenic agents. Drug News Perspect 13:99–104

Putnam J, Allshouse J, Kantor LS (2002) U.S. per capita supply trends: more calories, refined carbohydrates, and fats. Food Rev 25:2–15

Raben A (2002) Should obese patients be counselled to follow a low-glycaemic index diet? No. Obes Rev 3:245–256

Raben A, Holst JJ, Madsen J, Astrup A (1998) Diurnal metabolic profiles after 14d of an ad libidum high starch, high-sucrose, or high-fat diet in normal-weight never-obese and postobese women. Am J Clin Nutr 73:177–189

Rajnarayana K, Prabhakar MC, Krishna DR (2001) Influence of rice bran oil on serum lipid peroxides and lipids in human subjects. Indian J Physiol Pharmacol 45:442–444

Reaven G (2002) Metabolic syndrome: pathophysiology and implications for management of cardiovascular disease. Circulation 106:286–288

Reiser S, Powell AS, Scholfield DJ, Panda P, Ellwood KC, Canary JJ (1989) Blood lipids, lipoproteins, apoproteins, and uric acid in men fed diets containing fructose or high-amylose cornstarch. Am J Clin Nutr 49:832–839

Retzlaff BM, Walden CE, Dowdy AA, McCann BS, Anderson KV, Knopp RH (1995) Changes in plasma triacylglycerol concentrations among free-living hyperlipidemic men adopting different carbohydrate intakes over 2 y: the Dietary Alternatives Study. Am J Clin Nutr 62:988–995

Reusch JE (2002) Current concepts in insulin resistance, type 2 diabetes mellitus, and the metabolic syndrome. Am J Cardiol 90(5A):19G–26G

Rimm EB, Acherio A, Giovannucci E, Spiegleman D, Stampfer MJ, Willett WC (1996) Vegetable, fruit, and cereal fiber and risk of coronary heart disease among men. JAMA 275:447–451

Ripsin CM, Keenan JM, Jacobs DR, Elmer PJ, Welch RR, Van-Horn L, Liu K, Turnbull WH, Thye FW, Kestin M (1992) Oat products and lipid lowering. A meta-analysis. JAMA 267:3317–3325

Roberts CK, Vaziri ND et al. (2002) Effect of diet and exercise intervention on blood pressure, insulin, oxidative stress, and nitric oxide availability. Circulation 106:2530–2532

Roust LR, Kottke BA, Jensen MD (1994) Serum lipid responses to a eucaloric high-complex carbohydrate diet in different obesity phenotypes. Mayo Clin Proc 69:930–936

Sacks FM, Katan M (2002) Randomized clinical trials on the effects of dietary fat and carbohydrate on plasma lipoproteins and cardiovascular disease. Am J Med 113(Suppl 9B): 13S–24S

Sacks FM, Svetkey LP, Vollmer W. M., Appel LJ, Bray GA, Harsha D, Obarzanek E, Conlin PR, Miller ER, Simons-Morton DG (2001) Effects on blood pressure of reduced dietary sodium and the Dietary Approaches to Stop Hypertension (DASH) diet. N Engl J Med 344:3–10

Saito M, Ishimitsu T, Minami J, Ono H, Ohrui M, Matsuoka H (2003) Relations of plasma high-sensitivity C-reactive protein to traditional cardiovascular risk factors. Atherosclerosis 167:73–79

Salmeron J, Manson JE, Stampfer MJ, Colditz GA, Wing AL, Willett WC (1997) Dietary fiber, glycemic load and the risk of non-insulin-dependent diabetes mellitus. JAMA 277:472–477

Saris WH, Astrup A, Prentice AM, Zunft HJ, Formiguera X, Verboeket-van-de-Venne WP, Raben A, Poppitt SD, Seppelt B, Johnston S (2000) Randomized controlled trial of changes in dietary carbohydrate/fat ratio and simple vs complex carbohydrates on body weight and blood lipids: the CARMEN study. The Carbohydrate Ratio Management in European National diets. Int J Obes Relat Metab Disord 10:1310–1318

Schulze MB, Hu FB (2002) Dietary patterns and risk of hypertension, type 2 diabetes mellitus, and coronary heart disease. Curr Atheroscler Rep 4:462–467

Sciarrone SE, Strahan MT, Beilin LJ, Burke V, Rogers P, Rouse IR (1993) Ambulatory blood pressure and heart rate responses to vegetarian meals. J Hypertens 11:277–285

Sigman-Grant M, Morita J (2003) Defining and interpreting intakes of sugars. Am J Clin Nutr 78(Suppl):815S–826S

Slavin J (2003) Why whole grains are protective: biological mechanisms. Proceedings of the Nutrition Society 62:129–134

Solymoss BC, Bourassa MG, Campeau L, Lesperance J, Marcil M, Varga S (2003) Incidence, coronary risk profile and angiographic characteristics of prediabetic and diabetic patients in a population with ischemic heart disease. Can J Cardiol 19:1155–1160

Spiller GA (ed) (1993) Dietary fiber in human nutrition. CRC Press Inc., Boca Raton

Spiller GA (2002) Whole grains, whole wheat, and white flours in history. Whole grain foods in health and diseases. In: Marquart L, Slavin JL, Fulcher RG (eds) American Association of Cereal Chemists Inc., St. Paul (Minnesota, USA), pp 1–7

Stevens J, Ahn K, Juhaeri, Houston D, Steffan L, Couper D (2002) Dietary fiber intake and glycemic index and incidence of diabetes in African-American and White adults. Diabetes Care 25:1715–1721

Stolar MW, Chilton RJ (2003) Type 2 diabetes, cardiovascular risk, and the link to insulin resistance. Clin Ther 25(Suppl B):B4–B31

Suter PM, Gerritsen Zehnder M, , Häsler E, Gürtler M, Vetter W, Hänseler E (2001) Effect of alcohol on postprandial lipemia with and without preprandial exercise. J Am Coll Nutr 20:58–64

Trichopoulou A, Costacou T, Bamia C, Trichopoulos D (2003) Adherence to a Mediterranean diet and survival in a Greek population. N Engl J Med 348:2599–2608

Trichopoulou A, Naska A, Bamia C, Trichopoulos D (2003) Vegetable and fruit: the evidence in their favour and the public health perspective. Int J Vitam Nutr Res 73:63–69

Trowell H (1972) Ischemic heart disease and dietary fiber. Am J Clin Nutr 25:926–932

Truswell AS (2002) Cereal grains and coronary heart disease. Eur J Clin Nutr 56:1–14

Tucker KL, Dallal GE, Rush D (1992) Dietary pattern of elderly Boston-area residents defined by cluster analysis. J Am Diet Assoc 92:1487–1491

van-Dam RM, Visscher AW, Feskens EJ, Verhoef P, Kromhout D (2000) Dietary glycemic index in relation to metabolic risk factors and incidence of coronary heart disease: the Zutphen Elderly Study. Eur J Clin Nutr 54:726–731

van Dam RM, Rimm EB, Willett WC, Stampfer MJ, Hu FB (2002) Dietary patterns and risk for type 2 diabetes mellitus in U.S. men. Ann Intern Med 136:201–209

van-Dam RM, Grievink L, Feskens EJM (2003) Patterns of food consumption and risk factors for cardiovascular disease in the general Dutch population. Am J Clin Nutr 77:1156–1163

van Horn L (1997) Fiber, lipids, and coronary heart disease: A statement for health care professionals from the Nutrition Committee, American Heart Association. Circulation 95:2701–2704

Villaume C, Beck B, Gariot P, Desalme A, Debry G (1984) Long term evolution of the effect of bran ingestion on meal induced glucose and insulin responses in healthy man. Am J Clin Nutr 40:1023–1026

Walker AP, Walker BF, Adam F (2003) Nutrition, diet, physical activity, smoking, and longevity: from primitive hunter-gatherer to present passive consumer—how far can we go? Nutrition 19:169–173

Volek JS, Sharman MJ et al. (2003) An isoenergetic very low carbohydrate diet improves serum hdl cholesterol and triacylglycerol concentration, the total cholesterol to HDL cholesterol ratio and postprandial lipemic responses compared with a low fat diet in normal weight, normolipidemic women. J Nutr 133:2756–2761

Webster FH (2002) Whole-grain oats and oat products. Whole-grain foods in health and disease. In: Marquart L, Slavin JL, Fulcher RG. American Association of Cereal Chemists, Inc., St. Paul (Minnesota, USA), pp 83–123

Wirfält E, Hedblad B, Gullberg B, Mattisson I, Andrén C, Rosander U, Janzon L, Berglund G (2001) Food patterns and components of the metabolic syndrome in men and women: a cross-sectional study within the Malmö Diet and Cancer Cohort. Am J Epidemiol 154:1150–1159

Wolk AJ, Manson E, Stampfer MJ, Colditz GA, Hu FB, Speizer FE, Hennekens CH, Willett WC (1999) Long-term intake of dietary fiber and decreased risk of coronary heart disease among women. JAMA 281:1998–2004

Wood P, Stefanick M, Williams P, Haskell W (1994) The effects on plasma lipoproteins of a prudent weight reducing diet with or without exercise, in overweight men and women. N Engl J Med 325:461–466

Xie J, Liu L et al. (1998) Nutritional habits and serum lipid levels in low-fat intake Chinese population sample. Acta Cardiol 53:359–364

Yin W, Yuan Z, Wang Z, Yang B, Yang Y (2002) A diet high in saturated fat and sucrose alters glucoregulation and induces aortic fatty streaks in New Zealand White rabbits. Int J Exp Diabetes Res 3:179–184

Yudkin J (1960) Sugar and ischaemic heart disease. Practitioner 198:680–683

Yudkin J (1978) Dietary factors in atherosclerosis: sucrose. Lipids 13:370–372

Zilversmit DB (1979) Atherosclerosis: A postprandial phenomenon. Circulation 60:473–485

Zilversmit DB (1995) Atherogenic nature of triglycerides, postprandial lipidemia, and triglyceride-rich lipoproteins. Clin Chem 41:153–158

HEP (2005) 170:263–300

Dietary Antioxidants and Paraoxonases Against LDL Oxidation and Atherosclerosis Development

M. Aviram (✉) · M. Kaplan · M. Rosenblat · B. Fuhrman

The Lipid Research Laboratory, Technion Faculty of Medicin and Rambam Medical Center, 31096 Haifa, Israel
aviram@tx.technion.ac.il

Abstract Oxidative modification of low-density lipoprotein (LDL) in the arterial wall plays a key role in the pathogenesis of atherosclerosis. Under oxidative stress LDL is exposed to oxidative modifications by arterial wall cells including macrophages. Oxidative stress also induces cellular-lipid peroxidation, resulting in the formation of 'oxidized macrophages', which demonstrate increased capacity to oxidize LDL and increased uptake of oxidized LDL.

Macrophage-mediated oxidation of LDL depends on the balance between pro-oxidants and antioxidants in the lipoprotein and in the cells. LDL is protected from oxidation by antioxidants, as well as by a second line of defense—paraoxonase 1 (PON1), which is a high-density lipoprotein-associated esterase that can hydrolyze and reduce lipid peroxides in lipoproteins and in arterial cells. Cellular paraoxonases (PON2 and PON3) may also play an important protective role against oxidative stress at the cellular level. Many epidemiological studies have indicated a protective role for a diet rich in fruits and vegetables against the development and progression of cardiovascular disease. A large number of studies provide data suggesting that consumption of dietary antioxidants is associated with reduced risk for cardiovascular diseases. Basic research provides plausible mechanisms by which dietary antioxidants might reduce the development of atherosclerosis. These mechanisms include inhibition of LDL oxidation, inhibition of cellular lipid peroxidation and consequently attenuation of cell-mediated oxidation of LDL. An additional possible mechanism is preservation/increment of paraoxonases activity by dietary antioxidants. This review chapter presents recent data on the anti-atherosclerotic effects and mechanism of action of three major groups of dietary antioxidants—vitamin E, carotenoids and polyphenolic flavonoids.

Keywords Antioxidants · LDL · Oxidized-LDL · Paraoxonase · Flavonoids · Vitamin E · Carotenoids · Atherosclerosis

1
LDL Oxidation and Atherosclerosis

The 'oxidative modification of lipoproteins' hypothesis of atherosclerosis proposes that the oxidation of low-density lipoprotein (LDL) plays a pivotal role in early atherogenesis (Albertini et al. 2002; Aviram 1995, 1996, 2000; Berliner and Heinecke 1996; Glass and Witztum 2001; Hayek et al. 2005; Kaplan and Aviram 1999; Jialal and Devaraj 1996; Parthasarathy and Rankin 1992; Parthasarathy et al. 1998; Steinberg 1997; Witztum and Steinberg 1991). This hypothesis is supported by evidence that LDL oxidation occurs in vivo (Herttuala 1998) and contributes to the clinical manifestation of atherosclerosis. The early atherosclerotic lesion is characterized by the accumulation of arterial foam cells, which are initially derived mainly from cholesterol-loaded macrophages (Gerrity 1981; Schaffner et al. 1980). Most of the accumulated cholesterol in foam cells originates from plasma LDL. However, LDL has to undergo oxidative modification in order to be taken up by macrophages at an enhanced rate via the macrophage scavenger receptors pathway [scavenger receptors type A (SRA), CD-36], which, unlike the LDL receptor, are not subjected to downregulation by the cellular cholesterol content (Aviram 1993; Goldstein and Brown 1990; Steinberg et al. 1989). The uptake of oxidized LDL (Ox-LDL) via scavenger receptors promotes cholesterol accumulation and foam cell formation (Aviram 1991; Aviram and Rosenblat 2001; Steinberg et al. 1989; Parthasarathy and Rankin 1992), the hallmark of early atherosclerosis.

1.1
Oxidation of LDL in a Cell-Free System

Oxidation of LDL involves free radical attack on the lipoprotein components including cholesterol, phospholipids, fatty acids and apolipoprotein B-100. LDL oxidation results first in the consumption of its antioxidants (mainly vitamin E and carotenoids), and in a substantial loss of polyunsaturated fatty acids (PUFA) and of cholesterol, which are converted to oxidized PUFA and oxysterols.

During the oxidation of LDL, apolipoprotein B-100 also undergoes direct and indirect modifications. Direct attack of oxidants oxidizes amino acid side chains and fragments the polypeptide backbone.

1.2
Macrophage-Mediated Oxidation of LDL

Macrophage-mediated oxidation of LDL is considerably affected by the oxidative state in the cells, which depends on the balance between cellular oxidases and macrophage-associated antioxidants (Aviram and Fuhrman 1998a; Szuchmann et al. 2005). Macrophage binding of LDL to the LDL receptor initiates the activation of cellular oxygenases (Aviram and Rosenblat 1994; Aviram et al. 1996). When NADPH oxidase is activated, the cytosolic components of the NADPH oxidase complex, P-47 and P-67, translocate to the plasma membrane, where they form–together with the membrane bound cytochrome b558–the active NADPH oxidase complex. On the other hand, macrophage antioxidants also contribute to the extent of cell-mediated oxidation of LDL. Cellular reduced glutathione (GSH) is a most potent antioxidant (Meister and Anderson 1983; Rosenblat and Aviram 1997), and an inverse relationship has been shown between the extent of macrophage-mediated oxidation of LDL and the cellular GSH content (Rosenblat and Aviram 1997). Macrophage-mediated oxidation of LDL can also result from an initial cellular lipid peroxidation. When cultured macrophages were exposed to oxidants such as ferrous ions or angiotensin II, cellular lipid peroxidation took place (Fuhrman et al. 1994, 1997). These 'oxidized macrophages' could easily oxidize the LDL lipids, even in absence of any added transition metal ions. Furthermore, macrophage capacity to oxidize LDL increased during in vivo monocyte–to–macrophage differentation (Fuhrman et al. 2004a). Figure 1 summarizes our current view of macrophage-mediated oxidation of LDL and atherosclerosis.

2
Dietary Antioxidants and LDL Oxidation

For a compound to be defined as an antioxidant it must satisfy at least two basic conditions:

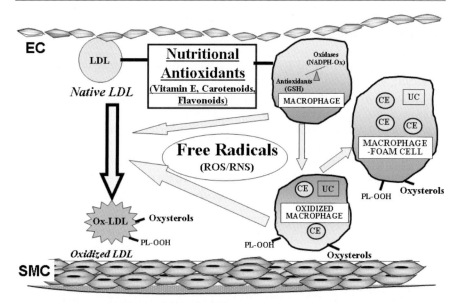

Fig. 1 Nutritional antioxidants and macrophage-foam cell formation. Nutritional antioxidants (vitamin E, carotenoids, flavonoids) can associate directly with LDL, resulting in the inhibition of LDL oxidation. Nutritional antioxidants can also associate with arterial cells such as macrophages, resulting in the inhibition of cellular oxygenases such as NADPH oxidase (*NADPH-Ox*), or in the activation of cellular antioxidants such as the glutathione (*GSH*) system. Reduction in the formation and the release of reactive oxygen/nitrogen species (*ROS/RNS*, respectively) in macrophages by antioxidants thus inhibits the formation of 'oxidized macrophages' and hence reduces cell-mediated oxidation of LDL. Altogether, these effects lead to a reduced formation of macrophage-foam cells, and thus attenuate the development of atherosclerotic lesion

- When present in low concentration relative to the substrate to be oxidized, it can delay, retard, or prevent auto-oxidation or free radical-mediated oxidation.

- The resulting radical formed after scavenging must be stable in order to interrupt the oxidation chain reaction.

The oxidation rate of LDL was shown to be reduced by dietary antioxidants intervention. Dietary antioxidants can inhibit LDL oxidation by several means:

- By scavenging free radicals, chelation of transition metal ions, or protection of the intrinsic antioxidants in the LDL particle (vitamin E and carotenoids) from oxidation.

- By protecting cells in the arterial wall against oxidative damage, and–as a result–inhibition of cell-mediated oxidation of LDL.

- By preservation of serum paraoxonase activity, and–as a result–promotion of the hydrolysis of LDL and arterial cell-associated lipid peroxides.

The beneficial health effects, attributed to the consumption of fruits and vegetables, are related at least in part, to their antioxidant activity.

Vitamin E (α-tocopherol) has been proposed to be the most important lipid-soluble radical-scavenging antioxidant in cellular and subcellular membranes and also in plasma lipoproteins (Burton et al. 1983). Vitamin E is synthesized by plants, and it is found primarily in plant products. Rich sources of vitamin E are vegetable oils, margarine, nuts, seeds and cereal grains. LDL is the major carrier of vitamin E in the circulation. It is estimated that for individuals who are not receiving any supplement, the LDL particle contains six molecules of vitamin E.

Carotenoids are natural pigments with lipophylic properties, widely distributed in fruits and vegetables, and possess some antioxidant characteristics (Krinsky 2001; Sies and Stahl 1995; Stahl and Sies 1997). β-Carotene and lycopene are the major carotenoids in human plasma. Lycopene is the open chain analog of β-carotene, and it is an acyclic carotenoid that contains 11 conjugated double bonds arranged linearly in the all-*trans* form. Carotenoids are transported in human blood complexed to plasma lipoproteins and mainly to the LDL particle. Lycopene, which lacks hydrophilic substituents, is extremely hydrophobic, is located within the hydrophobic core of LDL and thus, its free radical-scavenging ability is limited mostly to the interior of the lipoprotein.

Polyphenols constitute one of the largest category of phytochemicals, most widely distributed among plants, and are an integral part of the human diet. Flavonoids compose the largest and most studied group of plant polyphenols, and over 4,000 different flavonoids have been identified to date. Flavonoids are powerful antioxidants against LDL oxidation, and their activity is related to their localization in the LDL particle, as well as to their chemical structure (Rice-Evans et al. 1996). The free radical scavenging capability of flavonoids stems from the fact that their reducing potential is lower than that of the alkyl peroxyl radical and the superoxide radical and hence it results in free radicals inactivation. Flavonoids are effective scavengers of hydroxyl and peroxyl radicals, as well as superoxide anion (Yuting et al. 1999; Morel et al. 1993), and some of them act as antioxidants due to their potent chelation capacity to transition metal ions.

2.1
Vitamin E

Enrichment of LDL with vitamin E was reported to protect LDL against ex vivo oxidative modification (Dieber et al. 1991; Jialal et al. 1995; Reaven et al. 1993; Wen et al. 1999). However, recent mechanistic studies of the early stage of lipoprotein lipid peroxidation show that the role of vitamin E in this process is not simply that of a classical antioxidant (Stocker 1999a). It was demonstrated that vitamin E can display neutral, anti-, or even pro-oxidant activity under certain conditions (Noguchi and Niki 1998; Upston et al. 1999), depending on the fate of α-tocopheroxyl radical (α-TO˙) formed during the oxidation process. Unless the α-TO˙ is eliminated, it can replace the lipid peroxyl radical (LOO˙) as the peroxidation-chain carrying species. Effective protection of LDL lipids requires the presence of vitamin E plus a suitable reducing agent, which can reduce α-TO˙ and eliminate the resulting radical from interaction with the LDL particle. Vitamin E is regenerated by the water-soluble vitamin C (Sharma and Buttner 1993), and also by other co-antioxidants, including ubiquinol-10 or α-tocopheryl hydroquinone, which is obtained from the diet. Thus, the benefits of vitamin E supplementation together with other antioxidants that work in concert may explain why dietary vitamin E might be more beneficial against cardiovascular diseases than vitamin E supplements. Furthermore, we have recently demonstrated that vitamin E can act synergistically with lycopene, with β-carotene or with flavonoids, providing a better protection of LDL against oxidation (Fuhrman et al. 2000).

As our understanding of the antioxidant effect of vitamin E evolved, it became clear that vitamin E can also affect inhibition of cellular oxidative responses such as cell-mediated LDL oxidation. In vitro, cell supplementation with vitamin E did not influence their ability to oxidize LDL (Baoutina et al. 1998), whereas dietary supplementation of vitamin E to apolipoprotein E deficient (E^0) mice for a period of 6 weeks resulted in reduced capacity of their harvested macrophages to oxidize LDL (Rosenblat et al. 2002). This effect was associated with reduced cellular content of oxysterols, and inhibition of superoxide production by impairing the assembly of the NADPH–oxidase complex (Cachia et al. 1998; Rosenblat et al. 2002). One common mechanism to account for these effects is the inhibition of protein kinase C activation by vitamin E, which in turn maintains normal vascular homeostasis (Keany et al. 1999).

2.2
Carotenoids

We have previously demonstrated that LDL supplementation with β-carotene or with lycopene increases its resistance to oxidation, in some, but not all, LDL samples that were studied (Fuhrman et al. 1997a). This effect was further potentiated when the carotenoids were present in combination with vitamin E. When lycopene was supplemented as tomato oleoresin, which besides lycopene contains several other micronutrient antioxidants, including vitamin E, the inhibition of LDL oxidation was significantly greater than that of lycopene alone. Dietary antioxidants exist in nature in combination, and combinations of different antioxidants may act additively and even synergistically. Our study presented the first evidence that lycopene can indeed act as an effective antioxidant against LDL oxidation in synergism with several natural antioxidants, including vitamin E, the isoflavan glabridin and also the phenolics rosmarinic and carnosic acids (but not with tocotrienols) (Fuhrman et al. 2000a).

Enrichment of LDL with a mixture of vitamin E, β-carotene lycopene, anthaxanthin and lutein following a single oral supplementation resulted in the protection of LDL PUFA and of its cholesterol moieties against oxidative modification (Linseisen et al. 1998).

Lycopene was shown to react also with peroxynitrite, and to protect LDL against peroxynitrite-induced oxidation (Panasenko et al. 2000), suggesting that this carotenoid scavenges peroxynitrite in vivo. We have extended our studies to analyze the effect of lycopene on the susceptibility of LDL to oxidation in E^0 mice, as their LDL is highly susceptible to oxidation. Dietary supplementation of lycopene (50µg/mouse/week) for 6 weeks to E^0 mice resulted in a significant reduction in the susceptibility of their LDL to copper ion-induced oxidation. However, when lycopene was administered as Lycomato (the tomato's lipid extract where lycopene is present in combination with vitamin E, β-carotene and phytofluene), its antioxidative effect was substantially potentiated (Fuhrman et al. 1997a).

Dietary supplementation of β-carotene (180 mg/day) for 2 weeks to healthy volunteers resulted in enrichment of the subjects' LDL, as well as their monocyte derived macrophages (MDM) with β-carotene. However, β-carotene enrichment of MDM did not affect the capacity of the cells to oxidize LDL (Levy et al. 1996).

The impact of LDL carotenoid content on its oxidation by human aortic endothelial cells was also studied (Dugas et al. 1998, 1999) and the results showed that enrichment of LDL with β-carotene, but not with lycopene, or with lutein, in vivo or in vitro, protected it from oxidation by endothelial cells.

2.3
Flavonoids

The antioxidant capacity against LDL oxidation of a respective flavonoid or flavonoid-rich nutrient is determined by its quantity and its quality. This is evidenced by the observation that white wine, which is very poor in flavonoids in comparison to red wine, exhibits very limited antioxidant protection against LDL oxidation when studied in vitro, as well as in vivo (Fuhrman and Aviram 1996; Fuhrman et al. 2001; Tubaro et al. 1999; Vinson and Hontz 1995). However, enrichment of white wine with flavonoids (by incubation of whole squeezed grapes for 18 h with 18% alcohol) increased significantly the wine antioxidant capacity (inhibition by 87% of copper ion-induced LDL oxidation), almost similar to the antioxidant capacity of red wine, although the flavonoid content was still fourfold less than that found in red wine (Fuhrman et al. 2001). These results suggest that not only is the quantity of flavonoids an important determinant of the wine antioxidant capacity, but also that the diversity of flavonoid types plays an important role in this protective effect against LDL oxidation. This was further evidenced by the discrepancies in the results obtained in human intervention studies with red wine (Howard et al. 2002), which could be related to the variations in flavonoid composition of the various wines used. Different groups of flavonoids exhibit different extents of inhibitory activity against LDL oxidation at a similar concentration. Among the different groups of flavonoids, the flavonols, flavanols and isoflavans are most potent protectors of LDL against copper ion-induced oxidation. Furthermore, within each group of flavonoids, there are differences in the antioxidant capacity of the individual flavonoids, which is a function of their structure. Structure–function studies on the inhibitory effect of the licorice derived isoflavan glabridin on LDL oxidation, revealed that the antioxidant effect of glabridin on LDL oxidation resides mainly in the $2'$-hydroxyl group of the isoflavan B ring. The hydrophobic moiety of the isoflavan was also essential to obtain the inhibitory effect of glabridin on LDL oxidation, and the position of the hydroxyl groups at the B ring significantly affected the ability of glabridin to inhibit LDL oxidation (Belinky et al. 1998a).

Flavonoids can also protect LDL from oxidation by their ability to spare LDL-associated antioxidants. We have demonstrated that enrichment of LDL with glabridin prevented the consumption of β-carotene and that of lycopene by 41% and 50%, respectively, after 1 h of LDL oxidation in the presence of the free radical generator AAPH, but failed to protect vitamin E, the major LDL-associated antioxidant, from oxidation (Belinky et al. 1998b). On the contrary, other flavonoids (quercetin glycosides, as well as its aglycone form) were shown to inhibit the consumption of LDL-associated vitamin E during its oxidation (De-Whalley et al. 1990).

The beneficial effects of flavonoid consumption on LDL oxidation were studied in humans and in animal models. A substantial increase in the resistance of LDL to oxidation was obtained following red wine consumption by humans (Aviram and Fuhrman 1998; Fuhrman et al. 1995; Nigdikar et al. 1998) or by the atherosclerotic E^0 mice (Hayek et al. 1997). Flavonoids from red wine were shown to be absorbed following red wine ingestion, and to bind to the LDL particle, thus protecting it from oxidation. On the contrary, a recent study showed that although red wine consumption increased plasma phenols concentration, this increase was insufficient to protect LDL from oxidation (Caccetta et al. 2000). Red wine consumption increased the resistance of LDL to oxidation also in the postprandial state (Miyagi et al. 1997). Studies on the effect of the nonalcoholic components of red wine resulted in contradictory results. Dealcoholized red wine did not affect the susceptibility of LDL to copper ion-induced oxidation (de Rijke et al. 1996), whereas ingestion of purple grape juice was shown to reduce LDL susceptibility to oxidation in patients with coronary artery disease (CAD) (Stein et al. 1999). Following administration of pro-anthocyanidins-rich extract from grape seeds, these flavonoids protected LDL from oxidation, although they could be detected only in plasma but not in LDL (Yamakoshi et al. 1999). Potent antioxidant activities against LDL oxidation were also obtained following consumption of other groups of flavonoids. Consumption by humans or by E^0 mice of licorice extract or its major polyphenol glabridin, resulted in increased resistance of LDL to oxidation and to aggregation (Aviram et al. 2004b; Fuhrman et al. 1997; Belinky et al. 1998). This effect could also be related to the absorption of glabridin and it's binding to plasma LDL. Consumption by human volunteers of soy bars containing genistein and daidzein resulted in a marked increase in plasma flavonoid's level, and an increase in the resistance of the LDL to oxidation although LDL-associated flavonoids were not increased (Tikkanen et al. 1998). Tea flavonoids also inhibited LDL oxidation in some (Ishikawa et al. 1997; Serafini et al. 1996), but not in all studies (McAnlis et al. 1998; Princen et al. 1998; Van het Hof et al. 1997). Remarkable inhibition of LDL oxidation was observed following consumption of pomegranate juice (PJ) (Aviram et al. 2000a), ginger extract (Fuhrman et al. 2000b), or olive oil (Aviram and Eias 1993).

Consumption of PJ resulted in the inhibition of cellular lipid peroxidation and the formation of 'oxidized macrophages' (Aviram et al. 2000a). Consumption of nutrients rich in flavonoids such as PJ (Aviram et al. 2000), or red wine (Hayek et al. 1997), or the use of purified flavonoids such as glabridin, catechin or quercetin, by E^0 mice, resulted in a reduced capacity of the mice-harvested macrophages to oxidize LDL (Aviram and Fuhrman 1998b).

In an attempt to explore the mechanism by which flavonoids inhibit macrophage-mediated oxidation of LDL, cells were incubated in vitro with different flavonoids. Upon incubation of macrophages with the isoflavan glabridin, with the flavanol catechin, or with the flavonol quercetin, all of these flavonoids accumulated in the cells in a time- and dose-dependent manner, and this phenomenon was accompanied by a substantial reduction in the capacity of the flavonoid-enriched cells to oxidize LDL. We have shown that glabridin, which accumulated in the macrophages, inhibited cell-mediated oxidation of LDL via the inhibition of superoxide anions release due to the inhibition of the macrophage NADPH oxidase machinery (Rosenblat et al. 1999). Glabridin inhibited the activation of NADPH oxidase, secondary to its inhibitory effect on the translocation of the cytosolic component P-47 to the plasma membrane, and this effect was related to inhibition of the macrophage protein kinase C.

3
Dietary Antioxidants and Atherosclerosis Development

Epidemiological studies have demonstrated an association between increased intake of antioxidant vitamins and reduced morbidity and mortality from CAD (Chan 1998; Hertog et al. 1993; Kaul et al. 2001; Mayne 1996; Muldoon and Kritchevsky 1996). The beneficial health effects, attributed to the consumption of fruits and vegetables are related, at least in part, to their antioxidant activities (Frei 1999; Halliwel 1994; Sies and Sthal 1995; Stahl and Sies 1997; Stocker 1999b). Animal studies have shown that dietary antioxidant supplementation inhibits the progression of atherosclerosis development (Fuhrman and Aviram 2001a; Fuhrman et al. 2005a; Kaplan and Aviram 2004; Maor et al. 1997; Pratico et al. 1998). However, the results of randomized trials in human with antioxidants demonstrated inconsistent results (Chopra and Thurnham 1999; Futterman and Lemberg 1999; Jialal and Devaraj 2003; Paolisso et al. 1999; Rao 2002; Ursini et al. 1999; Visioli et al. 2002). There are several major issues that should be addressed when performing dietary antioxidant studies as illustrated in Table 1. For a dietary antioxidant to act against LDL oxidation in the arterial wall, it should be absorbed and reach the appropriate tissue, cell and subcellular localization, it should reach appropriate levels, and it also should be active and being able to be reactivated.

Table 1 Factors that determine the antioxidative capacity of an antioxidant

1. Biological absorption
2. Concentration
3. Rate constants for radical reactions
4. Location—aqueous or lipid domains (or in both phases)
5. Mobility in hydrophobic domains
6. Lifetime
7. Rate of regeneration or recycling activity
8. Metal scavenging (chelating, binding) activity
9. The presence of an additional (different) antioxidant
10. The extent of oxidative stress in the studied system

3.1
Vitamin E

3.1.1
Human Studies: Epidemiology

The role of vitamin E in the prevention of cardiovascular disease (CVD) is controversial and the subject of active debate (Chan 1998; Emmert and Kirchner 1999; Jialal and Devaraj 2003; Pryor 2000; Susukawa et al. 1998; Swain and Kaplan 1999; Visioli et al. 2002). Although, contradictory findings were reported in the literature regarding vitamin E supplementation, most of the studies demonstrated that populations using vitamin E supplementation are protected against CVD. Epidemiological data suggest that dietary consumption of vitamin E reduces the incidence of CVD. A substantial reduction in mortality generally correlates with elevated levels of vitamin E in plasma. A cross-sectional study of 16 European populations, the MONICA study, showed a significant inverse correlation between α-tocopherol concentrations and mortality from CAD (Gey et al. 1991). A 40% higher plasma vitamin E concentration was shown to be associated with an 84% lower mortality rate (Gey et al. 1991). Moreover, one longitudinal study involving 5133 Finnish men and women reported an inverse association between dietary α-tocopherol intake and coronary mortality with a 32% risk reduction (Knekt et al. 1994). Three large prospective epidemiologic studies that included the Nurses Health Study (Stampfer et al. 1993 which investigated 87,245 nurses), the Health Professionals Follow-Up Study (Rimm et al. 1993; which investigated 39,910 male health professionals), and an Elderly US population study (Losonczy 1996; composed of 11,178 elderly individuals), found that α-tocopherol supplementation reduced the risk of CAD. In the US Nurses' Health Study (Stampfer et al. 1993) vitamin E supplement, rather than dietary vitamin E, reduced the risk for CHD. Both the Nurses and the Health Professionals studies found that subjects in the highest quintile of α-tocopherol intake had about 40% reduction in CVD (Rimm et al. 1993; Stampfer et al. 1993). In the Elderly population study α-tocopherol supplement use was associated with a 41% reduction in CAD mortality and a 37% reduction in total mortality (Losonczy 1996). A Canadian study (of 2226 men) also reported a significant risk reduction for subjects using α-tocopherol (Meyer et al. 1994). Retrospective evaluation of clinical trials like the Cholesterol-Lowering Atherosclerosis Study (CLAS), a randomized placebo controlled study, provided additional support that coronary artery lesion progression was lowered with α-tocopherol (>100 IU/day) (Hodis et al.1995).

However, in the Iowa Womens' Health Study, Kushi et al. (1996) reported a risk reduction of coronary mortality (21,809 women) from food-derived α-tocopherol intake (>9.64 IU/day) but not from supplements.

3.1.2
Human Studies: Intervention

Prospective large-scale, randomized control clinical trials have been inconclusive regarding the protective role of vitamin E against atherosclerosis (Kaul et al. 2001).

Results from the Cambridge Heart Antioxidant Study (CHAOS) showed that vitamin E therapy (400–800 IU/day for 510 days) significantly reduced nonfatal myocardial infarction by 77% in 2002 patients with angiographically proven CAD (Stephen et al. 1996). Also, Steiner et al. (1995) showed in a double-blind randomized study in 100 patients with transient ischemic attacks, that the group receiving α-tocopherol (400 IU/day) in addition to aspirin, had significantly decreased platelet adhesion and lower incidence of recurrent transient ischemic attacks and ischemic strokes, than patients receiving aspirin alone.

The secondary prevention of CVD in end-stage renal disease (SPACE) with antioxidants, reported a significant reduction in composite CVD endpoints and myocardial infarction with vitamin E supplementation in patients with pre-existing CVD (Boaz et al. 2000). In this study only those patients with increased oxidative stress showed cardiovascular manifestation (Aviram 2003a; Boaz et al. 2003). It thus might be important to use vitamin E or an antioxidant treatment in general, only in those patients with enhanced oxidative stress (Aviram 2003a).

Two trials (ABTC and GSSI) demonstrated benefit for vitamin E supplementation on certain endpoints, despite the primary endpoint not being significant. The ATBC trial, which used α-tocopherol alone or in combination with β-carotene, failed to show any effect on coronary heart disease (CHD) (Rapola 1997). However, the ABTC trial did show that vitamin E supplementation significantly reduced cerebral infarction and onset of angina (Rapola 1997). Furthermore, the GISSI trial showed that in 2,830 patients who had prior myocardial infarction and were on a Mediterranean diet (which is enriched with antioxidants) supplementation with all rac-α-tocopherol (272 IU/day for 3.5 years) had no effect on the composite endpoint of death, nonfatal myocardial infarction and stroke (Investigators 1999). However, when a more appropriate four-way analysis was undertaken, the following significant effects were observed: 20% reduction in cardiovascular deaths, 23% reduction in cardiac death, 25% reduction in coronary death and 35% reduction in sudden death (Investigators 1999).

In the Heart Outcomes Prevention Evaluation (HOPE) study, 2,545 women and 6,696 men 55 years or older who were at high risk for CAD events, were enrolled. They were randomized to receive 400 IU of α-tocopherol from natural sources or placebo and either an angiotensin converting enzyme inhibitor or a matching placebo for a mean of 4.5 years (Hope Investigators 2000). Primary outcome was a composite of myocardial infarction, stroke, and CAD death. There were no significant differences in primary or secondary outcome variables in the subjects taking α-tocopherol. However, this study was undertaken in many countries where dietary intakes of antioxidants and objective measures of supplementation (e.g., plasma levels of vitamin E), were not reported.

The effects of vitamin E on regression of atherosclerotic lesions are also inconsistent. There is evidence to suggest that people on vitamin E supplements (>100 IU/day) demonstrate less atherosclerotic lesion progression in comparison to those who do not consume supplements (Hodis et al. 1995). Moreover, supplementation with antioxidant vitamins C and E retards the early progression of transplant-associated coronary arteriosclerosis given as average intimal index (plaque area divided by vessel area) and measured by intravascular ultrasonography (Fang et al. 2002). In the Antioxidant Supplementation in Atherosclerosis Prevention Study (ASAP) (Salonen et al. 2003), after 6 years of vitamin E supplementation (136 IU) twice daily plus 250 mg of slow-release vitamin C to 520 hypercholesterolemic subjects, a slowed progression of carotid atherosclerosis was found in men but not in women, thus confirming previous findings published after 3 years of supplementation (Salonen et al. 2000).

The vitamin E atherosclerosis prevention study (VEAPS) has shown that vitamin E supplementation (400 IU/day) had no effect on the progression of the common carotid artery far-wall intima-media thickness (IMT) assessed by computer image-processed B-mode ultrasonograms in healthy men and women at low risk for CVD (Hodis et al. 2002). Table 2 summarizes the results of human interventional trials with vitamin E supplementation.

Table 2 Human intervention trials with vitamin E or with carotenoid supplements

Study	Dose and duration	Population	Primary endpoint	Other endpoints	Reference
A. Vitamin E					
CHAOS	400 or 800 IU vit E/day for 510 days	CAD patients	↓77% in non fatal infarction		Stephens et al. 1996
SPACE	800 IU vit E/day for 519 days	Hemodialysis patients	↓ Myocardial infarction		Boaz et al. 2000
Transplant associated arteriosclerosis	800 IU vit E/day + 1,000 IU vit C/day for 1 year	Patients after cardiac transplantation (0–2 years)	↓ Coronary arteriosclerosis		Fang et al, 2002
Vitamin E administration plus aspirin	400 IU/day vit E with aspirin for 1 year	Patients with ischemic attacks	↓ Incidence of ischemic events		Steiner et al, 1995
ABTC	50 IU vit E/day for up to 8 years	Male smokers	↔ Lung cancer	↓ Cerebral infarction	Rapola 1997
GSSI	272 IU vit E (all rac)/day for up to 5 years	Patients with prior myocardial infarction	↔ Death, myocardial infarction	↓ Cardiovascular death	Investigators 1999
HOPE	400 IU vit E/day for up to 6 years	Patients with high risk for CAD	↔ Myocardial infarction, Stroke, cardiovascular death	↔ Death from any cause	Hope Investigators 2000
VEAPS	400 IU vit E/day for 3 years	Healthy men and women	↔ IMT thickness		Hodis et al, 2002
ASAP	272 IU/day vit E+ 500 mg vit C/day for 6 years	Hypercholesterolemic patients	↓ IMT thickness		Salonen et al. 2000, 2003
B. Carotenoids					
CARET	30 mg β-Carotene and 25,000 Vit A/day for 1 year	High risk for lung cancer	↑ 46% lung cancer	↑ 26% cardiovascular deaths	Redlich et al. 1999
Beta carotene prevention	50 mg β-carotene/day for 4.3 years	Patients enrolled for prevention of nonmelanoma skin cancer	↔ Death from all causes	↔ Cardiovascular death	Hennekens et al. 1996
Randomized trial of α-tocopherol and β-carotene	50 mg vit E and 20 mg β-carotene/day for 5.3 years	Smokers	↑ Death from coronary disease		Rapola 1997

vit, Vitamin.

3.1.3
Animal Studies

Animal studies allow a more direct investigation of the effect of vitamin E supplements on atherosclerosis. Although the earliest animal studies yielded ambivalent results (Kaul et al. 2001), most of the later studies described here have supported slow progression and prevention of atherosclerosis following vitamin E supplementation. We were the first to demonstrate that consumption of vitamin E by E^0 mice resulted in a 35% reduction in their aortic lesion area (Maor et al. 1997). Pratico et al. (1998) also reported that E^0 mice supplementation with vitamin E (2,000 IU/kg chow) significantly reduced aortic lesion. Cholesterol-fed macaques that were supplemented with vitamin E exhibited a 35% inhibition of atherosclerotic lesion formation as assessed by carotid Doppler studies over a 3-year period (Verlangieri and Buxh 1992). Moreover, in cholesterol-fed rabbits, a 70% inhibition of atherosclerotic lesion formation with 40 mg/kg/day vitamin E was reported (Prasad 1980). Reduced restenosis after angioplasty in rabbits with established experimental atherosclerosis was seen following vitamin E supplementation (Lafont et al. 1995). In another study (Williams et al. 1992), dietary vitamin E administered to modified Watanabe rabbits, led to reduced cholesterol levels and reduced LDL oxidation associated with the inhibition of early aortic lesion development. Also, chickens fed high doses of vitamin E had reduced concentrations of plasma peroxides and less aortic intimal thickening compared with controls (Smith and Kummerow 1989). Recently, administration of vitamin E-supplemented diet to LDL-deficient mice (Cyrus et al. 2003) as well as administration of a vitamin E water soluble to atherosclerotic rabbits (Yoshida et al. 2002), was also shown to reduce the progression of atherosclerosis. Table 3 summarizes the animal's trials with vitamin E supplementation.

At present, there is no conclusive evidence in epidemiological studies that vitamin E supplements provide the benefits observed for vitamin E rich nutrients.

The inconsistent results may be due to the various biological functions of vitamin E, including its role in protection of LDL against oxidation, as well as its other activities on cells of the vascular wall. The dosages of vitamin E administrated in the various studies varied considerably, and it seems that there might be a threshold dose of vitamin E (>800 IU/day) that is effective (Jialal and Devaraj 2003).

Most importantly, the problem of patient selection in human intervention trials has been highlighted recently (Jialal et al. 2001; Visioli et al. 2002). Several parameters must be taken into consideration when planning antioxidants clinical trials. These include the use of analyses, detailed information on the patient's dietary intake, reliable biological markers for oxidative stress and the selection of a population that is suitable for antioxidant treatment (Aviram 2003a).

Table 3 Animals supplementation with vitamin E, carotenoids or flavonoids and atherosclerotic lesions development

Study	Dose and duration	Animal population	Endpoint
A. Vitamin E			
Maor et al.	50 mg vit E/kg/day for 3 months	Apolipoprotein E deficient mice	↓ 33% Aortic lesion area
Prasad et al.	40 mg/kg/day vit E for 2 months	Hypercholesterolemic rabbits	↓ 70% Aortic lesion area
Lafont et al.	5 g/kg diet for 19 days	Hypercholesterolemic rabbits after angioplasty	↓ 43% Restenosis
Williams et al.	0.5% vit E for 12 weeks	Watanabe heritable hyperlipidemic rabbits	↓ 32% Aortic arch lesion area
Pratico et al.	2,000 IU/kg chow vit E for 16 weeks	Apolipoprotein E deficient mice	↓ 67% Aortic lesion area
Smith et al.	1,000 IU vit E /kg diet for 2 months	Hyperlipidemic hens	↓ 38% Intimal thickness
Cyrus et al.	2,000 IU vit E/kg diet for 3 months	LDL-receptor deficient mice	↓ 50% Aortic lesion area
Yoshida	0.8% water soluble vitamin E for 12 weeks	Watanabe heritable hyperlipidemic rabbits	↓ 20% Aortic lesion area
B. Carotenoids			
Shaish et al.	0.01% all trans β-carotene for 11 weeks	Hypercholesterolemic rabbits	↓ 38% Aortic arch lesion area
Dwyer et al.	0.2% Synthetic β-carotene /weight for 8 weeks	Apolipoprotein E deficient mice	↓ 43% Aortic lesion area
Sun et al.	Intravenous injection β-carotene (215 mg/kg/twice weekly)+0.5% vit E for 8 weeks	Hypercholesterolemic rabbits	↓ Atherosclerotic lesion area, intimal thickness
Crawford et al.	1,000 mg β-carotene/kg /day +200 mg vit E/kg /d+100 mg vit C/kg/day for 8weeks	LDL-receptor deficient mice	↓ 60% Aortic lesion area
Shaish A et al.	0.05% all-trans β-carotene +0.05% vit E for 16 weeks	Apolipoprotein E deficient mice	↔ Aortic sinus lesion ↔ aortic lesion area
C. Flavonoids			
Hayek et al.	0.5 ml Red wine/mouse /day for 12 weeks	Apolipoprotein E deficient mice	↓ 48% Atherosclerotic lesion area,
Aviram et al.	31 μl Pomegranate juice /mouse/day for 12 weeks	Apolipoprotein E deficient mice	↓ 44% Atherosclerotic lesion area
Fuhrman et al.	200 μg Licorice/mouse/day for 12 weeks	Apolipoprotein E deficient mice	↓ Atherosclerotic lesion area
Fuhrman et al.	250 μg ginger/mouse/day for 12 weeks	Apolipoprotein E deficient mice	↓ 44% Atherosclerotic lesion area

vit, Vitamin.

Table 3 continued

Study	Dose and duration	Animal population	Endpoint
Lee et al.	0.1% naringin or 0.05% naringenin for 8 weeks	New Zealand rabbits	↓ 18% Aortic fatty streak area
Vinson et al.	100 mg/kg/day grape seed proanthocyanidin extract for 10 weeks	Hypercholesterolemic hamsters	↓ 63% Atherosclerosis development
Yamakashi et al.	0.1% grape seed proanthocyanidin-rich extract for 8 weeks	Hypercholesterolemic rabbits	↓ 24% Aortic arch lesion
Wakabayashi et al.	7 ml red wine/kg/day for 14 months	Watanabe heritable hyperlypidemic rabbits	↔ Aortic and coronary atherosclerotic lesion size

vit, Vitamin.

3.2
Carotenoids

3.2.1
Human Studies: Epidemiology

Dietary carotenoid consumption was shown in epidemiological studies to be associated with reduced cardiovascular mortality (Kohlmeier and Hasting 1995; Pavia and Russell 1999). However, intervention trials with carotenoid supplements demonstrated no effect or even the opposite effects (Tavani and La Vecchia 1999). A Mediterranean diet rich in tomatoes, tomato products, lycopene, and other carotenoids is associated with the low incidence of atherosclerosis and CHD (Rao 2002). Low serum levels of carotenoids were associated with an increased risk of subsequent myocardial infarction among smokers (Street et al. 1994).

The cross-sectional association between intake of carotenoids with provitamin A activity and carotid artery plaques, as examined in 12,773 participants in the Atherosclerosis Risk in Communities Study, suggests that carotenoids may exert their influence later, rather than earlier, in the atherosclerotic process. It thus supports the hypothesis that carotenoids may play a role in preventing arterial plaque formation (Kritchevsky et al 1998). In a cross-sectional study comparing Lithuanian and Swedish populations showing diverging mortality rates from CHD, lower blood lycopene levels were associated with increased risk and mortality from CHD (Kritenson et al. 1997). In another study, a comparison of determinants for coronary heart disease was made among Czech, Bavarian and Israeli men (Bobak et al. 1999). The mortality rates, as well as the prevalence of CHD, were highest in Czech, intermediate in Bavarian and low in Israelis, and these observations correlated with the lycopene concentrations in plasma.

An inverse association between carotid IMT and lycopene was found in patients with essential hypertension and peripheral vascular disease (Gianetti et al. 2002). Low blood levels of lycopene were found to be associated with atherosclerosis risk in middle-aged men from eastern Finland. In women, however, the protective effect was weaker (Tiina et al. 2002).

The strongest population-based evidence comes from a multicenter case–control study (EURAMIC) that evaluated the relationship between adipose tissue antioxidant status and acute myocardial infarction (Kohlmeier et al. 1997). In subjects (662 cases and 717 controls) from ten European countries adipose tissue levels of α- and β-carotenes, lycopene, and α-tocopherol were measured shortly after myocardial infarction. After adjusting for age, body mass index, socioeconomic status, smoking, hypertension, and maternal and paternal history of the disease, only lycopene levels, but not β-carotene, were found to be protective.

3.2.2
Human Studies: Intervention

Several interventional trials (Greenberg et al.1996; Omenn et al. 1996; Rapola 1997; Redlich et al. 1999) using high dose of β-carotene supplements, showed an increase in CVD mortality in the supplemented groups, ranged from 12% to 26%, whereas in a trial among 11,036 healthy physicians, 12 years' supplementation with β-carotene (50 mg on alternate days) produced neither benefit not harm in terms of CVD or death from all causes (Hennekens et al. 1996). Rather, the high-risk population (smokers and asbestos workers) in these interventional trials showed an increase in cancer and angina cases. It appears that carotenoids (including β-carotene) can promote health when taken in small dosages, but may have adverse effects when taken in high dose by subjects who smoke or who have been exposed to asbestos (Pavia and Russell 1999). The Carotene and Retinol Efficacy Lung Cancer Chemoprevention Trial (CARET) (Redlich et al. 1999) ended prematurely due to the unexpected findings that the active treatment group on the combination of 30 mg β-carotene and 25,000 IU retinyl palmitate had a 46% increased lung cancer mortality and a 26% increased cardiovascular mortality compared with the placebo group (Redlich et al. 1999). Table 2 summarizes the results of human interventional trials with carotenoids.

3.2.3
Animals Studies

Supplementation of synthetic β-carotene (Shaish et al. 1995), or synthetic lutein (Dwyer et al. 2001) to atherosclerotic animals showed a protective effect on the progression of atherosclerosis . However, administration of dietary α-tocopherol in combination with β-carotene significantly inhibited the development of atherosclerotic lesion in some (Crawford et al. 1998; Sun et al. 1997) but not all studies (Shaish et al. 1999). Table 3 summarizes the results of animal trials with carotenoids.

The epidemiologic evidence is generally supportive of the notion that a diet rich in carotenoids is associated with a reduced risk for CHD. The clinical trials however show that supplementation of β-carotene does not prevent CHD, although the benefits of other carotenoids, such as lycopene, have not been ruled out.

It might be that serum β-carotene levels are confounded by one or more unmeasured factors that may correlate with reduced β-carotene levels and predict the risk of CHD risk (Kritchevsky 1999). Moreover, no trials have been conducted with lycopene, although its numerous antioxidative activities, mainly in combination with other antioxidants, were demonstrated (Fuhrman et al. 2000; Krinsky 2001; Levy et al. 1996).

3.3
Flavonoids

3.3.1
Human Studies

Consumption of flavonoids in the diet was shown to be inversely associated with morbidity and mortality from CHD (Hertog et al. 1995). Moreover, an inverse association between flavonoid intake and subsequent occurrence of ischemic heart disease, or cerebrovascular disease was shown (Knekt et al. 1996, 2002). Reduced risk for ischemic heart disease mortality was shown in individuals with high intake of apples and onions, which are rich with the flavonols quercetin and kaempferol (Knekt et al. 2002).

In most countries, a high intake of saturated fats is strongly correlated with high mortality from CHD, but this is not the case in some regions of France, the so-called 'French paradox' (Renaud and de Lorgeril 1992). This anomaly has been attributed to the regular intake of red wine (Fuhrman et al. 2001).

We investigated the effects of PJ consumption by patients with carotid artery stenosis (CAS) on carotid lesion development in association with changes in oxidative stress (Aviram et al. 2004a). Ten patients were supplemented with PJ for up to 1 year, and nine other patients that did not consume PJ served as a control group. Blood samples were collected before treatment and after 3, 6, 9 and 12 months of PJ consumption. Patients' carotid IMT was compared between the PJ group and the control group. While in the control group IMT increased by 10% during 1 year, PJ consumption resulted in a significant IMT reduction by up to 43%. Our results clearly demonstrate that PJ consumption by patients with CAS decrease lesion size and systolic blood pressure, and these effects could be related to the potent antioxidant characteristics of PJ.

3.3.2
Animal Studies

Dietary consumption of flavonoid-rich nutrients, as well as pure flavonoids, was shown to attenuate the progression of atherosclerosis in animals (Aviram 1996, 1999a, 2000a; Aviram and Fuhrman 1998b, 2003; Fuhrman and Aviram 2001b, 2001c). Reduced development of atherosclerotic lesion areas in the atherosclerotic E^0 mice was demonstrated following consumption of PJ (Aviram et al. 2000a; Kaplan et al. 2001), red wine (Hayek et al. 1997), grape powder (Fuhrman et al. 2005a), licorice root extract (Fuhrman et al. 1997), or ginger extract (Fuhrman et al. 2000b). Consumption of the flavonol quercetin or the isoflavan glabridin also showed a remarkable attenuation of lesion size in E^0 mice (Hayek et al. 1997).

In New Zealand white rabbits supplemented with 0.1% naringin or 0.05% naringenin, aortic fatty streak areas were significantly lower by 20% in comparison to the control group (Lee et al. 2001). In hamsters fed with hypercholesterolemic diet that was supplemented with grape seed proanthocyanidin extract (100 mg/kg/day), the atherosclerotic lesion size was reduced by up to 63% (Vinson et al. 2002). Ingestion of proanthocyanidin-rich extract from grape seeds also reduced severe atherosclerosis in the aorta of cholesterol-fed rabbits (Yamakoshi et al. 1999). In the Watanabe heritable hyperlipidemic rabbits however, administration of red wine reduced the susceptibility of LDL to oxidation, but it failed to prevent the progression of atherosclerotic lesion development (Wakabayashi 1999). Table 2 summarizes the results of the animal's trials with flavonoids.

The epidemiologic evidence, along with results observed in animal studies, clearly suggest that a diet rich in flavonoids may possess potent anti-atherosclerotic effects also in humans.

Figure 2 summarizes the effect of antioxidant nutrients consumption by the atherosclerotic E^0 mice on their LDL oxidation in a cell- free system (A), on macrophage-mediated LDL oxidation (B), and on atherosclerotic lesion development (C).

4
The Paraoxonase Gene Family

The paraoxonase (PON) gene family includes three members, PON1, PON2, and PON3 (Hegele 1999; Primo-Parmo et al. 1996). These PON genes appear to have arisen by gene duplication of a common evolutionary precursor because they share considerable structural homology and are located adjacently on chromosome 7 in humans, and on chromosome 6 in mice. Within a given species, PON1, PON2, and PON3 share about 70% identity at the nucleotide level.

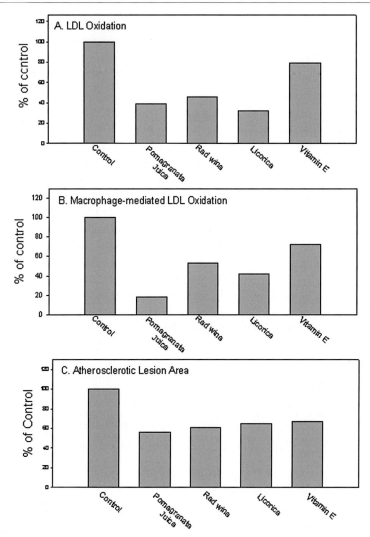

Fig. 2A–C Antioxidants consumption protects LDL from oxidation and attenuates atherosclerotic lesion development. Consumption of nutritional antioxidants (12.5 µl/day pomegranate juice, 0.5 ml/day red wine, 200µg/day licorice extract, or 1 mg/day vitamin E) by E^0 mice inhibits oxidation of LDL (**A**), macrophage-mediated oxidation of LDL (**B**), and the development of atherosclerotic lesion (**C**)

4.1
Serum Paraoxonase 1

Human serum paraoxonase (PON1) is an esterase of 354 amino acids and a molecular mass of 43 kDa (La Du et al. 1993; Mackness et al. 1996), which is physically associated with HDL (Mackness et al. 1996), and is also distributed in tissues such as liver, kidney and intestine (Rodrigo et al. 2001). PON1 is bound to the HDL phospholipids via its retained N-terminal leader sequence, and HDL-associated apolipoprotein A-I stabilized PON1 activity (Sorenson et al. 1999). PON1 was also present in postprandial chylomicrons (Fuhrman et al. 2005b).

4.1.1
PON1 and Atherosclerosis

Human serum PON1 activity was shown to be inversely related to the risk of CVD (Aviram 1999b; Aviram 2004; Durrington et al. 2001; Mackness et al. 2001), as shown in atherosclerotic, hypercholesterolemic and diabetic patients (Abbott et al. 1995; Boemi et al. 2001; Garin et al. 1997; Letellier et al. 2002; Mackness et al. 1991a), as well as in the atherosclerotic E^0 mice. PON1 activity was also decreased in rabbits fed a pro-atherogenic diet (Mackness et al. 2000a).

PON1/apolipoprotein E dual knockout mice exhibited accelerated atherosclerosis (Shih et al. 2000), and in human PON1 transgenic mice, a decreased lesion formation was shown in comparison to control mice (Rozenberg et al. 2005; Tward et al. 2002). This effect may be related to PON1 ability to enhance HDL-mediated macrphage cholesterol efflux via the ABCA1 transporter (Rosenblat et al. 2005).

4.1.2
PON1 and Oxidative Stress

An inverse relationship between serum PON1 activity and the extent of lipid peroxidation was indeed shown (La Du 1996). In PON1/apolipoprotein E dual knockout mice, increased lipoprotein oxidation was shown (Shih et al. 2000). Furthermore, HDL isolated from human PON1 transgenic mice was more protected from copper ion-induced oxidation than control HDL (Oda et al. 2002). PON1 protects both LDL and HDL against lipid peroxidation (Aviram et al 1998; Mackness et al. 1991b, 1993, 2000b; Navab et al. 1996). Inhibition of HDL oxidation by PON1 was shown to preserve the anti-atherogenic effects of HDL in reverse cholesterol transport. PON1 hydrolyzes oxidized cholesteryl esters, as well as specific oxidized phospholipids in oxidized lipoproteins and also in cells (macrophages) and in atherosclerotic tissue (Ahmed et al. 2001; Aviram et al. 2000b; Navab et al. 1996; Rozenberg et al. 2005). This mode of action resembles that of acetylcholine esterase (AChE), which share with PON1 the AChE-PON1 locus on chromosome 7 (Fuhrman et al. 2004b).

We have recently demonstrated that PON1 deficiency results in increased oxidative stress not only in serum, but also in tissues, as evident in arterial, as well as in peritoneal macrophages. This phenomenon may contribute to the accelerated atherosclerosis seen in PON1 knockout mice (Rozenberg et al. 2003). Incubation of macrophages from $PON1^0/E^0$ mice with purified human PON1 resulted in a reduction in the level of lipid peroxides, in the amount of superoxide anion release (Rozenberg et al. 2003), and in macrophage-mediated oxidation of LDL. This phenomenon may be related to the ability of PON1 to hydrolyze lipid peroxides in 'oxidized macrophages' obtained from the atherosclerotic E^0 mice (Fig. 3) (Kaplan and Aviram 2004b). While PON1 can hydrolyze lipid peroxides and thus protects against oxidative stress on the one hand, PON1 was shown to be inactivated by oxidative stress on the other hand. Furthermore, injection of oxidized phospholipid (oxidized 1-palmitoyol-2-arachidonyl-*sn*-glycerol-3-phosphoryl choline, Ox-PAPC) into C57BL/6J mice resulted in a marked reduction in PON1 activity.

4.1.3
Dietary Antioxidants and PON1

Consumption of antioxidant-rich nutrients, such as PJ or red wine, by healthy subjects or by atherosclerotic patients, as well as by the atherosclerotic E^0 mice was shown to preserve PON1 activity, probably by reducing the oxidative stress, thereby contributing to PON1 hydrolytic activity on lipid peroxides in oxidized lipoproteins and in atherosclerotic lesions (Aviram 2003b, 2004, Aviram and Rosenblat 2004, Aviram et al. 2000b, 2004, Fuhrman and Aviram 2002; Kaplan et al. 2001; Rosenblat and Aviram 2005). In a recent study it was demonstrated that vitamin C and vitamin E intake by patients with CAS was associated with increased PON1 activity (Jarvik et al. 2002).

We have shown that PJ consumption by patients with CAS significantly reduced their LDL oxidation rate, and that this was paralleled by a substantial increment in serum PON1 activity (Aviram et al. 2004a).

Intake of the monounsaturated fatty acid, oleic acid, by healthy subjects increased serum PON1 activity, especially in patients carrying the PON1-192R allele.

In another study, meals rich in olive oil (oleic acid rich) were associated with increased postprandial serum PON1 activity in middle-aged and older diabetic women (Tomas et al. 2001), whereas a diet rich in safflower oil had no such effect (Wallace et al. 2001).

In contrast, a high intake of vegetables, berries, and apples combined with a high intake of linoleic or oleic acid for 6 weeks only slightly affected markers of lipid peroxidation and paraoxonase activity (Freese et al. 2002), and in some studies even a reduction in PON1 activity was noted (Kleemola et al. 2002; Rantala et al. 2002). In vitro studies (Aviram et al. 1999) suggest that dietary antioxidants and antioxidant enzymes and PON1 showed a co-activity in protecting LDL from oxidation (Sozmen et al. 2001). Antioxidants, such as the flavonoids glabridin (from licorice root), or quercetin (from red wine) when present during LDL oxidation together with PON1, reduced the amount of lipoprotein-associated lipid peroxides and preserved PON1 activities, including its ability to hydrolyze Ox-LDL cholesteryl linoleate hydroperoxides (Aviram et al. 1999).

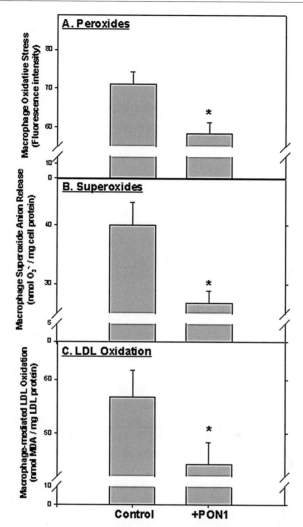

Fig. 3A–C Serum paraoxonase 1 (*PON1*) decreases macrophage oxidative stress. Mouse peritoneal macrophages (*MPM*) were harvested from PON1^0/E^0 mice, and incubated for 18 h at 37°C without or with purified PON1 (7.5 arylesterase Units/ml). Macrophage oxidative stress was expressed as cellular peroxide content (**A**), superoxide anions release (**B**) and cell capacity to oxidize LDL (**C**). **A** For cellular peroxide content, cells were incubated for 30 min at 37°C with DCFH-DA and cellular fluorescence was determined by flow cytometry. **B** Superoxide anions release from macrophage was measured after 1 h of cell incubation with cytochrome C at 37°C. **C** LDL oxidation was determined after cell incubation for 6 h at 37°C with LDL (100 mg protein/l), in the presence of 5 µmol/l of CuSO$_4$. At the end of the incubation, LDL oxidation was measured by the TBARS assay. All the results are given as mean percentage±SD (*n*=5). *P<0.01 (vs. control)

PONs possess lactonase activity, and they are capable of hydrolyzing statins (HMG-CoA reductase inhibitors, which are potent hypocholesterolmic drugs). Statin therapy can reduce the level of oxidized lipids (in the serum of hypercholesterolemic patients) and hence, preserves or even increases PON1 activity. Indeed, atorvastatin or simvastatin therapies increased serum PON1 activity (Fuhrman et al. 2002; Rosenblat et al 2004, Tomas et al. 2000,). In rats, cerivastatin decreased the level of oxidative stress, improved plasma antioxidant defense and also enhanced PON activity (Beltowski et al. 2002).

4.2
PON 2 and PON 3 and Oxidative Stress

By using PON3 specific peptide antibodies, human PON3 was detected as a 40-kDa protein, which, like PON1, is also associated with serum high-density lipoprotein (HDL) (La Du 2001; Reddy et al. 2001). In contrast to PON1, PON3 has very limited arylesterase activity, and no PON activity at all, but it rapidly hydrolyzes lactones such as statin pro-drugs like lovastatin (Draganov et al. 2000). While the mRNA expression of PON1 and PON3 is restricted primarily to the liver, PON2 mRNA is more widely expressed, and is found in a number of tissues, including brain, liver, kidney, testis, and also in white blood cells (Mochizuki et al. 1998).

PON2 overexpression was shown to lower the intracellular oxidative state of cells that were pretreated with either hydrogen peroxide or with Ox-PAPC (Ng et al. 2001). Minimally modified LDL (MM-LDL) that was incubated with cells overexpressing PON2 showed lower levels of lipid hydroperoxides, and was less able to induce monocyte chemotaxis than MM-LDL incubated with control cells (Ng et al. 2001). These data suggest that PON2 may act as a cellular antioxidant, and may thus play an antiatherogenic role by reducing the cellular oxidative stress.

We have recently demonstrated the presence (mRNA, protein, activity) of PON2 and PON3, but not PON1, in murine macrophages, whereas in human macrophages, only PON2 was expressed (Rosenblat et al. 2003). PON2 expression was shown to be upregulated via a NADPH oxidase-dependent mechanism during monocyte differentiation into macrophages (Shiner et al. 2004). Like serum PON 1, also macrophage PON3 (but not PON2) was shown to be inactivated, by up to 57%, under oxidative stress. Dietary antioxidants such as vitamin E or PJ significantly increased (23%–40%) macrophage PON3 activity.

5
Perspectives and Future Directions

LDL oxidation by arterial cells, including macrophages, and the uptake of Ox-LDL by arterial macrophages, leading to foam cell formation, the hallmark of early atherogenesis, is a seminal event in atherosclerosis development. Epidemiological studies, randomized clinical trials and basic research studies, support the hypothesis that changes in dietary patterns to increase dietary antioxidant consumption, will decrease the risk of atherosclerosis. However, clinical trials on antioxidants, mainly with vitamin E and β-carotene, were not supportive of the effects observed in epidemiological studies. There are several important issues that must be addressed prior to the use of an antioxidant. Because a combination of antioxidants can provide a wider range of free radical scavenging activity than an individual antioxidant, clinical and nutritional studies in humans should be directed towards the use of combinations of several types of dietary antioxidants, including combinations of flavonoids together with the other nutritional antioxidants, such as vitamin E and carotenoids. It is most important to use reliable biological markers of oxidative stress, and to identify populations suitable for antioxidant treatment, as antioxidant treatment may be beneficial only in subjects who are under oxidative stress.

Compounds called antioxidants may possess activity beside their antioxidant properties. Antioxidants differ in their ability to react with different reactive oxygen/nitrogen species (ROS/RNS). Some antioxidants exhibit additional anti-atherogenic activities beyond their antioxidant effects.

The exact roles of humoral (PON1) and cellular (PON2) PONs in macrophage foam cell formation under oxidative stress during the development of atherosclerosis is still not understood (Aviram 2003c, Aviram and Rosenblat 2004). Strategies to reduce LDL oxidation and to attenuate atherosclerosis may include appropriate antioxidant combinations that can, on the one hand, reduce oxidative stress as a first line of defense, and on the other hand increase PON activity as a second line of defense against CVDs.

References

Abbott CA, Mackness MI, Kumar S, Boulton AJ, Durrington PN (1995) Serum paraoxonase activity, concentration, and phenotype distribution in diabetes mellitus and its relationship to serum lipids and lipoproteins. Arterioscler Thromb Vasc Biol 15:1812–1818

Ahmed Z, Ravandi A, Maguire GF, Emili A, Draganov D, La Du BN, Kuksis A, Connelly PW (2001) Apolipoprotein A-I promotes the formation of phosphatidylcholine core aldehydes that are hydrolyzed by paraoxonase (pon-1) during high density lipoprotein oxidation with a peroxynitrite donor. J Biol Chem 276:24473–24481

Albertini R, Moratti R, De Luca G (2002) Oxidation of low-density lipoprotein in atherosclerosis from basic biochemistry to clinical studies. Curr Mol Med 6:579–592

Aviram M (1991) The contribution of the macrophage receptor for oxidized LDL to its cellular uptake. Biochem Biophys Res Commun 179:359–365

Aviram M (1993) Modified forms of low density lipoprotein and atherosclerosis. Atherosclerosis. 98:1–9

Aviram M (1995) Oxidative modification of low density lipoprotein and atherosclerosis. Isr J Med Sci 31:241–249

Aviram M (1996) Interaction of oxidized low density lipoprotein with macrophages in atherosclerosis and the antiatherogenicity of antioxidants. Eur J Clin Chem Clin Biochem 34:599–608

Aviram M (1999a) Antioxidants in restenosis and atherosclerosis. Curr Interven Cardiol Rep 1:66–78

Aviram M (1999b) Does paraoxonase play a role in susceptibility to cardiovascular disease? Mol Med 5:381–386

Aviram M (2000) Review of human studies on oxidative damage and antioxidant protection related to cardiovascular diseases. Free Radic Res 33:S85–S97

Aviram M. (2003a) Lipid peroxidation and atherosclerosis: the importance of selected patient groups analysis. Isr Med Assoc J 5:734–735

Aviram M (2003b) Dietary antioxidants stimulate the expression of paraoxonases which provides protection against atherosclerosis development. Curr Top Nutraceutical Res 1:183–191

Aviram M (2003c) Introduction to the serial review on paraoxonases, oxidative stress, and cardiovascular diseases. Free Radic Biol Med 37:1301–1303

Aviram M (2004) Introduction to the serial review on paraoxonases, oxidative stress, and cardiovascular diseases. Free Radic Biol Med 37:1301–1303

Aviram M, Eias K (1993) Dietary olive oil reduces low-density lipoprotein uptake by macrophages and decreases the susceptibility of the lipoprotein to undergo lipid peroxidation. Ann Nutr Metab 37:75–84

Aviram M, Fuhrman B (1998a) LDL Oxidation by arterial wall macrophages depends on the oxidative status in the lipoprotein and in the cells: Role of prooxidants vs. antioxidants. Mol Cell Biochem 188:149–159

Aviram M, Fuhrman B (1998b) Polyphenolic flavonoids inhibit macrophage-mediated oxidation of LDL and attenuate atherogenesis. Atherosclerosis 137 (Suppl): S45–S50

Aviram M, Fuhrman B (2003) Effects of flavonoids on the oxidation of LDL and atherosclerosis. In: Rich-Evans C, Packer L (eds) Flavonoids in health and disease, Vol II. Marcel Dekker, New York, pp 165–203

Aviram M, Rosenblat M (1994). Macrophage mediated oxidation of extracellular low density lipoprotein requires an initial binding of the lipoprotein to its receptor. J Lipid Res 35:385–398

Aviram M, Rosenblat M (2003) Oxidative stress in cardiovascular diseases: role of oxidized lipoproteins in macrophage foam cell formation and atherosclerosis. In: Fuchs J, Podda M, Packer L (eds) Redox genome interactions in health and disease. Marcel Dekker, New York, pp 557–590

Aviram M, Rosenblat M (2004) Paraoxonases 1, 2, and 3, oxidative stress, and macrophage foam cell formation during atherosclerosis development. Free Radic Biol Med 37:1304–1316

Aviram M, Rosenblat M, Etzioni A, Levy R (1996) Activation of NADPH oxidase is required for macrophage-mediated oxidation of low density lipoprotein. Metabolism 45:1069–1079

Aviram M, Rosenblat M, Bisgaier CL, Newton RS, Primo-Parmo SL, La Du BN. (1998) Paraoxonase inhibits high density lipoprotein (HDL) oxidation and preserves its functions: A possible peroxidative role for paraoxonase. J Clin Invest 101:1581–1590

Aviram M, Rosenblat M, Billecke S, Erogul J, Sorenson R, Bisgaier CL, Newton RS, La Du B (1999) Human serum paraoxonase (PON 1) is inactivated by oxidized low density lipoprotein and preserved by antioxidants. Free Radic Biol Med 26:892–904

Aviram M, Dorenfeld L, Rosenblat M, Volkova N, Kaplan M, Hayek T, Presser D, Fuhrman B (2000a) Pomegranate juice consumption reduces oxidative stress, atherogenic modifications to LDL, and platelet aggregation: studies in humans and in the atherosclerotic apolipoprotein E deficient mice. Am J Clin Nutr 71:1062–1076

Aviram M, Hardak E, Vaya J, Mahmood S, Milo S, Hoffman A, Billecke S, Draganov D, Rosenblat M (2000b) Human serum paraoxnases (PON 1), Q and R selectively decrease lipid peroxides in coronary and carotid atherosclerotic lesions: PON 1 esterase and peroxidase-like activities. Circulation 101:2510–2517

Aviram M, Rosenblat M, Gaitini D, Nitecki S, Hoffman A, Dornfeld L, Volkova N, Presser D, Attias J, Leiker H, Hayek T (2004a) Pomegranate juice consumption for 3 years by patients with carotid artery stenosis (CAS) reduces common carotid intima-media thickness (IMT), blood pressure and LDL oxidation. Clin Nutr 23:423–433

Aviram M, Vaya J, Fuhrman B (2004b) Licorice root flavonoid antioxidants reduce LDL oxidation and attenuate cardiovascular diseases. In: Packer L, Choon Nam O, Halliwell B (eds) Herbal and traditional medicine: Molecular aspects of health. CHIPS Texas, chap 27, pp595–614

Baoutina A, Dean RT, Jessup W (1998) Alpha-tocopherol supplementation of macrophages does not influence their ability to oxidize LDL. J Lipid Res. 39:114–130

Belinky PA., Aviram M, Mahmood S, Vaya J (1998a) Structural aspects of the inhibitory effect of glabridin on LDL oxidation. Free Radic Biol Med 24:1419–1429

Belinky PA, Aviram M, Fuhrman B, Rosenblat M, Vaya J (1998b) The antioxidative effects of the isoflavan glabridin on endogenous constituents of LDL during is oxidation. Atherosclerosis 137:49–61

Beltowski J, Wojcicka G, Mydlarcyk M, Jamroz A (2002) Cerivastatin modulates plasma paraoxonase/arylesterase activity and oxidant-antioxidant balance in the rat. Pol J Pharmacol 54:143–150

Berliner JA, Heinecke JW (1996) The role of oxidized lipoproteins in atherosclerosis. Free Radic Biol Med 20:707–727

Boaz M, Smetana S, Weinstein T, Matas Z, Gafter U, Iaina A, Knecht A, Weissgarten Y, Brunner D, Fainaru M, Green MS (2000) Secondary prevention with antioxidants of cardiovascular disease in endstage renal disease (SPACE): randomised placebo-controlled trial. Lancet 7:356(9237):1213–1218

Boaz M, Smetana S, Matas Z, Bor A, Pinchuk I, Fainaru M, Green MS, Lichtenberg D (2003) Lipid oxidation kinetics in hemodialysis patients with and without history of myocardial infarction. Isr Med Assoc J 10:692–696

Bobak M, Hense HW, Kark J, Kuch B, Vojtisek P, Sinnreich R, Gostomzyk J, Bui M von Eckardstein A, Junker R, Fobker M, Schulte H, Assmann G, Marmot M (1999) An ecological study of determinants of coronary heart disease rates: a comparison of Czech, Bavarian and Israeli men. Int J Epidemiol 28: 437–444

Boemi M, Leviev I, Sirolla C, Pieri C, Marra M, James RW (2001) Serum paraoxonase is reduced in type 1 diabetic patients compared to non-diabetic, first degree relatives; influence on the ability of HDL to protect LDL from oxidation. Atherosclerosis 155:229–235

Burton GW, Joyce A, Ingold KU (1983) Is vitamin E the only lipid-soluble, chain breaking antioxidant in human blood plasma and erythrocyte membranes? Arch Biochem Biophys 221:281–290

Caccetta RA, Croft KD, Beilin LJ, Puddey IB (2000) Ingestion of red wine significantly increases plasma phenolic acid concentrations but does not acutely affect ex vivo lipoprotein oxidizability. Am J Clin Nutr 71:67–74

Cachia O, Benna JE, Pedruzzi E, Descomps B, Gougerot-Pocidalo MA, Leger CL (1998) Alpha-tocopherol inhibits the respiratory burst in human monocytes. Attenuation of p47 (phox) membrane translocation and phosphorylation. J Biol Chem 273:32801–32805

Chan AC (1998) Vitamin E and atherosclerosis. J Nutr 128:1593–1596

Chopra M, Thurnham DI (1999) Antioxidants and lipoprotein metabolism. Proc Nutr Soc 58:663–671

Crawford RS, Kirk EA, Rosenfeld ME, LeBoeuf RC, Chait A (1998) Dietary antioxidants inhibit development of fatty streak lesions in the LDL receptor-deficient mouse. Arterioscler Thromb Vasc Biol 18:1506–1513

Cyrus T, Yao Y, Rokach J, Tang LX, Pratico D (2003) Vitamin E reduces progression of atherosclerosis in low-density lipoprotein receptor-deficient mice with established vascular lesions. Circulation 107:521–523

De Rijke YB, Demacker PN, Assen NA, Sloots LM, Katan MB, Stalenhoef AF (1996) Red wine consumption does not affect oxidizability of low-density lipoprotein volunteers. Am J Clin Nutr 63:329–334

De Whalley CV, Rankin SM, Hoult RS, Jessup W, Leake DS (1990) Flavonoids inhibit the oxidative modification of low density lipoproteins by macrophages. Biochem Pharmacol 39:1743–1750

Dieber RM, Puhl H, Waeg G, Striegl G, Esterbauer H (1991) Effect of oral supplementation with D-α-tocopherol on the vitamin E content of human LDLs and resistance to oxidation. J Lipid Res 32:1325–1332

Dugas TR, Morel DW, Harrison EH (1998) Impact of LDL carotenoid and alpha-tocopherol content on LDL oxidation by endothelial cells in culture. J Lipid Res 39:999–1007

Dugas TR, Morel DW, Harrison EH (1999) Dietary supplementation with beta-carotene, but not with lycopene, inhibits endothelial cell-mediated oxidation of low-density lipoprotein. Free Radic Biol Med 26:1238–1244

Durrington PN, Mackness B, Mackness MI (2001) Paraoxonase and atherosclerosis. Arterioscler Thromb Vasc Biol 21:473–480

Draganov D, Stetson PL, Watson C, Billecke S, La Du BN (2000) Rabbit serum paraoxonase 3 (PON3) is a high density lipoprotein-associated lactonase and protects low density lipoprotein against oxidation. J Biol Chem 275:33435–33442

Dwyer JH, Navab M, Dwyer KM, Hassan K, Sun P, Shircore A, Hama-Levy S, Hough G, Wang X, Drake T, Merz CN, Fogelman AM (2001) Oxygenated carotenoid lutein and progression of early atherosclerosis: the Los Angeles atherosclerosis study. Circulation 103:2922–2927

Emmert DH, Kirchner JT (1999) The role of vitamin E in the prevention of heart disease. Arch Fam Med 8:537–542

Fang JC, Kinlay S, Beltrame J, Hikiti H, Wainstein M, Behrendt D, Suh J, Frei B, Mudge GH, Selwyn AP, Ganz P (2002) Effect of vitamins C and E on progression of transplant-associated arteriosclerosis: a randomised trial. Lancet 359:1108–1113

Freese R, alfthan G, Jauhiainen M, Basu S, Erlund I, Salminen I, Aro A, Mutanen M (2002) High intake of vegetables, berries, and apples combined with a high intake of linoleic or oleic only slightly affect markers of lipid peroxidation and lipoprotein metabolism in healthy subjects. Am J Clin Nutr 76:950–960

Frei B (1999) On the role of vitamin C and other antioxidants in atherogenesis and vascular dysfunction. Proc Soc Exp Biol Med 222:196–204

Fuhrman B, Aviram M (1996) White wine reduces the susceptibility of low density lipoprotein to oxidation. Am J Clin Nutr 63:403–404

Fuhrman B, Aviram M (2001a) Flavonoids protect LDL from oxidation and attenuate atherosclerosis. Curr Opin Lipidol 12:41–48

Fuhrman B, Aviram M (2001b) Anti-atherogenicity of nutritional antioxidants. Idrugs 4:82–92

Fuhrman B, Aviram M (2001c) Polyphenols and flavonoids protect LDL against atherogenic modifications. In: Handbook of antioxidants: Biochemical, nutritional and clinical aspects, 2nd edn. Ch. 16, pp 303–336

Fuhrman B, Aviram M (2002) Preservation of paraoxonase activity by wine flavonoids : possible role in protection of LDL from lipid peroxidation. Ann NY Acad Sci 957:321–324

Fuhrman B Oiknine J, Aviram M (1994) Iron induces lipid peroxidation in cultured macrophages, increases their ability to oxidatively modify LDL, and affects their secretory properties. Atherosclerosis 111:65–78

Fuhrman B, Lavy A, Aviram M (1995) Consumption of red wine with meals reduces the susceptibility of human plasma and LDL to undergo lipid peroxidation. Am J Clin Nutr 61:549–554

Fuhrman B, Ben-Yaish L, Attias J, Hayek T, Aviram M (1997a) Tomato's lycopene and β-carotene inhibit low density lipoprotein oxidation and this effect depends on the lipoprotein vitamin E content. Nutr Metab Cardiovasc Dis 7:433–443

Fuhrman B, Oiknine J, Keidar S, Ben-Yaish L, Kaplan M, Aviram M (1997b) Increased uptake of LDL by oxidized macrophages is the result of an initial enhanced LDL receptor activity and of a further progressive oxidation of LDL. Free Radic Biol Med 23:34–46

Fuhrman B, Buch S, Vaya J, Belinky PA, Coleman R, Hayek T, Aviram M (1997c) Licorice extract and its major polyphenol glabridin protect low-density lipoprotein against lipid peroxidation: in vitro and ex vivo studies in humans and in atherosclerotic apolipoprotein E-deficient mice. Am J Clin Nutr 66:267–275

Fuhrman B, Volkova N, Rosenblat M, Aviram M (2000a) Lycopene synergistically inhibits LDL oxidation in combination with vitamin E, glabridin, rosmarinic acid, carnosic acid, or garlic. Antiox Redox Signal 2:491–506

Fuhrman B, Rosenblat M, Hayek T, Coleman R, Aviram M (2000b) Dietary consumption of ginger extract attenuates development of atherosclerosis in the atherosclerotic apolipoprotein E deficient mice: hypocholesterolemic and antioxidative effects. J Nutr 130:1124–1131

Fuhrman B, Volkova N, Aviram M (2001) White wine with red wine-like properties: increased extraction of grape skin polyphenols improves the antioxidant capacity of the derived white wine. J Agric Food Chem 49:3164–3168

Fuhrman B, Koren L, Volkova N, Hayek T, Aviram M (2002) Atorvastatin therapy in hypercholesterolemic patients suppresses cellular uptake of oxidized-LDL by differentiating monocytes. Atherosclerosis 164:179–185

Fuhrman B, Shiner M, Volova N, Aviram M (2004a) Cell-induced copper ion-mediated low density lipoprotein oxidation increases during in vivo monocyte-to-macrophage differentation. Free Radic Biol Med 37:259–271

Fuhrman B, Partoush A, Aviram M (2004b) Acetylcholine esterase protects LDL against oxidation. Biochem Biophys Res Commun 322:974–978

Fuhrman B, Volkova N, Aviram M (2005a) Paraoxonase 1 (PON1) is present in postprandial chylomicrons. Atherosclerosis (in press)

Fuhrman B, Volkova N, Coleman R, Aviram M (2005b) Grape powder polyphenols attenuate atherosclerosis development in apolipoprotein E deficient (E^0) mice and reduce macrophage atherogenicity. J Nutr (in press)

Futterman LG and Lemberg L (1999) The use of antioxidants in retarding atherosclerosis: fact or fiction? Am J Crit Care 8:130–133

Garin MC, James RW, Dussoix P, Blanche H, Passa P, Froguel P, Ruiz J (1997) Paraoxonase polymorphism Met-Leu54 is associated with modified serum concentrations of the enzyme. A possible link between the paraoxonase gene and increased risk of cardiovascular disease in diabetes. J Clin Invest 99:62–66

Gerrity RG (1981) The role of monocytes in atherogenesis. Am J Pathol 103:181–190

Gey K, Puska P, Jordan P, Moser UK (1991) Inverse correlation between plasma vitamin E and mortality from ischemic heart disease in cross-cultural epidemiology. Am J Clin Nutr 53(Suppl):326S–334S

Gianetti J, Pedrinelli R, Petrucci R, Lazzerini G, De Caterina M, Bellomo G, De Caterina R (2002) Inverse association between carotid intima-media thickness and the antioxidant lycopene in atherosclerosis. Am Heart J 143:467–474

Goldstein JL, Brown MS (1990) Regulation of the mevalonate pathway. Nature 343:425–430

Glass CK, Witztum JL (2001) Atherosclerosis: The road ahead. Cell 104:503–516

Greenberg ER, Baron JA, Karagas MR, Stukel TA, Nierenberg DW, Stevens MM, Mandel JS, Haile RW (1996) Mortality associated with low plasma concentration of beta carotene and the effect of oral supplementation. JAMA 275:699–703

Halliwell B (1994) Free radicals, antioxidants and human disease: Curiosity, cause, or consequence. Lancet 344:721–724

Hayek T, Fuhrman B, Vaya J, Rosenblat M, Belinky P, Coleman R, Elis A, Aviram M (1997) Reduced progression of atherosclerosis in the apolipoprotein E deficient mice following consumption of red wine, or its polyphenols quercetin or catechin, is associated with reduced susceptibility of LDL to oxidation and aggregation. Arterioscler Thromb Vasc Biol 17:2744–2752

Hayek T, Hussein K, Aviram M, Coleman R, Keidar S, Pavlotxky E, Kaplan M (2005) Macrophage-foam cell formation in streptozotocin-induced diabetic mice: Stimulatory effect of glucose. Curr Opin Liidol (in press)

Hegele RA (1999) Paraoxonase genes and disease. Ann Med 31:217–224

Hennekens CH, Buring JE, Manson JE, Stampfer M, Rosner B, Cook NR, Belanger C, LaMotte F, Gaziano JM, Ridker PM, Willett W, Peto R (1996) Lack of effect of long-term supplementation with beta carotene on the incidence of malignant neoplasms and cardiovascular disease. N Engl J Med 334:1145–1149

Hertog MG, Feskens EJ, Hollman PC, Katan MB, Kromhout D (1993) Dietary antioxidant flavonoids and risk of coronary heart disease: the Zutphen Elderly Study. Lancet 342:1007–1011

Hertog MG, Kromhout D, Aravanis C, Blackburn H, Buzina R, Fidanza F, Giampaoli S, Jansen A, Menotti A, Nedeljkovic S, et al (1995) Flavonoid intake and long-term risk of coronary heart disease and cancer in the seven countries study. Arch Intern Med 155:381–386

Herttuala SY (1998) Is oxidized low density lipoprotein present in vivo? Curr Opin Lipidol 9:337–344

Hodis HN, Mack WJ, LaBree L, Cashin-Hemphill L, Sevanian A, Johnson R, Azen SP (1995) Serial coronary angiographic evidence that antioxidant vitamin intake reduces progression of coronary artery atherosclerosis. JAMA 273:1849–1854

Hodis HN, Mack WJ, LaBree L, Mahrer PR, Sevanian A, Liu CR, Liu CH, Hwang J, Selzer RH, Azen SP (2002) VEAPS Research Group Alpha-tocopherol supplementation in healthy individuals reduces low-density lipoprotein oxidation but not atherosclerosis: the Vitamin E Atherosclerosis Prevention Study (VEAPS). Circulation 106:1453–1459

Howard A, Chopra M, Thurnham D, Strain J, Fuhrman B, Aviram M (2002) Red wine consumption and inhibition of LDL oxidation: What are the important components? Med Hypothesis 59:101–104

Investigators G (1999) Dietary supplementation with n-3PUFA and vitamin E after myocardial infarction: Results of the GISSI-Prevenzione trial. Lancet 354:447–455

Ishikawa T, Suzukawa M, Ito T, Yioshida H, Ayaori M, Nishiwaki M, Yonemura A, Hara Y, Nakamura H (1997) Effect of tea flavonoid supplementation on the susceptibility of low density lipoprotein to oxidative modification. Am J Clin Nutr 66:261–266

Jarvik GP, Tsai NT, McKinstry LA, Wani R, Brophy VH, Richter RJ, Schellenberg GD, Heagerty PJ, Hastsukami TS, Furlong CE (2002) Vitamin C and E intake is associated with increased paraoxonase activity. Arterioscler Thromb Vasc Biol 22:1329–1333

Jialal I, Fuller CJ, Huet BA (1995) The effect of α-tocopherol suplemetation on LDL oxidation. A dose-response study. Arterioscler Thromb Vasc Biol 15:190–198

Jialal I, Devaraj S (1996) The role of oxidized low density lipoprotein in atherogenesis. J Nutr 126:1053S–1057S

Jialal I, Devaraj S (2003) Antioxidants and atherosclerosis: don't throw out the baby with the bath water. Circulation 107:926–928

Jialal I, Traber M, Devaraj S (2001) Is there a vitamin E paradox. Curr Opin Lipidol 12:49–53

Kaplan M, Aviram M (1999) Oxidized low density lipoprotein: Atherogenic and proinflammatory characteristics during macrophage foam cell formation. An inhibitory role for nutritional antioxidants and serum paraoxonase. Clin Chem Lab Med 37:777–787

Kaplan M, Aviram M (2004a) Red wine administration to apolipoprotein E-deficient mice reduces their macrophage-derived extracellular matrix atherogenic properties. Biol Res 37:239–245

Kaplan M, Aviram M (2004b) Macrophage-mediated oxidation of LDL and atherogenesis: Protective role for paraoxonase. In: Cellular disfunction in atherosclerosis and diabetes – Reports from bench to bedside. Simionescu M, Sima A, Popov D (eds) Romanian Academy Publishing House, chap 25, pp336–351

Kaplan M, Hayek T, Raz A, Coleman R, Dornfeld L, Vaya J, Aviram M. (2001) Pomegranate juice supplementation to atherosclerotic mice reduces macrophages lipid peroxidation, cellular cholesterol accumulation and development of atherosclerosis. J Nutr 131:2082–2089

Kaul N, Devaraj S, Jialal I (2001) A-Tocopherol and atherosclerosis. Exp Biol Med 226:5–12

Keany JF, Simon DI, Freedman JE (1999) Vitamin E and vascular homeostasis: implications for atherosclerosis. FASEB J 13:965–975

Kleemola P, Freese R, Jauhiainen M, Pahlman R, Alfthan G, Mutanen M (2002) Dietary determinants of serum paraoxonase activity in healthy humans. Atherosclerosis 160:425–432

Knekt P, Reunanen A, Jarvinen R, Seppanen R, Heliovaara M, Aromaa A (1994) Antioxidant vitamin intake and coronary mortality in a longitudinal population study. Am J Epidemiol 139:1180–1189

Knekt P, Jarvinen R, Renuanen A, Maatela J (1996) Flavonoid intake and coronary mortality in Finland: a cohort study. BMJ 312:478–481

Knekt P, Kumpulainen J, Jarvinen R, Rissanen H, Heliovaara M, Reunanen A, Hakulinen T, Aromaa A (2002) Flavonoid intake and risk of chronic diseases. Am J Clin Nutr 76:560–568

Kohlmeier L, Hasting SB (1995) Epidemiologic evidence of a role of carotenoids in cardiovascular disease prevention. Am J Clin Nutr 62:137S–146S

Kohlmeier L, Kark JD, Gomez-Garcia E, Martin BC, Steck SE, Kardinaal AFM, Ringstad J, Thamm M, Masaev V, Riemersma R, Martin-Moreno JM, Huttunen JK, Kok F (1997) Lycopene and myocardial infarction risk in the EURAMIC study. Am J Epidemiol 146:618–626

Krinsky NI (2001) Carotenoids as antioxidants. Nutrition 17:815–817

Kritenson M, Zieden B, Kucinskiene Z, Elinder LS, Bergdahl B, Elwing B, Abaravicius A, Razinkoviene L, Calkauskas H, Olson A (1997) Antioxidant state and mortality from coronary heart disease in Lithuanian and Swedish men: concomitant cross sectional study of men aged 50. Br Med J 314:629–633

Kritchevsky SB, Tel GS, Shimakawa T, Dennis B I R, Kohlmeier L, Steere E, Heiss G (1998) Provitamin A carotenoid intake and carotid artery plaques: the atherosclerosis risk in communities study. Am J Clin Nutr 68:726–733

Kritchevsky SB (1999) β-carotene, carotenoids and the prevention of coronary heart disease. J Nutr 129: 5–8

Kushi LH, Folsom AR, Prineas RJ, Mink PJ, Wu Y, Bostick RM (1996) Dietary antioxidant vitamins and death from coronary heart disease in postmenopausal women. New Engl J Med 334:1156–1162

La Du BN, Adkins S, Kuo CL, Lipsig D (1993) Studies on human serum paraoxonase/arylesterase. Chem Biol Interact 87:25–34

La Du BN (1996) Structural and functional diversity of paraoxonases. Nat Med 2:1186–1187

La Du BN (2001) Is paraoxonase-3 another HDL-associated protein protective against atherosclerosis? Arterioscler Thromb Vasc Biol 21:467–468

Lafont AM, Chai YC, Cornhill JF, Whitlow PL, Howe PH, Chisolm GM (1995) Effect of α-tocopherol on restenosis after angioplasty in a model of experimental atherosclerosis. J Clin Invest 95:1018–1025

Lee CH, Jeong TS, Choi YK, Hyun BH, Oh GT, Kim EH, Kim JR, Han JI, Bok SH (2001) Anti-atherogenic effect of citrus flavonoids, naringin and naringenin, associated with hepatic ACAT and aortic VCAM and MCP-1 in high cholesterol-fed rabbits. Biochem Biophys Res Commun 15:681–688

Letellier C, Durou MR, Jouanolle AM, Le Gall JY, Poirier JY, Ruelland A (2002) Serum paraoxonase activity and paraoxonase gene polymorphism in type 2 diabetic patients with or without vascular complications. Diabetes Metab 28:297–304

Levy Y, Kaplan M, Ben-Amotz A, Aviram M (1996) Effect of dietary supplementation of beta-carotene on human monocyte-macrophage-mediated oxidation of low density lipoprotein. Isr J Med Sci 32:473–478

Linseisen J, Hoffmann J Riedl J, Wolfram G (1998) Effect of single oral dose of antioxidant mixture (vitamin E, carotenoids) on the formation of cholesterol oxidation products after ex vivo LDL oxidation in humans. Eur J Med Res 3: 5–12

Losonczy K (1996) Vitamin E and vitamin C supplement use and risk of all cause and coronary heart disease mortality in older persons: The established populations for epidemiologic studies of the elderly. Am J Clin Nutr 64:190–196

Mackness MI, Harty D, Bhatnagar D, Winocour PH, Arrol S, Ishola M, Durrington PN (1991a) Serum paraoxonase activity in familial hypercholesterolaemia and insulin-dependent diabetes mellitus. Atherosclerosis 86:193–197

Mackness MI, Arrol S, Durrington PN (1991b) Paraoxonase prevents accumulation of lipoperoxides in low- density lipoprotein. FEBS Lett 286: 152–154

Mackness Mi, Arrol S, Abbott CA, Durrington PN (1993) Protection of low-density lipoprotein against oxidative modification by high-density lipoprotein associated paraoxonase. Atherosclerosis 104:129–135

Mackness MI, Mackness B, Durrington PN, Connelly PW, Hegele RA (1996) Paraoxonases biochemistry, genetics and relationship to plasma lipoproteins. Curr Opin Lipidol 7:69–76

Mackness MI, Boullier H, Hennuyer M, Mackness B, Hall M, Tailleux A, Duriez P, Delfly b, Durrington PN, Fruchart JC, DuveragerN, Cailloud JM, Castro G, Bouiller A (2000a) Paraoxonase activity is reduced by a pro-atherogenic diet in rabbits. Biochem Biophys Res Commun 269:232–236

Mackness MI, Durrington PN, Mackness B (2000b) How high-density lipoprotein protects against the effects of lipid peroxidation. Curr Opin Lipidol 11:383–388

Mackness B, Davies GK, Turkie W, Lee E, Roberts DH, Hill E, Roberts C, Durrington PN, Mackness MI (2001) Paraoxonase status in coronary heart disease. Are activity and concentration more important than genotype? Arterioscler Thromb Vasc Biol 21:1451–1457

Maor I, Hayek T, Coleman R, Aviram M (1997) Plasma LDL oxidation leads to its aggregation in the atherosclerotic apolipoprotein E deficient mice. Arterioscler Thromb Vasc Biol 17:2995–3005

Mayne ST (1996) Beta-carotene, carotenoids, and disease prevention in humans. FASEB J 10:690–710

McAnlis GT, McEneny J, Pearce J, Young IS (1998) Black tea consumption does not protect low density lipoprotein from oxidative modification. Eur J Clin Nutr 52:202–206

Meyer F, Bairati I, Dagenais G (1994) Lower ischemic heart disease (IHD) incidence and mortality among vitamin supplement users in a cohort of 2226 men. 2nd International Conference. Antioxidant Vitamins and β-Carotene in Disease Prevention. Berlin

Meister A, Anderson ME (1983) Glutathione. Annu Rev Biochem 52:711–760

Miyagi Y, Miwa K, Inoue H (1997) Inhibition of human low density lipoprotein oxidation by flavonoids in red wine and grape juice. Am J Cardiol 80:1627–1631

Mochizuki H, Scherer SW, Xi T, Nickle DC, Majer M, Huizenga JJ, Tsui LC, Prochazka M (1998) Human PON2 gene at 7q21.3: cloning, multiple mRNA, and missense polymorphism in coding sequence. Gene 213:149–157

Morel I, Lescoat G, Cogrel P, et al. (1993) Antioxidant and iron-chelating activities of the flavonoids catechin, quercetin and diosmetin on iron-loaded rat hepatocyte cultures. Biochem Pharmacol 45:13–19

Muldoon MF and Kritchevsky SB (1996) Flavonoids and heart disease. BMJ 312:458–459

Navab M, Berliner JA, Watson AD, Hama SY, Territo MC, Lusis AJ, Shih DM, Van Lenten BJ, Frank JS, Demer LL, Edwards PA, Fogelman AM (1996) The yin and yang of oxidation in the development of the fatty streak : a review based on the 1004 George Lyman Duff Memorial Lecture. Arterioscler Thromb Vasc Biol 16:831–842

Ng CJ, Wadleigh DJ, Gangopadhyay A, Hama S,, Grijalva VR, Navab M, Fogelman AM, Reddy ST (2001) Paraoxonase-2 is an ubiquitously expressed protein with antioxidant properties, and is capable of preventing cell-mediated oxidative modification of low-density lipoprotein. J Biol Chem 276:44444–44449

Nigdikar SV, Williams N, Griffin BA, Howard AH (1998) Consumption of red wine polyphenols reduces the susceptibility of low density lipoproteins to oxidation in vivo. Am J Clin Nutr 68:258–265

Noguchi N, Niki E (1998) Dynamics of vitamin E action against LDL oxidation. Free Radic Res 28:561–572

Oda MN, Bielicki JK, Ho TT, Berger T, Rubin EM, Forte TM (2002) Paraoxonase 1 over-expression in mice and its effect on high-density lipoproteins. Biochem Biophys Res Commun 290:921–927

Omenn GS, Goodman GE, Thornquist MD, Balmes J, Cullen MR, Glass A, Keogh JP, Meyskens FL, Valanis B, Williams JH, Barnhart S, Hammar S (1996) Effects of a combination of beta carotene and vitamin A on lung cancer and cardiovascular disease. N Engl J Med 334:1150–1155

Panasenko OM, Sharov VS, Briviba K and Sies H (2000) Interaction of peroxynitrite with carotenoids in human low density lipoproteins. Arch Biochem Biophys 373:302–305

Paolisso G, Esposito R, D'Alessio MA, Barbieri M (1999) Primary and secondary prevention of atherosclerosis: is there a role for antioxidants? Diabetes Metab 25:298–306

Parthasarathy S, Rankin SM (1992) The role of oxidized LDL in atherogenesis. Prog Lipid Res 31:127–143

Parthasarathy S, Santanam N, Auge N (1998) Oxidized low-density lipoprotein, a two-faced janus in coronary artery disease? Biochem Pharmacol 56:279–284

Paiva SA, Russell RM (1999) Beta-carotene and other carotenoids as antioxidants. J Am Coll Nutr 18:426–433

Prasad J (1980) Effect of vitamin E supplementation on leukocyte function. Am J Clin Nutr 33:606–608

Pratico D, Tangirala RK, Rader DJ, Rokach J, FitzGerald GA (1998) Vitamin E suppresses isoprostane generation in vivo and reduces atherosclerosis in apoE-deficient mice. Nat Med 4:1189–1192

Primo-Parmo SL, Sorenson RC, Teiber J, La Du BN (1996) The human serum paraoxonase/arylesterase gene (PON1) is one member of a multigene family. Genomics 33: 498–507

Princen HM, van Duyvennvoorde W, Buytenhek R, Blonk C, Tijburg LB, Langius JA, Meinders AE, Pijl H (1998) No effect of consumption of green and black tea on plasma lipid and antioxidant levels and on LDL oxidation in smokers. Arterioscler Thromb Vasc Biol 18:833–841

Pryor WA (2000) Vitamin E and heart disease: basic science to clinical intervention trials. Free Radic Biol Med 28:141–164

Rantala M, Silaste ML, Tuominen A, Kaikkonen J, Salonen JT, Alfthan G, Aro A, Kesaniemi YA (2002) Dietary modifications and gene polymorphisms alter serum paraoxonase activity in healthy women. J Nutr 132:3012–3017

Rao AV (2002) Lycopene, tomatoes and the prevention of coronary heart disease. Exp Biol Med 227:908–913

Rapola J (1997) Randomized trial of α-tocopherol and β-carotene supplements on incidence of major coronary events in men with previous myocardial infarction. Lancet 349:1715–1720

Reaven PD, Khouw A, Beltz WF, Parthasarathy S, Witztum JL (1993) Effect of dietary antioxidant combinations in humans. Protection of LDL by vitamin E but not by β-carotene. Arterioscler Thromb 13:590–600

Reddy ST, Wadleigh DJ, Grijalva V, Ng C, Hama S, Gangopadhyay A, Shih DM, Lusis AJ, Navab M, Fogelman AM (2001) Human paraoxonase-3 is an HDL-associated enzyme with biological activity similar to paraoxonase-1 protein but is not regulated by oxidized lipids. Arterioscler Thromb Vasc Biol 21:542–547

Redlich CA, Chung JS, Cullen MR, Blaner WS, Van Bennekum AM, Berglund L (1999) Effect of long-term beta-carotene and vitamin A on serum cholesterol and triglyceride levels among participants in the Carotene and Retinol Efficacy Trial (CARET). Atherosclerosis 145:425–432

Renaud S, de Lorgeril M (1992) Wine alcohol, platelets and the French paradox for coronary heart disease. Lancet 339:1523–1526

Rice-Evans CA, Miller NJ, Paganga G (1996) Structure-antioxidant activity relationships of flavonoids and phenolic acids. Free Radic Biol Med 20:933–956

Rimm EB, Stampfer MJ, Ascherio A, Giovannucci E, Colditz GA, Willett WC (1993) Vitamin E consumption and the risk of coronary heart disease in men. N Engl J Med 328:1450–1456

Rodrigo L, Hernandez AF, Lopez-Caballero JJ, Gil F, Pla A (2001) Immunohistochemical evidence for the expression and induction of paraoxonase in rat liver, kidney, lung and brain tissue. Implications for its physiological role. Chem Biol Intreact 137:123–137

Rosenblat M, Aviram M (1997) Macrophage glutathione content and glutathione peroxidase activity are inversely related to cell-mediated oxidation of LDL. Free Radic Biol Med 24:305–313

Rosenblat M, Aviram M (2005) Nutritional and pharmacological influences on paraoxonases. Curr Opin Lipidol (in press)

Rosenblat M, Belinky P, Vaya J, Levy R, Hayek T, Coleman R, Merchav S, Aviram M (1999) Macrophage enrichment with the isoflavan glabridin inhibits NADPH oxidase-induced cell mediated oxidation of low density lipoprotein. J Biol Chem 274:13790–13799

Rosenblat M, Vaya J, Aviram M (2002) Oxysterols-induced activation of macrophage NADPH-oxidase enhances cell-mediated oxidation of LDL in the atherosclerotic apolipoprotein E deficient mouse: inhibitory role for vitamin E. Atherosclerosis 160:69–80

Rosenblat M, Draganov D, Watson CE, Bisgaier CL, La DU BN, Aviram M (2003) Mouse macrophage paraoxonase 2 (PON2) activity is increased whereas cellular PON3 activity is decreased under oxidative stress. Arterioscler Thromb Vasc Biol 23:468–474

Rosenblat M, Hayek T, Hussein K, Aviram M. (2004) Decreased macrophage paraoxonase 2 expression in patients with hypercholesterolemia is the result of their increased cellular cholesterol content: effect of atorvastatin therapy. Arterioscler Thromb Vasc Biol 24:175–180

Rosenblat M, Shih D, Vaya J, Aviram M (2005) Paraoxonase 1 (PON1) enhances HDL-mediated macrophage cholesterol efflux via the ABCA1 transporter in association with increased HDL binding to the cells: A possible role for lysophosphatidylcholine. Atherosclerosis 179:69–77

Rozenberg O, Rosenblat M, Coleman R, Shih DM, Aviram M (2003) Paraoxonase (PON1)-deficiency is associated with increased macrophage oxidative stress : studies in PON1-knockout mice. Free Radic Biol Med 34:774–784

Rozenberg O, Shih D, Aviram M (2005) Paraoxonase 1 (PON1) attenuates macrophage oxidative status: Studies in PON1 transfected cells and in PON1 transgenetic mice. Atherosclerosis (in press)

Salonen JT, Nyyssonen K, Salonen R, Lakka HM, Kaikkonen J, Porkkala-Sarataho E, Voutilainen S, Lakka TA, Rissanen T, Leskinen L, Tuomainen TP, Valkonen VP, Ristonmaa U, Poulsen HE (2000) Antioxidant Supplementation in Atherosclerosis Prevention (ASAP) study: a randomized trial of the effect of vitamins E and C on 3-year progression of carotid atherosclerosis. J Intern Med 248:377–386

Salonen RM, Nyyssonen K, Kaikkonen J, Porkkala-Sarataho E, Voutilainen S, Rissanen TH, Tuomainen TP, Valkonen VP, Ristonmaa U, Lakka HM, Vanharanta M, Salonen JT, Poulsen HE (2003) Antioxidant Supplementation in Atherosclerosis Prevention Study. Six-year effect of combined vitamin C and E supplementation on atherosclerotic progression: the Antioxidant Supplementation in Atherosclerosis Prevention (ASAP) Study. Circulation 107:947–953

Schaffner T, Taylor K, Bartucci EJ, Fischer-Dzoga K, Beenson JH, Glagov S, Wissler R (1980) Arterial foam cells with distinctive immuno-morphologic and histochemical features of macrophages. Am J Pathol 100:57–80

Serafini M, Ghiselli A, Ferro-Luzzi A (1996) In vivo antioxidant effect of green and black tea in man. Eur J Clin Nutr 50:28–32

Shaish A, Daugherty A, O'Sullivan F, Shnfeld G, Heinecke JW (1995) Beta-carotene inhibits atherosclerosis in hypercholesterolemic rabbits. J Clin Invest 96:2075–2082

Shaish A, George J, Giolburd B, Keren P, Levkovitz H, Harats D (1999) Dietary β-carotene and α-tocopherol combination does not inhibit atherogenesis in an apoE deficient mouse model. Arterioscler Thromb Vasc Biol 19:1470–1475

Sharma MK and Buttner GR (1993) Interaction of vitamin C and vitamin E during free radical stress in plasma: an ESR study. Free Radic Biol Med 14:649–653

Shih DM, Xia YR, Miller E, Castellani LW, Subbanagounder G, Cheroutre H, Faull KF, Berliner JA, Witztum JL, Lusis AJ (2000) Combined serum paraoxonase knockout/apolipoprotein E knockout mice exhibit increased lipoprotein oxidation and atherosclerosis. J Biol Chem 275:17527–17535

Shiner M, Fuhrman B, Aviram M (2004) Paraoxonase 2 (PON2) expression is upregulated via a reduced-nicotinamide-adenine-dinucleotide-phosphate (NADPH9)-oxidase-dependent mechanism during monocytes differentiation into macrophages. Free Radic Biol Med 37:2052–2063

Sies H and Stahl W (1995) Vitamins E and C, β-carotene, and other carotenoids as antioxidants. Am J Clin Nutr 62(Suppl 6): 1315S–1321S

Smith T, Kummerow F (1989) Effect of dietary vitamin E on plasma lipids and atherogenesis in restricted ovulator chicken. Atherosclerosis 75:105–109

Sorenson RC, Bisgaier CL, Aviram M, XSu C, Billecke S, La Du BN (1999) Human serum paraoxonase/arylesterase's retained hydrophobic N-terminal leader sequence associates with HDLs by binding phospholipids : apolipoprotein A-I stabilizes activity. Arterioscler Thromb Vasc Biol 19:2214–2225

Sozmen EY, sozmen B, Girgin FK, Delen Y, Azarsiz E, Erdener D, Ersoz B (2001) Antioxidant enzymes and paraoxonase show a co-activity in preserving low-density lipoprotein from oxidation. Clin Exp Med 1:195–199

Stahl W, Sies H (1997) Antioxidant defense: vitamins E and C and carotenoids. Diabetes 2: S14–S18

Stampfer MJ, Hennekens CH, Manson JE, Colditz GA, Rosner B, Willett WC (1993) A prospective study of vitamin E supplementation and risk of coronary disease in women. N Engl J Med 328:1444–1449

Stein JH, Keevil JG, Wiebe DA, Aeschlimann S, Folts JD (1999) Purple grape juice improves endothelial function and reduces the susceptibility of LDL cholesterol to oxidation in patients with coronary artery disease. Circulation 100:1050–1055

Steiner M, Glantz M, Lekos A (1995) Vitamin E plus aspirin compared to aspirin alone in patients with TIA. Am J Clin Nutr 62:1381–1384

Stephens NG, Parsons A, Schofield PM, Kelly F, Cheeseman K, Mitchinson MJ (1996) Randomized controlled trial of vitamin E in patients with coronary disease: Cambridge Heart Antioxidant Study (CHAOS). Lancet 347:781–786

Steinberg D (1997) Low density lipoprotein oxidation and its pathobiological significance. J Biol Chem 272:20963–20966

Steinberg D, Parthasarathy S, Carew TE, Khoo JC, Witztum JL (1989) Beyond cholesterol: modifications of low-density lipoprotein that increase its atherogenicity. N Engl J Med 320:915–924

Steiner M, Glantz M, Lekos A (1995) Vitamin E plus aspirin compared to aspirin alone in patients with TIA. Am J Clin Nutr 62:1381–1384

Stephens NG, Parsons A, Schofield PM, Kelly F, Cheeseman K, Mitchinson MJ (1996) Randomized controlled trial of vitamin E in patients with coronary disease: Cambridge Heart Antioxidant Study (CHAOS). Lancet 347:781–786

Stocker R (1999a) The ambivalence of vitamin E in atherogenesis. Trend Biochem Sci 24:219–223

Stocker R (1999b) Dietary and pharmacological antioxidants in atherosclerosis. Curr Opin Lipidol 10:589–597

Street DA, Comstock GW, Salkeld RM, Achuep W, Klag MJ (1994) Serum antioxidant and myocardial infarction: are low levels of carotenoids and α-tocopherol risk factors for myocardial infarction? Circulation 90:1154–1161

Sun J, Giraud SJ, Moxley RA, Driskell JA (1997) β-carotene and α-tocopherol inhibit the development of atherosclerotic lesions in hypercholesterolemic rabbits. Int J Vitam Nutr Res 67:155–163

Suzukawa M, Ayaori M, Shige H, Hisada T, Ishikawa T, Nakamura H (1998) Effect of supplementation with vitamin E on LDL oxidizability and prevention of atherosclerosis. Biofactors 7:51–54

Swain RA, Kaplan MB (1999) Therapeutic uses of vitamin E in prevention of atherosclerosis. Altern Med Rev 4:414–423

Szuchman A, Aviram M, Khatib S, Tamir S, Vaya J (2005) Exogenous tyrosine-linoleate marker as a tool of the characterization of cellular oxidatives stress in macrophages. Biochemistry (in press)

Tavani A, La Vecchia C (1999) Beta-carotene and risk of coronary heart disease. A review of observational and intervention studies. Biomed Pharmacother 53:409–416

Rissanen T, Voutilainen S, Nyyssönen K, Jukka T (2002) Salonen lycopene, atherosclerosis, and coronary heart disease. Exp Biol Med (Maywood) 227:900–907

The HOPE Investigators (2000) Vitamin E supplementation and cardiovascular events in high risk patients: HOPE. N Engl J Med 342:154–161

Tikkanen MJ, Wahala K, Ojala S, Vihma V, Adlercreutz H (1998) Effect of soybean phytoestrogen intake on low density lipoprotein oxidation resistance. Proc Natl Acad Sci USA 95:3106–3110

Tubaro FP, Rapuzzi F, Ursini U (1999) Kinetic analysis of antioxidant capacity of wine. Biofactors 9:37–47

Tomas M, Senti M, Garcia-Faria F, Vila J, Torrents A, Covas M, Marrugat J (2000) Effect of simvastatin therapy on paraoxonase activity and related proteins in familial hypercholesterolemic patients. Arterioscler Thromb Vasc Biol 20:2113–2119

Tomas M, Senti M, Elosua R, Vila J, Sala J, Masia R, Marrugat J (2001) Interaction between the Gln-Arg 192 variants of the paraoxonase gene and oleic acid intake as a determinant of high-density lipoprotein cholesterol and paraoxonase activity. Eur J Pharmacol 432:121–128

Tward A, Xia YR, Wang XP, Shi YS, Park C, Castellani LW, Lusis AJ, Shih DM (2002) Decreased atherosclerotic lesion formation in human serum paraoxonase transgenic mice. Circulation 106:484–490

Yuting C, Rongliang Z, Zhongjian J, Yong J (1999) Flavonoids as superoxide scavengers and antioxidants. Free Radic Biol Med 9:19–21

Upston JM, Terentis AC, Stocker R (1999) Tocopherol-mediated peroxidation of lipoproteins: implications for vitamin E as a potential antiatherogenic supplement. FASEB J 13:977–994

Ursini F, Tubaro F, Rong J, Sevanian A (1999) Optimization of nutrition: flavonoids and vascular protection. Nutr Rev 57:241–249

Van het Hof KH, de Boer HS, Wiseman SA, Lien N, Westrate JA, Tijburg LB (1997) Consumption of green or black tea does not increase resistance of low density lipoprotein to oxidation in humans. Am J Clin Nutr 66:1125–1132

Verlangieri A, Buxh M (1992) Effects of δ-tocopherol supplementation on experimentally induced primate atherosclerosis. J Am Coll Nutr 11:131–138

Vinson JA, Hontz BA (1995) Phenol antioxidant index: Comparative antioxidant effectiveness of red and white wines. J Agric Food Chem 43:401–403

Vinson JA, Mandarano MA, Shuta DL, Bagchi M, Bagchi D (2002) Beneficial effects of a novel IH636 grape seed proanthocyanidin extract and a niacin-bound chromium in a hamster atherosclerosis model. Mol Cell Biochem 240:99–103

Visioli F, Micheletta F, Iuliano L (2002) How to select patient candidates for antioxidant treatment? Circulation106:e195

Wallace AJ, Sutherland WH, Mann JI, Williams SM (2001) The effect of meals rich in thermally stressed olive oil and safflower oils on postprandial serum paraoxonase activity in patients with diabetes. Eur J Clin Nutr 55:951–958

Wen Y, Killalea S, Norris LA, Cooke T, Feely J (1999) Vitamin E supplementation in hyperlipidaemic patients: effect of increasing doses on in vitro and in vivo LDL oxidation. Eur J Clin Invest 29:1027–1034

Wakabayashi Y (1999) Effect of red wine consumption on low density lipoprotein oxidation and atherosclerosis in aorta and coronary artery in Watanabe heritable hyperlipidemic rabbits. J Agric Food Chem 47:4724–4730

Williams RJ, Motteram JM, Sharp CH, Gallagher PJ (1992) Dietary vitamin E and attenuation of early lesion development in modified Watanabe rabbits. Atherosclerosis 94:153–159

Witztum JL, and Steinberg D (1991) Role of oxidized low density lipoprotein in atherogenesis. J Clin Invest 88:1785–1792

Yamakoshi J, Kataoka S, Koga T, Ariga T (1999) Proanthocyanidin-rich extract from grape seeds attenuates the development of aortic atherosclerosis in cholesterol-fed rabbits. Atherosclerosis 142:139–149

Yoshida N, Murase H, Kunieda T, Toyokuni S, Tanaka T, Terao J, Naito Y, Tanigawa T, Yoshikawa T (2002) Inhibitory effect of a novel water-soluble vitamin E derivative on atherosclerosis in rabbits. Atherosclerosis 162:111–117

HEP (2005) 170:301–323

Soy, Isoflavones and Atherosclerosis

R. St. Clair (✉) · M. Anthony

Department of Pathology, Section on Comparative Medicine, Wake Forest University
School of Medicine, Winston-Salem NC, 27157, USA
rstclair@wfubmc.edu

Abstract Consumption of soy protein is associated with a lower risk of cardiovascular disease in man, and reduced atherosclerosis in a variety of experimental animals. Although a portion of the cardiovascular protective effects appears to be due to reductions in plasma lipoprotein concentration, in most people the magnitude of this effect is relatively small. In many, but not all studies using animal models, the reduction in atherosclerosis is in part independent of changes in plasma lipids and lipoproteins. This implies that there may be a direct effect on the arterial wall of one or more of the components in soy protein that reduces susceptibility to atherosclerosis. The most actively studied components of soy protein that may be responsible for these anti-atherogenic effects are the isoflavones and various protein factions. Extraction of isoflavones and other alcohol-soluble components from soy protein lowers, but does not eliminate its ability to reduce atherosclerosis. Surprisingly, in most studies, adding back the isoflavone-rich alcohol extract to the previously extracted soy protein, or to another protein, does not restore its lipoprotein lowering or anti-atherogenic properties. This implies that alcohol extraction either destroys an active component of soy, alters the structural integrity of the soy proteins, or disassociates a required isoflavone–soy protein complex. Understanding the mechanism of this effect is an important goal for future research. Likewise, the sites of action on the arterial wall, and the mechanisms by which various soy components act to reduce atherosclerosis are just now being studied. The recent demonstration that expression of estrogen receptor alpha is required for athero-protection by soy protein provides important new mechanistic insight. Other properties of soy, including antioxidant, anti-inflammatory and potentially antithrombogenic properties need to be explored more mechanistically before the full potential of dietary soy protein for the protection from cardiovascular disease will be known.

Keywords Risk factors · Compliance · Estrogen receptors · LDL receptors · Lipoproteins

1
Introduction

There is an inverse relationship between consumption of soy protein and car-diovascular disease (Nagata 2000; Nagata et al. 2002; Sasazuki et al. 2001; van der Schouw et al. 2002; Zhang et al. 2003). Asian populations, for example, consume 30 to 50 times more soy protein than Western populations and have a low prevalence of cardiovascular disease (Coward et al. 1993). This does not necessarily mean that there is a cause-and-effect relationship between soy con-sumption and lower cardiovascular disease rates, but it does suggest that this is a relationship that deserves additional study. The potential importance of soy protein in a healthful diet is supported by the action of the US Food and Drug Administration. In 1999, they authorized a health claim stating that "25 grams of soy protein per day, as part of a diet low in saturated fat and cholesterol, may reduce the risk of heart disease" (US Department of Health and Human Ser-vices 1999). The component(s) in soy protein responsible for these beneficial effects, and whether they target solely cardiovascular disease risk factors or also have direct effects on the arterial wall, remains to be determined. In this chapter we will review the effects of soy and some of its components on cardio-vascular risk factors and atherosclerosis, with a particular focus on the effects of soy protein and/or isoflavone that cannot be explained by improvements in risk factors, suggesting a direct effect on the arterial wall.

2
Epidemiology of Soy and Cardiovascular Disease

Several epidemiologic studies have explored the relationship between soy con-sumption and cardiovascular morbidity and mortality. One line of evidence is from cross-cultural studies. Asian populations with high soy consumption have coronary heart disease (CHD) rates that are lower than those of Western populations with low soy intakes. For example, the age-adjusted CHD mortality rates are about eight times higher for US men and women relative to Japanese men and women (Beaglehole 1990). Migrant studies, such as the Ni-Hon-San cohort study, provide evidence that the observed differences in CHD rates between the US and Japan are not entirely due to genetic factors. Robertson, et al. (1977) reported the incidence of myocardial infarction and death from CHD in Japanese men, 45–68 years of age, living in Japan, Hawaii and California. The lowest incidence rate was seen in Japanese men living in Japan, which was reported to be half that of the Japanese men living in Hawaii ($P<0.01$). For Japanese men in California the incidence rate was approximately 50% higher than that of the Japanese men in Hawaii ($P<0.05$). Thus, Japanese men who have emigrated from Japan to Hawaii and to California have increased CHD risk with increased westernization. This suggests that environmental factors, including diet, may play a key role in mediating some of the large differences in CHD risk observed among countries.

More recently, Nagata et al. (2000) did an ecologic study in Japan evaluating the relationship between soy and isoflavone intake (at a population level) with mortality from heart disease and cancer. Soy product and major nutrient intake was derived from the National Nutritional Survey in which dietary habits were surveyed annually by 3-day diet records in 6000 randomly selected households in 12 geographical districts covering 47 prefectures, from 1980 to 1985. The survey included the following four soy products: miso, tofu, fried tofu, soybeans, and other soy products (e.g., yuba, soy milk). Soy protein intake was estimated from food tables and isoflavone intake was derived from data published for Japanese foods. The mean values for soy and isoflavone intake were assigned to the prefectures forming the district.

Nagata et al. (2002) reported a significant inverse correlation between heart disease mortality rate and soy protein consumption in women ($r=-0.48$, $P<0.01$) and a modest correlation in men ($r=-0.25$, $P=$ns). For both men and women this association was attenuated (women: $r=-0.27$, men: $r=0.07$) when adjusted for differences in age, employment, smoking, animal fat intake, salt intake, and energy intake.

Somewhat more convincing evidence regarding the association between soy consumption and CHD derives from three large population-based observational studies. A population-based case–control study in Japanese men and women, age 40–79 years of age, (Sasazuki et al. 2001) included 660 incident cases of nonfatal acute myocardial infarction (MI) and 1,277 controls matched for age, sex, and residence. In women, but not men, there was a significantly lower risk of acute MI with more frequent consumption of tofu. Women who ate tofu four or more times per week had a 50% lower risk of acute MI (odds ratio=0.5, 95% confidence interval 0.3–0.9) than those women who ate tofu less than twice per week. There was a significant P-value for trend ($P=0.008$) across the tertiles of tofu consumption in women after adjusting for smoking, alcohol use, sedentary job, leisure time physical activity, hyperlipidemia, hypertension, diabetes mellitus, angina pectoris, obesity, and fish and fruit consumption. There was no trend in men.

In a cohort of 13,355 men and 15,724 women who were residents of Takayama, Gifu, Japan (Nagata et al. 2002), a semi-quantitative food frequency questionnaire was administered at baseline and follow-up was for 7 years. During that time 2,062 participants died, including 635 cardiovascular deaths. There was a significant trend for lower all-cause mortality with increasing quintile of soy intake in women (P for trend=0.04) and a marginally significant trend in men (P for trend=0.07) after adjustment for age, total energy, marital status, years of education (women only), body mass index, smoking, alcohol intake, coffee intake (men only), age at menarche (women only), menopausal status (women only), exercise, history of hypertension (men only) and diabetes. In the men with the highest soy product intake (median 166.4 g/day) there was a 17% lower risk of death compared to the lowest soy product intake (median 40.6 g/day, adjusted risk ratio 0.83, 95% confidence interval 0.69 to 1.01). In women with the highest level of soy product intake (median 148.6 g/day) the adjusted risk ratio was 0.83, the same as for men, with a 95% confidence interval of 0.68–1.02, compared to those with the lowest intake (median 38.5 g/day). For cardiovascular mortality, the adjusted risk ratio for men was 0.78 for the highest quintile of soy intake, a 22% lower risk compared to the lowest quintile; however, the P for trend was not significant (P=0.29) and the 95% confidence interval was 0.55–1.12, not statistically significant at the 5% level of confidence. For women, the adjusted risk ratio for cardiovascular mortality was 0.90 with 95% confidence interval 0.63–1.28 and the P for trend was not significant (P=0.57). The association between soy intake and cardiovascular mortality was not very robust in this analysis, but the trend for all-cause mortality was stronger.

In a report from the Shanghai Women's Health Study (Zhang et al. 2003), a cohort study involving about 75,000 Chinese women, aged 40–70 years at baseline, information regarding frequency and amount of soy food intake was collected at a baseline interview. Only women without previously diagnosed CHD, stroke, cancer and diabetes were included in this analysis (n=64,915 women contributing 162,277 person-years). After an average follow-up of 2.5 years, there were 62 incident cases of CHD (43 nonfatal MIs and 19 CHD deaths). There was a significant monotonic trend for lower total CHD across quartiles of soy consumption (P=0.003) after adjustment for age, smoking, body mass index, waist-to-hip ratio, hypertension, menopausal status, regular exercise, level of education, family income, alcohol consumption, season of recruitment, total energy intake, intake of fat, fiber, fruit, and vegetables. The women with the highest intake of soy protein ($\geq$11.2 g protein/day) had a 75% lower risk of total CHD (adjusted risk ratio=0.25, 95% confidence interval 0.10–0.63) compared to the quartile with the lowest soy protein consumption (<4.5 g/day). In this study, the association appeared to be stronger for nonfatal MI than CHD death. It is of interest that in most of these recent studies the association between soy intake and CHD appears to be more robust in women and for nonfatal MI.

3
Soy Bioactive Components

The components of soy responsible for the cardiovascular effects have been the subject of much research (Erdman and Fordyce 1989; Potter 1995, 1998). Beginning in the 1970s, the amino acid composition of soy protein was evaluated for its effect on plasma lipid and lipoprotein metabolism and its role in atherogenesis. More recently, other protein components, including specific protein fractions and globulins have been studied. Non-nutritive components of soy protein isolate have also been investigated, including the saponins, phytic acid, trypsin inhibitors, and isoflavones.

There is considerable evidence that the components of soy protein responsible for a portion of its hypocholesterolemic and atheroprotective effects are alcohol-extractable, or at least are affected by alcohol washing. Studies in both humans and nonhuman primates show that alcohol-washed soy protein, compared to unextracted soy protein isolate, is less beneficial for modulating plasma lipid and lipoprotein concentrations and is less effective at inhibiting atherosclerosis (Anthony et al. 1996, 1997; Clarkson et al. 2001; Crouse et al. 1999; Gardner et al. 2001; Merz-Demlow et al. 2000; Wangen et al. 2001).

Isoflavones (non-steroidal phytoestrogens), saponins, and phytosterols are all removed from soy protein isolate when it is alcohol-washed (Anderson and Wolf 1995). A recent study in nonhuman primates tested the effects of adding either a semi-purified isoflavone extract or the whole alcohol-extractable fraction back to alcohol-washed soy protein. These groups were compared to groups fed casein+lactalbumin, alcohol-washed soy protein isolate and unextracted soy protein isolate (Anthony et al. 2002b). While the isoflavone extract did not restore the benefits of alcohol-washed soy on plasma lipid concentrations, the whole alcohol-extracted fraction did restore a portion of the benefit. These findings suggest that both protein and alcohol-extractable material contribute to the plasma lipid benefits of soy; and further, that alcohol washing disrupts some component(s) preventing restoration of the full benefits of unextracted soy protein. Therefore, based on current knowledge, the unextracted soy protein appears to provide the greatest benefit for cardiovascular health.

4
Soy, Isoflavones and Their Effects on Lowering Plasma Lipids and Lipoproteins

4.1
Lipid and Lipoprotein Concentrations

In a meta-analysis conducted in 1995, Anderson et al. (1995) summarized the results of 38 controlled clinical trials in which the effects of soy protein on serum lipids was measured. Subjects ingested an average of 47 g of soy protein per day which resulted in a 9.3% lower total plasma cholesterol, a 12.9% decrease in low-density lipoprotein (LDL) cholesterol, a 10.5% decrease in triglycerides, and a nonsignificant 2.4% increase in high-density lipoprotein (HDL) cholesterol concentrations. The greatest effect on LDL cholesterol reduction was in those subjects having the highest plasma cholesterol concentrations at baseline (Anderson et al. 1995). As little as 20 g of soy protein per day has been shown to lower non-HDL cholesterol [LDL+ very-low-density lipoprotein (VLDL)] and apolipoprotein B (ApoB) in a well-controlled study in which the same amount of total protein was fed (50 g/day), but with different mixtures of isolated soy protein and casein (Teixeira et al. 2000). In the 10 years since this meta-analysis was published, their conclusions have been largely confirmed by others (Baum et al. 1998; Crouse et al. 1999; Duane 1999; Teede et al. 2001; Teixeira et al. 2000).

The effects of soy protein on lipoprotein(a) [Lp(a)], concentrations have been inconsistent (reviewed by Anthony 2002a). Three studies reported significantly higher Lp(a) concentrations with soy protein containing isoflavones (40–154 g protein/day) compared to casein (Nilausen and Meinertz 1999; Teede et al. 2001) or isoflavone-devoid soy protein (Meinertz et al. 2002), while at least five other studies reported no effect of soy containing isoflavones on Lp(a) concentrations at protein intake up to 63 g/day (Crouse, et al. 1999; Dent et al. 2001; Merz-Demlow et al. 2000; Teixeira et al. 2000; Wangen et al. 2001). In the two studies by Meinertz and colleagues (Meinertz et al. 2002; Nilausen and Meinertz, 1999), about 150 g/day of soy protein was consumed which is two- to threefold higher than most studies. However, in the study by Teede et al. (2001), the amount of soy protein (40 g/day) was comparable to other studies. This potentially adverse effect of soy protein on Lp(a) concentrations deserves further study.

4.2
Are Isoflavones Responsible for the Cholesterol Lowering Effects of Soy Proteins?

Although the hypocholesterolemic effects of soy protein have been known for many years (Carroll 1982), a major unanswered question is which of the many components in soy protein are responsible for the lipid lowering effect. The soy isoflavones have received the greatest attention recently, and are the subject of several recent reviews (Ghatge et al. 2003; Nestel 2003; Yeung and Yu 2003). Isoflavones (genistein, daidzein and glycetin) have been implicated due to the fact that soy protein depleted of isoflavones by extraction with alcohol is generally less effective in lowering plasma lipids than is the unextracted soy protein. This has been shown in man (Crouse et al. 1999; Merz-Demlow et al. 2000; Wangen et al. 2001), rodents (Blair et al. 2002; Kirk et al. 1998; Peluso et al. 2000), and monkeys (Anthony et al. 1996, 1997; Clarkson et al. 2001). As mentioned earlier, the problem with this approach is that alcohol extracts other lipid soluble components, and may alter the functional integrity of the remaining soy protein as well.

What is reasonably clear, however, is that the intake of isolated isoflavones has been largely disappointing with respect to lipid lowering. In people with intermediate levels of plasma cholesterol and nonhuman primates, the intake of 55–150 mg per day of isolated soy isoflavones has little effect on plasma lipids (Dewell et al. 2002; Greaves et al. 1999; Hodgson et al. 1998; Howes et al. 2000; Nestel et al. 1997, 1999; Simons et al. 2000). In contrast, when isoflavone concentrations were varied by using soy protein containing different amounts of isoflavones, from 3 to 62 mg per day in a soy protein beverage containing 25 g/day of total soy protein, an isoflavone dose–response effect on plasma lipids was shown, with the highest concentration of isoflavones (62 mg/day) showing the greatest effect (Crouse et al. 1999). For the entire study population, there was a small but significant lowering of total and LDL cholesterol by 4% and 6% respectively in the highest isoflavone group (62 mg/day). In patients with LDL cholesterol levels in the top half of the population at baseline, the total and LDL cholesterol reduction was 9% and 10% respectively in the 62 mg isoflavone group (Crouse et al. 1999). However, another study of soy protein containing different levels of isoflavones did not shown a clear isoflavone dose effect (Baum et al. 1998). Surprisingly isoflavones added back to the alcohol extracted soy protein from which they were removed did not produce a lipid lowering effect, even though the unextracted soy protein did (Anthony et al. 2002b). The reason for this discrepancy is not clear, but could be due to the inactivation of a component of soy protein, a protein–isoflavone complex, or some other component of isolated soy protein that is necessary for lipid lowering, but is lost or inactivated during the extraction process.

After extraction of soy protein with alcohol, the extracted protein, sometimes called soy(−), has been shown to still retain the ability to reduce plasma lipid and lipoprotein levels to some extent, when compared to a casein protein control (Blair et al. 2002; Song et al. 2003). This suggests that components in soy protein in addition to isoflavones, are responsible for some of its lipid lowering effects. The major storage protein fractions of soy protein are β-conglycinin (or 7S globulins), and glycinin (or 11S globulins). Sirtori et al. (1993) showed that the 7S globulin when fed to rats reduces plasma cholesterol concentrations by 35%. Thus, there is some evidence that one or more of the proteins in a soy protein mixture may be responsible for the residual cholesterol lowering properties of alcohol-extracted soy protein. In a recent study using ApoE null and LDLr null:ApoB transgenic mice, Adams et al. (2004) showed that a β-conglycinin-enriched protein fraction also has a marked inhibitory effect on atherosclerosis that was greater than the effects of a glycinin-enriched protein fraction and unfractionated soy protein, and independent of changes in plasma lipoprotein concentrations. Thus, additional studies are needed to identify the mechanisms by which β-conglycinin reduces atherosclerosis, as well as how it lowers plasma cholesterol concentrations.

5
Beneficial Effects of Soy and Isoflavones on Atherosclerosis

Because atherosclerosis is difficult to quantify noninvasively in human beings, most of the research on the effect of soy protein or isolated isoflavones on atherosclerosis has been done in animal models. In the first study to test directly the effect of soy with and without isoflavones on atherosclerosis Anthony, et al. (1997) compared the effect of intact soy protein [soy(+)] with that of alcohol-extracted soy(−) on atherosclerosis in cholesterol-fed male cynomolgus monkeys. A casein+lactalbumin-containing diet was used as a control. In all arterial beds studied, animals consuming the control diet (casein+lactalbumin) had the greatest atherosclerosis, with soy(+) having the least and soy(−) being intermediate (Fig. 1).

The difference in atherosclerosis could not be explained entirely by reductions in plasma lipoproteins, since total plasma cholesterol and LDL+VLDL concentrations in animals fed soy(−) were not different from the control group. This suggests that one or more of the components of soy has an effect on atherosclerosis that is independent of its lipoprotein lowering effect. This is an important concept since the cholesterol lowering effects of soy or isoflavones are much smaller or even nonexistent in human beings relative to most animal models. Although there is no doubt that some of the cardiovascular beneficial effects of soy protein can be explained by their plasma lipid and lipoprotein lowering effects when they are present (Anthony et al. 1996, 1997; Crouse et al. 1999), other studies to be discussed below suggest that the reduction in plasma cholesterol concentrations can explain only part of the athero-protective effects of soy protein.

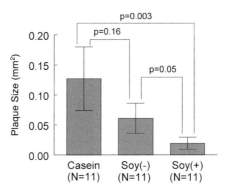

Fig. 1 Effect of unextracted and alcohol-extarcted soy protein isolate on coronary artery atherosclerosis (plaque size) in male cynomolgus monkeys. Animals were fed cholesterol-containing atherogenic diets that were matched except for protein. The dietary groups contained either casein+lactalbumin as the control (*Casein*), isolated soy protein (*Soy+*), or isolated protein that was extracted with alcohol to remove isoflavones (*Soy−*). After 14 months coronary artery atherosclerosis was evaluated. (Reproduced from Anthony et al. 1997, by permission of Lippincott Williams and Wilkins)

In a study in surgically postmenopausal nonhuman primates, the effects on atherosclerosis of unextracted soy protein and estrogen-replacement therapy (conjugated equine estrogens) were compared to an alcohol-extracted soy protein control group. In this study, the animals were fed an atherogenic diet for a 2-year premenopausal exposure period. Atherosclerosis was measured at the end of the premenopausal period (baseline) in an iliac artery biopsy. The animals were then ovariectomized and randomized either into a group fed soy(−), soy(+), or soy(−) with conjugated equine estrogens (CEE) for an additional 3 years. Some of the results of this study are shown in Fig. 2 and suggest beneficial effects of both unextracted soy protein and CEE for inhibition of progression of atherosclerosis in arteries with pre-existing atherosclerosis.

In a recent study by Wagner et al. (2003), a diet containing casein (casein+lactalbumin) as the source of protein was supplemented with a semi-purified alcohol extract of soy protein containing isoflavones and other alcohol soluble components, and effects on plasma lipids, lipoproteins and atherosclerosis were compared with those in animals receiving the same amount of isoflavones as unextracted soy protein. Plasma levels of total isoflavones were not different between the soy(+) group and the casein+isoflavones group, while there were no detectable isoflavones in the plasma of the casein control group. There was no reduction in plasma lipids or lipoproteins (Greaves et al. 1999), and no protection from atherosclerosis (Wagner et al. 2003) by addition of isoflavones to the casein diet (Fig. 3).

The intact soy protein diet showed a significant lowering in plasma ApoB containing lipoproteins, an increase in HDL-cholesterol, and a greater than 65% reduction in carotid artery esterified cholesterol content (a measure of atherosclerosis). The reduction in atherosclerosis by intact soy protein was associated with a 50% decrease in the degradation of LDL in the arterial wall. This could not be explained by a difference in permeability of the arterial wall to LDL, but instead was most likely the result of reduced delivery of LDL secondary to the reduction in plasma LDL concentrations. The possibility cannot be excluded, however, that some component of intact soy protein reduced the retention of LDL in the arterial wall, much as has been reported for estrogens (Wagner et al. 1991). If such a mechanism was working, it would be hard to attribute it to isoflavones as they were present in the plasma at the same concentration in the casein+isoflavones group as the group receiving the intact soy protein. Thus, this study is consistent with the conclusion that isolated isoflavones are not effective in reducing experimental atherosclerosis.

In addition to studies in monkeys, there are studies in other animal models suggesting a protective effect of soy protein on atherosclerosis. This includes an extensive literature going back nearly 40 years that substitution of soy protein for animal proteins will reduce experimental atherosclerosis in rabbits (Howard et al. 1965; Huff et al. 1977).

Studies using mouse models of atherosclerosis have not only strengthened the concept that soy protein or one of its components act independently of

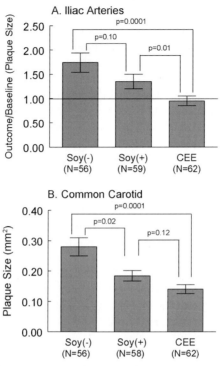

Fig. 2A, B Effect of soy phytoestrogens and conjugated equine estrogens on progression of iliac artery atherosclerosis, and on carotid artery atherosclerosis. Female cynomolgus monkeys were fed an atherogenic diet for 26 months to produce atherosclerosis similar to what would be present in premenopausal women. Animals were then ovarectomized, divided into three groups and fed one of three atherogenic diets that differed in the following treatments. The control group was fed a diet containing soy(−), the second group a diet containing soy(+), and the third group soy(−) plus CEE. **A** After the premenopausal phase (baseline) and again after the postmenopausal phase (outcome), atherosclerosis was evaluated by quantitative histomorphometry of the surgically removed right and left iliac arteries. The ratio of outcome/baseline iliac artery plaque size (mean±SEM) is shown. **B** Atherosclerosis in the common carotid arteries measured only after the outcome phase of the experiment. (Reproduced from Clarkson et al. 2001, by permission of The Endocrine Society, Stanford University Libraries)

the effects on plasma lipids or lipoproteins to reduce atherosclerosis, but also have provided important insight into potential mechanisms. In order to determine if the LDL receptor was required for the athero-protective effects of soy protein or isoflavones, the effect of soy(+) and soy(−) on plasma lipids, LDL oxidation and atherosclerosis were studied in LDL receptor (LDLr) null mice and C57BL/6 mice fed an atherogenic diet (Kirk et al. 1998). Plasma cholesterol concentrations in LDLr-null mice were unaffected by soy(+) relative to soy(−), but in the C57BL/6 mice soy(+)-fed animals had plasma cholesterol concen-

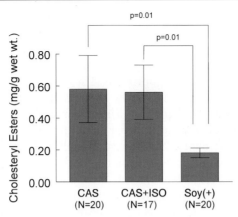

Fig. 3 Effect of isolated soy isoflavones on carotid artery atherosclerosis of surgically post-menopausal cynomolgus monkeys. Overectomized female cynomolgus monkeys were fed an atherogenic diet for 20 weeks. The control diet (*CAS*) contained casein+lactalbunim as the protein source. The CAS+ISO diet was identical except for the addition of isolated soy isoflavones (*ISO*) derived from an alcohol extract of soy protein containing similar amounts of isoflavones found in soy(+). Atherosclerosis was evaluated based on arterial cholesteryl ester content. Results are mean±SEM. (Reproduced from Wagner et al. 2003, , by permission of Lippincott Williams and Wilkins)

trations that were 30% lower. There was no effect on LDL oxidation. Dietary isoflavones did not protect against development of atherosclerosis in LDLr-null mice, but did reduce atherosclerosis in C57BL/6 mice fed an atherogenic diet. The authors suggest that this effect was due to stimulation by isoflavones of LDLr activity in the C57BL/6 mice, which lowered plasma cholesterol and in turn reduced atherosclerosis. This effect was not seen in LDLr-null mice. The authors suggest this was because they had no LDLrs to be stimulated and therefore LDL receptors were necessary for an isoflavone effects on plasma lipid concentrations and atherosclerosis.

Different results were found by Adams et al. (2002a) in a more recent study in which LDLr null:human ApoB transgenic mice and ApoE null mice were used. Although both develop atherosclerosis, the LDLr null:ApoB transgenic mice have a more human-like lipoprotein profile. At 6 weeks of age, male and ovarectomized female mice were assigned to one of three diets. A diet containing casein+lactalbubin as the control protein, a diet containing soy(+) (total isoflavone content=1.72 mg/g) and a diet containing the same amount of soy (−) containing only trace amounts of isoflavones (0.04 mg isoflavones/g). To equalize plasma cholesterol concentrations in the two types of mice, the diet fed to the ApoE null mice was supplemented with cholesterol. After 16 weeks, atherosclerosis was evaluated by measurement of aortic cholesteryl ester content. Both alcohol-washed and intact soy proteins produced a slight decrease in LDL and VLDL in male and overectomized female mice of both types.

Considering both types of mice, there was a significant 24% reduction in atherosclerosis in mice fed the soy(−) diet, and a 49% reduction in mice fed soy(+), relative to controls (Fig. 4).

The athero-inhibitory effects of the diets in both mouse models were independent of effects on plasma lipoproteins. These results are in contrast to the earlier report by Kirk et al. (1998), who showed that there was no difference in plasma lipids or atherosclerosis in LDLr null mice fed soy(+) or soy(−), but that soy(+) significantly lowered plasma lipids and reduced atherosclerosis in cholesterol-fed C57BL/6 mice. Since these animals had functioning LDLrs, the authors concluded that LDLrs were required for the athero-protective effects of soy(+). There is no obvious explanation for the differences in these two studies, other than the methods of quantification of atherosclerosis, the duration of the studies, and the much higher plasma cholesterol concentrations in the study by Kirk et al.

Given that isoflavones are phytoestrogens that can bind to estrogen receptors (ER), it is possible that ERs are required for the beneficial effects of soy proteins or isoflavones to be expressed. To test this possibility, Adams and coworkers (2002b) used ApoE null mice that were also devoid of either ERα or ERβ, to determine if the athero-protective effects of soy protein required either ER. Atherosclerosis was reduced 20%–27% by intact soy protein in ERβ wild-type, ERα wild-type, and ERβ null mice, but had no effect on ERα null mice. This study shows that the athero-inhibitory effect of soy protein was unrelated to the sex of the mice, or plasma lipoprotein concentrations, but requires the presence of ERα. This is similar to the requirement for ERα to mediate the athero-protective effects of 17β-estrodial, described by Hodgin et al. (2001) in ApoE null mice (Fig. 5).

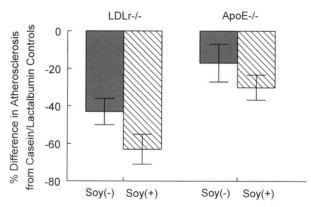

Fig. 4 Percentage decrease in atherosclerosis for LDLr null:ApoB transgenic (LDLr$^{-/-}$) and ApoE$^{-/-}$ mice consuming soy(+) or soy(−) protein for 16 weeks. There were 10–12 mice of each sex in each group. There were no sex differences in atherosclerosis. Results are mean±SD. (Reproduced from Adams et al. 2002a, by permission of the American Society for Nutritional Sciences)

There have been two studies that have found reductions in atherosclerosis with isoflavone extracts. In a study in rabbits, a dose-dependent reduction in atherosclerosis was seen in animals fed a soy isoflavone extract along with cholesterol (Yamakoshi et al. 2000). This was seen without any effect on plasma lipid concentrations, but a significant reduction was seen in measures of both arterial and LDL oxidation. More recently, Jiang et al. (2003) showed that 24 months of treatment of ApoE null mice consuming a Western diet with the daidzein metabolites dihydrodaidzein and dehydroequol, lowered plasma cholesterol levels, improved endothelial nitric oxide-mediated vasorelaxation, and reduced thickness of atherosclerotic plaques in the aortic arch, although the effect on atherosclerosis did not reach statistical significance.

There are several potential mechanisms by which one or more of the components of soy protein could act at the level of the arterial wall to reduce atherosclerosis. Some possibilities are summarized in the following sections.

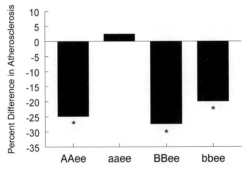

Fig. 5 Percent difference in atherosclerosis with a soy(+) diet versus a soy(−) control diet in Apo E null mice expressing ERα (AA) or ERβ (BB) versus controls not expressing ERα (*aa*) or ERβ (*bb*). All animals were bred to the ApoE null background as indicated by the ee genotype. Each *bar* represents data from approximately 50 mice, both intact males and ovarectomized females, in each genotype, after 16 weeks of cholesterol feeding. Aortic atherosclerosis was evaluated by measurement of aortic cholesteryl ester content/mg protein. *Significant difference between animals in the same genotype fed the soy(−) versus soy(+) diets at $P<0.05$. (Reproduced from Adams et al. 2002b, by permission of Lippincott Williams and Wilkins)

5.1
Antioxidant Properties of Isoflavones

Soy isoflavones can act as antioxidants reducing the formation of oxidized lipoproteins like LDL (Hwang et al. 2000). If this occurred in the arterial wall, it could result in less atherosclerosis even if there was no effect on plasma lipoprotein concentrations (Hwang et al. 2003), as was found in the study by Yamakoshi et al. (2000). There is a large body of evidence suggesting that lipoprotein oxidation is one of the early events in the pathogenesis of atherosclerosis (Witztum and Steinberg 2001). A number of authors have reported a reduced oxidative potential in the serum of people consuming soy protein (Jenkins et al. 2000; Tikkanen et al. 1998; Wiseman et al. 2000). This includes a reduction in the concentration of conjugated-dienes, copper-induced oxidation lag time, and cholesteryl ester hydroperoxides. Isoflavones have structural similarities to estrogens, which also can act as antioxidants at supraphysiological concentrations (Schwenke 1998). At high levels of intake, however, isoflavones can be present in the plasma at up to micromolar concentrations, which makes it more likely that they can function as physiologically important antioxidants in vivo (Hwang et al. 2000). The antioxidant properties of phytoestrogens are the result of their phenolic structure which resembles 17β-estradiol (Ruiz-Larrea et al. 1997), and the ability of specific phytoestrogens (e.g., genistein) to inhibit tyrosine kinases in a redox-sensitive manner (Akiyama et al. 1987). Phytoestrogens also have been reported to act synergistically with other antioxidants to inhibit LDL oxidation (Hwang et al. 2000). Like estrogens, isoflavones may be esterified to fatty acids, making them much more lipophilic and potentially able to partition into the hydrophobic core of lipoproteins where they could function more efficiently to protect the lipoprotein cholesteryl esters from oxidation (Tikkanen et al. 2002). Not all phytoestrogens are equivalent with respect to their antioxidant properties. Equol, for example, a metabolite of daidzein, has greater antioxidant activity than genistein or daidzein. Equol inhibits LDL oxidation in vitro, and LDL oxidative modification by J774 monocyte/macrophages (Hwang et al. 2003).

5.2
Inflammation

Inflammation coupled with dyslipidemia is believed to be a key component in the pathogenesis of atherosclerosis (Libby 2002). Since phytoestrogens bind to estrogen receptors, it is possible that they might act as do estrogens to modulate the immune response. In addition, genistein, a principle isoflavone of soy protein, has been implicated in the anti-inflammatory properties of isoflavones (Boersma et al. 2001; Verdrengh et al. 2003), including inhibition of adhesion molecule expression (Burke-Gaffney and Hellewell 1996; Weber 1996; Wolle et al. 1996), oxygen radical generation (Lim et al. 1997; Nagata et al. 1997), inhibition of chemotactic factor production (Tanabe et al. 1994), and cell-mediated immunity (Curran et al. 2004). The isoflavones have demonstrated anti-inflammatory properties in a variety of animal models of human disease, including chronic ileitis (Sadowska-Krowicka et al. 1998), inflammatory corneal neovascularization (Hayashi et al. 1997), ischemic reperfusion injury (Deodato et al. 1999), asthma (Regal et al. 2000), etc. Thus, a potential mechanism by which isoflavones may reduce the development of atherosclerosis is by modulation of one or more of these inflammatory processes.

5.3
Effects on Vascular Reactivity and Blood Pressure

Soy protein and phytoestrogens have been shown to improve vascular reactivity in response to acetylcholine and flow-mediated dilation (FMD). Both of these effects are secondary to the release of nitric oxide from arterial endothelial cells. These end points appear to be useful monitors of endothelial dysfunction in people, as there is a significant correlation between coronary endothelium-dependent vasoreactivity to acetylcholine and FMD of the brachial artery, and subsequent cardiac events (Schachinger et al. 2000; Suwaidi et al. 2000). Some (Cuevas et al. 2003; Honore et al. 1997; Squadrito et al. 2002, 2003; Steinberg et al. 2003; Walker et al. 2001; Yildirir et al. 2001), but not all studies (Hale et al. 2002; Nestel et al. 1997; Simons et al. 2000; Teede et al. 2001, 2003) show that isolated soy protein and isolated isoflavones improve endothelial function. Dysfunctional endothelial cells show a marked reduction in nitric oxide release in response to acetylcholine. An interesting development is the observation by Williams et al. (2001) showing that with in vivo treated ovarectomized cynomolgus monkeys, there was acetylcholine-induced coronary artery dilation of 5% with 17β-estradiol and 12% with soy protein plus 17β-estradiol, while there was no effect of the soy protein diet alone. This is consistent with the concept that in the absence of a critical level of 17β-estradiol, soy protein will not produce vasodilation. This may explain the failure of soy isoflavones to stimulate vasodilation in some studies of postmenopausal women (Nestel et al. 1997; Simons et al. 2000).

There are several reports suggesting that consumption of soy protein or isolated isoflavones also can influence other cardiovascular parameters. These include compliance (arterial stiffness) and blood pressure. Decreased compliance has been shown to be a risk factor for CHD (Kingwell and Gatzka 2002). Using pulse wave velocity measurements to assess aortic stiffness, van der Schouw et al. (2002) demonstrated an association between isoflavone intake estimated from food-frequency questionnaires and a decreased pulse wave velocity (i.e., reduced stiffness). Teede et al. (2001) reported on a 3-month double-blind, placebo-controlled intervention study with each subject consuming 40 g of isolated soy protein per day containing 118 mg of isoflavones or 40 g of casein. In these normotensive men and postmenopausal women, the soy protein group compared to the casein group had significantly improved peripheral pulse wave velocity and blood pressure, but central pulse wave velocity and systemic arterial compliance were not different (Teede et al. 2001). More recently, Teede and colleagues (2003) reported on another clinical trial in which 80 normotensive men and postmenopausal women were treated with 80 mg/day isoflavone tablets or placebo for 6 weeks and then crossed over to the alternate treatment for 6 weeks. The isoflavone intervention significantly improved systemic arterial compliance and central pulse wave velocity, but there was no significant effect on blood pressure or peripheral pulse wave velocity. Similarly, Nestel and colleagues reported significant improvements in systemic arterial compliance in peri- and postmenopausal women treated with 80 mg/day isoflavone tablets derived from soy (Nestel et al. 1997) or 80 mg isoflavones/day derived from red clover (Nestel et al. 1999). Thus, the effects on arterial elasticity appear to be relatively consistent and are likely to be due to the isoflavones, rather than to the soy protein. Due to the relatively short duration (a few weeks to a few months) of these studies, it is likely that this represents largely an effect on peripheral resistance. More long-term effects could be secondary to changes in the content or composition of connective tissue components of the arterial wall.

Several studies have evaluated the effects of soy protein or isoflavone tablets on blood pressure. Hodgson et al. (1999), found that 55 mg of isoflavanoids isolated from subterranean clover in patients with borderline hypertension did not lower blood pressure. A similar conclusion was reached by Teede et al. (2003) in another study in which isoflavone tablets prepared from red clover (80 mg/day) were administered for 6 weeks to postmenopausal women and men of the same age. In another study by this group (Teede et al. 2001) in which 118 mg/day of isoflavones were administered in soy protein, there was a significant reduction in both systolic and diastolic blood pressure (3.9 and 2.4 mmHg, respectively) when compared to a control group given casein. In a randomized double blind crossover trial with 51 perimenopausal women, 20 g of soy protein containing 34 mg of phytoestrogens split into two doses a day produced a significant 5 mmHg lowering in diastolic blood pressure (Washburn et al. 1999). There was no effect when the same total dose was given once a day (Washburn et al. 1999). Nestel and coworkers (1997, 1999) compared purified isoflavone supplements from soy and red clover, since the composition of the isoflavones is somewhat different. In neither study was there a significant effect on blood pressure. Thus, the effects of soy protein and/or isoflavones on blood pressure are inconsistent. This might be due to the variability in the measurement of blood pressure, or that most of the subjects of these studies were normotensive. Even where significant effects were seen, the reduction in blood pressure was small.

5.4
Thrombosis

In 1995, Wilcox and Blumenthal (1995) speculated that genistein could reduce thrombosis. This was based on in vitro studies showing that genistein, by virture of its tyrosine kinase inhibitionary action, could interfere with the action of growth factors, platelet activation and agonist-induced platelet aggregation. If similar effects occurred in vivo, genistein might be effective in reducing thrombosis associated with plaque rupture. Since that time little research in this area has been done. Dent et al (2001), in a double-blind study in perimenopausal women, showed that consumption of either isoflavone-poor or isoflavone-rich soy protein (40 g/day containing 80 mg isoflavones) had no effect on thrombotic or fibrinolytic markers. In contrast, in studies in young adult female rhesus monkeys fed an atherogenic diet for 6 months, intact soy protein reduced the constrictor response to intracoronary infusion of collagen compared to the animals consuming the isoflavone-poor soy protein diet (Williams and Clarkson 1998). In this same study, in vitro platelet aggregation to thrombin and serotonin were less in the animals receiving the isoflavone-rich soy protein. These studies suggest that dietary isoflavones may reduce platelet aggregation in vivo (Williams and Clarkson 1998). Similar results were found in a mouse femoral artery model of photochemical-induced arterial injury in which genistein reduced in vivo thrombogenesis and in vitro platelet aggregation (Kondo et al. 2002). Additional studies are needed in this area to determine the effect of soy protein and isoflavones on thrombosis associated with plaque rupture.

6
Summary

There are many mechanisms by which soy protein with its isoflavones might decrease CHD. There are the well-recognized improvements in plasma lipid and lipoprotein concentrations; i.e., lower LDL cholesterol, lower triglycerides, and possibly higher HDL cholesterol. There is also evidence that soy protein with isoflavones can have beneficial effects on arterial compliance, vascular function in women, LDL oxidatione, and atherosclerosis. The effects of alcohol-washed soy protein appear to be less robust than those of unextracted soy. Whether that is due entirely to the removal of active alcohol-extractable components, or adverse effects on the protein structures is unclear. Isolated isoflavones do not appear to be athero-protective, although they may have some cardiovascular beneficial effects secondary to improvements in arterial compliance.

There remain many questions surrounding soy/isoflavones and effects on cardiovascular disease risk. Minimal effective doses of soy and isoflavones, frequency of consumption, isoflavone metabolites (such as equol), and protein components; all remain to be clarified. Potential interactions with endogenous hormones is another area of important research for the future. The mechanisms by which soy and isoflavones might impact atherosclerosis and cardiovascular disease risk also are not well understood. Although some proportion of the athero-protective effects of soy can be explained by modification of risk factors, such as lowering of plasma LDL concentrations, in most people this effect appears to be rather small. An equivalent or perhaps even greater proportion of the athero-protective effects of soy is probably due to direct effects on the arterial wall, the nature of which are just beginning to be understood. Understanding the mechanisms by which this is mediated is a major challenge for the future. Whether the beneficial effects of soy and isoflavones on cardiovascular disease risk factors and on the arterial wall translate to reductions in cardiovascular morbidity and mortality requires further exploration.

References

Adams MR, Golden DL, Anthony MS, Register TC, Williams JK (2002a) The inhibitory effect of soy protein isolate on atherosclerosis in mice does not require the presence of LDL receptors or alteration of plasma lipoproteins. J Nutr 132:43–49

Adams MR, Golden DL, Franke AA, Potter SM, Smith HS, Anthony MS (2004) Dietary Soy beta-Conglycinin (7S Globulin) Inhibits Atherosclerosis in Mice. J Nutr 134:511–516

Adams MR, Golden DL, Register TC, Anthony MS, Hodgin JB, Maeda N, Williams JK (2002b). The atheroprotective effect of dietary soy isoflavones in apolipoprotein E-/- mice requires the presence of estrogen receptor-a. Arterioscler Thromb Vasc Biol 22:1859–1864

Akiyama T, Ishida J, Nakagawa S, Ogawara H, Watanabe S, Itoh N, Shibuya M, Fukami Y (1987). Genistein, a specific inhibitor of tyrosine-specific protein kinases. J Biol Chem 262:5592–5595

Anderson JW, Johnstone BM, Cook-Newell ME (1995) Meta-analysis of the effects of soy protein intake on serum lipids. N Engl J Med 333:276–282

Anderson RL, Wolf WJ (1995) Compositional Changes in Trypsin Inhibitors, Phytic Acid, Saponins and Isoflavones Related to Soybean Processing. J Nutr 125:581S–588S

Anthony MS (2002a) Soy/isoflavones and risk factors for cardiovascular disease. In: Gilani GS, Anderson JJB (eds) Phytoestrogens and health. AOCS Press, Champaign, IL, pp 268–289

Anthony MS, Blair RM, Clarkson TB (2002b) Neither isoflavones nor the alcohol-extracted fraction added to alcohol-washed soy protein isolate restores the lipoprotein effects of soy protein isolate. J Nutr 132:583S

Anthony MS, Clarkson TB, Bullock BC, Wagner JD (1997) Soy protein versus soy phytoestrogens in the prevention of diet-induced coronary artery atherosclerosis of male cynomolgus monkeys. Arterioscler Thromb Vasc Biol 17:2524–2531

Anthony MS, ClarksonTB, Hughes CL Jr, Morgan TM, Burke GL (1996) Soybean isoflavones improve cardiovascular risk factors without affecting the reproductive system of peripubertal rhesus monkeys. J Nutr 126:43–50

Baum JA, Teng H, Erdman JW Jr, Weigel RM, Klein BP, Persky VW, Freels S, Surya P, Bakhit RM, Ramos E, Shay NF, Potter SM (1998) Long-term intake of soy protein improves blood lipid profiles and increases mononuclear cell low-density-lipoprotein receptor messenger RNA in hypercholesterolemic, postmenopausal women. Am J Clin Nutr 68:545–551

Beaglehole R (1990) International trends in coronary heart disease mortality, morbidity, and risk factors. Epidemiol Rev 12:1–15

Blair RM, Appt SE, Bennetau-Pelissero C, Clarkson TB, Anthony MS, Lamothe V, Potter SM (2002) Dietary soy and soy isoflavones have gender-specific effects on plasma lipids and isoflavones in golden Syrian f(1)b hybrid hamsters. J Nutr 132:3585–3591

Boersma BJ, Patel RP, Botting N, White CR, Parks D, Barnes S, Darley-Usmar VM (2001) Formation of novel bioactive metabolites from the reactions of pro-inflammatory oxidants with polyphenolics. Biofactors 15:79–81

Burke-Gaffney A, Hellewell PG (1996) Tumour necrosis factor-alpha-induced ICAM-1 expression in human vascular endothelial and lung epithelial cells: modulation by tyrosine kinase inhibitors. Br. J Pharmacol. 119:1149–1158

Carroll KK (1982) Hypercholesterolemia and atherosclerosis: effects of dietary protein. Fed Proc 41:2792–2796

Clarkson TB, Anthony MS, Morgan TM. (2001) Inhibition of postmenopausal atherosclerosis progression: A comparison of the effects of conjugated equine estrogens and soy phytoestrogens. J Clin Endocrinol Metab 86:41–47.

Coward L, Barnes NC, Setchell KDR, Barnes S (1993) Genistein, daidzein, and their b-glycoside conjugates: antitumor isoflavones in soybean foods from American and Asian diets. J Agric Food Chem 41:1961–1967

Crouse JR III, Morgan T, Terry JG, Ellis J, Vitolins M, Burke GL (1999) A randomized trial comparing the effect of casein with that of soy protein containing varying amounts of isoflavones on plasma concentrations of lipids and lipoproteins. Arch Intern Med 159:2070–2076

Cuevas AM, Irribarra VL, Castillo OA, Yanez MD, Germain AM (2003) Isolated soy protein improves endothelial function in postmenopausal hypercholesterolemic women. Eur J Clin Nutr 57:889–894

Curran EM, Judy BM, Newton LG, Lubahn DB, Rottinghaus GE, Macdonald RS, Franklin C, Estes DM (2004) Dietary soy phytoestrogens and ERalpha signalling modulate interferon gamma production in response to bacterial infection. Clin Exp Immunol 135:219–225

Dent SB, Peterson CT, Brace LD, Swain JH, Reddy MB, Hanson KB, Robinson JG, Alekel DL (2001) Soy protein intake by perimenopausal women does not affect circulating lipids and lipoproteins or coagulation and fibrinolytic factors. J Nutr 131:2280–2287

Deodato B, Altavilla D, Squadrito G, Campo GM, Arlotta M, Minutoli L, Saitta A, Cucinotta D, Calapai G, Caputi AP, Miano M, Squadrito F (1999) Cardioprotection by the phytoestrogen genistein in experimental myocardial ischaemia-reperfusion injury. Br J Pharmacol 128:1683–1690

Dewell A, Hollenbeck CB, Bruce B (2002) The effects of soy-derived phytoestrogens on serum lipids and lipoproteins in moderately hypercholesterolemic postmenopausal women. J Clin Endocrinol Metab 87:118–121

Duane WC (1999) Effects of soybean protein and very low dietary cholesterol on serum lipids, biliary lipids, and fecal sterols in humans. Metabolism 48:489–494

Erdman JW, Fordyce EJ (1989) Soy Products and the Human Diet. Am J Clin Nutr 49:725–737

Gardner CD, Newell KA, Cherin R, Haskell WL (2001) The Effect of Soy Protein with or without Isoflavones Relative to Milk Protein on Plasma Lipids in Hypercholesterolemic Postmenopausal Women. Am J Clin Nutr 73:728–735

Ghatge S, Lee J, Smith I (2003) Sevoflurane: an ideal agent for adult day-case anesthesia? Acta Anaesthesiol Scand 47:917–931

Greaves KA, Parks JS, Williams JK, Wagner JD (1999) Intact dietary soy protein, but not adding an isoflavone-rich soy extract to casein, improves plasma lipids in ovariectomized cynomolgus monkeys. J Nutr 129:1585–1592

Hale G, Paul-Labrador M, Dwyer JH, Merz CN (2002) Isoflavone supplementation and endothelial function in menopausal women. Clin Endocrinol (Oxf) 56:693–701

Hayashi A, Popovich KS, Kim HC, de Juan E Jr (1997) Role of protein tyrosine phosphorylation in rat corneal neovascularization. Graefes Arch Clin Exp Ophthalmol 235:460–467

Hodgin JB, Krege JH, Reddick RL, Korach KS, Smithies O, Maeda N (2001) Estrogen receptor alpha is a major mediator of 17 beta-estradiol's atheroprotective effects on lesion size in Apoe(-/-) mice. J Clin Invest 107:333–340

Hodgson JM, Puddey IB, Beilin LJ, Mori TA, Croft KD (1998) Supplementation with isoflavonoid phytoestrogens does not alter serum lipid concentrations: A randomized controlled trial in humans. J Nutr 128:728–732

Hodgson JM, Puddey IB, Beilin LJ, Mori TA, Burke V, Croft KD, Rogers PB (1999) Effects of isoflavonoids on blood pressure in subjects with high-normal ambulatory blood pressure levels: a randomized controlled trial. Am J Hypertens 12:47–53

Honore EK, Williams JK, Anthony MS, ClarksonTB (1997) Soy isoflavones enhance coronary vascular reactivity in atherosclerotic female macaques. Fertil Steril 67:148–154

Howard AN, Gresham GA, Jones D, Jennings IW (1965) The prevention of rabbit atherosclerosis by soya bean meal. J Atheroscler Res 87:330–337

Howes JB, Sullivan D, Lai N, Nestel P, Pomeroy S, West L, Eden JA, Howes LG (2000) The effects of dietary supplementation with isoflavones from red clover on the lipoprotein profiles of post menopausal women with mild to moderate hypercholesterolaemia. Atherosclerosis 152:143–147

Huff M, Hamilton R, Carroll K (1977) Plasma cholesterol levels in rabbits fed low fat, cholesterol-free, semipurified diets: effects of dietary proteins, protein hydrolysates and amino acid mixtures. Atherosclerosis 28:187–195

Hwang J, Sevanian A, Hodis HN, Ursini F (2000) Synergistic inhibition of LDL oxidation by phytoestrogens and ascorbic acid. Free Radic Biol Med 29:79–89

Hwang J, Wang J, Morazzoni P, Hodis HN, Sevanian A (2003) The phytoestrogen equol increases nitric oxide availability by inhibiting superoxide production: an antioxidant mechanism for cell-mediated LDL modification. Free Radic Biol Med 34:1271–1282

Jenkins DJ, Kendall CW, Garsetti M, Rosenberg-Zand RS, Jackson CJ, Agarwal S, Rao AV, Diamandis EP, Parker T, Faulkner D, Vuksan V, Vidgen E (2000). Effect of soy protein foods on low-density lipoprotein oxidation and ex vivo sex hormone receptor activity–a controlled crossover trial. Metabolism 49:537–543

Jiang F, Jones GT, Husband AJ, Dusting GJ (2003) Cardiovascular protective effects of synthetic isoflavone derivatives in apolipoprotein e-deficient mice. J Vasc Res 40:276–284

Kingwell BA, Gatzka CD (2002) Arterial stiffness and prediction of cardiovascular risk. J Hypertens 20:2337–2340

Kirk EA, Sutherland P, Wang SA, Chait A, LeBoeuf RC (1998) Dietary isoflavones reduce plasma cholesterol and atherosclerosis in C57BL/6 mice but not LDL receptor-deficient mice. J Nutr 128:954–959

Kondo K, Suzuki Y, Ikeda Y, Umemura K (2002) Genistein, an isoflavone included in soy, inhibits thrombotic vessel occlusion in the mouse femoral artery and in vitro platelet aggregation. Eur J Pharmacol 455:53–57

Libby P (2002) Inflammation in atherosclerosis. Nature 420:868–874

Lim Y, Kim SH, Cho YJ, Kim KA, Oh MW, and Lee KH (1997) Silica-induced oxygen radical generation in alveolar macrophage. Ind Health 35:380–387

Meinertz H, Nilausen K, Hilden J (2002) Alcohol-extracted, but not intact, dietary soy protein lowers lipoprotein(a) markedly. Arterioscler Thromb Vasc Biol 22:312–316

Merz-Demlow BE, Duncan AM, Wangen KE, Xu X, Carr TP, Phipps WR, Kurzer MS (2000) Soy isoflavones improve plasma lipids in normocholesterolemic, premenopausal women. Am J Clin Nutr 71:1462–1469

Nagata C (2000) Ecological study of the association betweeen soy intake and mortality from cancer and heart disease in Japan. Int J Epidemiol 29:832–836

Nagata C, Takatsuka N, Shimizu H (2002) Soy and fish oil intake and mortality in a Japanese community. Am J Epidemiol 156:824–831

Nagata M, Sedgwick JB, Busse WW (1997) Synergistic activation of eosinophil superoxide anion generation by VCAM-1 and GM-CSF. Involvement of tyrosine kinase and protein kinase C. Int Arch Allergy Immunol 114 Suppl 1:78–80

Nestel P (2002) Role of soy protein in cholesterol-lowering—How good is it? Arterioscler Thromb Vasc Biol 22:1743–1744

Nestel P (2003) Isoflavones: their effects on cardiovascular risk and functions. Curr Opin Lipidol 14:3–8

Nestel PJ, Pomeroy S, Kay S, Komesaroff P, Behrsing J, Cameron JD, West L (1999) Isoflavones from red clover improve systemic arterial compliance but not plasma lipids in menopausal women. J Clin Endocrinol Metab 84:895–898

Nestel PJ, Yamashita T, Sasahara T, Pomeroy S, Dart A, Komesaroff P, Owen A, Abbey M (1997) Soy isoflavones improve systemic arterial compliance but not plasma lipids in menopausal and perimenopausal women. Arterioscler Thromb Vasc Biol 17:3392–3398

Nilausen K, Meinertz H (1999) Lipoprotein(a) and dietary proteins: Casein lowers lipoprotein(a) concentrations as compared with soy protein. Am J Clin Nutr 69:419–425

Peluso MR, Winters TA, Shanahan MF, Banz WJ. (2000) A cooperative interaction between soy protein and its isoflavone-enriched fraction lowers hepatic lipids in male obese Zucker rats and reduces blood platelet sensitivity in male Sprague-Dawley rats. J Nutr 130:2333–2342

Potter SM (1995) Overview of proposed mechanisms for the hypocholesterolemic effect of soy. J Nutr 125:606S–611S

Potter SM (1998) Soy protein and cardiovascular disease: the impact of bioactive components in soy. Nutr Rev 56:231–235

Regal JF, Fraser DG, Weeks CE, Greenberg NA (2000). Dietary phytoestrogens have anti-inflammatory activity in a guinea pig model of asthma. Proc Soc Exp Biol Med 223: 372–378

Robertson TL, Kato H, Rhoads A, Kagan M, Marmot M, Syme SL, GordonT, Worth RM, Belsky JL, Dock DS, Miyanishi M, Kawamoto S (1977) Epidemiologic studies of coronary heart disease and stroke in Japanese men living in Japan, Hawaii and California: Incidence of myocardial infarction and death from coronary heart disease. Am J Cardiol 39:239–243

Ruiz-Larrea MB, Mohan AR, Paganga G, Miller NJ, Bolwell GP, Rice-Evans CA (1997) Antioxidant activity of phytoestrogenic isoflavones. Free Radic Res 26:63–70

Sadowska-Krowicka H, Mannick EE, Oliver PD, Sandoval M, Zhang XJ, Eloby-Childess S, Clark DA, Miller MJ (1998) Genistein and gut inflammation: role of nitric oxide. Proc Soc Exp Biol Med 217:351–357

Sasazuki S, Fukuoka Heart Study Group (2001) Case-control study of nonfatal myocardial infarction in relation to selected foods in Japanese men and women. Jpn Circ J 65:200–206

Schachinger V, Britten MB, Zeiher AM (2000) Prognostic impact of coronary vasodilator dysfunction on adverse long-term outcome of coronary heart disease. Circulation 101:1899–1906

Schwenke DC (1998) Antioxidants and atherogenesis. J Nutr Biochem 9:424–445

Simons LA, von Konigsmark M, Simons J, Celermajer DS (2000) Phytoestrogens do not influence lipoprotein levels or endothelial function in healthy, postmenopausal women*1. Am J Cardiol 85:1297–1301

Sirtori CR, Even R, Lovati MR (1993) Soybean protein diet and plasma cholesterol: from therapy to molecular mechanisms. Ann NY Acad Sci 676:188–201

Song T, Lee SO, Murphy PA, Hendrich S (2003) Soy protein with or without isoflavones, soy germ and soy germ extract, and daidzein lessen plasma cholesterol levels in golden Syrian hamsters. Exp Biol Med (Maywood) 228:1063–1068

Squadrito F, Altavilla D, Morabito N, Crisafulli A, D'Anna R, Corrado F, Ruggeri P, Campo GM, Calapai G, Caputi AP, Squadrito G (2002) The effect of the phytoestrogen genistein on plasma nitric oxide concentrations, endothelin-1 levels and endothelium dependent vasodilation in postmenopausal women. Atherosclerosis 163:339–347

Squadrito F, Altavilla D, Crisafulli A, Saitta A, Cucinotta D, Morabito N, D'Anna R, Corrado F, Ruggeri P, Frisina N, Squadrito G (2003) Effect of genistein on endothelial function in postmenopausal women: a randomized, double-blind, controlled study. Am J Med 114:470–476

Steinberg FM, Guthrie NL, Villablanca AC, Kumar K, Murray MJ (2003) Soy protein with isoflavones has favorable effects on endothelial function that are independent of lipid and antioxidant effects in healthy postmenopausal women. Am J Clin Nutr 78:123–130

Suwaidi JA, Hamasaki S, Higano ST, Nishimura RA, Holmes DR Jr, Lerman A (2000) Long-term follow-up of patients with mild coronary artery disease and endothelial dysfunction. Circulation 101:948–954

Tanabe J, Watanabe M, Kondoh S, Mue S, Ohuchi K (1994) Possible roles of protein kinases in neutrophil chemotactic factor production by leucocytes in allergic inflammation in rats. Br J Pharmacol 113:1480–1486

Teede HJ, Dalais FS, Kotsopoulos D, Liang YL, Davis S, McGrath BP (2001) Dietary soy has both beneficial and potentially adverse cardiovascular effects: a placebo-controlled study in men and postmenopausal women. J Clin Endocrinol Metab 86:3053–3060

Teede HJ, McGrath BP, DeSilva L, Cehun M, Fassoulakis A, Nestel PJ (2003) Isoflavones reduce arterial stiffness—A placebo-controlled study in men and postmenopausal women. Arterioscler Thromb Vasc Biol 23:1066–1071

Teixeira SR, Potter SM, Weigel R, Hannum S, Erdman JW Jr, Hasler CM (2000) Effects of feeding 4 levels of soy protein for 3 and 6 wk on blood lipids and apolipoproteins in moderately hypercholesterolemic men. Am J Clin Nutr 71:1077–1084

Tikkanen MJ, Vihma V, Höckerstedt A, Jauhiainen M, Helisten H, Kaamanen M (2002) Lipophilic oestrogen derivatives contained in lipoprotein particles. Acta Physiol Scand 176:117–121

Tikkanen MJ, Wahala K, Ojala S, Vihma V, Adlercreutz H (1998). Effect of soybean phytoestrogen intake on low density lipoprotein oxidation resistance. Proc Natl Acad Sci USA 95:3106–3110

US Department of Health and Human Services, Food and Drug Administration (1999) Food labeling: health claims: soy protein and coronary heart disease. Fed Regist 64:21CFR part 101, 57700–57733

Van der Schouw YT, Pijpe A, Lebrun CE, Bots ML, Peeters PH, Van Staveren WA, Lamberts SW, Grobbee DE (2002). Higher usual dietary intake of phytoestrogens is associated with lower aortic stiffness in postmenopausal women. Arterioscler Thromb Vasc Biol 22:1316–1322

Verdrengh M, Jonsson IM, Holmdahl R, Tarkowski A (2003) Genistein as an anti-inflammatory agent. Inflamm Res 52:341–346

Wagner JD, Clarkson TB, StClair RW, Schwenke DC, Shively CA, Adams MR (1991) Estrogen and progesterone replacement therapy reduces LDL accumulation in the coronary arteries of surgically postmenopausal cynomolgus monkeys. J Clin Invest 88:1995–2002

Wagner JD, Schwenke DC, Greaves KA, Zhang L, Anthony MS, Blair RM, Shadoan MK, Williams JK (2003) Soy protein with isoflavones, but not an isoflavone-rich supplement, improves arterial low-density lipoprotein metabolism and atherogenesis. Arterioscler Thromb Vasc Biol 23:2241–2246

Walker HA, Dean TS, Sanders TA, Jackson G, Ritter JM, Chowienczyk PJ (2001) The phytoestrogen genistein produces acute nitric oxide-dependent dilation of human forearm vasculature with similar potency to 17ss-estradiol. Circulation 103:258–262

Wangen KE, Duncan AM, Xu X, Kurzer MS (2001) Soy isoflavones improve plasma lipids in normocholesterolemic and mildly hypercholesterolemic postmenopausal women. Am J Clin Nutr 73:225–231

Washburn S, Burke GL, Morgan T, Anthony M (1999) Effect of soy protein supplementation on serum lipoproteins, blood pressure, and menopausal symptoms in perimenopausal women. Menopause 6:7–13

Weber C (1996) Involvement of tyrosine phosphorylation in endothelial adhesion molecule induction. Immunol Res 15:30–37

Wilcox JN, Blumenthal BF (1995) Thrombotic mechanisms in atherosclerosis: Potential impact of soy proteins. J Nutr 125:S631–S638

Williams JK, Anthony MS, Herrington DM (2001). Interactive effects of soy protein and estradiol on coronary artery reactivity in atherosclerotic, ovariectomized monkeys. Menopause. 8:307–313

Williams JK, Clarkson TB (1998) Dietary soy isoflavones inhibit in-vivo constrictor responses of coronary arteries to collagen-induced platelet activation. Coron Artery Dis 9:759–764

Wiseman H, OReilly JD, Adlercreutz H, Mallet AI, Bowey EA, Rowland IR, Sanders TAB (2000) Isoflavone phytoestrogens consumed in soy decrease F-2-isoprostane concentrations and increase resistance of low-density lipoprotein to oxidation in humans. Am J Clin Nutr 72:395–400

Witztum JL, Steinberg D (2001) The oxidative modification hypothesis of atherosclerosis: does it hold for humans? Trends Cardiovasc Med 11:93–102

Wolle J, Hill RR, Ferguson E, Devall LJ, Trivedi BK, Newton RS, Saxena U (1996) Selective inhibition of tumor necrosis factor-induced vascular cell adhesion molecule-1 gene expression by a novel flavonoid. Lack of effect on transcription factor NF-kappa B. Arterioscler Thromb Vasc Biol 16:1501–1508

Yamakoshi J, Piskula MK, Izumi T, Tobe K, Saito M, Kataoka S, Obata A, Kikuchi M (2000) Isoflavone aglycone-rich extract without soy protein attenuates atherosclerosis development in cholesterol-fed rabbits. J Nutr 130:1887–1893

Yeung J, Yu TF (2003) Effects of isoflavones (soy phyto-estrogens) on serum lipids: a meta-analysis of randomized controlled trials. Nutr J 2:15

Yildirir A, Tokgozoglu SL, Oduncu T, Oto A, Haznedaroglu I, Akinci D, Koksal G, Sade E, Kirazli S, Kes S (2001) Soy protein diet significantly improves endothelial function and lipid parameters. Clin Cardiol 24:711–716

Zhang X, Shu XO, Gao YT, Yang G, Li Q, Li H, Jin F, Zheng W (2003) Soy food consumption is associated with lower risk of coronary heart disease in Chinese women. J Nutr 133:2874–2878

HEP (2005) 170:325–338

Homocysteine and B Vitamins

S. Cook · O.M. Hess (✉)

Swiss Cardiovascular Center, University Hospital, 3010 Bern, Switzerland
otto.hess@insel.ch

Abstract Homocysteine (tHcy) is an intermediate sulfur-containing amino acid which acts as a methyl group donor for methionine metabolism. Increased serum concentrations (=hyperhomocysteinemia, >10 µmol/l) have been associated with an increased cardiovascular risk. Homocystinuria, an infrequent genetic disease usually due to lack of cystathione beta-synthase, has been found with severely elevated serum homocysteine values (>150 µmol/l). Functional gene polymorphisms of key enzymes (e.g., N5,N10-methylene-tetrahydrofolate reductase) and dietary B-vitamin deficiencies in the elderly are, however, frequent in the 'Western' population. Hyperhomocysteinemia has been associated with other vascular effects such as atherothrombosis and endothelial dysfunction due to its auto-oxidative potential, thereby increasing the production of reactive oxygen species. Other effects may involve neurodegenerative diseases such as Alzheimer or dementia praecox of the elderly. Therapeutic interventions lowering tHcy may therefore offer novel tools for the prevention and treatment of atherosclerosis. B-vitamin supplementation (folic acid=vitamin B_9, vitamin B_6 and vitamin B_{12}) is an efficient and safe tHcy-lowering therapy, decreases tHcy by 30%–50% and has been shown to lower cardiovascular morbidity and mortality. Furthermore, folic acid supplementation has been shown to reduce or even almost eliminate neurotubular birth defects (spina bifida) and to markedly decrease the rate of megaloblastic anemia. Thus, fortification of flour with folic acid in the USA was advocated several years ago in order to prevent these entities.

Keywords Homocysteine · Homocystinuria · Hyperhomocysteinemia · Vitamin B · Folic acid

1
Introduction

Homocysteine (tHcy) has been identified as a risk factor for atherosclerosis only recently. It is an intermediate sulfur-containing amino acid produced from methionine during processing of dietary protein. It has gained considerable attention because elevated serum concentrations, even small, have been associated with an increased cardiovascular (CV) risk, including coronary artery, cerebrovascular, and peripheral vascular disease. Far from being a traditional CV risk factor, increased tHcy has also been associated with other entities such as thrombotic disease (den Heijer et al. 1996), congenital neural tube defects, (Kapusta et al. 1999, Rosenquist, 1996; Wenstrom et al. 2000) and Parkinson and Alzheimer diseases (Duan et al. 2002; Kruman et al. 2000, Seshadri et al. 2002).

The purpose of this chapter is to explore the current understanding of tHcy biology and to highlight its potential role in atherosclerosis, coronary artery and ischemic cerebrovascular disease. Furthermore, we will present evidence that decreasing plasma tHcy by B vitamins is both an effective treatment for major CV events and improves outcome.

2
Biology of tHcy

The methionine–tHcy–cysteine pathway is summarized in Fig. 1. Homocysteine accumulation (hyperhomocysteinemia) depends on a potential block in the metabolizing pathways. Three key vitamins (folate=vitamin B_9, pyridoxine=vitamin B_6, cobalamine=vitamin B_{12}) function as cofactors or substrates for methionine–homocysteine metabolism. Accordingly, a number of studies have demonstrated an inverse relationship between homocysteine concentration and B vitamins. Three key enzymes have been characterized in human pathology, namely cystathione beta-synthase, N_5,N_{10}-methylene-tetrahydrofolate reductase (MTHFR) and methionine synthase. Hyperhomocysteinemia can be due to a primary and/or secondary cause. Primary causes classically refer to enzymatic deficiency leading to homocystinuria, a dramatic but infrequent disorder usually due to a complete deficiency in cystathione beta-synthase . More frequent are gene polymorphisms or mutations of key enzyme. Secondary causes are frequent and often coexist with functional gene polymorphisms. Examples are smoking, heavy intake of coffee or alcohol, renal failure, vitamin deficiencies (or drugs impairing B vitamin metabolism, e.g., gemfibrozil) (Syvanne et al. 2004) malignant disease or hypothyroidism.

In plasma the major fraction of tHcy is oxidized and occurs as homocystine (5%–10%), homocysteine–cysteine mixed disulfide (5%–10%) and protein-bound homocysteine (70%–90%).

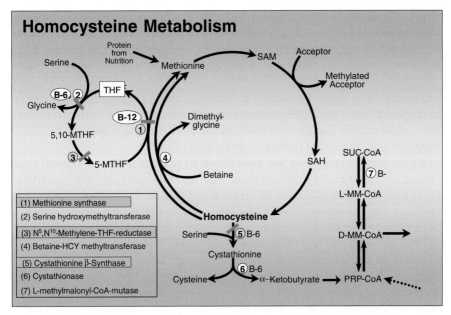

Fig. 1 Production of homocysteine from methionine, an essential amino acid. Homocysteine can be reconverted to methionine through the remethylation pathway. When methionine is in excess, Hcy is directed to the *trans*-sulfuration pathway that irreversibly converts Hcy to cysteine. The first step in this metabolic pathway is catalyzed by the vitamin B_6-dependent enzyme cystathionine s-synthase (*CBS*). Under methionine deprivation, Hcy is disposed via two methionine conserving pathways. In the liver, Hcy is remethylated by betaine–homocysteine methyltransferase (*BHMT*), whereas in other tissues the remethylation of Hcy is catalyzed by methionine synthase (*MS*), which uses vitamin B_{12} as cofactor and methyltetrahydrofolate as substrate

3
Homocysteine: A CV Risk Factor?

Moderate elevations of plasma tHcy were first identified as a risk factor for coronary artery disease (CAD) by McCully (1969) and later by Wilcken and Wilcken (1976). Compelling evidence has since then supported this theory. The majority of studies, but not all (Alfthan et al. 1994; Massy et al. 1994, Sharabi et al. 1999 Verhoef et al. 1996, 1997) have shown an association between tHcy concentration and classical risk factors (Nygard et al. 1995), angiographically documented CAD (Arnesen et al. 1995; Genest et al. 1990; Graham et al. 1997; Kang et al. 1986; Verhoef et al. 1997; Wilcken and Wilcken 1976), myocardial infarction (Israelsson et al. 1988; Stampfer et al. 1992; Verhoef et al. 1996) as well as CV mortality (Anderson et al. 2000; Nygard et al. 1997; Wald et al. 1998). The meta-analysis by Boushey et al. (1995) as well as the interventional study by Malinow et al. (1998) strongly suggested that tHcy is an independent risk factor for atherosclerosis and that between 15% and 50% of patients with symptomatic vascular disease have hyperhomocysteinemia. Increments of 5 µmol/l of tHcy have been estimated to correspond to an increase in CAD risk of approximately 60% in men and 80% in women (Boushey et al. 1995). As with serum cholesterol, the risk seems to be skewed, i.e., the risk rises with increasing tHcy level (Arnesen et al. 1995). Accordingly, in patients included in the *Swiss Heart Study*, tHcy levels (ranging from 9.1±3.2 µmol/l in controls to 12.4±5.4 µmol/l in patients with three-vessel disease) and the extent of CAD were strongly correlated (Schnyder et al. 2001) (Fig. 2).

Hyperhomocysteinemia has been found in siblings prone to familial CAD (Wu et al. 1994) raising the question whether special genotypes could trigger hyperhomocysteinemia in the general population. Stimulated by the study by Kang and colleagues (1988) who provided evidence consistent with this hypothesis, many subsequent investigators have looked for an association between functional gene polymorphisms, tHcy and CV diseases (Boers et al. 1985; Clarke et al. 1991; Gardemann et al. 1999; Kruger et al. 2000; Lalouschek et al. 1998; Streifler et al. 2001; Verhoef et al. 1997; Wu et al. 1994). For instance, the thermolabile variant of the MTHFR is due to a common mutation in the MTHFR gene (C677T), which can be observed up to 40% in Caucasians. Subjects with mutation of both alleles (TT-genotype) have a higher tHcy level than those who are heterozygous (Kang et al. 1988). Graham et al. (1997) estimated that 14% of

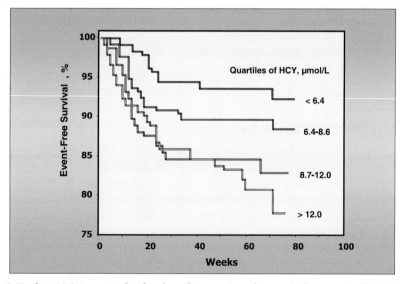

Fig. 2 Kaplan–Meier curves for freedom from major adverse cardiac events (MACE) according to homocysteine quartiles. As demonstrated by Schnyder et al., there is a strong dose–response relationship between homocysteine quartiles and the incidence of MACE. Hcy indicates plasma homocysteine levels, quartiles of tHcy are expressed in µmol/l. (Reproduced from Schnyder, et al. 2001, with permission)

patients with CAD have familial hyperhomocysteinemia. Parenthetically, but consistent with the theory of a key role of tHcy in atherosclerosis, the remarkable freedom from arteriosclerosis found in Down syndrome (Brattstrom et al. 1987; Murdoch et al. 1977) is attributed to increased activity of cystathionine synthase activity and therefore decreased tHcy levels (Kraus et al. 1986).

4
Mechanism of Action

Figure 3 summarizes the current understanding of the atherogenic effect of tHcy. At low plasma concentrations homocysteine is rapidly scavenged by nitric oxide (NO) (produced by endothelial NO synthase) resulting in *S*-nitroso-

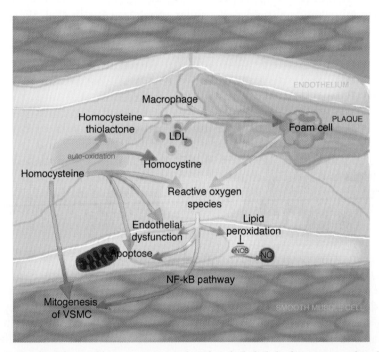

Fig. 3 Pathophysiology of homocysteine-induced endothelial dysfunction. In the plasma, homocysteine is rapidly auto-oxidized and forms homocysteine–thiolactone, homocystine, and mixed disulfides. Directly or by homocysteine–thiolactone-mediated mechanisms, homocysteine increase reactive oxygen species by oxidation of low-density lipoproteins (*LDL*) and formation of foam cells. These latter have been involved in a cluster of atherothrombogenic events such as vasoconstriction (and arterial hypertension), lipid peroxidation, proliferation of vascular smooth muscle cells and prothrombotic states. Moreover, homocysteine has other deleterious effects, such as stimulation of endothelial apoptosis and vascular smooth muscle cell proliferation (*VSMC*). *NO*, Nitric oxide; *eNOS*, endothelial NO synthase; *NF-κB*, nuclear factor kappa-B

homocysteine. This nitroso-compound has NO functionality, such as potent vasodilatation, regulation of glucose metabolism and oxidative modification of low-density lipoproteins, inhibition of proliferation of vascular smooth muscle cells, platelet aggregation and leukocyte adherence (Cook et al. 2002; Stamler et al. 1992). At higher plasma concentrations, hyperhomocysteinemia is responsible for endothelial dysfunction, platelet activation and thrombus formation in vivo (Celermajer et al. 1993; Harker et al. 1974; Van den Berg et al. 1995; Welch et al. 1998). When added to plasma, homocysteine is rapidly auto-oxidized and forms homocysteine–thiolactone, homocystine, mixed disulfides and, directly or indirectly, reactive oxygen species (Alvarez-Maqueda et al. 2004). The latter have been involved in a cluster of atherothrombogenic effects such as vasoconstriction, oxidation of low-density lipoproteins, lipid peroxidation, proliferation of vascular smooth muscle cells and prothrombotic states. Interestingly homocysteine appears also to alter mitochondrial function and to cause mitochondrial-mediated cellular apoptosis (Austin et al. 1998; Cook et al. 2002; Mercie et al. 2000; Olszewski et al. 1993).

5
Homocysteine and Stroke

Boers et al. (1985) found that one-third of patients with cerebrovascular and peripheral atherosclerosis had high tHcy levels after methionine exposure. Selhub and coworkers (1995) concluded that high plasma homocysteine concentrations and low concentrations of folate and vitamin B_6, through their role in homocysteine metabolism, are associated with an increased risk of extracranial carotid artery disease in the elderly. Perry et al. (1995) prospectively studied 5,661 patients to determine the relationship between tHcy and stroke risk. They found a direct correlation between the two.

Bots and coworkers (1999) compared 224 elderly patients with myocardial infarction or cerebrovascular stroke with 533 controls (Rotterdam Study) and found a direct relationship between the increase in tHcy and the risk of stroke. In order to demonstrate a causal relationship between increased tHcy and cerebral endothelial function, Lee et al. (2004) demonstrated that hyperhomocysteinemia induces endothelial dysfunction in brain arteries and that dietary folic acid supplementation lowers tHcy and restores endothelial function.

Major studies (Ay et al. 2003; Boers et al. 1985; Boysen et al. 2003; Brattstrom et al. 1984; Howard et al. 2002; Kittner et al. 1999; Meiklejohn et al. 2001; Perry et al. 1995; Petri et al. 1996; Sato et al. 2002; Selhub et al. 1995; Sen et al. 2002; Streifler et al.. 2001 Tanne et al. 2003; Verhoef et al. 1994; Vermeer et al. 2003) support a strong, dose-dependent association between plasma homocysteine, stroke (transient ischemic attack, recurrent stroke, silent brain infarcts) and classical risk factors for stroke, such as carotid stenosis, aortic atheroma or cardiac LV-thrombus.

6
Treatment of Hyperhomocysteinemia: The Role of B Vitamins

A growing body of evidence indicates tHcy as a major risk factor for CV morbidity and mortality (Alfthan et al. 1997; Anderson et al. 2000; Bostom et al. 1999; Moustapha et al. 1998; Retterstol et al. 2003; Wald et al. 1998) in Western countries. Functional gene polymorphisms have been associated with CAD, ischemic stroke and overall CV mortality. Some authors have suggested that polymorphisms could be responsible for 15%–20% of all patients with atherosclerotic disease. Thus, increased tHcy level accounts for a large proportion of CV events. Of particular interest is the prevalence of B-vitamin deficiencies, substrate or cofactors of the methionine–homocysteine–cysteine pathway. Although the recommended folate intake is approximately 300–400 µg/day in the young and 600–700 µg/day in the elderly, the mean folate intake is less than 300 µg/day in Europe (de Bree et al. 1997; Rydlewicz et al. 2002). In vivo and in vitro studies have shown in humans and experimental animals that high tHcy levels may cause–directly or indirectly–cellular and subcellular modifications responsible for the development of atherothrombosis. These findings open up the exciting possibility that tHcy-lowering therapies may represent novel tools for the prevention and treatment of atherosclerosis.

B-vitamin supplementation is an efficient and safe way to reduce an elevated tHcy levels. Brattstrom et al. (1988) showed that healthy subjects responded to high doses of folic acid (5 mg/day) with a marked reduction in tHcy levels. Since then, several studies have demonstrated that 0.20–10 mg/day of folic acid alone or together with vitamin B_{12} and/or B6 reduce the fasting and post-methionine loading tHcy levels by 25%–50%, in both healthy and 'vascular' patients. Vermeulen et al. (2000) studied healthy siblings of patients with premature atherothrombotic disease treated with folic acid (5 mg/day) plus vitamin B_6 (250 mg/day, vs. placebo). They showed a reduction in abnormal exercise stress tests in the B vitamin-treated group which was probably due to an improvement in endothelial function. Chambers and coworkers (2000) showed that tHcy was lowered and flow-mediated dilatation improved after 8 weeks treatment with folic acid (5 mg) and vitamin B_{12} (1 mg) daily in CAD patients. Title et al. (2000) demonstrated that folic acid alone (5 mg/day) reduced plasma tHcy and significantly improved brachial artery endothelium-dependent flow-mediated dilation.

Schnyder et al. (2002, 2003) conducted a prospective, double-blind, randomized trial, enrolling 205 consecutive patients who had undergone successful angioplasty. They found that 6 months of treatment with a combination of folic acid (1 mg), vitamin B_{12} (400 µg), and pyridoxine (10 mg) lowered plasma tHcy levels from 11.1±4.3 to 7.2±2.4 µM ($P<0.001$) and reduced the rate of restenosis (19.6% in treatment group vs. 37.6% in controls, $P=0.01$), as well as the need for target lesion revascularization (10.8% in treatment group vs. 22.3% in controls, $P<0.05$). Moreover, the homocysteine-lowering therapy decreased the incidence of major adverse cardiac events after a mean follow-up of 11 months (Fig. 4).

Folic acid fortification of food in the USA was shown to be sufficient to decrease spina bifida in newborns. Recently, Anderson et al. (2004) demonstrated that tHcy only marginally declined under substitution, which was associated with a minimal but significant reduction in mortality. Five milligrams of folic acid alone was also sufficient to decrease hyperhomocysteinemia and improve flow-mediated dilation of the brachial artery in patients with unstable angina (Guo et al. 2004). This apparent contradiction could be due to B-vitamin formulation. These data underline the importance of both dose and combination of B vitamins. A lowering of 16%–39% is expected by 0.2–5 mg of folic acid daily (Anonymous 1998). In order to avoid the so-called folate trap, in which vitamin B_{12} deficiency lead to a functional folate deficiency by trapping an increased proportion of folate as the 5-methyl derivative, combination with B_{12} vitamin supplementation is strongly recommended (Shane et al. 1985). Accordingly, in elderly patients with a 'normal' serum folate and low B_{12} vitamin (<350 pg/ml), B_{12} vitamin supplementation alone decreased tHcy and increased red blood cell folate (Flynn et al. 2003).

Alternatives to B vitamins include N-acetylcysteine, betain, tamoxifen, estrogen replacement therapy, and aminophil drugs. Scholze and coworkers

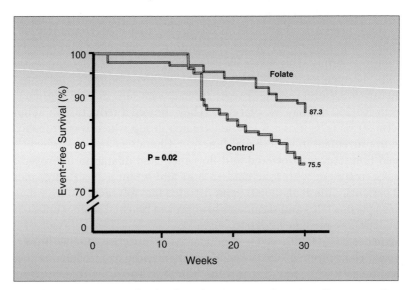

Fig. 4 Kaplan–Meier curves for freedom from major adverse cardiac events (MACE) after multivitamin therapy. Lowering plasma homocysteine levels (from 11.1±4.3 to 7.2±2.4 µmol/l) with B vitamins in patients following PCI decrease MACE. (Reproduced from Schnyder et al. 2001, with permission)

(2004) investigated effects of intravenous administration of acetylcysteine in 20 patients with end-stage renal failure and demonstrated a reduction of plasma tHcy, which was significantly correlated with a reduction in pulse pressure.

7
Conclusions

The question is how to address the relevance of these data to 'real-life' cardiology. Shall we treat all vascular patients with B vitamins or is the expected effect too small to be of significance? As the B-vitamin supplementation used in the *Swiss Heart Study* was shown to be safe, as well as cheap, and could have additional protective effects on other organs, we believe that it should be administered to all patients with vascular disease and increased tHcy plasma levels (>10 µmol/l). Similar recommendations have been made by the 'DACH-organization' against hyperhomocysteinemia (Anonymous 2003). In medical society, the debate of whether increased tHcy levels play a pivotal role—as does cholesterol—in the pathogenesis of atherosclerosis is ongoing (Cook et al. 2004). Future studies will show whether the beneficial effect of B vitamins, as outlined in this chapter, will be considered as important enough to be followed and to become a cornerstone in prevention and treatment of atherosclerosis.

References

Alfthan G, Pekkanen J, Jauhiainen M, Pitkaniemi J, Karvonen M, Tuomilehto J, Salonen JT, Ehnholm C (1994) Relation of serum homocysteine and lipoprotein(a) concentrations to atherosclerotic disease in a prospective Finnish population based study. Atherosclerosis 106:9–19

Alfthan G, Aro A, Gey KF (1997) Plasma homocysteine and cardiovascular disease mortality. Lancet 349:397

Alvarez-Maqueda M, El Bekay R, Monteseirin J, Alba G, Chacon P, Vega A, Santa Maria C, Tejedo JR, Martin-Nieto J, Bedoya FJ (2004) Homocysteine enhances superoxide anion release and NADPH oxidase assembly by human neutrophils. Effects on MAPK activation and neutrophil migration. Atherosclerosis 172:229–238

Anderson JL, Muhlestein JB, Horne BD, Carlquist JF, Bair TL, Madsen TE, Pearson RR (2000) Plasma homocysteine predicts mortality independently of traditional risk factors and C-reactive protein in patients with angiographically defined coronary artery disease. Circulation 102:1227–1232

Anderson JL, Jensen KR, Carlquist JF, Bair TL, Horne BD, Muhlestein JB (2004) Effect of folic acid fortification of food on homocysteine-related mortality. Am J Med 116:158–164

Anonymous (1998) Lowering blood homocysteine with folic acid based supplements: meta-analysis of randomised trials. Homocysteine Lowering Trialists' Collaboration. BMJ 316:894–898

Anonymous (2003) Konsensuspapier der D.A.C.H.-Liga Homocystein über den rationalen klinischen Umgang mit Homocystein, Folsäure und B-Vitaminen bei kardiovaskulären und thrombotischen Erkrankungen – Richtlinien und Empfehlungen. J Kardiol 10:190–199

Arnesen E, Refsum H, Bonaa KH, Ueland PM, Forde OH, Nordrehaug JE (1995) Serum total homocysteine and coronary heart disease. Int J Epidemiol 24:704–709

Austin RC, Sood SK, Dorward AM, Singh G, Shaughnessy SG, Pamidi S, Outinen PA, Weitz JI (1998) Homocysteine-dependent alterations in mitochondrial gene expression, function and structure. Homocysteine and H2O2 act synergistically to enhance mitochondrial damage. J Biol Chem 273:30808–30817

Ay H, Arsava EM, Tokgozoglu SL, Ozer N, Saribas O (2003) Hyperhomocysteinemia is associated with the presence of left atrial thrombus in stroke patients with nonvalvular atrial fibrillation. Stroke 34:909–912

Boers GH, Fowler B, Smals AG, Trijbels FJ, Leermakers AI, Kleijer WJ, Kloppenborg PW (1985) Improved identification of heterozygotes for homocystinuria due to cystathionine synthase deficiency by the combination of methionine loading and enzyme determination in cultured fibroblasts. Hum Genet 69:164–169

Bostom AG, Silbershatz H, Rosenberg IH, Selhub J, D'Agostino RB, Wolf PA, Jacques PF, Wilson PW (1999) Nonfasting plasma total homocysteine levels and all-cause and cardiovascular disease mortality in elderly Framingham men and women. Arch Intern Med 159:1077–1080

Bots ML, Launer LJ, Lindemans J, Hoes AW, Hofman A, Witteman JC, Koudstaal PJ, Grobbee DE (1999) Homocysteine and short-term risk of myocardial infarction and stroke in the elderly: the Rotterdam Study. Arch Intern Med 159:38–44

Boushey CJ, Beresford SA, Omenn GS, Motulsky AG (1995) A quantitative assessment of plasma homocysteine as a risk factor for vascular disease. Probable benefits of increasing folic acid intakes. JAMA 274:1049–1057

Boysen G, Brander T, Christensen H, Gideon R, Truelsen T (2003) Homocysteine and risk of recurrent stroke. Stroke 34:1258–1261

Brattstrom LE, Hardebo JE, Hultberg BL (1984) Moderate homocysteinemia–a possible risk factor for arteriosclerotic cerebrovascular disease. Stroke15:1012–1016

Brattstrom LE, Israelsson B, Jeppsson JO, Hultberg BL (1988) Folic acid–an innocuous means to reduce plasma homocysteine. Scand J Clin Lab Invest 48:215–221

Brattstrom L, Englund E, Brun A (1987) Does Down syndrome support homocysteine theory of arteriosclerosis? Lancet 1:391–392

Celermajer DS, Sorensen K, Ryalls M, Robinson J, Thomas O, Leonard JV, Deanfield JE (1993) Impaired endothelial function occurs in the systemic arteries of children with homozygous homocystinuria but not in their heterozygous parents. J Am Coll Cardiol 22:854–858

Chambers JC, Ueland PM, Obeid OA, Wrigley J, Refsum H, Kooner JS (2000) Improved vascular endothelial function after oral B vitamins: An effect mediated through reduced concentrations of free plasma homocysteine. Circulation 102:2479–2483

Clarke R, Daly L, Robinson K, Naughten E, Cahalane S, Fowler B, Graham I (1991) Hyperhomocysteinemia: an independent risk factor for vascular disease. N Engl J Med 324:1149–1155

Cook S, Scherrer U (2002) Insulin resistance, a new target for nitric oxide-delivery drugs. Fundam Clin Pharmacol 16:441–453

Cook S, Schnyder G, Hess OM (2004) Plasma Homocysteine and Cardiovascular Events: Hype, Myth or Truth? Eur Heart J 25:

de Bree A, van Dusseldorp M, Brouwer IA, van het Hof KH, Steegers-Theunissen RP (1997) Folate intake in Europe: recommended, actual and desired intake. Eur J Clin Nutr 51:643–660

den Heijer M, Koster T, Blom HJ, Bos GM, Briet E, Reitsma PH, Vandenbroucke JP, Rosendaal FR (1996) Hyperhomocysteinemia as a risk factor for deep-vein thrombosis. N Engl J Med 334:759–762

Duan W, Ladenheim B, Cutler RG, Kruman, II, Cadet JL, Mattson MP (2002) Dietary folate deficiency and elevated homocysteine levels endanger dopaminergic neurons in models of Parkinson's disease. J Neurochem 80:101–110

Flynn MA, Singh A, Slaughter J, King P, Krause G, Herbert V, Thomas W (2003) Interrelationship of homocysteine-cobalamin-folate indices in human subjects of various ages: can hyper-homocyteinemia be relieved with B-12 supplementation? Mol Med 100:155–158

Gardemann A, Weidemann H, Philipp M, Katz N, Tillmanns H, Hehrlein FW, Haberbosch W (1999) The TT genotype of the methylenetetrahydrofolate reductase C677T gene polymorphism is associated with the extent of coronary atherosclerosis in patients at high risk for coronary artery disease. Eur Heart J 20:584–592

Genest JJ, Jr., McNamara JR, Salem DN, Wilson PW, Schaefer EJ, Malinow MR (1990) Plasma homocyst(e)ine levels in men with premature coronary artery disease. J Am Coll Cardiol 16:1114–1119

Graham IM, Daly LE, Refsum HM, Robinson K, Brattstrom LE, Ueland PM, Palma-Reis RJ, Boers GH, Sheahan RG, Israelsson B, Uiterwaal CS, Meleady R, McMaster D, Verhoef P, Witteman J, Rubba P, Bellet H, Wautrecht JC, de Valk HW, Sales Luis AC, Parrot-Rouland FM, Tan KS, Higgins I, Garcon D, Andria G, et al. (1997) Plasma homocysteine as a risk factor for vascular disease. The European Concerted Action Project. JAMA 277:1775–1781

Guo H, Xing Y, Lee JD, Wang J, Hiroyasu U, Ueda T (2004) Changes of plasma homocysteine levels and arterial endothelial function in patients with unstable angina and interventional therapy of folic acid. Swiss Med Wkly. 134

Harker LA, Slichter SJ, Scott CR, Ross R (1974) Homocystinemia. Vascular injury and arterial thrombosis. N Engl J Med 291:537–543

Howard VJ, Sides EG, Newman GC, Cohen SN, Howard G, Malinow MR, Toole JF (2002) Changes in plasma homocyst(e)ine in the acute phase after stroke. Stroke 33:473–478

Homocysteine Lowering Trialists' Collaboration (1998) Lowering blood homocysteine with folic acid based supplements: meta-analysis of randomised trials. BMJ 316:894–898

Israelsson B, Brattstrom LE, Hultberg BL (1988) Homocysteine and myocardial infarction. Atherosclerosis 71:227–233

Kang SS, Wong PW, Cook HY, Norusis M, Messer JV (1986) Protein-bound homocyst(e)ine. A possible risk factor for coronary artery disease. J Clin Invest 77:1482–1486

Kang SS, Zhou J, Wong PW, Kowalisyn J, Strokosch G (1988) Intermediate homocysteinemia: a thermolabile variant of methylenetetrahydrofolate reductase. Am J Hum Genet 43:414–421

Kapusta L, Haagmans ML, Steegers EA, Cuypers MH, Blom HJ, Eskes TK (1999) Congenital heart defects and maternal derangement of homocysteine metabolism. J Pediatr 135:773–774

Kittner SJ, Giles WH, Macko RF, Hebel JR, Wozniak MA, Wityk RJ, Stolley PD, Stern BJ, Sloan MA, Sherwin R, Price TR, McCarter RJ, Johnson CJ, Earley CJ, Buchholz DW, Malinow MR (1999) Homocyst(e)ine and risk of cerebral infarction in a biracial population : the stroke prevention in young women study. Stroke 30:1554–1560

Kraus JP, Williamson CL, Firgaira FA, Yang-Feng TL, Munke M, Francke U, Rosenberg LE (1986) Cloning and screening with nanogram amounts of immunopurified mRNAs: cDNA cloning and chromosomal mapping of cystathionine beta-synthase and the beta subunit of propionyl-CoA carboxylase. Proc Natl Acad Sci USA 83:2047–2051

Kruger WD, Evans AA, Wang L, Malinow MR, Duell PB, Anderson PH, Block PC, Hess DL, Graf EE, Upson B (2000) Polymorphisms in the CBS gene associated with decreased risk of coronary artery disease and increased responsiveness to total homocysteine lowering by folic acid. Mol Genet Metab 70:53–60

Kruman, II, Culmsee C, Chan SL, Kruman Y, Guo Z, Penix L, Mattson MP (2000) Homocysteine elicits a DNA damage response in neurons that promotes apoptosis and hypersensitivity to excitoxicity. J Neurosci 20:6920–6926

Lalouschek W, Aull S, Korninger L, Mannhalter C, Pabinger-Fasching I, Schmid RW, Schnider P, Zeiler K (1998) 677C to T mutation in the 5,10-methylenetetrahydrofolate reductase (MTHFR) gene and plasma homocyst(e)ine levels in patients with TIA or minor stroke. J Neurol Sci 155:156–162

Lee H, Kim HJ, Kim J, Chang N (2004) Effects of dietary folic acid supplementation on cerebrovascular endothelial dysfunction in rats with induced hyperhomocysteinemia. Brain Res 996:139–147

Malinow MR, Duell PB, Hess DL, Anderson PH, Kruger WD, Phillipson BE, Gluckman RA, Block PC, Upson BM (1998) Reduction of plasma homocyst(e)ine levels by breakfast cereal fortified with folic acid in patients with coronary heart disease. N Engl J Med 338:1009–1015

Massy ZA, Chadefaux-Vekemans B, Chevalier A, Bader CA, Drueke TB, Legendre C, Lacour B, Kamoun P, Kreis H (1994) Hyperhomocysteinaemia: a significant risk factor for cardiovascular disease in renal transplant recipients. Nephrol Dial Transplant 9:1103–1108

McCully KS (1969) Vascular pathology of homocysteinemia: implications for the pathogenesis of arteriosclerosis. Am J Pathol 56:111–128

Meiklejohn DJ, Vickers MA, Dijkhuisen R, Greaves M (2001) Plasma homocysteine concentrations in the acute and convalescent periods of atherothrombotic stroke. Stroke 32:57–62

Mercie P, Garnier O, Lascoste L, Renard M, Closse C, Durrieu F, Marit G, Boisseau RM, Belloc F (2000) Homocysteine-thiolactone induces caspase-independent vascular endothelial cell death with apoptotic features. Apoptosis 5:403–411

Moustapha A, Naso A, Nahlawi M, Gupta A, Arheart KL, Jacobsen DW, Robinson K, Dennis VW (1998) Prospective study of hyperhomocysteinemia as an adverse cardiovascular risk factor in end-stage renal disease. Circulation 97:138–141

Murdoch JC, Rodger JC, Rao SS, Fletcher CD, Dunnigan MG (1977) Down's syndrome: an atheroma-free model? BMJ 2:226–228

Nygard O, Vollset SE, Refsum H, Stensvold I, Tverdal A, Nordrehaug JE, Ueland M, Kvale G (1995) Total plasma homocysteine and cardiovascular risk profile. The Hordaland Homocysteine Study. JAMA 274:1526–1533

Nygard O, Nordrehaug JE, Refsum H, Ueland PM, Farstad M, Vollset SE (1997) Plasma homocysteine levels and mortality in patients with coronary artery disease. N Engl J Med 337:230–236

Olszewski AJ, McCully KS (1993) Homocysteine metabolism and the oxidative modification of proteins and lipids. Free Radic Biol Med 14:683–693

Perry IJ, Refsum H, Morris RW, Ebrahim SB, Ueland PM, Shaper AG (1995) Prospective study of serum total homocysteine concentration and risk of stroke in middle-aged British men. Lancet 346:1395–1398

Petri M, Roubenoff R, Dallal GE, Nadeau MR, Selhub J, Rosenberg IH (1996) Plasma homocysteine as a risk factor for atherothrombotic events in systemic lupus erythematosus. Lancet 348:1120–1124

Retterstol L, Paus B, Bohn M, Bakken A, Erikssen J, Malinow MR, Berg K (2003) Plasma total homocysteine levels and prognosis in patients with previous premature myocardial infarction: a 10-year follow-up study. J Intern Med 253:284–292

Rydlewicz A, Simpson JA, Taylor RJ, Bond CM, Golden MH (2002) The effect of folic acid supplementation on plasma homocysteine in an elderly population. QJM 95:27–35

Rosenquist TH, Ratashak SA, Selhub J (1996) Homocysteine induces congenital defects of the heart and neural tube: effect of folic acid. Proc Natl Acad Sci USA 93:15227–15232

Sato Y, Kaji M, Kondo I, Yoshida H, Satoh K, Metoki N (2002) Hyperhomocysteinemia in Japanese patients with convalescent stage ischemic stroke: effect of combined therapy with folic acid and mecobalamine. J Neurol Sci 202:65–68

Schnyder G, Pin R, Roffi M, Flammer Y, Hess OM (2001) Association of plasma homocysteine with the number of major coronary arteries severely narrowed. Am J Cardiol 88:1027–1030

Schnyder G, Roffi M, Flammer Y, Pin R, Hess OM (2002) Effect of homocysteine-lowering therapy with folic acid, vitamin B12, and vitamin B6 on clinical outcome after percutaneous coronary intervention: the Swiss Heart study: a randomized controlled trial. JAMA 288:973–979

Seshadri S, Beiser A, Selhub J, Jacques PF, Rosenberg IH, D'Agostino RB, Wilson PW, Wolf PA (2002) Plasma homocysteine as a risk factor for dementia and Alzheimer's disease. N Engl J Med 346:476–383

Shane B, Stokstad EL (1985) Vitamin B12-folate interrelationships. Annu Rev Nutr 5:115–141

Sharabi Y, Doolman R, Rosenthal T, Grossman E, Rachima-Maoz C, Nussinovitch N, Sela B (1999). Homocysteine levels in hypertensive patients with a history of cardiac or cerebral atherothrombotic events. Am J Hypertens 12:766–771

Stamler JS, Jaraki O, Osborne J, Simon DI, Keaney J, Vita J, Singel D, Valeri CR, Loscalzo J (1992) Nitric oxide circulates in mammalian plasma primarily as an S-nitroso adduct of serum albumin. Proc Natl Acad Sci USA 89:7674–7677

Stampfer MJ, Malinow MR, Willett WC, Newcomer LM, Upson B, Ullmann D, Tishler PV, Hennekens CH (1992) A prospective study of plasma homocyst(e)ine and risk of myocardial infarction in US physicians. JAMA 268:877–881

Streifler JY, Rosenberg N, Chetrit A, Eskaraev R, Sela BA, Dardik R, Zivelin A, Ravid B, Davidson J, Seligsohn U, Inbal A (2001) Cerebrovascular events in patients with significant stenosis of the carotid artery are associated with hyperhomocysteinemia and platelet antigen-1 (Leu33Pro) polymorphism. Stroke 32:2753–2758

Syvanne M, Whittall RA, Turpeinen U, Nieminen MS, Frick MH, Kesaniemi YA, Pasternack A, Humphries SE, Taskinen M-R (2004) Serum homocysteine concentrations, gemfibrozil treatment, and progression of coronary atherosclerosis. Atherosclerosis 172:267–272

Tanne D, Haim M, Goldbourt U, Boyko V, Doolman R, Adler Y, Brunner D, Behar S, Sela BA (2003) Prospective study of serum homocysteine and risk of ischemic stroke among patients with preexisting coronary heart disease. Stroke 34:632–636

Title LM, Cummings PM, Giddens K, Genest JJ, Jr., Nassar BA (2000) Effect of folic acid and antioxidant vitamins on endothelial dysfunction in patients with coronary artery disease. J Am Coll Cardiol 36:758–765

Van den Berg M, Boers GH, Franken DG, Blom HJ, Van Kamp GJ, Jakobs C, Rauwerda JA, Kluft C, Stehouwert CD (1995) Hyperhomocysteinaemia and endothelial dysfunction in young patients with peripheral arterial occlusive disease. Eur J Clin Invest 25:176–181

Verhoef P, Hennekens CH, Malinow MR, Kok FJ, Willett WC, Stampfer MJ (1994) A prospective study of plasma homocyst(e)ine and risk of ischemic stroke. Stroke 25:1924–1930

Verhoef P, Stampfer MJ, Buring JE, Gaziano JM, Allen RH, Stabler SP, Reynolds RD, Kok FJ, Hennekens CH, Willett WC (1996) Homocysteine metabolism and risk of myocardial infarction: relation with vitamins B6, B12, and folate. Am J Epidemiol 143:845–859

Verhoef P, Kok FJ, Kruyssen DA, Schouten EG, Witteman JC, Grobbee DE, Ueland PM, Refsum H (1997) Plasma total homocysteine, B vitamins, and risk of coronary atherosclerosis. Arterioscler Thromb Vasc Biol 17:989–995

Verhoef P, Kok FJ, Kluijtmans LA, Blom HJ, Refsum H, Ueland PM, Kruyssen DA (1997) The 677C→T mutation in the methylenetetrahydrofolate reductase gene: associations with plasma total homocysteine levels and risk of coronary atherosclerotic disease. Atherosclerosis 132:105–113

Vermeer SE, Den Heijer T, Koudstaal PJ, Oudkerk M, Hofman A, Breteler MM (2003) Incidence and risk factors of silent brain infarcts in the population-based Rotterdam Scan Study. Stroke 34:392–396

Vermeulen EG, Stehouwer CD, Twisk JW, van den Berg M, de Jong SC, Mackaay AJ, van Campen CM, Visser FC, Jakobs CA, Bulterjis EJ, Rauwerda JA (2000) Effect of homocysteine-lowering treatment with folic acid plus vitamin B6 on progression of subclinical atherosclerosis: a randomised, placebo-controlled trial. Lancet 355:517–522

Wald NJ, Watt HC, Law MR, Weir DG, McPartlin J, Scott JM (1998) Homocysteine and ischemic heart disease: results of a prospective study with implications regarding prevention. Arch Intern Med 158:862–867

Welch GN, Loscalzo J (1998) Homocysteine and atherothrombosis. N Engl J Med 338:1042–1050

Wenstrom KD, Johanning GL, Owen J, Johnston KE, Acton S, Tamura T (2000) Role of amniotic fluid homocysteine level and of fetal 5, 10-methylenetetrahydrafolate reductase genotype in the etiology of neural tube defects. Am J Med Genet 90:12–16

Wilcken DE, Wilcken B (1976) The pathogenesis of coronary artery disease. A possible role for methionine metabolism. J Clin Invest 57:1079–1082

Wu LL, Wu J, Hunt SC, James BC, Vincent GM, Williams RR, Hopkins PN (1994) Plasma homocyst(e)ine as a risk factor for early familial coronary artery disease. Clin Chem 40:552–561

HEP (2005) 170:339–361

Alcohol

H.F.J. Hendriks[1] (✉) · A. van Tol[2]

[1] Physiological Sciences Department, TNO Nutrition and Food Research Institute, P.O. Box 360, 3700 AJ Zeist, The Netherlands
hendriks@voeding.tno.nl

[2] Departments of Biochemistry and Cell Biology and Genetics, Erasmus University Medical Center, Rotterdam, The Netherlands

Abstract Alcohol consumption affects overall mortality. Light to moderate alcohol consumption reduces the risk of coronary heart disease; epidemiological, physiological and genetic data show a causal relationship. Light to moderate drinking is also associated with a reduced risk of other vascular diseases and probably of type 2 diabetes. Mortality and disease risk increase at higher levels of alcohol consumption. A substantial portion of the benefit of moderate drinking is connected with the alcohol component. However, small differences in effects of various alcoholic beverages on minor risk factors may occur. Proposed protective mechanisms include improved vascular elasticity, anti-thrombotic and anti-inflammatory processes and most importantly, the stimulation of high-density lipoprotein-mediated processes such as reverse cholesterol transport and antioxidative effects.

Keywords Alcohol · Alcoholic beverages · Nutrition · HDL · Antioxidant · Reverse cholesterol transport · Inflammation · Diabetes · Haemostasis · Arterial stiffness

1
Introduction

Alcohol containing beverages play a prominent role in many societies. Alcoholic beverages, such as wine, were consumed as early as 8,000 B.C. Even in the first Bible, wine consumption and drunkenness are mentioned. In the early middle ages, alcoholic beverages (beer) became of vital importance as there was lack of clean drinking water. Nowadays alcohol is part of the diet in all industrialized countries, constituting about 5% of the energy intake (Scheig 1970; Mitchell and Herlong 1986).

Both the type of alcoholic beverage and the occasion at which alcohol is consumed often are based on cultural habits. However, over the past decades the marked national differences in the type of alcohol consumed are slowly disappearing (Hupkens et al. 1993). Also, the large differences in total per capita alcohol consumption between countries are evening out. For instance, in The Netherlands per capita alcohol consumption increased between 1945 and 1975, but then levelled off at about 8 l of pure alcohol per year. On the other hand in France, the country with Europe's highest per capita alcohol consumption, alcohol consumption is decreasing.

Alcohol is usually drunk for pleasure and relaxation. Alcohol consumption may however lead into alcoholism, a disease that includes alcohol craving and continued drinking despite repeated alcohol-related problems. Alcoholism is defined as a primary, chronic disease with genetic, psychosocial, and environmental factors influencing its development and manifestations. The disease is often progressive and fatal. It is characterized by (continuous or periodic) impaired control over drinking, preoccupation with the drug alcohol, use of alcohol despite adverse consequences, and distortions in thinking, most notably denial.

1.1
Moderate and Excessive Drinking

The literature contains widely different applications for the terms used to classify drinking. Research outcomes are often confusing when moderate and excessive drinking is expressed in 'standard drinks'. The term 'standard drink' was originally intended to apply to drinks of 'standard' strengths. However, nowadays the alcohol content varies greatly amongst different beers, wines and distilled spirits. Also, interpretations differ across countries of how much alcohol is contained in a standard drink. There may also be differences in the standard serving sizes depending on the type of beverage and on settings for drinking, e.g. larger sizes served at home. Another problem is lack of uniformity in the definition in which the alcohol content is measured—grams versus ounces of ethanol, American versus British fluid ounces, or measures of alcohol content as percentage by weight or by volume. So assessment and comparison of data from different countries would be greatly facilitated by the uniform expression of alcohol intakes and by the adoption of a uniform international definition of a standard drink (Kalant and Poikolainen 1999; De Vries et al. 1999).

Comparing average daily amounts defined as light, moderate and heavy in a sample of recent publications shows that the lower limit of moderate alcohol intakes ranges from 4.5 to 50 g/day, and the upper limit from about 24 to 80 g/day (Kalant and Poikolainen 1999). On a population basis, the optimal level for the average adult man may probably be in the range of 10 to 19 g alcohol/day and the non-injurious level may approximately be between 30 and 40 g/day. For a woman these levels may be less than 10 g per day and approximately 10–20 g per day, respectively. Gender effects are caused by differences in body weight and body composition which lead to marked differences in blood alcohol concentrations at the same level of intake (Pikaar et al. 1988). However, the individual differences in body size, age, and special situations that can increase the degree of risk (pregnancy, driving, diseases and medications) should also be taken into account.

Light and frequent drinking is suggested to be beneficial, whereas binge drinking (drinking large amounts drunk infrequently) is harmful with respect to disease. Chronic excessive drinking or alcoholism has several detrimental effects.

1.2
Nutritional Aspects of Alcohol Consumption

1.2.1
Nutritional Value

The nutritional value of alcoholic beverages is limited, because they contribute mainly to the caloric intake of the diet. The sugars in some alcoholic beverages may further add to the caloric intake. Alcohol contains calories and as a consequence alcohol consumption has been suggested to lead to overweight. However, the relationship between alcohol consumption and body weight is unclear. Experimental as well as epidemiological studies provide conflicting results. Intervention studies in healthy normal-weight men consuming moderate amounts of alcohol either result in no effect (Contaldo et al. 1989) or a small reduction in weight (McDonald and Margen 1976). Epidemiological studies on the relationship between alcohol and body weight are often inconclusive, because confounding factors, specifically smoking, are not taken into account (MacDonald et al. 1976; Muller 1999). In one study, Colditz et al. (1991) showed that in men, calories from alcohol were taken in addition to energy intake from other sources, whereas in women, energy from alcohol intake displaced energy intake from sucrose. An inverse correlation was observed between body mass index and alcohol consumption in women drinking up to 50 g per day. In contrast, in men body mass index varied little across levels of alcohol intake.

These data suggest that excess energy from alcohol consumption may not lead to an increased body weight. Several mechanistic explanations have been put forward. Possibly, the inverse correlation is spurious, because people with a higher body mass index tend to reduce their alcohol intake because of it supposedly being fattening, with women being more concerned about their weight than men (Veenstra et al. 1993).

Alternatively, loss of body heat increases after alcohol consumption. This increase, however, only partly offsets the caloric surplus due to alcohol consumption (Suter et al. 1992). It has therefore been hypothesized that alcohol enters a 'futile cycle' in which alcohol is catabolized with loss of energy (body heat) (Lands and Zakhari 1991). Also, subjects consuming alcohol may be habitually more active (Westerterp et al. 2004).

Alcohol consumption generally contributes little to the vitamin intake, with the exception of beer, which contributes to the folic acid intake (Mayer et al. 2001). Minerals and trace elements are present in both beer and wine. Consumption of two or three glasses of wine may significantly contribute to the intake of iron and potassium and, in the case of red wine, of copper. However, the overall contribution of alcoholic beverages to the intake of essential minerals and trace elements is relatively small.

1.2.2
Malnutrition

Chronic alcohol consumption may lead to primary and secondary malnutrition. In particular, protein energy malnutrition is not only aggravated by alcoholic liver disease but also correlates with impaired liver function. Clinical trials have shown that nutritional therapy, either enterally or parenterally, improves various aspects of alcohol-induced malnutrition, and there is increased evidence that it may also prolong survival.

Excessive alcohol consumption can result in mucosal injury resulting in an increased prevalence for bacterial overgrowth in the small intestine. The mucosal damage increases the permeability of the gut to macromolecules. This facilitates the translocation of endotoxin and other bacterial toxins from the lumen of the gut to the portal blood, thereby increasing the liver's exposure to these toxins and, consequently, the risk of liver injury (Bode and Bode 2003).

Micronutrient deficiencies typically encountered in alcoholics, such as for thiamine and folate, require specific supplementation. One of the most frequent deficiencies is thiamine deficiency, which may lead to the Wernicke–Korsakoff syndrome. Patients with hepatic encephalopathy may be treated with branched-chain amino acids in order to achieve a positive nitrogen balance (Stickel et al. 2003).

2
Alcohol Consumption and Total Mortality

Over the last few years the balance between benefits and adverse health effects has often been discussed and the effects of alcohol consumption on overall mortality were investigated in depth. Gaziano et al. (2000) recently confirmed the U-shaped relationship between alcohol consumption and total mortality described previously (Camargo et al. 1997; Keil et al. 1997; Renaud et al. 1998, 1999; White 1999). The reduction in total mortality is largely due to the reduction of cardiovascular diseases (CVD). The description of the overall disease burden due to alcohol consumption allows for the definition of that quantity of alcohol associated with the lowest mortality (nadir). The nadir appears to vary substantially between countries (in the USA, men: 69 g per week and in the UK, men: 116 g per week) and between sexes (USA women: 26 g per week), but is not affected by age (Fuchs et al. 1995). This was shown in a systematic review of 20 cohort studies with a total of more than 60,000 deaths in men and almost 75,000 deaths in women (White 1999).

Mortality risk or disease risk may increase at higher levels of alcohol consumption. The increase in mortality risk at high levels of intake is attributable to increased risks for accidents, cancers and cerebrovascular disease, but not for coronary heart disease. Other causes of death, typically associated with alcohol-related problems, such as liver cirrhosis, are also consistently increased. A Danish study confirmed the J-shaped relationship between alcohol consumption and total mortality. Surprisingly, the risk relationship appeared not to be modified by sex, age, body mass index or smoking (Gronbaek 1994).

3
Diseases of the Cardiovascular System

The effects of alcohol on the cardiovascular system are studied in relation to three main atherosclerotic diseases, which are coronary heart disease, cerebrovascular disease and peripheral artery disease.

3.1
Coronary Heart Disease

Epidemiological studies describing the relationship between alcohol consumption and coronary heart disease have been summarized recently (Grobbee et al. 1999). Some main conclusions are that light to moderate drinking is associated with a reduced risk for the development of coronary heart disease in middle-aged and elderly men and women living in western countries and that it is highly likely that the association is causal. Recent studies show a similar association in non-Western populations as well (Yuan et al. 1997; Kitamura et al. 1998). Moderate alcohol consumption could also protect after a first myocardial infarction (Muntwyler et al. 1998).

The inverse relationship between moderate alcohol consumption and coronary heart disease has now been studied both in men and women (Fuchs et al. 1995; Klatsky et al. 1997; Rehm et al. 1997; Thun et al. 1997; Nanchahal et al. 2000). Benefits for women are mostly found at lower quantities of alcohol and appear to be most pronounced in postmenopausal women. This is not surprising since this age group, like men over the age of 50, has a marked increase in cardiovascular risk.

Arrhythmias are associated with heavy alcohol consumption, even in men without CVD (Engstrom et al. 1999). The prevalence of sudden cardiac death may also be increased after heavy alcohol consumption (Wannamethee and Shaper 1992; Kadis et al. 1999), but appears to be decreased with light to moderate drinking (Albert et al. 1999).

3.1.1
Beverage-Specific Effects

Some reports have suggested that beverage type may be important (Renaud et al. 1999; Gronbaek et al. 1995), an issue which is discussed extensively in a comprehensive review (Rimm et al. 1996; Klatsky et al. 2003) of the effect of specific beverages on coronary hart disease risk. The study by Rimm et al. (1996) shows that observational studies, including only those that provide specific information on the consumption of beer, wine and spirits in relation to the risk of coronary heart disease, indicate that moderate consumption of all three alcohol-containing beverages is linked with lower risk. Thus, a substantial portion of the benefit is connected with the alcohol component, rather than with specific non-alcohol components present in the different types of beverages.

Also intervention studies directly comparing the effects of different alcoholic beverages in dietary controlled, randomized clinical trials have shown that the majority of the effect on coronary heart disease risk factors is alcohol-mediated (Van der Gaag et al. 1999). However, small differences in the effects of various alcohol-containing beverages on minor risk factor may occur (Van der Gaag et al. 2000a, 2000b).

3.1.2
Drinking Pattern

Drinking pattern is being recognized as an important factor determining the risk for diseases and drinking pattern is now being investigated more intensively. A recent study by Mukamal et al. (2003) indicates that consumption of alcohol at least 3–4 days per week was inversely associated with the risk of myocardial infarction. Neither the type of beverage nor the proportion consumed with meals substantially altered this association. This study suggests that the frequency of light and moderate drinking is an additional important factor in health benefits.

3.2
Cerebrovascular Diseases

Stroke is either characterized by an ischaemic necrosis of part of the brain, i.e. cerebral infarction, or by a haemorrhage in or at the base of the brain, i.e. haemorrhagic stroke. The association between alcohol consumption and all types of stroke appears to be J-shaped with a lower risk observed in light drinkers than in non-drinkers. Some evidence indicates that a modest excess risk for all types of stroke can only be observed in the highest category of alcohol intake, e.g. more than 60 g per day (Juvela et al. 1995; Kiyohara et al. 1995; Sacco et al. 1999).

Studies specifying the type of stroke indicate that individuals in the highest category of alcohol intake had an increased risk for haemorrhagic stroke (Hansagi et al. 1995). No statistically elevated relative risk was observed for ischaemic stroke. However, a borderline significant protective effect was found for ischaemic stroke after consumption of less than one drink per day. As 70%–85% of strokes are ischaemic, the J-shaped association for total stroke may result from a protective effect on ischaemic stroke and an elevated excess risk for haemorrhagic stroke.

While case reports suggest a direct relationship between binge drinking and stroke, epidemiological studies provide only meagre evidence for such a relationship (Hillbom et al. 1999).

3.3
Peripheral Artery Disease

Peripheral artery disease occurs when atherosclerosis affects the extremities. The disease causes pain due to insufficient blood flow into the extremities. The atherosclerotic plaques of peripheral artery disease are much more common in the legs than the arms. Although women do get peripheral artery disease, it is two to five times more common in men.

The association between alcohol consumption and peripheral artery disease has been investigated in several large studies (Vliegenthart et al. 2002; Djousse et al. 2000) reporting a protective effect of moderate drinking on the incidence of the disease in men as well as in women.

3.4
Dementia

Risk factors for vascular disease and stroke may also be associated with cognitive impairment and dementia (Breteler et al. 1998). There is evidence that excessive alcohol abuse in the long term may permanently affect cognitive abilities such as memory and reasoning (Bates and Tracy 1990; Elias et al. 1999). However, moderate alcohol consumption may be associated with a decreased risk for developing dementia (Orgogozo et al. 1997). The largest study using a well-defined population of more than 5,000 individuals of 55 years and older showed that moderate drinkers had a reduced incidence of dementia particularly dementia of the vascular type (Ruitenberg et al. 2002).

4
Hypertension

High blood pressure increases the risk of heart attacks, other heart diseases, and problems in other organs. A relationship between alcohol use and blood pressure has been noted since 1915, when it was described that French service men drinking 2.5 l of wine or more per day had an increased prevalence of high blood pressure (Lian 1915).

The relationship between alcohol consumption and blood pressure has been extensively investigated in a large number of population studies, including both observational and intervention studies (Keil et al. 1993). These studies have almost uniformly demonstrated that blood pressure increases with increasing levels of alcohol consumption in both men and women. A causal relationship is further substantiated by studies showing a fall in blood pressure when heavy drinkers abstain or restrict their alcohol intake (Howes et al. 1986; Maheswaran et al. 1992; Parker et al. 1990).

Some studies have found that blood pressure in people consuming low amounts of alcohol was not different from or was slightly lower than in those abstaining from alcohol. Yet other studies have suggested that blood pressure increases even at low levels of alcohol consumption. Therefore, there is no certainty as to the exact shape of the association and the exact level of consumption that will start to increase blood pressure. It seems likely that a threshold exists at 30–60 g of alcohol consumed per day, above which the risk of hypertension increases. This threshold may be lower for women than for men.

Data from population studies can be used to calculate the magnitude of the rise in blood pressure by heavier drinking. The contribution of alcohol consumption to the total number of people with high blood pressure in the population may also be estimated. It has been calculated that above a daily alcohol intake of 30 g per day, an increment of each 10 g per day (approximately one alcoholic beverage) will increase systolic blood pressure on average by 1–2 mmHg, and diastolic blood pressure by 1 mmHg (Keil et al. 1993).

Several mechanisms have been suggested to account for the relationship between heavy ethanol consumption and hypertension. Ethanol at high doses may activate the sympathetic nervous system resulting in constriction of blood vessels and in elevation of the contractile force of the heart. In addition, ethanol may affect the blood levels of several hormones and salts (catecholamines, epinephrine, norepinephrine, magnesium and calcium ions), which play an important role in cardiac function and vascular tone. Finally, it has been suggested that receptors in arteries monitoring blood pressure may become less sensitive, thus reducing regulation of arterial contraction and relaxation.

5
Physiological Mechanisms of Moderate Alcohol Consumption Related to CVD

It is important to examine the physiological changes occurring after moderate alcohol consumption in order to get a better understanding of how disease aetiology may be altered. However, well-controlled studies in humans describing these physiological changes are still scarce.

A meta-analysis assessed the effects of moderate alcohol intake on lipids and haemostatic factors (Rimm et al. 1999). Increases in high-density lipoprotein (HDL) cholesterol, apolipoprotein AI (apoAI) and total plasma triglycerides were quantified for an experimental dose of 30 g of alcohol/day. On the basis of published associations between these biomarkers and risk, this dose was estimated to reduce coronary heart disease risk by about 25%. This percentage is comparable to the relative risks reported in several large-scale prospective studies (Doll et al. 1994; Rimm et al. 1991; Klatsky 1994). Altogether these data strongly suggest that alcohol consumption may be causally related to a lower risk for coronary heart disease with HDL cholesterol increase being the most important factor (Van Tol and Hendriks 2001).

Causality of the association between moderate drinking and coronary heart disease risk reduction was further established by Hines et al. (2001) studying polymorphisms in one of the genes relevant for alcohol metabolism (alcohol dehydrogenase 3, ADH3) and the risk of myocardial infarction. Moderate alcohol consumption was associated with a decreased risk of myocardial infarction in all three genotype groups. However, the ADH3 genotype significantly modified this association; moderate drinkers who are homozygous for the slow-oxidizing *ADH3* allele have higher HDL levels and a substantially decreased risk of myocardial infarction.

5.1
Lipid and Lipoprotein Metabolism

Lipid and lipoprotein metabolism is affected by alcohol consumption in several ways. It is well known that moderate alcohol consumption increases HDL-cholesterol (Gaziano et al. 1993). Based on epidemiological findings it was estimated that more than 50% of the beneficial effect of alcohol is due to the increase in HDL-cholesterol (Langer et al. 1992).

In a diet-controlled cross-over study a moderate daily dose of alcohol consumed with the evening meal increased serum HDL-cholesterol already after 10 days (Sierksma et al. 2002). The average increase in HDL-cholesterol in middle-aged men and postmenopausal women after 3 weeks of moderate alcohol consumption in a diet-controlled condition is about 12% (Van der Gaag et al. 1999; Sierksma et al. 2002). These findings indicate that the increase in HDL-cholesterol is a true alcohol effect.

The mechanism responsible for the HDL-cholesterol increasing effect of alcohol is not completely clear, but different mechanisms may contribute. Hepatic lipase activity is reported to decrease within several hours of alcohol consumption (Goldberg et al. 1984; Taskinen et al. 1985). Another study suggests that elevated lipoprotein lipase contributes substantially to the alcohol-induced rise in HDL-cholesterol (Nishiwaki et al. 1994). Also, alcohol consumption may increase the transport rates of both apo A-I and apo A-II, the major apolipoproteins of HDL, without affecting their fractional catabolic rate (De Oliveira e Silva et al. 2000). The increased transport rates are most likely due to increased hepatic production of these apolipoproteins (Amarasuiya et al. 1992; De Oliveira e Silva et al. 2000; Tam et al. 1992). Other intervention studies show that at least part of the increase in plasma HDL-cholesterol concentrations may be due to increased activity of lecithin:cholesterol acyltransferase (LCAT) (Hendriks et al. 1998).

It was recently quantified how a moderate dose of alcohol (24 g) affects hepatic lipid metabolism. Using stable isotopes, Siler et al. (1999) confirmed and quantified that the bulk of a moderate dose of alcohol is metabolized into acetate. Only a minor portion (<5%) is used for de novo synthesis of fatty acids. The acetate produced is released into the circulation (Taskinen et al. 1985) and may inhibit whole body lipid and carbohydrate oxidation.

Moderate alcohol consumption, which leads to inhibition of the Krebs cycle, may inhibit hepatic oxidation of plasma free fatty acids, which are converted to triglycerides instead. The triglycerides are secreted by the liver as very-low-density lipoproteins (VLDL). In healthy normolipidaemic subjects this does not lead to elevated fasting plasma triglycerides, probably due to a compensatory increase in lipoprotein lipase activity. Increased VLDL turnover contributes to the formation of HDL precursors and thus results in elevated plasma HDL concentration (Van Tol et al. 1995). Interestingly, fasting plasma VLDL levels are hardly affected by moderate alcohol consumption but a moderate dose of alcohol transiently increases plasma triacylglycerol concentrations (Van der Gaag et al. 1999) and decreases plasma LDL cholesterol (Van Tol et al. 1998; Sierksma et al. 2001) when alcohol is consumed in combination with a meal. This post-prandial hypertriglyceridaemia after moderate alcohol consumption also profoundly affects the chemical composition of HDL (Van Tol et al. 1995; Hendriks et al. 2001). HDL triglycerides are elevated directly after the fat-containing meal, whereas HDL phospholipids are elevated several hours later (Nishiwaki et al.1994).

Not only HDL lipids are changed by alcohol consumption. Studies in healthy volunteers have shown that moderate alcohol consumption increases plasma HDL apolipoproteins and LCAT activity levels (Hendriks et al. 1998). It is likely that the rates of formation of plasma HDL apolipoproteins, HDL-phospholipids and HDL-cholesteryl esters are all increased, resulting in an elevation of the number of HDL particles per volume of plasma. In the fasting state, plasma cholesteryl ester transfer by the cholesteryl ester transfer protein (CETP) is not influenced by moderate alcohol consumption, due to normal plasma VLDL levels and unaffected CETP concentration and activity. However, net mass cholesteryl ester transfer is increased during alcohol consumption with an evening meal due to the elevation of triglyceride-rich lipoproteins in the post-prandial phase (Van Tol et al. 1998).

5.2
HDL Functions and Disease

Because moderate alcohol consumption is associated with coronary artery disease mainly via its HDL raising effect, it is crucial to study the functional consequences of this increase in plasma HDL concentration. Several properties of HDL may be important.

5.2.1
HDL and Reverse Cholesterol Transport

An important property of HDL is its capacity to take up excess cholesterol from peripheral cells and transport it to the liver for excretion and degradation to bile acids. Three mechanisms may be important in cholesterol efflux (Van der

Gaag et al. 2001). Firstly, a portion of cholesterol may leave the cell via aqueous diffusion. Secondly, cholesterol may be desorbed from the plasma membrane via the scavenger receptor BI (SRBI) and accepted by phospholipid-rich acceptors like HDL. Thirdly, cellular cholesterol (and phospholipid) efflux may be facilitated by the ABCA1 protein, directing the cholesterol and phospholipids to lipid-free or lipid-poor pre-β-HDL particles. The resulting lipoprotein particles are substrates for LCAT, which synthesizes cholesteryl esters from the unesterified cholesterol of cellular origin. Changes in lipoprotein metabolism allow for each of these mechanisms to be stimulated by moderate alcohol consumption (Van der Gaag et al. 1999).

In both middle-aged men and postmenopausal women moderate alcohol consumption increased cholesterol efflux (Sierksma et al. 2004; Van der Gaag et al. 2001). In middle-aged men there was also an alcohol-induced increase of cholesterol esterification (Van der Gaag et al. 2001). The increases were independent of the type of alcoholic beverage consumed, which suggests that the effects were due to alcohol rather than to other compounds of alcoholic drinks. The capacity of plasma to induce cholesterol efflux from Fu5AH cells in vitro is elevated after moderate alcohol consumption. As these cells have very high levels of SRBI, this effect is probably due to the raised plasma HDL-cholesterol and HDL-phospholipid concentrations. Unpublished data from our laboratory show that also the capacity of serum to stimulate ABCA1-mediated cholesterol efflux, evaluated using J774 macrophages, is also elevated after moderate alcohol consumption. (Beulens et al. 2004).

5.2.2
HDL as an Antioxidant

A good antioxidant status is considered important for human health. Low plasma levels of antioxidants as well as low intakes of dietary antioxidants have been associated with an increased risk for atherosclerotic disease in epidemiological studies. However, intervention studies have been disappointing (Gaziano 1999).

Alcohol abuse results in increased urinary lipid peroxides, indicating oxidative stress (Meagher et al. 1999). Red wine consumption has received much attention as a potential factor improving the antioxdant status (Kondo et al. 1994; Sharpe et al. 1995; Cao and Prior 1998). Increases in plasma antioxidant concentrations after consumption of red wine may (Cacetta et al. 2000; Bell et al. 2000) or may not (Van der Gaag et al. 2000) occur. It is unlikely, however, that the phenolic acids present in red wine, after consumption of moderate amounts, are able to raise the plasma levels enough to protect lipoproteins from oxidative modification. Also, ex vivo lipoprotein oxidation is not inhibited by these compounds (Cacetta et al. 2000).

Some time ago, the anti-oxidative properties of HDL were recognized (Mackness and Durrington 1995). Paraoxonase 1 (PON1) has been identified as a major contributor to these properties. HDL is associated with the enzyme PON, originally known for its ability to detoxify organophosphorus pesticides and nerve gases. Recently, evidence has been accumulating that PON may protect against atherosclerosis. It potently inhibits lipoprotein oxidation in vitro (Aviram et al. 1998: Mackness et al. 1997; Mackness et al. 1998), and protects human aortic endothelial cells against monocyte adhesion induced by mildly oxidized LDL (Watson et al. 1995). PON activity in human pericardial fluid is inversely related to the degree of coronary atherosclerosis (Hernandez et al. 1993), and lower serum PON activities occur in coronary heart disease patients as compared to healthy controls (McElveen et al. 1986; Mackness et al. 1998).

Both in middle-aged men and postmenopausal women PON activity is increased with moderate alcohol intake (Van der Gaag et al. 1999; Sierksma et al. 2002). Some studies suggest that there may be an association between PON gene polymorphisms and atherosclerotic diseases (Imai et al. 2000; Leus et al. 2000). However, the relative increase in PON activity after moderate alcohol consumption was essentially the same for different PON gene polymorphisms (Van der Gaag et al. 1999; Sierksma et al. 2002).

Interestingly, in addition to its protection against LDL oxidation, PON may also stimulate cellular cholesterol efflux (Aviram et al. 1998), the first step in reverse cholesterol transport.

We have shown that the activity of PON is increased by on average 8% after drinking moderate amounts of beer, wine and spirits (Van der Gaag et al. 1999). Consumption of moderate amounts of alcohol, rather than intake of non-alcohol components contained in alcoholic beverages, is likely to mediate antioxidant activity in vivo by PON raising mechanisms.

5.3
Alcohol Effects Not Mediated by HDL

Moderate alcohol consumption may not only protect by affecting HDL metabolism and functioning, but probably also via a whole range of other mechanisms. These include effects on haemostasis, inflammation and arterial stiffness.

5.3.1
Haemostasis

Haemostatic factors may play a role in the development of coronary heart disease mortality. Thrombotic factors may contribute to the development of atherosclerotic plaques; fibrin and platelet components are present in plaques, and platelets secrete chemotactic substances and growth factors in vitro. Also, at sites of destabilized atherosclerotic plaques, thrombotic factors are involved in occlusion, embolization, or both.

One of the main established haemostatic risk factors for coronary heart disease is fibrinogen (Hendriks and Van der Gaag 1998). In several epidemiological studies the level of fibrinogen has been found to be independently and significantly associated with the risk of coronary heart disease. Epidemiological studies have shown an inverse association between alcohol consumption and fibrinogen levels. In addition, in experimental studies fibrinogen levels were decreased with moderate alcohol consumption (Dimmitt et al. 1998; Sierksma et al. 2002).

In a cohort of 87,526 nurses, moderate drinkers had a lower risk of both coronary heart disease and ischaemic stroke but an increased risk of haemorrhagic stroke (Stampfer et al. 1988). Since occlusion of blood vessels occurs in both coronary heart disease and ischaemic stroke, and bleeding occurs in haemorrhagic stroke, effects on haemostatic factors might explain these different effects of moderate consumption of alcohol.

In both middle-aged men and postmenopausal women moderate alcohol consumption with evening meals affected the regulatory fibrinolytic factors, tissue-type plasminogen activator (tPA) and plasminogen activator inhibitor (PAI), temporarily. Fibrinolytic capacity decreased immediately after an evening meal with alcoholic beverage (increase in PAI and decrease in tPA), followed by an increased fibrinolytic capacity the following morning (increase in tPA) (Hendriks et al. 1994; Sierksma et al. 2001). This increase in fibrinolytic activity is mentioned as a possible protective effect against coronary heart disease, as a large proportion of heart attacks normally take place in the morning. Alcohol probably up-regulates tPA gene expression (Grenett et al. 1998; Booyse et al. 1999), as suggested in studies with cultured human endothelial cells.

5.3.2
Inflammation

A second category of recently discovered biochemical effects of moderate alcohol consumption that may act against atherosclerosis and CVD risk involves changes in inflammatory factors. Inflammation within the plaques contributes considerably to the initiation and progression of atherosclerosis.

C-reactive protein (CRP), a marker for systemic inflammation, predicts cardiovascular events among apparently healthy men and women. Even modest elevations of the concentration of CRP were predictive (Ridker et al. 1998). Epidemiological studies have suggested that CRP, an acute phase protein and sensitive marker of inflammation, decreases with moderate alcohol consumption (Koenig et al. 1999).

This hypothesis was tested in a randomized diet-controlled trial. Plasma CRP levels significantly decreased by about 35% after 3 weeks of moderate alcohol intake compared with no alcohol consumption (Sierksma et al. 2002). These findings support the epidemiological findings and indicate that an anti-inflammatory action of alcohol may help explain the link between moderate alcohol consumption and lower CVD risk.

The mechanism causing moderate alcohol consumption to reduce plasma CRP levels needs further investigation. The mechanism may involve nuclear factor-kappa B, which is a redox-sensitive transcription factor that activates genes involved in the immune, inflammatory, or acute-phase response, such as cytokines and tumour necrosis factor alpha, which regulate CRP production by the liver.

5.3.3
Homocysteine

Accumulating evidence indicates that plasma total homocysteine concentration is an independent risk factor for CVD (Bostom et al. 1999). It is suggested that homocysteine causes vascular damage, however the definite mechanism has not yet been identified. In vitro experiments with very high homocysteine concentrations have identified the stimulation of atherosclerosis and thrombosis through adverse effects on coagulation pathways, platelets, endothelial cells and vascular smooth muscle cells. Homocysteine concentrations are affected by lifestyle factors such as diet, e.g. inadequate intake of B vitamins involved in the homocysteine breakdown.

Van der Gaag et al. (2000) showed, in a 3-week randomized cross-over trial, that despite the equally administered amount of ethanol (four glasses per day) beer did not affect homocysteine concentration, whereas wine and spirits induced an increase. Homocysteine concentrations could rise by inhibition of its two major breakdown pathways, both dependent on B vitamins. The remethylation pathway depends on folate and vitamin B_{12}, whereas vitamin B_6 is essential in the breakdown via *trans*-sulphuration. No significant differences in vitamin B_{12} and folate were observed. Plasma vitamin B_6 increased by about 30% after beer consumption, whereas this increase was 17% and 15% after intake of wine and spirits, respectively. Changes in vitamin B_6 showed a significant inverse correlation with changes in homocysteine. This suggests that vitamin B_6 might be a rate-limiting factor for homocysteine breakdown after moderate alcohol consumption.

The increase in homocysteine after wine and spirits consumption could increase the CVD risk. However, moderate alcohol consumption is associated with a lowered CVD risk. There are several ways to explain this apparent contradiction. First the cardioprotective effects of moderate drinking could exceed the increase in risk caused by higher homocysteine concentrations. Alternatively, since vitamin B_6 is inversely associated with CVD risk, independently of homocysteine (Folsom et al. 1998), the increase in this vitamin might contribute to a lower CVD risk.

5.3.4
Arterial Stiffness

Several studies indicate that elevated levels of CVD risk factors are related to atherogenesis and vascular damage, such as stiffer arteries, specifically stiffness of the aorta (Van Popele et al. 2001). Pulse-wave velocity (PWV) is a non-invasive parameter of arterial stiffness. PWV is calculated from measurement of pulse transit time and the distance travelled by the pulse between the common carotid artery and one of the common femoral arteries. PWV increases with increasing arterial stiffness.

A cardioprotective effect of moderate alcohol consumption would be reflected in an inverse or U-shaped association between alcohol intake and PWV. A cross-sectional study in Japanese–American middle-aged and older men and women reported that the risk for high aortic PWV was lower among current drinkers and ex-drinkers than among non-drinkers (Namekata et al. 1997). In a follow-up study in middle-aged Japanese men the incidence of aortic stiffness was not related to alcohol intake (Nakanishi et al. 1998), whereas another longitudinal study in Japanese men suggested that alcohol is an important risk factor for development of aortic stiffness at an intake of more than 16 glasses of alcoholic beverage per week (Nakanishi et al. 2001).

Our research group also investigated the effect of alcohol consumption on PWV, using cross-sectional data of both young adults and middle-aged men and women. An inverse to J-shaped association between alcohol consumption and aortic PWV is reported in cross-sectional studies among post-menopausal women (Sierksma et al. 2004) and among men 40–80 years of age (Sierksma et al. 2004). The lowest PWV was observed with an alcoholic beverage intake of approximately 7–14 glasses (containing 10 g of pure alcohol) per week for both men and women.

These findings provide evidence for the view that moderate intake of alcohol may affect vascular elasticity. This is compatible with a vascular protective effect of alcohol that expresses itself well before symptomatic CVD becomes apparent.

6
Insulin Sensitivity

The results from recent studies on the association between alcohol consumption, insulin resistance (Facchini et al. 1994) and type 2 diabetes mellitus type (Conigrave et al. 2001; De Vegt et al. 2002) are very interesting. Resistance to the metabolic actions of insulin is not only associated with type 2 diabetes, but also plays an important role in the pathogenesis of obesity and CVD. Therefore the insulin-sensitizing effect of moderate alcohol consumption is another potential intermediary through which alcohol might exert its anti-atherogenic effect.

A systematic review of 32 studies on the relationship between alcohol consumption and the risk of type 2 diabetes showed that moderate alcohol consumption is associated with a 33%–56% lower incidence of diabetes and a 34%–55% lower incidence of diabetes-related coronary heart disease. Compared with moderate consumption, a consumption of more than 30 g of alcohol per day may be associated with up to a 43% increased incidence of diabetes. Moderate alcohol consumption does not acutely impair glycaemic control in persons with diabetes (Howard et al. 2004).

To date, the mechanism explaining the increased insulin sensitivity in moderate alcohol consumers is not well understood. Adiponectin is an adipocyte-derived plasma protein, which is closely related to increased insulin sensitivity (Cnop et al. 2003; Hotta et al. 2001) and associated with a risk of myocardial infarction (Pischon et al. 2004). The effect might be mediated through an alcohol-induced increase in adiponectin, as moderate alcohol intake increased adiponectin levels by 11% (Sierksma et al. 2004).

References

Albert CM, Manson JE, Cook NR, et al. (1999) Moderate alcohol consumption and the risk of sudden cardiac death among US male physicians. Circulation 100:944–950

Amarasuiya RN, Gupta AK, Civen M, et al. (1992) Ethanol stimulates apolipoprotein A-I secretion by human hepatocytes: implications for a mechanism for atherosclerosis protection. Metabolism 41:827–832

Aviram M, Rosenblat M, Bisgaire CL, et al. (1998) Paraoxonase inhibits high-density lipoprotein oxidation and preserves its functions. A possible peroxidative role for paraoxonase. J Clin Invest 101:1581–1590

Bates ME, Tracy JI (1990) Cognitive functioning in young 'social drinkers'. Is there impairment to detect? J Abnorm Psychol 99:242–249

Bell JRC, Donovan JL, Wong R, et al. (2000) (+)-Catechin in human plasma after ingestion of a single serving of reconstituted red wine. Am J Clin Nutr 71:103–108

Beulens JWJ, Sierksma A, Van Tol et al. (2004) Moderate alcohol consumption increases cholesterol efflux mediated by ABC AI. Accepted for publication in J Lipid Res 45:1716–1723

Bode C, Bode JC (2003) Effect of alcohol consumption on the gut. Best Pract Res Clin Gastroenterol 17:575–592

Booyse FM, Aikens ML, Grenett HE (1999) Endothelial cell fibrinolysis: transcriptional regulation of fibrinolytic protein gene expression (t-PA, u-PA, and PAI-1) by low alcohol. Alcohol Clin Exp Res 23:1119–1124

Bostom AG, Silbershatz H, Rosenberg IH, et al. (1999) Nonfasting plasma total homocysteine levels and all-cause and cardiovascular disease mortality in elderly Framingham men and women. Arch Int Med 159:1077–1080

Breteler MMB, Bots ML, Ott A, et al. (1998) Risk factors for vascular disease and dementia. Haemostasis 28:167–173

Caccetta RAA, Croft KD, Beilin LJ, et al. (2000) Ingestion of red wine significantly increases plasma phenolic acid concentrations but does not acutely affect ex vivo lipoprotein oxidizability. Am J Clin Nutr 71:67–74

Camargo CA, Stampfer MJ, Glynn RJ, et al. (1997) Moderate alcohol consumption and risk for angina pectoris or myocardial infarction in U.S. male physicians. Ann Intern Med 126:372–375

Cao G, Prior RL (1998) Comparison of different analytical methods for assessing total antioxidant capacity of human serum. Clin Chem 44:1309–1315

Cnop M, Havel PJ, Utzschneider KM, et al. (2003) Relationship of adiponectin to body fat distribution, insulin sensitivity and plasma lipoproteins: evidence for independent roles of age and sex. Diabetologia 46:459–469

Colditz GA, Giovannucci E, Rimm EB, et al. (1991) Alcohol intake in relation to diet and obesity in women and men. Am J Clin Nutr 54:49–55

Contaldo F, d'Arrigo E, Caradente V, et al. (1989) Short term effects of moderate alcohol consumption on lipid metabolism and energy balance in normal men. Metabolism 38:166–171

Conigrave KM, Hu BF, Camargo CA, et al. (2001) A prospective study of drinking patterns in relation to risk of type 2 diabetes among men. Diabetes 50:2390–2395

De Oliveira e Silva, ER, Foster D, McGee Harper M, et al. (2000) Alcohol consumption raises HDL cholesterol levels by increasing the transport rate of apolipoproteins A-I and A-II. Circulation 102:2347–2352

De Vegt F, Dekker JM, Groeneveld WJ, et al. (2002) Moderate alcohol consumption is associated with lower risk for incident diabetes and mortality: the Hoorn Study. Diabetes Res Clin Prac 57:53–60

De Vries JHM, Lemmens PHHM, Pietinen P, et al. (1999) Assessement of alcohol consumption. In: MacDonald I (ed) Health issues related to alcohol consumption. Blackwell Science, ILSI Europe, Brussel, pp 28–62

Dimmitt SB, Rakic V, Puddey IB, et al. (1998) The effects of alcohol on coagulation and fibrinolytic factors: a controlled trial. Blood Coagul Fibrinolysis 9:39–45

Djousse L, Levy D, Murabito JM, et al. (2000) Alcohol consumption and risk of intermittent claudication in the Framingham Heart Study. Circulation 102:3092–3097

Doll R, Peto R, Hall E, et al. (1994) Mortality in relation to consumption of alcohol: 13 years' observations on male British doctors. BMJ 309:911–918

Elias PK, Elias MF, D'Agostino RB, et al. (1999) Alcohol consumption and cognitive performance in the Framingham Heart Study. JAMA 150:580–589

Engstrom G, Hedblad B, Janzon L, et al. (1999) Ventricular arrhythmias during 24-h ambulatory ECG recording: incidence, risk factors and prognosis in men with and without a history of cardiovascular disease. J Intern Med 246:363–372

Facchini F, Chen YD, Reaven GM (1994) Light-to-moderate alcohol intake is associated with enhanced insulin sensitivity. Diabetes Care 17:115–119

Folsom AR, Nieto FJ, McGovern PG, et al. (1998) Prospective study of coronary heart disease incidence in relation to fasting total homocysteine, related genetic polymorphisms, and B vitamins: the Atherosclerosis Risk in Communities (ARIC) study. Circulation 98:204–210

Fuchs CS, Stampfer MJ, Colditz GA, et al. (1995) Alcohol consumption and mortality among women. N Engl J Med 332:1245–1250

Gaziano JM, Buring JE, Breslow JL, et al. (1993) Moderate alcohol intake, increased levels of high-density lipoprotein and its subfractions, and decreased risk of myocardial infarction. N Engl J Med 329:1829–1834

Gaziano JM (1999) Antioxidant vitamins and cardiovascular disease. Proc Assoc Am Phys 111:2–9

Gaziano JM, Gaziano TA, Glynn RJ, et al. (2000) Light-to-moderate alcohol consumption and mortality in the physicians' health study enrollment cohort. J Am Coll Card 35:96–105

Goldberg CS, Tall AR, Krumholz S (1984) Acute inhibition of hepatic lipase and increase in plasma lipoproteins after alcohol intake. J Lipid Res 25:714–720

Grenett HE, Aikens ML, Torres JA, et al. (1998) Ethanol transcriptionally upregulates t-PA and u-PA gene expression in cultured human endothelial cells. Alcohol Clin Exp Res 22:849–853

Grobbee DE, Rimm EB, Keil U, et al. (1999) Alcohol and the cardiovascular system. In: MacDonald I (ed) Health issues related to alcohol consumption. Blackwell Science, ILSI Europe, Brussel, pp 125–179

Gronbaek M, Deis A, SorensenTIA, et al. (1994) Influence of sex, age, body mass index, and smoking on alcohol intake and mortality. BMJ 308:302–306

Gronbaek M, Deis A, Sorensen TIA, et al. (1995) Mortality associated with moderate intakes of wine, beer, or spirits. BMJ 310:1165–1169

Hansagi H, Romelsjö A, Gerhardson de Verdier M, et al. (1995) Alcohol consumption and stroke mortality. 20 year follow-up of 15,077 men and women. Stroke 26:1768–1673

Hendriks HFJ, Veenstra J, Velthuis-te Wierik EJM, et al. (1994) Effect of moderate dose of alcohol with evening meal on fibrinolytic factors. BMJ 308:1003–1006

Hendriks HFJ, Veenstra J, van Tol A, et al. (1998) Moderate doses of alcoholic beverages with dinner and postprandial high density lipoprotein composition. Alcohol Alcoholism 33:403–410

Hendriks HFJ, Van der Gaag MS (1998) Alcohol, coagulation and fibrinolysis. In: Chadwick DJ, Goode JA (eds) Alcohol and cardiovascular diseases. Wiley, Chichester (Novartis Foundation Symposium 216) pp 111–124

Hendriks HFJ, Van Haaren MR, Leenen R, et al. (2001) Moderate alcohol consumption and postprandial lipids in men with different risks for coronary heart disease. Alcohol Clin Exp Res 25:563–570

Hernandez AF, Pla A, Valenzuela A, et al. (1993) Paraoxonase activity in human pericardial fluid: its relationship to coronary artery disease. Int J Legal Med 105:321–324

Hillbom M, Numminen H, Juvela S (1999) Recent heavy drinking of alcohol and embolic stroke. Stroke 30:2307–2312

Hines LM, Stampfer MJ, Ma J, et al. (2001) Genetic variation in alcohol dehydrogenase and the beneficial effect of moderate alcohol consumption on myocardial infarction. N Engl J Med 344:549–555

Hotta K, Funahashi T, Bodkin NL, et al. (2001) Circulating concentrations of the adipocyte protein adiponectin are decreased in parallel with reduced insulin sensitivity during the progression to type 2 diabetes in rhesus monkeys. Diabetes 50:1126–1133

Howes LG, Reid JL (1986) Changes in blood pressure and autonomy reflexes following regular moderate alcohol consumption. J Hypertension 4:421–425

Hupkens CLH, Knibbe RA, Drop MJ (1993) Alcohol consumption in the European Community: uniformity and diversity in drinking patterns. Addiction 88:1391–1404

Imai Y, Morita H, Kurihara H, et al. (2000) Evidence for association between paraoxonase gene polymorphisms and atherosclerotic diseases. Atherosclerosis 149:435–442

Juvela S, Hillbom M, Palomäki H (1995) Risk factors for spontaneous intracerebral hemorrhage. Stroke 26:1558–1564

Kadis P, Balazic J, Ferlan-Marolt V (1999) Alcoholic ketoacidiosis: a cause of sudden death of chronic alcoholics. Forensic Sci Int 103:S53–S59

Kalant H, Poikolainen K (1999). Moderate drinking: concepts, definitions and public health significance. In: MacDonald I (ed) Health issues related to alcohol consumption. Blackwell Science, ILSI Europe, Brussel, pp 1–27

Keil U, Swales JD, Grobbee, DE (1993) Alcohol intake and its relation to hypertension. In: Verschuren PM (ed) Health issues related to alcohol consumption. Blackwell Science, ILSI Europe, Brussel, pp 17–42

Keil U, Chambless LE, Döring A, et al. (1997) The relation of alcohol intake to coronary heart disease and all-cause mortality in a beer-drinking population. Epidemiology 8:150–156

Kitamura A, Iso H, Sankai T, et al. (1998) Alcohol intake and premature coronary heart disease in urban Japanese men. Am J Epidemiol 147:59–65

Kiyohara Y, Kato I, Iwamoto H, et al. (1995) The impact of alcohol and hypertension on stroke incidence in a general Japanese population. Stroke 26:368–372

Klatsky AL (1994) Epidemiology of coronary heart disease—influence of alcohol. Alcohol Clin Exp Res 18:88–96

Klatsky AL, Armstrong MA, Friedman GD (1997) Red wine, white wine, liquor, beer, and risk of coronary heart disease hospitalization. Am J Cardiol 80:416–420

Klatsky AL, Friedman GD, Armstrong MA et al. (2003) Wine, liquor, beer, and mortality. Am J Epidemiol 158:585–595

Koenig W, Sund M, Fröhlich M, et al. (1999) C-Reactive protein, a sensitive marker of inflammation, predicts future risk of coronary heart disease in initially healthy middle-aged men: results from the MONICA (Monitoring Trends and Determinants in Cardiovascular Disease) Augsburg Cohort Study, 1984 to 1992. Circulation 99:237–242

Kondo K, Matsumoto A, Kurata H, et al. (1994) Inhibition of oxidation of low-density lipoprotein with red wine. Lancet 344:1152

Lands WEM, Zakhari S (1991) The case of the missing calories. Am J Clin Nutr 54:47

Langer RD, Criqui MH, Reed DM (1992) Lipoproteins and blood pressure as biological pathways for effect of moderate alcohol consumption on coronary heart disease. Circulation 85:910–915

Leus FR, Wittekoek ME, Prins J, et al. (2000) Paraoxonase gene polymorphisms are associated with carotid arterial wall thickness in subjects with familial hypercholesterolemia. Atherosclerosis 149:371–377

Lian C (1915) L'alcoholisme, cause d'hypertension artérielle. Bull Acad Natl Méd Paris 74:525–528

MacDonald I, Debry G, Westerterp K (1993) Alcohol and overweight. In: Verschuren PM (ed) Health issues related to alcohol consumption. Blackwell Science, ILSI Europe, Brussel, pp 263–279

Mackness MI, Durrington PN (1995) HDL, its enzymes and its potential to influence lipid peroxidation. Atherosclerosis 115:243–253

Mackness MI, Arrol A, Mackness B et al. (1997) Alloenzymes of paraoxonase and effectiveness of high-density lipoproteins in protecting low-density lipoprotein against lipid peroxidation. Lancet 349:851–852

Mackness B, Mackness MI, Arrol S, et al. (1998) Effect of human serum paraoxonase 55 and 192 polymorphisms on the protection by high density lipoprotein against low density lipoprotein oxidative modification. FEBS Lett 423:57–60

Mackness MI, Mackness B, Durrington PN, et al. (1998) Paraoxonase and coronary heart disease. Curr Opin Lipidiol 9:319–324

Maheswaran R, Beevers M, Beevers DG (1992) Effectiveness of advice to reduce alcohol consumption in hypertensive patients. Hypertension 19:79–84

Mayer O Jr, Simon J, Rosolova H (2001) A population study of the influence of beer consumption on folate and homocsteine concentrations. Eur J Clin Nutr 55:605–609

McDonald JT, Margen S (1976) Wine versus ethanol in human nutrition. I. Nitrogen and calorie balance. Am J Clin Nutr 29:1093–1103

McElveen J, Mackness MI, Colley CM, et al. (1986) Distribution of paraoxon hydrolytic activity in the serum of patients after myocardial infarction. Clin Chem 32:671–673

Meagher EA, Barry OP, Burke A, et al. (1999) Alcohol-induced generation of lipid peroxidation products in humans. J Clin Invest 104:805–813

Mitchell MC, Herlong HF (1986) Alcohol and nutrition: caloric value, bioenergetics and relationship to liver damage. Ann Rev Nutr 6:457–474

Mukamal KJ, Conigrave KM, Mittleman MA, et al. (2003) Roles of drinking pattern and type of alcohol consumed in coronary heart disease in men. N Engl J Med 348:109–118

Muller MJ (1999) Alcohol and body weight. Z Gastroenterol 37:33–43

Muntwyler J, Hennekens CH, Buring JE, et al. (1998) Mortality and light to moderate alcohol consumption after myocardial infarction. Lancet 352:1882–1885

Nakanishi N, Kawashimo H, Nakamura K, et al. (2001) Association of alcohol consumption with increase in aortic stiffness: a 9-year longitudinal study in middle-aged Japanese men. Ind Health 39:24–28

Namekata T, Moore D, Suzuki K, et al. (1997) A study of the association between the aortic pulse wave velocity and atherosclerotic risk factors among Japanese Americans in Seattle, USA. Nippon Koshu Eisei Zasshi 44:942–951

Nanchahal K, Ashton WD, Wood DA (2000) Alcohol consumption, metabolic cardiovascular risk factors and hypertension in women. Int J Epidemiol 29:57–64

Nishiwaki M, Ishikawa T, Ito T et al. (1994) Effects of alcohol on lipoprotein lipase, hepatic lipase, cholesteryl ester transfer protein, and lecithin: cholesterol acyltransferase in high-density lipoprotein cholesterol elevation. Atherosclerosis 111:99–109

Orgogozo JM, Dartigues JF, Lafont S, et al. (1997) Wine consumption and dementia in the elderly: a prospective community study in the Bordeaux area. Rev Neurolog 153:185–192

Parker M, Puddey IB, Beilin LJ et al. (1990) A 2-way factorial study of alcohol and salt restriction in treated hypertensive men. Hypertension 16:398–406

Pikaar NA, Wedel M, Hermus RJJ (1988) Influence of several factors on blood alcohol concentrations after drinking alcohol. Alcohol Alcoholism 23:289–297

Pischon T, Girman CJ, Hotamisligil GS, et al. (2004) Plasma adiponectin levels and risk of myocardial infarction in men. JAMA 291:1730–1737

Rehm JT, Bondy SJ, Sempos CT, et al. (1997) Alcohol consumption and coronary heart disease morbidity and mortality. Am J Epidemiol 146:495–501

Renaud SC, Guéguen R, Schenker J, et al. (1998) Alcohol and mortality in middle-aged men from Eastern France. Epidemiology 9:184–188

Renaud SC, Gueguen R, Siest G, et al. (1999) Wine, beer, and mortality in middle-aged men from eastern France. Arch Int Med 159:1865–1870

Ridker PM, Buring JE, Shih J, et al. (1998) Prospective study of C-reactive protein and the risk of future cardiovascular events among apparently healthy women. Circulation 98:731–733

Rimm EB, Giovannuci EL, Willett WC, et al. (1991) A prospective study of alcohol consumption and the risk of coronary heart disease in men. Lancet 338:464–468

Rimm EB, Klatsky A, Grobbee D, et al. (1996) Review of moderate alcohol consumption and reduced risk of coronary heart disease: is the effect due to beer, wine, or spirits? BMJ 312:731–736

Rimm EB, Williams P, Fosher K, et al. (1999) Moderate alcohol intake and lower risk of coronary heart disease: meta-analysis of effects on lipids and haemostatic factors. BMJ 319:1523–1528

Ruitenberg A, Van Swieten JC, Witteman JC, et al. (2002) Alcohol consumption and risk of dementia: the Rotterdam Study. Lancet 359:281–286

Sacco RL, Elkind M, Boden-Albala B, et al. (1999) The protective effect of moderate alcohol consumption on ischemic stroke. JAMA 281:53–60

Scheig R (1970) Effects of ethanol on the liver. Am J Clin Nutr 23:467–473

Sharpe PC, McGrath LT, McClean E, et al. (1995) Effect of red wine consumption on lipoprotein (a) and other risk factors for atherosclerosis. Q J Med 88:101–108

Sierksma A, Van der Gaag MS, Schaafsma G, et al. (2001) Moderate alcohol consumption and fibrinolytic factors of pre- and postmenopausal women. Nutr Res 21:171–181

Sierksma A, Van der Gaag MS, Kluft C et al. (2002) Moderate alcohol consumption reduces plasma C-reactive protein and fibrinogen levels; a randomized, diet-controlled intervention study. Eur J Clin Nutr 56:1130–1136

Sierksma A, Van der Gaag MS, Van Tol, et al. (2002) Kinetics of HDL-cholesterol and paraoxonase activity in moderate alcohol consumers. Alcohol Clin Exp Res 26:1430–1435

Sierksma A, Lebrun CEI, Van der Schouw YT, et al. (2004) Alcohol consumption in relation to aortic stiffness and aortic wave reflections: a cross-sectional study in healthy postmenopausal women. Arterioscler Thromb Vasc Biol 24:342–348

Sierksma A, Muller M, Van der Schouw YT, et al. (2004) Alcohol consumption and arterial stiffness in men. J Hypertens 22:357–362

Sierksma A, Patel H, Ouchi N, et al. (2004) Effect of moderate alcohol consumption on adiponectin, tumor necrosis factor-α, and insulin sensitivity. Diabetes Care 27:184–189

Sierksma A, Vermunt SHF, Lankhuizen IM, et al. (2004) Effect of moderate alcohol consumption on parameters of reverse cholesterol transport in postmenopausal women. Alcohol Clin Exp Res 28:662–666

Siler SQ, Nees RA, Hellerstein MK (1999) De novo lipogenesis, lipid kinetics, and whole-body lipid balances in humans after acute alcohol consumption. Am J Clin Nutr 70:928–936

Stampfer MJ, Colditz GA, Willett WC, et al. (1988) A prospective study of moderate alcohol consumption and the risk of coronary disease and stroke in women. N Engl J Med 319:267–273

Stickel F, Hoehn B, Schuppan D, et al. (2003) Review article: nutritional therapy in alcoholic liver disease. Aliment Pharmacol Ther 18:357–373

Suter PM, Schutz Y, Jequier E (1992) The effect of ethanol on fat storage in healthy subjects, N Eng J Med 326:983–987

Tam SP (1992) Effect of ethanol on lipoprotein secretion in two human hepatoma cell lines, Hep G2 and Hep 3B. Alcohol Clin Exp Res 16:1021–1028

Taskinen M-R, Valimaki M, Nikkila EA, et al. (1985) Sequence of alcohol-induced initial changes in plasma lipoproteins (VLDL and HDL) and lipolytic enzymes in humans. Metabolism 34:112–119

Thun MJ, Peto R, Lopez AD, et al. (1997) Alcohol consumption and mortality among middle-aged and elderly US adults. N Engl J Med 337:1705–1714

Van der Gaag MS, Van Tol A, Scheek L, et al. (1999) Daily moderate alcohol consumption increases serum paraoxonase activity; a diet-controlled, randomised intervention study in middle-aged men. Atherosclerosis 147:405–410

Van der Gaag, M.S., Ubbink, J.B., Sillanaukee, P., Nikkari, S. and Hendriks, H.F.J. (2000a). Effect of consumption of red wine, spirits, and beer on serum homocysteine. Lancet 355, 1522

Van der Gaag MS, Van den Berg R, Van den Berg H, et al. (2000b) Moderate consumption of beer, red wine and spirits has counteracting effects on plasma antioxidants in middle-aged men. Eur J Clin Invest 54:586–591

Van der Gaag MS, Van Tol A, Vermunt SHF, et al. (2001) Alcohol consumption stimulates early steps in reverse cholesterol transport. J Lipid Res 42:2077–2083

Van Popele NM, Grobbee DE, Bots ML, et al. (2001) Association between arterial stiffness and atherosclerosis: the Rotterdam Study. Stroke 32:454–460

Van Tol A, Groener JEM, Scheek LM et al. (1995) Induction of net mass lipid transfer reactions in plasma by wine consumption with dinner. Eur J Clin Invest 25:390–395

Van Tol A, Van der Gaag MS, Scheek LM, et al. (1998) Changes in postprandial lipoproteins of low and high density caused by moderate alcohol consumption with dinner. Atherosclerosis 141:S101–S103

Van Tol A, Hendriks HFJ (2001) Moderate alcohol consumption: effects on lipids and cardiovascular disease risk. Curr Opin Lipidol 12:19–23

Veenstra J, Schenkel JAA, van Erp-Baart AMJ, et al. (1993) Alcohol consumption in relation to food intake and smoking habits in the Dutch National Food Consumption Survey, Eur J Clin Nutr 47:482–489

Vliegenthart R, Geleijnse JM, Hofman A, et al. (2002) Alcohol consumption and risk of peripheral arterial disease: the Rotterdam Study. Am J Epidemiol 155:332–338

Wannamethee G, Shaper AG. Alcohol and sudden cardiac death (1992) Br Heart J. 68:443–448

Watson AD, Berliner JA, Hama SY, et al. (1995) Protective effect of high density lipoprotein associated paraoxonase-inhibition of the biological activity of minimally oxidized low density lipoprotein. J Clin Invest 96:2882–2891

Westerterp KR, Meijer EP, Goris AH et al. (2004) Alcohol energy intake and habitual physical activity in older adults. Br J Nutr 91:149–152

Weyer C, Funahashi T, Tanaka S, et al. (2001) Hypoadiponectinemia in obesity and type 2 diabetes: close association with insulin resistance and hyperinsulinemia. J Clin Endocrinol Metab 86:1930–1935

White IR (1999) The level of alcohol consumption at which all-cause mortality is least. J Clin Epidemiol 52:967–975

Yuan J-M, Ross RK, Gao Y-T, et al. (1997) Follow up study of moderate alcohol intake and mortality among middle-aged men in Shanghai, China. BMJ 314:18–23

Part III

Evidence-Based Anti-Atherosclerotic Drug Therapy

HEP (2005) 170:365–388

Lipid and Non-lipid Effects of Statins

R. Paoletti (✉) · C. Bolego · A. Cignarella

Department of Pharmacological Sciences, University of Milan, via Balzaretti 9,
20133 Milan, Italy
rodolfo.paoletti@unimi.it

Abstract Long- and short-term trials with the 3-hydroxy-3-methylglutaryl coenzyme A reductase inhibitors (statins) have demonstrated significant reductions in cardiovascular events in patients with and without history of coronary heart disease. Statins are well-established low-density lipoprotein (LDL)-lowering agents, but their clinical benefit is believed to result from a number of lipid and non-lipid effects beyond LDL lowering, including a rise in plasma high-density lipoprotein levels. Beyond improving the lipid profile, statins have additional non-lipid effects including benefit on endothelial function, inflammatory mediators, intima-media thickening, prothombotic factors that ultimately result in plaque stabilization. These effects arise through the inhibition of several mevalonate-derived metabolites other than cholesterol itself, which are involved in the control of different cellular functions. Although statins represent the gold standard in the prevention and treatment of coronary heart disease, combination therapy with other lipid-lowering drugs, as well as novel therapeutic indications, may increase their therapeutic potential.

Keywords Statins · Coronary heart disease · LDL cholesterol · Pleiotropic effects ·
Plaque stabilization

1
Introduction

The direct correlation between plasma levels of low-density lipoprotein (LDL)-cholesterol (C) and the development of atherosclerosis is well established. Pharmacological lipid-lowering therapy is therefore a rational approach towards reduction of cardiovascular risk. The most significant achievements in this field came with the development of 3-hydroxy-3-methylglutaryl coenzyme A (HMG-CoA) reductase inhibitors (statins). By inhibiting the committed step in its biosynthetic pathway, statins prevent the intracellular synthesis of cholesterol and increase expression of LDL receptors particularly in the liver, whereby the plasma concentration of LDL particles is reduced. Several statins are currently available. All share an HMG-like moiety, which may be inactive in lacton form, to be hydrolysed in vivo, or in active hydroxyl-acid form. Lovastatin has been the first statin available for clinical use since 1987; thereafter simvastatin, pravastatin, fluvastatin and atorvastatin were introduced. Rosuvastatin and pitavastatin are the most recent additions to the group (Fig. 1; Bolego et al. 2002). Another compound, cerivastatin, was withdrawn from the market in August 2001 because of serious adverse effects arising especially when combined with gemfibrozil. This occurred because gemfibrozil (but not other fibrates) impairs the biotransformation of cerivastatin, in particular its glucuronidation (Thompson et al. 2003).

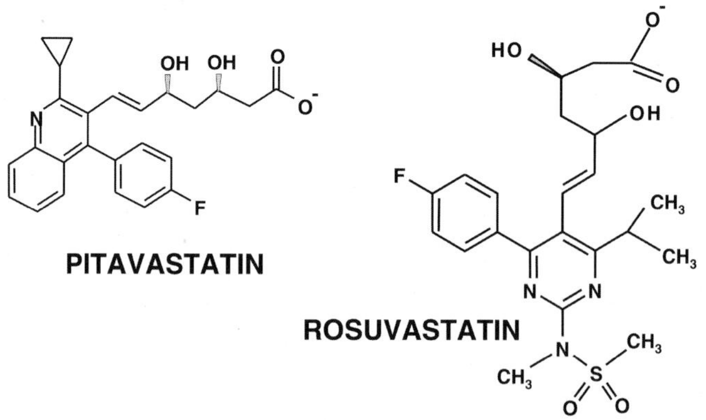

Fig. 1 The chemical structure of the newly introduced statins rosuvastatin and pitavastatin

Despite some differences in lipophilicity (Fig. 2) and pharmacokinetics (Table 1), statins may be regarded as a rather homogeneous class of drugs in terms of biological activity. Atorvastatin and rosuvastatin have longer half-lives. Atorvastatin, lovastatin and simvastatin are metabolized primarily by the cytochrome P450 3A4 isoenzyme, whereas fluvastatin and rosuvastatin appear to undergo little biotransformation via this pathway. By contrast, pravastatin and pitavastatin are scarcely biotransformed by liver microsomes. Pravastatin and rosuvastatin are rather hydrophilic compounds, in contrast to the other members of the group. Nevertheless, large-scale trials using four different statins so far (lovastatin, simvastatin, pravastatin, and atorvastatin) reported relative risk reductions for major coronary events between 24% and 37% in subjects with or without coronary heart disease (CHD) (Gotto 2003).

Statins reduce cardiovascular morbidity and mortality, as shown by large randomized clinical trials in selected types of high-risk patients over the last 10 years (Scandinavian Simvastatin Survival Study Group 1994; Shepherd et al. 1995; Sacks et al. 1996; Downs et al. 1998; The LIPID Study Group 1998; HPS Collaborative Group 2002; Athyros et al. 2002; Shepherd et al. 2002; Sever et al. 2003). The most recent large trials, however, are based on the novel

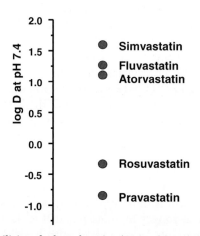

Fig. 2 The relative lipophilicity of selected statins (*D*, partition coefficient)

Table 1 Pharmacokinetic parameters of selected statins

	Lova	Simva	Prava	Fluva	Atorva	Rosuva
Absorption (%)	31	60–85	35	98	30	20
Half-life (h)	2–4	1–2	1–3	1–2	15–30	20
Protein binding (%)	95	98	40–50	99	98	90
Renal excretion (%)	30	13	60	6	2	10
Active metabolites	+	+	–	–	+	–

paradigm of global risk reduction, which overcomes and merges the previous distinction between primary and secondary prevention. Accordingly, the large 5-year MRC/BHF Heart Protection Study evaluated the effect of simvastatin in more than 20,000 patients considered at high risk for CHD death regardless of the nature of underlying risk factors. For instance, about 4,000 patients had no history of CHD and about 7,000 of them had LDL-C below 115 mg/dl (3 mmol/l). Treatment with 40 mg simvastatin daily reduced the rates of major vascular events across the board by about 25% (HPS Collaborative Group 2002). One of the most important lessons from this trial is that statin therapy produces significant clinical benefit regardless of baseline cholesterol values. Similar findings came from the LIPS trial carried out in 1,677 patients undergoing percutaneous transluminal coronary angioplasty (Serruys et al. 2002).

2
Statins and Cardiovascular Disease: LDL Lowering and Beyond

The clinical benefit associated with statin therapy has been ascribed to substantial reduction of serum LDL-C. Although this is the most popular interpretation of clinical trials' results, evidence now indicates that the lowering of LDL-C may not entirely account for the beneficial effects of statin treatment. In fact, a number of preclinical studies showed that statins improve vascular function in many respects without inducing major lipid changes. Further support to this notion is provided by clinical trials showing that reductions in cerebrovascular risk were achieved with lipid-lowering regimens that had limited effect on LDL-C levels (Rubins et al. 1999). This means that statins, beyond reducing LDL-C levels as a first-step result of their molecular mechanism, reduce non-LDL-C as well as non-lipid risk factors, although the clinical relevance of these pleiotropic effects still needs to be fully ascertained at the clinical level.

Statins lower LDL-C levels in a dose-dependent manner across the dose range tested (2.5–80 mg/day). A recent comparison among different statins indicated that rosuvastatin is more potent than atorvastatin, simvastatin and pravastatin across dose ranges at reducing LDL-C in more than 2,000 hypercholesterolaemic patients as compared with baseline (Jones et al. 2003). According to a meta-analysis of short-term trials of six statins and LDL-C reduction (Law et al. 2003), rosuvastatin 5 mg/day, atorvastatin 10 mg/day and lovastatin or simvastatin 40 mg/day reduced LDL concentrations by about 35%; fluvastatin and pravastatin produced smaller reductions even at the highest dose of 80 mg/day. The absolute reductions in LDL-C were greater in those with higher pre-treatment concentrations. The reduction in risk of fatal CHD events and non-fatal myocardial infarction for each 1 mmol/l (38.5 mg/dl) decrease in serum LDL concentrations was estimated by duration of treatment. Taking into account some 76,000 treated individuals, this reduction was 11% in the first year, 24% in the second, 33% in the third to fifth year combined and

36% in the sixth and subsequent years (Law et al. 2003). Thus, the longer one goes with statin treatment, the more LDL drops. This translates into a remarkable reduction in CHD associated with cholesterol reduction that can be more apparent from the third year of treatment on.

3
Effects of Statins on Lipid Classes Other Than LDL-C

Increasing knowledge of the pathophysiology of atherosclerosis has revealed other lipid risk factors beyond LDL-C and enhanced our understanding of how these risk factors affect disease. Recent advances in basic science focusing on the biochemical and functional heterogeneity of traditional lipoprotein classes have allowed definition of lipoprotein subfractions such as lipoprotein(a) [Lp(a)]), small, dense LDL particles, and subspecies of very-low-density lipoprotein (VLDL) and high-density lipoprotein (HDL). Recent studies indicated that HDL represents a heterogeneous group of particles differing in their biochemical function as well as anti-atherogenic potential. Today, rather than just lowering LDL-C, drug therapy should be endowed with widespread impact on a set of risk factors in high-risk individuals. Statins exhibit well established effects on circulating lipids and lipoprotein subclasses that are rounded off with an array of desirable additional effects on vascular function that are probably unrelated to lipid lowering.

3.1
HDL Levels

Low HDL is an important risk factor in CHD. It is well established that the CHD risk associated with low HDL-C is independent from other lipid and non-lipid risk factors (Gordon et al. 1977; Goldbourt et al. 1997). Low HDL-C with normal LDL-C occurs in large numbers of CHD patients. Many studies proved that low HDL concentrations often associated with elevated triglycerides predict premature CHD (Krauss 1998). In addition to the classical effect of increasing reverse cholesterol transport, HDL appears to improve the biology of the vessel wall in vivo (Nofer et al. 2002). This has been shown, for example, by enhanced endothelium-dependent vasodilation in hypercholesterolaemic patients after intravenous recombinant HDL infusion (Spieker et al. 2002) or by reduced cytokine-stimulated expression of adhesion molecules after injection of reconstituted HDL (Cockerill et al. 2001). These properties appear to be promoted by different components of HDL. Therefore, changes in HDL function along with mere changes in plasma HDL levels could be related to the benefit of pharmacological alterations in HDL metabolism. Much interest has been focused to HDL metabolism as a target for pharmacological intervention in atherosclerosis.

The aggregate evidence from a literature review on HDL response to therapy points to a 5%–10% increase in HDL following statin treatment. This modest HDL-raising effect is not dose dependent (Stein et al. 2000). The mechanism whereby statins affect HDL metabolism remains controversial (von Eckardstein and Assmann 2000). Both HDL production and HDL catabolism appear to be possible targets of the action of statins , therefore the above-mentioned rise in plasma levels of HDL may result from combined effects (Table 2). Statins have been shown to increase HDL-C by acting on lipoprotein lipase and hepatic lipase. In fact, HDL-C was positively associated with lipoprotein lipase activity and negatively associated with HL activity (Colvin et al. 1991). Statins may affect HDL-C metabolism also by selectively up-regulating the SR-BI receptor in the liver, which would facilitate the selective uptake of cholesteryl ester from circulating HDL (Tsuruoka et al. 2002). Finally, statins increase apolipoprotein (apo)A-I synthesis and secretion into plasma (Schaefer et al. 1999) probably by activating peroxisome proliferator-activated receptor alpha (PPARα) (Martin et al. 2001). It cannot be ruled out though that statins affect HDL metabolism and plasma HDL levels through modulation of ABCA1 or other transporters of the same family involved in cholesterol trafficking in the liver and in peripheral cells.

A recent meta-analysis of randomized comparative trials indicated that HDL-C and apoA-I were generally increased with doses of simvastatin ranging from 10 to 80 mg, but apparently exhibited a dose-dependent decrease with increasing doses of atorvastatin (Wierzbicki and Mikhailidis 2002) probably because of an enhanced turnover of apoA-I. At equivalent LDL-reducing doses, simvastatin appears to have a greater effect on HDL than atorvastatin at higher doses (Crouse et al. 1999, Kastelein et al. 2000). Higher doses of simvastatin have greater effects on reducing non-HDL cholesterol and increasing HDL-C and apo A-I (Stein et al. 2000) than the doses used, for example, in the 4S study (20–40 mg/day) (Scandinavian Simvastatin Survival Study Group 1994). Simvastatin at maximum dose (80 mg) increased HDL-C and apo A-I significantly more than did atorvastatin (80 mg) in 917 patients with hypercholesterolaemia at all baseline HDL level and with fewer effects on liver enzymes (Ballantyne et al. 2003). The CURVES study is the first trial to compare the effects of all statins in clinical use across their dose ranges in hypercholesterolaemic pa-

Table 2 Possible mechanisms underlying the effect of statins on HDL metabolism

Decreased cholesteryl ester transfer protein activity
Decreased lipoprotein lipase activity
Decreased hepatic lipase activity
Up-regulation of SR-BI in the liver
Increased synthesis and secretion of apoA-I

SR-BI, scavenger receptor BI.

tients after 8 weeks of treatment (Jones et al. 1998). Effects on HDL, ranging from 3% to 10%, were not different between atorvastatin and the other HMG-CoA reductase inhibitors except at the 40-mg dose, when simvastatin produced greater elevations in HDL-C than atorvastatin. Rosuvastatin has demonstrated increases in HDL-C as well as reductions in triglycerides across a dose range of up to 80 mg/day (Olsson et al. 2001), with no clear dose–response relationship. In a recent study in patients with type IIa or IIb hypercholesterolaemia, HDL-C levels were increased significantly in the rosuvastatin 5-mg group (13%) compared with atorvastatin (8%). Rosuvastatin proved effective even at lower doses, as shown in patients with primary hypercholesterolaemia (Yamamoto et al. 2002). HDL-C increased by 3% to 7% in patients receiving once-daily doses of 1, 2 or 4 mg rosuvastatin over 8 weeks of therapy. Although lacking the placebo group, this study indicated for the first time that rosuvastatin is effective on HDL as well as on total cholesterol, LDL-C and triglyceride levels at doses as low as 1–4 mg/day.

Statins are able to increase HDL levels but the magnitude of this effect is small compared to that on LDL and triglycerides. Some statins appear to be more effective than others, indicating that LDL and HDL response to statin treatment may occur through distinct pathways. Further, the mean absolute statin-related increment in HDL across a range of baseline values varies little, as shown by a subgroup analysis of patients included in the WOSCOPS trial (Streja et al. 2002). This implies that factors affecting the baseline values as well as the absolute increment of HDL could contribute to the ultimate modest HDL elevation following statin treatment.

In a cumulative analysis of the LIPID and CARE trials, HDL-C was a significantly stronger predictor of recurrent CHD events in patients with LDL below 125 mg/dl than in those with 125 mg/dl or greater (Sacks et al. 2002a). Increasing evidence suggests that HDL-raising effects should be considered to be as important as LDL-lowering, especially in high-risk individuals with features of the metabolic syndrome. Overall, although therapy with statins is effective in reducing the risk of CHD through lowering LDL-C levels, the remaining risk associated with a low HDL-C is still significant and is only mildly affected by the otherwise beneficial therapeutic effects of statins (Sacks et al. 2001, 2002b).

3.2
HDL Subclass Profile

As for LDL, not the concentration of HDL per se but that of specific HDL subclasses appears to contribute to the different functions of HDL. It is thought that only the larger HDL subclasses confer protection against CHD, with the smallest subclasses being associated with an increased CHD risk (von Eckardstein et al. 1994). The effects of atorvastatin, fluvastatin, lovastatin, pravastatin and simvastatin on HDL subclasses were compared in patients with established CHD (Asztalos et al. 2002a). All five statins had comparable effects with regard to changes in the concentrations of HDL-C and apoA-I. However, atorvastatin was the most effective statin at increasing the large LpA-I α_1-HDL particles, which in turn were significantly lower in CHD patients with respect to controls, and decreasing the concentration of the small, triglyceride-rich, LpA-I:A-II α_3-HDL subpopulations. In a further subgroup analysis (Asztalos et al. 2002b), atorvastatin significantly increased the large LpA-I α_1 and pre-α_1 HDL particles at both 40 and 80 mg/day. The responses of HDL-C and HDL subpopulation profile were not dose dependent, but were rather dependent on baseline lipid profiles. Thus, atorvastatin beneficially modifies the HDL subclass profile towards the patterns of healthy individuals. It will be interesting to determine whether specific HDL subclasses isolated from statin-treated subjects are more resistant to degradation by cell-derived proteolytic enzymes. Consequently, selective modulation of HDL subclasses may be the way ahead for the pharmacological management of CHD.

3.3
Small Dense LDL

Over the past several years, the importance of specific lipoprotein subclasses in the pathogenesis of cardiovascular disease has become more apparent. Certain lipoprotein phenotypes, such as small, dense LDL and VLDL particles, have been identified that are associated with increased risk of CHD events, independent of absolute LDL-C levels. Numerous studies provide evidence of the ability of statins to beneficially modify LDL subfraction concentrations. A recent study in hyperlipidaemic patients (Sasaki et al. 2002) showed that 3 months of treatment with atorvastatin 10–20 mg/day markedly decreased the proportion of small, dense LDL particles, with a shift to larger, less atherogenic particles. In patients with atherogenic dyslipidaemia (small, dense LDL particles, low HDL-C and elevated triglycerides), 12 weeks of treatment with atorvastatin 10 mg/day significantly increased the mean size of LDL particles and decreased concentrations of small LDL, intermediate-density lipoprotein (IDL), and VLDL subclass particles (McKenney et al. 2001). Increasing doses of atorvastatin (10–40 mg/day) preferentially reduced atherogenic small, dense LDL, IDL and the VLDL-2 subclass in patients with type IIb hyperlipidaemia and significantly enhanced the ability of plasma to promote cholesterol efflux, the first step in reverse cholesterol transport (Guerin et al. 2002). In patients with diabetic dyslipidaemia, atorvastatin 80 mg/day for 2 months significantly increased the mean LDL particle diameter from small, dense (25.29 nm) to intermediate (26.51 nm; Pontrelli et al. 2002). In patients with moderate combined hyperlipidaemia on atorvastatin and simvastatin 40 mg/day, both drugs markedly decreased all LDL subfractions. In particular, the concentration of small dense LDL (LDL-III) fell 64% on atorvastatin and 45% on simvastatin

(Forster et al. 2002). A similar action applied across the spectrum of apoB-containing lipoproteins, leading to substantial reductions in plasma triglyceride and LDL cholesterol.

3.4
Lipoprotein(a)

Elevated plasma levels of Lp(a) are a well-established risk factor for premature atherosclerosis and CHD (von Eckardstein et al. 2001; The Expert Panel 2002). Although statins have not had reliably beneficial effects on Lp(a) levels, a double-blind study of high-risk hypercholesterolaemic patients treated with atorvastatin 10 mg/day or simvastatin 20 mg/day for 6 weeks showed that both statins significantly reduced Lp(a) levels (Gonbert et al. 2002). Similarly, treatment with 80 mg atorvastatin or 40 mg simvastatin for 2 years significantly lowered Lp(a) in familial hypercholesterolaemic patients, but this change in Lp(a) concentrations was not correlated with change in intima-media thickness (IMT) over the time span of the trial (van Wissen et al. 2003). Overall, despite the inconsistency of the effects of statins on Lp(a) levels, the improvement of multiple risk factors with statins warrants their use in persons with elevated Lp(a).

4
Non-lipid Effects of Statins

There is no doubt that the beneficial effects of statins involve their hypolipidaemic activity. However, the HMG-CoA reductase product mevalonate is a precursor not only of cholesterol, but also of a number of key metabolites involved in the control of several cellular functions (Fig. 3). In particular, statins prevent the biosynthesis of the isoprenoids geranyl-geraniol and farnesol that are responsible for post-translational isoprenylation of a number of proteins regulating cell growth, membrane targeting and other key functions. Members of the *ras* and *rho* GTPase family are major substrates for post-translational modification by isoprenylation and may be important targets for inhibition by statins (Liao 2002; Laufs and Liao 2003). It is therefore conceivable that statins exert an anti-atherosclerotic action also through mechanisms other than lipid lowering, currently referred to as pleiotropic effects, affecting vascular cells such as macrophages, endothelial cells and smooth muscle cells (Corsini et al. 1999). Such effects may thus result in control of the main processes underlying clinical manifestations of atherosclerosis (Vaughan et al. 1996).

The pleiotropic effects of statins include the modulation of different factors of non-lipid nature. These include plasma markers of endothelial function and inflammation, particularly C-reactive protein (CRP), and morphological parameters of the arterial wall, such as IMT. An increasing number of in vitro

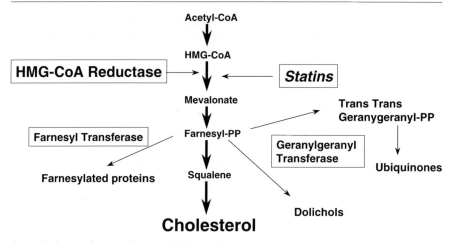

Fig. 3 The biosynthetic pathway of cholesterol and other biologically active isoprenoids (*PP*, pyrophosphate)

and in vivo studies indicate that statins have direct anti-inflammatory effects that appear not to be related to their hypocholesterolaemic activity (Weitz-Schmidt 2002).

4.1
Endothelial Function

Statins affect not only circulating lipoprotein levels and their composition, but also the function of a number of cell types, such as endothelial cells, involved in the pathogenesis of atherosclerosis. Endothelial dysfunction has been regarded as 'the risk of the risk factors' (Bonetti et al. 2003). These cellular effects may contribute to the clinical benefit of statins.

Recent findings indicate that simvastatin may accelerate endothelial regeneration after balloon injury and decrease restenosis in the rat carotid model (Walter et al. 2002). This activity may be related to an enhanced turnover of intact endothelial cells from the bone marrow. Data from in vitro experiments indicate that statins attenuate adhesion of monocytes to the endothelium, which is an early event in atherosclerosis (Teupser et al. 2001). Pre-treatment with atorvastatin (10 μM) reduced the adhesion of U937 monocytes to endothelial cells activated with interleukin 1β (Kawakami et al. 2002). This activity of atorvastatin appears to be unrelated to its cholesterol-lowering effects. Similarly, endothelial cell activation induced by anti-β2-glycoprotein I antibodies in vitro was prevented by treatment with simvastatin and fluvastatin (Meroni et al. 2001), thus suggesting a potential therapeutic role for statins in anti-phospholipid-syndromes.

Endothelial dysfunction is one of the first steps in the pathogenesis of atherosclerosis and may occur even in the absence of angiographic evidence of disease. One important consequence of endothelial dysfunction is the reduced biosynthesis of nitric oxide (NO), a key mediator of vascular tone. Statins have been shown to increase blood flow and reduce ischaemic areas in the brain of normolipidaemic mice by upregulating endothelial NO synthase function (Endres et al. 1998; Laufs et al. 2002). This protective effect, however, is reversed upon acute termination of statin treatment (Gertz et al. 2003). Regional haemo-dynamics improved with rosuvastatin in different models of hypertensive rats, as evidenced by increased blood flow and decreased vascular resistances in the absence of plasma lipid effects (Susic et al. 2003).

Flow-mediated vasodilation of the brachial artery is commonly used to measure endothelial function in humans. Endothelium-dependent vasodila-tion improved significantly after 24 weeks of fluvastatin therapy (40 mg twice a day) compared with baseline and placebo in hypercholesterolaemic patients on account of increased bioavailability of NO (John et al. 1998). In patients with diabetes, in whom endothelial dysfunction often appears early, statins have demonstrated beneficial effects. In 84 young adults with uncomplicated type 1 (insulin-dependent) diabetes and normal LDL-C levels, 6 weeks of treatment with atorvastatin 40 mg/day improved endothelial function (Mullen et al. 2000). In a study of patients with type 2 diabetes, atorvastatin 10 and 20 mg/day for 6 months significantly improved endothelium-dependent vasodilation com-pared with placebo. The reversal of endothelial dysfunction achieved with atorvastatin therapy in this study was correlated not with plasma lipids but with a significant decrease in CRP levels, suggesting an anti-inflammatory effect of atorvastatin (Tan et al. 2002).

The Diabetes Atorvastatin Lipid Intervention (DALI) study (The DALI Study Group 2001) was conducted in patients with type 2 (non-insulin-dependent) diabetes and diabetic dyslipidaemia. Atorvastatin 10 or 80 mg/day for 30 weeks effectively lowered triglycerides, LDL-C and apoB levels and increased HDL-C levels in these patients (The DALI Study Group 2001). However, no significant effects were reported on flow-mediated vasodilatation or response to sublin-gual nitro-glycerine, despite the observed improvement in lipid profile (van Venrooij et al. 2002; van Etten et al. 2002). By contrast, additional evidence for a protective effect of statins on the endothelium comes from a study in patients with type 2 diabetes treated with 40 mg/day simvastatin for 12 weeks (Ceriello et al. 2002). Despite the lack of significant lipid changes, statin treatment had acute beneficial effects on oxidative stress and improved flow-mediated vasodi-lation and endothelial dysfunction associated with post-prandial hypertriglyc-eridaemia and hyperglycaemia. In CHD patients treated with atorvastatin or simvastatin (20 mg/day) for 1 year, statin treatment reduced proinflammatory markers of endothelial dysfunction, such as intercellular adhesion molecule-1 (ICAM-1) and P-selectin, thereby attenuating the activated state of the en-dothelium (Seljeflot et al. 2002).

4.2
Inflammation

Considerable evidence suggests that vascular inflammation is involved in the development, progression and clinical expression of atherosclerosis (Ross 1999).

Atorvastatin was shown to inhibit in vitro the activation of cytokine-induced transcription factors, such as signal transducer and activator of transcription-1 and nuclear factor kappa B (NF-κB), in endothelial cells, preventing the expression of inducible NO synthase, an enzyme implicated in vascular inflammation (Wagner et al. 2002). Evidence for statin anti-inflammatory effects comes also from animal studies. Of note, rosuvastatin reduced the expression of the inflammation parameters monocyte chemoattractant protein-1 and tumour necrosis factor-α in the vessel wall and lowered plasma concentrations of serum amyloid A and fibrinogen in apoE3-Leiden mice on atherogenic diet, independently of its cholesterol-lowering effect (Kleemann et al. 2003).

The prototypic marker of inflammation, CRP, binds to oxidized LDL and apoptotic cells, but not to native LDL or viable cells, suggesting a key role for CRP in the early development of atherosclerotic plaques (Chang et al. 2002). Furthermore, elevated levels of CRP have been associated with increased CHD risk (Ridker et al. 2001) and with the development of type 2 diabetes (Festa et al. 2002). The clinical benefits on levels of CRP observed with statin treatment result, at least in part, from plaque stabilization produced by associated anti-inflammatory mechanisms. Wiklund et al. (2002) reported that atorvastatin, but not simvastatin, decreased the liver-derived acute phase reactants CRP and serum amyloid A in hypercholesterolaemic patients. The two statins reduced markers of local inflammation (soluble phospholipase A_2, ICAM-1 and interleukin 6) to a similar degree. In addition, simvastatin 20 mg/day, pravastatin 40 mg/day, and atorvastatin 10 mg/day produced similar reductions in high-sensitive CRP levels in patients with combined hyperlipidaemia (Jialal et al. 2001). In a substudy of the DALI trial, atorvastatin 10 and 80 mg/day for 30 weeks lowered median CRP levels by 15% and 47%, respectively, in patients with type 2 diabetes (van de Ree et al. 2003). Recently, high-dose atorvastatin treatment was shown to reduce CRP and serum amyloid A, but not interleukin 6, in 2402 subjects with acute coronary syndromes enrolled in the Myocardial Ischemia Reduction with Aggressive Cholesterol Lowering (MIRACL) study (Kinlay et al. 2003). From a clinical perspective, it is important to note that statins appear to have a rapid onset of anti-inflammatory activity (Plenge et al. 2002). All statins are effective at lowering CRP levels (Balk et al. 2003; Cignarella et al, 2003). No studies reported significant correlation between statin dose and CRP effects. By contrast, the studies that assessed changes in the concentration of homocysteine, a possible risk marker, with statin use indicated that statins have minor effects on homocysteine levels

(Balk et al. 2003). Overall it appears that stable inflammatory biomarkers are not related to lipid levels, yet both are critically involved in the atherothrombotic process.

4.3
LDL Oxidation

Oxidation of LDL is an important event in the atherosclerotic process. The susceptibility of LDL to oxidation can be evaluated using different in vitro methods, although it is not clear whether any method accurately reflects LDL oxidation in vivo. Fluvastatin has been shown to reduce LDL oxidation by binding to the phospholipid moiety of LDL (Hussein et al. 1997). Simvastatin reduces superoxide production from macrophages with a mevalonate-dependent mechanism, suggesting that isoprenylated proteins contribute to this effect (Giroux et al. 1993). Atorvastatin and fluvastatin generate potent anti-oxidant metabolites upon biotransformation (Aviram et al. 1998; Suzumura et al. 2000). However, the evidence from trials supporting a beneficial effect of statins overall on LDL susceptibility to oxidation is not consistent (Balk et al. 2003).

4.4
Athero-thrombotic Tendency

It has been demonstrated that CRP causes aortic endothelial cells to produce higher levels of plasminogen activator inhibitor-1 (PAI-1), a marker of atherothrombosis, especially when hyperglycaemia exists, thus suggesting a critical role for inflammation as a prothrombotic factor in diabetes and the metabolic syndrome (Devaraj et al. 2003). Statins have been reported to control a variety of prothrombotic factors even without major effects on plasma lipids. These effects include, for instance, decreased expression of tissue factor, the main activator of the coagulation cascade, in macrophages incubated with lipophilic statins (Colli et al. 1997). Treatment with fluvastatin reduced lipid accumulation, tissue factor overexpression, NF-κB activation and platelet deposition in hypercholesterolaemic rabbits (Camera et al. 2002). Similar findings came from the ATROCAP study in patients with bilateral carotid stenosis, in which atorvastatin (20 mg/day) decreased tissue factor antigen immunostaining and macrophage infiltration compared with placebo (Cortellaro et al. 2002). A large number of trials has been carried out to determine the effects of statins on the functional expression of tissue plasminogen activator, PAI-1 and fibrinogen as well as on platelet aggregation. There is convincing evidence for a lack of effect of any statin on fibrinogen level. While it appears that pravastatin is the only statin effective at reducing tissue plasminogen activator antigen levels (Avellone et al. 1994; Dangas et al. 1999), the effects of statins on PAI-1 antigen or activity levels reported in human trials are not consistent (Balk et al. 2003). The evidence supporting a beneficial role of statins in reducing platelet aggregation is limited. Claims that concomitant use of statins could block the anti-platelet activity of clopidogrel in patients with stable angina on aspirin therapy have not been confirmed (Müller et al. 2003).

4.5
Plaque Stabilization

Local and systemic factors contribute to make plaques vulnerable over time. Unstable plaques feature increased levels of lipids mainly in form of modified LDL, decreased amount of connective tissue, greater presence of macrophages and T cells with fewer smooth muscle cells, and high rate of apoptosis. Shear stress affects the morphology and organization of endothelial cells and supports deposition of modified LDL in the subendothelial space. Shear stress is particularly active at plaque shoulder, where the fibrous cap is thinner and may be gradually eroded until thrombogenic plaque components underneath the fibrous cap are exposed to blood flow, resulting in platelet activation and ultimately thrombus formation.

Macrophage-derived foam cells, a hallmark of early atherosclerotic lesions, store large amounts of cholesteryl ester in cytoplasm droplets. This uncontrolled uptake of cholesterol carried by modified LDL and its subsequent esterification ultimately leads to cell death and release of a number of inflammatory mediators. Statins have been shown to hamper cholesterol esterification, thereby preventing foam cell formation (Kempen et al. 1991; Bernini et al. 1993; Cignarella et al. 1998). In addition, fluvastatin and simvastatin reduce functional expression of macrophage metalloproteinase 9, a proteolytic enzyme affecting plaque stability (Bellosta et al. 1998).

Statins elicit morphological changes in the arterial wall and in plaque composition that enhance plaque stabilization. In preclinical studies, fluvastatin prevented the formation of neointimal lesions and tissue factor over-expression in the carotid artery of rabbits on hypercholesterolaemic diet without major lipid-lowering effects (Baetta et al. 2002). This negative regulation of smooth muscle cell growth and proliferation achieved with statins is of great interest, given the significant contribution of smooth muscle cells to the progression of atherosclerotic lesions. Impaired prenylation of proteins involved in signal transduction, such as those from the *ras* family, accounts for statin-induced inhibition of smooth muscle cell proliferation (Negre-Aminou et al. 1997).

Statins appear to be unique among drugs affecting plaque stabilization in that they control several aspects of plaque activation (Libby and Aikawa 2003). In a study using intravascular ultrasound, it was observed that the changes in plaque composition induced by atorvastatin therapy (more fibrosis, smaller lipid pool) led to less progression of plaque size and to significant different changes in plaque echogenicity in minor coronary lesions (Schartl et al. 2001).

These mechanisms are associated with the well-established reduction of serum LDL-C, which remains the most widely accepted explanation for the clinical benefit of statins.

Morphological parameters of the arterial wall, such as IMT, correlate with severity and future risk of clinical events. B-mode ultrasonography of IMT in the carotid artery has been shown to be correlated with existing cardiovascular disease and predictive of major events in individuals without clinically evident disease (Hodis et al. 1998; Baldassarre et al. 2000a). Carotid IMT is now widely used as a surrogate marker for atherosclerotic disease and has been proposed as an independent risk factor for myocardial infarction and stroke (O'Leary et al. 1999).

The Carotid Atherosclerosis Italian Ultrasound Study (CAIUS) (Mercuri et al. 1996) was designed to determine the efficacy of pravastatin 40 mg/day on carotid plaque progression in asymptomatic patients. Over the 3-year study period, pravastatin significantly delayed the rate of carotid IMT progression. A later analysis of the CAIUS data (Baldassarre et al. 2000b) indicated that the beneficial changes in IMT observed with pravastatin treatment occurred independently of LDL-C lowering. A further study (Youssef et al. 2002) demonstrated that atorvastatin 20 mg/day significantly reduced IMT in the carotid and femoral arteries after 8 weeks of treatment, with a significant trend detectable as early as 4 weeks. Similarly, results of the Arterial Biology for the Investigation of the Treatment Effects of Reducing Cholesterol (ARBITER) trial (Taylor et al. 2002) suggest that lowering LDL-C below than 2.59 mmol/l (100 mg/dl) with atorvastatin 80 mg/day is more effective than pravastatin 40 mg/day in reducing carotid IMT. The change in the mean carotid IMT at 12 months with atorvastatin was significantly greater than that with pravastatin. Whether or not LDL lowering and its apparent effects on IMT translate into a reduction in clinical events, however, remains to be clarified in ongoing clinical trials (Kastelein et al. 2003).

4.6
Lipid or Non-lipid: Is That the Question?

Several large randomized controlled trials using statins have shown reductions in mortality and CHD events in a variety of clinical settings. Statins are very effective in lowering total cholesterol and LDL-C levels. As the Heart Protection Study taught us, however, the high-risk patient for CHD does not match a single phenotype and may have normal cholesterol levels. By contrast, such patients featured multiple predisposing causes of cardiac events and yet could benefit from treatment with statins, which appear to reduce an array of risk factors. It seems therefore advisable to integrate the classical view of reducing LDL-C for prevention and treatment of CHD. Beyond LDL-C, a number of novel risk markers are emerging in the clinical arena and their role in vascular disease is supported by increasingly convincing evidence. Endothelial function and vascular inflammation, for example, claim further attention as primary targets of therapy, because of their crucial involvement in the regulation of progression and stability of atherosclerotic lesions (Szmitko et al. 2003; Bonetti et al. 2003). Today, rather than just lowering LDL-C, pharmacological therapy of CHD should be endowed with beneficial impact on the whole set of risk factors in high-risk individuals. Accordingly, statins exhibit well established effects on circulating lipids and lipoprotein subclasses that are rounded off with an array of desirable additional effects on vascular function that are probably unrelated to lipid lowering (all summarized in Table 3). Yet current evidence in humans suggests that the lipid-lowering effects pave the way for further effects of statins. The clinical relevance, if any, of non-lipid effects of statins shall be determined in clinical trials that would allow the cholesterol-dependent and -independent effects of statins to be evaluated separately.

Table 3 Potential effects of statins beyond LDL lowering

Lipoprotein subfractions
Beneficially modify HDL particles
Decrease proportion of small, dense LDL particles
Shift small, dense to larger LDL particles
Markers of endothelial function
Attenuate adhesion of monocytes to endothelium
Up-regulate endothelial NO synthase
Decrease oxidative stress
Vascular inflammation
Reduce levels of CRP
Reduce markers of local inflammation
Plaque stabilization
Inhibit macrophage foam cell formation
Prevent smooth muscle cell proliferation
Decrease plaque thrombogenicity
Delay carotid IMT progression

CRP, C-reactive protein; HDL, high-density lipoprotein; IMT, intima-media thickness; LDL, low-density lipoprotein; NO, nitric oxide.

5
Future Directions of Statin Therapy

The array of statin effects associated with lipid-lowering have led investigators to test their therapeutic potential in clinical settings other than vascular disease. Despite the lack of clinical evidence, preclinical results or observational studies are encouraging and warrant further investigation. For instance, simvastatin reduced collagen-induced arthritis in mice (Leung et al. 2003). Statins also attenuate transplant graft arterial disease in murine heart transplants, showing a potential immunosuppressive activity (Shimizu et al. 2003). Similarly, much interest has arisen whether statins might prove effective in the treatment of central nervous system autoimmune and neuroinflammatory disorders including multiple sclerosis and related disease (Stuve et al. 2003). Moreover, observational studies point to beneficial effects of statins in depression and anxiety (Young-Xu et al. 2003). An over-enthusiastic interpretation of these preliminary studies, however, should be avoided. The clinical benefits of statins in CHD are well established and are associated with remarkable safety and risk to benefit ratio. Beyond seeking further therapeutic indications for statins, attention should be focused on the at least 60% of CHD events continuing to occur despite lipid-lowering therapy. In this regard, combination therapy with statins and other lipid-lowering drugs such as ezetimide or nicotinic acid may prove a rewarding strategy. In addition, statins could be associated with other drugs acting on the cardiovascular system, such as ACE inhibitors or calcium channel blockers.

6
Conclusion

From the above considerations, successful therapeutic approaches in atherosclerosis should allow control of multiple aspects of vascular biology. Statins fulfil such a requirement in that they show well-established lipid-lowering properties along with direct effects on the vessel wall. The latter might contribute to the eventual clinical benefit. Yet combination therapy may be of use in specific clinical settings to extend clinical benefit to a larger proportion of patients.

References

Asztalos BF, Horvath KV, McNamara JR et al. (2002a) Comparing the effects of five different statins on the HDL subpopulation profiles of coronary heart disease patients. Atherosclerosis 164:361–369

Asztalos BF, Horvath KV, McNamara JR et al. (2002b) Effects of atorvastatin on the HDL subpopulation profile of coronary heart disease patients. J Lipid Res 43:1701–1707

Athyros VG, Papageorgiou AA, Mercouris BR et al. (2002) Treatment with atorvastatin to the National Cholesterol Educational Program goal versus 'usual' care in secondary coronary heart disease prevention: the GREek Atorvastatin and Coronary-heart-disease Evaluation (GREACE) study. Curr Med Res Opin 18:220–228

Avellone G, Di Garbo V, Cordova R et al. (1994) Changes induced by pravastatin treatment on hemostatic and fibrinolytic patterns in patients with type IIB hyperlipoproteinemia. Curr Ther Res 55:1335–1344

Aviram M, Rosenblat M, Bisgaier CL, Newton RS (1998) Atorvastatin and gemfibrozil metabolites, but not the parent drugs, are potent antioxidants against lipoprotein oxidation. Atherosclerosis 138:271–280

Baetta R, Camera M, Comparato C et al. (2002) Fluvastatin reduces tissue factor expression and macrophage accumulation in carotid lesions of cholesterol-fed rabbits in the absence of lipid lowering. Arterioscler Thromb Vasc Biol 22:692–698

Baldassarre D, Amato M, Bondioli A, Sirtori CR, Tremoli E (2000a) Carotid artery intima-media thickness measured by ultrasonography in normal clinical practice correlates well with atherosclerosis risk factors. Stroke 31:2426–2430

Baldassarre D, Veglia F, Gobbi C et al. (2000b) Intima-media thickness after pravastatin stabilizes also in patients with moderate to no reduction in LDL-cholesterol levels: the Carotid Atherosclerosis Italian Ultrasound Study. Atherosclerosis 151:575–583

Balk EM, Lau J, Goudas LC et al. (2003) Effects of statins on nonlipid serum markers associated with cardiovascular disease: a systematic review. Ann Intern Med 139:670–682

Ballantyne CM, Blazing MA, Hunninghake DB et al. (2003) Effect on high-density lipoprotein cholesterol of maximum dose simvastatin and atorvastatin in patients with hypercholesterolemia: results of the Comparative HDL Efficacy and Safety Study (CHESS). Am Heart J 146:862–869

Bellosta S, Via D, Canavesi M et al. (1998) HMG-CoA reductase inhibitors reduce MMP-9 secretion by macrophages. Arterioscler Thromb Vasc Biol 18:1671–1678

Bernini F, Didoni G, Bonfadini G, Bellosta S, Fumagalli R (1993) Requirement for mevalonate in acetylated LDL induction of cholesterol esterification in macrophages. Atherosclerosis 104:19–26

Bolego C, Poli A, Cignarella A, Catapano AL, Paoletti R (2002) Novel statins: pharmacological and clinical results. Cardiovasc Drugs Ther 16:251–257

Bonetti PO, Lerman LO, Lerman A (2003) Endothelial dysfunction – a marker of atherosclerotic risk. Arterioscler Thromb Vasc Biol 23:168–175

Camera M, Toschi V, Comparato C et al. (2002) Cholesterol-induced thrombogenicity of the vessel wall: inhibitory effect of fluvastatin. Thromb Haemost 87:748–755

Ceriello A, Taboga C, Tonutti L et al. (2002) Evidence for an independent and cumulative effect of postprandial hypertriglyceridemia and hyperglycemia on endothelial dysfunction and oxidative stress generation: effects of short- and long-term simvastatin treatment. Circulation 106:1211–1218

Chang MK, Binder CJ, Torzewski M, Witztum JL (2002) C-reactive protein binds to both oxidized LDL and apoptotic cells through recognition of a common ligand: phosphorylcholine of oxidized phospholipids. Proc Natl Acad Sci USA 99:13043–13048

Cignarella A, Bolego C, Paoletti R (2003) Impact of statins on novel risk markers. Cardiovasc Drugs Ther 17:361–366

Cignarella A, Brennhausen B, von Eckardstein A et al. (1998) Differential effects of lovastatin on the trafficking of endogenous and lipoprotein-derived cholesterol in human monocyte-derived macrophages. Arterioscler Thromb Vasc Biol 18:1322–1329

Cockerill GW, Huehns TY, Weerasinghe A et al. (2001) Elevation of plasma high-density lipoprotein concentration reduces interleukin-1-induced expression of E-selectin in an in vivo model of acute inflammation. Circulation 103:108–112

Colli S, Eligini S, Lalli M et al. (1997) Vastatins inhibit tissue factor in cultured human macrophages – a novel mechanism of protection against atherothrombosis. Arterioscler Thromb Vasc Biol 17:265–272

Colvin PL Jr, Auerbach BJ, Case LD, Hazzard WR, Applebaum-Bowden D (1991) A dose-response relationship between sex hormone-induced change in hepatic triglyceride lipase and high-density lipoprotein cholesterol in postmenopausal women. Metabolism 40:1052–1056

Corsini A, Bellosta S, Baetta R et al. (1999) New insights into the pharmacodynamic and pharmacokinetic properties of statins. Pharmacol Ther 84:413–428

Cortellaro M, Cofrancesco E, Arbustini E, et al. (2002) Atorvastatin and thrombogenicity of the carotid atherosclerotic plaque: the ATROCAP study. Thromb Haemost 88:41–47

Crouse JR 3rd, Frohlich J, Ose L, Mercuri M, Tobert JA (1999) Effects of high doses of simvastatin and atorvastatin on high-density lipoprotein cholesterol and apolipoprotein A-I. Am J Cardiol 83:1476–1477

Dangas G, Badimon JJ, Smith DA et al. (1999) Pravastatin therapy in hyperlipidemia: effects on thrombus formation and the systemic hemostatic profile. J Am Coll Cardiol 33:1294–1304

Devaraj S, Xu DY, Jialal I (2003) C-reactive protein increases plasminogen activator inhibitor-1 expression and activity in human aortic endothelial cells: implications for the metabolic syndrome and atherothrombosis. Circulation 107:398–404

Downs JR, Clearfield M, Weis S et al. (1998) Primary prevention of acute coronary events with lovastatin in men and women with average cholesterol levels: results of AF-CAPS/TexCAPS. JAMA 279:1615–1622

Endres M, Laufs U, Huang Z et al. (1998) Stroke protection by 3-hydroxy-3-methylglutaryl (HMG)-CoA reductase inhibitors mediated by endothelial nitric oxide synthase. Proc Natl Acad Sci USA 95:8880–8885

Festa A, D'Agostino R Jr, Tracy RP, Haffner SM (2002) Elevated levels of acute-phase proteins and plasminogen activator inhibitor-1 predict the development of type 2 diabetes: the Insulin Resistance Atherosclerosis Study. Diabetes 51:1131–1137

Forster LF, Stewart G, Bedford D et al. (2002) Influence of atorvastatin and simvastatin on apolipoprotein B metabolism in moderate combined hyperlipidemic subjects with low VLDL and LDL fractional clearance rates. Atherosclerosis 164:129–145

Gertz K, Laufs U, Lindauer U et al. (2003) Withdrawal of statin treatment abrogates stroke protection in mice. Stroke 34:551–557

Giroux LM, Davignon J, Naruszewicz M (1993) Simvastatin inhibits the oxidation of low-density lipoproteins by activated human monocyte-derived macrophages. Biochim Biophys Acta 1165:335–338

Goldbourt U, Yaari S, Medalie JH (1997) Isolated low HDL cholesterol as a risk factor for coronary heart disease mortality – a 21-year follow-up of 8000 men. Arterioscler Thromb Vasc Biol 17:107–113

Gonbert S, Malinsky S, Sposito AC et al. (2002) Atorvastatin lowers lipoprotein(a) but not apolipoprotein(a) fragment levels in hypercholesterolemic subjects at high cardiovascular risk. Atherosclerosis 164:305–311

Gordon T, Castelli WP, Hjortland MC, Kannel WB, Dawber TR (1977) High density lipoprotein as a protective factor against coronary heart disease – the Framingham Study. Am J Med 62:707–714

Gotto AM Jr. (2003) Safety and statin therapy: reconsidering the risks and benefits. Arch Intern Med 163:657–659

Guerin M, Egger P, Soudant C et al. (2002) Dose-dependent action of atorvastatin in type IIB hyperlipidemia: preferential and progressive reduction of atherogenic apoB-containing lipoprotein subclasses (VLDL-2, IDL, small dense LDL) and stimulation of cellular cholesterol efflux. Atherosclerosis 163:287–296

Heart Protection Study Collaborative Group (2002) MRC/BHF Heart Protection Study of cholesterol lowering with simvastatin in 20 536 high-risk individuals: a randomised placebo-controlled trial. Lancet 360:7–22

Hodis HN, Mack WJ, LaBree L et al. (1998). The role of carotid arterial intima-media thickness in predicting clinical coronary events. Ann Intern Med 128:262–269

Hussein O, Schlezinger S, Rosenblat M, Keidar S, Aviram M (1997) Reduced susceptibility of low density lipoprotein (LDL) to lipid peroxidation after fluvastatin therapy is associated with the hypocholesterolemic effect of the drug and its binding to the LDL. Atherosclerosis 128:11–18

Jialal I, Stein D, Balis D et al. (2001) Effect of hydroxymethyl glutaryl coenzyme A reductase inhibitor therapy on high sensitive C-reactive protein levels. Circulation 103:1933–1935

John S, Schlaich M, Langenfeld M et al. (1998) Increased bioavailability of nitric oxide after lipid-lowering therapy in hypercholesterolemic patients: a randomized, placebo-controlled, double-blind study. Circulation 98:211–216

Jones P, Kafonek S, Laurora I, Hunninghake D (1998) Comparative dose efficacy study of atorvastatin versus simvastatin, pravastatin, lovastatin, and fluvastatin in patients with hypercholesterolemia (the CURVES study). Am J Cardiol 81:582–587

Jones PH, Davidson MH, Stein EA (2003) Comparison of the efficacy and safety of rosuvastatin versus atorvastatin, simvastatin, and pravastatin across doses (STELLAR* Trial). Am J Cardiol 92:152–160

Kastelein JJ, Isaacsohn JL, Ose L et al. (2000) Comparison of effects of simvastatin versus atorvastatin on high-density lipoprotein cholesterol and apolipoprotein A-I levels. Am J Cardiol 86:221–223

Kastelein JJ, Wiegman A, de Groot E (2003) Surrogate markers of atherosclerosis: impact of statins. Atheroscler Suppl 4:31–36

Kawakami A, Tanaka A, Nakajima K, Shimokado K, Yoshida M (2002) Atorvastatin attenuates remnant lipoprotein-induced monocyte adhesion to vascular endothelium under flow conditions. Circ Res 91:263–271

Kempen HJ, Vermeer M, de Wit E, Havekes LM (1991) Vastatins inhibit cholesterol ester accumulation in human monocyte-derived macrophages. Arterioscler Thromb 11:146–153

Kinlay S, Schwartz GG, Olsson AG et al. (2003) High-dose atorvastatin enhances the decline in inflammatory markers in patients with acute coronary syndromes in the MIRACL study. Circulation 108:1560–1566

Kleemann R, Princen HM, Emeis JJ et al. (2003) Rosuvastatin reduces atherosclerosis development beyond and independent of its plasma cholesterol-lowering effect in APOE*3-Leiden transgenic mice: evidence for antiinflammatory effects of rosuvastatin. Circulation 108:1368–1374

Krauss RM (1998) Triglycerides and atherogenic lipoproteins: rationale for lipid management. Am J Med 105:58S–62S

Laufs U, Gertz K, Dirnagl U et al. (2002) Rosuvastatin, a new HMG-CoA reductase inhibitor, upregulates endothelial nitric oxide synthase and protects from ischemic stroke in mice. Brain Res 942:23–30

Laufs U, Liao JK (2003) Isoprenoid metabolism and the pleiotropic effects of statins. Curr Atheroscler Rep 5:372–378

Law MR, Wald NJ, Rudnicka AR (2003) Quantifying effect of statins on low density lipoprotein cholesterol, ischaemic heart disease, and stroke: systematic review and meta-analysis. BMJ 326:1423

Leung BP, Sattar N, Crilly A et al. (2003) A novel anti-inflammatory role for simvastatin in inflammatory arthritis. J Immunol 170:1524–1530

Liao JK (2002) Isoprenoids as mediators of the biological effects of statins. J. Clin. Invest 110:285–288

Libby P, Aikawa M (2003) Mechanisms of plaque stabilization with statins. Am J Cardiol 91:4B–8B

Martin G, Duez H, Blanquart C et al. (2001) Statin-induced inhibition of the Rho-signaling pathway activates PPARα and induces HDL apoA-I. J Clin Invest 107:1423–1432

McKenney JM, McCormick LS, Schaefer EJ, Black DM, Watkins ML (2001) Effect of niacin and atorvastatin on lipoprotein subclasses in patients with atherogenic dyslipidemia. Am J Cardiol 88:270–274

Mercuri M, Bond MG, Sirtori CR et al. (1996) Pravastatin reduces carotid intima-media thickness progression in an asymptomatic hypercholesterolemic Mediterranean population: the Carotid Atherosclerosis Italian Ultrasound Study. Am J Med 101:627–634

Meroni PL, Raschi E, Testoni C et al. (2001) Statins prevent endothelial cell activation induced by antiphospholipid (anti-beta2-glycoprotein I) antibodies: effect on the proadhesive and proinflammatory phenotype. Arthritis Rheum 44:2870–2878

Mullen MJ, Wright D, Donald AE et al. (2000) Atorvastatin but not L-arginine improves endothelial function in type I diabetes mellitus: a double-blind study. J Am Coll Cardiol 36:410–416

Müller I, Besta F, Schulz C et al. (2003) Effects of statins on platelet inhibition by a high loading dose of clopidogrel. Circulation 108:2195–2197

Negre-Aminou P, van Vliet AK, van Erck M et al. (1997) Inhibition of proliferation of human smooth muscle cells by various HMG-CoA reductase inhibitors; comparison with other human cell types. Biochim Biophys Acta 1345:259–268

Nofer JR, Kehrel B, Fobker M et al. (2002) HDL and arteriosclerosis: beyond reverse cholesterol transport. Atherosclerosis 161:1–16

O'Leary DH, Polak JF, Kronmal RA et al. (1999) Carotid-artery intima and media thickness as a risk factor for myocardial infarction and stroke in older adults. N Engl J Med 340:14–22

Olsson AG, Pears J, McKellar J, Mizan J, Raza A (2001) Effect of rosuvastatin on low-density lipoprotein cholesterol in patients with hypercholesterolemia. Am J Cardiol 88:504–508

Plenge JK, Hernandez TL, Weil KM et al. (2002) Simvastatin lowers C-reactive protein within 14 days: an effect independent of low-density lipoprotein cholesterol reduction. Circulation 106:1447–1452

Pontrelli L, Parris W, Adeli K, Cheung RC (2002) Atorvastatin treatment beneficially alters the lipoprotein profile and increases low-density lipoprotein particle diameter in patients with combined dyslipidemia and impaired fasting glucose/type 2 diabetes. Metabolism 51:334–342

Ridker PM (2001) High sensitivity C-reactive protein: potential adjunct for global risk assessment in the primary prevention of cardiovascular disease. Circulation 103:1813–1818

Ross R (1999) Atherosclerosis: an inflammatory disease. N Engl J Med 340:115–126

Rubins HB, Robins SJ, Collins D et al. (1999) Gemfibrozil for the secondary prevention of coronary heart disease in men with low levels of high-density lipoprotein cholesterol. Veterans Affairs High-Density Lipoprotein Cholesterol Intervention Trial Study Group. N Engl J Med 341:410–418

Sacks FM (2001) The relative role of low-density lipoprotein cholesterol and high-density lipoprotein cholesterol in coronary artery disease: evidence from large-scale statin and fibrate trials. Am J Cardiol 88:14N–18N

Sacks FM for the Expert Group on HDL cholesterol (2002b) The role of high-density lipoprotein (HDL) cholesterol in the prevention and treatment of coronary heart disease: expert group recommendations. Am J Cardiol 90:139–143

Sacks FM, Pfeffer MA, Moyé LA et al. (1996) The effect of pravastatin on coronary events after myocardial infarction in patients with average cholesterol levels. N Engl J Med 335:1001–1009

Sacks FM, Tonkin AM, Craven T et al. (2002a) Coronary heart disease in patients with low LDL-cholesterol: benefit of pravastatin in diabetics and enhanced role for HDL-cholesterol and triglycerides as risk factors. Circulation 105:1424–1428

Sasaki S, Kuwahara N, Kunitomo K et al. (2002) Effects of atorvastatin on oxidized low-density lipoprotein, low-density lipoprotein subfraction distribution, and remnant lipoprotein in patients with mixed hyperlipoproteinemia. Am J Cardiol 89:386–389

Scandinavian Simvastatin Survival Study Group (1994) Randomised trial of cholesterol lowering in 4444 patients with coronary heart disease: the Scandinavian Simvastatin Survival Study (4S). Lancet 344:1383–1389

Schaefer JR, Schweer H, Ikewaki K et al. (1999) Metabolic basis of high density lipoproteins and apolipoprotein A-I increase by HMG-CoA reductase inhibition in healthy subjects and a patient with coronary artery disease. Atherosclerosis 144:177–184

Schartl M, Bocksch W, Koschyk DH et al. (2001) Use of intravascular ultrasound to compare effects of different strategies of lipid-lowering therapy on plaque volume and composition in patients with coronary artery disease. Circulation 104:387–392

Seljeflot I, Tonstad S, Hjermann I, Arnesen H (2002) Reduced expression of endothelial cell markers after 1 year treatment with simvastatin and atorvastatin in patients with coronary heart disease. Atherosclerosis 162:179–185

Serruys PW, de Feyter P, Macaya C et al. (2002) Fluvastatin for prevention of cardiac events following successful first percutaneous coronary intervention: a randomized controlled trial. JAMA 287:3215–3222

Sever PS, Dahlof B, Poulter NR et al. (2003) Prevention of coronary and stroke events with atorvastatin in hypertensive patients who have average or lower-than-average cholesterol concentrations, in the Anglo-Scandinavian Cardiac Outcomes Trial – Lipid Lowering Arm (ASCOT-LLA): a multicentre randomised controlled trial. Lancet 361:1149–1158

Shepherd J, Blauw GJ, Murphy MB et al. (2002) Pravastatin in elderly individuals at risk of vascular disease (PROSPER): a randomised controlled trial. Lancet 360:1623–1630

Shepherd J, Cobbe SM, Ford I et al. (1995) Prevention of coronary heart disease with pravastatin in men with hypercholesterolemia. N Engl J Med 333:1301–1307

Shimizu K, Aikawa M, Takayama K, Libby P, Mitchell RN (2003) Direct anti-inflammatory mechanisms contribute to attenuation of experimental allograft arteriosclerosis by statins. Circulation 108:2113–2120

Spieker LE, Sudano I, Hurlimann D et al. (2002) High-density lipoprotein restores endothelial function in hypercholesterolemic men. Circulation 105:1399–1402

Stein E, Plotkin D, Bays H et al. (2000) Effects of simvastatin (40 and 80 mg/day) in patients with mixed hyperlipidemia. Am J Cardiol 86:406–411

Streja L, Packard CJ, Shepherd J, Cobbe S, Ford I (2002) Factors affecting low-density lipoprotein and high-density lipoprotein cholesterol response to pravastatin in the West Of Scotland Coronary Prevention Study (WOSCOPS). Am J Cardiol 90:731–736

Stuve O, Youssef S, Steinman L, Zamvil SS (2003) Statins as potential therapeutic agents in neuroinflammatory disorders. Curr Opin Neurol 16:393–401

Susic D, Varagic J, Ahn J, Slama M, Frohlich ED (2003) Beneficial pleiotropic vascular effects of rosuvastatin in two hypertensive models. J Am Coll Cardiol 42:1091–1097

Suzumura K, Tanaka K, Yasuhara M, Narita H (2000) Inhibitory effects of fluvastatin and its metabolites on hydrogen peroxide-induced oxidative destruction of hemin and low-density lipoprotein. Biol Pharm Bull 23:873–878

Szmitko PE, Wang CH, Weisel RD et al. (2003) New markers of inflammation and endothelial cell activation – part I. Circulation 108:1917–1923

Tan KC, Chow WS, Tam SC et al. (2002) Atorvastatin lowers C-reactive protein and improves endothelium-dependent vasodilation in type 2 diabetes mellitus. J Clin Endocrinol Metab 87:563–568

Taylor AJ, Kent SM, Flaherty PJ et al. (2002) ARBITER: Arterial Biology for the Investigation of the Treatment Effects of Reducing Cholesterol: a randomized trial comparing the effects of atorvastatin and pravastatin on carotid intima medial thickness. Circulation 106:2055–2060

Teupser D, Bruegel M, Stein O, Stein Y, Thiery J (2001) HMG-CoA reductase inhibitors reduce adhesion of human monocytes to endothelial cells. Biochem Biophys Res Commun 289:838–844

The Diabetes Atorvastatin Lipid Intervention (DALI) Study Group (2001) The effect of aggressive versus standard lipid lowering by atorvastatin on diabetic dyslipidemia – the DALI study: a double-blind, randomized, placebo-controlled trial in patients with type 2 diabetes and diabetic dyslipidemia. Diabetes Care 24:1335–1341

The Expert Panel (2002) Third Report of the National Cholesterol Education Program (NCEP) Expert Panel on Detection, Evaluation, and Treatment of High Blood Cholesterol in Adults (Adult Treatment Panel III) – Final Report. Circulation 106:3143–3421

The Long-Term Intervention with Pravastatin in Ischaemic Disease (LIPID) Study Group (1998) Prevention of cardiovascular events and death with pravastatin in patients with coronary heart disease and a broad range of initial cholesterol levels. N Engl J Med 339:1349–1357

Thompson PD, Clarkson P, Karas RH (2003) Statin-associated myopathy. JAMA 289:1681–1690

Tsuruoka H, Khovidhunkit W, Brown BE et al. (2002) Scavenger receptor class B type I is expressed in cultured keratinocytes and epidermis – regulation in response to changes in cholesterol homeostasis and barrier requirements. J Biol Chem 277:2916–2922

van de Ree MA, Huisman MV, Princen HMG, Meinders AE, Kluft C (2003) Strong decrease of high sensitivity C-reactive protein with high-dose atorvastatin with type 2 diabetes mellitus. Atherosclerosis 166:129–135

van Etten RW, de Koning EJP, Honing ML et al. (2002) Intensive lipid lowering by statin therapy does not improve vasoreactivity in patients with type 2 diabetes. Arterioscler Thromb Vasc Biol 22:799–804

van Venrooij FV, van de Ree MA, Bots ML et al. (2002) Aggressive lipid lowering does not improve endothelial function in type 2 diabetes – the Diabetes Atorvastatin Lipid Intervention (DALI) Study: a randomized, double-blind, placebo-controlled trial. Diabetes Care 25:1211–1216

van Wissen S, Smilde TJ, Trip MD et al. (2003) Long term statin treatment reduces lipoprotein(a) concentrations in heterozygous familial hypercholesterolaemia. Heart 89:893–896

Vaughan CJ, Murphy MB, Buckley BM (1996) Statins do more than just lower cholesterol. Lancet 348:1079–1082

von Eckardstein A, Assmann G (2000) Prevention of coronary heart disease by raising high-density lipoprotein cholesterol? Curr Opin Lipidol 11:627–637

von Eckardstein A, Huang Y, Assmann G (1994) Physiological role and clinical relevance of high-density lipoprotein subclasses. Curr Opin Lipidol 5:404–416 von Eckardstein A, Schulte H, Cullen P, Assmann G (2001) Lipoprotein(a) further increases the risk of coronary events in men with high global cardiovascular risk. J Am Coll Cardiol 37:434–439

Wagner AH, Schwabe O, Hecker M (2002) Atorvastatin inhibition of cytokine-inducible nitric oxide synthase expression in native endothelial cells in situ. Br J Pharmacol 136:143–149

Walter DH, Rittig K, Bahlmann FH et al. (2002) Statin therapy accelerates reendothelialization: a novel effect involving mobilization and incorporation of bone marrow-derived endothelial progenitor cells. Circulation 105:3017–3024

Weitz-Schmidt G (2002) Statins as anti-inflammatory agents. Trends Pharmacol Sci 23:482–486

Wierzbicki AS, Mikhailidis DP (2002) Dose-response effects of atorvastatin and simvastatin on high-density lipoprotein cholesterol in hypercholesterolaemic patients: a review of five comparative studies. Int J Cardiol 84:53–57

Wiklund O, Mattsson-Hultén L, Hurt-Camejo E, Oscarsson J (2002) Effects of simvastatin and atorvastatin on inflammation markers in plasma. J Intern Med 251:338–347

Yamamoto A, Arakawa K, Sasaki J et al. (2002) Clinical effects of rosuvastatin, a new HMG-CoA reductase inhibitor, in Japanese patients with primary hypercholesterolemia: an early phase II study. J Atheroscler Thromb 9:48–56

Young-Xu Y, Chan KA, Liao JK, Ravid S, Blatt CM (2003) Long-term statin use and psychological well-being. J Am Coll Cardiol 42:690–697

Youssef F, Seifalian AM, Jagroop IA et al. (2002) The early effect of lipid-lowering treatment on carotid and femoral intima media thickness (IMT). Eur J Vasc Endovasc Surg 23:358–364

HEP (2005) 170:389–406

Fibrates

R. Robillard · C. Fontaine · G. Chinetti · J.-C. Fruchart · B. Staels (✉)

UR545 INSERM, Département d'Athérosclérose, Institut Pasteur, 1 rue Calmette,
59019 Lille, France
e-mail Bart.Staels@pasteur-lille.fr

Abstract Atherosclerosis of the large arteries is the main origin of cerebro- and cardiovascular diseases, the leading causes of mortality and morbidity in industrialized countries. The pathophysiology of coronary and cerebrovascular atherosclerosis is multifactorial and complex. Fibrates are hypolipidemic drugs that lower progression of atherosclerotic lesions mainly through activation of the nuclear receptor peroxisome-proliferator activated receptor-α. In addition, fibrates exert pleiotropic and anti-inflammatory actions. In this chapter, we will focus on the different effects of fibrates impacting on the development of atherosclerosis.

Keywords Fibrates · PPARα · Atherosclerosis

1
Introduction

Atherosclerosis is a chronic disease of the large arteries characterized by a local inflammatory response and the accumulation of lipids and fibrous connective tissue in the subendothelial space resulting in formation of the neointima

(Lusis 2000). Atherosclerosis is the main origin of vascular diseases of the heart and brain, leading to clinical endpoints such as myocardial infarction and stroke, the major causes of mortality and morbidity in industrialized countries. Epidemiological studies have revealed several genetic and environmental risk factors predisposing to atherosclerosis.

Fibrates are drugs used in the management of hypertriglyceridemia, combined hyperlipidemia, diabetic dyslipidemia and transplant dyslipidemias either as monotherapy or as a component of combination therapy (Guay 2002). Fibrates are activators of the peroxisome proliferator-activated receptor alpha (PPARα), a transcription factor belonging to the superfamily of nuclear receptors, that modulates several metabolic risk factors.

The PPAR subfamily consists of three distinct subtypes termed α (NR1C1), β/δ (NR1C2) and γ (NR1C3) which display tissue-selective expression patterns reflecting their biological functions (Barbier et al. 2002). PPARα is expressed preferentially in tissues where fatty acids are catabolized (Barbier et al. 2002; Duval et al. 2002). PPARα is furthermore expressed in most cell types of the vascular wall as well as in atherosclerotic lesions (for a review see Chinetti et al. 2000a), where it affects atherogenic processes. Numerous studies have illustrated the role of PPARs in the control of glucose homeostasis, insulin resistance and hypertension (Barbier et al. 2002; Torra et al. 2001; Willson et al. 2001).

Most of the physiological functions of PPARα can be explained by its activity as transcription factor, modulating the expression of specific target genes (Barbier et al. 2002; Duval et al. 2002). Upon ligand activation, PPARα regulates gene transcription by dimerizing with the retinoid X receptor (RXR) and binding to PPAR response elements (PPREs) within the regulatory regions of target genes (Barbier et al. 2002). These PPREs usually consist of a direct repeat of the hexanucleotide sequence, AGGTCA, separated by one or two nucleotides (DR1 or DR2) (Fig. 1). PPARα can also repress gene transcription in a DNA binding-independent manner by interfering with the nuclear factor-kappa B (NF-κB), signal transducer and activator of transcription (STAT), activator protein-1 (AP-1), CCAAT/enhancer binding protein and other signaling pathways via protein–protein interactions and cofactor competition (Chinetti et al. 2000a; Delerive et al. 2000b; Gervois et al. 2001). Such *trans*-repression mechanism is likely to participate in the anti-inflammatory actions of PPARα (Chinetti et al. 2000a).

Fatty acids (FA) and FA-derived compounds are natural ligands for PPARα. Natural eicosanoids derived from arachidonic acid via the lipoxygenase pathway, such as 8-S-hydroxytetraenoic acid and leukotriene B4 activate PPARα (Barbier et al. 2002). Oxidized phospholipids derived from oxidized lipoproteins are also natural ligands for PPARα (Davies et al. 2001; Delerive et al. 2000a). In addition, PPARα is activated by lipolysis products (Ziouzenkova et al. 2003) and mediates some of the effects of eicosapentaenoic acid (EPA) and docosahexaenoic acid on the vascular wall (Sethi et al. 2002).

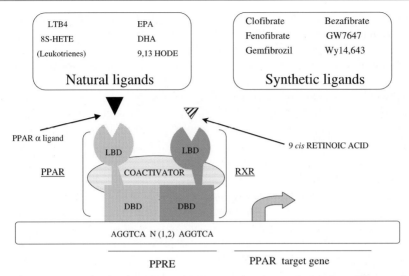

LTB4	EPA
8S-HETE	DHA
(Leukotrienes)	9,13 HODE

Natural ligands

Clofibrate	Bezafibrate
Fenofibrate	GW7647
Gemfibrozil	Wy14,643

Synthetic ligands

Fig. 1 Target gene activation by PPARα. PPARα acts in a transcriptional complex as a heterodimer with RXR. The PPAR/RXR complex is activated by natural or synthetic agonists that bind to PPARα. Both RXR and PPARα possess a ligand-binding domain (*LBD*) and a DNA-binding domain (*DBD*)

PPARs are promising therapeutic targets not only for the treatment of metabolic disorders predisposing to atherosclerosis but acting also on the atherosclerosis process itself. Synthetic agonists of PPARs are used in the treatment of metabolic diseases, such as dyslipidemia and type 2 diabetes. The antidiabetic glitazones, which are insulin sensitizers, are synthetic high affinity ligands for PPARγ (Lehmann et al. 1995; Martens et al. 2002; Raji and Plutzky 2002). The hypolipidemic fibrate drugs are low affinity PPARα ligands (Willson et al. 2000). Recently, novel high affinity subtype-specific PPAR agonists have been synthesized, such as the human PPARα ligand GW7647 (Brown et al. 2001), the PPARγ activators GW1929 and GW7845 (Brown et al. 1999; Li et al. 2000) and the PPARβ/δ specific agonist GW501516 (Oliver et al. 2001). Recently, novel dual PPAR α/ γ agonists were designed in an attempt to obtain simultaneously synergistic and complementary effects on lipid metabolism, insulin sensitivity and glucose utilization. Dual activation of PPARα/ γ decreases circulating triglyceride levels and improves glucose homeostasis in insulin resistant animal models (Lohray et al. 2001) (Table 1).

As a regulator of lipid and lipoprotein metabolism, PPARα controls plasma concentrations of lipoproteins, major risk factors for coronary heart disease (CHD) (Staels et al. 1998). Angiography intervention studies, such as the LOCAT, BECAIT, and DAIS trials, indicate that fibrate treatment lowers progression of atherosclerotic lesions in humans (Ericsson et al. 1996 ; Frick et al.

Table 1 Transactivation affinities of novel PPARα/γ agonists and activation activities of classical fibrates

Name	Chemical class	Clinical tests	EC50 (μM) mouse		EC50 (μM) human	
			PPARα	PPARγ	PPARα	PPARγ
Ragaglitazar (NNC 61–0029, DRF-2725)	Propanoic acid derivative	Investigations stopped in phase III	–	–	3.21	0.57
GW-409544	Tyrosine derivative	Phase III	–	–	0.002	0.0003
Tesaglitazar/AZ-242	Tyrosine derivative	Phase III	32	0.25	9.44	1.82
MK-767/KRP-297	TZD	Investigations stopped in phase III	10	0.14	0.85	0.083
LY-465608	Non-TZD	Preclinical	0.003	–	0.15	0.882
NC-2100	TZD	Preclinical	40	30	–	–
Farglitazar/GI-262570	Tyrosine derivative	Stopped	–	–	0.4	0.0003
Wy-14643	Close to fibrate	Not clinically used	0.63	32	5	60
Clofibrate	Fibrate	Rarely clinically used	50	500	55	500
Fenofibrate	Fibrate	Clinically used	18	250	30	300
Bezafibrate	Fibrate	Clinically used	90	55	50	60

EC_{50}, The molar concentration of an agonist, which produces 50% of the maximum response for that agonist as tested in a cell-based transactivation assay; TZD, thiazolidinedione, PPAR, peroxisome proliferator-activated receptor (based on Willson et al. 2000 and Duran-Sandoval et al. 2003); –, unknown.

1997; Guay 2002). Moreover, the effects of gemfibrozil resulted in decreased mortality and morbidity of cardiovascular disease and stroke in the VA-HIT Trial (Robins 2003). In this chapter, we will focus on the role of fibrates as cardio-protective agents.

2
The Fibrate Family

Fibrates are amphiphatic carboxylic acids that have been proven useful in the treatment of hypertriglyceridemia. Studies performed using PPARα-deficient mice have demonstrated the obligatory role of PPARα in mediating most of the effects of fibrates on lipid and lipoprotein metabolism (Peters et al. 1997). The prototypical members of this compound class were developed prior to the identification of PPARs, using in vivo assays in rodents to assess lipid-lowering efficacy (Thorp and Waring 1962). Clofibrate, gemfibrozil and fenofibrate activate PPARα with a tenfold selectivity over PPARγ. On the contrary, bezafibrate is a pan-agonist that shows similar potency on all three isoforms (Fig. 2). In humans, all the fibrates must be used at high doses (200–1,200 mg/day) to achieve efficacious lipid-lowering activity (Berger and Wagner 2002). Pharmacological activation of PPARα by fibrates decreases plasma triglyceride concentrations by acting on different metabolic pathways (Staels et al. 1998). Fibrates increase FA uptake and catabolism resulting in decreased triglyceride and very-low-density lipoprotein (VLDL) production by the liver (Staels et al. 1998). Fibrate treatment induces FA transport protein 1 and FA translocase mRNA levels in rodent liver (Martin et al. 1997; Motojima et al. 1998). In addition, hepatic expression of intracellular FA binding protein is regulated by fibrates. Fibrate-induced PPARα activation also controls FA uptake and catabolism in mitochondria via stimulation of muscle and liver carnitine palmitoyltransferase I and II (Brandt et al. 1998; Guerre-Millo et al. 2000; Louet et al. 2001; Mascaro et al. 1998) and several mitochondrial FA-catabolizing enzymes (Djouadi et al. 1998). Simultaneously, fibrates enhance intravascular triglyceride metabolism. Intravascular lipolysis activity is controlled by the activity of lipoprotein lipase (LPL). Fibrates control LPL activity by inducing its expression in the liver and by regulating the hepatic expression of apolipoprotein (apo)C-III, LPL activity and remnant catabolism inhibitor (Hertz et al. 1995; Schoonjans et al. 1996; Staels et al. 1995), and apoA-V, a stimulator of triglyceride catabolism (Vu-Dac et al. 2003). These effects promote lipolysis and catabolism of triglyceride-rich lipoproteins, thus contributing to the decrease of plasma triglycerides. Interestingly, combination treatment of fenofibrate with simvastatin significantly increased high-density lipoprotein (HDL) cholesterol levels (Vega et al. 2003). Thus, combination treatment appears to be a promising means of combating atherosclerosis (for a review see Black 2003).

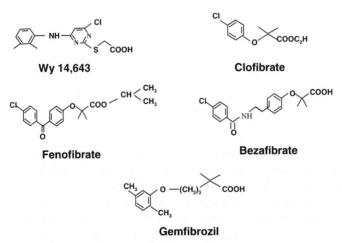

Fig. 2 Chemical structures of fibrates and PPARα agonists

3
Fibrates, Early Stages of Atherogenesis and Endothelial (Dys)Function

Under normal conditions, the endothelium forms a relatively impermeable barrier between circulating blood and the vessel wall. Endothelial injury is thought
to be a primary event in atherosclerosis which leads to the attraction, recruitment and activation of different cell types, including monocytes/macrophages,
T lymphocytes, endothelial cells (ECs) and smooth muscle cells (SMCs).

The recruitment of monocytes to the intima requires the interaction of locally produced chemokines with specific cell surface receptors, such as CCR2,
the receptor for monocyte chemoattractant protein-1 (MCP-1). The effects
of PPARα on monocyte recruitment are controversial. Indeed, whereas both
natural and certain synthetic, but not clinically used, PPARα ligands stimulate basal expression of MCP-1 in human aortic ECs (Lee et al. 2000; Pasceri
et al. 2001), it has been demonstrated that C-reactive protein -induced MCP-
1 expression in human ECs is inhibited by synthetic PPARα ligands such as
fenofibrate (Pasceri et al. 2001). Moreover fenofibric acid abrogated MCP-1
mRNA expression in glycoxidized low-density lipoprotein (LDL)-stimulated
human ECs (Sonoki et al. 2003). It has also been demonstrated that oxidized,
but not unoxidized EPA significantly inhibits human monocyte adhesion to
ECs through a PPARα-dependent mechanism (Sethi et al. 2002).

The activation of ECs, macrophages and T lymphocytes leads to the release
of pro-inflammatory molecules, such as cytokines, and the onset of a chronic
inflammatory response. In inflammation, the transcription factor NF-κB is
activated and increases the expression of multiple pro-inflammatory genes.
PPARα activation by fibrates results in a negative crosstalk with inflammatory
transcription factors, such as NF-κB, STAT-1 and AP-1, to block their downstream target genes (for a review see Chinetti et al. 2000a). T-cell recruitment to
inflammation sites may be modulated by PPARα. Indeed, PPARα ligands may
induce the expression of interleukin (IL)-8, a cytokine exerting chemotactic
effects on T-lymphocytes (Lee et al. 2000). Activation of T lymphocytes and
their ensuing elaboration of proinflammatory cytokines, such as interferon
(IFN)-γ, represents a critical step in atherogenesis. Fibrates may influence the
expression of proinflammatory cytokines in human CD4-positive T cells. Different synthetic PPARα activators reduced anti-CD3-induced IFNγ secretion
(Marx et al. 2002), and inhibited tumor necrosis factor (TNF)α and IL-2 protein expression (Jones et al. 2002; Marx et al. 2002). In clinics, TNFα release is
inhibited by gemfibrozil in peripheral blood mononuclear cells from both CHD
patients and controls (Zhao et al. 2003). Thus, activation of PPARα in human
CD4-positive T cells limits the expression of proinflammatory cytokines, such
as IFN-γ (Jones et al. 2002; Marx et al. 2002). PPARα-dependent suppression
of the adaptive immune response has also been reported in vivo by studying
the PPARα-deficient mouse model (Yang et al. 2002). Rolling and adhesion of
circulating leukocytes to the ECs is a critical early step in atherogenesis, and

several cell adhesion molecules are involved in this process, including intercellular adhesion molecule-1 and vascular cell adhesion molecule-1 (VCAM-1). Fibrate-activated PPARα inhibits VCAM-1 transcription, in part, by inhibiting the NF-κB pathway (Marx et al. 1999; Rival et al. 2002).

In addition, the expression and secretion (Kandoussi et al. 2002; Martin-Nizard et al. 2002) of endothelin-1 (ET-1), a vasoconstrictor peptide, monocyte chemoattractant and potent inducer of cell adhesion molecules (for review see Agapitov and Haynes 2002), is repressed by different PPARα ligands in ECs. PPARα appears to act indirectly by blocking the AP-1 signaling pathway (Delerive et al. 1999). Iglarz et al. have recently extended these observations in vivo by studying the effects of fenofibrate in deoxycorticosterone acetate -salt treated rats, a model of endothelin-dependent hypertension (Iglarz et al. 2003). Moreover, an inhibition of ET-1 by PPARα activators has also been observed in rats with overload induced cardiac hypertrophy (Ogata et al. 2002).

Under basal conditions, endothelium-derived nitric oxide (NO), produced by endothelial NO synthase, inhibits leukocyte attachment and promotes vascular relaxation (Napoli 2002; Russo et al. 2002). Recently it has also been demonstrated that the combination of fenofibrate and coenzyme Q(10) markedly improves endothelial function in dyslipidemic type 2 diabetic patients. The favorable vascular effect of this therapeutic combination could be due to an increase in the bioactivity of and/or responses to endothelium-derived relaxing factors, including NO (Playford et al. 2003).

However, NO may also present pro-atherogenic effects, since it promotes oxidative stress and inflammation when produced at high concentration by inducible NO synthase (iNOS). PPARα ligands inhibit iNOS expression in macrophages, and as such reduce inflammatory NO production (Colville-Nash et al. 1998). Zuckerman et al. have recently shown that the synthesis of both NO, iNOS dependent and β-2 integrin CD11 induced by IFN-γ is inhibited in peritoneal macrophages from apoE deficient mice treated with a PPARα/γ coagonist, thus leading to the inhibition of macrophage activation (Zuckerman et al. 2002).

Thus, the effects of PPARα on chemokines, adhesion molecules and NO production suggests that fibrates may influence the early stages of atherosclerosis characterized by chemo-attraction and leukocyte adhesion to ECs.

4
Fibrates, Lipid Accumulation and Reverse Cholesterol Transport

After recruitment into the subendothelial space, monocytes differentiate into macrophages. Accumulation of cholesterol by macrophages leads to the formation of foam cells. These cells are characteristic of the early atherosclerotic lesion and participate in the chronic inflammation associated with lesion progression (Lee et al. 2003).

Before uptake by macrophages, atherogenic lipoproteins undergo modifications, such as oxidation, glycosylation and aggregation. In ECs, PPARα modulates the generation of free radicals, which contribute to oxidized LDL (OxLDL) formation. For instance, bezafibrate increases the expression of the Cu^{2+}, Zn^{2+} superoxide dismutase, a superoxide scavenger enzyme, which protects arteries from the deleterious effects of reactive oxygen species (Inoue et al. 2001). Fenofibrate treatment decreases oxidant stress in the brains of mice that were submitted to ischemia (Deplanque et al. 2003). PPARα activation by OxLDL, fenofibrate and Wy14643 also results in the downregulation of platelet-activating factor (PAF)-receptor gene expression in human monocytes and macrophages (Hourton et al. 2001). PAF is a potent pro-inflammatory substance playing an important role in LDL oxidation and whose effects are mediated by a specific cell receptor (PAF-receptor).

In addition, PPARα plays an important role in regulating cholesterol uptake and homeostasis in macrophages. Overall, PPARα does not promote LDL accumulation in macrophages. Moreover, PPARα inhibits apoB48 receptor expression, which mediates lipid accumulation of triglyceride-rich lipoproteins (Haraguchi et al. 2003) and decreases glycated LDL uptake (Gbaguidi et al. 2002).

Cholesterol efflux is the first step of the reverse cholesterol transport pathway, the centripetal transport of cholesterol from peripheral cells back to the liver. Macrophage cholesterol efflux to HDL occurs either via passive diffusion facilitated or not by proteins, such as SR-B1/CLA-1, or via active efflux mediated by the ATP-binding cassette (ABC) transporters directed towards apoA-I. In human macrophages, PPARα activators induce expression of SR-B1/CLA-1 (Chinetti et al. 2000b) and ABCA-1 (Chinetti et al. 2001) and, as such, stimulate cholesterol efflux from macrophages. Fibrates regulate ABCA-1 by an indirect mechanism via induction of the liver X receptor α (LXRα) (Chinetti et al. 2001). Finally, PPARα activation by fibrates decreases the cholesteryl ester/free cholesterol ratio in macrophages resulting in an enhanced availability of free cholesterol for efflux through the ABCA-1 pathway (Chinetti et al. 2003). In type 2 diabetic patients, fenofibrate treatment increases expression of both LXRα and ABCA-1 genes in isolated monocytes, thus demonstrating the relevance of these findings in the clinical setting (Forcheron et al. 2002).

PPARα influences HDL-cholesterol metabolism also by regulating its major apolipoproteins as well as a number of HDL remodeling enzymes. Fibrates induce the expression of phospholipid transfer protein (Bouly et al. 2001), an enzyme that transfers phospholipids from VLDL/LDL to HDL, and decrease lecithin/cholesterol acyl transferase (Staels et al. 1992), in mice and rats respectively. The molecular mechanisms behind this induction and the relevance for the human situation remain to be clarified.

ApoA-I and apoA-II, the major HDL apolipoproteins, are induced by fibrates in humans, via PPARα binding to PPREs in their promoters (Vu-Dac et al. 1994, 1995). Interestingly, fenofibrate treatment increased plasma and hepatic expression levels of apoA-I in apoE-deficient mice expressing the human apoA-I transgene resulting in a decrease of atherosclerotic lesion size (Duez et al. 2002). Although the increase of plasma apoA-I is undoubtedly beneficial, as has recently been shown in patients infused with apoA-I Milano (Nissen et al. 2003), substantial controversy exists on the role of apoA-II in atherosclerosis. Indeed, whereas transgenic mice over-expressing murine apoA-II are more prone to develop atherosclerosis (Warden et al. 1993), over-expression of human apoA-II protects against atherogenesis (Tailleux et al. 2000).

Thus, PPARα appears to protect against accumulation of cholesterol in macrophages and to promote cholesterol efflux, to decrease cholesterol esterification in macrophages and to increase HDL production.

5
Fibrates, Plaque Progression and Plaque Stability

Formation of the fibrous plaque is due to SMC migration and proliferation in the intima. SMCs participate in the production of the extracellular matrix (ECM), which gives rise to a fibrous cap. Inhibition of SMC proliferation may thus be beneficial to prevent early plaque formation. However, in advanced plaques, these cells may play an important role in maintaining plaque stability. Factors influencing SMC proliferation and apoptosis probably influence atherosclerosis–albeit with opposite outcomes–depending on the stage of plaque development. Inhibition of ET-1 secretion, a potent inducer of SMC proliferation, by PPARα agonists (Delerive et al. 1999; Iglarz et al. 2003; Kandoussi et al. 2002; Martin-Nizard et al. 2002) might represent one mechanism by which PPARα may interfere with SMC proliferation. Gemfibrozil influences the development of early fibrinogen-rich vascular lesions in a porcine model of atherosclerosis by decreasing platelet–fibrinogen binding (Royo et al. 2000). Gemfibrozil also significantly decreases vascular biosynthesis of proteoglycan and glucosaminoglycan (Nigro et al. 2002), two important components of the ECM.

Plaque rupture is the end-stage of the atherogenic process, leading to thrombus formation, occlusion and the clinical sequels of atherosclerosis. Plaque instability is partly due to the degradation of the extracellular matrix. PPARα ligands inhibit secretion and gelatinolytic activity (Shu et al. 2000) of MMP-9, a matrix degrading protein secreted in response to inflammatory activation. In addition, PPARα agonists decrease the expression of PAF receptor in macrophages (Hourton et al. 2001). PAF stimulates the secretion of elastase-type enzymes, which contribute to plaque instability and rupture.

Angiogenesis also participates in plaque instability. Fenofibrate inhibits EC proliferation induced by angiogenic factors, and at high concentrations increases apoptosis, inhibits capillary tube formation in vitro, and inhibits angiogenesis in vivo (Varet et al. 2003).

Finally, plaque stability is also influenced by apoptosis of SMCs and macrophages (Boitier et al. 2003; Kockx et al. 1998; Roberts et al. 2002). Apoptosis occurring in atherosclerotic areas is potentially involved in necrotic core formation and plaque rupture which may trigger atherothrombotic events (for a review see Chinetti et al. 1998). The significance of apoptosis in atherosclerosis remains unclear. Although it has been proposed that apoptotic cell death contributes to plaque instability, rupture and thrombus formation, macrophage apoptosis also decreases inflammation of macrophage origin and avoids the disruption of ECM collagen which maintains the elasticity of the plaque (Martinet and Kockx 2001). Once activated, PPARα controls apoptosis via negative cross-talk with the anti-apoptotic NF-κB pathway in macrophages (Chinetti et al. 1998).

6
Fibrates and Thrombosis

Fibrates also modulate platelet aggregation. Tissue factor (TF) is a major factor in thrombus formation and blood coagulation at the site of the ruptured plaque. PPARα agonists inhibit TF expression in monocytes and macrophages (Marx et al. 2001; Neve et al. 2001). In addition, fenofibrate and gemfibrozil also modulate the secretion of plasminogen activator inhibitor-1 (PAI-1) which is an important pro-thrombotic factor (Durrington et al. 1998). Low concentrations of clofibric acid and bezafibrate increase PAI-1 transcription and secretion. In contrast, both fenofibrate and gemfibrozil markedly decreased PAI-1 transcription and secretion from human umbilical vein endothelial cells and EA.hy926 cells (Nilsson et al. 1999). PPARα agonists also decrease production of fibrinogen by hepatocytes (Gervois et al. 2001).

On the whole, PPARα activation by fibrates could be protective against atherothrombosis. However, the exact mechanisms and effects of different fibrates are still unclear and consequences for atherothrombosis remain to be clarified.

7
Anti-atherosclerotic Effects of Fibrates: Results from In Vivo Studies

Compelling evidence for a regulatory role of fibrates on atherogenesis in vivo comes from studies in animal models of atherosclerosis and human clinical trials.

Various animals models presenting accelerated atherosclerosis have been developed to study the pathophysiology of the disease and/or the evaluation of potential therapeutic strategies (for a review see Tailleux et al. 2003).

Protection against myocardial ischemic injury and improvement of endothelial vasodilatation by activation of PPARα by fenofibrate was demonstrated in mice (Tabernero et al. 2002). In addition, fenofibrate reduces lesion surface area in the aortic sinus of apoE-deficient mice expressing the human apoA-I transgene (Duez et al. 2002). However, surprisingly, PPARα-deficiency in the apoE null background results in lowered atherosclerosis (Tordjman et al. 2001). These double knockout mice are characterized by higher concentrations of atherogenic lipoproteins, but also higher insulin sensitivity, lower blood pressure and fewer intimal lesions. Paradoxically, it has been recently demonstrated that mice lacking apoE treated with ciprofibrate and other PPARα agonists (fenofibrate, bezafibrate and WY14,643) developed a three to fourfold increase in their plasma cholesterol levels resulting in a considerably more advanced development of atherosclerotic lesions than untreated animals (Fu et al. 2003). This pro-atherogenic effect has been recently shown to be due to the downregulation of hepatic SR-BI expression in these mice (Mardones et al. 2003).

A number of clinical studies have revealed that fibrates improve the cardiovascular risk profile. Several angiographic intervention trials, including the Lipid Coronary Angiography Trial (LOCAT), the Diabetes Atherosclerosis Intervention Study (DAIS) and the Bezafibrate Coronary Atherosclerosis Intervention Trial (BECAIT), have demonstrated beneficial effects of fibrates on atherosclerotic lesion progression (Ericsson et al. 1996; Frick et al. 1997; Steiner 2001). Furthermore, secondary prevention trials, such as the Veterans Administration-HDL-Cholesterol Intervention Trial (VA-HIT) (Rubins et al. 1999) and the Helsinki Heart Study (HSS) (Frick et al. 1987), demonstrated a decreased incidence of cardiovascular events following fibrate treatment. In patients with type 2 diabetes, who are characterized by moderate hypertriglyceridemia and low HDL-cholesterol concentrations, fibrates decrease the incidence of myocardial infarction, as observed in the Mary's Ealing, Northwick Park Diabetes (SENDCAP) study (Elkeles et al. 1998).

Running trials, such as the Fenofibrate Intervention and Event Lowering in Diabetes (FIELD), will provide additional evidence for possible clinical cardiovascular benefits of PPARα agonists, such as fibrates, in the diabetic population. Several PPARα/γ co-agonists are currently in phase 3 development for the treatment of patients with type 2 diabetes (Ebdrup et al. 2003).

8
Conclusion

Considerable evidence indicates that PPARα activation by fibrates has beneficial effects on inflammatory diseases, including atherosclerosis. Although the molecular mechanisms are not yet fully established and the pathophysiological complexity is important, PPARα interferes at different steps of atherogenesis by blocking vascular cell recruitment, by modulating foam cell formation, by interfering with the inflammatory response and by inhibiting fibrous plaque development. Its implication in plaque stability and atherothrombosis is less clear, and its understanding requires further studies.

In conclusion, synthetic PPARα agonists are pharmacological drugs with high potential. Combination treatment with statins (for example) and development of PPARα/γ co-agonists appear to be promising future options for an optimal treatment of atherosclerosis.

Acknowledgements Support by grants from Fonds Européens de Développement Régional, Conseil Régional Région Nord/Pas-de-Calais 'Genopole Project 01360124' and grants from the Leducq Foundation are kindly acknowledged.

References

Agapitov AV, Haynes WG (2002) Role of endothelin in cardiovascular disease. J Renin Angiotensin Aldosterone Syst 3:1–15

Barbier O, Torra IP, Duguay Y, Blanquart C, Fruchart JC, Glineur C, Staels B (2002) Pleiotropic actions of peroxisome proliferator-activated receptors in lipid metabolism and atherosclerosis. Arterioscler Thromb Vasc Biol 22:717–726

Berger J, Wagner JA (2002) Physiological and therapeutic roles of peroxisome proliferator-activated receptors. Diabetes Technol Ther 4:163–174

Black DM (2003) The development of combination drugs for atherosclerosis. Curr Atheroscler Rep 5:29–32

Boitier E, Gautier JC, Roberts R (2003) Advances in understanding the regulation of apoptosis and mitosis by peroxisome-proliferator activated receptors in pre-clinical models: relevance for human health and disease. Comp Hepatol 2:3

Bouly M, Masson D, Gross B, Jiang XC, Fievet C, Castro G, Tall AR, Fruchart JC, Staels B, Lagrost L, Luc G (2001) Induction of the phospholipid transfer protein gene accounts for the high density lipoprotein enlargement in mice treated with fenofibrate. J Biol Chem 276:25841–2587

Brandt JM, Djouadi F, Kelly DP (1998) Fatty acids activate transcription of the muscle carnitine palmitoyltransferase I gene in cardiac myocytes via the peroxisome proliferator-activated receptor alpha. J Biol Chem 273:23786–23792

Brown KK, Henke BR, Blanchard SG, Cobb JE, Mook R, Kaldor I, Kliewer SA, Lehmann JM, Lenhard JM, Harrington WW, Novak PJ, Faison W, Binz JG, Hashim MA, Oliver WO, Brown HR, Parks DJ, Plunket KD, Tong WQ, Menius JA, Adkison K, Noble SA, Willson TM (1999) A novel N-aryl tyrosine activator of peroxisome proliferator-activated receptor-gamma reverses the diabetic phenotype of the Zucker diabetic fatty rat. Diabetes 48:1415–1424

Brown PJ, Stuart LW, Hurley KP, Lewis MC, Winegar DA, Wilson JG, Wilkison WO, Ittoop OR, Willson TM (2001) Identification of a subtype selective human PPARalpha agonist through parallel-array synthesis. Bioorg Med Chem Lett 11:1225–1227

Chinetti G, Fruchart JC, Staels B (2000a) Peroxisome proliferator-activated receptors (PPARs): nuclear receptors at the crossroads between lipid metabolism and inflammation. Inflamm Res 49:497–505

Chinetti G, Gbaguidi FG, Griglio S, Mallat Z, Antonucci M, Poulain P, Chapman J, Fruchart JC, Tedgui A, Najib-Fruchart J, Staels B (2000b) CLA-1/SR-BI is expressed in atherosclerotic lesion macrophages and regulated by activators of peroxisome proliferator-activated receptors. Circulation 101:2411–2417

Chinetti G, Griglio S, Antonucci M, Torra IP, Delerive P, Majd Z, Fruchart JC, Chapman J, Najib J, Staels B (1998) Activation of proliferator-activated receptors alpha and gamma induces apoptosis of human monocyte-derived macrophages. J Biol Chem 273:25573–25580

Chinetti G, Lestavel S, Bocher V, Remaley AT, Neve B, Torra IP, Teissier E, Minnich A, Jaye M, Duverger N, Brewer HB, Fruchart JC, Clavey V, Staels B (2001) PPAR-alpha and PPAR-gamma activators induce cholesterol removal from human macrophage foam cells through stimulation of the ABCA1 pathway. Nat Med 7:53–58

Chinetti G, Lestavel S, Fruchart JC, Clavey V, Staels B (2003) Peroxisome proliferator-activated receptor alpha reduces cholesterol esterification in macrophages. Circ Res 92:212–217

Colville-Nash PR, Qureshi SS, Willis D, Willoughby DA (1998) Inhibition of inducible nitric oxide synthase by peroxisome proliferator-activated receptor agonists: correlation with induction of heme oxygenase 1. J Immunol 161:978–984

Davies SS, Pontsler AV, Marathe GK, Harrison KA, Murphy RC, Hinshaw JC, Prestwich GD, Hilaire AS, Prescott SM, Zimmerman GA, McIntyre TM (2001) Oxidized alkyl phospholipids are specific, high affinity peroxisome proliferator-activated receptor gamma ligands and agonists. J Biol Chem 276:16015–16023

Delerive P, Furman C, Teissier E, Fruchart J, Duriez P, Staels B (2000a) Oxidized phospholipids activate PPARalpha in a phospholipase A2-dependent manner. FEBS Lett 471:34–38

Delerive P, Gervois P, Fruchart JC, Staels B (2000b) Induction of IkappaBalpha expression as a mechanism contributing to the anti-inflammatory activities of peroxisome proliferator-activated receptor-alpha activators. J Biol Chem 275:36703–36707

Delerive P, Martin-Nizard F, Chinetti G, Trottein F, Fruchart JC, Najib J, Duriez P, Staels B (1999) Peroxisome proliferator-activated receptor activators inhibit thrombin-induced endothelin-1 production in human vascular endothelial cells by inhibiting the activator protein-1 signaling pathway. Circ Res 85:394–402

Deplanque D, Gele P, Petrault O, Six I, Furman C, Bouly M, Nion S, Dupuis B, Leys D, Fruchart JC, Cecchelli R, Staels B, Duriez P, Bordet R (2003) Peroxisome proliferator-activated receptor-alpha activation as a mechanism of preventive neuroprotection induced by chronic fenofibrate treatment. J Neurosci 23:6264–6271

Djouadi F, Weinheimer CJ, Saffitz JE, Pitchford C, Bastin J, Gonzalez FJ, Kelly DP (1998) A gender-related defect in lipid metabolism and glucose homeostasis in peroxisome proliferator- activated receptor alpha- deficient mice. J Clin Invest 102:1083–1091

Duez H, Chao YS, Hernandez M, Torpier G, Poulain P, Mundt S, Mallat Z, Teissier E, Burton CA, Tedgui A, Fruchart JC, Fievet C, Wright SD, Staels B (2002) Reduction of atherosclerosis by the peroxisome proliferator-activated receptor alpha agonist fenofibrate in mice. J Biol Chem 277:48051–48057

Duran-Sandoval D, Thomas AC, Bailleul B, Fruchart JC, Staels B (2003) Pharmacology of PPARalpha, PPARgamma and dual PPARalpha/gamma agonists in clinical development. Med Sci (Paris) 19:819–825

Durrington PN, Mackness MI, Bhatnagar D, Julier K, Prais H, Arrol S, Morgan J, Wood GN (1998) Effects of two different fibric acid derivatives on lipoproteins, cholesteryl ester transfer, fibrinogen, plasminogen activator inhibitor and paraoxonase activity in type IIb hyperlipoproteinaemia. Atherosclerosis 138:217–225

Duval C, Chinetti G, Trottein F, Fruchart JC, Staels B (2002) The role of PPARs in atherosclerosis. Trends Mol Med 8:422–430

Ebdrup S, Pettersson I, Rasmussen HB, Deussen HJ, Frost Jensen A, Mortensen SB, Fleckner J, Pridal L, Nygaard L, Sauerberg P (2003) Synthesis and biological and structural characterization of the dual-acting peroxisome proliferator-activated receptor alpha/gamma agonist ragaglitazar. J Med Chem 46:1306–1317

Elkeles RS, Diamond JR, Poulter C, Dhanjil S, Nicolaides AN, Mahmood S, Richmond W, Mather H, Sharp P, Feher MD (1998) Cardiovascular outcomes in type 2 diabetes. A double-blind placebo-controlled study of bezafibrate: the St. Mary's, Ealing, Northwick Park Diabetes Cardiovascular Disease Prevention (SENDCAP) Study. Diabetes Care 21:641–648

Ericsson CG, Hamsten A, Nilsson J, Grip L, Svane B, de Faire U (1996) Angiographic assessment of effects of bezafibrate on progression of coronary artery disease in young male postinfarction patients. Lancet 347:849–853

Forcheron F, Cachefo A, Thevenon S, Pinteur C, Beylot M (2002) Mechanisms of the triglyceride- and cholesterol-lowering effect of fenofibrate in hyperlipidemic type 2 diabetic patients. Diabetes 51:3486–3491

Frick MH, Elo O, Haapa K, Heinonen OP, Heinsalmi P, Helo P, Huttunen JK, Kaitaniemi P, Koskinen P, Manninen V, et al. (1987) Helsinki Heart Study: primary-prevention trial with gemfibrozil in middle-aged men with dyslipidemia. Safety of treatment, changes in risk factors, and incidence of coronary heart disease. N Engl J Med 317:1237–1245

Frick MH, Syvanne M, Nieminen MS, Kauma H, Majahalme S, Virtanen V, Kesaniemi YA, Pasternack A, Taskinen MR (1997) Prevention of the angiographic progression of coronary and vein-graft atherosclerosis by gemfibrozil after coronary bypass surgery in men with low levels of HDL cholesterol. Lopid Coronary Angiography Trial (LOCAT) Study Group. Circulation 96:2137–2143

Fu T, Kozarsky KF, Borensztajn J (2003) Overexpression of SR-BI by adenoviral vector reverses the fibrate-induced hypercholesterolemia of ApoE-deficient mice. J Biol Chem

Gbaguidi FG, Chinetti G, Milosavljevic D, Teissier E, Chapman J, Olivecrona G, Fruchart JC, Griglio S, Fruchart-Najib J, Staels B (2002) Peroxisome proliferator-activated receptor (PPAR) agonists decrease lipoprotein lipase secretion and glycated LDL uptake by human macrophages. FEBS Lett 512:85–90

Gervois P, Vu-Dac N, Kleemann R, Kockx M, Dubois G, Laine B, Kosykh V, Fruchart JC, Kooistra T, Staels B (2001) Negative regulation of human fibrinogen gene expression by peroxisome proliferator-activated receptor alpha agonists via inhibition of CCAAT box/enhancer-binding protein beta. J Biol Chem 276:33471–33477

Guay DR (2002) Update on fenofibrate. Cardiovasc Drug Rev 20:281–302

Guerre-Millo M, Gervois P, Raspe E, Madsen L, Poulain P, Derudas B, Herbert JM, Winegar DA, Willson TM, Fruchart JC, Berge RK, Staels B (2000) Peroxisome proliferator-activated receptor alpha activators improve insulin sensitivity and reduce adiposity. J Biol Chem 275:16638–16642

Haraguchi G, Kobayashi Y, Brown ML, Tanaka A, Isobe M, Gianturco SH, Bradley WA (2003) PPAR(alpha) and PPAR(gamma) activators suppress the monocyte-macrophage poB-48 receptor. J Lipid Res 44:1224–1231

Hertz R, Bishara-Shieban J, Bar-Tana J (1995) Mode of action of peroxisome proliferators as hypolipidemic drugs. Suppression of apolipoprotein C-III. J Biol Chem 270:13470–13475

Hourton D, Delerive P, Stankova J, Staels B, Chapman MJ, Ninio E (2001) Oxidized low-density lipoprotein and peroxisome-proliferator-activated receptor alpha down-regulate platelet-activating-factor receptor expression in human macrophages. Biochem J 354: 225–232

Iglarz M, Touyz RM, Amiri F, Lavoie MF, Diep QN, Schiffrin EL (2003) Effect of peroxisome proliferator-activated receptor-alpha and -gamma activators on vascular remodeling in endothelin-dependent hypertension. Arterioscler Thromb Vasc Biol 23:45–51

Inoue I, Goto S, Matsunaga T, Nakajima T, Awata T, Hokari S, Komoda T, Katayama S (2001) The ligands/activators for peroxisome proliferator-activated receptor alpha (PPARalpha) and PPARgamma increase Cu2+,Zn2+-superoxide dismutase and decrease p22phox message expressions in primary endothelial cells. Metabolism 50:3–11

Jones DC, Ding X, Daynes RA (2002) Nuclear receptor peroxisome proliferator-activated receptor alpha (PPARalpha) is expressed in resting murine lymphocytes. The PPARalpha in T and B lymphocytes is both transactivation and transrepression competent. J Biol Chem 277:6838–6845

Kandoussi A, Martin F, Hazzan M, Noel C, Fruchart JC, Staels B, Duriez P (2002) HMG-CoA reductase inhibition and PPAR- alpha activation both inhibit cyclosporin A induced endothelin-1 secretion in cultured endothelial cells. Clin Sci (Lond) 103 Suppl 48:81S–83S

Kockx MM, De Meyer GR, Muhring J, Jacob W, Bult H, Herman AG (1998) Apoptosis and related proteins in different stages of human atherosclerotic plaques. Circulation 97:2307–2315

Lee CH, Chawla A, Urbiztondo N, Liao D, Boisvert WA, Evans RM (2003) Transcriptional repression of atherogenic inflammation: modulation by PPARdelta. Science 302:453–457

Lee H, Shi W, Tontonoz P, Wang S, Subbanagounder G, Hedrick CC, Hama S, Borromeo C, Evans RM, Berliner JA, Nagy L (2000) Role for peroxisome proliferator-activated receptor alpha in oxidized phospholipid-induced synthesis of monocyte chemotactic protein-1 and interleukin-8 by endothelial cells. Circ Res 87:516–521

Lehmann JM, Moore LB, Smith-Oliver TA, Wilkison WO, Willson TM, Kliewer SA (1995) An antidiabetic thiazolidinedione is a high affinity ligand for peroxisome proliferator-activated receptor gamma (PPAR gamma). J Biol Chem 270:12953–12956

Li AC, Brown KK, Silvestre MJ, Willson TM, Palinski W, Glass CK (2000) Peroxisome proliferator-activated receptor gamma ligands inhibit development of atherosclerosis in LDL receptor-deficient mice. J Clin Invest 106:523–531

Lohray BB, Lohray VB, Bajji AC, Kalchar S, Poondra RR, Padakanti S, Chakrabarti R, Vikramadithyan RK, Misra P, Juluri S, Mamidi NV, Rajagopalan R (2001) (-)-3-[4-[2-(Phenoxazin-10-yl)ethoxy]phenyl]-2-ethoxypropanoic acid [(-)DRF 2725]: a dual PPAR agonist with potent antihyperglycemic and lipid modulating activity. J Med Chem 44:2675–2678

Louet JF, Chatelain F, Decaux JF, Park EA, Kohl C, Pineau T, Girard J, Pegorier JP (2001) Long-chain fatty acids regulate liver carnitine palmitoyltransferase I gene (L-CPT I) expression through a peroxisome-proliferator-activated receptor alpha (PPARalpha)-independent pathway. Biochem J 354:189–197

Lusis AJ (2000) Atherosclerosis. Nature 407:233–241

Mardones P, Pilon A, Bouly M, Duran D, Nishimoto T, Arai H, Kozarsky KF, Altayo M, Miquel JF, Luc G, Clavey V, Staels B, Rigotti A (2003) Fibrates down-regulate hepatic scavenger receptor class B type I protein expression in mice. J Biol Chem 278:7884–7890

Martens FM, Visseren FL, Lemay J, de Koning EJ, Rabelink TJ (2002) Metabolic and additional vascular effects of thiazolidinediones. Drugs 62:1463–1480

Martin G, Schoonjans K, Lefebvre AM, Staels B, Auwerx J (1997) Coordinate regulation of the expression of the fatty acid transport protein and acyl-CoA synthetase genes by PPARalpha and PPARgamma activators. J Biol Chem 272:28210–28217

Martinet W, Kockx MM (2001) Apoptosis in atherosclerosis: focus on oxidized lipids and inflammation. Curr Opin Lipidol 12:535–541

Martin-Nizard F, Furman C, Delerive P, Kandoussi A, Fruchart JC, Staels B, Duriez P (2002) Peroxisome proliferator-activated receptor activators inhibit oxidized low-density lipoprotein-induced endothelin-1 secretion in endothelial cells. J Cardiovasc Pharmacol 40:822–831

Marx N, Kehrle B, Kohlhammer K, Grub M, Koenig W, Hombach V, Libby P, Plutzky J (2002) PPAR activators as antiinflammatory mediators in human T lymphocytes: implications for atherosclerosis and transplantation-associated arteriosclerosis. Circ Res 90:703–710

Marx N, Mackman N, Schonbeck U, Yilmaz N, Hombach VV, Libby P, Plutzky J (2001) PPA-Ralpha Activators Inhibit Tissue Factor Expression and Activity in Human Monocytes. Circulation 103:213–219

Marx N, Sukhova GK, Collins T, Libby P, Plutzky J (1999) PPARalpha activators inhibit cytokine-induced vascular cell adhesion molecule-1 expression in human endothelial cells. Circulation 99:3125–3131

Mascaro C, Acosta E, Ortiz JA, Marrero PF, Hegardt FG, Haro D (1998) Control of human muscle-type carnitine palmitoyltransferase I gene transcription by peroxisome proliferator-activated receptor. J Biol Chem 273:8560–8563

Motojima K, Passilly P, Peters JM, Gonzalez FJ, Latruffe N (1998) Expression of putative fatty acid transporter genes are regulated by peroxisome proliferator-activated receptor alpha and gamma activators in a tissue- and inducer-specific manner. J Biol Chem 273:16710–16714

Napoli C (2002) Nitric oxide and atherosclerotic lesion progression: an overview. J Card Surg 17:355–362

Neve BP, Corseaux D, Chinetti G, Zawadzki C, Fruchart JC, Duriez P, Staels B, Jude B (2001) PPARalpha Agonists Inhibit Tissue Factor Expression in Human Monocytes and Macrophages. Circulation 103:207–212

Nigro J, Dilley RJ, Little PJ (2002) Differential effects of gemfibrozil on migration, proliferation and proteoglycan production in human vascular smooth muscle cells. Atherosclerosis 162:119–129

Nilsson L, Takemura T, Eriksson P, Hamsten A (1999) Effects of fibrate compounds on expression of plasminogen activator inhibitor-1 by cultured endothelial cells. Arterioscler Thromb Vasc Biol 19:1577–1581

Nissen SE, Tsunoda T, Tuzcu EM, Schoenhagen P, Cooper CJ, Yasin M, Eaton GM, Lauer MA, Sheldon WS, Grines CL, Halpern S, Crowe T, Blankenship JC, Kerensky R (2003) Effect of recombinant ApoA-I Milano on coronary atherosclerosis in patients with acute coronary syndromes: a randomized controlled trial. JAMA 290:2292–2300

Ogata T, Miyauchi T, Sakai S, Irukayama-Tomobe Y, Goto K, Yamaguchi I (2002) Stimulation of peroxisome-proliferator-activated receptor alpha (PPAR alpha) attenuates cardiac fibrosis and endothelin-1 production in pressure-overloaded rat hearts. Clin Sci (Lond) 103 Suppl 48:284S–288S

Oliver WR, Jr., Shenk JL, Snaith MR, Russell CS, Plunket KD, Bodkin NL, Lewis MC, Winegar DA, Sznaidman ML, Lambert MH, Xu HE, Sternbach DD, Kliewer SA, Hansen BC, Willson TM (2001) A selective peroxisome proliferator-activated receptor delta agonist promotes reverse cholesterol transport. Proc Natl Acad Sci USA 98:5306–5311

Pasceri V, Cheng JS, Willerson JT, Yeh ET, Chang J (2001) Modulation of C-reactive protein-mediated monocyte chemoattractant protein-1 induction in human endothelial cells by anti-atherosclerosis drugs. Circulation 103:2531–2534

Peters JM, Hennuyer N, Staels B, Fruchart JC, Fievet C, Gonzalez FJ, Auwerx J (1997) Alterations in lipoprotein metabolism in peroxisome proliferator-activated receptor alpha-deficient mice. J Biol Chem 272:27307–27312

Playford DA, Watts GF, Croft KD, Burke V (2003) Combined effect of coenzyme Q(10) and fenofibrate on forearm microcirculatory function in type 2 diabetes. Atherosclerosis 168:169–179

Raji A, Plutzky J (2002) Insulin resistance, diabetes, and atherosclerosis: thiazolidinediones as therapeutic interventions. Curr Cardiol Rep 4:514–521

Rival Y, Beneteau N, Taillandier T, Pezet M, Dupont-Passelaigue E, Patoiseau JF, Junquero D, Colpaert FC, Delhon A (2002) PPARalpha and PPARdelta activators inhibit cytokine-induced nuclear translocation of NF-kappaB and expression of VCAM-1 in EAhy926 endothelial cells. Eur J Pharmacol 435:143–151

Roberts RA, Chevalier S, Hasmall SC, James NH, Cosulich SC, Macdonald N (2002) PPAR alpha and the regulation of cell division and apoptosis. Toxicology 181/182:167–170

Robins SJ (2003) Cardiovascular disease with diabetes or the metabolic syndrome: should statins or fibrates be first line lipid therapy? Curr Opin Lipidol 14:575–583

Royo T, Alfon J, Berrozpe M, Badimon L (2000) Effect of gemfibrozil on peripheral atherosclerosis and platelet activation in a pig model of hyperlipidemia. Eur J Clin Invest 30:843–852

Rubins HB, Robins SJ, Collins D, Fye CL, Anderson JW, Elam MB, Faas FH, Linares E, Schaefer EJ, Schectman G, Wilt TJ, Wittes J (1999) Gemfibrozil for the secondary prevention of coronary heart disease in men with low levels of high-density lipoprotein cholesterol. Veterans Affairs High-Density Lipoprotein Cholesterol Intervention Trial Study Group. N Engl J Med 341:410–418

Russo G, Leopold JA, Loscalzo J (2002) Vasoactive substances: nitric oxide and endothelial dysfunction in atherosclerosis. Vascul Pharmacol 38:259–269

Schoonjans K, Peinado-Onsurbe J, Lefebvre AM, Heyman RA, Briggs M, Deeb S, Staels B, Auwerx J (1996) PPARalpha and PPARgamma activators direct a distinct tissue-specific transcriptional response via a PPRE in the lipoprotein lipase gene. Embo J 15:5336–5348

Sethi S, Ziouzenkova O, Ni H, Wagner DD, Plutzky J, Mayadas TN (2002) Oxidized omega-3 fatty acids in fish oil inhibit leukocyte-endothelial interactions through activation of PPAR alpha. Blood 100:1340–1346

Shu H, Wong B, Zhou G, Li Y, Berger J, Woods JW, Wright SD, Cai TQ (2000) Activation of PPARalpha or gamma reduces secretion of matrix metalloproteinase 9 but not interleukin 8 from human monocytic THP-1 cells. Biochem Biophys Res Commun 267:345–349

Sonoki K, Iwase M, Iino K, Ichikawa K, Yoshinari M, Ohdo S, Higuchi S, Iida M (2003) Dilazep and fenofibric acid inhibit MCP-1 mRNA expression in glycoxidized LDL-stimulated human endothelial cells. Eur J Pharmacol 475:139–147

Staels B, Dallongeville J, Auwerx J, Schoonjans K, Leitersdorf E, Fruchart JC (1998) Mechanism of action of fibrates on lipid and lipoprotein metabolism. Circulation 98:2088–2093

Staels B, van Tol A, Skretting G, Auwerx J (1992) Lecithin:cholesterol acyltransferase gene expression is regulated in a tissue-selective manner by fibrates. J Lipid Res 33:727–735

Staels B, Vu-Dac N, Kosykh VA, Saladin R, Fruchart JC, Dallongeville J, Auwerx J (1995) Fibrates downregulate apolipoprotein C-III expression independent of induction of peroxisomal acyl coenzyme A oxidase. A potential mechanism for the hypolipidemic action of fibrates. J Clin Invest 95:705–712

Steiner G (2001) The use of fibrates and of statins in preventing atherosclerosis in diabetes. Curr Opin Lipidol 12:611–617

Tabernero A, Schoonjans K, Jesel L, Carpusca I, Auwerx J, Andriantsitohaina R (2002) Activation of the peroxisome proliferator-activated receptor alpha protects against myocardial ischaemic injury and improves endothelial vasodilatation. BMC Pharmacol 2002 Apr 09; 2(1):10

Tailleux A, Bouly M, Luc G, Castro G, Caillaud JM, Hennuyer N, Poulain P, Fruchart JC, Duverger N, Fievet C (2000) Decreased susceptibility to diet-induced atherosclerosis in human apolipoprotein A-II transgenic mice. Arterioscler Thromb Vasc Biol 20:2453–2458

Tailleux A, Torpier G, Mezdour H, Fruchart JC, Staels B, Fievet C (2003) Murine models to
investigate pharmacological compounds acting as ligands of PPARs in dyslipidemia and
atherosclerosis. Trends Pharmacol Sci 24:530–534

Thorp JM, Waring WS (1962) Modification of metabolism and distribution of lipids by ethyl
chlorophenoxyisobutyrate. Nature 194:948–949

Tordjman K, Bernal-Mizrachi C, Zemany L, Weng S, Feng C, Zhang F, Leone TC, Coleman T,
Kelly DP, Semenkovich CF (2001) PPARalpha deficiency reduces insulin resistance and
atherosclerosis in apoE-null mice. J Clin Invest 107:1025–1034

Torra IP, Chinetti G, Duval C, Fruchart JC, Staels B (2001) Peroxisome proliferator-activated
receptors: from transcriptional control to clinical practice. Curr Opin Lipidol 12:245–254

Varet J, Vincent L, Mirshahi P, Pille JV, Legrand E, Opolon P, Mishal Z, Soria J, Li H, Soria C
(2003) Fenofibrate inhibits angiogenesis in vitro and in vivo. Cell Mol Life Sci 60:810–819

Vega GL, Ma PT, Cater NB, Filipchuk N, Meguro S, Garcia-Garcia AB, Grundy SM (2003)
Effects of adding fenofibrate (200 mg/day) to simvastatin (10 mg/day) in patients with
combined hyperlipidemia and metabolic syndrome. Am J Cardiol 91:956–960

Vu-Dac N, Gervois P, Jakel H, Nowak M, Bauge E, Dehondt H, Staels B, Pennacchio LA,
Rubin EM, Fruchart-Najib J, Fruchart JC (2003) Apolipoprotein A5, a crucial determinant
of plasma triglyceride levels, is highly responsive to peroxisome proliferator-activated
receptor alpha activators. J Biol Chem 278:17982–17985

Vu-Dac N, Schoonjans K, Kosykh V, Dallongeville J, Fruchart JC, Staels B, Auwerx J (1995)
Fibrates increase human apolipoprotein A-II expression through activation of the peroxisome proliferator-activated receptor. J Clin Invest 96:741–750

Vu-Dac N, Schoonjans K, Laine B, Fruchart JC, Auwerx J, Staels B (1994) Negative regulation
of the human apolipoprotein A-I promoter by fibrates can be attenuated by the interaction
of the peroxisome proliferator-activated receptor with its response element. J Biol Chem
269:31012–31018

Warden CH, Hedrick CC, Qiao JH, Castellani LW, Lusis AJ (1993) Atherosclerosis in transgenic mice overexpressing apolipoprotein A-II. Science 261:469–472

Willson TM, Brown PJ, Sternbach DD, Henke BR (2000) The PPARs: from orphan receptors
to drug discovery. J Med Chem 43:527–550

Willson TM, Lambert MH, Kliewer SA (2001) Peroxisome proliferator-activated receptor
gamma and metabolic disease. Annu Rev Biochem 70:341–367

Yang Q, Xie Y, Alexson SE, Nelson BD, DePierre JW (2002) Involvement of the peroxisome
proliferator-activated receptor alpha in the immunomodulation caused by peroxisome
proliferators in mice. Biochem Pharmacol 63:1893–1900

Zhao SP, Ye HJ, Zhou HN, Nie S, Li QZ (2003) Gemfibrozil reduces release of tumor necrosis
factor-alpha in peripheral blood mononuclear cells from healthy subjects and patients
with coronary heart disease. Clin Chim Acta 332:61–67

Ziouzenkova O, Perrey S, Asatryan L, Hwang J, MacNaul KL, Moller DE, Rader DJ, Sevanian
A, Zechner R, Hoefler G, Plutzky J (2003) Lipolysis of triglyceride-rich lipoproteins
generates PPAR ligands: evidence for an antiinflammatory role for lipoprotein lipase.
Proc Natl Acad Sci U S A 100:2730–2735

Zuckerman SH, Kauffman RF, Evans GF (2002) Peroxisome proliferator-activated receptor
alpha,gamma coagonist LY465608 inhibits macrophage activation and atherosclerosis in
apolipoprotein E knockout mice. Lipids 37:487–494

HEP (2005) 170:407–442
© Springer-Verlag Berlin Heidelberg 2005

ACE Inhibitors and Angiotensin II Receptor Antagonists

A. Dendorfer · P. Dominiak · H. Schunkert (✉)

Medizinische Klinik II, Universitätsklinikum Schleswig-Hostein, Ratzeburger Allee 160,
23538 Lübeck, Germany
Heribert.schunkert@innere2.uni-luebeck.de

Abstract The biological actions of angiotensin II (ANG), the most prominent hormone of the renin–angiotensin–aldosterone system (RAAS), may promote the development of atherosclerosis in many ways. ANG aggravates hypertension, metabolic syndrome, and endothelial dysfunction, and thereby constitutes a major risk factor for cardiovascular disease. The formation of atherosclerotic lesions involves local uptake, synthesis and oxidation of lipids, inflammation, as well as cellular migration and proliferation—mechanisms that may all be enhanced by ANG via its AT_1 receptor. ANG may also increase the risk of acute thrombosis by destabilizing atherosclerotic plaques and enhancing the activity of thrombocytes and coagulation. After myocardial infarction, ANG promotes myocardial remodeling and fibrosis, and its many pathological mechanisms deteriorate the prognosis of these high-risk patients in particular. Therapeutically, inhibitors of the angiotensin I-converting enzyme (ACEI) and AT_1 receptor blockers (ARB) are available to suppress the generation and cellular signaling of ANG, respectively. Despite major differences in the efficacy of ANG suppression and the modulation of other hormones and receptors, both classes of drugs are generally effective in attenuating numerous pathomechanisms of ANG in vitro, and in diminishing the development of atherosclerotic lesions and restenosis after angioplasty in various animal models. In clinical therapy, ACEI and ACE are well-tolerated antihypertensive drugs that also improve the prognosis of heart failure patients. After myocardial infarction and in stable coronary heart disease, ACEI have been shown to reduce mortality in a manner independent of hemodynamic alterations. However, there is little evidence that inhibitors of the RAAS may be effective against arterial restenosis, and a possible benefit of these substances compared to other antihypertensive drugs in the primary prevention of coronary heart disease in hypertensive patients is still a matter of debate, possibly depending on the specific substance and condition being investigated. As such, the general clinical efficacy of ACEI and ARB may be due to a positive influence on hemodynamic load, vascular function, myocardial remodeling, and neuro-humoral regulation, rather than to a direct attenuation of the atherosclerotic process. Further therapeutic advances may be achieved by identifying optimum drugs, patient populations, and treatment protocols.

Keywords Renin-angiotensin-aldosterone system · Angiotensin I · Angiotensin I-converting enzyme · ACE inhibitor · Angiotensin AT_1-receptor

Abbreviations

RAAS	Renin-angiotensin-aldosterone system
ANG	Angiotensin II
ACE	Angiotensin I-converting enzyme
SHR	Spontaneously hypertensive rat
oxLDL	Oxidized low-density lipoprotein
LOX-1	Lectin-like oxidized low-density lipoprotein receptor-1
CRP	C-reactive protein
ARB	Angiotensin AT_1-receptor blocker
ACEI	ACE inhibitor
IMT	Intimal medial thickness
MCP-1	Monocyte chemoattractant protein-1
PDGF	Platelet derived growth factor
MMP	Matrix metallo-proteinase
EGF	Epidermal growth factor

1
Introduction

Research over the past decades has drawn a complex picture of the pathophysiology of human vascular disease. Intrinsic risk factors have been described–such as hypertension, dyslipidemia, and endothelial dysfunction–that have paved the way to understanding the cellular pathomechanisms involved in the initiation or promotion of atherosclerotic plaque formation (Ross 1999). This disease is now understood primarily as an inflammatory process of the vascular wall that includes dysfunctional regulation, invasion of white blood cells, cellular proliferation, and at the molecular level activation of cytokines, adhesion factors, growth hormones, as well as oxygen radicals. Usually, this process proceeds over years until it culminates in an acute vascular occlusion, frequently initiated by plaque rupture and activation of thrombocyte aggregation and coagulation. With the occurrence of ischemic episodes or an acute atherothrombotic event, cardiovascular disease becomes clinically manifest and launches additional pathophysiological mechanisms. Recurrent thrombosis now becomes threatening and must be prevented by antiplatelet or anticoagulant drugs. In the case of a negotiated myocardial infarction, the sequel of scar formation, myocardial remodeling and physical impairment entails the risk of severe clinical complications, e.g., cardiac arrhythmias and heart failure, which ultimately determine the prognosis of cardiovascular disease.

The discovery and investigation of the renin–angiotensin–aldosterone system (RAAS) is intimately intertwined with scientific advances in the field of

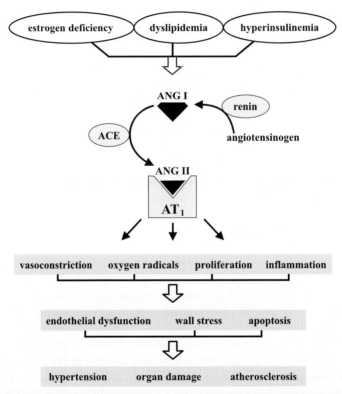

Fig. 1 Major risk factors of atherosclerosis target the RAAS which provides a link to numerous pathophysiologic events. Components of the renin-angiotensin systen, e.g., angiotensinogen [the parent peptide of angiotensin I (*ANG I*)], angiotensin I converting-enzyme (*ACE*), and AT$_1$ receptors are upregulated by common metabolic and hormonal alterations. Via its AT$_1$ receptor, ANG promotes a variety of pathomechanisms that are significant in the initiation, progression, and clinical prognosis of cardiovascular disease

atherosclerosis. Originally, circulating angiotensin II (ANG) was recognized as a major factor causing hypertension, and was therefore regarded as a risk factor of atherosclerosis. More recently, evidence has accumulated that the RAAS is acting as a pathogenic factor at virtually all stages of cardiovascular disease. Many pathophysiological details have been revealed about the function of ANG as a mediator of lipid alterations and inflammation in the initiation phase of atherosclerosis. Conversely, major risk factors of atherosclerosis modulate the expression of angiotensinogen, angiotensin I converting-enzyme (ACE) and AT_1 receptors, so that the RAAS provides an important functional link between the risk factors and pathomechanisms of this disease (Fig. 1). Angiotensin II also appears to contribute significantly to the progression and clinical prognosis of cardiovascular disease which will be decided by acute atherothrombosis and by ischemia related cardiovascular pathophysiology. This review attempts to differentiate the implications of the RAAS in the individual pathomechanisms of cardiovascular disease, and will focus on the experimental and clinical experiences obtained with its pharmacological suppression.

2
Pathogenic Mechanisms Linking RAAS and Atherosclerosis

2.1
Physiology and Localization of ANG Formation

Hypertension has long been known as a risk factor for the development of atherosclerosis, and its association with kidney disease has shown that circulating ANG can constitute a decisive pathogenic factor. With the identification of endothelial dysfunction and vascular inflammation as prominent pathomechanisms of vascular disease, the significance of multiple local, tissue-based RAAS has been disclosed more and more. Numerous organs, including heart, blood vessels, kidneys and brain express the components of ANG synthesis (Dzau et al. 2002), so that locally released ANG can act as an autocrine and paracrine hormone which is not only of major significance for blood pressure regulation, but also for proliferation, growth and inflammatory processes (Fig. 2). The local restriction of such ANG actions has been demonstrated using transgenic rats overexpressing angiotensinogen in the myocardium in a tissue-specific manner. These animals develop myocardial hypertrophy in the absence of an increase in blood pressure or circulating ANG levels (Mazzolai et al. 1998). On the other hand, deletion of the membrane-bound form of ACE in mice resulted in a cardiovascular phenotype very closely resembling that of completely ACE-deficient animals (Esther et al. 1997). These mice also show less generation of oxygen radicals by macrophages and less lipid peroxidation, and are protected from the development of atherosclerosis when deletion of apolipoprotein (apo) E is introduced as a pathogenic factor (Hayek et al. 2003).

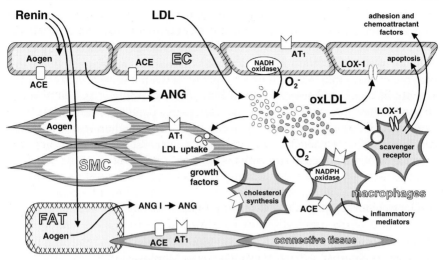

Fig. 2 Local generation and actions of angiotensin II (*ANG*) in the vascular wall. Components like angiotensinogen (*Aogen*) and angiotensin I converting-enzyme (*ACE*) are expressed in endothelial cells (*EC*), vascular smooth muscle cells (*SMC*), fat cells (*FAT*) and macrophages that combine with incorporated renin to form local systems of ANG synthesis. Circulating renin can be taken up by some of these cells. This system is activated in diseases like hypertension and hyperinsulinemia, and also in the inflammatory environment of atherosclerotic plaques. Angiotensin II promotes atherogenesis by stimulating cholesterol synthesis in macrophages, as well as by vascular and cellular uptake of LDL. Stimulation of all vascular cell types by ANG induces vasoconstriction, hypertrophy, proliferation and generation of the superoxide radical (O_2^-) that further promotes endothelial dysfunction and LDL oxidation. The product of this reaction (*oxLDL*) is avidly taken up by macrophages via scavenger receptors, but also by the lectin-like receptor LOX-1 whose expression is induced by ANG among other mediators

For local ANG forming systems, the only external requirement appears to be active renin that must be taken up from the circulation despite the fact that prorenin can be expressed in the myocardium and vascular wall under pathophysiological conditions (Dostal et al. 1999; Endo-Mochizuki et al. 1995; Hilgers et al. 2001). This puts into perspective the significance of the last step of ANG synthesis that is conferred by ACE, chymase, or enzymes forming ANG directly from angiotensinogen such as cathepsin G and other chymostatin-sensitive enzymes (Danser 2003; Dostal et al. 1999). These enzymes are predominantly membrane bound and occur with a wide organ distribution in many tissues. ACE is most prominently expressed by the endothelium, from which its circulating activity originates as a result of shedding; it is also present in fibrocytes, leukocytes and parenchymal cells of various tissues (Kim et al. 2000; Ruiz-Ortega et al. 2001; Zhuo et al. 1998). Most importantly, the myocardial activity of ACE is upregulated in cardiac hypertrophy, in infarcted myocardium, and also in atherosclerotic vessels, where ACE has been localized to macrophages and foam cells of atherosclerotic plaques and myofibroblasts of the neointima (Fig. 2) (Diet et al. 1996; Rakugi et al. 1994a; Schunkert et al. 1990). While the role of ACE in ANG formation is convincingly established, uncertainty exists as to the relative contribution by chymase. Whereas the vascular activity of this enzyme is negligible in the rabbit, it represents the majority of ANG forming activity in human myocardium (Akasu et al. 1998; Wolny et al. 1997), and it is upregulated in arteries of hypercholesteremic patients (Ihara et al. 1999; Uehara et al. 2000). However, chymase in the intima of atheromatous plaques was found to be restricted to the cytosol of mast cells, and its location in the vascular wall did not correlate with that of ANG (Ohishi et al. 1999).

2.2
Cardiovascular Pathophysiology: Role of the Genetic Variability of ACE

The chromosomal loci of the ACE and angiotensinogen genes have been linked to the variabilities of respective protein levels. Moreover, ACE activity and angiotensinogen levels appear to modulate arterial blood pressure, as well as left ventricular mass (independently of blood pressure) as demonstrated in several rodent breeding experiments (Harris et al. 1995; Jacob et al. 1991). Particularly, a deletion/insertion (D/I) polymorphism of intron 16 of the human ACE gene appears to be functionally relevant as it is associated with 14%–50% of the interindividual variance of serum and cardiac ACE activity (Danser et al. 1995; Schunkert 1997). Plasma levels, as well as the deletion allele of the polymorphism, have been associated with the risk of developing myocardial infarction or left ventricular hypertrophy (Cambien et al. 1994, 1995; Schunkert et al. 1995, 1997). These results, although largely reproducible, have not been duplicated by all investigators (Lindpaintner et al. 1995, 1996; Schunkert 1997). It has been suggested that in healthy subjects, negative feedback inhibition may neutralize the genetically enhanced expression of singular components in the ANG synthetic cascade (Danser et al. 1998). By contrast, the ACE DD genotype appears to play a permissive role in the development of left ventricular hypertrophy when the cardiac growth machinery is activated. This hypothesis is impressively illustrated by recent data from Montgomery et al. in which young healthy subjects were studied before and after a rigorous exercise protocol (Montgomery et al. 1997). Only those participants who carried the ACE deletion allele displayed an increase in left ventricular mass. Thus, the ACE genotype may act only under specific conditions suggesting an interaction between altered hemodymanics, ACE, and/or other genetic cofactors in the modulation of left ventricular mass. In agreement with this notion are the observations of Pinto et al. and Ohmichi et al. who both found that pathological remodeling early after myocardial infarction occurs predominantly in those subjects with the ACE DD genotype (Ohmichi et al. 1996; Pinto et al. 1995). Even more strikingly, transgenic rats with high levels of cardiac ACE expression have normal hearts as long as these animals are housed under physiological conditions. However, cardiac growth and diastolic dysfunction were augmented in the same ACE transgenic rats when the animals were stressed by abdominal aortic banding and subsequent cardiac pressure overload (Pinto et al. 1997).

2.3
Role of RAAS in the Pathogenesis of Atherosclerosis

2.3.1
Risk Factors and Endothelial Dysfunction

The development of atherosclerotic disease is a multifactorial process and ANG may be implicated in all of its pathomechanisms. In the following, we will discuss the significance of the molecular actions of ANG in the multifaceted pathomechanisms of atherosclerosis, as summarized in Fig. 3. Before going into the molecular details of local vascular processes, attention should be called to the fact that ANG may contribute to most of the general risk factors for atherosclerosis. This connection is evident in the case of renal hypertension which is provoked by ANG as a monogenic factor, and which clearly fosters the development of atherosclerosis (Weiss et al. 2001). Similar considerations may apply to some of the pathomechanisms of primary hypertension. Increased sympathetic tone is found in hypertensive patients and in the spontaneously hypertensive rat model, and is mutually connected with the RAAS. AT_1 receptors are located in central nervous nuclei of autonomic

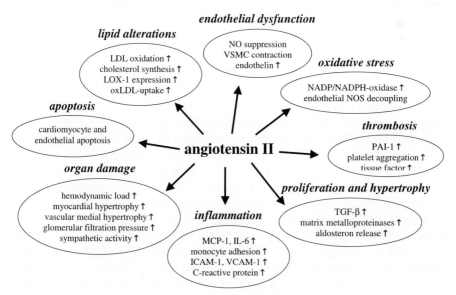

Fig. 3 Pathogenic mechanisms of angiotensin II with potential relevance in atherosclerosis

regulation, in sympathetic ganglia, and at the prejunctional membranes of peripheral adrenergic neurons (Palatini 2001; Veerasingham et al. 2003). At these locations, ANG may stimulate central nervous sympathetic tone, the firing rate of peripheral adrenergic nerves, as well as the amount of catecholamines released with each action potential (Brasch et al. 1993; Dendorfer et al. 2002). Conversely, renin release from the iuxtaglomerular cells is under strict control of sympathetic innervation in a manner mediated by β_1 receptors. Denervation of the kidneys of spontaneously hypertensive rats at a prehypertensive age delays the establishment of hypertension (DiBona 2002). The RAAS is also known as a pathogenic contributor to the metabolic syndrome. Plasma renin activity is negatively correlated with insulin sensitivity in hypertensive patients and normotensive subjects (Townsend et al. 1994; Wheatcroft et al. 2003), and insulin has the potential to activate the RAAS by upregulating the expression of AT_1 receptors (Fig. 1) (Nickenig et al. 1998).

One common denominator of vascular, autonomic and metabolic dysregulation fostered by ANG can be addressed as endothelial dysfunction (Fig. 1). This describes the impaired ability of the endothelium to provoke vasodilation, and to suppress leukocyte adhesion, platelet aggregation, and proliferation of media cells, due to a reduced synthesis of mediators such as nitric oxide (NO), prostacyclin, and endothelium-derived hyperpolarizing factor. Endothelial dysfunction is detectable in patients with hypertension, hypercholesterolemia, or hyperinsulinemia, and represents the first functional abnormality present at the initiation of atherosclerosis (Mancini 1998; Wheatcroft et al. 2003). Besides a variety of hormonal, autonomic, and metabolic conditions, endothelial dysfunction may also be provoked by ANG, as has been demonstrated in ANG-infused rats and rabbits (Rajagopalan et al. 1996). One hallmark in the suppression of endothelial function by ANG is constituted by an increased generation of oxygen radicals which react with and inactivate NO (Fig. 4). ANG activates NADH/NADPH-oxidases of endothelial and smooth muscle cells via AT_1 receptors, and thereby induces the formation of superoxide anion (O_2^-) and hydrogen peroxide (H_2O_2) (Griendling et al. 1997; Lassegue et al. 2003; Seshiah et al. 2002). Reaction of NO with superoxide in particular will not only inactivate the vasodilator, but will give rise to peroxynitrite ($ONOO^-$) which is considered as a more cytotoxic radical because it readily oxidizes free and protein-associated tyrosine (Droge 2002; Dusting et al. 1998; Napoli et al. 2001). Oxygen radicals trigger a variety of redox-sensitive intracellular signaling pathways that further impair the functional capacity of endothelial cells. Endothelial NO synthase is upregulated and decoupled in response to ANG infusion, so that it contributes to vascular superoxide formation (Mollnau et al. 2002). Finally, oxygen radicals increase the expression of the vasoconstrictor endothelin, and may trigger the cascade resulting in apoptosis (Feuerstein et al. 2000; Herizi et al. 1998; Schiffrin 2001).

ANG induces the described detrimental effects via its AT_1 receptor subtype. These actions may be balanced by stimulation of AT_2 receptors that are

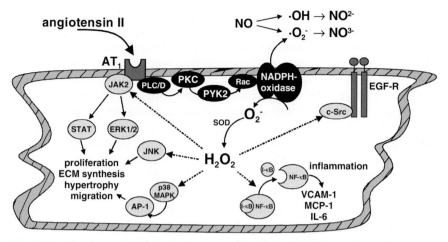

Fig. 4 Role of oxygen radicals in the suppression of NO availability and in the signaling of inflammatory and proliferative actions of angiotensin II. Reactions are summarized that provoke the stimulation of NADH/NADPH-oxidase by AT_1 receptors (*black*), or that mediate the growth and inflammatory responses to the intracellular generation of H_2O_2 (*gray*). Stimulation of NADH/NADPH oxidases via the AT_1 receptor results in the generation of superoxide anion (O_2^-) which, after conversion to H_2O_2 by superoxide dismutase (*SOD*), constitutes an important intracellular signaling molecule, and also inactivates the vasodilator NO

greatly expressed during fetal development, but restricted to certain organs (e.g., brain, kidney, adrenal medulla) in adults. In particular, AT_2 receptors represent the main subtype in human myocardium, whereas their expression is low in rodents (Regitz-Zagrosek et al. 1995). Cardiovascular AT_2 receptors are present at endothelium, fibroblasts, cardiomyocytes and smooth muscle cells and are upregulated in pathophysiological conditions such as heart failure and myocardial infarction (Matsubara 1998). In general, AT_2 receptors may counteract the signal transduction of AT_1 receptors by activating protein phosphatases, thereby reverting the signaling of AT_1-activated protein kinases (Cui et al. 2001; Sohn et al. 2000). Furthermore, AT_2 receptors promote the generation of bradykinin, a nonapeptide that stimulates the release of endothelial autacoids via B_2 receptors, thereby alleviating the vasopressor and fibrogenic actions of ANG (Kurisu et al. 2003; Siragy et al. 1999). This physiological significance of AT_2 receptors has mainly been derived from studies with AT_2-deficient mice. These mice show a slight elevation of blood pressure, vascular hypertrophy and enhanced sensitivity to ANG (Brede et al. 2001), and are prone to neointima formation in vascular lesions (Suzuki et al. 2002). Blockade of AT_2 receptors has been shown to promote the formation of aneurysms in ANG-infused $apoE^{-/-}$ mice, and to diminish the protective action of an AT_1 antagonist after myocardial infarction (Daugherty et al. 2001; Liu et al. 1997). In the latter situation, both an AT_1 antagonist and an ACE inhibitor attenuated remodeling, but AT_2 receptor stimulation appeared to be functional during AT_1 blockade, exclusively (Xu et al. 2002). Suppression of proliferation via AT_2 receptors has been clearly demonstrated in neointima formation after balloon injury of carotid artery which was significantly attenuated by local gene transfer and overexpression of these receptors (Nakajima et al. 1995). However, under certain conditions, AT_2 receptors mediate effects that may be detrimental in cardiovascular diseases. Myocardial hypertrophy and fibrosis induced by ANG infusion were abolished in $AT_2^{-/-}$ mice (Ichihara et al. 2001). AT_2 receptors may trigger apoptosis in cardiomyocytes and may impair the proliferation of endothelial cells (Dimmeler et al. 1997; Goldenberg et al. 2001). Evidence has also been obtained that AT_2 receptors activate nuclear factor κB (NF-κB) in smooth muscle cells, an effect resembling the prominent inflammatory actions of AT_1 receptors (Ruiz-Ortega et al. 2000). As such, the contribution of AT_2 receptors in processes relevant for atherosclerosis has not been conclusively characterized, and there is no in vivo evidence of any anti-atherosclerotic influence of overexpression or exogenous stimulation of AT_2 receptors. Overall, most pathophysiological mechanisms of ANG appear to be mediated by the AT_1 subtype.

2.3.2
Plaque Formation

Early in the development of atheromatous plaques, cholesterol accumulates in the vascular wall due to either enhanced invasion, stimulated cellular uptake, or exaggerated synthesis by tissue macrophages. Locally formed ANG may accelerate all of these processes. Atherosclerosis in ANG-infused apoE$^{-/-}$ mice is related to an increase in cholesterol synthesis that is provoked in macrophages by transcriptional upregulation of 3-hydroxy-3-methylglutaryl coenzyme A (HMG-CoA) reductase via the AT_1 receptor (Fig. 2) (Keidar et al. 1999). Diffusion of low-density lipoprotein (LDL) into the vascular wall is greatly enhanced by the vasopressor effects of ANG (Nielsen et al. 1994), and may proceed unrestrictedly when the integrity of the endothelium is locally disturbed. LDL also binds ANG and this complex is taken up at an enhanced rate by the macrophage scavenger receptor (Keidar 1998). Oxidation is another modification of lipoproteins that fosters their uptake into the vessel wall. ANG promotes LDL oxidation by increasing radical production via activation of NADH/NADPH oxidases in macrophages and endothelial cells, as described above. Strong interactions exist between these effects of ANG and hypercholesterolemia. In the aorta of cholesterol-fed rabbits, superoxide production was about doubled as a result of endothelial NADH oxidase activity (Warnholtz et al. 1999). Interestingly, administration of an AT_1 antagonist normalized lipid oxidation, suggesting an at least local activation of the RAAS by lipid alteration. This activation is based on several molecular mechanisms. The ANG generating enzymes, ACE and chymase, have been found to be upregulated in atherosclerotic lesions of hypercholesterolemic animals (Mitani et al. 1996; Takai et al. 1997). The vascular responsiveness to ANG is increased in hyper-cholesteremia due to post-translational enhancement of AT_1 receptor density in vascular smooth muscle (Nickenig et al. 1997). The oxidized forms of LDL (oxLDL) also promote AT_1 mRNA expression in human coronary endothe-lial cells via activation of NF-κB (Li et al. 2000). Within this setting, it is not surprising that hypercholesterolemic patients respond with exaggerated blood pressure increases to infused ANG (Nickenig et al. 1999). The interaction be-tween ANG and vascular lipids is further confirmed by the observation that enhanced vascular sensitivity to ANG as well as AT_1 receptor expression in vas-cular smooth muscle and endothelial cells could be normalized by HMG-CoA reductase inhibitors (Nickenig et al. 1999; Wassmann et al. 2001).

OxLDL exerts a certain atherogenic toxicity (Steinberg et al. 1989) that arises not only from its uncontrolled uptake by macrophages via scavenger receptors, but also from its stimulation of the lectin-like oxidized low-density lipoprotein receptor-1 (LOX-1) (Fig. 2) . This receptor has been described as a specific uptake mechanism for oxLDL in endothelial cells, but it is also present in macrophages and smooth muscle cells (Chen et al. 2002; Kume et al. 2000). Binding of oxLDL to this receptor not only triggers its internalization, but also activates pathophysiological signal pathways. In endothelial cells, LOX-1 activation induces apoptosis and expression of monocyte chemoattractant protein-1 (MCP-1) as well as further cell adhesion molecules [vascular cell adhesion molecule-1 (VCAM), intercellular adhesion molecule-1 (ICAM-1), P-selectin] (Li et al. 2000) in a manner involving increased generation of oxygen radicals and subsequent activation of NF-κB as signaling pathways (Cominacini et al. 2000). The vascular expression of LOX-1 is upregulated in the conditions of hypercholesterolemia, hypertension and diabetes (Mehta et al. 2002), where it is mediated by vasoconstrictors and cytokines such as ANG, endothelin and tumor necrosis factor-α (Morawietz et al. 1999, 2001; Moriwaki et al. 1998). In hypercholesterolemic rabbits, the RAAS seems to be responsible for the induction of LOX-1 expression in artherosclerotic plaques, since it was largely prevented by losartan treatment (Chen et al. 2000). Conversely, LOX-1 contributes to the local activation of the RAAS by enhancing the expression of ACE and AT_1 receptors in endothelial cells (Li et al. 2003)

2.4
Role of RAAS in the Pathogenesis of Atherothrombosis

2.4.1
Inflammation and Proliferation

Propagation of atherosclerosis is characterized by foam cell formation, in-flammation, and proliferation of smooth muscle cells (Ross 1999). Again, there is ample evidence for an involvement of ANG in these processes. The

AT_1 receptor activates a variety of redox-sensitive signaling pathways that promote inflammation and growth whereby accumulating oxygen radicals mediate many of these processes (Fig. 4). ANG activates NF-κB in monocytes, vascular smooth muscle cells, and endothelial cells (Brand et al. 1996; Kranzhofer et al. 1999). Expression of interleukin (IL)-6, MCP-1, and VCAM-1 and ICAM-1 can be attributed to this transcription factor (Collins et al. 2001; Schieffer et al. 2000; Tummala et al. 1999). As a consequence, these mediators promote invasion of the vascular wall by monocytes, T lymphocytes, and mast cells, and thereby create the conditions for cellular inflammation and the release of further inflammation factors, such as tumor necrosis factor-α. In vascular smooth muscle cells, the AT_1 receptor induces contraction by stimulating phospholipase C, but growth responses depend on a variety of protein kinases and their targets, including ERK, p90RSK, JAK2, STAT1, JNK, p38, and AP-1 (Griendling et al. 1997). The essential signaling of ANG-induced hypertrophy in these cells seems to be related to p70S6K, MEK and ERK, and ultimately to ANG-induced tyrosine phosphorylation of the epidermal growth factor receptor that results in trans-activation (Fig. 4) (Eguchi et al. 1998). These messengers stimulate vascular smooth muscle hypertrophy and the synthesis of extracellular matrix proteins (fibronectin, collagen, laminin, tenascin) in a manner that is at least partially independent of increased physical stress in hypertension (Griffin et al. 1991; Kato et al. 1991; Sharifi et al. 1992). Smooth muscle cells respond to ANG with proliferation, particularly when further stimulatory conditions are present, e.g., during neointima formation after balloon injury (Su et al. 1998). This action of ANG seems to be related to the activation of PI3-kinase and to the autocrine release of basic fibroblast growth factor (Saward et al. 1997). However, ANG induces the release of various additional growth factors such as tumor growth factor-β_1, platelet-derived growth factor, vascular endothelial growth factor, and insulin-like growth factor whose roles in the redifferentiation and proliferation of vascular smooth muscle cells are not yet established (Delafontaine et al. 1993; Gibbons et al. 1992; Naftilan et al. 1989; Williams et al. 1995).

Disruption of vulnerable atherosclerotic plaques is considered as a major trigger of thrombosis and ultimate infarction. Destabilization of plaques concurs with a high lipid content and a high inflammatory activity. ANG, ACE, the AT_1 receptor and IL-6 are colocalized in the lesion zones bearing the highest risk of rupture (Schieffer et al. 2000). The acute-phase C-reactive protein (CRP) represents a strong predictor of cardiovascular death (Ridker 2001). Besides the predictive value of CRP, its functional involvement in the process of atherosclerosis has also recently been recognized. CRP acts as a mediator of inflammation by itself, and provokes various pathophysiological events, including activation of NF-κB and expression of AT_1 receptors in vascular smooth muscle cells (Hattori et al. 2003; Wang et al. 2003). The RAAS further contributes to plaque destabilization by provoking smooth muscle apoptosis which is highly prevalent in culprit lesions (Mallat et al. 2000), and by inducing matrix metallo-proteinases (MMPs) that degrade the fibrous cap (Chen et al. 2002). The collagen-cleaving MMP-9 is particularly involved in the degradation of the basal membrane that is necessary for smooth muscle cell migration and proliferation. Excessive activation of MMP-9 is able to destabilize atherosclerotic plaques (Morishige et al. 2003). Finally, the RAAS should also support the pathomechanisms of thrombosis. Platelets possess ANG receptors that alleviate aggregation by promoting the effects of other platelet agonists (Ding et al. 1985). The RAAS increases the production and release of plasminogen activator inhibitor-1 (PAI-1) from endothelial cells and vascular smooth muscle cells (Nakamura et al. 2000; Vaughan 2002), and is apparently also involved in the accumulation of tissue factor in atherosclerotic plaques, that was found to be reduced in ACE inhibitor-treated patients (Soejima et al. 1999).

2.5
Role of RAAS in the Pathogenesis of Cardiovascular Disease

2.5.1
Secondary Events and Restenosis

When vascular disease proceeds to manifest ischemia or even infarction, the RAAS becomes involved in multiple pathophysiologic mechanisms that lead to hemodynamic and neurohumoral dysbalance, and ultimately organ damage. Based on the multiple studies demonstrating protective effects of ACEI, it is tempting to hypothesize that ANG sets the basis for ischemia by promoting vascular and ventricular hypertrophy. Furthermore, ANG aggravates myocardial infarction, the risk of cardiac arrhythmias, and post-ischemic myocardial stunning by impairing reperfusion and by increasing oxygen radical generation, leukocyte emigration, wall stress, and sympathetic activity. In the infarcted myocardium, ANG may foster myocardial remodeling by induction of inflammation, myocyte apoptosis, and cardiac fibrosis. The sequels of these pathomechanisms will ultimately precipitate heart failure, supported by multiple interactions of ANG with neurohumoral homeostasis and by hemodynamic alterations in the kidney. It needs to be stated that the causal role of the RAAS is not proven in any of these processes, but is reflected by the therapeutic spectrum of RAAS inhibitors. However, this includes effects that are not restricted to the suppression of ANG actions. For ACEI, potentiation of preconditioning, reduction of infarct size, attenuation of fibrosis, and improved perfusion of the kidney may be attributed to the potentiation of bradykinin actions (Linz et al. 1995). Stimulation of AT_2 receptors may contribute to the attenuation of postinfarct myocardial remodeling achieved with AT_1 receptor blockers (ARB) (Liu et al. 1997). The various implications of the RAAS in ischemic cardiac disease and heart failure have been reviewed recently (Brewster et al. 2003), and will not be gone into further because they occur subsequently to the atherosclerotic process, which is the main focus of the present review. However, it should be kept in mind that these actions of the RAAS will determine the clinical prognosis of cardiovascular disease which constitutes the most relevant endpoint assessed in clinical studies.

Restenosis is a major complication occurring after angioplasty of diseased vessels. The tissue trauma induces migration and proliferation of medial smooth muscle cells that ultimately occlude the vessel by forming a neointima. Local activation of the RAAS by this process has been demonstrated in terms of an enhanced expression of ACE and AT_1 receptors in the neointima of rat arteries after balloon injury (Fernandez-Alfonso et al. 1997; Viswanathan et al. 1992). Endogenous ANG appears to be involved in the activation of mitogenic protein kinases (JNK, ERK, AP-1) after vascular trauma, since this signaling was attenuated by ACEI and ARB treatment (Kim et al. 1998). ANG appeared to be of highest significance for initiating proliferation and migration of medial smooth muscle cells (Fingerle et al. 1995). Accordingly, treatment with ACEI has been shown to reduce neointima formation in rat and porcine models (Matsumoto et al. 2001; Wong et al. 1997). Accumulation of bradykinin has been implicated in the antiproliferative action of ACEI (Farhy et al. 1993). Reduction of neointima formation has also been achieved with ARBs (Igarashi et al. 2001), whereby the beneficial action of valsartan in a mouse model appeared to be contributed by AT_2 receptor stimulation (Wu et al. 2001). It has been pointed out that a highly efficient RAAS inhibition is required to exert antiproliferative actions. ACE inhibition in plaques was observed only at a substantially higher dose of quinapril than needed for inhibition of plasma ACE or for blood pressure reduction in rats (Rakugi et al. 1994b). The clinical potential of RAAS blockade may also be limited by the finding that ANG suppression will only remove a trigger of the proliferation response, whereas further growth factors are more relevant for the long-term development of restenosis (Fingerle et al. 1995; Wong et al. 1997).

3
Actions of ACEI and ARB in Experimental Atherosclerosis

3.1
Pharmacodynamic Differences Between ACEI and ARB

The general ability of ACE inhibitors (ACEI) and of angiotensin AT_1-receptor blockers (ARB) to attenuate virtually all of the cardiovascular actions of the RAAS is commonly accepted. The differences between the two drug classes comprise a differential impact on the affected angiotensin receptor subtypes, a different involvement of peptide hormones other than ANG, and possible differences in the efficacy of RAAS suppression (Fig. 5). ACEI reduce the

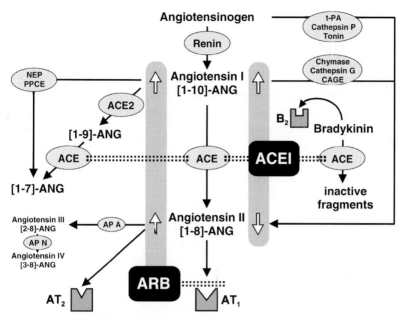

Fig. 5 Differential interaction of ACE inhibitors (*ACEI*) and AT_1 receptor blockers (*ARB*) on hormone levels and pathways within the renin–angiotensin and the kinin–kallikrein systems. By blocking the degradation of angiotensin I, ACEI decrease the availability of angiotensin II (*[1–8]-ANG*) and promote accumulation of angiotensin I (*[1–10]-ANG*) (indicated by *arrows* at the *right* side of the angiotensin metabolic pathway). Blockade of bradykinin degradation by ACEI also efficaciously potentiates the actions of bradykinin at its B_2 receptors. Despite blockade of ACE, angiotensin II can be generated by alternative pathways. Alleviation of negative feedback on renin activity induces accumulation of angiotensin I under therapy with both, ACEI and ARB. This may be of functional significance since this peptide enables the generation of active metabolites, e.g., [1–7]-ANG. Increased levels of angiotensin II are observed during AT_1 blockade, a condition leading to enhanced stimulation of the AT_2 receptor subtype, and to the generation of further angiotensin fragments, such as angiotensins III and IV whose biological significance has not yet been clarified

stimulation of AT_1 and AT_2 receptors, but inhibition may be overcome by activation of renin, by induction of ACE, and by alternative ANG-forming enzymes, such as chymase. Inhibition of ACE blocks the degradation of various peptides, the most important of which is the vasodilator bradykinin. ACEI produce a marginal increase in circulating concentrations of bradykinin, but increase the functional potency of bradykinin by factors of 3–50 (Bonner et al. 1990). Bradykinin stimulates NO release from endothelial cells via B_2 receptors, and exerts a variety of beneficial actions that have been implicated in the organ-protective actions of ACEI (Linz et al. 1995). Within their class, ACEI may be differentiated according to their lipophilicity which may foster preferential inhibition of tissue vs. plasma ACE, and according to their ability to form high affinity complexes with ACE. Clinically approved ACEI do not differentiate between the two catalytic centers of ACE, and nonspecific properties, e.g., a radical scavenging ability of sulfhydryl-containing substances, do not appear to be of therapeutic significance.

Therapeutically used ARB are highly selective for the AT_1 subtype of ANG receptors, so that during therapy AT_2 receptors will be stimulated by the reflective activation of the RAAS (Fig. 5). The therapeutic impact of AT_2 receptor stimulation is not clearly established, as described above. It has been demonstrated experimentally that AT_2 receptor stimulation enhances bradykinin generation, so that some vasodilatory or diuretic actions of ARB may arise through this pathway (Carey et al. 2001). However, bradykinin potentiation by ARB is inferior to that of ACEI, a fact that may limit some of the therapeutically desired actions, but that also lowers the incidence of unwanted angioedema. ACEI and ARB have in common that they enhance renin activity by interruption of negative feedback, and thus increase the generation of angiotensin I. This peptide accumulates during ACE inhibition, while ARB increase both angiotensin I and ANG. As such, both therapies increase the levels of potentially active cleavage fragments that are derived from angiotensin I (e.g., the fragments [1–7]-ANG, and [1–9]-angiotensin I), whereas those resulting from cleavage of ANG (angiotensin III and angiotensin IV) will be enhanced only by ARB treatment. Functional differences between approved ARB may arise from their propensity to form high-affinity receptor complexes which varies greatly between the individual substances. The slow dissociation rates of such complexes implicate an 'insurmountable' binding of the antagonists that results in a noncompetitive mode of antagonism. This may be reflected by a higher efficacy of inhibition under conditions of RAAS activation and, eventually, by a higher maximum efficacy of insurmountable substances for reducing blood pressure in hypertensive patients (Elmfeldt et al. 2002).

3.2
Anti-atherosclerotic Efficacy of ACEI and ARB in Experimental Models

With so many implications of the RAAS in the pathomechanisms of atherosclerosis, it is tempting to speculate about the therapeutic success of pharmacological RAAS suppression. Indeed, in the classical model of atherosclerosis (the cholesterol-fed rabbit), an impressive reduction of area and of cholesterol content of aortic lesions could be achieved with enalapril treatment (Schuh et al. 1993). Similar results with different ACE inhibitors were obtained in the Watanabe heritable hyperlipidemic rabbit, in cholesterol-fed hamster, mini-pig, and cynomolgus monkey, as well as in apoE-deficient mice (Candido et al. 2002; Hayek et al. 2002; Miyazaki et al. 1999). Corresponding experiments could be successfully reproduced using ARB (Hope et al. 1999; Keidar et al. 2000; Li et al. 1999; Miyazaki et al. 1999; Strawn et al. 2000). The anti-atherosclerotic actions of both types of RAAS antagonists appeared to be unrelated to their hypotensive or metabolic effects, because most studies performed in normotensive animals disproved an alteration of blood pressure or plasma cholesterol in the treatment groups (Keidar et al. 2000; Miyazaki et al. 1999). In some rabbit models, an ARB failed to reduce atheroma formation, was less effective than an ACEI, or was active only at a blood pressure reducing dosage (Hope et al. 1999; Li et al. 1999; Schuh et al. 1993). Thus, it was tested whether a superior efficacy of ACEI might be related to the potentiation of the known protective actions of bradykinin. Cotreatment with the B_2 antagonist HOE 140 did not suppress the salutary effect of ACE inhibition on aortic atheroma formation in cholesterol-fed rabbits, or in apoE-deficient mice (Fennessy et al. 1996; Keidar et al. 2000), however the functional reactivity of the endothelium was better restored by ACEI than by ARB treatment (Sun et al. 2001). As such, only minor differences between both groups of drugs have been recognized, which cannot permit a prediction of therapeutic success in humans.

Many of the pathophysiological events outlined above could be identified as targets of RAAS suppressive therapies in vivo. AT_1 antagonism improved endothelial function and decreased oxidative stress in cholesterol-fed rabbits (Warnholtz et al. 1999). This was paralleled by enhanced oxidation resistance of plasma lipoproteins and by reduced levels of oxLDL in plasma (Napoli et al. 1999; Strawn et al. 2000). AT_1 blockade also reduced expression of LOX-1, uptake of oxLDL, and cholesterol synthesis in macrophages isolated from ANG-injected or apoE-deficient mice (Keidar et al. 1995; Keidar et al. 1999). Expression of inflammation markers NF-κB, IL-8, MCP-1 was reduced by quinapril in a rabbit model of accelerated atherosclerosis (Hernandez-Presa et al. 1997, 1998). The suppression of PDGF, fibronectin, PAI-1 and of many signaling protein kinases (c-fos, c-jun, p46-JNK, p55-JNK) by ACEI or ARB was demonstrated in rat arteries after balloon injury (Abe et al. 1997; Hamdan et al. 1996; Kim et al. 1995; Kim et al. 1998).

4
Clinical Efficacy of RAAS Inhibitors in Thromboembolic Disease

4.1
Modulation of Risk Factors and Surrogate Parameters

A variety of surrogate parameters of atherosclerotic activity determined in experimental studies could also be assessed as effects of clinical therapy. A comparison of antihypertensive treatments with hydrochlorothiazide or the ARB eprosartan revealed reduced levels of MCP-1 and of soluble cell adhesion molecules, and an increased oxidation resistance of LDL only in the ARB-treated patients (Rahman et al. 2002). AT_1 receptor blockade reduced the expression of a NADH/NADPH oxidase subunit, gp91-phox, in human internal mammary artery (Rueckschloss et al. 2002). Treatment with enalapril after myocardial infarction lowered the circulating levels of MCP-1 and tissue factor (Soejima et al. 1999).

Major functional improvements of endothelial vasodilation were achieved by RAAS inhibition. The TREND study was the first to demonstrate that treatment with quinapril, an ACEI, for 6 months can abolish acetylcholine-induced coronary vasoconstriction in normotensive patients (Mancini et al. 1996). These findings were confirmed by the BANFF study which compared quinapril, enalapril, losartan and amlodipin in their efficacies to enhance flow-mediated brachial artery vasodilation in patients with coronary disease (Anderson et al. 2000). Amongst these treatments, only quinapril alleviated endothelial dysfunction significantly, and this effect was restricted to patients with the II- or I/D-genotype of *ACE*. Quinapril also exerted greater efficacy on endothelial function in comparison to enalapril in heart failure patients (Hornig et al. 1998). In the BANFF study, however, measurements were taken 72 h after the last application of drugs, so that the duration of action of the individual drugs may have decisively influenced their efficacies. In further studies, enalapril augmented acetylcholine-provoked vasodilation in coronary arteries, where improvement of endothelial function was greatest in patients with hypercholesterolemia, in patients bearing at least one D-allele of ACE, and in smokers (Prasad et al. 2000a). Similarly, losartan improved endothelial function of femoral arteries in patients with vascular disease (Prasad et al. 2000b). Interestingly, ramipril (ACEI) and losartan (an ARB) appeared to be equivalent in their potential for improving endothelial vasodilation and reducing vascular stress due to oxygen radicals (Hornig et al. 2001). Correspondingly, even the improvement of flow-dependent vasodilation provoked acutely by the ARB candesartan was shown to be related to an enhanced activity of bradykinin (Hornig et al. 2003). In general, ACEI and ARB improve endothelial function in diseased, but not in healthy vessels, and eventually with preference for the coronary vascular bed and for certain ACE genotypes (Mancini 2002). Differences between specific ACEI may be related to their selectivity for tissue ACE, which may not be regarded as a predictor of clinical efficacy.

4.2
Retardation or Regression of Manifest Vascular Disease

Although RAAS inhibitors positively influence many biochemical and functional parameters of atherosclerosis, the assessment of morphological alterations in existing vascular lesions has rarely been successful. An outstanding positive example is given in the SECURE study that was designed as a substudy of the HOPE trial (Lonn et al. 2001; Yusuf et al. 2000b). This study randomized 693 patients with vascular disease or diabetes mellitus and at least one additional risk factor to treatment with ramipril (2.5 or 10 mg/day), vitamin E (400 IU/day) or corresponding placebos, and followed the development of intimal medial thickness (IMT) in carotid arteries for 4.5 years. IMT in the placebo group increased by 0.0217 mm per year, which was significantly more rapid than it was in the ramipril-treated groups (0.018 mm/year at 2.5 mg/day, and 0.0137 mm/year at 10 mg/day). Supplementation with vitamin E failed to retard atherosclerosis, a finding that corresponds to the reduction of mortality and various cardiovascular events with ramipril, but not with vitamin E in the overall HOPE study (Yusuf et al. 2000b, 2000a). In contrast, a similarly designed study, PART-2, failed to confirm such protection (MacMahon et al. 2000). In PART-2, 617 patients suffering from coronary, carotid, or peripheral vascular disease were treated with ramipril (5–10 mg/day) or placebo for 4 years. Carotid IMT in the placebo group showed only a slight progression from 0.79 to 0.81 mm over this time, which was not intercepted by ramipril (final IMT 0.83 mm) (MacMahon et al. 2000). A further study failed to detect retardation of coronary atherosclerosis by ACE inhibition. The SCAT trial compared enalapril and simvastatin in 460 normocholesterolemic patients with coronary heart disease. After 4 years, coronary diameters and the stenosis to lumen ratio were reduced by simvastatin, but not by enalapril. However, enalapril effectively reduced blood pressure and lowered the combined incidence of death, myocardial infarction and stroke, by more than 40% (Teo et al. 2000). The fact that SECURE remained the only study demonstrating morphological retardation of plaque progression by an ACEI may be related to the type and dose of the ACEI used, and to differing sensitivities of techniques for carotid ultrasound measurement (Lonn et al. 2001). Due to the improved clinical outcome of coronary heart disease in ACEI-treated patients, however, the effect of treatment on the process of restenosis per se cannot be ascertained further.

The promotion of growth by ANG has also been implicated in the proliferation of smooth muscle cells after vascular trauma, a pathomechanism that emerges clinically as restenosis after angioplasty. As such, clinical studies have evaluated the potential of ACEI to prevent this complication. The trials QUIET (1,750 patients treated for 27 months with quinapril after coronary angioplasty or atherectomy), MARCATOR (1436 patients treated with cilazapril for 6 months after coronary angioplasty) and PARIS (79 patients with the DD genotype of ACE treated with quinapril for 6 months after coronary stenting) consistently denied any beneficial effect of an ACEI on the morphology of coronary atherosclerosis and on the risk of cardiovascular events (Cashin-Hemphill et al. 1999; Faxon 1995; Meurice et al. 2001; Pitt et al. 2001). It has been discussed whether certain ACE genotypes or the mode of angioplasty with or without stenting may impair the therapeutic efficacy of ACE inhibitors. However, lack of clinical success with ACEI has been confirmed in patients bearing the DD genotype of ACE after interventional stenting (Koch et al. 2003). The efficacy of ACEI in this situation may be limited by the fact that in-stent restenosis occurs as a purely proliferative process with high expression of AT_1 receptors by myofibroblasts, but little accumulation of ACE in the neointima (Wagenaar et al. 2003). This observation suggests a higher efficacy of AT_1 antagonists in this indication. Indeed, treatment with valsartan after coronary stenting reduced the incidence of in-stent restenosis by 50% in an open-label study (Peters et al. 2001), however this therapeutic approach awaits further confirmation.

4.3
Endpoint Studies of Secondary Prevention

Therapies of secondary prevention aim to reduce vascular ischemic events in patients with preexistent symptomatic cardiovascular disease. The use of antihypertensive agents in this situation is based on several pathophysiologic considerations. First, reduction of blood pressure lowers mechanical stress in the vascular wall, which constitutes a first-line risk for the promotion and rupture of atherosclerotic plaques. Second, reduction of hemodynamic load reduces oxygen consumption, wall stress, hypertrophy, remodeling and ultimately fibrosis in the diseased heart so that myocardial protection results. Third, lower perfusion pressure may protect further organs, e.g., the kidney, which play a key role in determining cardiovascular mortality (Hillege et al. 2002). Fourth, vasodilators may improve blood supply in post-stenotic areas, thereby alleviating symptoms and complications of ischemia such as inflammation, venous thrombosis and necrosis. The success of therapeutically targeting these pathomechanisms has been demonstrated for vasodilators in severe heart failure, and the many implications of the RAAS have been confirmed with the demonstration of superior improvements by ACEI in the prognosis of severe, moderate, and asymptomatic heart failure (The CONSENSUS Trial Study Group 1987; The SOLVD Investigators 1992). These positive findings have been extended to the use of losartan, valsartan and candesartan in heart failure (Cohn et al. 2001; Pfeffer et al. 2003; Pitt et al. 2000), and to the treatment of heart failure following myocardial infarction (Rutherford et al. 1994; The Acute Infarction Ramipril Efficacy Study Investigators 1993).

A difficulty, however, remains to discern the influence that RAAS inhibition exerts directly on the process or complications of atherosclerosis, rather than on its risk factors or on sequels of ischemia. The first landmark study in this regard was the HOPE study, performed on 9297 patients suffering from either manifest vascular disease or type 2 diabetes and featuring at least one additional risk factor, but no sign of heart failure (Yusuf et al. 2000b). The prevalence of cardiovascular disease or diabetes in the study population was 88% and 38%, respectively. Treatment with ramipril (10 mg/day) reduced the occurrence of the combined endpoint (myocardial infarction, stroke, or cardiovascular death) by 22% within the 5-year observation period. In parallel, ramipril reduced the individual risks of myocardial infarction, stroke, revascularization, cardiac arrest, heart failure, diabetic complications, and all-cause mortality by 15%–37%.

This profound benefit could not be explained by the minor reduction in blood pressure (−3 mmHg systolic blood pressure) occurring in the ramipril-treated group, and was evenly distributed amongst the study population, including patients unaffected by diabetes or preceding infarction. These results strongly suggest a delay of the atherosclerotic process by ramipril therapy. However, due to the high prevalence of patients with preceding myocardial infarction in this study (53%), the possible significance of protective hemodynamic or myocardial influences could not be denied. Indeed, the PART-2 study demonstrated in a comparable population that ramipril (5–10 mg/day) reduced left ventricular mass by 5%, thus indicating either direct or blood pressure-dependent actions of ramipril on the myocardium. The clinical implications of the HOPE study were strengthened by the recently completed EUROPA trial that confirmed the success of HOPE in 12,218 patients with stable coronary heart disease and no apparent heart failure (Fox 2003). Treatment with perindopril (8 mg/day) over 4.2 years reduced the combined cardiovascular endpoint by 20%, and provoked a blood pressure reduction similar to the HOPE study (−5 mmHg systolic blood pressure). Generalized to the whole class of drugs, these data mandate the application of an ACEI after myocardial infarction and for any kind of coronary heart disease, regardless of the morphological status of atherosclerosis, blood pressure, or cardiac performance.

4.4
Endpoint Studies of Primary Prevention

Primary prevention aims to attenuate an anticipated atherosclerotic process, whereby at this early stage organ protection is unlikely to affect clinical outcome. Antihypertensive therapy reduces one common pathogenic factor of vascular disease and is generally effective for primary prevention. On the basis of the vast experimental evidence implicating the RAAS in the development of atherosclerosis, RAAS-suppressing drugs were expected to reduce the incidence of ischemic vascular disease in a manner superior to other antihypertensive drugs. The first approaches for direct evaluation of ACEI therapy were the 'UK Prospective Diabetes Study' (UKPDS, 1,148 hypertensive patients with type-2 diabetes treated with captopril or atenolol) and the 'Captopril Prevention Project' (CAPPP, 10,985 hypertensive patients treated with captopril or alternative antihypertensives) (Hansson et al. 1999; UK Prospective Diabetes Study Group 1998). These studies did not find significant advantages of captopril with regard to the prevention of diabetic complications, myocardial infarction, or cardiovascular mortality.

Two recent studies set out to clarify the prospects of ACEI as a first-line therapy for the reduction of mortality in hypertensive patients. In the ALLHAT study, 33,357 patients with hypertension and at least one additional risk factor for coronary heart disease were randomized to treatment with either amlodipine, lisinopril, doxazosin, or chlorthalidone (The ALLHAT Collaborative

Research Group 2002). The study population had a considerable prevalence of cardiovascular disease (52%) and diabetes (36%). The doxazosin arm of the study was terminated prematurely because of a higher incidence of clinical signs of heart failure, as compared to the chlorthalidone arm. After a mean follow-up of 4.9 years, the risk of the primary endpoint (cardiovascular death or nonfatal myocardial infarction), as well as total mortality did not differ between the remaining three treatment groups. Lisinopril proved to be inferior to chlorthalidone with regard to the relative risks of stroke (1.15) and heart failure (1.19). These negative results for lisinopril may have resulted from a less effective reduction of blood pressure compared to the chlorthalidone group (−2 mmHg systolic blood pressure vs. lisinopril). Alternatively, the inclusion of a high percentage of Black patients, a group known to be less responsive to ACE inhibition, may explain this unexpected finding. Indeed, African–Americans had high incidences of both complications (relative risks of 1.4 and 1.32, respectively) and more pronounced differences in achieved blood pressure levels during lisinopril treatment (systolic blood pressure higher by 4 mmHg). Interestingly, a very similar 'Comparison of Outcomes with ACEI and Diuretics for Hypertension in the Elderly' (Second Australian National Blood Pressure Study, ANBP 2) obtained different results (Wing et al. 2003). This study involved 6,083 mainly Caucasian hypertensive patients, 65–84 years of age, and with a low prevalence of coronary heart disease (8%). Treatment was performed with ACEI or diuretics as primary medications, using substances chosen by the contributing practitioners (enalapril or hydrochlorothiazide were recommended). After a mean follow-up of 4.1 years, identical blood pressure levels were achieved in both groups, and ACEI treatment reduced the primary endpoint (all cardiovascular events or death from any cause) by 11%, but did not affect total mortality. In the ACEI group, the risk of myocardial infarction was decreased (relative risk 0.68), and a corresponding tendency was also observed for heart failure. Total strokes were evenly distributed in both groups, however fatal strokes occurred more frequently under ACEI treatment. Although these treatment effects apply to the total study population, any differences between the treatments were confined to the subgroup of male patients.

Definite reasons for the discrepancies between ALLHAT and the ANBP 2 study (The ALLHAT Collaborative Research Group 2002; Wing et al. 2003) are not evident. Regarding the therapy of non-Black patients, both studies concur that an ACEI in comparison with a thiazide diuretic will not negatively affect the risks of all-cause mortality, coronary events, or heart failure. However, potential therapeutic advantages of ACEI are limited to an 11% reduction in the combined risk of cardiovascular events and all-cause mortality, which was derived mainly from a reduced risk of nonfatal cardiovascular events (Wing et al. 2003). On the negative side, both studies indicate that ACEI may not be optimally effective to decrease the risk of stroke, particularly that of fatal stroke, and furthermore that diuretics should be preferred for the treatment of Black patients. The lack of clinical advantages of ACEI was even more surprising, since plasma cholesterol and fasting glucose levels, as well as the incidence of diabetes were lowered by lisinopril in the ALLHAT study, thus confirming the similar metabolic findings of the HOPE study (Yusuf et al. 2000b). It could be said that the follow-up of ALLHAT was too short for this reduction of risk factors to translate into clinical outcomes. However, even in patients followed for up to 7 years, there was no evident decline in the yearly rate of combined cardiovascular disease, whereas a tendency for a delayed benefit occurred after 4 years of lisinopril treatment with regard to the development of heart failure (The ALLHAT Collaborative Research Group 2002). It is important to note that the findings of ALLHAT and of ANBP 2 were obtained in patients of higher age (mean age 67 and 72 years, respectively) and should not be extrapolated to patients with uncomplicated hypertension in which treatment is usually initiated. It is plausible to assume that prophylactic measures will be more effective when they are started at a less advanced stage of disease.

In contrast, the first primary prevention study evaluating an ARB revealed positive aspects of the novel treatment. The LIFE study compared losartan against the β-receptor blocker atenolol in 9,193 hypertensive patients (mean age 67 years) with proven left ventricular hypertrophy, of which 25% had any kind of vascular disease (Dahlof et al. 2002). Within 4 years of equieffective treatment, losartan reduced the combined risk of cardiovascular death, myocardial infarction or stroke by 14%, and the risk of stroke by 25%, whereas cardiovascular mortality and the incidence of myocardial infarction were not affected. These differences were even more pronounced in the diabetic patients of the LIFE study (1,195 patients), who benefited from losartan with a 23% lower incidence of cardiovascular events, and with a reduced risk of cardiovascular and total mortality (Lindholm et al. 2002). In nondiabetic patients, losartan reduced the risk of newly diagnosed diabetes by 25%, thus extending the antidiabetic action of ramipril, as documented in the HOPE study, to the ARB losartan. An overview over ALLHAT, LIFE, and ANBP 2 suggests that antihypertensive treatment with RAAS inhibitors is effective at preventing the onset of diabetes, and will more positively influence cardiovascular events in patients who have lower prevalence of cardiovascular disease at the onset of therapy. However, the risk of strokes will not be lowered more effectively than with diuretics or β-blockers provided that comparable antihypertensive effects have been achieved. This seems to contradict the HOPE study, where ramipril prevented ischemic events including stroke in high-risk patients. As such, clinical evidence seems to suggest a therapeutic differentiation between secondary prevention which mandates the use of an ACEI for organ protection, and primary antihypertensive treatment that favors diuretics or ARB, the two drugs representing the extremes of economic choice. Although a direct comparison of both drugs is lacking, ARB should be beneficial in hypertensive patients if they are either diabetic or at risk of developing diabetes.

5
Conclusion

It can be concluded that despite enormous biochemical and experimental evidence for strong implications of the RAAS in the pathogenesis of atherosclerosis, there is little proof that the clinical benefits of RAAS inhibitors arise from direct actions on the atherosclerotic process. ACE inhibitors and AT_1 receptor antagonists are successfully applied in the treatment of hypertension, heart failure, diabetes, as well as coronary heart disease. However, their principle efficacy after myocardial infarction or in stable coronary heart disease appears to be related to their influence on neuro-humoral regulation, blood supply, myocardial hypertrophy and remodeling, and perhaps on the vulnerability of existing atherosclerotic plaques. The earliest conditions in which ACEI have been evaluated for primary prevention of atherosclerosis was in high-risk patients with established hypertension. Although the comparative data on ACEI and diuretics in this application are controversial, a superiority of ACEI, if existent, is certainly limited in extent. On the other hand, the excellent tolerability of these agents, their potential to prevent the onset of diabetes and the profound knowledge of the functional implications of an activated RAAS support a widespread use. Future prospects may focus on the possibility that ARB might perform better than ACEI in primary prevention. Furthermore, the prophylactic activities of RAAS inhibitors may arise more clearly when treatment is started at the onset of disease, and when combined treatments will target more efficaciously the alternative pathomechanisms of atherosclerosis, such as lipid disorders, inflammation and thrombosis.

References

Abe J, Deguchi J, Matsumoto T, Takuwa N, Noda M, Ohno M, Makuuchi M, Kurokawa K, Takuwa Y (1997) Stimulated activation of platelet-derived growth factor receptor in vivo in balloon-injured arteries: a link between angiotensin II and intimal thickening. Circulation 96:1906–1913

Akasu M, Urata H, Kinoshita A, Sasaguri M, Ideishi M, Arakawa K (1998) Differences in tissue angiotensin II-forming pathways by species and organs in vitro. Hypertension 32:514–520

Anderson TJ, Elstein E, Haber H, Charbonneau F (2000) Comparative study of ACE-inhibition, angiotensin II antagonism, and calcium channel blockade on flow-mediated vasodilation in patients with coronary disease (BANFF study). J Am Coll Cardiol 35:60–66

Bonner G, Preis S, Schunk U, Toussaint C, Kaufmann W (1990) Hemodynamic effects of bradykinin on systemic and pulmonary circulation in healthy and hypertensive humans. J Cardiovasc Pharmacol 15 Suppl 6:S46–S56

Brand K, Page S, Rogler G, Bartsch A, Brandl R, Knuechel R, Page M, Kaltschmidt C, Baeuerle PA, Neumeier D (1996) Activated transcription factor nuclear factor-kappa B is present in the atherosclerotic lesion. J Clin Invest 97:1715–1722

Brasch H, Sieroslawski L, Dominiak P (1993) Angiotensin II increases norepinephrine release from atria by acting on angiotensin subtype 1 receptors. Hypertension 22:699–704

Brede M, Hadamek K, Meinel L, Wiesmann F, Peters J, Engelhardt S, Simm A, Haase A, Lohse MJ, Hein L (2001) Vascular hypertrophy and increased P70S6 kinase in mice lacking the angiotensin II AT(2) receptor. Circulation 104:2602–2607

Brewster UC, Setaro JF, Perazella MA (2003) The renin-angiotensin-aldosterone system: cardiorenal effects and implications for renal and cardiovascular disease states. Am J Med Sci 326:15–24

Cambien F, Costerousse O, Tiret L, Poirier O, Lecerf L, Gonzales MF, Evans A, Arveiler D, Cambou JP, Luc G, . (1994) Plasma level and gene polymorphism of angiotensin-converting enzyme in relation to myocardial infarction. Circulation 90:669–676

Cambien F, Evans A (1995) Angiotensin I converting enzyme gene polymorphism and coronary heart disease. Eur Heart J 16 Suppl K:13–22

Candido R, Jandeleit-Dahm KA, Cao Z, Nesteroff SP, Burns WC, Twigg SM, Dilley RJ, Cooper ME, Allen TJ (2002) Prevention of accelerated atherosclerosis by angiotensin-converting enzyme inhibition in diabetic apolipoprotein E-deficient mice. Circulation 106:246–253

Carey RM, Howell NL, Jin XH, Siragy HM (2001) Angiotensin type 2 receptor-mediated hypotension in angiotensin type-1 receptor-blocked rats. Hypertension 38:1272–1277

Cashin-Hemphill L, Holmvang G, Chan RC, Pitt B, Dinsmore RE, Lees RS (1999) Angiotensin-converting enzyme inhibition as antiatherosclerotic therapy: no answer yet. QUIET Investigators. QUinapril Ischemic Event Trial. Am J Cardiol 83:43–47

Chen H, Li D, Sawamura T, Inoue K, Mehta JL (2000) Upregulation of LOX-1 expression in aorta of hypercholesterolemic rabbits: modulation by losartan. Biochem Biophys Res Commun 276:1100–1104

Chen M, Masaki T, Sawamura T (2002) LOX-1, the receptor for oxidized low-density lipoprotein identified from endothelial cells: implications in endothelial dysfunction and atherosclerosis. Pharmacol Ther 95:89–100

Cohn JN, Tognoni G (2001) A randomized trial of the angiotensin-receptor blocker valsartan in chronic heart failure. N Engl J Med 345:1667–1675

Collins T, Cybulsky MI (2001) NF-kappaB: pivotal mediator or innocent bystander in atherogenesis? J Clin Invest 107:255–264

Cominacini L, Pasini AF, Garbin U, Davoli A, Tosetti ML, Campagnola M, Rigoni A, Pastorino AM, Lo C, V, Sawamura T (2000) Oxidized low density lipoprotein (ox-LDL) binding to ox-LDL receptor-1 in endothelial cells induces the activation of NF-kappaB through an increased production of intracellular reactive oxygen species. J Biol Chem 275:12633–12638

Cui T, Nakagami H, Iwai M, Takeda Y, Shiuchi T, Daviet L, Nahmias C, Horiuchi M (2001) Pivotal role of tyrosine phosphatase SHP-1 in AT2 receptor-mediated apoptosis in rat fetal vascular smooth muscle cell. Cardiovasc Res 49:863–871

Dahlof B, Devereux RB, Kjeldsen SE, Julius S, Beevers G, Faire U, Fyhrquist F, Ibsen H, Kristiansson K, Lederballe-Pedersen O, Lindholm LH, Nieminen MS, Omvik P, Oparil S, Wedel H (2002) Cardiovascular morbidity and mortality in the Losartan Intervention For Endpoint reduction in hypertension study (LIFE): a randomised trial against atenolol. Lancet 359:995–1003

Danser AH (2003) Local renin-angiotensin systems: the unanswered questions. Int J Biochem Cell Biol 35:759–768

Danser AH, Derkx FH, Hense HW, Jeunemaitre X, Riegger GA, Schunkert H (1998) Angiotensinogen (M235T) and angiotensin-converting enzyme (I/D) polymorphisms in association with plasma renin and prorenin levels. J Hypertens 16:1879–1883

Danser AH, Schalekamp MA, Bax WA, van den Brink AM, Saxena PR, Riegger GA, Schunkert H (1995) Angiotensin-converting enzyme in the human heart. Effect of the deletion/insertion polymorphism. Circulation 92:1387–1388

Daugherty A, Manning MW, Cassis LA (2001) Antagonism of AT2 receptors augments angiotensin II-induced abdominal aortic aneurysms and atherosclerosis. Br J Pharmacol 134:865–870

Delafontaine P, Lou H (1993) Angiotensin II regulates insulin-like growth factor I gene expression in vascular smooth muscle cells. J Biol Chem 268:16866–16870

Dendorfer A, Thornagel A, Raasch W, Grisk O, Tempel K, Dominiak P (2002) Angiotensin II induces catecholamine release by direct ganglionic excitation. Hypertension 40:348–354

DiBona GF (2002) Sympathetic nervous system and the kidney in hypertension. Curr Opin Nephrol Hypertens 11:197–200

Diet F, Pratt RE, Berry GJ, Momose N, Gibbons GH, Dzau VJ (1996) Increased accumulation of tissue ACE in human atherosclerotic coronary artery disease. Circulation 94:2756–2767

Dimmeler S, Rippmann V, Weiland U, Haendeler J, Zeiher AM (1997) Angiotensin II induces apoptosis of human endothelial cells. Protective effect of nitric oxide. Circ Res 81:970–976

Ding YA, MacIntyre DE, Kenyon CJ, Semple PF (1985) Potentiation of adrenaline-induced platelet aggregation by angiotensin II. Thromb Haemost 54:717–720

Dostal DE, Baker KM (1999) The cardiac renin-angiotensin system: conceptual, or a regulator of cardiac function? Circ Res 85:643–650

Droge W (2002) Free radicals in the physiological control of cell function. Physiol Rev 82:47–95

Dusting GJ, Fennessy P, Yin ZL, Gurevich V (1998) Nitric oxide in atherosclerosis: vascular protector or villain? Clin Exp Pharmacol Physiol Suppl 25:S34–S41

Dzau VJ, Bernstein K, Celermajer D, Cohen J, Dahlof B, Deanfield J, Diez J, Drexler H, Ferrari R, Van Gilst W, Hansson L, Hornig B, Husain A, Johnston C, Lazar H, Lonn E, Luscher T, Mancini J, Mimran A, Pepine C, Rabelink T, Remme W, Ruilope L, Ruzicka M, Schunkert H, Swedberg K, Unger T, Vaughan D, Weber M (2002) Pathophysiologic and therapeutic importance of tissue ACE: a consensus report. Cardiovasc Drugs Ther 16:149–160

Eguchi S, Numaguchi K, Iwasaki H, Matsumoto T, Yamakawa T, Utsunomiya H, Motley ED, Kawakatsu H, Owada KM, Hirata Y, Marumo F, Inagami T (1998) Calcium-dependent epidermal growth factor receptor transactivation mediates the angiotensin II-induced mitogen-activated protein kinase activation in vascular smooth muscle cells. J Biol Chem 273:8890–8896

Elmfeldt D, Olofsson B, Meredith P (2002) The relationships between dose and antihypertensive effect of four AT1-receptor blockers. Differences in potency and efficacy. Blood Press 11:293–301

Endo-Mochizuki Y, Mochizuki N, Sawa H, Takada A, Okamoto H, Kawaguchi H, Nagashima K, Kitabatake A (1995) Expression of renin and angiotensin-converting enzyme in human hearts. Heart Vessels 10:285–293

Esther CR, Marino EM, Howard TE, Machaud A, Corvol P, Capecchi MR, Bernstein KE (1997) The critical role of tissue angiotensin-converting enzyme as revealed by gene targeting in mice. J Clin Invest 99:2375–2385

Farhy RD, Carretero OA, Ho KL, Scicli AG (1993) Role of kinins and nitric oxide in the effects of angiotensin converting enzyme inhibitors on neointima formation. Circ Res 72:1202–1210

Faxon DP (1995) Effect of high dose angiotensin-converting enzyme inhibition on restenosis: final results of the MARCATOR Study, a multicenter, double-blind, placebo-controlled trial of cilazapril. The Multicenter American Research Trial With Cilazapril After Angioplasty to Prevent Transluminal Coronary Obstruction and Restenosis (MARCATOR) Study Group. J Am Coll Cardiol 25:362–369

Fennessy PA, Campbell JH, Mendelsohn FA, Campbell GR (1996) Angiotensin-converting enzyme inhibitors and atherosclerosis: relevance of animal models to human disease. Clin Exp Pharmacol Physiol 23:S30–S32

Fernandez-Alfonso MS, Martorana PA, Licka I, van Even P, Trobisch D, Scholkens BA, Paul M (1997) Early induction of angiotensin I-converting enzyme in rat carotid artery after balloon injury. Hypertension 30:272–277

Feuerstein GZ, Young PR (2000) Apoptosis in cardiac diseases: stress- and mitogen-activated signaling pathways. Cardiovasc Res 45:560–569

Fingerle J, Muller RM, Kuhn H, Pech M, Baumgartner HR (1995) Mechanism of inhibition of neointimal formation by the angiotensin-converting enzyme inhibitor cilazapril. A study in balloon catheter-injured rat carotid arteries. Arterioscler Thromb Vasc Biol 15:1945–1950

Fox KM (2003) Efficacy of perindopril in reduction of cardiovascular events among patients with stable coronary artery disease: randomised, double-blind, placebo-controlled, multicentre trial (the EUROPA study). Lancet 362:782–788

Gibbons GH, Pratt RE, Dzau VJ (1992) Vascular smooth muscle cell hypertrophy vs. hyperplasia. Autocrine transforming growth factor-beta 1 expression determines growth response to angiotensin II. J Clin Invest 90:456–461

Goldenberg I, Grossman E, Jacobson KA, Shneyvays V, Shainberg A (2001) Angiotensin II-induced apoptosis in rat cardiomyocyte culture: a possible role of AT1 and AT2 receptors. J Hypertens 19:1681–1689

Griendling KK, Ushio-Fukai M, Lassegue B, Alexander RW (1997) Angiotensin II signaling in vascular smooth muscle. New concepts. Hypertension 29:366–373

Griffin SA, Brown WC, MacPherson F, McGrath JC, Wilson VG, Korsgaard N, Mulvany MJ, Lever AF (1991) Angiotensin II causes vascular hypertrophy in part by a non-pressor mechanism. Hypertension 17:626–635

Hamdan AD, Quist WC, Gagne JB, Feener EP (1996) Angiotensin-converting enzyme inhibition suppresses plasminogen activator inhibitor-1 expression in the neointima of balloon-injured rat aorta. Circulation 93:1073–1078

Hansson L, Lindholm LH, Niskanen L, Lanke J, Hedner T, Niklason A, Luomanmaki K, Dahlof B, de Faire U, Morlin C, Karlberg BE, Wester PO, Bjorck JE (1999) Effect of angiotensin-converting-enzyme inhibition compared with conventional therapy on cardiovascular morbidity and mortality in hypertension: the Captopril Prevention Project (CAPPP) randomised trial. Lancet 353:611–616

Harris EL, Phelan EL, Thompson CM, Millar JA, Grigor MR (1995) Heart mass and blood pressure have separate genetic determinants in the New Zealand genetically hypertensive (GH) rat. J Hypertens 13:397–404

Hattori Y, Matsumura M, Kasai K (2003) Vascular smooth muscle cell activation by C-reactive protein. Cardiovasc Res 58:186–195

Hayek T, Kaplan M, Raz A, Keidar S, Coleman R, Aviram M (2002) Ramipril administration to atherosclerotic mice reduces oxidized low-density lipoprotein uptake by their macrophages and blocks the progression of atherosclerosis. Atherosclerosis 161:65–74

Hayek T, Pavlotzky E, Hamoud S, Coleman R, Keidar S, Aviram M, Kaplan M (2003) Tissue angiotensin-converting-enzyme (ACE) deficiency leads to a reduction in oxidative stress and in atherosclerosis. Studies in ACE-knockout mice type 2. Arterioscler Thromb Vasc Biol 23:2090–2096

Herizi A, Jover B, Bouriquet N, Mimran A (1998) Prevention of the cardiovascular and renal effects of angiotensin II by endothelin blockade. Hypertension 31:10–14

Hernandez-Presa M, Bustos C, Ortego M, Tunon J, Renedo G, Ruiz-Ortega M, Egido J (1997) Angiotensin-converting enzyme inhibition prevents arterial nuclear factor-kappa B activation, monocyte chemoattractant protein-1 expression, and macrophage infiltration in a rabbit model of early accelerated atherosclerosis. Circulation 95:1532–1541

Hernandez-Presa MA, Bustos C, Ortego M, Tunon J, Ortega L, Egido J (1998) ACE inhibitor quinapril reduces the arterial expression of NF-kappaB-dependent proinflammatory factors but not of collagen I in a rabbit model of atherosclerosis. Am J Pathol 153:1825–1837

Hilgers KF, Veelken R, Muller DN, Kohler H, Hartner A, Botkin SR, Stumpf C, Schmieder RE, Gomez RA (2001) Renin uptake by the endothelium mediates vascular angiotensin formation. Hypertension 38:243–248

Hillege HL, Fidler V, Diercks GF, van Gilst WH, de Zeeuw D, van Veldhuisen DJ, Gans RO, Janssen WM, Grobbee DE, de Jong PE (2002) Urinary albumin excretion predicts cardiovascular and noncardiovascular mortality in general population. Circulation 106:1777–1782

Hope S, Brecher P, Chobanian AV (1999) Comparison of the effects of AT1 receptor blockade and angiotensin converting enzyme inhibition on atherosclerosis. Am J Hypertens 12:28–34

Hornig B, Arakawa N, Haussmann D, Drexler H (1998) Differential effects of quinaprilat and enalaprilat on endothelial function of conduit arteries in patients with chronic heart failure. Circulation 98:2842–2848

Hornig B, Kohler C, Schlink D, Tatge H, Drexler H (2003) AT1-receptor antagonism improves endothelial function in coronary artery disease by a bradykinin/B2-receptor-dependent mechanism. Hypertension 41:1092–1095

Hornig B, Landmesser U, Kohler C, Ahlersmann D, Spiekermann S, Christoph A, Tatge H, Drexler H (2001) Comparative effect of ace inhibition and angiotensin II type 1 receptor antagonism on bioavailability of nitric oxide in patients with coronary artery disease: role of superoxide dismutase. Circulation 103:799–805

Ichihara S, Senbonmatsu T, Price E Jr, Ichiki T, Gaffney FA, Inagami T (2001) Angiotensin II type 2 receptor is essential for left ventricular hypertrophy and cardiac fibrosis in chronic angiotensin II-induced hypertension. Circulation 104:346–351

Igarashi M, Hirata A, Yamaguchi H, Tsuchiya H, Ohnuma H, Tominaga M, Daimon M, Kato T (2001) Candesartan inhibits carotid intimal thickening and ameliorates insulin resistance in balloon-injured diabetic rats. Hypertension 38:1255–1259

Ihara M, Urata H, Kinoshita A, Suzumiya J, Sasaguri M, Kikuchi M, Ideishi M, Arakawa K (1999) Increased chymase-dependent angiotensin II formation in human atherosclerotic aorta. Hypertension 33:1399–1405

Jacob HJ, Lindpaintner K, Lincoln SE, Kusumi K, Bunker RK, Mao YP, Ganten D, Dzau VJ, Lander ES (1991) Genetic mapping of a gene causing hypertension in the stroke-prone spontaneously hypertensive rat. Cell 67:213–224

Kato H, Suzuki H, Tajima S, Ogata Y, Tominaga T, Sato A, Saruta T (1991) Angiotensin II stimulates collagen synthesis in cultured vascular smooth muscle cells. J Hypertens 9:17–22

Keidar S (1998) Angiotensin, LDL peroxidation and atherosclerosis. Life Sci 63:1–11

Keidar S, Attias J, Coleman R, Wirth K, Scholkens B, Hayek T (2000) Attenuation of atherosclerosis in apolipoprotein E-deficient mice by ramipril is dissociated from its antihypertensive effect and from potentiation of bradykinin. J Cardiovasc Pharmacol 35:64–72

Keidar S, Attias J, Heinrich R, Coleman R, Aviram M (1999) Angiotensin II atherogenicity in apolipoprotein E deficient mice is associated with increased cellular cholesterol biosynthesis. Atherosclerosis 146:249–257

Keidar S, Kaplan M, Hoffman A, Aviram M (1995) Angiotensin II stimulates macrophage-mediated oxidation of low density lipoproteins. Atherosclerosis 115:201–215

Kim S, Iwao H (2000) Molecular and cellular mechanisms of angiotensin II-mediated cardiovascular and renal diseases. Pharmacol Rev 52:11–34

Kim S, Izumi Y, Yano M, Hamaguchi A, Miura K, Yamanaka S, Miyazaki H, Iwao H (1998) Angiotensin blockade inhibits activation of mitogen-activated protein kinases in rat balloon-injured artery. Circulation 97:1731–1737

Kim S, Kawamura M, Wanibuchi H, Ohta K, Hamaguchi A, Omura T, Yukimura T, Miura K, Iwao H (1995) Angiotensin II type 1 receptor blockade inhibits the expression of immediate-early genes and fibronectin in rat injured artery. Circulation 92:88–95

Koch W, Mehilli J, von Beckerath N, Bottiger C, Schomig A, Kastrati A (2003) Angiotensin I-converting enzyme (ACE) inhibitors and restenosis after coronary artery stenting in patients with the DD genotype of the ACE gene. J Am Coll Cardiol 41:1957–1961

Kranzhofer R, Schmidt J, Pfeiffer CA, Hagl S, Libby P, Kubler W (1999) Angiotensin induces inflammatory activation of human vascular smooth muscle cells. Arterioscler Thromb Vasc Biol 19:1623–1629

Kume N, Moriwaki H, Kataoka H, Minami M, Murase T, Sawamura T, Masaki T, Kita T (2000) Inducible expression of LOX-1, a novel receptor for oxidized LDL, in macrophages and vascular smooth muscle cells. Ann N Y Acad Sci 902:323–327

Kurisu S, Ozono R, Oshima T, Kambe M, Ishida T, Sugino H, Matsuura H, Chayama K, Teranishi Y, Iba O, Amano K, Matsubara H (2003) Cardiac angiotensin II type 2 receptor activates the kinin/NO system and inhibits fibrosis. Hypertension 41:99–107

Lassegue B, Clempus RE (2003) Vascular NAD(P)H oxidases: specific features, expression, and regulation. Am J Physiol Regul Integr Comp Physiol 285:R277–R297

Li D, Mehta JL (2000) Antisense to LOX-1 inhibits oxidized LDL-mediated upregulation of monocyte chemoattractant protein-1 and monocyte adhesion to human coronary artery endothelial cells. Circulation 101:2889–2895

Li D, Singh RM, Liu L, Chen H, Singh BM, Kazzaz N, Mehta JL (2003) Oxidized-LDL through LOX-1 increases the expression of angiotensin converting enzyme in human coronary artery endothelial cells. Cardiovasc Res 57:238–243

Li DY, Zhang YC, Philips MI, Sawamura T, Mehta JL (1999) Upregulation of endothelial receptor for oxidized low-density lipoprotein (LOX-1) in cultured human coronary artery endothelial cells by angiotensin II type 1 receptor activation. Circ Res 84:1043–1049

Lindholm LH, Ibsen H, Dahlof B, Devereux RB, Beevers G, de Faire U, Fyhrquist F, Julius S, Kjeldsen SE, Kristiansson K, Lederballe-Pedersen O, Nieminen MS, Omvik P, Oparil S, Wedel H, Aurup P, Edelman J, Snapinn S (2002) Cardiovascular morbidity and mortality in patients with diabetes in the Losartan Intervention For Endpoint reduction in hypertension study (LIFE): a randomised trial against atenolol. Lancet 359:1004–1010

Lindpaintner K, Lee M, Larson MG, Rao VS, Pfeffer MA, Ordovas JM, Schaefer EJ, Wilson AF, Wilson PW, Vasan RS, Myers RH, Levy D (1996) Absence of association or genetic linkage between the angiotensin-converting-enzyme gene and left ventricular mass. N Engl J Med 334:1023–1028

Lindpaintner K, Pfeffer MA, Kreutz R, Stampfer MJ, Grodstein F, LaMotte F, Buring J, Hennekens CH (1995) A prospective evaluation of an angiotensin-converting-enzyme gene polymorphism and the risk of ischemic heart disease. N Engl J Med 332:706–711

Linz W, Wiemer G, Gohlke P, Unger T, Scholkens BA (1995) Contribution of kinins to the cardiovascular actions of angiotensin-converting enzyme inhibitors. Pharmacol Rev 47:25–49

Liu YH, Yang XP, Sharov VG, Nass O, Sabbah HN, Peterson E, Carretero OA (1997) Effects of angiotensin-converting enzyme inhibitors and angiotensin II type 1 receptor antagonists in rats with heart failure. Role of kinins and angiotensin II type 2 receptors. J Clin Invest 99:1926–1935

Lonn E, Yusuf S, Dzavik V, Doris C, Yi Q, Smith S, Moore-Cox A, Bosch J, Riley W, Teo K (2001) Effects of ramipril and vitamin E on atherosclerosis: the study to evaluate carotid ultrasound changes in patients treated with ramipril and vitamin E (SECURE). Circulation 103:919–925

MacMahon S, Sharpe N, Gamble G, Clague A, Mhurchu CN, Clark T, Hart H, Scott J, White H (2000) Randomized, placebo-controlled trial of the angiotensin-converting enzyme inhibitor, ramipril, in patients with coronary or other occlusive arterial disease. PART-2 Collaborative Research Group. Prevention of Atherosclerosis with Ramipril. J Am Coll Cardiol 36:438–443

Mallat Z, Tedgui A (2000) Apoptosis in the vasculature: mechanisms and functional importance. Br J Pharmacol 130:947–962

Mancini GB (1998) Role of angiotensin-converting enzyme inhibition in reversal of endothelial dysfunction in coronary artery disease. Am J Med 105:40S–47S

Mancini GB (2002) Emerging role of angiotensin II type 1 receptor blockers for the treatment of endothelial dysfunction and vascular inflammation. Can J Cardiol 18:1309–1316

Mancini GB, Henry GC, Macaya C, O'Neill BJ, Pucillo AL, Carere RG, Wargovich TJ, Mudra H, Luscher TF, Klibaner MI, Haber HE, Uprichard AC, Pepine CJ, Pitt B (1996) Angiotensin-converting enzyme inhibition with quinapril improves endothelial vasomotor dysfunction in patients with coronary artery disease. The TREND (Trial on Reversing ENdothelial Dysfunction) Study. Circulation 94:258–265

Matsubara H (1998) Pathophysiological role of angiotensin II type 2 receptor in cardiovascular and renal diseases. Circ Res 83:1182–1191

Matsumoto K, Morishita R, Moriguchi A, Tomita N, Aoki M, Sakonjo H, Matsumoto K, Nakamura T, Higaki J, Ogihara T (2001) Inhibition of neointima by angiotensin-converting enzyme inhibitor in porcine coronary artery balloon-injury model. Hypertension 37:270–274

Mazzolai L, Nussberger J, Aubert JF, Brunner DB, Gabbiani G, Brunner HR, Pedrazzini T (1998) Blood pressure-independent cardiac hypertrophy induced by locally activated renin-angiotensin system. Hypertension 31:1324–1330

Mehta JL, Li D (2002) Identification, regulation and function of a novel lectin-like oxidized low-density lipoprotein receptor. J Am Coll Cardiol 39:1429–1435

Meurice T, Bauters C, Hermant X, Codron V, VanBelle E, Mc Fadden EP, Lablanche J, Bertrand ME, Amouyel P (2001) Effect of ACE inhibitors on angiographic restenosis after coronary stenting (PARIS): a randomised, double-blind, placebo-controlled trial. Lancet 357:1321–1324

Mitani H, Bandoh T, Kimura M, Totsuka T, Hayashi S (1996) Increased activity of vascular ACE related to atherosclerotic lesions in hyperlipidemic rabbits. Am J Physiol 271:H1065–H1071

Miyazaki M, Sakonjo H, Takai S (1999) Anti-atherosclerotic effects of an angiotensin converting enzyme inhibitor and an angiotensin II antagonist in Cynomolgus monkeys fed a high-cholesterol diet. Br J Pharmacol 128:523–529

Mollnau H, Wendt M, Szocs K, Lassegue B, Schulz E, Oelze M, Li H, Bodenschatz M, August M, Kleschyov AL, Tsilimingas N, Walter U, Forstermann U, Meinertz T, Griendling K, Munzel T (2002) Effects of angiotensin II infusion on the expression and function of NAD(P)H oxidase and components of nitric oxide/cGMP signaling. Circ Res 90:E58–E65

Montgomery HE, Clarkson P, Dollery CM, Prasad K, Losi MA, Hemingway H, Statters D, Jubb M, Girvain M, Varnava A, World M, Deanfield J, Talmud P, McEwan JR, McKenna WJ, Humphries S (1997) Association of angiotensin-converting enzyme gene I/D polymorphism with change in left ventricular mass in response to physical training. Circulation 96:741–747

Morawietz H, Duerrschmidt N, Niemann B, Galle J, Sawamura T, Holtz J (2001) Induction of the oxLDL receptor LOX-1 by endothelin-1 in human endothelial cells. Biochem Biophys Res Commun 284:961–965

Morawietz H, Rueckschloss U, Niemann B, Duerrschmidt N, Galle J, Hakim K, Zerkowski HR, Sawamura T, Holtz J (1999) Angiotensin II induces LOX-1, the human endothelial receptor for oxidized low-density lipoprotein. Circulation 100:899–902

Morishige K, Shimokawa H, Matsumoto Y, Eto Y, Uwatoku T, Abe K, Sueishi K, Takeshita A (2003) Overexpression of matrix metalloproteinase-9 promotes intravascular thrombus formation in porcine coronary arteries in vivo. Cardiovasc Res 57:572–585

Moriwaki H, Kume N, Kataoka H, Murase T, Nishi E, Sawamura T, Masaki T, Kita T (1998) Expression of lectin-like oxidized low density lipoprotein receptor-1 in human and murine macrophages: upregulated expression by TNF-alpha. FEBS Lett 440:29–32

Naftilan AJ, Pratt RE, Dzau VJ (1989) Induction of platelet-derived growth factor A-chain and c-myc gene expressions by angiotensin II in cultured rat vascular smooth muscle cells. J Clin Invest 83:1419–1424

Nakajima M, Hutchinson HG, Fujinaga M, Hayashida W, Morishita R, Zhang L, Horiuchi M, Pratt RE, Dzau VJ (1995) The angiotensin II type 2 (AT2) receptor antagonizes the growth effects of the AT1 receptor: gain-of-function study using gene transfer. Proc Natl Acad Sci U S A 92:10663–10667

Nakamura S, Nakamura I, Ma L, Vaughan DE, Fogo AB (2000) Plasminogen activator inhibitor-1 expression is regulated by the angiotensin type 1 receptor in vivo. Kidney Int 58:251–259

Napoli C, Cicala C, D'Armiento FP, Roviezzo F, Somma P, de Nigris F, Zuliani P, Bucci M, Aleotti L, Casini A, Franconi F, Cirino G (1999) Beneficial effects of ACE-inhibition with zofenopril on plaque formation and low-density lipoprotein oxidation in watanabe heritable hyperlipidemic rabbits. Gen Pharmacol 33:467–477

Napoli C, Ignarro LJ (2001) Nitric oxide and atherosclerosis. Nitric Oxide 5:88–97

Nickenig G, Baumer AT, Temur Y, Kebben D, Jockenhovel F, Bohm M (1999) Statin-sensitive dysregulated AT1 receptor function and density in hypercholesterolemic men. Circulation 100:2131–2134

Nickenig G, Roling J, Strehlow K, Schnabel P, Bohm M (1998) Insulin induces upregulation of vascular AT1 receptor gene expression by posttranscriptional mechanisms. Circulation 98:2453–2460

Nickenig G, Sachinidis A, Michaelsen F, Bohm M, Seewald S, Vetter H (1997) Upregulation of vascular angiotensin II receptor gene expression by low-density lipoprotein in vascular smooth muscle cells. Circulation 95:473–478

Nielsen LB, Stender S, Kjeldsen K, Nordestgaard BG (1994) Effect of angiotensin II and enalapril on transfer of low-density lipoprotein into aortic intima in rabbits. Circ Res 75:63–69

Ohishi M, Ueda M, Rakugi H, Naruko T, Kojima A, Okamura A, Higaki J, Ogihara T (1999) Relative localization of angiotensin-converting enzyme, chymase and angiotensin II in human coronary atherosclerotic lesions. J Hypertens 17:547–553

Ohmichi N, Iwai N, Maeda K, Shimoike H, Nakamura Y, Izumi M, Sugimoto Y, Kinoshita M (1996) Genetic basis of left ventricular remodeling after myocardial infarction. Int J Cardiol 53:265–272

Palatini P (2001) Sympathetic overactivity in hypertension: a risk factor for cardiovascular disease. Curr Hypertens Rep 3 (Suppl 1):S3–S9

Peters S, Gotting B, Trummel M, Rust H, Brattstrom A (2001) Valsartan for prevention of restenosis after stenting of type B2/C lesions: the VAL-PREST trial. J Invasive Cardiol 13:93–97

Pfeffer MA, Swedberg K, Granger CB, Held P, McMurray JJ, Michelson EL, Olofsson B, Ostergren J, Yusuf S, Pocock S (2003) Effects of candesartan on mortality and morbidity in patients with chronic heart failure: the CHARM-Overall programme. Lancet 362:759–766

Pinto YM, Tian X, Costerousse O, Stula M, Franz WM, Paul M (1997) Cardiac overexpression of angiotensin-converting enzyme in transgenic rats augments cardiac hypertrophy. Circulation 96:I-629;abstract 3521

Pinto YM, van Gilst WH, Kingma JH, Schunkert H (1995) Deletion-type allele of the angiotensin-converting enzyme gene is associated with progressive ventricular dilation after anterior myocardial infarction. Captopril and Thrombolysis Study Investigators. J Am Coll Cardiol 25:1622–1626

Pitt B, O'Neill B, Feldman R, Ferrari R, Schwartz L, Mudra H, Bass T, Pepine C, Texter M, Haber H, Uprichard A, Cashin-Hemphill L, Lees RS (2001) The QUinapril Ischemic Event Trial (QUIET): evaluation of chronic ACE inhibitor therapy in patients with ischemic heart disease and preserved left ventricular function. Am J Cardiol 87:1058–1063

Pitt B, Poole-Wilson PA, Segal R, Martinez FA, Dickstein K, Camm AJ, Konstam MA, Riegger G, Klinger GH, Neaton J, Sharma D, Thiyagarajan B (2000) Effect of losartan compared with captopril on mortality in patients with symptomatic heart failure: randomised trial–the Losartan Heart Failure Survival Study ELITE II. Lancet 355:1582–1587

Prasad A, Narayanan S, Husain S, Padder F, Waclawiw M, Epstein N, Quyyumi AA (2000a) Insertion-deletion polymorphism of the ACE gene modulates reversibility of endothelial dysfunction with ACE inhibition. Circulation 102:35–41

Prasad A, Tupas-Habib T, Schenke WH, Mincemoyer R, Panza JA, Waclawin MA, Ellahham S, Quyyumi AA (2000b) Acute and chronic angiotensin-1 receptor antagonism reverses endothelial dysfunction in atherosclerosis. Circulation 101:2349–2354

Rahman ST, Lauten WB, Khan QA, Navalkar S, Parthasarathy S, Khan BV (2002) Effects of eprosartan versus hydrochlorothiazide on markers of vascular oxidation and inflammation and blood pressure (renin-angiotensin system antagonists, oxidation, and inflammation). Am J Cardiol 89:686–690

Rajagopalan S, Kurz S, Munzel T, Tarpey M, Freeman BA, Griendling KK, Harrison DG (1996) Angiotensin II-mediated hypertension in the rat increases vascular superoxide production via membrane NADH/NADPH oxidase activation. Contribution to alterations of vasomotor tone. J Clin Invest 97:1916–1923

Rakugi H, Kim DK, Krieger JE, Wang DS, Dzau VJ, Pratt RE (1994a) Induction of angiotensin converting enzyme in the neointima after vascular injury. Possible role in restenosis. J Clin Invest 93:339–346

Rakugi H, Wang DS, Dzau VJ, Pratt RE (1994b) Potential importance of tissue angiotensin-converting enzyme inhibition in preventing neointima formation. Circulation 90: 449–455

Regitz-Zagrosek V, Friedel N, Heymann A, Bauer P, Neuss M, Rolfs A, Steffen C, Hildebrandt A, Hetzer R, Fleck E (1995) Regulation, chamber localization, and subtype distribution of angiotensin II receptors in human hearts. Circulation 91:1461–1471

Ridker PM (2001) Role of inflammatory biomarkers in prediction of coronary heart disease. Lancet 358:946–948

Ross R (1999) Atherosclerosis–an inflammatory disease. N Engl J Med 340:115–126

Rueckschloss U, Quinn MT, Holtz J, Morawietz H (2002) Dose-dependent regulation of NAD(P)H oxidase expression by angiotensin II in human endothelial cells: protective effect of angiotensin II type 1 receptor blockade in patients with coronary artery disease. Arterioscler Thromb Vasc Biol 22:1845–1851

Ruiz-Ortega M, Lorenzo O, Ruperez M, Esteban V, Suzuki Y, Mezzano S, Plaza JJ, Egido J (2001) Role of the renin-angiotensin system in vascular diseases: expanding the field. Hypertension 38:1382–1387

Ruiz-Ortega M, Lorenzo O, Ruperez M, Konig S, Wittig B, Egido J (2000) Angiotensin II activates nuclear transcription factor kappaB through AT(1) and AT(2) in vascular smooth muscle cells: molecular mechanisms. Circ Res 86:1266–1272

Rutherford JD, Pfeffer MA, Moye LA, Davis BR, Flaker GC, Kowey PR, Lamas GA, Miller HS, Packer M, Rouleau JL (1994) Effects of captopril on ischemic events after myocardial infarction. Results of the Survival and Ventricular Enlargement trial. SAVE Investigators. Circulation 90:1731–1738

Saward L, Zahradka P (1997) Angiotensin II activates phosphatidylinositol 3-kinase in vascular smooth muscle cells. Circ Res 81:249–257

Schieffer B, Schieffer E, Hilfiker-Kleiner D, Hilfiker A, Kovanen PT, Kaartinen M, Nussberger J, Harringer W, Drexler H (2000) Expression of angiotensin II and interleukin 6 in human coronary atherosclerotic plaques: potential implications for inflammation and plaque instability. Circulation 101:1372–1378

Schiffrin EL (2001) Role of endothelin-1 in hypertension and vascular disease. Am J Hypertens 14:83S–89S

Schuh JR, Blehm DJ, Frierdich GE, McMahon EG, Blaine EH (1993) Differential effects of renin-angiotensin system blockade on atherogenesis in cholesterol-fed rabbits. J Clin Invest 91:1453–1458

Schunkert H (1997) Polymorphism of the angiotensin-converting enzyme gene and cardiovascular disease. J Mol Med 75:867–875

Schunkert H, Dzau VJ, Tang SS, Hirsch AT, Apstein CS, Lorell BH (1990) Increased rat cardiac angiotensin converting enzyme activity and mRNA expression in pressure overload left ventricular hypertrophy. Effects on coronary resistance, contractility, and relaxation. J Clin Invest 86:1913–1920

Schunkert H, Sadoshima J, Cornelius T, Kagaya Y, Weinberg EO, Izumo S, Riegger G, Lorell BH (1995) Angiotensin II-induced growth responses in isolated adult rat hearts. Evidence for load-independent induction of cardiac protein synthesis by angiotensin II. Circ Res 76:489–497

Seshiah PN, Weber DS, Rocic P, Valppu L, Taniyama Y, Griendling KK (2002) Angiotensin II stimulation of NAD(P)H oxidase activity: upstream mediators. Circ Res 91:406–413

Sharifi BG, LaFleur DW, Pirola CJ, Forrester JS, Fagin JA (1992) Angiotensin II regulates tenascin gene expression in vascular smooth muscle cells. J Biol Chem 267:23910–23915

Siragy HM, Inagami T, Ichiki T, Carey RM (1999) Sustained hypersensitivity to angiotensin II and its mechanism in mice lacking the subtype-2 (AT2) angiotensin receptor. Proc Natl Acad Sci USA 96:6506–6510

Soejima H, Ogawa H, Yasue H, Kaikita K, Takazoe K, Nishiyama K, Misumi K, Miyamoto S, Yoshimura M, Kugiyama K, Nakamura S, Tsuji I (1999) Angiotensin-converting enzyme inhibition reduces monocyte chemoattractant protein-1 and tissue factor levels in patients with myocardial infarction. J Am Coll Cardiol 34:983–988

Sohn HY, Raff U, Hoffmann A, Gloe T, Heermeier K, Galle J, Pohl U (2000) Differential role of angiotensin II receptor subtypes on endothelial superoxide formation. Br J Pharmacol 131:667–672

Steinberg D, Parthasarathy S, Carew TE, Khoo JC, Witztum JL (1989) Beyond cholesterol. Modifications of low-density lipoprotein that increase its atherogenicity. N Engl J Med 320:915–924

Strawn WB, Chappell MC, Dean RH, Kivlighn S, Ferrario CM (2000) Inhibition of early atherogenesis by losartan in monkeys with diet-induced hypercholesterolemia. Circulation 101:1586–1593

Su EJ, Lombardi DM, Siegal J, Schwartz SM (1998) Angiotensin II induces vascular smooth muscle cell replication independent of blood pressure. Hypertension 31:1331–1337

Sun YP, Zhu BQ, Browne AE, Pulukurthy S, Chou TM, Sudhir K, Glantz SA, Deedwania PC, Chatterjee K, Parmley WW (2001) Comparative effects of ACE inhibitors and an angiotensin receptor blocker on atherosclerosis and vascular function. J Cardiovasc Pharmacol Ther 6:175–181

Suzuki J, Iwai M, Nakagami H, Wu L, Chen R, Sugaya T, Hamada M, Hiwada K, Horiuchi M (2002) Role of angiotensin II-regulated apoptosis through distinct AT1 and AT2 receptors in neointimal formation. Circulation 106:847–853

Takai S, Shiota N, Kobayashi S, Matsumura E, Miyazaki M (1997) Induction of chymase that forms angiotensin II in the monkey atherosclerotic aorta. FEBS Lett 412:86–90

Teo KK, Burton JR, Buller CE, Plante S, Catellier D, Tymchak W, Dzavik V, Taylor D, Yokoyama S, Montague TJ (2000) Long-term effects of cholesterol lowering and angiotensin-converting enzyme inhibition on coronary atherosclerosis: The Simvastatin/Enalapril Coronary Atherosclerosis Trial (SCAT). Circulation 102:1748–1754

The Acute Infarction Ramipril Efficacy (AIRE) Study Investigators (1993) Effect of ramipril on mortality and morbidity of survivors of acute myocardial infarction with clinical evidence of heart failure. Lancet 342:821–828

The ALLHAT Collaborative Research Group (2002) Major outcomes in high-risk hypertensive patients randomized to angiotensin-converting enzyme inhibitor or calcium channel blocker vs diuretic: The Antihypertensive and Lipid-Lowering Treatment to Prevent Heart Attack Trial (ALLHAT). JAMA 288:2981–2997

The CONSENSUS Trial Study Group (1987) Effects of enalapril on mortality in severe congestive heart failure. Results of the Cooperative North Scandinavian Enalapril Survival Study (CONSENSUS). N Engl J Med 316:1429–1435

The SOLVD Investigattors (1992) Effect of enalapril on mortality and the development of heart failure in asymptomatic patients with reduced left ventricular ejection fractions. N Engl J Med 327:685–691

Townsend RR, Zhao H (1994) Plasma renin activity and insulin sensitivity in normotensive subjects. Am J Hypertens 7:894–898

Tummala PE, Chen XL, Sundell CL, Laursen JB, Hammes CP, Alexander RW, Harrison DG, Medford RM (1999) Angiotensin II induces vascular cell adhesion molecule-1 expression in rat vasculature: A potential link between the renin-angiotensin system and atherosclerosis. Circulation 100:1223–1229

Uehara Y, Urata H, Sasaguri M, Ideishi M, Sakata N, Tashiro T, Kimura M, Arakawa K (2000) Increased chymase activity in internal thoracic artery of patients with hypercholesterolemia. Hypertension 35:55–60

UK Prospective Diabetes Study Group (1998) Efficacy of atenolol and captopril in reducing risk of macrovascular and microvascular complications in type 2 diabetes: UKPDS 39. BMJ 317:713–720

Vaughan DE (2002) Angiotensin and vascular fibrinolytic balance. Am J Hypertens 15:3S–8S

Veerasingham SJ, Raizada MK (2003) Brain renin-angiotensin system dysfunction in hypertension: recent advances and perspectives. Br J Pharmacol 139:191–202

Viswanathan M, Stromberg C, Seltzer A, Saavedra JM (1992) Balloon angioplasty enhances the expression of angiotensin II AT1 receptors in neointima of rat aorta. J Clin Invest 90:1707–1712

Wagenaar LJ, van Boven AJ, van der Wal AC, Amoroso G, Tio RA, van der Loos CM, Becker AE, van Gilst WH (2003) Differential localisation of the renin-angiotensin system in de-novo lesions and in-stent restenotic lesions in in-vivo human coronary arteries. Cardiovasc Res 59:980–987

Wang CH, Li SH, Weisel RD, Fedak PW, Dumont AS, Szmitko P, Li RK, Mickle DA, Verma S (2003) C-reactive protein upregulates angiotensin type 1 receptors in vascular smooth muscle. Circulation 107:1783–1790

Warnholtz A, Nickenig G, Schulz E, Macharzina R, Brasen JH, Skatchkov M, Heitzer T, Stasch JP, Griendling KK, Harrison DG, Bohm M, Meinertz T, Munzel T (1999) Increased NADH-oxidase-mediated superoxide production in the early stages of atherosclerosis: evidence for involvement of the renin-angiotensin system. Circulation 99:2027–2033

Wassmann S, Laufs U, Baumer AT, Muller K, Ahlbory K, Linz W, Itter G, Rosen R, Bohm M, Nickenig G (2001) HMG-CoA reductase inhibitors improve endothelial dysfunction in normocholesterolemic hypertension via reduced production of reactive oxygen species. Hypertension 37:1450–1457

Weiss D, Kools JJ, Taylor WR (2001) Angiotensin II-induced hypertension accelerates the development of atherosclerosis in apoE-deficient mice. Circulation 103:448–454

Wheatcroft SB, Williams IL, Shah AM, Kearney MT (2003) Pathophysiological implications of insulin resistance on vascular endothelial function. Diabet Med 20:255–268

Williams B, Baker AQ, Gallacher B, Lodwick D (1995) Angiotensin II increases vascular permeability factor gene expression by human vascular smooth muscle cells. Hypertension 25:913–917

Wing LM, Reid CM, Ryan P, Beilin LJ, Brown MA, Jennings GL, Johnston CI, McNeil JJ, Macdonald GJ, Marley JE, Morgan TO, West MJ (2003) A comparison of outcomes with angiotensin-converting–enzyme inhibitors and diuretics for hypertension in the elderly. N Engl J Med 348:583–592

Wolny A, Clozel JP, Rein J, Mory P, Vogt P, Turino M, Kiowski W, Fischli W (1997) Functional and biochemical analysis of angiotensin II-forming pathways in the human heart. Circ Res 80:219–227

Wong J, Rauhoft C, Dilley RJ, Agrotis A, Jennings GL, Bobik A (1997) Angiotensin-converting enzyme inhibition abolishes medial smooth muscle PDGF-AB biosynthesis and attenuates cell proliferation in injured carotid arteries: relationships to neointima formation. Circulation 96:1631–1640

Wu L, Iwai M, Nakagami H, Li Z, Chen R, Suzuki J, Akishita M, de Gasparo M, Horiuchi M (2001) Roles of angiotensin II type 2 receptor stimulation associated with selective angiotensin II type 1 receptor blockade with valsartan in the improvement of inflammation-induced vascular injury. Circulation 104:2716–2721

Xu J, Carretero OA, Liu YH, Shesely EG, Yang F, Kapke A, Yang XP (2002) Role of AT2 receptors in the cardioprotective effect of AT1 antagonists in mice. Hypertension 40:244–250

Yusuf S, Dagenais G, Pogue J, Bosch J, Sleight P (2000a) Vitamin E supplementation and cardiovascular events in high-risk patients. The Heart Outcomes Prevention Evaluation Study Investigators. N Engl J Med 342:154–160

Yusuf S, Sleight P, Pogue J, Bosch J, Davies R, Dagenais G (2000b) Effects of an angiotensin-converting-enzyme inhibitor, ramipril, on cardiovascular events in high-risk patients. The Heart Outcomes Prevention Evaluation Study Investigators. N Engl J Med 342: 145–153

Zhuo J, Moeller I, Jenkins T, Chai SY, Allen AM, Ohishi M, Mendelsohn FA (1998) Mapping tissue angiotensin-converting enzyme and angiotensin AT1, AT2 and AT4 receptors. J Hypertens 16:2027–2037

HEP (2005) 170:443–462

Inhibition of Platelet Activation and Aggregation

I. Ahrens (✉) · C. Bode · K. Peter

Abteilung für Innere Medizin III (Kardiologie u. Angiologie), Universitätsklinikum Freiburg, Medizinische Universitätsklinik und Poliklinik, Hugstetter Strasse 55, 79106 Freiburg, Germany
ahrens@medizin.ukl.uni-freiburg.de

Abstract It has recently been established that platelets are involved at all stages of atherosclerotic disease. A major platelet mediated process is the acute vessel closure at the site of atherosclerotic plaque rupture and there is emerging evidence for platelet adhesion to endothelial cells in the early stage of atherosclerotic disease. This, through engagement of other cells, leads to the development of the atherosclerotic plaque. Beside dietary, cholesterol- and lipid-lowering, and other pharmaceutical approaches antiplatelet therapy plays an important part in the treatment of atherosclerosis and its multifarious clinical manifestations. Antiplatelet therapy and the currently approved substances for oral (acetylsalicylic acid, dipyridamole, cilostazol, ticlopidin and clopidogrel) and parenteral (acetylsalicylic acid, abciximab, eptifibatide and tirofiban) administration are discussed in the following section. Attention is given to each single agent and its mechanism of action. Differences in pharmacodynamic and pharmacokinetic properties are elucidated and outlook on future antiplatelet strategies is discussed.

Keywords Atherosclerosis · Antiplatelet drugs · Acetylsalicylic acid · Clopidogrel · Dipyridamole · GPIIb/IIIa inhibitors · Platelet activation

1
The Role of Platelet Adhesion and Aggregation in Atherosclerosis

The intact endothelium helps to prevent platelets from adhering to vessel walls. Both the secretion of inhibitory substances, such as nitric oxide and prostacycline, and the intact mechanical barrier to adhesive substrates of the subendothelial matrix are crucial to keep circulating platelets in their nonreactive state. It is well known that in the late stage of atherogenesis platelets adhere to denuded vessel wall areas via exposed matrix proteins. Less well known is the fact that already very early in atherogenesis platelets stick to endothelial cells that express an 'atherogenic' profile of cell membrane-bound adhesion molecules. The adhering platelets recruit other cells (platelets and white blood cells) and deliver growth signals to the neighboring vessel wall cells, such as smooth muscle cells and fibroblasts. Aggregating platelets and other blood cells are incorporated into the growing atherosclerotic plaque. Finally, after acute plaque rupture, the formation of platelet aggregates leads to acute vessel closure and severe clinical sequelae. Coronary artery disease and acute coronary syndromes (ACS) are some of the manifold manifestations of atherosclerosis. Considering the central role of platelets in the pathogenesis described above, it is clearly justified to administer a therapy aiming at the inhibition of platelet function to treat acute and chronic atherosclerosis and their clinical sequelae.

1.1
Receptors That Mediate Platelet Adhesion, Stimulation and Aggregation

Disruption of the endothelium in atherosclerosis allows platelets to interact with the subendothelial matrix. The release of subendothelial von Willebrand factor and the exposure of collagen lead, at conditions of high shear rates, to the adhesion of unactivated platelets (Turrito et al. 1985, Kehrel et al. 1998). GPIb-IX-V is the platelet receptor binding von Willebrand factor, and glycoprotein VI (GPVI) is the major collagen receptor on the platelet surface. Besides binding to platelet GPVI, collagen also serves as a binding site for von Willebrand factor in the subendothelial matrix and therefore contributes to the adhesion of unactivated platelets via GPIb-IX-V (Savage et al 1998). The more or less passive process of adhesion is followed by an active metabolic process of platelet activation leading to platelet aggregation by binding the activated integrin $\alpha IIb\beta3$ (the platelet receptor for fibrinogen, also termed GPIIb/IIIa) to soluble fibrinogen or von Willebrand factor. Both fibrinogen and von Willebrand factor, bound to activated GPIIb/IIIa, crosslink platelets, which contributes to the formation of a thrombus.

Collagen and thrombin are the most potent physiological activators of platelets. Thrombin is an agonist for two platelet receptors the protease activated receptors 1 (PAR1) and 4 (PAR4) (Kahn et al. 1998). These receptors belong to the family of the G-protein coupled receptors. PAR1 mediates platelet activation at low concentrations of thrombin while PAR4 is activated at higher concentrations. A blockade of PAR4 has little effect on platelet aggregation, whereas a blockade of both PAR1 and PAR4 virtually ablates platelet aggregation even at high concentrations of thrombin (Kahn et al. 1999).

Exposed to ADP, platelets undergo shape changes, activate the fibrinogen receptor GPIIb/IIIa, aggregate, release the contents of their granules and produce thromboxane (TX) A_2. The receptors binding extracellular nucleotides such as ADP have been classified as P2 receptors. P2 receptors are subdivided into P2X intrinsic ion channels and P2Y G-protein-coupled receptors. Three different types of P2 receptors have been identified on platelets: P2X1, P2Y1 and PTY12. P2X1 has been identified as an ADP-stimulated calcium channel that enables fast calcium entry into the platelet upon ADP binding (MacKenzie et al. 1996). P2Y1 is a G-protein-coupled seven-transmembrane domain receptor that changes the platelet shape and mobilizes calcium from intracellular stores by activating phospholipase C (Jin et al. 1998). The P2Y12 receptor inhibits the platelet adenylate cyclase and seems to be responsible for a positive feedback mechanism that amplifies platelet stimulation especially by weak agonists (Hollopeter et al. 2001). Therefore, this receptor plays a central part in the final step of platelet aggregation and stabilization of aggregates (Gachet 2001).

Epinephrin and other catecholamines stimulate the platelet α2A-adrenergic receptor coupled to a G-protein and inhibit adenylate cyclase activity (Keularts et al. 2000), thereby antagonizing the cAMP-elevating effect of agents like prostacyclin and prostaglandin E_1 (Paul et al. 1998). Other G-protein coupled receptors expressed on the platelet surface are the serotonin receptor 5-HT$_{2a}$ (Hourani and Cusack 1991), the vasopressin receptor V_1 (Siess et al. 1986), and the receptor for platelet activating factor (Chao and Olson 1993).

Active phospholipase A2 mediates the release of arachidonic acid from membrane phospholipids of activated platelets. The arachidonic acid is then converted to the prostaglandin endoperoxide intermediates PGG_2 and PGH_2 by action of cyclooxygenase-1 (COX-1). The prostaglandin endoperoxide intermediates are subsequently converted to TXA_2 by the TX synthase (Smith et al. 1996). TXA_2, when released from the platelets, binds to the G-protein-coupled TX receptor TP and functions as an agonist for platelet stimulation (Hirata et al. 1991).

After stimulation, the platelet releases the contents of granules in the platelet cytoplasm. This process has been termed platelet secretion. Platelets contain several dense granules (δ-granules) and around 50 α-granules. δ-granules mainly contain ADP, ATP, calcium, pyrophosphate and serotonin. α-granules contain a variety of plasma proteins including fibrinogen, von Willebrand factor, Factor V and albumin. Other proteins are synthesized by the megakaryocyte itself, for example platelet-derived growth factor, thrombospondin, β-thromboglobulin, and platelet factor 4. The α-granule membrane also contains the platelet integrin αIIbβ3, the von Willebrand receptor GPIb-IX-V, P-selectin, and osteonectin. These receptors reflect the platelet pool of receptors that, once activated, can be translocated to and incorporated into the platelet membrane during the process of secretion. The newly incorporated receptors may contribute to some of the pharmacological effects of antiplatelet drugs such as inconsistence in platelet aggregation inhibition.

2
Clinically Approved Antiplatelet Drugs

To date, various orally and intraveneously administered agents have been made available for antiplatelet therapy. Some of them do act synergistically by inhibiting different steps of platelet adhesion and aggregation. In the following chapter, the four now clinically approved strategies for platelet function inhibition are discussed: (1) inhibition of cyclooxygenase; (2) phosphodiesterase inhibition; (3) blockade of the $P2Y_{12}$ ADP receptor; and (4) blockade of the GP IIb/IIIa receptor.

2.1
Inhibition of Cyclooxygenase with Acetylicsalicylic Acid (Aspirin)

2.1.1
Mechanism of Action

Acetylsalicylic acid inhibits the enzymes COX-1[prostaglandin (PG)H-synthase-1] and cyclooxygenase-2 (COX-2, PGH-synthase-2) in their conversion of arachidonic acid to PGG_2 and PGH_2 (Patrono 1994). COX-1 is constitutively expressed in most cell types, whereas COX-2 is detectable after induction in inflammatory, endothelial and other cells. It is generally believed that platelets express only COX-1, although in one study COX-2 was found in platelets too (Weber et al. 1999). Aspirin selectively acetylates the serine residue at position 529 of COX-1, which results in the steric hindrance of arachidonic acid to access the catalytic center and thereby in a permanent loss of cyclooxygenase activity. COX-2 is inhibited by the same mechanism; however, higher doses of aspirin are needed for inhibition. In human platelets PGH_2, the product of COX 1, is predominantly metabolized to TXA_2. Through its release and binding to the TXA_2-receptor, TXA_2 represents an amplification system of the platelets that is active after stimulation with divergent primary platelet agonists (ADP, collagen, thrombin, epinephrin, etc.). Since platelets cannot re-synthesize COX-1, the irreversible blockade of COX-1 results in irreversible platelet inhibition. Thus, although aspirin is detectable in plasma only for a limited time (plasma half-life, 15 min), platelet inhibition can be demonstrated for about 7–10 days (Patrono et al. 2001).

2.1.2
Clinical Use of Acetylsalicylic Acid as an Antiplatelet Drug

The pivotal role of platelets in arterial thrombosis has been established essentially by the beneficial effects of aspirin in patients with myocardial infarction (MI). In the ISIS-2 trial, the administration of aspirin reduced the 5-week mortality of patients with MI by 23%. The effect of platelet inhibition equaled and added to the effect of thrombolysis by streptokinase (ISIS-2 Collaborative Group 1988). In the 10-year-follow-up, the original benefit of aspirin was still present (Baigent et al. 1998). Unstable angina is also associated with platelet activation (Fitzgerald et al. 1986) and, in fact, aspirin does reduce the rate of death and MI in patients with unstable angina (Lewis et al. 1983; Cairns et al. 1985; Theroux et al. 1988). Coronary angioplasty is linked to platelet activation, and aspirin significantly reduces the rate of acute vessel closure (Barnathan et al. 1987; Gawaz et al. 1996). In all these acute clinical situations, the administration of aspirin is a therapeutic necessity. Nevertheless, aspirin saved most lives in the secondary prevention of cardiovascular events—and as a single drug it probably saved the most lives in all. In the Antiplatelet Trialists' meta-analysis of approximately 70,000 patients with coronary artery disease, TIA, stroke or peripheral arterial vascular disease, aspirin showed a risk reduction of 25% for MI, stroke or vascular death (Antiplatelet Trialists' Collaboration 1994). Just recently, a meta-analysis of 200,000 patients treated with antiplatelet drugs confirmed the benefits and even showed additional advantages of antiplatelet therapy for the secondary prevention of cardiovascular complications in patients with stable angina pectoris, intermittent claudication, and (if oral anticoagulants are unsuitable) atrial fibrillation (Antiplatelet Trialists' Collaboration 2002). In the primary prevention of cardiovascular events, the increase of hemorrhagic strokes—a severe side effect of aspirin—seems to counteract the beneficial effects of aspirin on the rate of MI (Peto et al. 1988; Steering Committee of the Physicians' Health Study Research Group 1989; ETDRS Investigators 1992). In the Physicians' Health Study, the rate of stroke increased by 21% and the rate of MI decreased by 44% (Peto et al. 1988). Nevertheless, a reduction of mortality from all cardiovascular causes was not associated with aspirin (Peto et al. 1988). When extrapolated from the data of aspirin treatment in primary and secondary prevention, the cut point at which the benefit in the prevention of ischemic cardiovascular events outweighs the increase of the risk of stroke has to be determined with caution. A higher cardiovascular risk seems to correlate with a higher benefit conferred by aspirin. However, patients with clear cardiovascular risk factors, especially with diabetes mellitus, may indeed profit from aspirin treatment in the primary prevention of cardiovascular events (Hansson et al. 1998; The Medical Research Council's General Practice Research Framework 1998; Avanzini et al. 2000).

For a long time, the dosing of aspirin has been debated controversially. There is no doubt that aspirin-induced gastrointestinal toxicity is dose dependent (Roderick et al. 1993). On the other hand, an increase in dose does not correlate with an increase in the antiplatelet effects of aspirin. The results of the recent Antithrombotic Trialists' Collaborations' meta-analysis convincingly demonstrate that high daily doses of aspirin (500–1500 mg) are not more effective than medium doses (160–325 mg) or low doses (75–150 mg). (Antithrombotic Trialists' Collaboration 2002). Thus, low-dose aspirin seems to exert the full antiplatelet efficiency with the lowest risk of side effects.

2.2
Inhibition of the Phosphodiesterase

2.2.1
Mechanism of Action

The phosphodiesterases (PDE) are a family of enzymes catalyzing the hydrolysis of cyclic nucleoside monophosphates, namely cyclic adenosine monophosphate (cAMP) and cyclic guanosine monophosphate (cGMP) (Beavo 1995). At least nine different isoforms termed PDE1 through PDE9 have been identified in mammalian tissues (Soderling et al. 1998). Platelets have been found to express PDE2, PDE3 and PDE5 isoenzymes. Two substances acting by inhibition of PDE—dipyridamole and cilostazol—are now clinically approved. Dipyridamole primarily inhibits the degradation of cGMP (Ziegler et al. 1995) by PDE5 inhibition, but it also elevates platelet cAMP levels. The increased platelet cAMP and cGMP concentrations lead to a reduced platelet reactivity by decreasing the cytoplasmic calcium and inhibiting platelet prostaglandin synthesis. Another nonplatelet-specific effect of dipyridamole is the elevation of extracellular adenosine levels by reducing their uptake and metabolism (Newsholme 1978). Dipyridamole also enhances the release and prevents the metabolic degradation of endothelial prostaglandin PGI_2 (Moncada and Korbut 1978; Neri et al. 1981), a potent inhibitor of platelet aggregation.

Cilostazol potently inhibits the PDE3 and adenosine uptake, thereby increasing platelet and vascular smooth muscle cell cAMP levels, which ultimately helps to inhibit platelet aggregation (Schror 2002). Additional beneficial effects of cilostazol have been observed and cannot be explained solely by the elevation of cAMP-levels. Lipid metabolism seems to be influenced in a positive way, as cilostazol facilitates the removal of triglycerides and increases high-density lipoprotein (HDL) cholesterol levels (Elam et al. 1998; Thompson et al. 2002).

2.2.2
Dipyridamole (Persantin)

Since the first introduction of dipyridamole as an antianginal medication in 1959, there has been a lot of controversy about the clinical relevance of dipyridamole as an antithrombotic agent. Two major studies were performed to elucidate the role of dipyridamole in the secondary prevention of MI: first, the Persantine-Aspirin Reinfarction Study (PARIS I) (The Persantine-Aspirin Reinfarction Study research group 1980) and second, the PARIS II study (Klimt et al. 1986). PARIS I directly compared aspirin 324 mg three times daily to the same dose of aspirin plus dipyridamole 75 mg three times daily in a total of 2,026 patients. Primary endpoints were total mortality, coronary mortality, and fatal plus nonfatal MI. The average follow-up was 41 months. There was no statistical significant difference between the two treatment groups. In PARIS II, patients were randomized to aspirin plus dipyridamole or placebo. A 24% reduction of coronary adverse events was found in the group treated with aspirin plus dipyridamole. However, a group receiving aspirin only was not included in this trial, so that a direct beneficial effect of dipyridamole added to aspirin could not be proven.

Furthermore, other clinical trials failed to show consistent benefit of dipyridamole added to aspirin in patients having undergone coronary artery bypass surgery (Sanz et al. 1990), in patients with peripheral vascular disease (Kohler et al. 1984), or in patients with prosthetic heart valves (Stein et al. 1986). However there is evidence that dipyridamole plays an important part in the prevention of stroke. The European Stroke Prevention Study 2 (ESPS-2) was a randomized placebo-controlled double-blind trial examining aspirin 50 mg daily, dipyridamole 400 mg daily, a regimen of both drugs together or placebo. The combined treatment with aspirin 50 mg and dipyridamole 400 mg daily reduced the relative risk of major vascular events by 22% compared to a treatment with aspirin alone (The ESPS-2 Group 1997). The mechanism by which dipyridamole prevents stroke still needs to be determined. A recent study failed to establish a link between dipyridamole and a permanent reduction of blood pressure. This link would have explained how strokes are prevented (De Schryver 2003).

2.2.3
Cilostazol (Pletal)

The quinolinone derivative cilostazol has been shown to inhibit platelet activation (Kimura et al. 1985) and increase vasodilation (Tanaka et al. 1988). Cilostazol inhibits the proliferation of vascular smooth muscle cells (Takahashi et al. 1992). After oral administration, cilostazol is extensively metabolized by hepatic cytochrome P-450 enzymes. Two metabolites of cilostazol are active and account for the pharmacologic effects observed in patients treated with cilostazol 100 mg or 50 mg (when administered together with other antiplatelet drugs) twice daily. The elimination half-lives of cilostazol and its active metabolites amount to 11–13 h. The substance has been extensively studied in patients with peripheral vascular disease and intermittent claudication. A meta-analysis of placebo controlled trials with cilostazol in the treatment of peripheral artery disease showed that cilostazol therapy (administered for 12–

24 weeks) increased the maximal and pain-free walking distance in patients with intermittent claudication by 50% and 67%, respectively (Thompson et al. 2002). In addition to the enhancement of quality of life, treatment with cilostazol reduced plasma triglyceride levels by 15.8% and increased HDL by 12.8% (Thompson et al. 2002). Cilostazol is primarily used for the treatment of symptomatic peripheral artery disease. The role of cilostazol in the treatment of other diseases secondary to atherosclerosis needs to be carefully investigated in larger scale placebo-controlled clinical trials.

2.3
P2Y$_{12}$ ADP Receptor Antagonists Ticlopidin and Clopidogrel

2.3.1
Mechanism of Action

The thienonyridines ticlopidin and clopidogrel are prodrugs metabolized in the liver by cytochrome P450. The short-lived active metabolite of clopidogrel was recently identified as being a thiol derivate of the parent agent clopidogrel (Savi et al. 2000). The selectivity of thienopyridines for the P2Y$_{12}$ ADP receptor is thought to be caused by covalent modification of the four cystein residues in the P2Y$_{12}$ receptor via the thiol metabolites (Hollopeter et al. 2001; Savi et al. 2000).

2.3.2
Ticlopidin (Ticlid) and Clopidogrel (Plavix/Iscover)

The inhibition of platelet aggregation by the thienopyridine ticlopidine was already reported by Thebault et al. (1975). Rather recently, clopidogrel, also belonging to the thienopyridines, replaced ticlopidine in its clinical use, as ticlopidine showed significant adverse effects such as skin rash, gastrointestinal symptoms and bone marrow toxicity with severe and fatal neutropenia. Treatment with clopidogrel, however, caused none or many fewer of these problems (CAPRIE Steering Committee 1996; Bennett et al. 2000; Bertrand et al. 2000; Bhatt et al. 2002). The breakthrough study for the widespread clinical use of clopidogrel was the CAPRIE trial (CAPRIE Steering Committee 1996). In this study, clopidogrel proved to be slightly more effective than aspirin for the secondary prevention of thrombembolic complications in patients with atherosclerotic disease (prior MI, ischemic stroke or peripheral vascular disease). In addition, safety and tolerability of clopidogrel and aspirin were similar. In interventional cardiology the combinational therapy of aspirin and clopidogrel after stent placement has become a widespread standard (Bhatt et al. 2002). In particular, the risk of a subacute stent thrombosis after stent placement could be reduced substantially by the combination of aspirin and thienopyridines (Bhatt et al. 2002; Schomig et al. 1996; Moussa et al. 1999;

Cosmi et al. 2001). Finally, just recently evolving has been the concept of long-term treatment of coronary syndromes with the combination of aspirin and clopidogrel (Yusuf et al. 2001).

The specific abundance of the $P2Y_{12}$ ADP receptor limited to platelets and potentially to the brain makes this receptor an interesting pharmacological target, promising nearly ideal selectivity (Hollopeter et al. 2001). Clopidogrel has been shown to block all available $P2Y_{12}$ receptors on the platelet and thus demonstrates highest efficiency (Gachet 2001). Clopidogrel presents an almost ideal safety and tolerability profile (CAPRIE Steering Committee 1996; Bertrand et al. 2000; Bhatt et al. 2002). In fact, clopidogrel is a remarkable pharmaceutical agent. Nevertheless, two characteristics of clopidogrel justify the search for other $P2Y_{12}$ ADP receptor inhibitors. First, even with a loading dose of 300 mg at least two, but probably up to 12 h are needed for the full antiplatelet effect of clopidogrel to develop (Savcic et al. 1999). The data of the ISAR REACT study suggest that with a loading dose of 600 mg, a steady state can be reached in less time than with 300 mg, and that the higher dose may lead to a better outcome in the setting of percutaneous coronary interventions (PCI) (ACC 2003, late breaking trials). However, in acute MI or urgent coronary interventions for example, the antiplatelet effect of clopidogrel comes too late. Second, the $P2Y_{12}$ receptor is irreversibly blocked and thus the effect persists for the entire platelet life span (Weber et al. 2001). Since there is no antagonist available, needed for example when urgent operations are performed, bleeding complications may occur. To overcome these problems, a new class of $P2Y_{12}$ ADP receptor inhibitors has been developed (Story 2001), based on the fact that ATP is a competitive antagonist of ADP. Structural homologues were screened for selectivity against the $P2Y_{12}$ receptor, and there were indeed several agents found, some of them already having been tested in clinical trials. The advantage of these agents consists in their immediate antiplatelet effects after intravenous application that, because of their short half-life, are rapidly reversible (Storey 2001). Some of these agents can be used as intravenous, some as oral drugs (Storey 2001).

2.4
GP IIb/IIIa Inhibitors

2.4.1
Mechanism of Action

GPIIb/IIIa, or integrin $\alpha IIb\beta 3$, is the platelet receptor for fibrinogen and mediates the final step in platelet aggregation. As the default state of $\alpha IIb\beta 3$ is a nonactivated and resting state, it needs to become activated in order to bind its major ligand, i.e., soluble fibrinogen. This occurs after the activation of platelets by physiological agonists (e.g., thrombin, ADP, collagen) stimulate intracellular signal pathways and thereby induce conformational changes of $\alpha IIb\beta 3$. This process is termed 'inside-out' signaling (Shattli 1999). It switches the receptor into an activated state with high affinity for fibrinogen and numerous other ligands (Phillips et al. 1998). As a result of αIIbβ3-mediated binding to the bivalent molecule fibrinogen, platelets aggregate and form a thrombus rich in platelets. To date, two binding sites have been well characterized in αIIbβ3: an Arg-Gly-Asp (RGD)-binding site and a Lys-Glu-Ala-Gly-Asp-Val (KQAGDV)-binding site (Tcheng 2000). Other binding sites have been described as well, with yet unknown functional properties (Lin et al. 1997; Basani et al 2000). Interestingly, fibrinogen binds via the KQAGDV-binding site. Agents that bind within the ligand-binding region of αIIbβ3 and block the binding of its natural ligands have been developed and termed GPIIb/IIIa inhibitors. Of the three clinically approved parenteral GPIIb/IIIa inhibitors, one (abciximab; ReoPro, Lilly, IN, USA) is based on an antibody structure, and the two others (eptifibatide; Integrilin, Millennium/Schering-Plough, NJ, USA and tirofiban; Aggrastat, Merck, NJ, USA) are described as small-molecule GPIIb/IIIa inhibitors. All of them bind to αIIbβ3 either in the resting or activated conformation and inhibit fibrinogen binding and, consequently platelet aggregation. The first substance to be developed was a murine monoclonal antibody (mAb) that blocked αIIbβ3 (Coller et al. 1989). The immunogenicity of this mAb could be reduced by its humanization, i.e., by the exchange of the constant regions of the mouse antibody with the constant regions of human immunoglobulin IgG1 to produce a chimeric Fab fragment called abciximab. The other two GPIIb/IIIa inhibitors belong to the group of small molecules and can be subdivided into synthetic peptide inhibitors (eptifibatide) and synthetic nonpeptide inhibitors (tirofiban).

2.4.2
Abciximab (ReoPro)

The Fab fragment abciximab, with a molecular mass of 48 kDa and a reported equilibrium dissociation constant (K_D) of 5 nM is a high-affinity GPIIb/IIIa inhibitor for parenteral use only (Scarborough et al. 1999). The high receptor affinity and low K_D characterize the antagonist–receptor binding as noncompetitive, rendering a low plasma concentration of unbound abciximab that is eliminated through protein metabolism. Besides binding to αIIbβ3, abciximab has been reported to bind to with equal affinity to integrin αVβ3 (Tam et al. 1998) and with lower affinity (K_D, 160 nM) to the activated integrin αMβ2 (Mac-1) on monocytes and granulocytes (Coller 1999). The blockade of Mac-1 by abciximab inhibits leukocyte adhesion and aggregation and thus directly attenuates inflammatory reactions (Schwarz et al. 2002). Furthermore, since abciximab inhibits the binding of Factor X and its conversion to Factor Xa, it attenuates the cell-based initiation of the coagulation cascade (Schwarz et al. 2002). However, the clinical relevance of the cross-reactivity of abciximab against αVβ3 and Mac-1 remains to be determined. Interestingly, abciximab competes with heparin for binding to Mac-1 (Peter et al. 1999) and may thereby prolong the activated clotting time. This has been observed in patients treated with unfractionated heparin and abciximab (Moliterno et al. 1995; Ammar et al. 1997). The cross-reactivity of abciximab with the endothelial cell integrin $\alpha V\beta 3$ and the leukocyte integrin Mac-1 provides a possible explanation for abciximab-related effects on the coronary microcirculation. Microvascular coronary resistance decreased after abciximab bolus administration in patients with unstable refractory angina pectoris and hemodynamic-relevant coronary artery stenosis (Marzilli et al. 2002). Abciximab is currently approved for the use in patients undergoing PCI. It has also been studied as first-line medical treatment in patients with ACS in the absence of PCI, but for up to 48 h no benefit of abciximab treatment could be reported in this setting (The GUSTO IV-ACS Investigators 2001). Initial dose-finding trials were performed to identify the dosage leading to over 80% inhibition of platelet aggregation in humans or to less than 20% of baseline ADP-induced platelet aggregation. The findings led to the current administration as a bolus of 0.25 mg/kg followed by a 12-h infusion of 0.125 µg/kg/min (Tcheng et al. 1994). This dosing regimen has been kept constant in several clinical trials with a huge number of patients. The trials proved the benefit of abciximab treatment in the setting of acute MI and PCI. A newer study using the current dosing regimen showed that although most of the abciximab-treated patients achieved a platelet inhibition of 95% or higher 10 min after bolus administration, as assessed with the Ultegra Rapid Platelet Function Assay, the level of platelet inhibition 8 h after bolus administration and during continuous infusion of 0.125µg/kg/min was only 90%±11%. Patients showed a significant higher rate of major cardiac adverse events if platelet inhibition was less than 95% 10 min after bolus administration (Steinhubl et al. 2001). This result may lead to further dose-adjustment trials monitoring the platelet function inhibition. The high affinity and the low half-time rate of dissociation from the receptor led to prolonged platelet inhibition lasting for up to 7 days and distinguished abciximab from the small-molecule inhibitors with a lower affinity and more rapid dissociation (Mascelli et al. 1998; Peter et al. 2000). Due to the rapid plasma clearance of unbound abciximab and the high receptor affinity, a dose reduction in patients with renal disease does not seem to be necessary and platelet inhibition can be reversed rapidly by platelet transfusion. A rare adverse event of abciximab administration is the development of acute, severe thrombocytopenia with platelet counts of less than 20,000 platelets/µl. This condition develops within 24 h in approximately 0.7% of patients (Berkowitz et al. 1997). The pathogenesis of this thrombocytopenia is unknown. One of the most often discussed theories states that pre-existing antibodies against $\alpha IIb\beta 3$ conformations induced by abciximab or other antagonists can induce thrombocytopenia (Bednar et al. 1999). There was one patient described who presented with severe thrombocytopenia and in whom abciximab treatment resulted in direct platelet activation. It has been hypothesized that the sequestration of these activated platelets caused thrombocytopenia (Peter et al. 1999).

2.4.3
Eptifibatide (Integrilin)

Eptifibatide is a synthetic heptapeptide with a mass of 800 Da, modeled on the active site of barbourin, a peptide from the disintegrin family found in the venom of the southeastern pigmy rattlesnake. Unlike other disintegrins that have an RGD sequence and block all integrins that recognize this sequence, barbourin mediates its high affinity to αIIbβ3 through a Lys-Gly-Asp (KGD) sequence (Phillips and Scarborough 1997). Eptifibatide contains a modified KGD sequence and binds with high specificity to αIIbβ3, but with a lower affinity (K_D, 120 nM) than abciximab.

Despite its initially proposed specificity for αIIbβ3, binding of eptifibatide to αV integrins has been reported (Thibault et al. 2001) and inhibition of αVβ3 on different cell types, including smooth muscle and endothelial cells, has been demonstrated (Lele et al. 2001). The low affinity of the drug accounts for the high plasma concentration of unbound eptifibatide with only 25% of eptifibatide bound to plasma proteins. As eptifibatide is eliminated through the kidney, dose reductions in patients with severe renal disease or renal failure are necessary. Eptifibatide is currently approved for patients with ACS and patients undergoing PCI. The Integrilin to Minimize Platelet Aggregation and Coronary Thrombosis (IMPACT II) trial (IMPACT-II Investigators 1997) showed that eptifibatide, given as a 0.135 µg/kg bolus followed by a 0.75-µg/kg/min infusion, reduced the rate of ischemic events during the 24-h treatment period in patients undergoing elective, urgent or emergency PCI. It was found that the calcium-chelating property of the anticoagulant sodium citrate used for platelet aggregation assays in the IMPACT II trial led to an overestimation of the inhibitory effect of eptifibatide (Phillips et al. 1997). The dosing regimen was re-evaluated in the Posicor Reduction of Ischemia During Exercise (PRIDE) trial (Tcheng et al. 2001), with the direct thrombin inhibitor Phe-Pro-Arg chloromethyl ketone (PPACK) as an anticoagulant for platelet aggregation assays. In the PRIDE trial, the dose of 180µg/kg bolus followed by a 2.0-µg/kg/min infusion proved to be sufficient to achieve and maintain over 90% inhibition of 20 µM ADP-induced platelet aggregation. This dosing regimen was confirmed in the Platelet Glycoprotein IIb/IIIa in Unstable Angina trial [Receptor Suppression Using Integrilin Therapy (PURSUIT) trial]. Compared to a treatment with placebo, patients with unstable angina or non-ST-segment elevation MI (NSTEMI) had a significantly lower incidence of death or MI when treated with eptifibatide 180 µg/kg bolus followed by 2.0-µg/kg/min infusion (The PURSUIT trial investigators 1998).

The plasma elimination half-life of eptifibatide is approximately 2.5 h. The level of platelet aggregation inhibition 4 h after cessation of the infusion is less than 50% and the bleeding time 6 h after cessation is not remarkably prolonged. As an early peak level with a small decline within 4–6 h after the bolus administration was observable, a double bolus of 180µg/kg followed by another 180µg/kg 10 min later was considered safe in patients undergoing PCI in the Enhanced Suppression of the Platelet IIb/IIIa Receptor with Integrilin Therapy (ESPRIT) trial (The ESPRIT trial investigators 2000). Data from patients who underwent PCI suggest that the decline in platelet aggregation inhibition could be overcome by the double bolus administration of eptifibatide (Gilchrist et al. 2001).

2.4.4
Tirofiban (Aggrastat)

The synthetic nonpeptide tirofiban is a small-molecule (500 Da) GPIIb/IIIa inhibitor that mimics the RGD sequence (Egbertson et al. 1994). Tirofiban is a competitive antagonist with a receptor affinity higher than eptifibatide but lower than abciximab (K_D, 15 mM). To date, no cross-reactivity of tirofiban with other integrins has been reported. The fraction of unbound tirofiban in human plasma is 35%, the plasma elimination half-life of 2 h is comparable with eptifibatide. Normal hemostatic function is restored within 4 h of cessation of the drug infusion. The renal clearance of tirofiban accounts for 39%–69% of the plasma clearance. Patients with creatinine clearance of less than 30 ml/min present a significantly decreased plasma clearance (>50%) of tirofiban. For these patients, the manufacturer recommends a weight-adjusted reduction of the dose by 50%. Tirofiban is licensed for the treatment of ACS and in the setting of PCI. The dosing regimen for the use in ACS is a bolus infusion of 0.4 µg/kg/min over 30 min, followed by an infusion of 0.1 µg/kg/min. In patients undergoing PCI, a bolus dose of 10 µg/kg given 10 min prior to PCI followed by a 0.15-µg/kg/min infusion for 18 h has been used in the Randomized Efficacy Study of Tirofiban for Outcomes and Restenosis (RESTORE) trial (RESTORE Investigators 1997). Sufficient and consistent platelet aggregation inhibition of more than 80% in the response to 20 µM ADP has been reported with either dosing regimen during the time of infusion (Batchelor et al. 2002). However, an inhibition of platelet aggregation exceeding 80% after a bolus of 10 µg/kg (RESTORE regimen) was not achieved in all patients at 15 and 30 min, but could be observed after 4 h (Batchelor et al. 2002). The same dosing regimen for tirofiban was used in the Tirofiban and ReoPro Give Similar Efficacy Outcomes trial (TARGET) (The Target Investigators 2001). This trial, intended to asses the noninferiority of tirofiban compared to abciximab, was the first direct comparison of the two GPIIb/IIIa inhibitors abciximab and tirofiban in the setting of PCI. The 30-day results demonstrated the superiority of abciximab. The primary end point occurred in 7.6% of patients treated with tirofiban versus 6% of patients treated with abciximab. A possible explanation for this phenomenon is the incomplete inhibition of platelet aggregation by tirofiban. Platelet aggregation measurements were not incorporated in the study protocol. Therefore, this issue has to be addressed by further investigations.

2.4.5
Oral GPIIb/IIIa Inhibitors

The rationale behind the development of oral GPIIb/IIIa antagonist was the assumption that long-term inhibition of αIIbβ3 would provide a new therapeutic approach for the prevention of recurrent ischemic events in patients with cardiovascular disease. Four oral GPIIb/IIIa antagonists (lotrafiban, orbofiban, sibrafiban and xemilofiban), all of which are nonpeptide prodrugs, have been examined in large Phase III clinical trials. None of them fulfilled the high expectations. Therapies applying these substances have not proven to be superior to aspirin therapy. Furthermore, a meta-analysis of four major Phase III trials [Evaluation of Oral Xemilofiban in Controlling Thrombotic Events (EXCITE), Orbofiban Post Unstable Coronary Syndromes (OPUS), Sibrafiban versus Aspirin to Yield Maximum Protection from Ischemic Heart Events Post-acute Coronary Syndromes (SYMPHONY) and 2nd SYMPHONY] including 33,326 patients showed a statistically significant increase in mortality in patients treated with the oral GPIIb/IIIa antagonists (Chew et al. 2001). The short plasma half-life of these drugs that causes undulating plasma levels and pro-aggregatory effects especially at low concentrations of the GPIIb/IIIa blockers is discussed as a potential reason for the disappointing outcomes of these large Phase III trials (Peter et al. 1998).

References

Ammar T, Scudder LE, Coller BS (1997) In vitro effects of the platelet glycoprotein IIb/IIIa receptor antagonist c7E3 Fab on the activated clotting time. Circulation 95:614–617

Antiplatelet Trialists' Collaboration (1994) Collaborative overview of randomised trials of antiplatelet therapy-I: Prevention of death, myocardial infarction, and stroke by prolonged antiplatelet therapy in various categories of patients. BMJ 308:81–106

Antithrombotic Trialists' Collaboration (2002) Collaborative meta-analysis of randomised trials of antiplatelet therapy for prevention of death, myocardial infarction, and stroke in high risk patients. BMJ 324:71–86

Avanzini F, Palumbo G, Alli C, Roncaglioni MC, Ronchi E, Cristofari M, Capra A, Rossi S, Nosotti L, Costantini C, Pietrofeso R (2000) Effects of low-dose aspirin on clinic and ambulatory blood pressure in treated hypertensive patients. Collaborative Group of the Primary Prevention Project (PPP)–Hypertension study. Am J Hypertens≥ 13:611–616

Baigent C, Collins R, Appleby P, Parish S, Sleight P, Peto R (1998) ISIS-2:10 year survival among patients with suspected acute myocardial infarction in randomised comparison of intravenous streptokinase, oral aspirin, both, or neither. The ISIS-2 (Second International Study of Infarct Survival) Collaborative Group. BMJ 316:1337–1343

Barnathan ES, Schwartz JS, Taylor L, Laskey WK, Kleaveland JP, Kussmaul WG, Hirshfeld JW Jr (1987) Aspirin and dipyridamole in the prevention of acute coronary thrombosis complicating coronary angioplasty. Circulation 76:125–134

Basani RB, French DL, Vilaire G, Brown DL, Chen F, Coller BS, Derrick JM, Gartner TK, Bennet JS, Poncz M (2000) A naturally occuring mutation near the amino terminus of alphaIIb defines a new region involved in ligand binding to alphaIIbbeta3. Blood 95:180–188

Batchelor WB, Tolleson TR, Huang Y, Larsen RL, Mantell RM, Dillard P, Davidian M, Zhang D, Cantor WJ, Sketch MH Jr, Ohman EM, Zidar JP, Gretler D, DiBattiste PM, Tcheng JE, Califf RM, Harrington RA (2002) Randomized COMparison of platelet inhibition with abciximab, tirofiban and eptifibatide during percutaneous coronary intervention in acute coronary syndromes. The COMPARE trial. Circulation 106:1470–1476

Beavo JA (1995) Cyclic nucleotide phosphodiesterases: functional implications of multiple isoforms. Physiol Rev 75:725–748

Bednar B, Cook JJ, Holahan MA, Cunnigham ME, Jumes PA, Bednar RA, Hartman GD, Gould RJ (1999) Fibrinogen receptor antagonist-induced thrombocytopenia in chimpanzee and rhesus monkey associated with preexisting drug-dependent antibodies to platelet glycoprotein IIb/IIIa. Blood 94:587–599

Bennett CL, Conners JM, Carwile JM, Moake JL, Bell WR, Tarantolo SR, McCarthy LJ, Sarode R, Hatfiled AJ, Feldman MD, Davidson CJ, Tsai HM (2000) Thrombotic thrombocytopenic purpura associated with clopidogrel. New Engl J Med 342:1773–1777

Berkowitz SD, Harrington RA, Rund MM, Tcheng JE (1997) Acute profound thrombocytopenia after C7E3 Fab (abciximab) therapy. Circulation 95:809–813

Bertrand ME, Rupprecht HJ, Urban P, Gershlick AH (2000) Double-blind study of the safety of clopidogrel with and without a loading dose in combination with aspirin compared with ticlopidine in combination with aspirin after coronary stenting: the clopidogrel aspirin stent international cooperative study (CLASSICS). Circulation 102:624–629

Bhatt DL, Bertrand ME, Berger PB, L'Allier PL, Moussa I, Moses JW, Dangas G, Taniuchi M, Lasala JM, Holmes DR, Ellis SG, Topol EJ (2002) Meta-analysis of randomized and registry comparisons of ticlopidine with clopidogrel after stenting. J Am Coll Cardiol 39:9–14

Cairns JA, Gent M, Singer J, Finnie KJ, Froggatt GM, Holder DA, Jablonsky G, Kostuk WJ, Melendez LJ, Myers MG, et al. (1985) Aspirin, sulfinpyrazone, or both in unstable angina. Results of a Canadian multicenter trial. N Engl J Med 313:1369–1375

CAPRIE Steering Committee (1996) A randomised, blinded, trial of clopidogrel versus aspirin in patients at risk of ischaemic events (CAPRIE). Lancet 348:1329–1339

Chao W, Olson MS (1993) Platelet-activating factor: receptors and signal transduction. Biochem J 292:617–629

Chew DP, Bhatt DL, Sapp S, Topol EJ (2001) Increased mortality with oral platelet glycoprotein IIb/IIIa antagonists. A meta-analysis of phase III multicenter randomized trials. Circulation 103:201–216

Coller BS (1999) Binding of abciximab to $\alpha V \beta 3$ and activated $\alpha M \beta 2$ receptors: with a review of platelet–leukocyte interactions. Thromb Haemost 82:326–336

Coller BS, Folts JD, Smith SR, Scudder LE, Jordan R (1989) Abolition of in vivo platelet thrombus formation in primates with monoclonal antibodies to the platelet GPIIb/IIIa receptor: correlation with bleeding time, platelet aggregation, and blockade of GPIIb/IIIa receptors. Circulation 80:1766–1774

Cosmi B, Rubboli A, Castelvetri C, Milandri M (2001) Ticlopidine versus oral anticoagulation for coronary stenting (Cochrane Review) [CD002133]. Cochrane Database Syst Rev 2001:4

De Schryver ELLM for the ESPRIT study group (2003) Dipyridamole in stroke prevention. Effect of dipyridamole on blood pressure. Stroke 34:2339–2342

Egbertson MS, Chang CT, Duggan ME, Gould RJ, Halczenko W, Hartman GD, Laswell WL, Lynch JJ Jr, Lynch RJ, Manno PD, et al. (1994) Non-peptide fibrinogen receptor antagonists. 2. Optimization of a tyrosine template as a mimic for arg–gly–asp. J Med Chem 37:2537–2551

Elam MB, Heckman J, Crouse JR, Hunninghake DB, Herd JA, Davidson M, Gordon IL, Bortey EB, Forbes WP (1998) Effect of the novel antiplatelet agent cilostazol on plasma lipoproteins in patients with intermittent claudication. Arterioscler Thromb Vasc Biol 18:1942–1947

ETDRS Investigators (1992) Aspirin effects on mortality and morbidity in patients with diabetes mellitus. Early Treatment Diabetic Retinopathy Study report 14. JAMA 268:1292–1300

Fitzgerald DJ, Roy L, Catella F, FitzGerald GA (1986) Platelet activation in unstable coronary disease. N Engl J Med 315:983–989

Gachet C (2001) ADP receptors of platelets and their inhibition. Thromb Haemost 86:222–232

Gawaz M, Neumann FJ, Ott I, May A, Schomig A (1996) Platelet activation and coronary stent implantation. Effect of antithrombotic therapy. Circulation 94:279–285

Gilchrist IC, O'Shea JC, Kosoglou T, Jennings LK, Lorenz TJ, Kitt MM, Kleimann NS, Talley D, Aguirre F, Davidson C, Runyon J, Tcheng JE (2001) Pharmacodynamics and pharmacokinetics of higher-dose, double-bolus eptifibatide in percutaneous coronary intervention. Circulation 104:406–411

Hansson L, Zanchetti A, Carruthers SG, Dahlof B, Elmfeldt D, Julius S, Menard J, Rahn KH, Wedel H, Westerling S (1998) Effects of intensive blood-pressure lowering and low-dose aspirin in patients with hypertension: principal results of the Hypertension Optimal Treatment (HOT) randomised trial. HOT Study Group. Lancet 35:1755–1762

Hirata M, Hayashi Y, Ushikubi F, Yokota Y, Kageyama R, Nakanishi S, Narumiya S (1991) Cloning and expression of cDNA for a human thromboxane A2 receptor. Nature 349:617–620

Hollopeter G, Jantzen HM, Vincent D, Li G, England L, Ramakrishnan V, Yang RB, Nurden P, Nurden A, Julius D, Conley PB (2001) Identification of the platelet ADP receptor targeted by antithrombotic drugs. Nature 409:202–207

Hourani SM, Cusack NJ (1991) Pharmacological receptors on blood platelets. Pharmacol Rev 43:243–298

IMPACT-II investigators (1997) Randomized placebo-controlled trial of effect of eptifibatide on complications of percutaneous coronary intervention: IMPACT-II. Integrilin to Minimize Platelet Aggregation and Coronary Thrombosis-II. Lancet 349:1422–1428

ISIS-2 (Second International Study of Infarct Survival) Collaborative Group (1988) Randomised trial of intravenous streptokinase, oral aspirin, both, or neither among 17'187 cases of suspected acute myocardial infarction: ISIS-2. Lancet 2:349–360

Jin J, Daniel JL, Kunapuli SP (1998) Molecular basis for ADP-induced platelet aggregation. II. The P2Y1 receptor mediates ADP-induced intracellular calcium mobilization and shape change in platelets. J Biol Chem 273:2030–2034

Kahn ML, Zheng YW, Huang W, Bigornia V, Zeng D, Moff S, Farese RV, Tam C, Coughlin SR (1998) A dual thrombin receptor system for platelet activation. Nature 394:690–694

Kahn ML, Nakanishi-Matsui M, Shapiro MJ, Ishihara H, Coughlin SR (1999) Protease-activated receptors 1 and 4 mediate activation of human platelets by thrombin. J Clin Invest 103:879–887

Kehrel B, Wierwille S, Clemetson KJ, Anders O, Steiner M, Knight G, Farndale RW, Okuma M, Barnes MJ (1998) Glycoprotein VI is a major collagen receptor for platelet activation: it recognizes the platelet-activating quarternary structure of collagen whereas CD36, Glycoprotein IIb/IIIa, and von Willebrand factor do not. Blood 91:491–499

Keularts IMLW, van Gorp RMA, Feijge MAH, Vuist WMJ, Heemskerk JWM (2000) α2A-adrenergic receptor stimulation potentiates calcium release in platelets by modulating cAMP levels. J Biol Chem 275:1763–1772

Kimura Y, Tani T, Kambe T, Watanabe K (1985) Effect of cilostazol on platelet aggregation and experimental thrombosis. Arzneimittelforschung 35:1144–1149

Klimt CR, Knatterud OL, Stamler J, Meier P (1986) Persantine-Aspirine Reinfarction Study II. Secondary prevention with Persantine and Aspirin. J Am Coll Cardiol 7:251–269

Kohler TR, Kaufman JL, Kacoyanis G, Clowes A, Donaldson MC, Kelly E, Skillman J, Couch NP, Whittemore AD, Mannick JA, et al. (1984) Effect of aspirin and dipyridamole on the patency of lower extremity bypass grafts. Surgery 96:462–466

Lele M, Sajid M, Wajih N, Stouffer GA (2001) Eptifibatide and 7E3, but not tirofiban, inhibit αVβ3 integrin mediated binding of smooth muscle cells to thrombospondin and prothrombin. Circulation 104:582–587

Lewis HD Jr, Davis JW, Archibald DG, Steinke WE, Smitherman TC, Doherty JE 3rd, Schnaper HW, LeWinter MM, Linares E, Pouget JM, Sabharwal SC, Chesler E, DeMots H (1983) Protective effects of aspirin against acute myocardial infarction and death in men with unstable angina. Results of a Veterans Administration Cooperative Study. N Engl J Med 309:396–403

Lin EC, Ratnikov BI, Tsai PM, Carron CP, Myers DM, Barbas CF, Smith JM (1997) Identification of a region in the integrin β3 subunit that confers ligand binding specificity. J Biol Chem 272:23912–23920

MacKenzie AB, Mahaut-Smith MP, Sage SO (1996) Activation of receptor-operated cation channels via P2X1 not P2T purinoceptors in human platelets. J Biol Chem 271:2879–2881

Marzilli M, Sambuceti G, Testa R, Fedele S (2002) Platelet glycoprotein IIb/IIIa receptor blockade and coronary resistance in unstable angina. J Am Coll Cardiol 40:2102–2109

Mascelli MA, Lance ET, Damaraju L, Wagner CL, Weisman HF, Jordan RE (1998) Pharmacodynamic profile of short-term abciximab treatment demonstrates prolonged platelet inhibition with gradual recovery from GP IIb/IIIa receptor blockade. Circulation 97:1680–1688

Moliterno DJ, Califf RM, Aguirre FV, Anderson K, Sigmon KN, Weisman HF, Topol EJ (1995) Effect of platelet glycoprotein IIb/IIIa integrin blockade on activated clotting time during percutaneous transluminal coronary angioplasty or directional atherectomy (the EPIC trial). Evaluation of c7E3 Fab in the Prevention of Ischemic Complications trial. Am J Cardiol 75:559–562

Monocada S, Korbut R (1978) Dipyridamole and other phosphodiesterase inhibitors act as antithrombotic agents by potentiating endogenous prostacyclin. Lancet 1:1286–1289

Moussa I, Oetgen M, Roubin G, Colombo A, Wang X, Iyer S, Maida R, Collins M, Kreps E, Moses JW (1999) Effectiveness of clopidogrel and aspirin versus ticlopidine and aspirin in preventing stent thrombosis after coronary stent implantation. Circulation 99:2364–2366

Neri Serneri GG, Masotti G, Poggesi L, Galanti G, Morettini A (1981) Enhanced prostacyclin production by dipyridamole in man. Eur J Clin Pharmacol 21:9–15

Newsholme EA (1978) The control of the mechanism and the hormonal control of adenosine. Essays Biochem 14:82–123

Patrono C (1994) Aspirin as an antiplatelet drug. N Engl J Med 330:1287–294

Patrono C, Coller B, Dalen JE, FitzGerald GA, Fuster V, Gent M, Hirsh J, Roth G (2001) Platelet-active drugs. The relationships among dose, effectiveness, and side effect. Chest 119(1 Suppl):S39–S63

Paul BZS, Ashby B, Sheth SB (1998) Distribution of prostaglandin IP and EP receptor subtypes and isoforms in platelets and human umbilical artery smooth muscle cells. Br J Haematol 102:1204–1211

Peter K, Schwarz M, Ylanne J, Kohler B, Moser M, Nordt T, Salbach P, Kubler W, Bode C (1998) Induction of fibrinogen binding and platelet aggregation as a potential intrinsic property of various glycoprotein IIb/IIIa inhibitors. Blood 92:3240–3249

Peter K, Schwarz M, Conradt C, Nordt T, Moser M, Kubler W, Bode C (1999) Heparin inhibits ligand binding to the leukocyte integrin Mac-1 (CD11b/CD18). Circulation 100:1533–1539

Peter K, Straub A, Kohler B, Volkmann M, Schwarz M, Kubler W, Bode C (1999) Platelet activation as a potential mechanism of GP IIb/IIIa inhibitor-induced thrombocytopenia. Am J Cardiol 84:519–524

Peter K, Kohler B, Straub A, Ruef J, Moser M, Nordt T, Olschewski M, Ohman ME, Kubler W, Bode C (2000) Flow cytometric monitoring of glycoprotein IIb/IIIa blockade and platelet function in patients with acute myocardial infarction receiving reteplase, abciximab, and ticlopidine: continuous platelet inhibition by the combination of abciximab and ticlopidine. Circulation 102:1490–1496

Peto R, Gray R, Collins R, Wheatley K, Hennekens C, Jamrozik K, Warlow C, Hafner B, Thompson E, Norton S, et al. (1988) Randomised trial of prophylactic daily aspirin in British male doctors. Br Med J 296:313–316

Phillips DR, Scarborough RM (1997) Clinical pharmacology of eptifibatide. Am J Cardiol 80:11B–20B

Phillips DR, Teng W, Arfsten A, Nannizzi-Alaimo L, White MM, Longhurst C, Shattil SJ, Randolph A, Jakubowski JA, Jennings LK, Scarborough RM (1997) Effect of Ca 2+ on GPIIb-IIIa interactions with integrilin: enhanced GPIIb-IIIa binding and inhibition of platelet aggregation by reductions in the concentration of ionized calcium in plasma anticoagulated with citrate. Circulation 96:1488–1498

Phillips DR, Charo IF, Parise LV, Fitzgerald LA (1998) The platelet membrane glycoprotein IIb/IIIa complex. Blood 71:831–843

RESTORE investigators (1997) Effects of platelet glycoprotein IIb/IIIa blockade with tirofiban on adverse cardiac events in patients with unstable angina or acute myocardial infarction undergoing coronary angioplasty. The RESTORE investigators. Randomized Efficacy Study of Tirofiban for Outcomes and Restenosis. Circulation 96:1445–1453

Roderick PJ, Wilkes HC, Meade TW (1993) The gastrointestinal toxicity of aspirin: an overview of randomised controlled trials. Br J Clin Pharmacol 35:219–226

Sanz G, Pajaron A, Alegria E, Coello I, Cardona M, Fournier JA, Gomez-Recio M, Ruano J, Hidalgo R, Medina A, et al. (1990) Prevention of early aorto-coronary bypass occlusion by low dose aspirin and dipyridamole. Circulation 82:765–773

Savage B, Almus-Jacobs F, Ruggeri ZM (1998) Specific synergy of multiple substrate-receptor interactions in platelet thrombus formation under flow. Cell 94:657–666

Savcic M, Hauert J, Bachmann F, Wyld PJ, Geudelin B, Cariou R (1999) Clopidogrel loading dose regimens: kinetic profile of pharmacodynamic response in healthy subjects. Semin Thromb Hemost 25:15–19

Savi P, Pereillo JM, Uzabiaga MF, Combalbert J, Picard C, Maffrand JP, Pascal M, Herbert JM (2000) Identification and biological activity of the active metabolite of clopidogrel. Thromb Haemost 84:891–896

Scarborough RM, Kleiman N, Phillips DR (1999) Platelet glycoprotein IIb/IIIa antagonists. What are the relevant issues concerning their pharmacology and clinical use? Circulation 100:437–444

Schomig A, Neumann FJ, Kastrati A, Schuhlen H, Blasini R, Hadamitzky M, Walter H, Zitzmann-Roth EM, Richardt G, Alt E, Schmitt C, Ulm K (1996) A randomized comparison of antiplatelet and anticoagulant therapy after the placement of coronary-artery stents. N Engl J Med 334:1084–1089

Schror K (2002) The pharmacology of cilostazol. Diabetes Obes Metab 4:S14–S19

Schwarz M, Nordt T, Bode C, Peter K (2002) The GP IIb/IIIa inhibitor abciximab (c7E3) inhibits the binding of various ligands to the leukocyte integrin Mac-1 (CD11b/CD18, $\alpha M\beta 2$). Thromb Res 107:121–128

Shattil S (1999) Signaling through platelet integrin $\alpha IIb\beta 3$: inside-out, outside-in, and sideways. Thromb Haemost 82:318–325

Siess W, Stifel M, Binder H, Weber PC (1986) Activation of V1-receptors by vasopressin stimulates inositol phospholipid hydrolysis and arachidonate metabolism in human platelets. Biochem J 233:83–91

Smith WL, Garavito RM, DeWitt DL (1996) Prostaglandin endoperoxide H synthases (cyclooxygenases)-1 and -2. J Biol Chem 271:33157–33160

Soderling SH, Bayuga SJ, Beavo JA (1998) Identification and characterization of a novel family of cyclic nucleotide phosphodiesterases. J Biol Chem 273:15553–15558

Steering Committee of the Physicians' Health Study Research Group (1989) Final report on the aspirin component of the ongoing Physicians' Health Study. N Engl J Med 321:129–135

Stein PD, Collins JJ, Kantrowitz A (1986) Antithrombotic therapy in mechanical and biological prosthetic heart valves and saphenous vein bypass grafts. Arch intern Med 146:468–469

Steinhubl SR, Talley JD, Braden GA, Tcheng JE, Casterella PJ, Moliterno DJ, Navetta FI, Berger PB, Popma JJ, Dangas G, Gallo R, Sane DC, Saucedo JF, Jia G, Lincoff AM, Theroux P, Holmes DR, Teirstein PS, Kereiakes DJ (2001) Point-of-care measured platelet inhibition correlates with a reduced risk of an adverse cardiac event after percutaneous coronary intervention. Results of the GOLD (AU-Assessing Ultegra) multicenter study. Circulation 103:2572–2578

Storey F (2001) The P2Y12 receptor as a therapeutic target in cardiovascular disease. Platelets 12:197–209

Takahashi S, Oida K, Fujiwara R, Maeda H, Hayashi S, Takai H, Tamai T, Nakai T, Miyabo S (1992) Effect of cilostazol, a cyclic AMP phosphodiesterase inhibitor, on the proliferation of rat aortic smooth muscle cells in culture. J Cardiovasc Pharmacol 20:900–906

Tam SH, Sassoli PM, Jordan RE, Nakada MT (1998) Abciximab (ReoPro), chimeric 7E3 Fab demonstrates equivalent affinity and functional blockade of glycoprotein IIb/IIIa and $\alpha V\beta 3$ integrins. Circulation 98:1085–1092

Tanaka T, Ishikawa T, Hagiwara M, Onoda K, Itoh H, Hidaka H (1988) Effects of cilostazol, a selective cAMP phosphodiesterase inhibitor on the concentration of vascular smooth muscle. Pharmacology 36:313–320

Tcheng JE (2000) Clinical challenges of platelet glycoprotein IIb/IIIa receptor inhibitor therapy: bleeding, reversal thrombocytopenia, and retreatment. Am Heart J 139:S38–S45

Tcheng JE, Ellis SG, George BS, Kereiakes DJ, Kleiman NS, Talley JD, Wang AL, Weisman HF, Califf RM, Topol EJ (1994) Pharmacodynamics of chimeric glycoprotein IIb/IIIa integrin antiplatelet antibody FAB 7E3 in high-risk coronary angioplasty. Circulation 90:1757–1764

Tcheng JE, Talley JD, O'Shea JC, Gilchrist IC, Kleiman NS, Grines CL, Davidson CJ, Lincoff AM, Califf RM, Jennings LK, Kitt MM, Lorenz TJ (2001) Clinical pharmacology of higher dose eptifibatide in percutaneous coronary intervention (the PRIDE study). Am J Cardiol 88:1097–1102

The ESPRIT trial investigators (2000) Novel dosing regimen of eptifibatide in planned coronary stent implantation (ESPRIT): a randomized, placebo-controlled trial. Lancet 356:2037–2044

The ESPS-2 Group (1997) European Stroke Prevention Study 2: efficacy and safety data. J Neurol Sci 151:S1–S77

The GUSTO IV-ACS investigators (2001) Effect of glycoprotein IIb/IIIa receptor blocker abciximab on outcome in patients with acute coronary syndromes without early coronary revascularisation: the GUSTO IV-ACS randomised trial. Lancet 357:1915–1924

The Medical Research Council's General Practice Research Framework (1998) Thrombosis prevention trial: randomised trial of low-intensity oral anticoagulation with warfarin and low-dose aspirin in the primary prevention of ischaemic heart disease in men at increased risk. Lancet 351:233–241

The Persantine-Aspirin Reinfarction Study research group (1980) Persantine and Aspirin in coronary heart disease. Circulation 3:449–460

The PURSUIT trial investigators (1998) Inhibition of platelet glycoprotein IIb/IIIa with eptifibatide in patients with acute coronary syndromes. Platelet glycoprotein IIb/IIIa in unstable angina: receptor suppression using integrilin therapy. N Engl J Med 339:436–443

The TARGET investigators (2001) Comparison of two platelet glycoprotein IIb/IIIa inhibitors, tirofiban and abciximab, for the prevention of ischemic events with percutaneous coronary revascularisation. N Engl J Med 344:1888–1894

Thebault JJ, Blatrix CE, Blanchard JF, Panak EA (1975) Effects of ticlopidine, a new platelet aggregation inhibitor in man. Clin Pharmacol Ther 18:485–490

Theroux P, Ouimet H, McCans J, Latour JG, Joly P, Levy G, Pelletier E, Juneau M, Stasiak J, deGuise P, et al. (1988) Aspirin, heparin, or both to treat acute unstable angina. N Engl J Med 319:1105–1111

Thibault G, Tardiff P, Lapalme G (2001) Comparative specificity of platelet αIIbβ3 integrin antagonists. J Pharmacol Exp Therapy 296:690–696

Thompson PD, Zimet R, Forbes WP, Zhang P (2002) Meta-Analysis of results from eight randomized, placebo-controlled trials on the effect of cilostazol on patients with intermittent claudication. Am J Cardiol 90:1314–1319

Turrito VT, Weiss HJ, Zimmerman TS, Sussman II (1985) Factor VIII/von Willebrand factor in subendothelium mediates platelet adhesion. Blood 65:823–831

Weber AA, Zimmermann KC, Meyer-Kirchrath J, Schror K (1999) Cyclooxygenase-2 in human platelets as a possible factor in aspirin resistance. Lancet 353:900

Weber AA, Braun M, Hohlfeld T, Schwippert B, Tschope D, Schror K (2001) Recovery of platelet function after discontinuation of clopidogrel treatment in healthy volunteers. Br J Clin Pharmacol 52:333–336

Yusuf S, Zhao F, Mehta SR, Chrolavicius S, Tognoni G, Fox KK (2001) Effects of clopidogrel in addition to aspirin in patients with acute coronary syndromes without ST-segment elevation. N Engl J Med 345:494–502

Ziegler JW, Ivy DD, Fox JJ, Kinsella JP, Clarke WR, Abman SH (1995) Dipyridamole, a cGMP phosphodiesterase inhibitor, causes pulmonary vasodilation in the ovine fetus. Am J Physiol 269:H473–H479

Part IV

Targets of Future Anti-Atherosclerotic Drug Therapy

HEP (2005) 170:465–482

The ABC of Hepatic and Intestinal Cholesterol Transport

T. Plösch[1] · A. Kosters[2] · A.K. Groen[2] · F. Kuipers[1] (✉)

[1]Laboratory of Pediatrics, Center for Liver, Digestive and Metabolic Diseases, University Medical Center Groningen, Hanzeplein 1, 9713 GZ Groningen, The Netherlands
f.kuipers@med.umcg.nl

[2]Department of Experimental Hepatology, Academic Medical Center, Amsterdam, The Netherlands

Abstract The liver and (small) intestine are key organs in maintenance of cholesterol homeostasis: both organs show active de novo cholesterogenesis and are able to transport impressive amounts of newly synthesized and diet-derived cholesterol via a number of distinct pathways. Cholesterol trafficking involves the concerted action of a number of transporter proteins, some of which have been identified only recently. In particular, several ATP-binding cassette (ABC) transporters fulfil critical roles. For instance, the ABCG5/ABCG8 couple is crucial for hepatobiliary and intestinal cholesterol excretion, while ABCA1 is essential for high-density lipoprotein formation and, hence, for inter-organ trafficking of the highly water-insoluble cholesterol molecules. Very recently, the Niemann–Pick C1-like 1 protein has been identified as a key player in cholesterol absorption by the small intestine and may represent a target of the cholesterol absorption inhibitor ezetimibe. Alterations in hepatic and intestinal cholesterol transport affect circulating levels of atherogenic lipoproteins and thus the risk for cardiovascular disease. This review specifically deals with the processes of hepatobiliary cholesterol excretion and intestinal cholesterol absorption as well as the interactions between these important transport routes. During the last few years, insight into the mechanisms of hepatic and intestinal cholesterol transport has greatly increased not in the least by the identification of involved transporter proteins and the (partial) elucidation of their mode of action. In addition, information has become available on (transcription) factors regulating expression of the encoding genes. This knowledge is of great importance for the development of a tailored design of novel plasma cholesterol-lowering strategies.

Keywords Hepatocyte · Enterocyte · ABC transporters · Niemann–Pick C1-like 1 protein · Lipoproteins

1
Introduction

Elevated plasma cholesterol concentrations comprise a major risk factor for the development of atherosclerosis; cardiovascular disease remains the leading cause of morbidity and mortality in Western societies. This, in combination with the fact that a relatively high proportion of hypercholesterolaemic patients fail to reach their target low-density lipoprotein (LDL)-cholesterol concentrations on 'standard' (diet, statins) therapy alone, provides the basis for a quest for more effective treatment modalities and/or supportive strategies. The development of ezetimibe, a specific and potent inhibitor of intestinal cholesterol absorption (van Heek et al. 1997) that reduces plasma LDL-cholesterol by approximately 20% in mildly hypercholesteroleamic patients (Sudhop et al. 2002), and the established LDL-lowering effects of dietary plant sterols/stanols (Ostlund 2002) that interfere with cholesterol absorption has focused attention on the intestine as a promising site of action. As a consequence, there is an increased interest in achieving a better understanding of the molecular mechanisms involved in control of intestinal cholesterol absorption. Uptake from the intestine represents a major source for cholesterol entry into the body pools (Turley and Dietschy 2003). However, it should be realized that although the intestine is an important station in cholesterol trafficking, the liver is the dominant regulatory unit. Therefore, the plasma cholesterol-lowering effects of cholesterol absorption inhibitors are primarily brought about by metabolic adaptations in the liver, i.e. the organ in which diet-derived cholesterol ends up via the chylomicron remnant pathway. Furthermore, it must be kept in mind that the major part of cholesterol that is taken up by the intestine on a daily basis is not derived from the diet but is actually biliary cholesterol that comes directly from the liver. A comprehensive and integrated picture of intestinal and hepatic cholesterol metabolism is therefore required to design more effective strategies for prevention or treatment of cardiovascular disease. During the last few years, there have been highly significant advances in our understanding of specific areas of cholesterol transport, particularly concerning mechanisms of hepatobiliary cholesterol excretion and the actual cholesterol absorption process. This chapter reviews these recent developments and addresses some of the still unresolved issues.

1.1
Quantitative Estimates of Cholesterol Transport Rates

The total turnover of body cholesterol pools in adult humans ($\sim$70 kg) equals about 1–1.5 g/day, i.e. in the order of 1% of the whole body cholesterol content (Turley and Dietschy 2003). A major part of this turnover reflects the conversion of cholesterol to bile salts by the liver and their subsequent loss via the faeces (Stellaard et al. 1983). Under steady-state conditions, the loss of cholesterol from the body is compensated for by de novo synthesis and absorption from the diet. De novo synthesis in adults amounts up to 0.6–1 g/day, as revealed by careful balance studies and confirmed by direct measurements using stable isotope techniques (e.g. Neese et al. 1993). A "typical Western diet" provides 0.3–0.5 g/day of cholesterol which mixes with an even larger amount of biliary cholesterol, i.e. approximately 1 g/day, in the upper small intestine. There are data to indicate that biliary cholesterol is absorbed from the intestine with greater efficacy than is dietary cholesterol (see Wilson and Rudel 1994), because it is delivered in mixed micelles and thus is readily available for absorption. Cholesterol therefore undergoes extensive enterohepatic circulation, which represents an important yet often ignored factor in the control of cholesterol homeostasis. Most studies showed that humans absorb about 50% of all cholesterol entering the intestine (e.g. Ostlund et al. 1999). These figures clearly demonstrate that the intestine processes a considerable amount of cholesterol each day, which, via the chylomicron remnant pathway, is directly delivered to the liver. Because the liver is the principal site for the production as well as the clearance of LDL-cholesterol (Dietschy et al. 1993), alterations in the delivery of intestine-derived cholesterol to the liver can potentially have a significant impact on plasma LDL-cholesterol concentrations through interference with hepatocytic cholesterol metabolism.

The massive enterohepatic circulation of cholesterol has important but often underestimated methodological implications when evaluating cholesterol absorption in experimental settings. In most recent studies in humans as well as in experimental animals, dual (radioactive or stable) isotope tracer techniques are used to estimate fractional cholesterol absorption. Principally, two approaches can be discerned, i.e., the dual-isotope faecal collection method and the dual-isotope plasma ratio method. In the first, labelled cholesterol is given orally together with a labelled non-absorbable marker, in most cases sitostanol or sitosterol, and faeces are collected for a given period of time. The faecal ratio of labelled cholesterol over marker provides an estimate of the fractional absorption rate. The second method requires simultaneous administration of exact amounts of (differently) labelled cholesterol both intravenously and orally/intragastrically, and plasma ratios over time provide a value for the fractional absorption rate. The pros and cons of these two methods have recently been discussed by Turley and Dietschy (2003) and Wang and Carey (2003): the important issue with respect to interpretation of the data is that the cholesterol absorption rates obtained always reflect a fractional (percent) value and are, therefore by definition, not a measure of the absolute amount of cholesterol that is delivered to the liver from the intestine. For the latter, one needs to know the mass of the intraluminal cholesterol pool and this is usually not the case since the contribution from bile and other endogenous sources (e.g. sloughing of intestinal cells) is unknown in most situations. Hence, a direct translation of changes in fractional absorption rates to absolute changes in the amounts of chylomicron remnant cholesterol reaching the liver is sometimes difficult to make.

2
Mechanisms of Hepatobiliary Cholesterol Transport

Bile formation is an important function of the liver, which is performed by the parenchymal liver cells or hepatocytes. Hepatocytes are polarized cells with their basolateral (sinusoidal) membrane facing the blood and their apical (canalicular) membrane facing the bile canaliculus. Both membrane domains are separated from each other by tight junctions. Bile is an aqueous solution that contains, apart from a variety of other organic molecules, bile salts, phospholipids and free cholesterol in millimolar concentrations. These bile components are present mainly in the form of aggregates, i.e. mixed micelles, simple micelles or vesicular structures (see Verkade et al. 1995). Formation of bile is an osmotic process. Bile salt secretion, which is mediated by the so-called Bile Salt Export Pump (BSEP) or ABCB11, provides the major driving force for bile formation and, in addition, stimulates the secretion of cholesterol (see below).

2.1
Dependency of Biliary Cholesterol Secretion on Bile Salt and Phospholipid Secretion

It has been known for decades that biliary cholesterol and phospholipid secretion is tightly coupled to that of bile salts. Infusion of bile salts into different animal species as well as in humans invariably leads to induction of biliary cholesterol (and phospholipid) secretion (see Verkade et al. 1995 for review). The stimulatory actions of bile salts on biliary lipid secretion depend to a large extent on their relative hydrophobicity: the more hydrophobic the higher their efficacy to induce lipid secretion. When bile salts are incubated with isolated cells or erythrocytes, release of cholesterol and phospholipid is readily induced (Billington and Coleman 1978a, 1978b). Hence, biliary lipid secretion that occurs at the canalicular pole of the hepatocyte could be a passive process fully controlled by the detergent actions of bile salts. It therefore came as a great surprise when it was found that biliary lipid secretion is fully abrogated in mice lacking the gene encoding Mdr2 P-glycoprotein (*Mdr2*), now known as *ABCB4*

(Smit et al. 1993). This ABC transporter supposedly mediates transport of phosphatidylcholine from the inner leaflet to the external leaflet of the canalicular membrane where, in concert with bile salts, phospholipid/cholesterol-containing vesicles are formed that are subsequently secreted into the canalicular lumen. The most convincing evidence for this concept came from studies of the group of Crawford (Crawford et al. 1995a, 1995b, 1995c) demonstrating the presence of vesicle-like structures expanding from the canalicular membrane using ultra-rapid fixation of liver tissue. As far as we know, reconstitution of this system in cultured polarized cell systems has not succeeded. Therefore, formal proof of this mechanism of lipid secretion is still lacking. ABCB4 is supposed to provide the driving force for vesicle formation since in the absence of this protein no vesicles could be detected (Crawford et al. 1995b). Since the *Abcb4*-null mice, in addition to a complete absence of phospholipid, also show a virtually complete absence of biliary cholesterol secretion (Oude Elferink et al. 1995, 1996; Smit et al. 1993), the sterol was supposed to follow phospholipids passively. However, this concept has appeared to be too simplistic, because in later studies it was shown that cholesterol secretion can be restored to almost normal levels when *Abcb4*-null mice are infused with hydrophobic bile salts (Oude Elferink et al. 1996). A clear uncoupling of cholesterol secretion into bile from that of phospholipids and bile salts has also been shown in a number of other conditions (Verkade et al. 1993, 1995). Biliary cholesterol secretion shows great species-to-species variation whereas the cholesterol content in the liver seems much less variable (Kuipers et al. 1997).

2.2
The Abcg5/Abcg8 Heterodimer as Mediator of Biliary Cholesterol Secretion

Very recently, candidate proteins that may account for the phenomena described in Sect. 1.2.1 have been identified. In 2002, the groups of Hobbs (Berge et al. 2000) and Patel (Lee et al. 2001) almost simultaneously identified mutations in the genes that encode two ABC half-transporters, i.e. *ABCG5* and *ABCG8*, that underlie the inborn error of metabolism called sitosterolaemia. Patients suffering from this disease accumulate large amounts of plant sterols in their bodies, have an increased cholesterol absorption, a decreased bile cholesterol secretion, and, finally, a complete abrogation of secretion of plant sterols into the bile (Patel et al. 1998; Berger et al. 1998; Salen et al. 2002). ABCG5 and G8 were postulated to function as exporters of sterols in the form of a heterodimer at the apical membranes of small intestinal epithelial cells (see below) and of hepatocytes. A defect in either of the two proteins is sufficient to cause the full phenotype of sitosterolaemia, suggesting that expression of only one of the two proteins does not salvage the transport function.

ABCG5/Abcg5 and *ABCG8/Abcg8* are predominantly expressed in hepatocytes and in small intestinal enterocytes in humans and mice. The two genes are arranged in a head-to-head configuration in the human (Remaley et al.

2002) and mouse (Lu et al. 2002) genome. Expression of both genes is co-ordinately regulated and highly induced in mice kept on a high-cholesterol diet (Repa et al. 2002a). LXRα, a nuclear receptor activated by oxysterols and that plays a crucial role in regulating genes involved in cholesterol traffick-ing (Repa et al. 2002b), is required for induction of murine *Abcg5* and *Abcg8* expression upon cholesterol feeding (Repa et al. 2002a). Treatment of mice with synthetic LXR agonists induces the expression of both genes in liver and intestine (Plösch et al. 2002; Repa et al. 2002a).

Via adenoviral over-expression of the human genes in cell lines it was re-cently found that both proteins are required to ensure proper processing from the endoplasmic reticulum (ER) through the Golgi and subsequently to the apical membrane. ABCG5 or G8 expressed singly remained in the ER. These studies by Graf et al. (2002) were carried out with tagged proteins which still leaves the possibility open that the tags may have disrupted the normal routing of the proteins. The proposed concept that simultaneous expression of ABCG5 and G8 is at least essential for proper transport via the secretory pathway could explain why mutations in either gene induce the full phenotype in sitostero-laemia patients. The group of Hobbs has subsequently constructed transgenic *ABCG5/G8* over-expressing mice as well as double knock-out mice (Yu et al. 2002a; Yu et al. 2002b). In the transgenics, a P1 clone containing both human genes with the connecting promoter region was inserted, leading to up to 14 times over-expression of both genes exclusively in liver and intestine (Yu et al. 2002b). In gallbladder bile of these mice, the cholesterol content was fivefold increased while bile salt content was unchanged. This supported an important role of the heterodimer in biliary cholesterol secretion. Detailed analysis of *Abcg5/g8* double knock-out mice confirmed the role of the heterodimer in bil-iary sterol secretion. The cholesterol content of gallbladder bile was decreased by more than 90% in these mice whereas no significant effects on bile salt con-tent were observed. Interestingly, also plasma and liver cholesterol contents were decreased in the *Abcg5/g8* knock-out mice. Since the content of plant sterols was increased dramatically, secondary effects caused by these sterols may underlie this phenomenon. Heterozygous *Abcg5/g8* mice showed a 30%–40% decrease in biliary cholesterol concentration, indicating that the biliary phenotype is not due to a secondary effect induced by massive amounts of plant sterols in the liver. Feeding these mice a high-cholesterol diet induced a massive increase of cholesterol in the liver but had little effect on biliary cholesterol secretion, again indicating a crucial role of ABCG5 and ABCG8 in biliary cholesterol secretion (Yu et al. 2002a).

The molecular mechanism by which the ABCG5/ABCG8 heterodimer medi-ates cholesterol secretion is still an enigma. It is generally assumed that choles-terol readily flips between the lipid bilayers in biological membranes. Studies in model membranes invariably show high rates of flipping, making a role for ABCG5/G8 as a cholesterol flippase unlikely. Recently, Small (2003) advanced an alternative hypothesis. In his view, ABCG5/G8 activity decreases the activation energy for cholesterol efflux out of the outer leaflet of the canalicular membrane. If Small's hypothesis is true, current schemes of the mechanism of biliary cholesterol secretion need substantial revision. Presently, co-secretion of the two lipids in the form of vesicles is the most favoured mechanism, based on the rather strict coupling of cholesterol and phospholipid that has been observed in a large variety of studies. However, when ABCG5 and G8 indeed serve to lower activation energy for cholesterol efflux, one might assume that mixed micelles would be the preferred carrier to capture this activated cholesterol rather than to assume that cholesterol diffuses laterally into phospholipid domains before their combined secretion in the form of vesicles.

Based on the genetics of sitosterolaemia, i.e. no phenotypic differences in humans with defects in either *ABCG5* or *ABCG8*, mouse studies and in vitro studies as described above, it was hypothesized that Abcg5 and Abcg8 function as obligate heterodimers. In line herewith, quantitative trait locus analysis identified *Abcg5/Abcg8* as important genes for the genetic susceptibility and pathogenesis of cholesterol cholelithiasis in inbred strains of mice (Wittenburg et al. 2003). Kosters et al. (2003) found a close relationship between biliary cholesterol secretion rates normalized to phospholipid secretion and both hepatic *Abcg5* and *Abcg8* expression levels normalized to *Abcb4* expression, when various mouse models of cholesterol hypo- and hypersecretion were included in the analysis. It should be noted, however, that there was one exception to the rule: the 15-fold induction of biliary cholesterol secretion induced by diosgenin feeding occurred without any change in *Abcg5/Abcg8* expression. Very recently, Klett et al. (2004) reported a mouse model of sitosterolaemia created by a targeted disruption of the *Abcg8* gene alone. These mice showed very significantly elevated levels of plasma and tissue plant sterols (sitosterol, campesterol) consistent with sitosterolaemia. These mice also showed an impaired ability to secrete cholesterol into bile (−70%), as determined after gallbladder canulation. Heterozygous $Abcg8^{+/-}$ mice that were not sitosterolaemic showed an intermediate phenotype with respect to biliary cholesterol secretion (−34%). In a separate study, Plösch et al. (2004) reported that the cholesterol content of gallbladder bile was decreased by approximately 60% in sitosterolaemic mice in which the *Abcg5* gene alone was disrupted: no heterozygous mice were included in this particular study. It is of interest to note that hepatic expression levels of *Abcg5* and of *Abcg8* were reduced in the mice in which the respective partner gene was selectively disrupted (Klett et al. 2004; Plösch et al. 2004), possibly as a consequence of the close proximity of the two genes.

All together, these data support an important role of the Abcg5/Abcg8 heterodimer in control of biliary cholesterol secretion. However, some issues warrant further evaluation to establish its exact role in the secretory process. First, Kosters et al. (2003) observed that diosgenin-induced hypersecretion of cholesterol into bile does not require induction of *Abcg5/Abcg8* expression. In addition, it should be noted that cholesterol secretion is not completely abrogated in the *Abcg5/Abcg8* double knock-out mouse and that there is still a considerable amount (30%–40%) of biliary cholesterol secretion left in both the *Abcg5* and *Abcg8* single knock-outs (Klett et al. 2004; Plösch et al. 2004). Surprisingly, the cholesterol content of gallbladder bile of Abcg5-deficient mice was remarkably enhanced by treatment of these animals with a synthetic LXR agonist, to a similar extent as observed in wild-type mice (Plösch et al. 2004), in spite of the fact that hepatic *Abcg8* mRNA level was not induced. Combined, these data suggest that alternative secretory mechanisms, possibly independent of Abcg5/Abcg8, may exist.

3
Mechanisms of Intestinal Cholesterol Absorption

Intestinal cholesterol absorption has long been considered to primarily represent a passive process, in spite of the fact that it was recognized decades ago that the process is selective in the sense that dietary cholesterol is absorbed relatively efficiently while structurally similar plant sterols and other noncholesterol sterols are not. After hydrolysis of the small portion of dietary cholesterylester and solubilization by mixed bile salt/(phospho)lipid micelles, cholesterol was supposed to traverse the unstirred water layer where the micelles subsequently disintegrated in the local acid microclimate to deliver their cargo at the enterocytic membrane. Size and composition of the bile salt pool (Wang et al. 1999; Schwarz et al. 2001) as well as the amount of phospholipids present in the intestinal lumen (Voshol et al. 1998; Eckhardt et al. 2002) were shown to exert regulatory actions on the amount of cholesterol that is ultimately absorbed. During the last few years, however, the paradigm of passive enterocytic cholesterol uptake has changed considerably. Cholesterol absorption has been shown to be saturable and to display very large person-to-person variation. Several groups have worked intensely to identify and characterize the proteins involved. Scavenger receptor (SR)-B1 appeared to be a good candidate. This protein was shown to be expressed at the apical membranes of enterocytes of mainly duodenum and jejunum, exactly the sites where most cholesterol is likely to be absorbed (Voshol et al. 2001). In isolated brush border membrane vesicles cholesterol uptake could be inhibited by the SR-B1 ligand apoA-I and also by antibodies against SR-B1 (Werder et al. 2001; Schulthess et al. 2000). In addition, the recently developed specific inhibitor of cholesterol absorption, ezetimibe, was found to bind to SR-B1 (Altmann et al. 2002). However, SR-B1 null mice absorbed even more cholesterol than the corresponding wild-type mice did, indicating that SR-B1, if indeed involved in transport, is at least redundant. It cannot be excluded that the SR-B1 null mice have compensated for their defect by up-regulation of other cholesterol transporters, but as far as we know this has not yet been studied in detail.

3.1
Has the "Real Cholesterol Transporter" Been Identified?

In a very recent paper (Altmann et al. 2004), the identity of a prime candidate for the putative cholesterol uptake transporter has been revealed. Altmann and his colleagues searched human and rodent expressed sequence tag databases for sequences highly expressed in the intestine that contained several characteristic 'transporter' features, i.e. transmembrane domains, extracellular signal sequences, sites for N-linked glycosylation, but, in addition, also a sterol-sensing domain. These domains are found in a number of important proteins involved in cholesterol metabolism, including HMGCoA reductase, Niemann–Pick C1 (NPC1) and sterol regulatory element binding protein cleavage-activating protein. From their analysis only a single credible candidate gene emerged: the rat homologue of *Niemann–Pick C1 Like 1 protein* (NPC1L1). NPC1L1 has approximately 50% amino acid homology to NPC1 (Davies et al. 2000). The latter protein functions in intracellular cholesterol trafficking and is defective in the inborn cholesterol storage disease Niemann–Pick Type C. In contrast to *NPC1*, which is ubiquitously expressed, *NPC1L1* appeared to be predominantly expressed in the small intestine in humans, rats and mice. Much lower expression levels were observed in liver, gallbladder, testis and stomach. In the rat small intestine, *NPC1L1* mRNA levels varied along the duodenum–ileum axis with peak expression in the proximal jejunum, i.e. the site were most of the cholesterol is thought to be absorbed. NPC1L1 protein levels showed a similar distribution pattern along the length of the small intestine. In the jejunum, *NPC1L1* mRNA was confined to enterocytes and the protein appeared to be predominantly localized apically, i.e. close to or at the plasma membrane facing the intestinal lumen.

NPC1L1-null ($Npc1l1^{-/-}$) mice were created to establish the actual role of the protein in cholesterol absorption. NPC1L1-deficiency did not affect development, fertility or any hematological or plasma parameter that was measured. Intestinal morphology was normal. Plasma cholesterol and triglyceride levels were similar in knock-out and wild-type littermates while a significantly lower hepatic cholesterylester content was observed in the $Npc1l1^{-/-}$ mice. Fractional cholesterol absorption rates, determined by a faecal dual isotope method, were 51%±3% and 45%±4% in wild-type ($Npc1l1^{+/+}$) and heterozygous $Npc1l1^{+/-}$ mice, respectively, but only 16%±0.4% in $Npc1l1^{-/-}$ mice. Addition of cholate to the diet did not improve cholesterol absorption in the latter, indicating that bile salt deficiency is not the cause of cholesterol malabsorption in these animals. Interestingly, ezetimibe treatment reduced cholesterol absorption efficiency in wild-type mice to exactly the value seen in non-treated $Npc1l1^{-/-}$ mice while the drug had no additional effect in these knock-outs. Together, these data indicate that NPC1L1 plays an essential role in ezetimibe-sensitive cholesterol absorption and that part of the absorption process ($\sim$ 30% of total in this particular mouse strain) is NPC1L1-independent. Acute experiments using radiolabelled cholesterol demonstrated that uptake by the enterocytes was drastically reduced in the $Npc1l1^{-/-}$ mice, supporting a role of the protein in the uptake of cholesterol across the apical membrane of the enterocytes. These data are of great importance for our understanding of the cholesterol absorption process. Obviously, identification of NPC1L1 as a bona fide cholesterol transporter awaits demonstration of actual transport activity in appropriate systems. In addition, a number of other issues remain to be addressed. For instance, it should be demonstrated that ezetimibe really binds to or interacts with the NPC1L1 protein. It was reported that attempts in this direction have been unsuccessful so far.

In this context it is highly interesting that Smart et al. (2004) very recently identified annexin2 (ANX2) and caveolin1 (CAV1) as potential important components of the intestinal sterol transport machinery that may also be targeted by ezetimibe. Complexes of CAV1 and ANX2 with cyclophilins A and 40 have been implicated in trafficking of exogenous cholesterol from caveolae at the plasma membrane to the ER. Studies in zebrafish larvae using morpholino oligonucleotide antisense technology revealed that deletion of $ANX2$ prevented complex formation as well as processing of a fluorescent cholesterol reporter and results in reduced sterol mass. Exposure of fish embryos to ezetimibe completely disrupted the complex, with CAV1 and ANX2 detected only as monomers. Feeding of ezetimibe to chow-fed C57BL/6 mice did not affect complex stability in enterocytes but, intriguingly, when mice were fed a cholesterol-containing Western-type diet the complex did become sensitive to disruption by ezetimibe. Likewise, ezetimibe treatment disrupted the CAV2–ANX2 complex in hypercholesterolaemic LDL receptor-deficient mice. Furthermore, it was shown by immunopreciptitation on enterocytes followed by mass spectrometry that cholesterol selectively co-precipitated with the complex, and that this could be prevented by pretreatment of the enterocytes with ezetimibe. Experiments in CaCo2 cells revealed that ezetimibe itself co-precipitated with CAV1 but not with ANX2 or with cyclophilin A. Thus, these data suggest that ezetimibe disrupts the CAV1–ANX2 complex through a direct interaction with CAV1 protein, implying an intracellular site of action of the drug. Whether or not interactions between NPC1L1 and CAV1-ANX2 are operational at some stage of the cholesterol absorption process remains elusive for the moment.

3.2
Controlled Efflux to the Intestinal Lumen as a Determinant of Cholesterol Absorption Efficacy?

In addition to a role of proteins in cholesterol uptake, there is good evidence now that ABC transporter proteins are involved in efflux of sterol from the enterocytes to the intestinal lumen and that the efficiency of the absorption process is, at least in part, governed by this 'reflux' system. The function of

ABCG5/G8 in biliary cholesterol secretion has been discussed above. Both proteins are also expressed in the intestine, mainly in jejunal sections, where they are responsible for the efflux of plant sterols as indicated by the greatly increased absorption of plant sterols in patients with sitosterolaemia (Berge et al. 2000; Lee et al. 2001). Since these proteins mediate cholesterol secretion from liver to bile one may assume that they have similar activity in the intestine. Indeed, over-expression of both human proteins reduced cholesterol absorption efficiency and greatly increased faecal neutral sterol loss (Yu et al. 2002a). The role of the intestine in cholesterol homeostasis has long been confined to its absorptive function towards bile- and diet-derived cholesterol. However, the notion that the intestine itself may function as an important secretory organ for cholesterol is novel. Plösch et al. (2002) studied the effect of dietary administration of the LXR agonist T0901317 in C57BL/6 and in DBA/1 mice. By determination of biliary cholesterol secretion and faecal neutral sterol loss, the net intestinal transport could be estimated. In C57Bl/6 mice, the intestine secreted more cholesterol than was (re)absorbed and this net secretion tripled during treatment with T0901317. A similar conclusion can be drawn from the work of Yu et al. (2002a; 2002b; 2003). In the *Abcg5/g8* double knock-out mice, biliary cholesterol secretion is almost absent, yet their endogenous neutral sterol excretion is barely affected. Conversely in the *ABCG5/G8* over-expressor neutral sterol output was strongly increased. In these mice faecal neutral sterol output was increased more than fivefold to reach a value of about 110 μmol/day/100 g body weight. Unfortunately, biliary output was not quantified making a direct comparison with the data of Plösch et al. (2002) impossible. The increase in faecal neutral sterol excretion of about 90 μmol/day/100 g body weight is equivalent to 60 nmol/min/100 g body weight of biliary cholesterol flow on the assumption that no biliary cholesterol is reabsorbed. This underestimated value is about threefold higher than the (already very high) total T0901317-induced biliary cholesterol secretion reported by Plösch et al. (2002). Accordingly, one has to conclude that also in the experiments of Yu et al. (2002b) substantial net cholesterol secretion from the intestine occurs.

The origin of this net intestinal cholesterol secretion is an intriguing issue. It is generally assumed that there is no appreciable cholesterol flux from the circulation to the enterocyte. When this assumption would hold in the now rapidly changing understanding of cholesterol fluxes, the cholesterol secreted into the intestine can only be derived directly from the enterocytes. In the experiments of Plösch *et al.* (2002) intestinal HMG-CoA reductase expression did not change. So, either the enzyme in the intestine is regulated post-transcriptionally or the extra cholesterol is not derived from de novo synthesis. Yu et al. (2003) did not find any effect of the LXR agonist on intestinal neutral sterol output in the Abcg5/g8 double knock-out mouse indicating that the heterodimer is fully responsible for the LXR-mediated effect on neutral sterol excretion. There have been reports for a role of other genes in regulation of sterol uptake (Schwarz et al. 2001; Sehayek et al. 2002). Whether these genes are involved in cholesterol uptake or in additional efflux pathways is not clear at the moment and requires further investigation.

3.3
Intestinal Lipoprotein Formation as Part of the Cholesterol Absorption Cascade

Cholesterol that has entered the enterocyte traffics to the ER to be esterified by acylCoA:cholesterol acyltransferase-2 (ACAT2), the ACAT isoform that is highly expressed in intestine and liver. The mechanisms by which cholesterol and plant sterols move to the ER are largely unknown but, as outlined above, several chaperones of vesicular transport have been implicated in the process. Studies in ACAT2-deficient mice (Buhman et al. 2000) revealed that the fractional absorption of dietary cholesterol was not affected as compared to wild-type controls when the animals were fed a low-cholesterol chow diet. Yet, when animals were fed a high-fat, high-cholesterol diet, fractional cholesterol absorption was much less in ACAT2-deficient mice than in controls. As a consequence, these animals were protected from diet-induced hypercholesterolaemia and gallstone formation. Thus, ACAT2 seems to be of regulatory importance in cholesterol absorption in mice only when cholesterol intake is at an appreciable level, as also appeared to be the case for ABCG5/ABCG8 (Yu et al. 2002). It has been postulated that selectivity of intestinal sterol absorption is, at least in part, related to sterol selectivity of ACAT2: the enzyme shows a strong preference for cholesterol rather than sitosterol (Temel et al. 2003). In this scenario, microsomal sterols not esterified by the actions of ACAT2 would be transported back to the apical plasma membrane to be effluxed by the ABCG5/ABCG8 heterodimer. The nature of this apical transport process is still unresolved. Nonselective ACAT inhibitors, exemplified by the sulfamic acid phenyl ester avasimibe, have been developed and were shown to reduce the absorption of dietary cholesterol, to impair the secretion of very-low-density lipoprotein (VLDL) particles by liver cells and to reduce the extent of atherosclerosis in animal models (e.g. Delsing et al. 2001). Avasimibe is currently in clinical trials and has, for instance, been shown to induce a modest reduction of triglycerides and VLDL-cholesterol with no significant changes in LDL-cholesterol in subjects with combined hyperlipidaemia (Insull et al. 2001). Avasimibe monotherapy was not effective in subjects with homozygous familial hypercholesterolaemia (Raal et al. 2003), and showed only a modest synergistic effect on total cholesterol levels when given with atorvastatin. Thus, the clinical benefit of this particular drug appears limited for the moment: it may be that increasing selectivity of novel drugs towards ACAT2, perhaps with an intestine-specific profile, will improve the effectiveness of this approach.

A final crucial event in the cholesterol absorption process involves the incorporation of newly esterified cholesterol molecules, together with a small amount of unesterified sterol, triglycerides and phospholipids, along with apolipoprotein B48 into nascent chylomicrons that are delivered into the lymphatics. The availability of apoB48 is essential for cholesterol absorption: mice lacking functional apoB48 in their intestine do not absorb measurable quantities of cholesterol (Young et al. 1995). The assembly of chylomicrons, like that of VLDL in hepatocytes, is facilitated by the microsomal triglyceride transfer protein (MTP). The remarkable effects of MTP inhibitors on plasma lipid concentrations may involve consequences of reduced cholesterol absorption but there are safety concerns with respect to the use of these drugs that need to be solved (Sudhop and von Bergmann 2002).

It has been known for decades that the intestine is an important source of high-density lipoprotein (HDL) but whether or not intestinal HDL serves specific physiological functions, for instance in cholesterol absorption, is not clear. ABCA1, crucial for HDL formation, is highly expressed in enterocytes of the small intestine and present at the basolateral plasma membrane (Wellington et al. 2002). In a chicken model of ABCA1 dysfunction, Mulligan et al. (2003) showed that the percentage of orally administered ^{14}C cholesterol appearing in plasma was reduced by 79% and that radiolabelled cholesterol accumulated in the intestinal wall. From these data, the authors concluded that ABCA1 regulates the efflux of cholesterol from the basolateral membrane during absorption of dietary cholesterol in chicken which, unlike mammals, lack lymphatic contribution to intestinal lipid absorption. The quantitative importance of this pathway in overall absorption in mammals remains, therefore, to be established. Measurement of fractional cholesterol absorption in ABCA1-deficient mice by different dual isotope measurements revealed no marked differences in comparison to wild-type controls when animals were kept on low cholesterol diets (McNeish et al.2000; Drobnick et al. 2001). Since biliary cholesterol content is not affected in ABCA1-deficient mice (Groen et al. 2001), it is likely that absolute amounts of cholesterol absorbed were also not strongly affected in the absence of ABCA1 under these experimental conditions. Likewise, measurement of fractional cholesterol absorption in a single patient with Tangier disease revealed a value in the 'normal range' (Schaeffer et al. 2001). Interestingly, fractional cholesterol absorption was significantly higher in $ABCA1^{-/-}$ mice than in wild-type mice when fed a high-cholesterol Western type diet (McNeish et al. 2000). Evidently, the mechanisms of action of and the interactions between the various pathways involved in cholesterol absorption, that may be different under various dietary conditions, need further exploration.

4
Concluding Remarks

Since the beginning of this century insight into mechanisms involved in regulation of cholesterol handling in liver and intestine has increased considerably, as summarized in Fig. 1. Separate proteins active in cholesterol import and

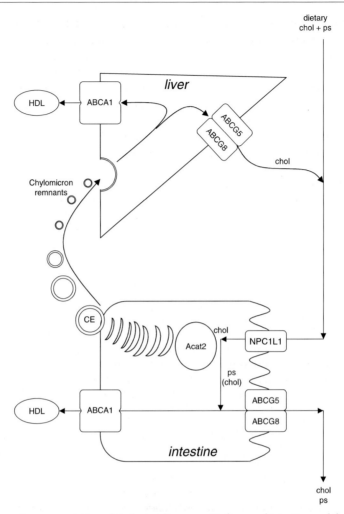

Fig. 1 Schematic representation of cholesterol transport in liver and intestine and the proteins involved (chol: cholesterol; ps: plant sterol; ce cholesterol ester)

efflux have been characterized in the intestine, constituting a so-called substrate cycle. It has been known for many years that in humans the responses to dietary cholesterol and cholesterol-lowering medication as well as several parameters of cholesterol metabolism (fractional absorption rate, conversion to bile salts, biliary secretion rates) show wide inter-individual variations. Subtle difference in the activity of one or both of the arms of the substrate cycle may account for these variations. Although most of the regulatory modulators active in vivo have not yet been elucidated, the available knowledge allows development of drugs specifically targeted to these transport systems. Ezetimibe and dietary plant sterols probably already fulfil these criteria. In this chapter we have shown that biliary secretion may not be the only pathway via which cholesterol can be excreted from the body. A direct route has to exist as well although it is not yet clear which carriers and transcellular mechanism account for this activity. Nevertheless elucidation of the steps involved may provide attractive additional targets to stimulate cholesterol disposal from the body. Such strategies potentially would be powerful complements to the traditional therapies aimed at decreasing cholesterol synthesis and together with statins may lead to potent regression of atherosclerotic lesions.

Acknowledgements Work by Folkert Kuipers and Albert Groen on cholesterol transport is supported by the Netherlands Organisation for Scientific Research and the Netherlands Heart Foundation.

References

Altmann SW, Davis HR, Yao X et al. (2002) The identification of intestinal scavenger receptor class B, type I (SR- BI) by expression cloning and its role in cholesterol absorption. Biochim Biophys Acta 1580:77–93

Altmann SW, Davis HR, Zhu LJ et al. (2004) Niemann–Pick C1 Like 1 Protein is critical for intestinal cholesterol absorption. Science 303:1201–1204

Berge KE, Tian H, Graf GA et al. (2000) Accumulation of dietary cholesterol in sitosterolemia caused by mutations in adjacent ABC transporters. Science 290:1771–1775

Berger GM, Pegoraro RJ, Patel SB et al. (1998) HMG-CoA reductase is not the site of the primary defect in phytosterolemia. J Lipid Res 39:1046–1054

Billington D, Coleman R (1978) Effects of bile salts of human erythrocytes. Plasma membrane vesiculation, phospholipid solubilization and their possible relationships to bile secretion. Biochim Biophys Acta 509:33–47

Billington D, Coleman R (1978) The removal of membrane components from human erythrocytes by glycocholate. Biochem Soc Trans 6:286–288

Buhman KK, Accad M, Novak S et al. (2000) Resistance to diet-induced hypercholesterolemia and gallstone formation in ACAT2-deficient mice. Nat Med 6:1341–1347

Crawford J, Crawford A R, Hatch V C et al. (1995) Hepatocellular secretion of biliary lipid: bile salt-induced vesiculation of the canalicular membrane outer leaflet. In: Hofmann AF, Paumgartner G, Stiehl A (eds) Bile acids in gastroenterology. Basic and clinical advances, Kluwer Academic Publishers, Dordrecht. pp 254–257

Crawford J, Hatch VC, Groen AK et al. (1995) Bile canalicular vesicles are markedly decreased in mdr2 knockout mice: electron microscopy of cryofixed liver. Hepatology 22:316A

Crawford J, Möckel GM, Crawford AR et al. (1995). Imaging biliary lipid secretion in the rat: ultrastructural evidence for vesiculation of the hepatocyte canalicular membrane. J Lipid Res 36:2147–2163

Davies JP, Levy B, Ioannou YA (2000) Evidence for a Niemann-Pick C (NPC) gene family: identification and characterization of NPC1L1. Genomics 65:137–145

Delsing DJ, Offerman EH, van Duyvenvoorde W et al. (2001) Acyl-CoA: cholesterol acyltransferase inhibitor avasimibe reduces atherosclerosis in addition to its cholesterol-lowering effect in ApoE*3-Leiden mice. Circulation 103:1778–1786

Dietschy JM, Turley SD, Spady DK (1993) Role of liver in maintenance of cholesterol and low density lipoprotein homeostasis in different animal species, including humans. J Lipid Res 34:1637–1659

Drobnik W, Lindenthal B, Lieser B et al. (2001) ATP-binding cassette transporter A1 (ABCA1) affects total body sterol metabolism. Gastroenterology 120:1203–1211

Eckardt ERM, Wang DQ, Donovan JM et al. (2002) Dietary sphingomyelin suppresses intestinal cholesterol absorption by decreasing thermodynamic avtivity of cholesterol monomers. Gastroenterology 122:948–956

Groen AK, Bloks VW, Bandsma RHJ et al. (2001) Hepatobiliary cholesterol transport is not impaired in ABCA1 null mice lacking high density lipoproteins. J Clin Invest 108:843–850

Insull W, Koren M, Davignon J et al. (2001) Efficacy and short-term safety of a new ACAT inhibitor, avasimibe, on lipids, lipoproteins, and apolipoproteins, in patients with combined hyperlipidemia. Atherosclerosis 157:137–144

Klett EL, Lu K, Kosters A et al. (2004) A mouse model of sitosterolemia: absence of Abcg8/sterolin-2 results in failure to secrete biliary cholesterol. BMC Med 2:5

Kosters A, Frijters RJMM, Vink E et al. (2003) Relation between hepatic expression of ATP-binding cassette transporters G5 and G8 and biliary cholesterol secretion in mice. J Hepatol 38:710–716

Kuipers F, Oude Elferink RPJ, Verkade HJ, Groen AK (1997) Mechanisms and (patho)physiological significance of biliary cholesterol secretion. Sub-Cell Biochem 28:295–318

Lee MH, Lu K, Hazard S et al. (2001) Identification of a gene, ABCG5, important in the regulation of dietary cholesterol absorption. Nat Genet 27:79–83

Lu K, Lee MH, Zhou Y et al. (2002) Molecular cloning, genomic organization, genetic variations, and characterization of murine sterolin genes Abcg5 and Abcg8. J Lipid Res 43:565–578

McNeish J, Aiello RJ, Gyot D et al. (2000) High density lipoprotein deficiency and foam cell accumulation in mice with targeted disruption of ATP-binding cassette transporter-1. Proc Natl Acad Sci USA 97:4245–4250

Mulligan JD, Flowers MT, Tebon A et al. (2003) ABCA1 is essential for efficient basolateral cholesterol efflux during the absorption of dietary cholesterol in chickens. J Biol Chem 278:13356–13366

Neese RA, Faix D, Kletke C et al. (1993) Measurement of endogenous synthesis of plasma cholesterol in rats and humans using MIDA. Am J Physiol 264: E136–E147

Ostlund RE (2002) Phytosterols in human nutrition. Annu Rev Nutr 22:533–549

Ostlund RE, Bosner MS, Stenson WF (1999) Cholesterol absorption efficiency declines at moderate dietary intake in normal human subjects. J Lipid Res 40:1453–1458

Oude Elferink RPJ, Bakker CTM, Roelofsen H et al. (1993). Accumulation of organic anion in intracellular vesicles of cultured rat hepatocytes is mediated by the canalicular multispecific organic anion transporter. Hepatology 17:434–444

Oude Elferink RPJ, Ottenhoff R, van Wijland M et al. (1996) Uncoupling of biliary phospholipid and cholesterol secretion in mice with reduced expression of mdr2 P-glycoprotein. J Lipid Res 37:1065–1075

Oude Elferink RPJ, Ottenhoff R, van Wijland MJA et al. (1995) Regulation of biliary lipid secretion by mdr2-P-glycoprotein in the mouse. J Clin Invest 95:31–38

Patel SB, Honda A, Salen G (1998) Sitosterolemia: exclusion of genes involved in reduced cholesterol biosynthesis. J Lipid Res 39:1055–1061

Plösch T, Bloks VW, Terasawa Y et al. (2004) Sitosterolemia in ABC-transporter G5-deficient mice is aggravated on activation of the liver X receptor. Gastroenterology 126:290–300

Plösch T, Kok T, Bloks VW et al. (2002) Increased hepatobiliary and fecal cholesterol excretion upon activation of the liver X receptor (LXR) is independent of ABCA1. J Biol Chem 277:33870–33877

Raal FJ, Marais DA, Klepack E et al. (2003) Avasimibe, an ACAT inhibitor, enhances the lipid lowering effect of atorvastatin in subjects with homozygous familial hypercholesterolemia. Atherosclerosis 171:273–279

Remaley AT, Bark S, Walts AD et al. (2002) Comparative genome analysis of potential regulatory elements in the ABCG5-ABCG8 gene cluster. Biochem Biophys Res Commun 295:276–282

Repa JJ, Berge KE, Pomajzl C et al. (2002) Regulation of ATP-Casette sterol transporters ABCG5 and ABCG8 by the liver X receptors α and β. J Biol Chem 277:18793–18800

Repa JJ, Mangelsdorf DJ (2002) The liver X receptor gene team: potential new players in atherosclerosis. Nat Med 8:1243–1248

Salen G, Patel SB, Batta AK (2002) Sitosterolemia. Cardiovasc Drug Rev 20:255–270

Graf GA, Li WP, Gerard RD et al. (2002) Coexpression of ATP-binding cassette proteins ABCG5 and ABCG8 permits their transport to the apical surface. J Clin Invest 110:659–669

Schaeffer EJ, Bruosseau ME, Diffenderfer MR et al. (2001) Cholesterol and apolipoprotein B metabolism in Tangier disease. Atherosclerosis 159:231–236

Schulthess G, Compassi S, Werder M et al. (2000) Intestinal sterol absorption mediated by scavenger receptors is competitively inhibited by amphipathic peptides and proteins. Biochemistry 39:12623–12631

Schwarz M, Davis DL, Vick BR et al. (2001) Genetic analysis of intestinal cholesterol absorption in inbred mice. J Lipid Res 42:1801–1811

Schwarz M, Russell DW, Dietschy JM et al. (2001) Alternate pathways of bile acid synthesis in the cholesterol 7α-hydroxylase knock out mouse are not upregulated by either cholesterol or cholestyramine feeding. J Lipid Res 42:1594–1603

Sehayek E, Duncan EM, Lütjohann D, et al. (2002) Loci on chromosomes 14 and 2, distinct from ABCG5/ABCG8, regulate plasma plant sterol levels in a C57BL/6 J x CASA/Rk intercross. Proc Natl Acad Sci USA 99:16215–16219

Small DM (2003) Role of ABC transporters in secretion of cholesterol from liver into bile. Proc Natl Acad Sci USA 100:4–6

Smart EJ, De Rose RA, Farber SA (2004) Annexin2-caveolin1 complex is a target of ezetimibe and regulates intestinal cholesterol transport. Proc Natl Acad Sci USA 101:3450–3455

Smit JJ, Schinkel AH, Oude Elferink RPJ et al. (1993). Homozygous disruption of the murine mdr2 P-glycoprotein gene leads to a complete absence of phospholipid from bile and to liver disease. Cell 75:451–462

Stellaard F, Sackmann M, Sauerbruch T et al. (1984) Simultaneous determination of cholic acid and chenodeoxycholic acid pool sizes and fractional turnover rates in human serum using labeled bile acids. J Lipid Res 25:1313–1319

Sudhop T, von Bergmann K (2002) Cholesterol absorption inhibitors for the treatment of hypercholesterolemia. Drugs 62:2333–2347

Sudhop T, Lütjohann D, Kodal A et al. (2002) Inhibition of cholesterol absorption by ezetimibe in humans. Circulation 106:1943–1948

Temel RE, Gebre AK, Parks JS et al. (2003) Compared with acyl-CoA:cholesterol O-acyltransferase (ACAT) 1 and lecithin:cholesterol acyltransferase, ACAT2 displays the greatest capacity to differentiate cholesterol from sitosterol. J Biol Chem 278:47594–47601

Turley SD, Dietschy J (2003) Sterol absorption by the small intestine. Curr Opin Lipidol 14:233–240

Van Heek M, France CF, Compton DS et al. (1997) In vivo metabolism-based discovery of a potent cholesterol absorption inhibitor, SCH58235, in the rat and rhesus monkey through the identification of the active metabolites of SCH48461. J Pharmacol Exp Ther 283:157–163

Verkade HJ, Havinga R, Gerding A et al. (1993) Mechanism of Bile Acid-Induced Biliary Lipid Secretion in the Rat: Effect of Conjugated Bilirubin. Am J Physiol 264: G462–G469

Verkade HJ, Vonk RJ, Kuipers F (1995). New insights into the mechanism of bile acid induced biliary lipid secretion. Hepatology 21:1174–1189

Voshol PJ, Minich DM, Havinga R et al. (2000) Postprandial chylomicron formation and fat absorption in multidrug resistance gene 2 P-glycoprotein-deficient mice. Gastroenterology 118:173–182

Voshol PJ, Schwarz M, Rigotti A et al. (2001) Down-regulation of intestinal scavenger receptor class B, type I (SR-BI) expression in rodents under conditions of deficient bile delivery to the intestine. Biochem J 356:317–325

Wang DQ, Carey MC (2003) Measurement of intestinal cholesterol absorption by plasma dual-isotope ratio, mass balance, and lymph fistula methods in the mouse: an analysis of direct versus indirect methodologies. J Lipid Res 44:1042–1059

Wang DQ, Tazuma S, Cohen DE (1999) Natural hydrophilic bile acids profoundly inhibit intestinal cholesterol absorption in mice. Hepatology 30:395A

Wellington CL, Walker EK, Suarez A et al. (2002) ABCA1 mRNA and protein distribution patterns predict multiple different roles and levels of regulation. Lab Invest 82:273–283

Werder M, Han CH, Wehrli E et al. (2001) Role of scavenger receptors SR-BI and CD36 in selective sterol uptake in the small intestine. Biochemistry 40:11643–11650

Wilson MD, Rudel LL (1994) Review of cholesterol absorption with emphasis on dietary and biliary cholesterol. J Lipid Res 35:943–955

Wittenburg H, Lyons MA, Li R (2003) FXR and ABCG5/ABCG8 as determinants of cholesterol gallstone formation from quantitative trait locus mapping in mice. Gastroenterology 125:868–881

Young SG, Cham CM, Pitas RE et al. (1995) A genetic model for absent chylomicron formation: mice producing apolipoprotein B48 in the liver, but not in the intestine. J Clin Invest 96:2932–2946

Yu L, Hammer RE, Li-Hawkins J et al. (2002A) Disruption of Abcg5 and Abcg8 in mice reveals their crucial role in biliary cholesterol secretion. Proc Natl Acad Sci USA 99:16237–16242

Yu L, Li-Hawkins J, Hammer RE et al. (2002B) Overexpression of ABCG5 and ABCG8 promotes biliary cholesterol secretion and reduces fractional absorption of dietary cholesterol. J Clin Invest 110:671–680

Yu L, York J, von Bergmann K et al. (2003) Stimulation of cholesterol excretion by the liver X receptor agonist requires ATP-binding cassette transporters G5 and G8. J Biol Chem 278:15565–15570

HEP (2005) 170:483–517

Inhibition of the Synthesis of Apolipoprotein B-Containing Lipoproteins

J. Greeve

Klinik für Allgemeine Innere Medizin, Inselspital-Universitätsspital Bern, 3010 Bern, Switzerland
jobst.greeve@insel.ch

Abstract Increased serum concentrations of low density lipoproteins represent a major cardiovascular risk factor. Low-density lipoproteins are derived from very low density lipoproteins secreted by the liver. Apolipoprotein (apo)B that constitutes the essential structural protein of these lipoproteins exists in two forms, the full length form apoB-100 and the carboxy-terminal truncated apoB-48. The generation of apoB-48 is due to editing of the apoB mRNA which generates a premature stop translation codon. The editing of apoB mRNA is an important regulatory event because apoB-48-containing lipoproteins cannot be converted into the atherogenic low density lipoproteins. The apoB gene is constitutively expressed in liver and intestine, and the rate of apoB secretion is regulated post-transcriptionally. The translocation of apoB into the endoplasmic reticulum is complicated by the hydrophobicity of the nascent polypeptide. The assembly and secretion of apoB-containing lipoproteins within the endoplasmic reticulum is strictly dependent on the microsomal tricylceride transfer protein which shuttles triglycerides onto the nascent lipoprotein particle. The overall synthesis of apoB lipoproteins is regulated by proteosomal and nonproteosomal degradation and is dependent on triglyceride availability. Noninsulin dependent diabetes mellitus, obesity and the metabolic syndrome are characterized by an increased hepatic synthesis of apoB-containing lipoproteins. Interventions aimed to reduce the hepatic secretion of apoB-containing lipoproteins are therefore of great clinical importance. Lead targets in these pathways are discussed.

Keywords Apolipoprotein B · mRNA editing · Translocation · Lipoprotein assembly · Proteosomal degradation

1
Introduction

Arteriosclerotic cardiovascular disease (CVD) is the major cause for morbidity and mortality in industrialized societies and an emerging disease in the developing world. Large prospective cohort studies identified four major risk factors for arteriosclerosis and CVD: (a) hypertension; (b) elevated levels of low-density lipoprotein (LDL) cholesterol; (c) smoking; and (d) diabetes mellitus (Wilson and Culleton 1998). A reduction of these risk factors through changes in nutrition, behavior or life style or by using drug therapy can lower morbidity and mortality of arteriosclerotic CVD (Levine et al. 1995). The accumulation of LDL particles in the subendothelial matrix is the causal event in the initiation and progression of arteriosclerosis, and is dependent on interactions between the sole protein constituent apolipoprotein (apo) B-100 and matrix proteoglycans (Boren et al. 1998, Skalen et al. 2002). The regulation of synthesis and metabolism of the triglyceride-rich very-low-density lipoproteins (VLDL) as the precursors of LDL formation is therefore of outstanding importance (Glass and Witztum 2001). Prevalent disorders such as non-insulin-dependent diabetes mellitus (NIDDM), obesity and the metabolic syndrome are characterized by an increase of VLDL secretion (Brunzell and Hokanson 1999; Ginsberg 2000). This chapter describes the molecular basis of the assembly and secretion of apoB lipoproteins and discusses obvious targets for nutritional and/or pharmaceutical interventions to reduce VLDL secretion. Since apoB is the essential protein core component of VLDL and the only protein constituent of LDL, the regulation of apoB transcription, mRNA processing, translation and secretion is described in detail.

2
Transcription and Editing of ApoB mRNA

2.1
Genomic Organization and Transcription of the ApoB Gene

The apoB gene encoded on chromosome 2 (2p23) covers approximately 43 kb with 29 exons and is expressed constitutively in liver and intestine, and also in placenta (Knott et al 1985; Blackhart et al. 1986, Demmer et al. 1986). The tissue-specific expression of the apoB gene is controlled by distinct enhancer and control regions for efficient transcription in the liver or in the intestine, respectively (Levy-Wilson et al. 1992; Levy-Wilson et al. 2000; Antes et al. 2000). While the amount of apoB secreted varies in parallel with the rate of lipogenesis and the nutritional supply, apoB mRNA levels in the liver in vivo remain nearly constant despite of a coordinate increase of lipoprotein assembly and secretion (Borchard and Davis 1987; Leighton et al. 1990). Similarly, in hepatoma cells in vitro the apoB mRNA levels remain unchanged even when the amount of apoB secreted is modulated seven-fold by addition of oleate or albumin to the culture medium (Pullinger et al. 1989). Thus, the transcription of the apoB gene is not influenced by nutritional or hormonal stimuli, and the post-transcriptional processing of apoB is of central importance for the coordinate control of VLDL assembly and secretion in the liver (Davis and Hui 2001).

2.2
Editing of ApoB mRNA

2.2.1
Metabolic Differences of ApoB100 and ApoB48

apoB exists in two different forms, the full-length protein apoB-100 and the carboxy-terminal truncated apoB-48 (Kane 1983). ApoB-100, with a molecular weight of 512 kDa is one of the largest proteins in humans, is the essential protein core component of VLDL that are secreted by the liver (Kane 1983). After triglyceride hydrolysis most of the VLDL remnants are rapidly removed by the liver, but some are further metabolized to LDL which circulate with an approximate half-life of 20 h (Brown and Goldstein 1986). LDL consist mainly of cholesterol and apoB-100 and contain approximately 60%–70% of the total cholesterol of human plasma (Kane 1983, Brown and Goldstein 1986). Mutations in the ligand binding domain in the carboxy-terminal half of apoB-100 result in retarded clearance of LDL and are the basis of the genetic syndrome Familial Defective ApoB, a phenocopy of Familial Hypercholesterolemia (FH) that is caused by defective LDL receptors (Innerarity et al. 1987, Boren et al. 1998). ApoB-100 contains an unpaired cysteine residue in its carboxy-terminal half that can link apoB-100 to apo(a) via a disulfide bond to generate lipoprotein (a) (McLean et al. 1987, Young 1990, Brunner et al. 1993). Lipoprotein (a) is a second atherogenic lipoprotein and is emerging as an important risk factor for arteriosclerotic CVD (Marcovina et al. 2003).

ApoB-48 consists only of the amino-terminal 48% of apoB-100 and is lacking both the LDL receptor domain as well as the linkage site for apo(a) (Kane 1983; Knott et al. 1986, Powell et al. 1987). In humans, apoB-48 is synthesized exclusively in the intestine and serves as the integral protein component of chylomicrons that transport dietary lipids (Kane et al. 1983, Greeve et al. 1993). The large chylomicrons are secreted into the mesenteric lymph vessels and enter the blood stream via the thoracic lymph duct (Kane 1983). After triglyceride hydrolysis, chylomicron remnants are completely removed by the liver via interaction of apoE with the LDL receptor related protein (Herz and Willnow 1995). In contrast to the hepatic derived VLDL, chylomicrons do not serve as precursors of LDL formation and are cleared from the plasma very rapidly with an average half-life of less than 10 min (Windler et al. 1988). The existence of apoB-48 is the sole explanation for this complete hepatic removal of intestinal derived lipoproteins, and apoB-48 can be viewed as a biochemical portal vein that channels lipophilic nutrients directly and rapidly to the liver (Greeve et al. 1993). Generally, apoB-48 is referred to as the exogenous and apoB-100 as the endogenous lipoprotein pathway (Brown and Goldstein 1986).

2.2.2
mRNA Editing Leads to ApoB48 and Prevents LDL Formation

A single post-transcriptional base change at nucleotide 6666 in the apoB mRNA from C to U, termed editing of apoB mRNA, generates a premature stop translation codon and explains the translation of the truncated apoB-48 in the intestine (Powell et al. 1987; Chen et al. 1987) (Fig. 1). In contrast to humans and other mammalian species that edit the apoB mRNA only in the intestine, but not in liver, some species such as dog, horse, rat and mouse do edit also the hepatic apoB mRNA (Greeve et al. 1993). The synthesis of apoB-48-containing VLDL by the liver of these species correlates to very low concentrations of LDL in plasma (Greeve et al. 1993). Thus, editing of apoB mRNA in the liver is a genetic mechanism to prevent the accumulation of the atherogenic LDL (Greeve et al. 1993).

2.2.3
Regulation of ApoB mRNA Editing

In the rat liver, apoB mRNA editing remains low until the third postnatal week when it increases strongly and attains adult levels (Funahashi et al. 1995). The editing of apoB mRNA in the small intestine increases sharply before birth, resulting in editing of 90%–95% of the intestinal apoB mRNA post-

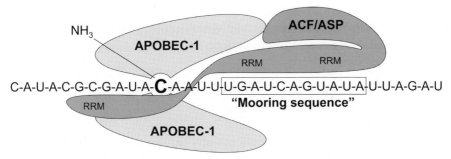

Fig. 1 Illustration of the apoB mRNA editing enzyme-complex

natally (Patterson et al. 1992). Both in rat and human small intestine, the complete editing of apoB mRNA is sustained throughout life and increases with the differentiation of the enterocytes along the crypt-to-villus functional unit (Teng et al 1990, Patterson et al. 2003). In rat liver, editing of apoB mRNA increases after feeding carbohydrates or ethanol (Baum et al. 1990, Lau et al. 1995), after administration of thyroid hormones (Davidson et al. 1988), growth hormone (Sjöberg et al. 1992), or insulin (Thorngate et al. 1994), and decreases during starvation (Baum et al. 1990) or after estrogen administration (Seishima et al. 1991).

2.2.4
Familial Hypobetalipoproteinemia Due to Truncated Apoforms

In subjects with familial hypobetalipoproteinemia (FHBL) various heterozygous point mutations in the apoB gene lead to premature termination of apoB translation (Linton et al. 1993; Young 1996, Schonfeld 2003). In a subject with homozygous FHBL, the identical C to T mutation at codon 2252 in both apoB alleles generated a premature stop translation codon with the subsequent synthesis of only apoB-50 and led to the complete absence of LDL in plasma (Hardman et al. 1991). In patients with heterozygous FHBL, low LDL levels below the 5th percentile were observed (Schonfeld 2003). Two mechanisms lead to these low LDL levels: first, the truncated apoB forms are not converted to LDL, but are rapidly metabolized (Parhofer et al. 1990, 1992). Second, the truncated apoB forms inhibit the synthesis and secretion of apoB-100 encoded by the normal apoB allele (Aguilar-Salinas et al. 1995, Kim et al. 1998, Schonfeld 2003). Kinetic studies have shown that the production rates of apoB-100 are reduced by 70%–80% in heterozygous FHBL instead of the expected 50% (Aguilar-Salinas et al. 1995, Welty et al. 1997, Schonfeld 2003). The inhibition of apoB-100 production by the truncated apoB-38.9 has been demonstrated most elegantly in transgenic mice that express only apoB-100 and a truncated apoB-38.9 transgene (Chen et al. 2003). Moreover, freshly isolated primary horse hepatocytes that edit approximately 40%–50% of the apoB mRNA secrete predominantly apoB-48 (Greeve et al. 1993). In rat hepatoma McArdle7777 cells, apoB-48 is preferentially translated over apoB-100 when apoB mRNA is increased by stable expression of betaine-homocysteine S-methyltransferase (Collins et al. 2000).

2.2.5
The ApoB mRNA Editing Enzyme Complex

The editing of apoB mRNA occurs co- or post-transcriptionally coincident with splicing and polyadenylation of the apoB pre-mRNA, and is mediated by an enzyme complex that deaminates C_{6666} to uridine (Greeve et al. 1991, Hodges et al. 1991, Lau et al. 1991, Johnson et al. 1993). An 11-nucleotide 'mooring' motif (nt 6,671–6,681) immediately downstream of the editing site C_{6666} is absolutely required for editing (Shah et al. 1991). Sequences located upstream and downstream of this indispensable mooring sequence enhance editing, indicating that the essential elements for physiological editing at C_{6666} consist of upstream efficiency elements, the mooring sequence and a 3'-efficiency element, encompassing approximately 139 nucleotides (Hersberger and Innerarity 1998). Phylogenetic analyses, computer predictions and ribonuclease probing predict a stem–loop structure around the editing site (Richardson et al. 1998, Hersberger et al. 1999).

The catalytic subunit APOBEC-1 (apoB mRNA editing enzyme catalytic component 1) of this enzyme-complex was cloned by Davidson and colleagues (Teng et al. 1993). APOBEC-1 is a cytidine deaminase and related in quaternary and tertiary structure to *Escherichia coli* cytidine deaminase (ECCDA) as both enzymes form homodimers in a head-to-tail configuration (Navaratnam et al. 1993, 1998; Lau et al. 1994). Molecular modelling by superimposing the primary sequence of APOBEC-1 on the crystal structure of ECCDA proposes that the active-site residues of the deaminase domain recognize the target C, whereas the opposite 'pseudoactive' site binds a downstream U and targets the active site for deamination (Navaratnam et al. 1998).

APOBEC-1 alone although it contains a novel, albeit weak, RNA binding motif cannot edit the apoB mRNA by cytidine deamination, but requires additional 'auxiliary' components for activity (Teng et al. 1993, Yamanaka et al. 1994, Navaratnam et al. 1995). The second essential component of the apoB mRNA editing enzyme complex was purified and cloned simultaneously by our group (Lellek et al. 2000) and Driscoll and colleges (Mehta et al. 2000). This protein, termed APOBEC-1 complementing factor (ACF) or APOBEC-1 stimulating protein (ASP), is a novel type of RNA-binding protein with three nonidentical RNA recognition motifs for single-stranded RNA and an additional putative binding domain for double-stranded RNA (Lellek et al. 2000; Mehta et al. 2000). Recombinant ACF/ASP and APOBEC-1 reconstitute efficient apoB mRNA editing activity in vitro and in yeast in vivo (Lellek et al. 2000, 2002; Mehta et al. 2000). Thus, APOBEC-1 and ACF/ASP constitute the apoB mRNA editing-holoenzyme. The specificity of editing is due to the specific binding of ACF/ASP to the apoB mRNA (Mehta et al. 2002).

Coexpression of ACF/ASP and APOBEC-1 leads to an entirely nuclear localization of APOBEC-1 that without ACF/ASP is also found in the cytoplasm (Blanc et al. 2001). A novel nuclear localization signal has been identified in the auxiliary domain of ACF/ASP that regulates nucleo-cytoplasmic shuttling of ACF/ASP (Blanc et al. 2003). Apparently, both APOBEC-1 and ACF/ASP shuttle as a complex associated with the apoB mRNA and prevent nonsense-mediated decay of edited apoB mRNA (Chester et al. 2003).

2.2.6
Expression of APOBEC-1 in Liver to Reduce LDL Plasma Levels

APOBEC-1 is the only missing component of the apoB mRNA editing enzyme complex in the liver of species without hepatic apoB mRNA editing (Giannoni et al. 1994; Greeve et al. 1996; Kozarsky et al. 1996). The hepatic expression of APOBEC-1 in mice or rats is mediated by an additional promoter at the 5'end of the APOBEC-1 gene that confers low level expression in extra-intestinal tissues including the liver (Nakamuta et al. 1995; Qian et al. 1997; Hirano et al. 1997; Greeve et al. 1998). The lack of this additional promoter in the human APOBEC-1 gene explains the absence of APOBEC-1 and apoB mRNA editing in the human liver (Hirano et al. 1997; Fujino et al. 1998). Homozygous APOBEC-1 deficient mice are healthy and fertile and have only slightly elevated LDL levels (Morrison et al. 1996; Hirano et al. 1996; Nakamuta et al. 1996). However, LDL-receptor$^{-/-}$ and APOBEC-1$^{-/-}$ double knock-out mice have strongly elevated LDL levels as compared to LDL-receptor$^{-/-}$ mice (Powell-Braxton et al. 1998). The markedly less severe phenotype in LDL-receptor deficient mice as compared to patients with homozygous FH or to the homozygous LDL-receptor deficient Watanabe heritable hyperlipidemic (WHHL) rabbits is explained by the editing of the hepatic apoB mRNA in mice (Powell-Braxton et al. 1998).

We and Davidson and colleges demonstrated by adenovirus-mediated hepatic gene transfer of APOBEC-1 that induction of hepatic apoB mRNA editing reduces the elevated LDL levels of WHHL rabbits by up to 70% (Greeve et al. 1996; Kozarsky et al. 1996). These experiments provide the proof of principle that induction of editing in the liver has the capacity to reduce elevated plasma LDL levels irrespective of their metabolic or genetic basis (Greeve et al. 1996; Kozarsky et al. 1996).

An alternative approach for the delivery of APOBEC-1 used TAT-mediated protein transduction in primary rat hepatocytes and rat hepatoma McArdle cells (Yang et al. 2002). The effects, however, were rather small, and most importantly the antigenic properties of the protein adducts make their reiterated use in humans in vivo rather unlikely.

2.2.7
APOBEC-1 Genes Can Act as DNA Mutators

Innerarity and colleges expressed APOBEC-1 in transgenic animals using the strong apoE promoter and observed hepatocellular dysplasias and carcinomas in several independent transgenic lines (Yamanaka et al. 1995). This oncogenic potential of APOBEC-1 is related to the over-expression as transgenic lines with low APOBEC-1 expression do not develop carcinomas (Qian et al. 1998). Initially, the oncogenic effect of APOBEC-1 was attributed to aberrant hyper-editing of other mRNAs apart from apoB such as the translational repressor NAT-1 (Yamanaka et al. 1997). Recent findings, however, suggest a different view on the oncogenic potential of APOBEC-1.

In 1999, activation-induced cytidine deaminase (AID), a close homologue of APOBEC-1, was identified in a murine lymphoma cell line (Muramatsu et al. 1999). In homozygous AID deficient mice, immunoglobulin class switch recombination and somatic hypermutations of the immunoglobulin genes (SHM) are complete abolished (Muramatsu et al. 2000). In human patients with the autosomal recessive form of the hyper-IgM syndrome various mutations in the human AID gene cripple AID function (Revy et al. 2000). In chicken B cells, AID is required for immunoglobulin gene conversion that provides the genetic diversification of the immunoglobulin genes in chicken, rabbits, cattle and pigs by retrotransposition of pseudogene V elements into the functional VDJ exon (Arakawa et al. 2002). Thus, AID is of central importance for antibody diversity and represents a point of convergence for these seemingly separate genetic mechanisms.

A series of recent studies indicate that AID acts by cytidine deamination directly in the DNA. Over-expression of AID in bacteria leads to a hypermutator phenotype with nucleotide transitions at dC/dG in a context dependent manner (Petersen-Mahrt et al. 2002). In eukaryotic cells, uracils in the DNA generated by either enzymatic or nonenzymatic cytosine deamination are removed by base excision repair with the uracil being cleaved from the ribose moiety by uracil-DNA-gylcosylase (Di Noia and Neuberger 2002). Replication of the DNA over the abasic site without base repair should result in random incorporation of nucleotides with a predominance of transversions over transitions at a 2:1 ratio (Di Noia and Neuberger 2002). Indeed, expression of a bacteriophage derived inhibitor protein of uracil-DNA glycosylase in chicken DT40 cells that are deficient in the repair gene *XRCC2* shifts the pattern of SHM from transversions to transitions (Di Noia and Neuberger 2002). Similarly, in uracil-DNA glycosylase deficient mice the mutations at the dC/dG sites in the variable region exons of the immunoglobulin genes are shifted toward transitions (Rada et al. 2002). Moreover, both AID and APOBEC-1 have been shown to exert cytidine deamination activity on DNA in vitro (Pham et al. 2003; Bransteitter et al. 2003; Dickerson et al. 2003; Petersen-Mahrt and Neuberger 2003) and also in bacteria in vivo (Petersen-Mahrt et al. 2002; Harris et al. 2003).

We have demonstrated recently that AID mRNA is constitutively expressed in germinal center B-NHL, while during normal B cell maturation the expression of AID is restricted a discrete period of 24–36 h during the development of the B cell germinal center (Greeve et al. 2003). Thus, a deregulation of AID expression may predispose to the development of germinal center B-NHL (Greeve et al. 2003). Indeed, AID transgenic mice with a constitutive and ubiquitous AID expression by the β-actin promoter develop T-cell lymphomas and lung adenocarcinomas (Okazaki et al. 2003).

In 2002, a cluster of five APOBEC-1 related genes and two probable pseudogenes designated APOBEC3A-G were identified on chromosome 22 (Jarmuz et al. 2002). Most recently, APOBEC3G was shown to be responsible for the failure of Vif-deficient HIV strains to replicate in nonpermissive cell lines (Sheehy et al. 2002). The first hint that APOBEC3G deaminates DNA came from a study demonstrating that APOBEC-1, APOBEC3C and APOBEC3G induce mutations in bacteria at a more frequent rate as compared to AID (Harris et al. 2002). A series of recent studies demonstrated that APOBEC3G mediates innate immunity to various retroviruses including HIV by deamination of cytidines in the retroviral first (minus)-strand cDNA (Harris et al. 2003; Mangeat et al. 2003; Mariani et al. 2003; Zhang et al. 2003). The HIV Vif protein binds APOBEC3G and induces its degradation by the proteasome, thus enabling HIV to replicate in T cells in the presence of APOBEC3G (Marin et al. 2003; Sheehy et al. 2003; Stopak et al. 2003).

Taken together, these results suggest that all members of the APOBEC gene family including APOBEC-1 have DNA mutator activity and therefore potentially can exert oncogenic effects. The RNA editing activity of APOBEC-1 might be the exception rather than the rule for these proteins

3
Translation of ApoB and Lipoprotein Assembly

3.1
Translation of ApoB and Translocation Across the ER Membranes

ApoB contains a signal peptide that directs the translated apoB into the lumen of the ER (Taskinen et al. 1988). The translocation of secretory proteins occurs cotranslationally via a tight junction between the ribosome and the ER membrane, and once initiated the polypeptide chain translocation into the ER progresses to completion (Hedge and Lingappa 1996; Liao et al. 1997). Unlike most other secretory proteins, apoB is not translocated entirely, but appears to be exposed during translation both to the ER lumen as well as to the cytosol (Davis et al. 1990; Furukawa et al. 1992). In isolated microsomes, domains of apoB are accessible for exogenous proteases, indicating that apoB, although it lacks a classical transmembrane domain, is exposed to the cytosol at some points during synthesis or intracellular transport (Chen et al. 1998; Linnik et Herscovitz 1998). Studies in cell free translation systems demonstrated putative 'pause-transfer' sequences in apoB that can interrupt translocation across the ER membrane without pausing translation (Chuck et al. 1990). Alternatively, pausing is explained by transient translocation difficulties due to the apoB secondary structure or to the β-sheet domains in the apoB protein structure (Pease et al. 1991; Liang et al. 1998). Inefficient translocation, regardless of its molecular basis, apparently results in the escape of the nascent apoB polypeptide from the translocon into the cytosol, and completion of translation is delayed until a lipid-associated signal for secretion occurs (Mitchell et al. 1998; Pariyarath and Fisher 2001).

3.2
Lipoprotein Assembly

3.2.1
Two-Step Lipidation Model of ApoB Lipoprotein Assembly

In rat liver, apoB-48 VLDL and also apoB-100 VLDL are assembled in the ER in two discontinuous lipidation steps (Boren et al. 1994; Stillemark et al. 2000; Rustaeus et al. 1995, 1998). In the first step, apoB-48 is associated cotranslationally with a small amount of lipid to form a 'high-density' apoB lipoprotein particle. This HDL-like particle is further lipidated in a second step that is expanding its triglyceride content to form a VLDL particle. The assembly of apoB-48-containing chylomicrons in the enterocytes also occurs as a two-step process: The first step produces dense apoB-48 phospholipid-rich particles which accumulate in the smooth ER. In the second step, these dense particles rapidly acquire the bulk of triglycerides and additional phospholipid (Cartwright and Higgins 2000). Similarly, the assembly of apoB-100 VLDL in hepatoma cells involves a two-step pathway in which without adequate supply of lipids most of the apoB-100 is degraded intracellularly (Rustaeus et al. 1995, 1998; Stillemark et al. 2000).

3.2.2
Microsomal Triglyceride Transfer Protein

The assembly of apoB-containing lipoproteins requires, in addition to the translocation of the nascent apoB polypeptide, a number of molecular chaperones: heat-shock-protein70 (hsp70) in the cytosol, calnexin in the ER membranes, and most importantly, microsomal triglyceride transfer protein (MTP) within the ER lumen (Zhou et al. 1995; Wu et al. 1996; Wang et al. 1996; Linnik et Herscovitz 1998). MTP is a heterodimer that consists of the ubiquitous ER-localized chaperone protein-disulfide isomerase and a unique 97-kDa subunit (Wetterau et al. 1990). The genetic syndrome abetalipoproteinemia, that is characterized by the inability to secrete intestinal or hepatic apoB lipoproteins, is caused by mutations in the gene encoding the large 97-kDa subunit (Sharp et al. 1993). Thus, abetalipoproteinemia illustrates the outstanding importance of MTP for apoB lipoprotein assembly. MTP has the capacity to transport neutral and amphipathic lipids between membranes and vesicles (Wetterau et al. 1997). During the cotranslational phase of lipoprotein assembly ('first step') MTP transfers lipids from the ER membrane or other donor sites onto the nascent apoB particle (Wetterau et al. 1997). This process requires a physical interaction between MTP and the amino terminus of apoB (Patel and Grundy 1996; Hussain et al. 1998; Bradbury et al. 1999). The interaction of MTP with apoB is also required for initiation of translocation (Fleming et al. 1999; Liang and Ginsburg 2001). The cotranslational lipid transfer mediated by MTP prevents the early proteosomal degradation of apoB (Benoist and Grand-Perret 1997; Zhou et al. 1998).

The 'second-step' in apoB lipoprotein assembly that provides bulk lipid addition to the HDL-like apoB precursor lipoprotein is less well defined. MTP is required for the availability of triglyceride-rich droplets in the ER lumen (Wang et al. 1997, 1999; Hebbachi et al. 1999; Raabe et al. 1999). The final step in lipoprotein assembly that involves the fusion of the HDL-like apoB precursor lipoprotein with this triglyceride-rich droplet can occur independently of MTP activity or of triglyceride synthesis (Olofson et al. 1999; Raabe et al. 1999; Pan et al. 2002). This step in lipoprotein synthesis requires the exit of apoB from the ER, is dependent on COPII vesicles, and is concluded in a post-ER compartment (Gusarova et al. 2003).

Studies using MTP deficient mice have contributed substantially to the insight of the role of MTP in apoB lipoprotein assembly. Homozygote deficiency of MTP results in embryonic lethality in mice, most probably due to an impaired capacity of the yolk sac to export lipids to the developing embryo (Raabe et al. 1998). Heterozygote MTP deficiency in mice reduces the apoB lipoprotein secretion without any adverse effect by about 50% (Raabe et al. 1998, Leung et al. 2000). Thus, the activity of MTP is rate limiting for the production of VLDL in the liver. This important conclusion is underscored by studies using adenovirus-mediated overexpression of MTP that lead to increased VLDL production (Liao et al. 1999; Tietge et al. 1999). A liver-specific conditional gene knock-out of MTP abolishes apoB-100 lipoprotein secretion by the liver completely (Raabe et al. 1999; Chang et al. 1999). Interestingly, these two studies differed in the extent of the inhibition of hepatic apoB48 secretion by the conditional MTP knock-out. While Chang et al. (1999) found a complete inhibition of both apoB-100 and apoB-48, Raabe et al. (1999) reported that only the apoB-100 secretion was completely abolished, while the apoB-48 secretion was almost unaffected. Young and coworkers have recently generated a mouse model ('reversa mice') that is homozygous deficient for the LDL-receptor ($Ldlr^{-/-}$), expresses only apoB-100 ($ApoB^{100/100}$), and harbors a homozygous conditional MTP gene knock-out that can be executed by liver-specific expression of a Cre-transgene from the inducible Mx1-promoter

(Lieu et al. 2003). The severe hypercholesterolemia with strongly elevated LDL plasma levels in the Ldlr$^{-/-}$, ApoB$^{100/100}$ mice can completely be reversed by inactivation of MTP in the liver (Lieu et al. 2003). The inactivation of hepatic apoB lipoprotein synthesis does not only correct the hyperlipidemia in these 'reversa mice', but also prevents the development of premature arteriosclerosis (Lieu et al. 2003).

Besides MTP, other unconditional cofactor(s) for apoB lipoprotein secretion from the small intestine must be required. This is demonstrated by autosomal recessive disorders of chylomicron secretion that are characterized by a selective defect in chylomicron production with little impact on hepatic VLDL synthesis (Kane and Havel 1995). Chylomicron retention disease (CMRD), Anderson disease and CMRD with the neuromuscular disorder Marinseco–Sjogren syndrome are all characterized by deficiency in fat-soluble vitamins, low blood cholesterol levels and the complete absence of chylomicrons (Jones et al. 2003). Obvious candidate genes for these genetic disorders such as intestinal apoproteins, MTP or fatty acid binding proteins could be excluded by linkage studies (Dannoura et al. 1999; Davidson and Shelness 2000). By carrying out a genome-wide scan the group of James Scott and Carol Shoulders identified a region of apparent homozygosity in four affected families and could pin-point homozygous coding sequence variants of *SARA2* in 11 affected individuals from eight different families with CMRD or Anderson disease (Jones et al. 2003). *SARA2* belongs to the Sar1-ADP-ribosylation factor family of small GTPases which govern the intracellular trafficking of proteins in COPII (coat protein)-coated vesicles (Schekman and Orci 1996; Takai et al. 2001). All five missense mutations associated with CMRD or Anderson disease cause damage the GTP-binding pocket of the *SARA2* gene product (Sar1b) as deduced from alignment to the crystal structure of hamster Sar1 that shares 99% amino-acid sequence identity with Sar1b (Jones et al. 2003). The three amino acid changes associated with CMRD or Anderson disease are expected to profoundly compromise the ability of SAR1b to bind GTP, while a homozygous splice site mutation abolishes the production of functional Sar1b (Jones et al. 2003). This study therefore establishes a link between chylomicron secretion and the COPII transport machinery. The precise function of Sar1b in the intracellular trafficking of chylomicrons, however, remains to be established.

3.2.3
Regulated Intracellular Degradation of ApoB

In the liver, a major proportion of newly synthesized apoB is degraded intracellularly as first demonstrated in HepG2 cells and primary rat hepatocytes (Bostrom et al. 1986; Borchard and Davis 1987). Numerous subsequent studies have since shown that apoB is degraded both by proteasomal and nonproteasomal pathways.

3.2.3.1
Proteosomal Degradation of ApoB

When apoB translation and translocation is arrested, the translocation-arrested apoB is targeted by ubiquitinylation for degradation by the proteasome (Benoist and Grand-Perret 1997; Yeung et al. 1996; Fisher et al. 1997). The lack of co-translational lipid association with the nascent β-sheets of apoB results in an increased cytosolic exposure of apoB domains and targets apoB to the ubiquitin–proteosome pathway. This degradation is facilitated by the cytosolic chaperones hsp70 and hsp90, involves the chymotrypsin-like activity of the proteasome, and begins co-translationally (Zhou et al. 1998; Benoist and Grand-Perret 1997; Yeung et al. 1996; Fisher et al. 1997; Gusarova et al. 2001, Fisher and Ginsburg 2002). In contrast to most other proteins that are retrotranslocated into the cytosol for proteosomal degradation after being fully translocated into the ER, apoB is targeted co-translationally for degradation while it is still bound to the ribosome (Liao et al. 1998; Fisher et al. 1997; Mitchell et al. 1998; Pariyarath et al. 2001; Zhou et al. 1998; Chen et al. 1998; Liang et al. 2000). The degradation of apoB by the proteasome is regulated by various metabolic factors. A lack of triglycerides or low activity of MTP are the most important conditions that lead to an increased proteosomal degradation of apoB. The total lack of apoB secretion in humans with abetalipoproteinemia and in MTP deficient mice proves the central role of MTP in the regulation of proteosomal degradation of nascent apoB.

Increased lipogenesis induced by SREBP-1 protects apoB from proteosomal degradation and results in increased hepatic apoB lipoprotein secretion (Wang et al. 1997). Besides hsp70, hsp90 promotes apoB degradation by the ubiquitin–proteasome pathway by unfolding the apoB substrate into the narrow mouth of the 19S cap subunit of the proteasome (Verma et al. 2000; Gustarova et al. 2001). Ubiquitinylation of apoB is, at least partly, mediated by GP78, a ubiquitin protein ligase (Liang et al. 2003). Taken together, insufficient lipid association of the nascent apoB polypeptide initiates the targeting of apoB to cotranslational quality control mechanisms that are designed to prevent the exit of misfolded proteins from the ER (Ellgard et al. 1999).

3.2.3.2
Non-proteosomal Degradation of ApoB

Both n-3 (omega-3) fatty acids of fish oil and insulin stimulate apoB degradation and decrease the secretion of buoyant apoB lipoproteins, yet this type of apoB degradation is insensitive to proteosomal inhibitors (Fisher et al. 2001; Fisher and Ginsburg 2002). Most probably, these stimuli induce apoB degradation after lipoprotein assembly and exit from the ER (Phung et al. 1997; Fisher et al. 2001). Inhibition of phosphatidylinositol 3-kinase reduces this non-proteosomal degradation of apoB (Sparks et al. 1996; Fisher et al. 2001). The increased rate of apoB lipoprotein secretion that develops frequently in NIDDM as a consequence of insulin resistance thus might be explained by a decrease of the non-proteosomal degradation of apoB (Fisher and Ginsburg 2002).

A further potential important regulation of apoB lipoprotein production by the liver is related to the activity of hepatic LDL receptors. In FH not only the clearance of LDL is decreased, but the hepatic secretion of VLDL is increased substantially (Packard et al. 1976; Soutar et al. 1977). Statin therapy can effectively lower LDL plasma levels even without affecting LDL clearing rates, and therefore at least a proportion of the LDL lowering effect can be attributed to a decreased production rate of VLDL (Huff and Burnett 1997). The LDL receptor mediates presecretory degradation of apoB-100 within the secretory pathway in primary mice hepatocytes (Twisk et al. 2000). A naturally occurring mutant LDL receptor as well an engineered LDL receptor mutant consisting of only the ligand-binding domains and a carboxy-terminal endoplasmic retention sequence both of which are retained within the ER abolish apoB secretion in primary hepatocytes of $Ldlr^{-/-}$ mice (Gillian-Daniel et al. 2002). When the ligand-binding domain of the truncated receptor was disrupted, this receptor was unable to block apoB secretion (Gillian-Daniel et al. 2002). These findings establish LDL receptor-mediated pre-secretory degradation as a pathway distinct from the re-uptake of nascent apoB-lipoproteins at the cell surface. However, these results are not undisputed as Millar et al. (2002) did not find an effect of the LDL receptor on apoB lipoprotein secretion in the mouse liver in vivo when they measured hepatic triglyceride and apoB production in LDL receptor$^{-/-}$ mice in comparison to wild-type mice.

ApoB degradation is rapid and complete in HepG2 cells after addition of oleate to facilitate apoB translocation (Fig. 2), of brefeldin A to inhibit the vesicular transport from the ER to the Golgi apparatus, and of N-acetyl-leucinyl-leucinyl-norleucinal (ALLN) to inhibit neutral cysteine proteases and the proteasome (Wu et al. 1997). Additional treatment with dithiothreitol (DTT) prevents this degradation (Wu et al. 1997). Thus, the co- and post-translational degradation of apoB involves a DTT-sensitive protease within the ER lumen in addition to proteosomal degradation (Wu et al. 1997). A candidate protease for nonproteosomal degradation of apoB within the ER lumen is the ER-60 protease that has been shown to interact physically with apoB (Adeli et al. 1997). In addition, dexamethasone decreases the activity of a cysteine protease that degrades apoB in a post-ER compartment (Wang et al. 1995). In a cell-free assay system a major proportion of the intracellular degradation of newly synthesized apoB occurs in a post-ER compartment, possibly the Golgi apparatus, mediated by this dexamethasone inducible cysteine protease (Wang et al. 1995).

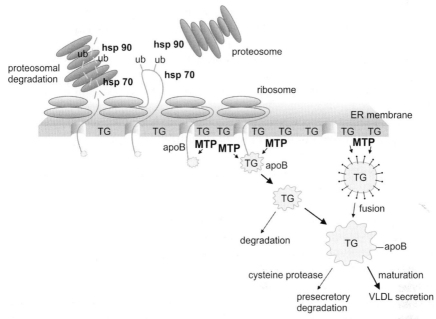

Fig. 2 Illustration of apoB translocation, lipoprotein assembly and proteosomal and non-proteosomal degradation

3.2.4
Bulk Lipidation and Maturation of ApoB Lipoproteins

The cascades in the final assembly of mature, triglyceride-enriched apoB lipoproteins are less well defined. As outlined above, the addition of bulk lipids requires the fusion of dense, 'HDL'-like apoB lipoproteins with preformed triglyceride-rich droplets either in a specialized ER compartment or in a pre-Golgi compartment (Pan et al. 2002). This 'second-step' occurs independently of MTP, yet MTP is required for the formation of the triglyceride-rich droplet that reside preformed within the secretory pathway (Pan et al. 2002). The dense nascent apoB lipoproteins are still associated with the ER membranes and the translocon (Hebbachi et al. 1999; Pan et al. 2002). This transmembrane conformation of apoB persists until apoB is transported to the Golgi-apparatus (Liao et al. 2003). The bulk lipidation occurs just prior to secretion of the mature apoB lipoproteins and may be linked to the generation of oleoyl-enriched phospholipids and associated membrane changes that are necessary for the formation of triglyceride-rich droplets within the ER lumen or their fusion with the lipoprotein particle (Tran et al. 2000). Therefore, oleate stimulation of apoB lipoprotein secretion by cultured cells may act as a signalling molecule rather than serving merely as a lipid source (Tran et al. 2000; Fisher and Ginsberg 2002). This second-step in lipoprotein formation occurs at the distal end of the secretory pathway, and is probably most active in a distal Golgi compartment adjacent to the site of secretion (Tran et al. 2002). This process does not require palmitylation of apoB, but palmitylation may influence the partitioning of apoB between microsomal membranes and the microsomal lumen (Vukmirica et al. 2003).

4
Lead Targets for the Inhibition of ApoB Lipoprotein Synthesis

Prevalent disorders such as NIDDM, obesity and the metabolic syndrome are characterized by an increase of VLDL secretion that results in hyperlipidemia and leads to accelerated atherosclerosis (Brunzell and Hokanson 1999; Ginsberg 2000). Means to reduce hepatic apoB lipoprotein production are therefore of great clinical significance. First, in some species, but notably not in humans, the hepatic synthesis of apoB-48 as a consequence of mRNA editing in the liver represents the physiological response to high-caloric diet. The proven mutator activity of APOBEC-1, however, precludes its use a therapeutic gene in humans for the treatment of hyperlipidemia and atherosclerosis. Second, the activity of MTP is the rate-limiting step in apoB lipoprotein secretion and therefore the most obvious target for medical intervention. Strategies aimed to directly increase apoB degradation without affecting MTP activity represent a valuable alternative. Approaches to reverse the insulin resistance in the liver to inhibit the hepatic lipoprotein secretion are a further alternative.

4.1
Inhibition of MTP

4.1.1
Nutritional Effects on MTP Activity

The restriction of calorie intake and of dietary lipids is the most straightforward approach to reduce the hepatic secretion of apoB lipoproteins. As outlined above, lipid deprivation slows the 'first-step' in the lipidation process mediated by MTP and leads to increased proteosomal degradation of the nascent apoB polypeptide. In addition, some nutritional ingredients affect hepatic apoB lipoprotein secretion and lower LDL plasma levels. Flavonoids are naturally occurring molecules abundantly present in fruits, vegetables, nuts, seeds and beverages such as tea and wine. The roles of naringenin and the related citrus flavonoid, hesperetin, in prevention and treatment of hyperlipidemia and atherosclerosis as well as cancer has recently attracted a great deal of attention. Narigenin and hespertin are found largely as the glycosides, naringin and hesperidin, in grapefruit and oranges, respectively (Wilcox et al. 2001). These glycosides are hydrolyzed to their active forms, narigenin and hespertin, by intestinal bacteria (Wilcox et al. 2001). Studies in animal models have demonstrated that diets supplemented with grapefruit juice, orange juice or narigenin or hespertin lead to a reduction of plasma cholesterol levels (Choi et al. 1991; Monforte et al. 1995; Shin et al. 1999; Bok et al. 1999; Kurowska et al. 2000). Naringenin and hesperitin have been shown not only to lower plasma lipids in rodent models, but also to reduce atherosclerosis (Lee et al. 2001). Studies in hepatoma cells in vitro have shown that hepatocyte apoB secretion is inhibited by naringenin and hesperitin via a reduced expression of ACAT2 and also MTP (Wilcox et al. 2001). Recent studies have demonstrated that the decrease of apoB secretion induced by naringenin and hesperitin is caused by the inhibition of MTP and the subsequent limitation of microsomal triglycerides within the ER, not by limiting cholesteryl-esters in the ER lumen as a consequence of the ACAT inhibition (Borradaile et al. 2002, 2003).

Many epidemiological studies have demonstrated that a high intake of fruits and vegetables is associated with lower plasma levels of LDL and a reduced risk of coronary artery disease (Bazzano et al. 2002). A reduced rate of apoB lipoprotein secretion due to flavonoid-induced MTP inhibition may contribute to this inverse association between fruit intake and CVD.

4.1.2
Hormonal Influences on MTP Activity

4.1.2.1
Effects of Insulin on MTP Activity

Insulin decreases the hepatic secretion of apoB lipoproteins, and this effect requires the activation of phosphatidylinositol 3-kinase (PI3-K) (Sparks and Sparks 1990; Phung et al. 1997). The inhibition of the hepatic apoB secretion by insulin is mediated by an increase of apoB degradation (Sparks and Sparks 1990; Phung et al. 1997). Emerging evidence from studies in animals indicates that the dsylipidemia associated with insulin resistance in NIDDM is associated with an increased hepatic expression of MTP mRNA (Kuriyama et al. 1998; Taghibiglou et al. 2000, 2002; Bartels et al. 2002). The mRNA expression of MTP in hepatocytes is increased by carbohydrate-rich diets and is decreased by insulin (Lin et al. 1994, 1995; Hagan et al. 1994). Insulin lowers MTP mRNA levels mainly through transcriptional repression of the MTP gene that is mediated through the MAPK^{erk} cascade, but not through the PI3-K pathway (Hagan et al. 1994; Au et al. 2003). Cellular MAPK^{p38} has a counterbalancing role in fine-tuning MTP activity in the liver through an inhibition of MEK1/2 by cross-talk between MEK1/2 and MAPK^{p38} (Au et al. 2003). Specific MAPK^{p38} inhibitors such as SB202190 or SB203580 lead to reduced MTP mRNA levels in human hepatoma HepG2 cells even in the absence of insulin, and can further augment the extent of insulin-mediated inhibition of MTP expression (Au et al. 2003). On the contrary, stimulating MAPK^{P38} in HepG2-cells by the constitutively activated MKK6-EE increases the MTP promoter activity (Singh et al. 1999; Au et al. 2003). Therefore, approaches to inhibit MAPK^{P38} activity have considerable potential to lower the activity of MTP in liver and to decrease the hepatic secretion of apoB lipoproteins.

An alternative pharmacological approach to lower MTP activity is through interference with peroxisome proliferator-activated receptors (PPARs). The PPARs are members of the nuclear receptor superfamily, and exist in three subtypes: PPARα, PPARγ and PPARδ (Lee et al. 2003). The thiazolidinediones (i.e., rosiglitazone or pioglitazone) are agonists of PPARγ and improve the insulin sensitivity both in the adipose tissue as well as in the liver (Stumvoll 2003). The fructose-fed golden Syrian hamster develops a syndrome of insulin resistance with mild hypertriglyceridemia, VLDL-apoB overproduction, increased intracellular apoB-particle stability and an increased expression of hepatic MTP similar as observed in patients with NIDDM (Taghibiglou et al. 2000). Treatment of fructose-fed golden Syrian hamsters with rosiglitazone ameliorated the defect in hepatic insulin-stimulated tyrosine phosphorylation of the insulin receptor and of the insulin-receptor substrate 1 and 2, reduced MTP protein in the liver and resulted in a significant reduction of intracellular apoB stability (Carpentier et al. 2002). Thus, PPARγ agonists lead to a reduction of hepatic VLDL assembly and secretion as a consequence of a decrease in MTP expression and a concomitant increase in intracellular apoB degradation (Carpentier et al. 2002).

4.1.2.2
Effects of Growth Hormone on MTP Activity

Growth hormone (GH) increases hepatic VLDL production (Elam et al. 1992; Linden et al. 2000). Studies in rats demonstrated a higher MTP expression in female rats that could be explained by the feminine GH secretory pattern (Ameen and Oscarsson. 2003). GH appears to be a central regulator for MTP expression (Ameen and Oscarsson. 2003). The signal transduction pathways induced by GH that ultimately lead to the increase in MTP expression are still not well defined, but offer possibilities for pharmacological interventions to decrease hepatic MTP expression for lowering of VLDL secretion.

4.1.3
Pharmacological Inhibition of MTP Activity

Due to the central role of MTP in the regulation of VLDL secretion by the liver, the pharmaceutical industry has devised both screening protocols as well as drug-design strategies to identify potent MTP inhibitors. Independent efforts have yielded strikingly similar series of lipophilic amide inhibitors (Chang et al. 2002).

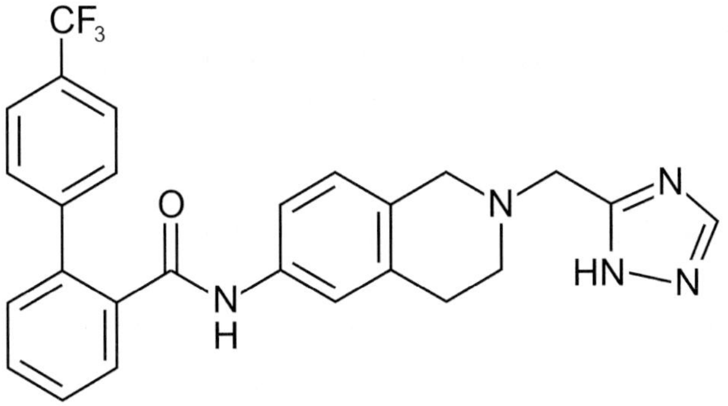

Fig. 3 Structure of the MTP inhibitor CP-346086 (Pfizer)

In rat hepatoma McArdle7777 cells and in primary rat hepatocytes a decrease in MTP activity by addition of the MTP inhibitor BMS-200150 (Bristol-Myers Squibb) leads to a proportional decrease in the secretion of apoB lipoproteins (Jamil et al. 1998). The inhibition of MTP activity in rat hepatoma McArdle7777 cells by BMS-197636 (Bristol-Myers Squibb) promotes both proteasomal and non-proteasomal degradation of apoB-100 (Cardozo et al. 2002). In HepG2-cells, the MTP inhibitor CP-10447 (Pfizer) leads to a specific reduction of apoB synthesis due to reduced rates of apoB elongation even in the presence of proteasomal inhibitors such as ALLN (Pan et al. 2000). Treatment of LDL receptor deficient mice with the MTP inhibitor 8aR (Novartis) for 7 days lowered plasma lipids to normal control values, while liver triglyceride levels were increased only about fourfold (Liao et al. 2003). Similarly, administration of the MTP inhibitor Implitapide (Bayer) to LDL receptor deficient WHHL rabbits decreased the plasma cholesterol and triglyceride levels by 70% and 45%, respectively, and the VLDL secretion rate by 80% (Shiomi and Ito 2001). Recently, the first report of the MTP inhibitor CP-346086 (Pfizer) in humans was made (Chandler et al. 2003) (Fig. 3). After 2 weeks of treatment, CP-346086 reduced plasma total and LDL cholesterol, and triglycerides by 47%, 72% and 75%, respectively, with little change in HDL cholesterol (Chandler et al. 2003). Significant toxicity was not observed in the healthy human volunteers, nor in experimental animals treated with CP-34086.

The most important side effect of MTP inhibitors is the increase of intestinal and hepatic triglyceride content, ultimately the induction of a fatty liver. The dosing of MTP inhibitors appears to be critical in this respect. In experimental animals, MTP inhibition by CP-34086 resulted in increases in both liver and intestinal triglyceride content when CP-34086 was administered in close temporal proximity to feeding. However, when dosed away from feeding, only hepatic triglycerides were increased (Chandler et al. 2003).

The pharmacological inhibition of MTP activity in the liver is a promising approach for the treatment of hyperlipidemia and arteriosclerosis, especially in patients with NIDDM and increased VLDL production. It is eagerly awaited whether or not any of the currently explored compounds will meet the expectations and can pass the necessary safety requirements to finally make it to the market.

4.2
Stimulation of Intracellular ApoB Degradation

The unique features of post-translational apoB proteolytic degradation offer targets for inhibition of the hepatic assembly and secretion of apoB lipoproteins. Most notably, the lipid lowering potential of some forms of fatty acids appears to be due to stimulation of presecretory degradation of apoB.

4.3
Nutritional Effects on Intracellular ApoB Degradation

4.3.1
Effects of Omega-3 Fatty Acids

Omega-3 fatty acids are associated with a lipid-lowering effect in vivo (Harris 1989) and with reduced rates of CVD (von Schacky 1999). Two specific omega-3 fatty acids, eicosapentaenoic acid (EPA, 20:5) and docosahexanoid acid (22:6) have been shown to stimulate the degradation of newly synthesized apoB by cultured rat hepatocytes and rat hepatoma McArdle7777 cells (Wang et al. 1993, 1994). Because omega-3 fatty acids can enhance the expression of the LDL receptor in hepatocytes, an enhanced LDL receptor-mediated re-uptake of secreted VLDL could explain this effects that is most pronounced for the most buoyant lipoproteins (Wang et al. 1993). In primary rat hepatocytes and rat hepatoma cells, however, EPA inhibited apoB secretion even when re-uptake was completely inhibited (Fisher et al. 2001). Inhibition of proteosomal degradation by lactocystin produced little if any inhibition of EPA-induced apoB degradation (Fisher et al. 2001). However, the specific PI3-K inhibitor wortmannin nearly completely inhibited EPA-induced apoB degradation (Fisher et al. 2001). These results establish that the treatment of hepatic cells with omega-3 fatty acids induces the degradation of newly synthesized apoB by a third pathway distinct from re-uptake or proteosomal degradation within in the ER (Fisher et al. 2001). On the contrary, saturated fatty acids such as myristic acid reduce the intracellular degradation of apoB and induce the secretion of dense apoB lipoproteins (Kummrow et al. 2002). For this type of apoB degradation the term 'post-ER presecretory proteolysis' (PERPP) has been proposed (Fisher et al. 2001). The protease and the potential signal transduction pathways involved in PERPP are currently unknown, but they represent excellent targets for pharmacological interventions. Most importantly, a diet that is rich in omega-3 fatty acids is a simple mode to reduce hepatic VLDL secretion.

4.3.2
Effects of PPARα on ApoB Secretion

PPARα has a central role in the regulation of hepatic lipid metabolism. Long-chain fatty acids are amongst the natural ligands for PPARα, and PPARα is also activated by the so-called peroxisome-proliferators, a group of compounds that includes the lipid-lowering fibrates (Schoonjans et al. 1996). The PPARα agonist WY14,643 (Chemsyn Co.) increased the secretion of apoB-100-containing lipoproteins from primary rat hepatocytes, and simultaneously decreased the biosynthesis of triglycerides (Linden et al. 2002). WY14,643 also increased the expression and biosynthesis of liver fatty acid-binding protein (LFABP), while transfected LFABP increased apoB-100 secretion, decreased triglyceride biosynthesis and increased PPARα mRNA (Linden et al. 2002). These findings indicate that PPARα and LFABP synergistically induce the hepatic synthesis of apoB lipoproteins. Thus, both PPARα and LFABP are potential targets for pharmacological interventions of hepatic lipoprotein synthesis and secretion. A partial antagonist of PPARα that reduces its stimulating effect on lipoprotein assembly while retaining its inhibitory effect on triglyceride biosynthesis would be an ideal substance to reduce hepatic VLDL secretion.

References

Adeli K, Macri J, Mohammadi A, Kito M, Urade R, Cavallo D (1997) Apolipoprotein B is intracellularly associated with an ER-60 protease homologue in HepG2 cells. J Biol Chem 272:22489–22494

Aguilar-Salinas CA, Barrett PH, Parhofer KG, Young SG, Tessereau D, Bateman J, Quinn C, Schonfeld G (1995) Apoprotein B-100 production is decreased in subjects heterozygous for truncations of apoprotein B. Arterioscler Thromb Vasc Biol 15:71–80

Ameen C, Oscarsson J (2003) Sex difference in hepatic microsomal triglyceride transfer protein expression is determined by the growth hormone secretory pattern in the rat. Endocrinology 144:3914–3921

Antes TJ, Goodart SA, Huynh C, Sullivan M, Young SG, Levy-Wilson B (2000) Identification and characterization of a 315-base pair enhancer, located more than 55 kilobases 5' of the apolipoprotein B gene, that confers expression in the intestine. J Biol Chem 275:26637–26648

Arakawa H, Hauschild J, Buerstedde JM (2002) Requirement of the activation-induced deaminase (AID) gene for immunoglobulin gene conversion. Science 295:1301–1306

Au WS, Kung HF, Lin MC (2003) Regulation of microsomal triglyceride transfer protein gene by insulin in HepG2 cells: roles of MAPKerk and MAPKp38. Diabetes 52:1073–1080

Bartels ED, Lauritsen M, Nielsen LB (2002) Hepatic expression of microsomal triglyceride transfer protein and in vivo secretion of triglyceride-rich lipoproteins are increased in obese diabetic mice. Diabetes 51:1233–1239

Baum CL, Teng BB, Davidson NO (1990) Apolipoprotein B messenger RNA editing in the rat liver. Modulation by fasting and refeeding a high carbohydrate diet. J Biol Chem 265:19263–19270

Bazzano LA, He J, Ogden LG, Loria CM, Vupputuri S, Myers L, Whelton PK (2002) Fruit and vegetable intake and risk of cardiovascular disease in US adults: the first National Health and Nutrition Examination Survey Epidemiologic Follow-up Study. Am J Clin Nutr 76:93–99

Benoist F, Grand-Perret T (1997) Co-translational degradation of apolipoprotein B100 by the proteasome is prevented by microsomal triglyceride transfer protein. Synchronized translation studies on HepG2 cells treated with an inhibitor of microsomal triglyceride transfer protein. J Biol Chem 272:20435–20442

Blackhart BD, Ludwig EM, Pierotti VR, Caiati L, Onasch MA, Wallis SC, Powell L, Pease R, Knott TJ, Chu ML, et al. (1986) Structure of the human apolipoprotein B gene. J Biol Chem 261:15364–15367

Blanc V, Henderson JO, Kennedy S, Davidson NO (2001a) Mutagenesis of apobec-1 complementation factor reveals distinct domains that modulate RNA binding, protein-protein interaction with apobec-1, and complementation of C to U RNA-editing activity. J Biol Chem 276:46386–46393

Blanc V, Kennedy S, Davidson NO (2003) A novel nuclear localization signal in the auxiliary domain of apobec-1 complementation factor regulates nucleocytoplasmic import and shuttling. J Biol Chem 278:41198–41204

Blanc V, Navaratnam N, Henderson JO, Anant S, Kennedy S, Jarmuz A, Scott J, Davidson NO (2001b) Identification of GRY-RBP as an apolipoprotein B RNA-binding protein that interacts with both apobec-1 and apobec-1 complementation factor to modulate C to U editing. J Biol Chem 276:10272–10283

Bok SH, Lee SH, Park YB, Bae KH, Son KH, Jeong TS, Choi MS (1999) Plasma and hepatic cholesterol and hepatic activities of 3-hydroxy-3-methyl-glutaryl-CoA reductase and acyl CoA: cholesterol transferase are lower in rats fed citrus peel extract or a mixture of citrus bioflavonoids. J Nutr 129:1182–1185

Borchardt RA, Davis RA (1987) Intrahepatic assembly of very low density lipoproteins. Rate of transport out of the endoplasmic reticulum determines rate of secretion. J Biol Chem 262:16394–16402

Boren J, Lee I, Zhu W, Arnold K, Taylor S, Innerarity TL (1998a) Identification of the low density lipoprotein receptor-binding site in apolipoprotein B100 and the modulation of its binding activity by the carboxyl terminus in familial defective apo-B100. J Clin Invest 101:1084–1093

Boren J, Olin K, Lee I, Chait A, Wight TN, Innerarity TL (1998b) Identification of the principal proteoglycan-binding site in LDL. A single-point mutation in apo-B100 severely affects proteoglycan interaction without affecting LDL receptor binding. J Clin Invest 101:2658–2664

Boren J, Rustaeus S, Olofsson SO (1994) Studies on the assembly of apolipoprotein B-100- and B-48-containing very low density lipoproteins in McA-RH7777 cells. J Biol Chem 269:25879–25888

Borradaile NM, de Dreu LE, Barrett PH, Behrsin CD, Huff MW (2003a) Hepatocyte apoB-containing lipoprotein secretion is decreased by the grapefruit flavonoid, naringenin, via inhibition of MTP-mediated microsomal triglyceride accumulation. Biochemistry 42:1283–1291

Borradaile NM, de Dreu LE, Barrett PH, Huff MW (2002a) Inhibition of hepatocyte apoB secretion by naringenin: enhanced rapid intracellular degradation independent of reduced microsomal cholesteryl esters. J Lipid Res 43:1544–1554

Borradaile NM, De Dreu LE, Huff MW (2003b) Inhibition of net HepG2 cell apolipoprotein b secretion by the citrus flavonoid naringenin involves activation of phosphatidylinositol 3-kinase, independent of insulin receptor substrate-1 phosphorylation. Diabetes 52:2554–2561

Borradaile NM, de Dreu LE, Wilcox LJ, Edwards JY, Huff MW (2002b) Soya phytoestrogens, genistein and daidzein, decrease apolipoprotein B secretion from HepG2 cells through multiple mechanisms. Biochem J 366:531–539

Bostrom K, Wettesten M, Boren J, Bondjers G, Wiklund O, Olofsson SO (1986) Pulse-chase studies of the synthesis and intracellular transport of apolipoprotein B-100 in Hep G2 cells. J Biol Chem 261:13800–13806

Bradbury P, Mann CJ, Kochl S, Anderson TA, Chester SA, Hancock JM, Ritchie PJ, Amey J, Harrison GB, Levitt DG, Banaszak LJ, Scott J, Shoulders CC (1999) A common binding site on the microsomal triglyceride transfer protein for apolipoprotein B and protein disulfide isomerase. J Biol Chem 274:3159–3164

Bransteitter R, Pham P, Scharff MD, Goodman MF (2003) Activation-induced cytidine deaminase deaminates deoxycytidine on single-stranded DNA but requires the action of RNase. Proc Natl Acad Sci USA 100:4102–4107

Brown MS, Goldstein JL (1986) A receptor-mediated pathway for cholesterol homeostasis. Science 232:34–47

Brunner C, Kraft HG, Utermann G, Muller HJ (1993) Cys4057 of apolipoprotein(a) is essential for lipoprotein(a) assembly. Proc Natl Acad Sci USA 90:11643–11647

Brunzell JD, Hokanson JE (1999) Dyslipidemia of central obesity and insulin resistance. Diabetes Care 22 Suppl 3: C10–C13

Cardozo C, Wu X, Pan M, Wang H, Fisher EA (2002) The inhibition of microsomal triglyceride transfer protein activity in rat hepatoma cells promotes proteasomal and nonproteasomal degradation of apoprotein b100. Biochemistry 41:10105–10114

Carpentier A, Taghibiglou C, Leung N, Szeto L, Van Iderstine SC, Uffelman KD, Buckingham R, Adeli K, Lewis GF (2002) Ameliorated hepatic insulin resistance is associated with normalization of microsomal triglyceride transfer protein expression and reduction in very low density lipoprotein assembly and secretion in the fructose-fed hamster. J Biol Chem 277:28795–28802

Cartwright IJ, Plonne D, Higgins JA (2000) Intracellular events in the assembly of chylomicrons in rabbit enterocytes. J Lipid Res 41:1728–1739

Chandler CE, Wilder DE, Pettini JL, Savoy YE, Petras SF, Chang G, Vincent J, Harwood HJ, Jr. (2003) CP-346086: an MTP inhibitor that lowers plasma cholesterol and triglycerides in experimental animals and in humans. J Lipid Res 44:1887–1901

Chang BH, Liao W, Li L, Nakamuta M, Mack D, Chan L (1999) Liver-specific inactivation of the abetalipoproteinemia gene completely abrogates very low density lipoprotein/low density lipoprotein production in a viable conditional knockout mouse. J Biol Chem 274:6051–6055

Chen SH, Habib G, Yang CY, Gu ZW, Lee BR, Weng SA, Silberman SR, Cai SJ, Deslypere JP, Rosseneu M, et al. (1987) Apolipoprotein B-48 is the product of a messenger RNA with an organ-specific in-frame stop codon. Science 238:363–366

Chen X, Sparks JD, Yao Z, Fisher EA (1993) Hepatic polysomes that contain apoprotein B mRNA have unusual physical properties. J Biol Chem 268:21007–21013

Chen Y, Le Caherec F, Chuck SL (1998) Calnexin and other factors that alter translocation affect the rapid binding of ubiquitin to apoB in the Sec61 complex. J Biol Chem 273:11887–11894

Chester A, Somasekaram A, Tzimina M, Jarmuz A, Gisbourne J, O'Keefe R, Scott J, Navarat-
    nam N (2003) The apolipoprotein B mRNA editing complex performs a multifunctional
    cycle and suppresses nonsense-mediated decay. EMBO J 22:3971–3982
Choi JS, Yokozawa T, Oura H (1991) Antihyperlipidemic effect of flavonoids from Prunus
    davidiana. J Nat Prod 54:218–224
Chuck SL, Yao Z, Blackhart BD, McCarthy BJ, Lingappa VR (1990) New variation on the
    translocation of proteins during early biogenesis of apolipoprotein B. Nature 346:382–
    385
Collins HL, Sparks CE, Sparks JD (2000) B48 is preferentially translated over B100 in cells
    with increased endogenous apoB mRNA. Biochem Biophys Res Commun 273:1156–1160
Dannoura AH, Berriot-Varoqueaux N, Amati P, Abadie V, Verthier N, Schmitz J, Wetterau JR,
    Samson-Bouma ME, Aggerbeck LP (1999) Anderson's disease: exclusion of apolipopro-
    tein and intracellular lipid transport genes. Arterioscler Thromb Vasc Biol 19:2494–2508
Davidson NO, Powell LM, Wallis SC, Scott J (1988) Thyroid hormone modulates the in-
    troduction of a stop codon in rat liver apolipoprotein B messenger RNA. J Biol Chem
    263:13482–13485
Davidson NO, Shelness GS (2000) APOLIPOPROTEIN B: mRNA editing, lipoprotein assem-
    bly, and presecretory degradation. Annu Rev Nutr 20:169–193
Davis RA, Hui TY (2001) 2000 George Lyman Duff Memorial Lecture: atherosclerosis is
    a liver disease of the heart. Arterioscler Thromb Vasc Biol 21:887–898
Davis RA, Thrift RN, Wu CC, Howell KE (1990) Apolipoprotein B is both integrated into and
    translocated across the endoplasmic reticulum membrane. Evidence for two functionally
    distinct pools. J Biol Chem 265:10005–10011
Demmer LA, Levin MS, Elovson J, Reuben MA, Lusis AJ, Gordon JI (1986) Tissue-specific
    expression and developmental regulation of the rat apolipoprotein B gene. Proc Natl
    Acad Sci USA 83:8102–8106
Di Noia J, Neuberger MS (2002) Altering the pathway of immunoglobulin hypermutation
    by inhibiting uracil-DNA glycosylase. Nature 419:43–48
Dickerson SK, Market E, Besmer E, Papavasiliou FN (2003) AID mediates hypermutation
    by deaminating single stranded DNA. J Exp Med 197:1291–1296
Elam MB, Wilcox HG, Solomon SS, Heimberg M (1992) In vivo growth hormone treatment
    stimulates secretion of very low density lipoprotein by the isolated perfused rat liver.
    Endocrinology 131:2717–2722
Ellgaard L, Molinari M, Helenius A (1999) Setting the standards: quality control in the
    secretory pathway. Science 286:1882–1888
Fisher EA, Ginsberg HN (2002) Complexity in the secretory pathway: the assembly and
    secretion of apolipoprotein B-containing lipoproteins. J Biol Chem 277:17377–17380
Fisher EA, Pan M, Chen X, Wu X, Wang H, Jamil H, Sparks JD, Williams KJ (2001) The triple
    threat to nascent apolipoprotein B. Evidence for multiple, distinct degradative pathways.
    J Biol Chem 276:27855–27863
Fisher EA, Zhou M, Mitchell DM, Wu X, Omura S, Wang H, Goldberg AL, Ginsberg HN
    (1997) The degradation of apolipoprotein B100 is mediated by the ubiquitin-proteasome
    pathway and involves heat shock protein 70. J Biol Chem 272:20427–20434
Fleming JF, Spitsen GM, Hui TY, Olivier L, Du EZ, Raabe M, Davis RA (1999) Chinese
    hamster ovary cells require the coexpression of microsomal triglyceride transfer protein
    and cholesterol 7alpha-hydroxylase for the assembly and secretion of apolipoprotein
    B-containing lipoproteins. J Biol Chem 274:9509–9514
Fujino T, Navaratnam N, Scott J (1998) Human apolipoprotein B RNA editing deaminase
    gene (APOBEC1). Genomics 47:266–275

Funahashi T, Giannoni F, DePaoli AM, Skarosi SF, Davidson NO (1995) Tissue-specific, developmental and nutritional regulation of the gene encoding the catalytic subunit of the rat apolipoprotein B mRNA editing enzyme: functional role in the modulation of apoB mRNA editing. J Lipid Res 36:414–428

Furukawa S, Sakata N, Ginsberg HN, Dixon JL (1992) Studies of the sites of intracellular degradation of apolipoprotein B in Hep G2 cells. J Biol Chem 267:22630–22638

Giannoni F, Bonen DK, Funahashi T, Hadjiagapiou C, Burant CF, Davidson NO (1994) Complementation of apolipoprotein B mRNA editing by human liver accompanied by secretion of apolipoprotein B48. J Biol Chem 269:5932–5936

Gillian-Daniel DL, Bates PW, Tebon A, Attie AD (2002) Endoplasmic reticulum localization of the low density lipoprotein receptor mediates presecretory degradation of apolipoprotein B. Proc Natl Acad Sci USA 99:4337–4342

Ginsberg HN (2000) Insulin resistance and cardiovascular disease. J Clin Invest 106:453–458

Glass CK, Witztum JL (2001) Atherosclerosis. the road ahead. Cell 104:503–516

Greeve J, Altkemper I, Dieterich JH, Greten H, Windler E (1993) Apolipoprotein B mRNA editing in 12 different mammalian species: hepatic expression is reflected in low concentrations of apoB-containing plasma lipoproteins. J Lipid Res 34:1367–1383

Greeve J, Axelos D, Welker S, Schipper M, Greten H (1998) Distinct promoters induce APOBEC-1 expression in rat liver and intestine. Arterioscler Thromb Vasc Biol 18:1079–1092

Greeve J, Chowdhury JR, Chowdhury NR (1996a) Induction of hepatic apolipoprotein B mRNA editing for reducing serum cholesterol levels: a breakthrough or a disaster? Hepatology 24:964–966

Greeve J, Jona VK, Chowdhury NR, Horwitz MS, Chowdhury JR (1996b) Hepatic gene transfer of the catalytic subunit of the apolipoprotein B mRNA editing enzyme results in a reduction of plasma LDL levels in normal and watanabe heritable hyperlipidemic rabbits. J Lipid Res 37:2001–2017

Greeve J, Navaratnam N, Scott J (1991) Characterization of the apolipoprotein B mRNA editing enzyme: no similarity to the proposed mechanism of RNA editing in kinetoplastid protozoa. Nucl Acids Res 19:3569–3576

Greeve J, Philipsen A, Krause K, Klapper W, Heidorn K, Castle BE, Janda J, Marcu KB, Parwaresch R (2003) Expression of activation-induced cytidine deaminase in human B-cell non-Hodgkin lymphomas. Blood 101:3574–3580

Gusarova V, Brodsky JL, Fisher EA (2003) Apolipoprotein B100 exit from the ER is COPII dependent and its lipidation to very low density lipoprotein occurs post-ER. J Biol Chem

Gusarova V, Caplan AJ, Brodsky JL, Fisher EA (2001) Apoprotein B degradation is promoted by the molecular chaperones hsp90 and hsp70. J Biol Chem 276:24891–24900

Hagan DL, Kienzle B, Jamil H, Hariharan N (1994) Transcriptional regulation of human and hamster microsomal triglyceride transfer protein genes. Cell type-specific expression and response to metabolic regulators. J Biol Chem 269:28737–28744

Hardman DA, Pullinger CR, Hamilton RL, Kane JP, Malloy MJ (1991) Molecular and metabolic basis for the metabolic disorder normotriglyceridemic abetalipoproteinemia. J Clin Invest 88:1722–1729

Harris RS, Bishop KN, Sheehy AM, Craig HM, Petersen-Mahrt SK, Watt IN, Neuberger MS, Malim MH (2003a) DNA deamination mediates innate immunity to retroviral infection. Cell 113:803–809

Harris RS, Petersen-Mahrt SK, Neuberger MS (2002a) RNA editing enzyme APOBEC1 and some of its homologs can act as DNA mutators. Mol Cell 10:1247–1253

Harris RS, Sale JE, Petersen-Mahrt SK, Neuberger MS (2002b) AID is essential for immunoglobulin V gene conversion in a cultured B cell line. Curr Biol 12:435–438

Harris RS, Sheehy AM, Craig HM, Malim MH, Neuberger MS (2003b) DNA deamination: not just a trigger for antibody diversification but also a mechanism for defense against retroviruses. Nat Immunol 4:641–643

Harris WS (1989) Fish oils and plasma lipid and lipoprotein metabolism in humans: a critical review. J Lipid Res 30:785–807

Hebbachi AM, Brown AM, Gibbons GF (1999) Suppression of cytosolic triacylglycerol recruitment for very low density lipoprotein assembly by inactivation of microsomal triglyceride transfer protein results in a delayed removal of apoB-48 and apoB-100 from microsomal and Golgi membranes of primary rat hepatocytes. J Lipid Res 40:1758–1768

Hegde RS, Lingappa VR (1996) Sequence-specific alteration of the ribosome-membrane junction exposes nascent secretory proteins to the cytosol. Cell 85:217–228

Hersberger M, Innerarity TL (1998) Two efficiency elements flanking the editing site of cytidine 6666 in the apolipoprotein B mRNA support mooring-dependent editing. J Biol Chem 273:9435–9442

Hersberger M, Patarroyo-White S, Arnold KS, Innerarity TL (1999) Phylogenetic analysis of the apolipoprotein B mRNA-editing region. Evidence for a secondary structure between the mooring sequence and the 3' efficiency element. J Biol Chem 274:34590–34597

Herz J, Willnow TE (1995) Lipoprotein and receptor interactions in vivo. Curr Opin Lipidol 6:97–103

Hirano K, Min J, Funahashi T, Davidson NO (1997) Cloning and characterization of the rat apobec-1 gene: a comparative analysis of gene structure and promoter usage in rat and mouse. J Lipid Res 38:1103–1119

Hirano K, Young SG, Farese RV, Jr., Ng J, Sande E, Warburton C, Powell-Braxton LM, Davidson NO (1996) Targeted disruption of the mouse apobec-1 gene abolishes apolipoprotein B mRNA editing and eliminates apolipoprotein B48. J Biol Chem 271:9887–9890

Hodges PE, Navaratnam N, Greeve JC, Scott J (1991) Site-specific creation of uridine from cytidine in apolipoprotein B mRNA editing. Nucl Acids Res 19:1197–1201

Huff MW, Burnett JR (1997) 3-Hydroxy-3-methylglutaryl coenzyme A reductase inhibitors and hepatic apolipoprotein B secretion. Curr Opin Lipidol 8:138–145

Hussain MM, Bakillah A, Nayak N, Shelness GS (1998) Amino acids 430–570 in apolipoprotein B are critical for its binding to microsomal triglyceride transfer protein. J Biol Chem 273:25612–25615

Innerarity TL, Weisgraber KH, Arnold KS, Mahley RW, Krauss RM, Vega GL, Grundy SM (1987) Familial defective apolipoprotein B-100: low density lipoproteins with abnormal receptor binding. Proc Natl Acad Sci USA 84:6919–6923

Jamil H, Chu CH, Dickson JK, Jr., Chen Y, Yan M, Biller SA, Gregg RE, Wetterau JR, Gordon DA (1998) Evidence that microsomal triglyceride transfer protein is limiting in the production of apolipoprotein B-containing lipoproteins in hepatic cells. J Lipid Res 39:1448–1454

Jarmuz A, Chester A, Bayliss J, Gisbourne J, Dunham I, Scott J, Navaratnam N (2002) An anthropoid-specific locus of orphan C to U RNA-editing enzymes on chromosome 22. Genomics 79:285–296

Johnson DF, Poksay KS, Innerarity TL (1993) The mechanism for apo-B mRNA editing is deamination. Biochem Biophys Res Commun 195:1204–1210

Jones B, Jones EL, Bonney SA, Patel HN, Mensenkamp AR, Eichenbaum-Voline S, Rudling M, Myrdal U, Annesi G, Naik S, Meadows N, Quattrone A, Islam SA, Naoumova RP, Angelin B, Infante R, Levy E, Roy CC, Freemont PS, Scott J, Shoulders CC (2003) Mutations in a Sar1 GTPase of COPII vesicles are associated with lipid absorption disorders. Nat Genet 34:29–31

Kane JP (1983) Apolipoprotein B: structural and metabolic heterogeneity. Annu Rev Physiol 45:637–650

Kim E, Cham CM, Veniant MM, Ambroziak P, Young SG (1998) Dual mechanisms for the low plasma levels of truncated apolipoprotein B proteins in familial hypobetalipoproteinemia. Analysis of a new mouse model with a nonsense mutation in the Apob gene. J Clin Invest 101:1468–1477

Knott TJ, Pease RJ, Powell LM, Wallis SC, Rall SC, Jr., Innerarity TL, Blackhart B, Taylor WH, Marcel Y, Milne R, et al. (1986) Complete protein sequence and identification of structural domains of human apolipoprotein B. Nature 323:734–738

Kozarsky KF, Bonen DK, Giannoni F, Funahashi T, Wilson JM, Davidson NO (1996) Hepatic expression of the catalytic subunit of the apolipoprotein B mRNA editing enzyme (apobec-1) ameliorates hypercholesterolemia in LDL receptor-deficient rabbits. Hum Gene Ther 7:943–957

Kummrow E, Hussain MM, Pan M, Marsh JB, Fisher EA (2002) Myristic acid increases dense lipoprotein secretion by inhibiting apoB degradation and triglyceride recruitment. J Lipid Res 43:2155–2163

Kuriyama H, Yamashita S, Shimomura I, Funahashi T, Ishigami M, Aragane K, Miyaoka K, Nakamura T, Takemura K, Man Z, Toide K, Nakayama N, Fukuda Y, Lin MC, Wetterau JR, Matsuzawa Y (1998) Enhanced expression of hepatic acyl-coenzyme A synthetase and microsomal triglyceride transfer protein messenger RNAs in the obese and hypertriglyceridemic rat with visceral fat accumulation. Hepatology 27:557–562

Kurowska EM, Spence JD, Jordan J, Wetmore S, Freeman DJ, Piche LA, Serratore P (2000) HDL-cholesterol-raising effect of orange juice in subjects with hypercholesterolemia. Am J Clin Nutr 72:1095–1100

Lau PP, Cahill DJ, Zhu HJ, Chan L (1995) Ethanol modulates apolipoprotein B mRNA editing in the rat. J Lipid Res 36:2069–2078

Lau PP, Xiong WJ, Zhu HJ, Chen SH, Chan L (1991) Apolipoprotein B mRNA editing is an intranuclear event that occurs posttranscriptionally coincident with splicing and polyadenylation. J Biol Chem 266:20550–20554

Lau PP, Zhu HJ, Baldini A, Charnsangavej C, Chan L (1994) Dimeric structure of a human apolipoprotein B mRNA editing protein and cloning and chromosomal localization of its gene. Proc Natl Acad Sci USA 91:8522–8526

Lee CH, Jeong TS, Choi YK, Hyun BH, Oh GT, Kim EH, Kim JR, Han JI, Bok SH (2001) Anti-atherogenic effect of citrus flavonoids, naringin and naringenin, associated with hepatic ACAT and aortic VCAM-1 and MCP-1 in high cholesterol-fed rabbits. Biochem Biophys Res Commun 284:681–688

Lee CH, Olson P, Evans RM (2003a) Minireview: lipid metabolism, metabolic diseases, and peroxisome proliferator-activated receptors. Endocrinology 144:2201–2207

Lee MK, Moon SS, Lee SE, Bok SH, Jeong TS, Park YB, Choi MS (2003b) Naringenin 7-O-cetyl ether as inhibitor of HMG-CoA reductase and modulator of plasma and hepatic lipids in high cholesterol-fed rats. Bioorg Med Chem 11:393–398

Leighton JK, Joyner J, Zamarripa J, Deines M, Davis RA (1990) Fasting decreases apolipoprotein B mRNA editing and the secretion of small molecular weight apoB by rat hepatocytes: evidence that the total amount of apoB secreted is regulated post-transcriptionally. J Lipid Res 31:1663–1668

Lellek H, Kirsten R, Diehl I, Apostel F, Buck F, Greeve J (2000) Purification and molecular cloning of a novel essential component of the apolipoprotein B mRNA editing enzyme-complex. J Biol Chem 275:19848–19856

Lellek H, Welker S, Diehl I, Kirsten R, Greeve J (2002) Reconstitution of mRNA editing in yeast using a Gal4-apoB-Gal80 fusion transcript as the selectable marker. J Biol Chem 277:23638–23644

Leung GK, Veniant MM, Kim SK, Zlot CH, Raabe M, Bjorkegren J, Neese RA, Hellerstein MK, Young SG (2000) A deficiency of microsomal triglyceride transfer protein reduces apolipoprotein B secretion. J Biol Chem 275:7515–7520

Levine GN, Keaney JF, Jr., Vita JA (1995) Cholesterol reduction in cardiovascular disease. Clinical benefits and possible mechanisms. N Engl J Med 332:512–521

Levy-Wilson B, Paulweber B, Antes TJ, Goodart SA, Lee SY (2000) An open chromatin structure in a liver-specific enhancer that confers high level expression to human apolipoprotein b transgenes in mice. Mol Cell Biol Res Commun 4:206–211

Levy-Wilson B, Paulweber B, Nagy BP, Ludwig EH, Brooks AR (1992) Nuclease-hypersensitive sites define a region with enhancer activity in the third intron of the human apolipoprotein B gene. J Biol Chem 267:18735–18743

Liang J, Ginsberg HN (2001) Microsomal triglyceride transfer protein binding and lipid transfer activities are independent of each other, but both are required for secretion of apolipoprotein B lipoproteins from liver cells. J Biol Chem 276:28606–28612

Liang J, Wu X, Jiang H, Zhou M, Yang H, Angkeow P, Huang LS, Sturley SL, Ginsberg H (1998) Translocation efficiency, susceptibility to proteasomal degradation, and lipid responsiveness of apolipoprotein B are determined by the presence of beta sheet domains. J Biol Chem 273:35216–35221

Liang JS, Kim T, Fang S, Yamaguchi J, Weissman AM, Fisher EA, Ginsberg HN (2003) Overexpression of the tumor autocrine motility factor receptor Gp78, a ubiquitin protein ligase, results in increased ubiquitinylation and decreased secretion of apolipoprotein B100 in HepG2 cells. J Biol Chem 278:23984–23988

Liang S, Wu X, Fisher EA, Ginsberg HN (2000) The amino-terminal domain of apolipoprotein B does not undergo retrograde translocation from the endoplasmic reticulum to the cytosol. Proteasomal degradation of nascent apolipoprotein B begins at the carboxyl terminus of the protein, while apolipoprotein B is still in its original translocon. J Biol Chem 275:32003–32010

Liao S, Lin J, Do H, Johnson AE (1997) Both lumenal and cytosolic gating of the aqueous ER translocon pore are regulated from inside the ribosome during membrane protein integration. Cell 90:31–41

Liao W, Chang BH, Mancini M, Chan L (2003a) Ubiquitin-dependent and -independent proteasomal degradation of apoB associated with endoplasmic reticulum and Golgi apparatus, respectively, in HepG2 cells. J Cell Biochem 89:1019–1029

Liao W, Hong SH, Chan BH, Rudolph FB, Clark SC, Chan L (1999a) APOBEC-2, a cardiac- and skeletal muscle-specific member of the cytidine deaminase supergene family. Biochem Biophys Res Commun 260:398–404

Liao W, Hui TY, Young SG, Davis RA (2003b) Blocking microsomal triglyceride transfer protein interferes with apoB secretion without causing retention or stress in the ER. J Lipid Res 44:978–985

Liao W, Kobayashi K, Chan L (1999b) Adenovirus-mediated overexpression of microsomal triglyceride transfer protein (MTP): mechanistic studies on the role of MTP in apolipoprotein B-100 biogenesis. Biochemistry 38:10215

Liao W, Yeung SC, Chan L (1998) Proteasome-mediated degradation of apolipoprotein B targets both nascent peptides cotranslationally before translocation and full-length apolipoprotein B after translocation into the endoplasmic reticulum. J Biol Chem 273:27225–27230

Lieu HD, Withycombe SK, Walker Q, Rong JX, Walzem RL, Wong JS, Hamilton RL, Fisher EA, Young SG (2003) Eliminating atherogenesis in mice by switching off hepatic lipoprotein secretion. Circulation 107:1315–1321

Lin MC, Arbeeny C, Bergquist K, Kienzle B, Gordon DA, Wetterau JR (1994) Cloning and regulation of hamster microsomal triglyceride transfer protein. The regulation is independent from that of other hepatic and intestinal proteins which participate in the transport of fatty acids and triglycerides. J Biol Chem 269:29138–29145

Lin MC, Gordon D, Wetterau JR (1995) Microsomal triglyceride transfer protein (MTP) regulation in HepG2 cells: insulin negatively regulates MTP gene expression. J Lipid Res 36:1073–1081

Linden D, Lindberg K, Oscarsson J, Claesson C, Asp L, Li L, Gustafsson M, Boren J, Olofsson SO (2002) Influence of peroxisome proliferator-activated receptor alpha agonists on the intracellular turnover and secretion of apolipoprotein (Apo) B-100 and ApoB-48. J Biol Chem 277:23044–23053

Linden D, Sjoberg A, Asp L, Carlsson L, Oscarsson J (2000) Direct effects of growth hormone on production and secretion of apolipoprotein B from rat hepatocytes. Am J Physiol Endocrinol Metab 279: E1335–E1346

Linnik KM, Herscovitz H (1998) Multiple molecular chaperones interact with apolipoprotein B during its maturation. The network of endoplasmic reticulum-resident chaperones (ERp72, GRP94, calreticulin, and BiP) interacts with apolipoprotein b regardless of its lipidation state. J Biol Chem 273:21368–21373

Linton MF, Farese RV, Jr., Young SG (1993) Familial hypobetalipoproteinemia. J Lipid Res 34:521–541

Mangeat B, Turelli P, Caron G, Friedli M, Perrin L, Trono D (2003) Broad antiretroviral defence by human APOBEC3G through lethal editing of nascent reverse transcripts. Nature 424:99–103

Marcovina SM, Koschinsky ML, Albers JJ, Skarlatos S (2003) Report of the National Heart, Lung, and Blood Institute Workshop on Lipoprotein(a) and Cardiovascular Disease: Recent Advances and Future Directions. Clin Chem 49:1785–1796

Mariani R, Chen D, Schrofelbauer B, Navarro F, Konig R, Bollman B, Munk C, Nymark-McMahon H, Landau NR (2003) Species-specific exclusion of APOBEC3G from HIV-1 virions by Vif. Cell 114:21–31

Marin M, Rose KM, Kozak SL, Kabat D (2003) HIV-1 Vif protein binds the editing enzyme APOBEC3G and induces its degradation. Nat Med

McLean JW, Tomlinson JE, Kuang WJ, Eaton DL, Chen EY, Fless GM, Scanu AM, Lawn RM (1987) cDNA sequence of human apolipoprotein(a) is homologous to plasminogen. Nature 330:132–137

Mehta A, Driscoll DM (2002) Identification of domains in apobec-1 complementation factor required for RNA binding and apolipoprotein-B mRNA editing. RNA 8:69–82

Mehta A, Kinter MT, Sherman NE, Driscoll DM (2000) Molecular cloning of apobec-1 complementation factor, a novel RNA-binding protein involved in the editing of apolipoprotein B mRNA. Mol Cell Biol 20:1846–1854

Millar JS, Maugeais C, Fuki IV, Rader DJ (2002) Normal production rate of apolipoprotein B in LDL receptor-deficient mice. Arterioscler Thromb Vasc Biol 22:989–994

Mitchell DM, Zhou M, Pariyarath R, Wang H, Aitchison JD, Ginsberg HN, Fisher EA (1998) Apoprotein B100 has a prolonged interaction with the translocon during which its lipidation and translocation change from dependence on the microsomal triglyceride transfer protein to independence. Proc Natl Acad Sci USA 95:14733–14738

Monforte MT, Trovato A, Kirjavainen S, Forestieri AM, Galati EM, Lo Curto RB (1995)
    Biological effects of hesperidin, a Citrus flavonoid. (note II): hypolipidemic activity on
    experimental hypercholesterolemia in rat. Farmaco 50:595–599

Morrison JR, Paszty C, Stevens ME, Hughes SD, Forte T, Scott J, Rubin EM (1996) Apolipopro-
    tein B RNA editing enzyme-deficient mice are viable despite alterations in lipoprotein
    metabolism. Proc Natl Acad Sci USA 93:7154–7159

Muramatsu M, Kinoshita K, Fagarasan S, Yamada S, Shinkai Y, Honjo T (2000) Class
    switch recombination and hypermutation require activation-induced cytidine deam-
    inase (AID), a potential RNA editing enzyme. Cell 102:553–563

Muramatsu M, Sankaranand VS, Anant S, Sugai M, Kinoshita K, Davidson NO, Honjo
    T (1999) Specific expression of activation-induced cytidine deaminase (AID), a novel
    member of the RNA-editing deaminase family in germinal center B cells. J Biol Chem
    274:18470–18476

Nakamuta M, Chang BH, Hoogeveen R, Li WH, Chan L (1996a) Mouse microsomal triglyc-
    eride transfer protein large subunit: cDNA cloning, tissue-specific expression and chro-
    mosomal localization. Genomics 33:313–316

Nakamuta M, Chang BH, Zsigmond E, Kobayashi K, Lei H, Ishida BY, Oka K, Li E, Chan L
    (1996b) Complete phenotypic characterization of apobec-1 knockout mice with a wild-
    type genetic background and a human apolipoprotein B transgenic background, and
    restoration of apolipoprotein B mRNA editing by somatic gene transfer of Apobec-1.
    J Biol Chem 271:25981–25988

Nakamuta M, Oka K, Krushkal J, Kobayashi K, Yamamoto M, Li WH, Chan L (1995) Al-
    ternative mRNA splicing and differential promoter utilization determine tissue-specific
    expression of the apolipoprotein B mRNA-editing protein (Apobec1) gene in mice. Struc-
    ture and evolution of Apobec1 and related nucleoside/nucleotide deaminases. J Biol
    Chem 270:13042–13056

Navaratnam N, Bhattacharya S, Fujino T, Patel D, Jarmuz AL, Scott J (1995) Evolutionary
    origins of apoB mRNA editing: catalysis by a cytidine deaminase that has acquired
    a novel RNA-binding motif at its active site. Cell 81:187–195

Navaratnam N, Fujino T, Bayliss J, Jarmuz A, How A, Richardson N, Somasekaram A,
    Bhattacharya S, Carter C, Scott J (1998) Escherichia coli cytidine deaminase provides
    a molecular model for ApoB RNA editing and a mechanism for RNA substrate recogni-
    tion. J Mol Biol 275:695–714

Navaratnam N, Morrison JR, Bhattacharya S, Patel D, Funahashi T, Giannoni F, Teng BB,
    Davidson NO, Scott J (1993) The p27 catalytic subunit of the apolipoprotein B mRNA
    editing enzyme is a cytidine deaminase. J Biol Chem 268:20709–20712

Okazaki I, Yoshikawa K, Kinoshita K, Muramatsu M, Nagaoka H, Honjo T (2003a) Activation-
    induced cytidine deaminase links class switch recombination and somatic hypermuta-
    tion. Ann NY Acad Sci 987:1-8

Okazaki IM, Hiai H, Kakazu N, Yamada S, Muramatsu M, Kinoshita K, Honjo T (2003b)
    Constitutive expression of AID leads to tumorigenesis. J Exp Med 197:1173–1181

Olofsson SO, Asp L, Boren J (1999) The assembly and secretion of apolipoprotein B-
    containing lipoproteins. Curr Opin Lipidol 10:341–346

Packard CJ, Third JL, Shepherd J, Lorimer AR, Morgan HG, Lawrie TD (1976) Low density
    lipoprotein metabolism in a family of familial hypercholesterolemic patients. Metabolism
    25:995–1006

Pan M, Liang J, Fisher EA, Ginsberg HN (2000) Inhibition of translocation of nascent
    apolipoprotein B across the endoplasmic reticulum membrane is associated with selec-
    tive inhibition of the synthesis of apolipoprotein B. J Biol Chem 275:27399–27405

Pan M, Liang Js JS, Fisher EA, Ginsberg HN (2002) The late addition of core lipids to nascent apolipoprotein B100, resulting in the assembly and secretion of triglyceride-rich lipoproteins, is independent of both microsomal triglyceride transfer protein activity and new triglyceride synthesis. J Biol Chem 277:4413–4421

Parhofer KG, Barrett PH, Bier DM, Schonfeld G (1992) Lipoproteins containing the truncated apolipoprotein, ApoB-89, are cleared from human plasma more rapidly than ApoB-100-containing lipoproteins in vivo. J Clin Invest 89:1931–1937

Parhofer KG, Daugherty A, Kinoshita M, Schonfeld G (1990) Enhanced clearance from plasma of low density lipoproteins containing a truncated apolipoprotein, apoB-89. J Lipid Res 31:2001–2007

Pariyarath R, Wang H, Aitchison JD, Ginsberg HN, Welch WJ, Johnson AE, Fisher EA (2001) Co-translational interactions of apoprotein B with the ribosome and translocon during lipoprotein assembly or targeting to the proteasome. J Biol Chem 276:541–550

Patel SB, Grundy SM (1996) Interactions between microsomal triglyceride transfer protein and apolipoprotein B within the endoplasmic reticulum in a heterologous expression system. J Biol Chem 271:18686–18694

Patterson AP, Chen Z, Rubin DC, Moucadel V, Iovanna JL, Brewer HB, Jr., Eggerman TL (2003) Developmental regulation of apolipoprotein B mRNA editing is an autonomous function of small intestine involving homeobox gene Cdx1. J Biol Chem 278:7600–7606

Patterson AP, Tennyson GE, Hoeg JM, Sviridov DD, Brewer HB, Jr. (1992) Ontogenetic regulation of apolipoprotein B mRNA editing during human and rat development in vivo. Arterioscler Thromb 12:468–473

Pease RJ, Harrison GB, Scott J (1991) Cotranslocational insertion of apolipoprotein B into the inner leaflet of the endoplasmic reticulum. Nature 353:448–450

Petersen-Mahrt SK, Harris RS, Neuberger MS (2002) AID mutates E. coli suggesting a DNA deamination mechanism for antibody diversification. Nature 418:99–103

Petersen-Mahrt SK, Neuberger MS (2003) In vitro deamination of cytosine to uracil in single-stranded DNA by apolipoprotein B editing complex catalytic subunit 1 (APOBEC1). J Biol Chem 278:19583–19586

Pham P, Bransteitter R, Petruska J, Goodman MF (2003) Processive AID-catalysed cytosine deamination on single-stranded DNA simulates somatic hypermutation. Nature 424:103–107

Phung TL, Roncone A, Jensen KL, Sparks CE, Sparks JD (1997) Phosphoinositide 3-kinase activity is necessary for insulin-dependent inhibition of apolipoprotein B secretion by rat hepatocytes and localizes to the endoplasmic reticulum. J Biol Chem 272:30693–30702

Powell LM, Wallis SC, Pease RJ, Edwards YH, Knott TJ, Scott J (1987) A novel form of tissue-specific RNA processing produces apolipoprotein-B48 in intestine. Cell 50:831–840

Powell-Braxton L, Veniant M, Latvala RD, Hirano KI, Won WB, Ross J, Dybdal N, Zlot CH, Young SG, Davidson NO (1998) A mouse model of human familial hypercholesterolemia: markedly elevated low density lipoprotein cholesterol levels and severe atherosclerosis on a low-fat chow diet. Nat Med 4:934–938

Pullinger CR, North JD, Teng BB, Rifici VA, Ronhild de Brito AE, Scott J (1989) The apolipoprotein B gene is constitutively expressed in HepG2 cells: regulation of secretion by oleic acid, albumin, and insulin, and measurement of the mRNA half-life. J Lipid Res 30:1065–1077

Qian X, Balestra ME, Innerarity TL (1997) Two distinct TATA-less promoters direct tissue-specific expression of the rat apo-B editing catalytic polypeptide 1 gene. J Biol Chem 272:18060–18070

Qian X, Balestra ME, Yamanaka S, Boren J, Lee I, Innerarity TL (1998) Low expression of the apolipoprotein B mRNA-editing transgene in mice reduces LDL levels but does not cause liver dysplasia or tumors. Arterioscler Thromb Vasc Biol 18:1013–1020

Raabe M, Flynn LM, Zlot CH, Wong JS, Veniant MM, Hamilton RL, Young SG (1998) Knockout of the abetalipoproteinemia gene in mice: reduced lipoprotein secretion in heterozygotes and embryonic lethality in homozygotes. Proc Natl Acad Sci USA 95:8686–8691

Raabe M, Veniant MM, Sullivan MA, Zlot CH, Bjorkegren J, Nielsen LB, Wong JS, Hamilton RL, Young SG (1999) Analysis of the role of microsomal triglyceride transfer protein in the liver of tissue-specific knockout mice. J Clin Invest 103:1287–1298

Rada C, Williams GT, Nilsen H, Barnes DE, Lindahl T, Neuberger MS (2002) Immunoglobulin isotype switching is inhibited and somatic hypermutation perturbed in UNG-deficient mice. Curr Biol 12:1748–1755

Revy P, Muto T, Levy Y, Geissmann F, Plebani A, Sanal O, Catalan N, Forveille M, Dufourcq-Labelouse R, Gennery A, Tezcan I, Ersoy F, Kayserili H, Ugazio AG, Brousse N, Muramatsu M, Notarangelo LD, Kinoshita K, Honjo T, Fischer A, Durandy A (2000) Activation-induced cytidine deaminase (AID) deficiency causes the autosomal recessive form of the Hyper-IgM syndrome (HIGM2). Cell 102:565–575

Richardson N, Navaratnam N, Scott J (1998) Secondary structure for the apolipoprotein B mRNA editing site. Au-binding proteins interact with a stem loop. J Biol Chem 273:31707–31717

Rustaeus S, Lindberg K, Boren J, Olofsson SO (1995) Brefeldin A reversibly inhibits the assembly of apoB containing lipoproteins in McA-RH7777 cells. J Biol Chem 270:28879–28886

Rustaeus S, Stillemark P, Lindberg K, Gordon D, Olofsson SO (1998) The microsomal triglyceride transfer protein catalyzes the post-translational assembly of apolipoprotein B-100 very low density lipoprotein in McA-RH7777 cells. J Biol Chem 273:5196–5203

Schekman R, Orci L (1996) Coat proteins and vesicle budding. Science 271:1526–1533

Schonfeld G (2003) Familial hypobetalipoproteinemia: a review. J Lipid Res 44:878–883

Schoonjans K, Peinado-Onsurbe J, Lefebvre AM, Heyman RA, Briggs M, Deeb S, Staels B, Auwerx J (1996) PPARalpha and PPARgamma activators direct a distinct tissue-specific transcriptional response via a PPRE in the lipoprotein lipase gene. EMBO J 15:5336–5348

Seishima M, Bisgaier CL, Davies SL, Glickman RM (1991) Regulation of hepatic apolipoprotein synthesis in the 17 alpha-ethinyl estradiol-treated rat. J Lipid Res 32:941–951

Shah RR, Knott TJ, Legros JE, Navaratnam N, Greeve JC, Scott J (1991) Sequence requirements for the editing of apolipoprotein B mRNA. J Biol Chem 266:16301–16304

Sharp D, Blinderman L, Combs KA, Kienzle B, Ricci B, Wager-Smith K, Gil CM, Turck CW, Bouma ME, Rader DJ, et al. (1993) Cloning and gene defects in microsomal triglyceride transfer protein associated with abetalipoproteinaemia. Nature 365:65–69

Sheehy AM, Gaddis NC, Choi JD, Malim MH (2002) Isolation of a human gene that inhibits HIV-1 infection and is suppressed by the viral Vif protein. Nature 418:646–650

Sheehy AM, Gaddis NC, Malim MH (2003) The antiretroviral enzyme APOBEC3G is degraded by the proteasome in response to HIV-1 Vif. Nat Med

Shin YW, Bok SH, Jeong TS, Bae KH, Jeoung NH, Choi MS, Lee SH, Park YB (1999) Hypocholesterolemic effect of naringin associated with hepatic cholesterol regulating enzyme changes in rats. Int J Vitam Nutr Res 69: 341–347

Shiomi M, Ito T (2001) MTP inhibitor decreases plasma cholesterol levels in LDL receptor-deficient WHHL rabbits by lowering the VLDL secretion. Eur J Pharmacol 431:127–131

Singh RP, Dhawan P, Golden C, Kapoor GS, Mehta KD (1999) One-way cross-talk between p38(MAPK) and p42/44(MAPK). Inhibition of p38(MAPK) induces low density lipoprotein receptor expression through activation of the p42/44(MAPK) cascade. J Biol Chem 274:19593–19600

Sjoberg A, Oscarsson J, Bostrom K, Innerarity TL, Eden S, Olofsson SO (1992) Effects of growth hormone on apolipoprotein-B (apoB) messenger ribonucleic acid editing, and apoB 48 and apoB 100 synthesis and secretion in the rat liver. Endocrinology 130:3356–3364

Skalen K, Gustafsson M, Rydberg EK, Hulten LM, Wiklund O, Innerarity TL, Boren J (2002) Subendothelial retention of atherogenic lipoproteins in early atherosclerosis. Nature 417:750–754

Soutar AK, Myant NB, Thompson GR (1977) Simultaneous measurement of apolipoprotein B turnover in very-low-and low-density lipoproteins in familial hypercholesterolaemia. Atherosclerosis 28:247–256

Sparks JD, Phung TL, Bolognino M, Sparks CE (1996) Insulin-mediated inhibition of apolipoprotein B secretion requires an intracellular trafficking event and phosphatidylinositol 3-kinase activation: studies with brefeldin A and wortmannin in primary cultures of rat hepatocytes. Biochem J 313: 567–574

Sparks JD, Sparks CE (1990) Insulin modulation of hepatic synthesis and secretion of apolipoprotein B by rat hepatocytes. J Biol Chem 265:8854–8862

Stillemark P, Boren J, Andersson M, Larsson T, Rustaeus S, Karlsson KA, Olofsson SO (2000) The assembly and secretion of apolipoprotein B-48-containing very low density lipoproteins in McA-RH7777 cells. J Biol Chem 275:10506–10513

Stopak K, de Noronha C, Yonemoto W, Greene WC (2003) HIV-1 Vif blocks the antiviral activity of APOBEC3G by impairing both its translation and intracellular stability. Mol Cell 12:591–601

Stumvoll M (2003) Thiazolidinediones – some recent developments. Expert Opin Investig Drugs 12:1179–1187

Taghibiglou C, Carpentier A, Van Iderstine SC, Chen B, Rudy D, Aiton A, Lewis GF, Adeli K (2000) Mechanisms of hepatic very low density lipoprotein overproduction in insulin resistance. Evidence for enhanced lipoprotein assembly, reduced intracellular ApoB degradation, and increased microsomal triglyceride transfer protein in a fructose-fed hamster model. J Biol Chem 275:8416–8425

Taghibiglou C, Rashid-Kolvear F, Van Iderstine SC, Le-Tien H, Fantus IG, Lewis GF, Adeli K (2002) Hepatic very low density lipoprotein-ApoB overproduction is associated with attenuated hepatic insulin signaling and overexpression of protein-tyrosine phosphatase 1B in a fructose-fed hamster model of insulin resistance. J Biol Chem 277:793–803

Takai Y, Sasaki T, Matozaki T (2001) Small GTP-binding proteins. Physiol Rev 81:153–208

Taskinen MR, Kuusi T, Helve E, Nikkila EA, Yki-Jarvinen H (1988) Insulin therapy induces antiatherogenic changes of serum lipoproteins in noninsulin-dependent diabetes. Arteriosclerosis 8:168–177

Teng B, Black DD, Davidson NO (1990) Apolipoprotein B messenger RNA editing is developmentally regulated in pig small intestine: nucleotide comparison of apolipoprotein B editing regions in five species. Biochem Biophys Res Commun 173:74–80

Teng B, Burant CF, Davidson NO (1993) Molecular cloning of an apolipoprotein B messenger RNA editing protein. Science 260:1816–1819

Thorngate FE, Raghow R, Wilcox HG, Werner CS, Heimberg M, Elam MB (1994) Insulin promotes the biosynthesis and secretion of apolipoprotein B-48 by altering apolipoprotein B mRNA editing. Proc Natl Acad Sci USA 91:5392–5396

Tietge UJ, Bakillah A, Maugeais C, Tsukamoto K, Hussain M, Rader DJ (1999) Hepatic overexpression of microsomal triglyceride transfer protein (MTP) results in increased in vivo secretion of VLDL triglycerides and apolipoprotein B. J Lipid Res 40:2134–2139

Tran K, Thorne-Tjomsland G, DeLong CJ, Cui Z, Shan J, Burton L, Jamieson JC, Yao Z (2002) Intracellular assembly of very low density lipoproteins containing apolipoprotein B100 in rat hepatoma McA-RH7777 cells. J Biol Chem 277:31187–31200

Tran K, Wang Y, DeLong CJ, Cui Z, Yao Z (2000) The assembly of very low density lipoproteins in rat hepatoma McA-RH7777 cells is inhibited by phospholipase A2 antagonists. J Biol Chem 275:25023–25030

Twisk J, Gillian-Daniel DL, Tebon A, Wang L, Barrett PH, Attie AD (2000) The role of the LDL receptor in apolipoprotein B secretion. J Clin Invest 105:521–532

Verma R, Chen S, Feldman R, Schieltz D, Yates J, Dohmen J, Deshaies RJ (2000) Proteasomal proteomics: identification of nucleotide-sensitive proteasome-interacting proteins by mass spectrometric analysis of affinity-purified proteasomes. Mol Biol Cell 11:3425–3439

von Schacky C, Angerer P, Kothny W, Theisen K, Mudra H (1999) The effect of dietary omega-3 fatty acids on coronary atherosclerosis. A randomized, double-blind, placebo-controlled trial. Ann Intern Med 130:554–562

Vukmirica J, Tran K, Liang X, Shan J, Yuan J, Miskie BA, Hegele RA, Resh MD, Yao Z (2003) Assembly and secretion of very low density lipoproteins containing apolipoprotein B48 in transfected McA-RH7777 cells. Lack of evidence that palmitoylation of apolipoprotein B48 is required for lipoprotein secretion. J Biol Chem 278:14153–14161

Wang CN, Hobman TC, Brindley DN (1995) Degradation of apolipoprotein B in cultured rat hepatocytes occurs in a post-endoplasmic reticulum compartment. J Biol Chem 270:24924–24931

Wang H, Chen X, Fisher EA (1993) N-3 fatty acids stimulate intracellular degradation of apoprotein B in rat hepatocytes. J Clin Invest 91:1380–1389

Wang H, Yao Z, Fisher EA (1994) The effects of n-3 fatty acids on the secretion of carboxyl-terminally truncated forms of human apoprotein B. J Biol Chem 269:18514–18520

Wang S, McLeod RS, Gordon DA, Yao Z (1996) The microsomal triglyceride transfer protein facilitates assembly and secretion of apolipoprotein B-containing lipoproteins and decreases cotranslational degradation of apolipoprotein B in transfected COS-7 cells. J Biol Chem 271:14124–14133

Wang SL, Du EZ, Martin TD, Davis RA (1997a) Coordinate regulation of lipogenesis, the assembly and secretion of apolipoprotein B-containing lipoproteins by sterol response element binding protein 1. J Biol Chem 272:19351–19358

Wang Y, McLeod RS, Yao Z (1997b) Normal activity of microsomal triglyceride transfer protein is required for the oleate-induced secretion of very low density lipoproteins containing apolipoprotein B from McA-RH7777 cells. J Biol Chem 272:12272–12278

Wang Y, Tran K, Yao Z (1999) The activity of microsomal triglyceride transfer protein is essential for accumulation of triglyceride within microsomes in McA-RH7777 cells. A unified model for the assembly of very low density lipoproteins. J Biol Chem 274:27793–27800

Welty FK, Lichtenstein AH, Barrett PH, Dolnikowski GG, Ordovas JM, Schaefer EJ (1997) Decreased production and increased catabolism of apolipoprotein B-100 in apolipoprotein B-67/B-100 heterozygotes. Arterioscler Thromb Vasc Biol 17:881–888

Wetterau JR, Combs KA, Spinner SN, Joiner BJ (1990) Protein disulfide isomerase is a component of the microsomal triglyceride transfer protein complex. J Biol Chem 265:9801–9807

Wetterau JR, Lin MC, Jamil H (1997) Microsomal triglyceride transfer protein. Biochim Biophys Acta 1345:136–150

Wilcox LJ, Borradaile NM, de Dreu LE, Huff MW (2001) Secretion of hepatocyte apoB is inhibited by the flavonoids, naringenin and hesperetin, via reduced activity and expression of ACAT2 and MTP. J Lipid Res 42:725–734

Wilson PW, Culleton BF (1998) Epidemiology of cardiovascular disease in the United States. Am J Kidney Dis 32: S56–S65

Windler EE, Greeve J, Daerr WH, Greten H (1988) Binding of rat chylomicrons and their remnants to the hepatic low-density-lipoprotein receptor and its role in remnant removal. Biochem J 252:553–561

Wu X, Sakata N, Lele KM, Zhou M, Jiang H, Ginsberg HN (1997) A two-site model for ApoB degradation in HepG2 cells. J Biol Chem 272:11575–11580

Wu X, Zhou M, Huang LS, Wetterau J, Ginsberg HN (1996) Demonstration of a physical interaction between microsomal triglyceride transfer protein and apolipoprotein B during the assembly of ApoB-containing lipoproteins. J Biol Chem 271:10277–10281

Yamanaka S, Balestra ME, Ferrell LD, Fan J, Arnold KS, Taylor S, Taylor JM, Innerarity TL (1995) Apolipoprotein B mRNA-editing protein induces hepatocellular carcinoma and dysplasia in transgenic animals. Proc Natl Acad Sci USA 92:8483–8487

Yamanaka S, Poksay KS, Arnold KS, Innerarity TL (1997) A novel translational repressor mRNA is edited extensively in livers containing tumors caused by the transgene expression of the apoB mRNA-editing enzyme. Genes Dev 11:321–333

Yamanaka S, Poksay KS, Balestra ME, Zeng GQ, Innerarity TL (1994) Cloning and mutagenesis of the rabbit ApoB mRNA editing protein. A zinc motif is essential for catalytic activity, and noncatalytic auxiliary factor(s) of the editing complex are widely distributed. J Biol Chem 269:21725–21734

Yang Y, Ballatori N, Smith HC (2002) Apolipoprotein B mRNA editing and the reduction in synthesis and secretion of the atherogenic risk factor, apolipoprotein B100 can be effectively targeted through TAT-mediated protein transduction. Mol Pharmacol 61:269–276

Yeung SJ, Chen SH, Chan L (1996) Ubiquitin-proteasome pathway mediates intracellular degradation of apolipoprotein B. Biochemistry 35:13843–13848

Young SG (1990) Recent progress in understanding apolipoprotein B. Circulation 82:1574–1594

Young SG, Krul ES, McCormick S, Farese RV, Jr., Linton MF (1996) Identification and characterization of truncated forms of apolipoprotein B in hypobetalipoproteinemia. Methods Enzymol 263:120–145

Zhang H, Yang B, Pomerantz RJ, Zhang C, Arunachalam SC, Gao L (2003) The cytidine deaminase CEM15 induces hypermutation in newly synthesized HIV-1 DNA. Nature 424:94–98

Zhou M, Fisher EA, Ginsberg HN (1998) Regulated Co-translational ubiquitination of apolipoprotein B100. A new paradigm for proteasomal degradation of a secretory protein. J Biol Chem 273:24649–24653

Zhou M, Wu X, Huang LS, Ginsberg HN (1995) Apoprotein B100, an inefficiently translocated secretory protein, is bound to the cytosolic chaperone, heat shock protein 70. J Biol Chem 270:25220–25224

HEP (2005) 170:519–536

Therapy of Hyper-Lp(a)

K.M. Kostner[1] (✉) · G.M. Kostner[2]

[1] Research Wing Level 3, Princess Alexandra Hospital, O'Keefe Roads,
4102 Woolloongabba,Queensland , Australia
KKostner@soms.pa.uq.edu.au

[2] Institute of Medical Biochemistry and Molecular Biology, Medical University of Graz,
8010 Graz, Austria

Abstract Lipoprotein (a) [Lp(a)] appears to be one of the most atherogenic lipoproteins. It consists of a low-density lipoprotein (LDL) core in addition to a covalently bound glycoprotein, apolipoprotein (a) [apo(a)]. Apo(a) exists in numerous polymorphic forms. The size polymorphism is mediated by the variable number of kringle-4 Type-II repeats found in apo(a). Plasma Lp(a) levels are determined to more than 90% by genetic factors. Plasma Lp(a) levels in healthy individuals correlate significantly high with apo(a) biosynthesis and not with its catabolism. There are several hormones known to have a strong impact on Lp(a) metabolism. In certain diseases, such as kidney disease, Lp(a) catabolism is impaired leading to up to fivefold elevations. Lp(a) levels rise with age but are otherwise influenced only little by diet and lifestyle. There is no safe and efficient way of treating individuals with elevated plasma Lp(a) concentrations. Most of the lipid-lowering drugs have either no significant influence on Lp(a) or exhibit a variable effect in patients with different forms of primary and secondary hyperlipoproteinemia. There is without doubt a strong need to concentrate on the development of specific medications to selectively target Lp(a) biosynthesis, Lp(a) assembly and Lp(a) catabolism. So far only anabolic steroids were found to drastically reduce Lp(a) plasma levels. This class of substance cannot, of course, be used for treatment of patients with hyper-Lp(a). We recommend that the mechanism of action of these drugs be studied in more detail and that the possibility of synthesizing derivatives which may have a more specific effect on Lp(a) without having any side effects be pursued. Other strategies that may be of use in the development of drugs for treatment of patients with hyper-Lp(a) are discussed in this review.

Keywords Atherosclerosis · Risk factor · Fibrinolysis · Metabolism · Hormones

1
Introduction

Lipoprotein(a) [Lp(a)] was first described in 1963 as a genetic variant of β-lipoprotein (Berg 1963). Despite intensive research the physiological function of Lp(a) remains elusive. In the late 1970s several research groups including our own suggested that Lp(a) might be a highly atherogenic lipoprotein. This was based on case–control studies with only few patients and on observational reports of single families. Based on the results of numerous more recent prospective studies with large sample sizes it became clear that the risk of developing coronary artery diseases in the Western population is more than two times higher in individuals with increased plasma Lp(a) levels (Marcovina et al. 2003).

Unfortunately we are still left in the dark concerning Lp(a) biosynthesis and catabolism and have therefore so far not reached our target to reduce plasma Lp(a) levels in patients who are at an increased coronary risk. Today, there is no safe medication known to selectively reduce plasma Lp(a) except for Lp(a) apheresis. Current therapies concentrate on reducing other risk factors such as low-density lipoprotein (LDL), which have been shown to potentiate the adverse effect of Lp(a).

2
Lp(a) Structure

Lp(a) is a complex particle which disintegrates upon treatment with reducing agents into apolipoprotein (a) [apo(a)], a highly glycosylated protein, and a lipoprotein particle which is chemically and structurally indistinguishable from LDL. A disulfide bridge links Cys4326 in apoB-100 with the only free Cys in apo(a), i.e., Cys4057 located in kringle four Type-9. Chemically, Lp(a) consists of approximately 30% protein, 10% carbohydrates, 37% cholesterol + cholesteryl esters, 18% phospholipids and 5% triglycerides (Fig. 1).

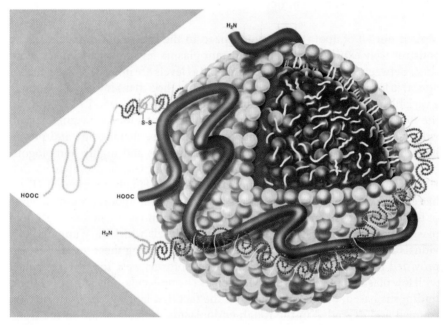

Fig. 1 Schematic view of an Lp(a) particle

Apo(a), the characteristic glycoprotein component of Lp(a) has a rather unique structure. It consists of repetitive protein segments, which are highly homologous to structures in plasminogen (Plg), so-called kringles, i.e., stretches of approximately 110 amino acids forming a secondary structure, which resembles 'Danish kringles' (McLean et al. 1987). The major part of apo(a) consists of numerous repetitive copies of Plg-like kringle-IVs (K-IV). In addition, one copy of a K-V like kringle and a protease like domain of Plg are found. In humans there exist in excess of 30 genetically determined apo(a) isoforms giving rise to a great size heterogeneity. The smallest apo(a) isoform contains the protease domain, K-V and 11 K-IVs of which K-IV Type-1 (T-1) and T-(3-10) are unique in their primary structure, whereas K-IV T-2 is present in two identical copies. Larger isoforms differ by the number of K-IV T-2s; the largest apo(a) described so far had 52 K-IVs. Between the K-IV domains there are linker regions, which are highly glycosylated by N- and O-linked sugars. Although the majority of apo(a) is complexed to LDL, there are small and variable amounts present in plasma in the free form (Gries et al. 1987). It is assumed that this fraction of free apo(a) plays an important role in Lp(a) metabolism and its physiological function.

3
Lp(a) Metabolism and Genetics

Most if not all of apo(a) is biosynthesized in the liver. Apo(a) appears to be constitutively expressed yielding constant plasma levels over long periods of time. Between 90 and 95% of the plasma Lp(a) levels are inherited. The gene for apo(a) is located on chromosome 6q26-q27 and the 5' flanking region contains a variable number of tandem repeats with the pentanucleotide TTTTA. Within the 40-kilobase pair apo(a)–plasminogen intergenic region, two segments with enhancer sequences have been characterized. These include Sp1 and peroxisome proliferator-activated receptors binding sites and highly homologous binding sites for AP-1, NF-κB, GATA-1, C/EBP and GR. It also appears that HNF-1 is crucial for mediating apo(a) expression. Finally interleukin (IL)-6 like and sex hormone binding sites are abundant in the apo(a) promoter. None of these elements so far provide any clue for the non-Gaussian distribution of plasma Lp(a) concentrations, and the plasma levels which vary among individuals by a factor of 1000. The basis for understanding these variations was provided by Utermann et al. (1987). Large isoforms were found to correlate with low plasma Lp(a) levels and vice versa. The molecular mechanism of these findings is based, on the one hand, on the fact that large apo(a) isoforms are trapped and degraded in the rough endoplasmic reticulum and in the Golgi compartment to a much greater extent than small isoforms (White et al. 1994). On the other hand the +93 C/T polymorphism of the untranslated region in the apo(a) gene in addition to several other mutations and polymorphisms in unique K-IVs have an additional impact on Lp(a) plasma levels. All together 90%–95% of the plasma Lp(a) levels are inherited, the rest is caused by environmental factors.

3.1
Assembly of Lp(a)

Apo(a) binds with high affinity to LDL, a process that may be observed in vitro by mixing these two components in a test tube. In vivo, the assembly probably occurs on the surface of liver cells. The final assembly to Lp(a) proceeds in two steps (reviewed in Frank et al. 1994). In the first step, a loose association between apo(a) and LDL is formed which is competitively inhibited by Lys-analogs. This association brings free–SH groups of apo(a) and apoB into close vicinity which in turn form a stable covalent disulfide bond. For the first assembly step the unique K-IV T-6 or T-7 and for the second K-IV T-9 are essential. The binding of apo(a) to LDL occurs in close vicinity of the LDL-receptor (LDL-R) binding site, which in turn yields a particle with low LDL-R binding. On the other hand, particles with low affinity to the LDL-R such as very-low-density lipoprotein (VLDL) do not form stable complexes with apo(a); this is also true for lipoproteins that contain apo B-48. It must be emphasized however that in vivo turnover studies in man using stable isotopes strongly suggest that the assembly of Lp(a) occurs intracellularly.

The pathways responsible for the catabolism of Lp(a) in humans are mostly unexplored. We have shown previously that the apo(a) antigen of Lp(a) in blood is cleaved by metalloproteinases yielding fragments of variable size. Only a small fraction of these fragments is secreted into urine, yet the majority is rapidly cleared from the circulation by various tissues and organs in transgenic mice (Frank et al. 2001). Yet, less than 1% of Lp(a) catabolism is accounted for by the urinary secretion of apo(a) fragments (Kostner et al. 1996). The majority of Lp(a) in animal experiments is taken up by the liver yet the specific role of various receptors in Lp(a) catabolism is controversial and not fully explored for the in vivo situation (Wo et al. 1997). It was suggested that LDL-R related protein, megalin and the VLDL-receptor all might be involved in Lp(a) catabolism. In addition we have demonstrated that the galactose specific asialo glycoprotein receptor (ASGPR) might play a crucial role as well (Hrzenjak et al. 2003). ASGPR knock-out mice exhibited a slower catabolism and a reduced uptake of native freshly isolated Lp(a). COS-7 cells transfected with ASGPR on the other hand showed an increased binding of Lp(a). Thus we suggest that some of the newly synthesized Lp(a) might be devoid of terminal sialic acids or alternatively, a sialidase might be active in human plasma which in turn leads to the catabolism of Lp(a) by the ASGPR pathway.

4
Nongenetic Factors Affecting Plasma Lp(a) Levels

Epidemiologic studies have revealed that at given apo(a) isoform size there are striking differences in plasma Lp(a) concentrations among different ethnic groups. In the black population for example, Lp(a) levels are approximately twice as high as compared to the white population. In the Asian population on the other hand Lp(a) is much lower than in Caucasians. Although it cannot be excluded that variations in the apo(a) gene might be responsible for these observations it is generally believed that other as yet unknown factors might be operative.

Within a given individual, the plasma Lp(a) concentration is rather constant over time. On the other hand, Lp(a) rises quite significantly with age. This is particularly true for the first weeks immediately after birth. An increase however, has also been found in each decade of life. There are in addition numerous nongenetic factors leading to significant modifications of plasma Lp(a) levels including alcohol abuse, various types of dietary fatty acids, smoking, obesity, hypercholesterolemia and more.

4.1
Major Factors and Conditions Affecting Plasma Lp(a) Levels

Cholestatic liver diseases, particularly patients with the occurrence of high lipoprotein-X concentrations, are also linked to very low plasma Lp(a) levels. This may be caused, in part, by an impairment of the Lp(a) assembly due to the lack of normal LDL.

Chronic alcohol intake has a very drastic effect and reduces plasma Lp(a) by 60% and more. Serum Lp(a) is inversely and dose dependently related with alcohol intake and this relationship is independent of the size distribution of apo(a) isoforms (Catena et al. 2003). The mode by which alcohol reduces Lp(a) is not completely understood, however the effect might be caused by its action on insulin-like growth factor (IGF) binding protein. Furthermore, cigarette smoking also lowers plasma Lp(a) by 10%–20%.

Patients suffering from cancer of different locations and origin exhibit up to twofold elevated plasma Lp(a) concentrations (Wright et al. 1989). Patients with acute myelotic leukemia have very high Lp(a) levels that normalize upon chemotherapy with immune suppressive agents. These changes in Lp(a) are associated with fluctuations in plasma IL-6, suggesting that the IL-6 elements in the apo(a) promoter are functional.

Increased Lp(a) levels in acute phases, such as after surgery, inflammation, pregnancy, myocardial infarction, psoriasis, gout and others have been reported. These increased Lp(a) levels normalize after the stimulus for the acute phase disappears. It is also worth mentioning here that Lp(a) has been shown to be a potent chemoattractant for human peripheral monocytes (Syrovets et al. 1997).

The anti-diabetic drug rosiglitazone has been shown to increase plasma Lp(a) levels by about 15% in one study (Ko et al. 2003). There are also numerous reports that individuals with familial hypercholesterolemia (FH) exhibit significantly higher Lp(a) levels than control individuals despite the assumption that LDL-R does not catabolize Lp(a). The pathomechanism of this phenomenon remains to be elucidated.

Under certain circumstances, diet has also a measurable effect on Lp(a) levels. Polyunsaturated fatty acids, e.g., fish oils were found to reduce plasma Lp(a) particularly in physically active individuals. It has also been reported that saturated fatty acids found in palm oil reduce Lp(a). Obese individuals or overweight patients unsurprisingly have lower plasma Lp(a) levels than control individuals and weight loss is accompanied by a measurable rise in Lp(a). It would be of importance to elucidate the pathomechanisms involved in all the phenomena described above.

4.2
Hormonal Influences on Plasma Lp(a) Levels

Hormonal effects on plasma Lp(a) levels are divergent and not coupled to their effect on other plasma lipids or lipoproteins. It appears that steroid hormones or derivatives thereof have the most profound reducing effect on plasma Lp(a) concentrations. Of all of the other hormones known to significantly affect Lp(a) levels, human growth hormone (HGH) is the only one that increases plasma levels significantly.

4.2.1
Sex Hormones

The only substance known so far to drastically reduce Lp(a) levels are anabolic sterols such as stanazolol and danazolol. These hormones lower plasma Lp(a) by more than 70%. Much lower effects are found with estradiol and testosterone. The latter effects may be caused by an increase in Lp(a) catabolism by endocrine organs, e.g., the gonads. In support of this is the finding that gonadotropin releasing hormone analogs reduce plasma Lp(a) by up to 50%. It is also important to note that tamoxifen treatment reduced plasma Lp(a) by 30%–40%. Finally, Lp(a) levels rise by a factor of two and more during pregnancy and normalize post-partum.

4.2.2
Corticoid Hormones

Adrenocorticotrophic hormone administration has a profound effect on Lp(a) concentrations and yields reductions of up to 30%–40%.

4.2.3
Thyroid Hormones

Hypothyroid patients have increased, while hyperthyroid patients have decreased plasma Lp(a) levels in comparison to euthyroid controls. Treatment of hypothyroid patients with T4 drastically reduces elevated plasma Lp(a) levels.

4.2.4
Insulin

The effect of insulin on plasma Lp(a) is highly controversial. Type-I diabetics appear to have Lp(a) levels comparable to controls. Improvement of metabolic control in these patients has little impact on Lp(a). Type-II [noninsulin dependent diabetes mellitus (NIDDM)] patients, on the other hand, revealed increased plasma Lp(a) levels compared to controls. One possibility for these elevated levels is the finding that NIDDM patients with decreased kidney function excrete significantly less apo(a) fragments into their urine compared to controls, which could lead to increased plasma Lp(a) levels (Clodi et al. 1997). There are, however, numerous studies which show opposite results with respect to plasma Lp(a) levels in Type-II diabetics. This most probably relates to the type of hyperlipoproteinemia associated in such collectives.

4.2.5
IGF-I and HGH

The administration of these two hormones has opposing effects on serum Lp(a) (Laron et al. 1997) While HGH drastically increases Lp(a) by up to 120%, IGF-I was found to decrease Lp(a) levels by 60%.

5
Is There a Physiological Function of Lp(a)?

Early studies carried out in the group of Berg (1963) suggest that individuals who were 'Lp(a) negative' do not suffer from any defect whatsoever. As the sensitivity of the Lp(a) assays increased, it turned out that these 'Lp(a) negative' individuals might have Lp(a) values up to 25 mg/dl. We have studied probands with background plasma Lp(a) levels (<0.5 mg/dl) and to our surprise their urinary excretion of apo(a) fragments was comparably high. Thus it appears that bona fide Lp(a) negative individuals rarely exist, and the old dogma that Lp(a) has no function needs to be reiterated. It is hard to rationalize that nature has designed such a complex molecule without any physiological function.

5.1
Lp(a) and Angiogenesis

Several groups including our own suggested that Lp(a) interferes with angiogenesis and vessel outgrowth. The rationale behind this is the fact that angiogenesis starts with the remodeling of matrix proteins and the activation of matrix metalloproteinases (MMPs). MMPs are normally synthesized as inactive zymogens, which need to be activated by proteases. Here plasmin was found to play a key role. As Lp(a) interferes with the activation of plasminogen it appears quite plausible that Lp(a) might have an anti-angiogenic effect. Recently we have demonstrated that apo(a) and also apo(a) fragments secreted into urine are highly effective inhibitors in the tube-forming assay, an in vitro surrogate assay for angiogenesis (Schulter et al. 2001). Apo(a) had no effect on plasminogen activator inhibitor (PAI-I)-1 accumulation and only little effect on urokinase activation in our test system suggesting that alternative pathways must be operative. Other investigators found that apo(a) inhibits angiogenesis dependent colon tumor outgrowth in nude mice (Kim et al. 2003). Another observation which is noteworthy here is the fact that among the older population (80+ years) there is a relatively high proportion of individuals with increased Lp(a) plasma levels. We therefore rationalize that those individuals who escape from premature cardiac death might be partially protected from cancer, the second most important life threatening disease in humans.

5.2
Lp(a) and Hemostasis

Due to the striking homology between apo(a) and plasminogen it was suggested that Lp(a) interferes with fibrinolysis in several ways (Harpel et al. 1995). Lp(a) competitively inhibited plasminogen binding to fibrinogen and fibrin. Lp(a) is postulated also to interfere with plasminogen conversion to plasmin. Furthermore it was found that PAI-I biosynthesis in endothelial cells is stimulated by Lp(a). Lp(a) also up-regulated PAI-2 expression in blood monocytes (Buechler et al. 2001). Another link between Lp(a) and thrombosis is the binding and inactivation of tissue factor pathway inhibitor (Caplice et al. 2001). All of these pro-thrombotic effects of Lp(a) are counteracted by the finding that Lp(a) binds platelet activating factor acetyl hydrolase with high affinity and specificity. Thus it not only inactivates one of the strongest factors known for platelet aggregation, PAF, but also hydrolyses short chain phospholipids which are generated during lipid peroxidation (Blencowe et al. 1995). Furthermore Lp(a) also attenuated collagen mediated platelet aggregation and in turn thromboxane secretion. Taken together it appears that many of the proposed prothrombotic properties of Lp(a) are counterbalanced by some quite significant anti-thrombotic effects and it remains to be determined which effect prevails under different in vivo situations.

6
Lp(a) and Atherosclerosis

Numerous case–control and prospective studies have revealed that Lp(a) is an independent risk factor for coronary artery disease (CAD), stroke and peripheral artery disease. Animal studies of the past and present underline this association. Recently Fan et al. (2001) showed that increased levels of Lp(a) enhanced the development of atherosclerosis in the setting of hypercholes- terolemia in Watanabe heritable hyperlipidemic transgenic rabbits expressing human apolipoprotein(a). The combination of high Lp(a) plasma concentra- tions with other cardiovascular risk factors, in particular low levels of high- density lipoprotein (HDL), strongly increases the risk for CAD. In a prospective population study in 788 male participants of the PROCAM study von Eckard- stein et al. (2001) reported that Lp(a) increases coronary risk, especially in men with high LDL-cholesterol, low HDL-cholesterol, hypertension and high global cardiovascular risk. In a subanalysis of participants in the prospective Multiple Risk Factor Intervention Trial (MRFIT), small apo(a) isoforms were significantly associated with coronary heart disease deaths among smokers (Evans et al. 2001). Polymorphisms in the promoter and coding regions of the apo(a) gene have also been associated with an increased risk for myocardial infarction (MI) (Holmer et al. 2003).

It should be mentioned however, that other prospective studies in the past, such as the Physicians Health Study, have shown contrasting results (Ridker et al. 1993). In some of these reports, Lp(a) was measured in long term, frozen samples with insufficiently evaluated test kits. Moreover, due to the extremely wide range of plasma Lp(a) levels from less than 0.1 mg/dl to more than 300 mg/dl and the highly skewed distribution, studies that include a small number of cases/controls are prone to random deviations. Another reason why studies on Lp(a) are sometimes controversial is the fact that due to its heterogeneity it is difficult to standardize the measurement of Lp(a).

Another aspect, which has been brought up recently, is that Lp(a) may play a role in acute coronary syndromes. Shindo et al (2001) found significantly higher apo(a) and PAI-1 stainable areas in atherectomy specimens of patients with unstable than in those with stable angina. Interesting in this context is the fact that Fu et al. (2001) found mRNA of apo(a) but not of apoB within the vessel wall. Cerebral vascular disease, peripheral vascular disease and more recently carotid atherosclerosis have also been associated with elevated Lp(a) levels. Lp(a) may also be involved as a cofactor in essential hypertension (Antonicelli et al. 2001).

There are several hundreds reports in the literature dealing with one or the other aspect of atherosclerosis, MI, stroke and peripheral vascular diseases in relation to elevated plasma levels or various isoforms of apo(a). The majority of them strongly suggest that Lp(a) in fact is a severe risk factor—in several studies even the best discriminator for the atherogenic risk. Since Lp(a) is metabolically not related to any other plasma lipoprotein it is not surprising that the atherogenic risk of Lp(a) is independent of other factors.

7
Treatment of Elevated Lp(a) Levels

Even though Lp(a) has been established as an independent risk factor for coronary artery disease and cerebrovascular disease, it is still not clear whether lowering of Lp(a) is beneficial. This is mainly due to the fact that to date no practical treatment is available to reduce elevated Lp(a) levels. Furthermore most effective treatments like LDL-apheresis also affect LDL levels. Most lipidologists and clinicians recommend lowering LDL cholesterol more aggressively to levels below 100 mg/dl in cases of elevated Lp(a) levels above 30 mg/dl, even though the hard evidence for this is also lacking.

7.1
Diet

Dietary influences on plasma Lp(a) levels are variable and moderate, yet measurable. Polyunsaturated fatty acids and saturated fatty acids found in palm oil, have a mild, although significant, reducing effect. Dietary intake of omega-3 fatty acids has been shown to decrease plasma Lp(a) levels in some studies. A diet rich in coconut oil has also been shown to reduce plasma Lp(a) levels (Muller et al. 2003). In a similar way trans fatty acids were suggested to have a lowering effect on Lp(a).

Taking all published studies on dietary treatment of hyper-Lp(a) patients together it is fair to say that the effects are moderate and transient in many cases and appear to vary among individuals depending on their type of hyperlipoproteinemia. Long-term studies on this topic in fact are lacking.

7.2
Lipid-Lowering Drugs

7.2.1
Statins

Statin treatment may have a variable effect on plasma Lp(a) concentrations. In most studies Lp(a) remains unchanged after treatment with HMG CoA reductase inhibitors. Treatment of hypercholesterolemic patients for 6 weeks revealed that approximately one-third responded with a reduction of plasma Lp(a), in one-third there was no change and in the remaining third Lp(a) was significantly increased (Kostner et al. 1989). Some studies have shown lowering of Lp(a) by long-term treatment of FH patients with statins (Van Wissen et al. 2003).

7.2.2
Nicotinic Acid

Nicotinic acid and its derivatives can reduce Lp(a) levels by up to 30%, however hypertriglyceridemic patients may respond with an increase of Lp(a) (Carlson et al. 1989). Niceritrol, a nicotinic acid derivative has also been shown to reduce plasma Lp(a) levels in patients with chronic renal disease and hyperlipidemia. Of all the lipid-lowering drugs described so far, nicotinic acid and its derivatives appear to be the most efficient in lowering Lp(a). However, there are no studies addressing the questions of dose–response and long term efficacy.

7.2.3
Fibrates

There are numerous reports in the literature concerning the influence of fibrates, which include clofibrate, fenofibrate and gemfibrocil on plasma Lp(a) levels. In essence it appears that there is no uniform response as some treated patients respond with approximate 25% decreases in plasma Lp(a), in some there are no changes and there are also numerous individuals whose plasma Lp(a) increases upon fibrate therapy. The latter group of patients is characterized by rather high plasma triglycerides and VLDL, and respond to fibrate therapy with elevations of LDL in addition to elevations of Lp(a). The pathomechanism of this phenomenon remains to be elucidated.

7.2.4
Other Agents

All angiotensin I-converting enzyme (ACE) inhibitors in monotherapy lower elevated Lp(a) plasma concentrations in proteinuric patients by reversing proteinuria and in turn enhanced Lp(a) production by the liver (Schlueter et al. 1993). Fosinopril seems to be the only ACE inhibitor to reduce Lp(a) concentrations also in nonproteinuric patients, probably by increasing apo(a) fragmentation and excretion into the urine (K. Kostner and G. Kostner, unpublished results).

Lp(a)-lowering steroid hormones are not indicated for treatment due to side effects. Likewise, tranexamic acid is able to lower Lp(a) plasma concentrations in vivo, but cannot be used in the majority of patients due to possible side effects. The anti-estrogen tamoxifen has also an interesting Lp(a)-lowering effect (Shewmon et al. 1994). The synthetic steroid tibolone reportedly reduced Lp(a) by about 35%, however this was accompanied by a concomitant reduction of the anti-atherogenic HDLs by about 20%. Raloxifene is a selective estrogen receptor modulator and an alternative to estrogen replacement as it obviates the need for a progestin and does not increase C-reactive protein levels. In a recent study it was reported that raloxifene significantly reduced Lp(a) by 18% (Sbarouni et al. 2003).

As mentioned previously ACTH has been found to decrease Lp(a) by more than 50% and also resulted in lower total cholesterol, LDL and apoB levels in hemodialysis patients and steroid treated healthy and hyperlipidemic individuals.

Recently L-carnitine was shown to reduce elevated Lp(a) levels by about 10% in patients with and without diabetes mellitus (Derosa et al. 2003). There are also reports indicating that aspirin and vitamin C lower elevated Lp(a) levels.

7.2.5
Apheresis

The most effective therapy for lowering Lp(a) known to date is extracorporal elimination with apheresis. LDL-apheresis and selective Lp(a)-apheresis using antibody coupled columns, precipitation and complex formation at low pH, double filtration and direct absorption have been demonstrated to lower plasma Lp(a) to the same extent as LDL-cholesterol (up to 80%). However these treatments are expensive and accessible only to a small number of high-risk patients (Kostner 1999). Lp(a) apheresis has also been shown to have a rebound effect, i.e., if the intervals between treatment are more than 4 days, Lp(a) plasma concentrations in some patients increase to above pre-treatment levels.

7.3
Future Targets for the Development of Lp(a)-Lowering Medication

There are several possible strategies to design drugs, which may either interfere with Lp(a) biosynthesis, Lp(a) assembly from LDL and apo(a), with the hydrolytic cleavage of apo(a) into fragments, or with Lp(a) catabolism. As it appears that the apo(a) gene is constitutively expressed, the most straightforward strategy certainly would be to interfere with apo(a) biosynthesis. A very interesting approach which so far has been proven to be successful only in cell cultures or in animal studies is the inhibition of apo(a) synthesis by adenovirus mediated apo(a) antisense RNA expression, as shown in mice (Frank et al. 2001). Future research will tell whether this approach might be also feasible in humans.

The mechanism of action of anabolic steroids on the reduction of plasma Lp(a) levels is unknown. However it appears that these compounds interfere with Lp(a) biosynthesis. With respect to that, the observations in transgenic mice containing a YAC clone with the whole genomic DNA and including the promoter region of human apo(a) are noteworthy: female animals exhibited by far higher plasma apo(a) levels than males. Thus we strongly suggest that steroids might be the target to focus on in searching for drugs with high efficacy. It is suggested to evaluate derivatives of anabolic steroids for specific effect, on Lp(a) biosynthesis without the class specific side effects.

Many regulatory elements and transactivating factors have been characterized in the apo(a) gene, yet it is unknown how they may be influenced by medication. We definitely need more mechanistic studies related to the biosynthesis of apo(a) to design new drugs for Lp(a). The inhibition of Lp(a) assembly is another promising approach. A synthetic apoB peptide has recently been shown to be an effective inhibitor of Lp(a) assembly (Sharp et al. 2003).

An alternative approach of course is to speed up Lp(a) catabolism. Liver is the major organ in which Lp(a) is degraded. This has been proven in many laboratory animals including mice, rats, rabbits and even hedgehogs. We therefore believe that also in man the liver may account for the removal of more than 50% of the Lp(a) from circulation. In a recent study we have demonstrated that the asialo glycoprotein receptor specific for galactose not only avidly binds and catabolizes neuraminidase treated Lp(a) but certainly also 'native' Lp(a) isolated form fresh plasma (Hrzenjak et al 2003). Thus there might be a strategy to activate this pathway by stimulating endogenous neuraminidases specific for lipoproteins, or alternatively to increase artificially the galactose content of Lp(a), a task which proved to be successful in animals studies for removal of other atherogenic lipoproteins (Bijsterbosch et al. 1992).

Patients with elevated LDL-C—in particular FH patients exhibit significantly higher Lp(a) levels than control individuals. This is not due to the inefficient action of the LDL-R, because drugs that strongly increase the number of this receptor in the liver are without significant effect on plasma Lp(a) levels. Thus it appears that derivatives of statins or resins (e.g., cholestyramine) will be ineffective in the future. Nevertheless it is feasible that other lipid-lowering agents might be effective also for Lp(a). This has been postulated for nicotinic acid and some of the fibrates, yet their action is restricted only to patients with certain subtypes of hyperlipidemia. Once it is known why FH patients have such high Lp(a) levels it will be possible to think about mechanisms to interfere therapeutically with increased Lp(a). One possibility is that this relates to a faster or more efficient assembly of Lp(a); an alternative explanation would be that during the assembly of Lp(a) on the surface of liver cells, as suggested by White (1994), the binding of LDL to LDL-competes with apo(a) binding and assembly. If the binding of LDL to its receptor is low, there might be more LDL available to assemble with apo(a). This theory is purely speculative at the present time.

We also know from in vivo and in vitro studies that free apo(a) not complexed to LDL is effectively bound to a variety of cells including liver cells, and is then internalized and degraded. So if LDL is structurally altered as, for example, in patients with liver diseases, lecithin/cholesterol acyl transferase deficiency and others, it assembles only slowly to form Lp(a), and degradation prevails over release of Lp(a) into the circulation. One therapeutic strategy might therefore be to take advantage of this phenomenon and interfere with Lp(a) assembly by altering the structure of LDL. In fact many well-known lipid-lowering drugs do alter VLDL/LDL structure or cause a redistribution of the pattern of lipoproteins with d<1.063. As this varies significantly between patients and depends on the hyperlipoproteinemic phenotype, it may explain the diverging effects of almost any lipid lowering drug on plasma Lp(a) concentrations among individuals.

As pointed out above, there are apo(a) fragments found in the circulation which are removed very effectively and extremely quickly from the circulation; a portion of them is found in urine. The actual protease leading to this type of Lp(a) fragmentation is not known at present. It might therefore be worthwhile to put more emphasis on the characterization of that protease and in turn evaluate the possibility of speeding up Lp(a)catabolism by activating that system.

Patients with many forms of kidney disease exhibit striking elevations of plasma Lp(a) levels. In patients with end-stage renal disease (ESRD), Lp(a) and the apo(a) phenotype are predictors for both the degree of preclinical atherosclerosis and atherosclerotic events. In ESRD and nephrotic syndrome elevations of Lp(a) are not only due to overproduction of Lp(a) by the liver but also to diminished excretion of apo(a) fragments into the urine (Kostner and Kostner 2002). This opens up the possibility to aim at activating renal processes, which are linked to the catabolism of Lp(a), e.g., by increasing urinary apo(a) secretion. It is well established that upon successful treatment of kidney diseases plasma Lp(a) returns back to pre-treatment values. This is true also for patients who undergo kidney transplantation. Thus, it appears that the kidney may be one target organ for reducing Lp(a) values.

Without doubt, the liver is the most efficient organ for uptake and degradation not only of Lp(a) but also for apo(a). The actual mechanism by which liver achieves this has not been unambiguously elucidated. All of the receptors that bind Lp(a) in vitro need to be studied in more detail in experiments in vivo to clearly establish their significance for Lp(a) catabolism. Modulation of their activity will, without doubt, have an impact on plasma Lp(a) levels.

What remains for now is to concentrate on risk factors for atherosclerosis and MI other than Lp(a), in particular on LDL. We believe that the most important therapeutic measure for the time being in patients with elevated Lp(a) (>30 mg/dl) is to reduce LDL-cholesterol to values below 100 mg/dl, especially in patients with additional cardiovascular risk factors.

Acknowledgements Work cited in this article has been supported by the Austrian Research Foundation, Project S-47-02.

References

Antonicelli R, Testa R, Bonfigli AR, Sirolla C, Pieri C, Marra M, Marcovina SM (2001) Relationship between lipoprotein (a) levels, oxidative stress and blood pressure levels in patients with essential hypertension. Clin Exp Med 1:145–150

Berg K (1963) A new serum type system in man: the Lp system. Acta Pathol Microbiol Scand 59:362–382

Blencowe C, Hermetter A, Kostner GM, Deigner HP (1995) Enhanced association of platelet activating factor acetylhydrolase with Lipoprotein(a) in comparison to Low Density Lipoprotein. J Biol Chem 270:31151–31157

Bijsterbosch MK, Bakkeren HF, Kempen HJ, Roelen HC, vanBoom JH, vanBerkel TJ (1992) A monogalactosylated cholesterol derivative that specifically induces uptake of LDL by the liver. Arterioscler Thromb 12:1153–1160

Buechler C, Ullrich H, Ritter M, Porsch-Oezcueruemez M, Lackner KJ, Barlage S, Friedrich SO, Kostner GM, Schmitz G (2001) Lipoprotein(a) upregulates the expression of the plasminogen activator inhibitor 2 in human blood monocytes. Blood 97:981–986

Caplice NM, Panetta C, Peterson TE, Kleppe LS, Mueske CS, Kostner GM, Broze GJ, Simari RD (2001) Lipoprotein(a) binds and inactivates tissue factor pathway inhibitor. A novel link between lipoproteins and thrombosis. Blood 98:2980–2987

Carlson LA, Hamsten A, Asplund A (1989) Pronounced lowering of serum levels of Lp(a) in hyperlipidemic subjects with nicotinic acid. J Intern Med 226:271–276

Catena C, Novello M, Dotto L, De Marchi S, Sechi LA (2003) Serum Lp(a) concentrations and alcohol consumption in hypertension: possible relevance for cardiovascular damage. J Hypertens 2:281–288

Clodi M, Oberbauer R, Waldhäusl W, Maurer G, Kostner GM, Kostner K (1997) Urinary excretion of apo(a) fragments in NIDDM patients. Diabetologia 40:1455–1460

Derosa G, Cicero AF, Gaddi A, Muggelini A, Ciccarelli L, Fogari R (2003) The effect of L-carnitine on plasma Lp(a) levels in hypercholesteremic patients with type 2 diabetes mellitus. Clin Ther 25:1429–1439

Evans RW, Spielberg O, Shaten BJ (2001) Prospective association of lipoprotein (a) concentrations and apo(a) size with coronary heart disease among men in the Multiple Risk Factor Intervention Trial. J Clin Epidemiol 54:51–7

Fan J, Sun H, Unoki H, Shiomi M, Watanabe T (2001) Enhanced atherosclerosis in Lp(a) WHHL transgenic rabbits. Ann N Y Acad Sci 947:362–365

Fu L, Jamieson DG, Usher DC, Lavi E (2001) Gene expression of apolipoprotein (a) within the wall of human aorta and carotid arteries. Atherosclerosis 158:303–311

Frank S, Durovic S, Kostner GM (1994) Structural requirements of apo-a for the lipoprotein-a assembly. Biochem J 304:27–30

Frank S, Gauster M, Strauss J, Hrzenjak A, Kostner GM (2001) Adenovirus-mediated apo(a)-antisense-RNA expression efficiently inhibits apo(a) synthesis in vitro and in vivo. Gene Therapy 6:425–430

Frank S, Hrzenjak A, Blaschitz A, Dohr G,Kostner GM (2001) Role of various tissues in apo(a) fragmentation and excretion of fragments by the kidney. Eur J Clin Invest 31:504–512

Gries A, Nimpf J, Nimpf M, Wurm H, Kostner GM (1987) Free and apoB-associated Lp(a) specific protein in human serum. Clin Chim Acta 164:93–100

Harpel P, Hermann A, Zhang X Ostfeld I, Borth W (1995) Lipoprotein (a), plasmin modulation and atherogenesis. Thromb Haemost 74:382–386

Holmer SR, Hengstenberg C, Kraft HG, Mayer B, Poll M, Kurzinger S, Fischer M, Lowel H, Klein G, Riegger GA, Schunkert H (2003) Associations of polymorphisms of the apo(a) gene with Lp(a) and myocardial infarction. Circulation 107:696–701

Hrzenjak A, Frank S, Wo X, Zhou Y, Van Berkel T, Kostner GM (2003) Galactose-specific asialoglycoprotein receptor is involved in lipoprotein (a) catabolism. Biochem J 376:765–771

Kim JS, Chang JH, Yu HK, Ahn JH, Yum JS, Lee SK, Jung KH, Park DH, Yoon Y, Byun SM, Chung SI (2003) Inhibition of angiogenesis and angiogenesis dependent tumor growth by the cryptic kringle fragments of human apolipoprotein(a). J Biol Chem 278:29000–29008

Ko SH, Song KH, Ahn YB, Yoo SJ, Son HS, Yoon KH, Cha BY, Lee KW, Son HY, Kang SK (2003) The effect of rosiglitazone on serum lipoprotein(a) levels in Korean patients with type 2 diabetes mellitus. Metabolism 52:731–734

Kostner GM, Gavish D, Leopold B, Bolzano K, Weintraub MS, Breslow JL (1989) HMG CoA reductase inhibitors lower LDL cholesterol without reducing Lp(a) levels. Circulation 80:1313–1319

Kostner K (1999) Aggressive Therapie und Kombinationstherapie von Hypercholester-inämien. Wien Med Wochenschr 149:146–148

Kostner KM, Kostner GM (2002) Lipoprotein (a): Still an enigma? Curr Opin Lipidol 13:391–396

Kostner KM, Maurer G, Huber, K, Stefenelli T, Dieplinger H, Steyrer E, Kostner GM (1996) Urinary excretion of Apo(a) Fragments: role in Apo(a) catabolism. Arterioscler Throm Vas Biol 16:905–911

Laron Z, Klinger B, Silbergeld A,Wang XL (1997) Opposing effects of growth hormone and insulin-like growth factor I on serum lipoprotein(a). J Pediatr Endocr Met 10:143–149

Marcovina SM, Koschinsky ML, Albers JJ, Skarlatos S (2003) Recent Advances and Future Directions. In: Report of the National Heart, Lung, and Blood Institute Workshop on Lipoprotein(a) and Cardiovascular Disease. Clin Chem 49:1785–1796

McLean JW, Tomlinson JE, Kuang WJ, Eaton DL, Chen EY, Fless GM, Scanu AM, Lawn RM (1987) cDNA sequence of human apolipoprotein(a) is homologous to plasminogen. Nature 330:132–127

Muller H, Lindman AS, Blomfeldt A, Seljeflot I, Pedersen JI (2003) A diet rich in coconut oil reduces diurnal postprandial variations in circulating tissue plasminogen activator antigen and fasting lipoprotein (a) levels compared to a diet rich in unsaturated fat in women. J Nutr 133:3422–3427

Ridker PM, Hennekens CA, Stampfer MJ (1993) A prospective study of Lp(a) and the risk of myocardial infarction. JAMA 270:2195–2199

Sbarouni E, Flevari P, Kroupis C, Kyriakides ZS, Koniavitou K, Kremastinos DT (2003) The effects of raloxifene and simvastatin on plasma lipids and endothelium. Cardiovasc Drugs Ther 17:319–323

Schlueter W, Keilani T, Batlle DC (1993) Metabolic effects of ACE inhibitors: focus on the reduction of cholesterol and lipoprotein (a) by fosinopril. Am J Cardiol 72:37H–44H

Schulter V, Koolwijk P, Peters E, Frank S, Hrzenjak A, Graier WF, van Hinsbergh VWM, Kostner GM (2001) The Impact of apolipoprotein(a) on in vitro angiogenesis. Arterioscl Throm Vas Biol 21:433–438

Sharp RJ, Perugini MA, Marcovina SM, McCormick SP (2003) A synthetic peptide that inhibits lipoprotein(a) assembly. Arterioscler Thromb Vasc Biol 23:502–507

Shewmon DA, Stock JL, Rosen CJ, Heiniluoma KM, Hogue MM, Morrison A, Doyle EM, Ukena T, Weale V, Baker S(1994) Tamoxifen and estrogen lower circulating Lp(a) concentrations in healthy postmenopausal women. Arterioscl Thromb 14:1586–1593

Shindo J, Ishibashi T, Kijima M, Nakazato K, Nagata K, Yokoyama K, Hirosaka A, Sato E, Kunii H, Yamaguchi N, Watanabe N, Saito T, Maehara K, Maruyama Y (2001) Increased plasminogen activator inhibitor-1 and apolipoprotein (a) in coronary atherectomy specimens in acute coronary syndromes. Coron Artery Dis 12:573–579

Syrovets T, Thillet J, Chapman J, Simmet T (1997) Lp(a) is a potent chemoattractant for human peripheral monocytes. Blood 90:2027–2036

Utermann G, Menzel HJ, Kraft HG, Duba HC, Kemmler HG, Seitz C (1987) Lp(a) glycoprotein phenotypes: inheritance and relation to Lp(a)- lipoprotein concentrations in plasma. J Clin Invest 80:458–465

Von Eckardstein A, Schulte H, Cullen P, Assmann G (2001) Lipoprotein(a) further increases the risk of coronary events in men with high global cardiovascular risk. J Am Coll Cardiol 37:434–439

Van Wissen S, Smilde TJ, Trip MD, De Boo T, Kastelein JJ, Stalenhoef AF (2003) Long term statin treatment reduces lipoprotein(a) concentrations in heterozygous FH. Heart 89:893–896

White AL, Hixon JE, Rainwater DL, Lanford RE (1994) Molecular basis for "null" lipoprotein(a) phenotypes and the influence of apolipoprotein(a) size on plasma lipoprotein(a) level in the baboon. J Biol Chem 269:9060–9066

White AL, Lanford RE (1994) Cell surface assembly of lipoprotein(a) in primary cultures of baboon hepatocytes. J Biol Chem 269:28716–28723

Wo X, Kostner K, Frank S, Kostner GM (1997) Assembly and catabolism of Lipoprotein(a). In: Jacotot B, Mathe D, Fruchart JC (eds) Proceedings of the 11th International Symposium on Atherosclerosis. Paris, 5–9 October, pp 567–574

Wright LC, Sullivan DR, Muller M, Dyne M, Tattersall MH, Mounford, CE (1989) Elevated apolipoprotein(a) levels in cancer patients. Int J Cancer 43:241–244

HEP (2005) 170:537–561

Modulation of High-Density Lipoprotein Cholesterol Metabolism and Reverse Cholesterol Transport

M. Hersberger · A. von Eckardstein (✉)

Institute of Clinical Chemistry, University and University Hospital Zurich, Raemistrasse 100, 8091 Zurich, Switzerland
arnold.voneckardstein@ikc.usz.ch

Abstract Low high-density lipoprotein (HDL)-cholesterol (C) is an important risk factor for coronary heart disease. In vitro, HDL exerts several potentially anti-atherogenic effects including reverse cholesterol transport (RCT) from peripheral cells to the liver. Hence, raising HDL-C has become an interesting target for anti-atherosclerotic drug therapy. Levels of HDL-C and the composition of HDL subclasses in plasma are regulated by apolipoproteins, lipolytic enzymes, lipid transfer proteins, receptors, and cellular transporters. The interplay of these factors leads to RCT and determines the composition and thereby the anti-atherogenic properties of HDL. Recent findings suggest that the mechanism of HDL modification rather than a sole increase in HDL-C determines the efficacy of anti-atherosclerotic drug therapy. In several controlled and prospective intervention studies, patients with low HDL-C and additional risk factors benefited from treatment with fibrates or statins. However, in only some of the fibrate trials was prevention of coronary events in patients with low HDL-C and hypertriglyceridaemia related to an increase in HDL-C. This may be because currently available drugs increase HDL-C levels only moderately and because HDL levels per se do not necessarily correlate with the functionality of HDL. However, several novel targets to modify RCT have emerged from the recent understanding of HDL synthesis, maturation and catabolism. The four major targets for an anti-atherogenic strategy in HDL metabolism include stimulation of apoA-I synthesis and secretion, the stimulation of ABCA1 expression, the inhibition of cholesterol ester transfer protein, and the up-regulation of scavenger receptor BI. These and other modulations of HDL metabolism are thought to result in improved RCT making them attractive targets for the development of new regimens of anti-atherogenic drug therapy.

Keywords High-density lipoprotein · HDL · Drug · Medication · Reverse cholesterol transport

1
Introduction

Numerous clinical and epidemiological studies have demonstrated the inverse association of high-density lipoprotein (HDL) cholesterol (C) with the risk of coronary heart disease (CHD) events (Hersberger and von Eckardstein 2003). HDL exerts various potentially anti-atherogenic properties and increasing HDL-C was found to protect from atherosclerosis in several genetic animal models (Hersberger and von Eckardstein 2003). In vitro, HDL exerts several potentially anti-atherogenic activities. HDLs mediate the reverse cholesterol transport (RCT) from peripheral cells to the liver, inhibit oxidation of low-density lipoprotein (LDL), adhesion of monocytes to the endothelium, apoptosis of vascular endothelial and smooth muscle cells and platelet activation, and stimulate the endothelial secretion of vasoactive substances as well as smooth muscle cell proliferation. These anti-atherogenic properties have been reviewed in detail previously (Hersberger and von Eckardstein 2003; Nofer et al. 2002; von Eckardstein and Assmann 2000). Therefore and since the vascular, anti-inflammatory and anti-oxidative targets of pleiotropic HDL effects are covered in other articles of this volume (see chapters by Aviram et al., Spieker and Lüscher, Cynshi and Stocker in this volume) we focus in this article on the modulation of HDL metabolism and RCT.

2
HDL Metabolism and RCT

RCT describes both the metabolism and an important anti-atherogenic function of HDL, namely the HDL-mediated efflux of cholesterol from non-hepatic cells and its subsequent delivery to the liver and steroidogenic organs where it is used for the synthesis of lipoproteins, bile acids, vitamin D, and steroid hormones.

Approximately 9 mg cholesterol/kg body weight is synthesized by peripheral tissues every day and has to be delivered to the liver for effective catabolism (von Eckardstein et al. 2001b). Distortion of RCT contributes to the deposition of cholesterol within the arterial wall and thereby to the development of atherosclerosis.

Lipid-poor HDL-precursors are produced either as nascent HDL by hepatocytes and the intestinal mucosa, or dissociate from chylomicrons and very-low-density lipoprotein (VLDL) during lipoprotein lipase (LPL) mediated hydrolysis of triglycerides, or are generated by the conversion of HDL_2 and HDL_3 by cholesteryl ester transfer protein (CETP), hepatic lipase (HL), scavenger receptor BI (SR-BI), and endothelial lipase (EL) (Barter 2002; Hersberger and von Eckardstein 2003) (Fig. 1). Lipid-free apolipoproteins or lipid-poor particles (i.e. preβ1-LpA-I) acquire phospholipids and unesterified cholesterol from hepatic and non-hepatic cells (Hersberger and von Eckardstein 2003) and develop into the lipid-rich α-HDLs which contain the cholesterol quantified in the routine analysis for HDL-C (Barter 2002). This initial step of HDL formation is interrupted in patients with Tangier disease and in mice lacking the ATP binding cassette transporter A1 (ABCA1). In Tangier disease patients and in gene-targeted mice, cellular lipid efflux is drastically reduced which causes absence of lipid-rich α-HDL in plasma and macrophage foam cell formation (Oram 2002). Since ABCA1 is expressed in many cells including hepatocytes and enterocytes, this cellular lipid transporter probably plays an important role not only in lipid efflux from peripheral cells but also in the hepatic and intestinal generation of HDL.

HDL precursors generated by ABCA1-mediated lipid efflux become mature, lipid-rich and spherical α-HDL_3 by acquisition of additional phospholipids and unesterified cholesterol either from cells or apolipoprotein B (apoB)-containing lipoproteins (at least partially phospholipid transfer protein (PLTP)-mediated), by the lecithin (LCAT)-mediated esterification of cholesterol, and by the association of additional apolipoproteins (Barter 2002). Ongoing LCAT-mediated cholesterol esterification and PLTP-mediated fusion with other HDL_3 further increases the size of these initially small HDL_3 (Rye et al. 1999). In addition, lipolysis of VLDL and chylomicrons by LPL generates surface remnants of triglyceride-rich lipoproteins which, again with the help of PLTP, are transferred onto HDL (Fig. 1).

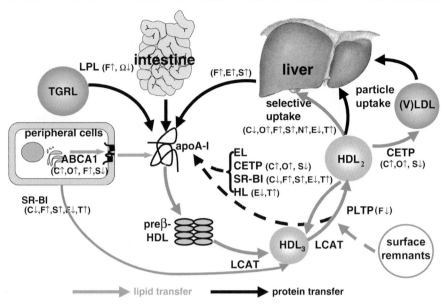

Fig. 1 Pathways of HDL metabolism and regulation by metabolites, drugs and hormones. Mature HDL_3 and HDL_2 are generated from lipid-free apoA-I or lipid-poor preβ_1-HDL as the precursors. These precursors are produced as nascent HDL by the liver or intestine or are released from lipolysed VLDL and chylomicrons, or by interconversion of HDL_3 and HDL_2. ABCA1-mediated lipid efflux from cells is important for initial lipidation; LCAT-mediated esterification of cholesterol generates spherical particles that continue to grow after undergoing cholesterol esterification, PLTP-mediated particle fusion and surface remnant transfer. Larger HDL_2 are converted into smaller HDL_3 upon CETP-mediated export of cholesteryl esters from HDL onto apoB-containing lipoproteins, SR-B1-mediated selective uptake of cholesterol esters into liver and steroidogenic organs, and HL- and endothelial lipase-mediated hydrolysis of phospholipids. HDL lipids are catabolized either separately from HDL proteins, i.e. by selective uptake or via CETP-transfer, or together with HDL proteins, i.e. via uptake through as yet unknown HDL receptors or apoE receptors. Both the conversion of HDL_2 to HDL_3 and the PLTP-mediated conversion of HDL_3 to HDL_2 liberate lipid-free or poorly lipidated apoA-I. For further details see text. *Grey arrows* represent lipid transfer processes, *black arrows* represent protein transfer processes. *Letters* refer to metabolites, drugs and hormones which regulate HDL metabolism: C, cholesterol: O, oxysterols; F, fibrates; S, statins; N, nicotinic acid; Ω, fish oil; E, estradiol; T, testosterone. ↑ Denotes stimulatory effects, ↓ inhibitory effects. Other abbreviations: *ABCA1*, ATP binding cassette transporter A1; *CETP*, cholesteryl ester transfer protein; *EL*, endothelial lipase; *HL*, hepatic lipase; *LCAT*, lecithin: cholesterol-acyltransferase; *LPL*, lipoprotein lipase; *PLTP*, phospholipid transfer protein; *SR-B1*, scavenger receptor B1; *TGRL*, triglyceride-rich lipoproteins

Lipids or proteins of α-HDL are removed from the circulation by at least two direct pathways which involve the selective uptake of lipids and the holoparticle-uptake by the apoE-receptors and possibly apoA-I-receptors. Furthermore, two indirect pathways which involve the actions of CETP, HL, and

EL were shown to play a role in HDL catabolism (Fig. 1) (Krieger 1999; Trigatti et al. 2000; Curtiss and Boisvert 2000; Tall et al. 2000; Cohen et al. 1999; Thuren 2000; Rader and Jaye 2000). The selective uptake of cholesterol esters from HDL into hepatocytes and steroidogenic cells is mediated by the binding of HDL to SR-BI (Silver and Tall 2001). SR-BI appears to internalize HDL into a cellular compartment of hepatocytes from where apolipoproteins are directed to the basolateral site for resecretion and lipids to apical membranes for secretion into the bile (Silver et al. 2001). Selective uptake by SR-BI may depend on the presence of cofactors such as HL which hydrolyses phospholipids on the surface of both HDL and plasma membranes and thereby enables the flux of cholesteryl esters from the lipoprotein core into the plasma membrane (Cohen et al. 1999; Thuren 2000).

Whereas SR-BI internalizes HDL lipids but not HDL-apolipoproteins, the apoE-receptors and the as yet unknown apoA-I receptors, such as the recently described beta-chain of ATP-synthase, mediate holoparticle uptake of HDL (Martinez et al. 2003). CETP exchanges cholesteryl esters of α-HDL with triglycerides of VLDL, intermediate density lipoprotein (IDL), and LDL which are then removed via the LDL-receptor pathway (Tall et al. 2000). EL hydrolyses phospholipids and generates free fatty acids taken up by endothelial cells (Rader and Jaye 2000).

The removal of lipids from HDL_2 by SR-BI, CETP, and HL and the subsequent conversion of HDL_2 to HDL_3 as well as the conversion of HDL_3 to HDL_2 by PLTP regenerate $pre\beta_1$-LpA-I or lipid-free apoA-I (Silver et al. 2001). These small apolipoproteins or particles can leave the plasma into the extravascular space where they serve as acceptors of cellular lipids and thus again initiate the generation of HDL. In the kidney, these small particles are filtered and removed from the plasma. Again, apoA-I is recycled in the proximal tubulus lumen by a cubilin-mediated re-uptake (Christensen and Birn 2002).

3
Peripheral Cholesterol Efflux

In contrast to most other cells of the body, which regulate their cholesterol content by a finely tuned interplay of LDL-receptor mediated lipoprotein uptake and endogenous cholesterol synthesis, macrophages—including those of the arterial wall—can accumulate large amounts of cholesterol by uncontrolled scavenger receptor-mediated (SR-A) uptake of modified lipoproteins and phagocytosis. This process turns macrophages into activated foam cells, which produce various growth factors, cytokines and proteases and thereby influence the course of atherosclerosis (Glass and Witztum 2001).

Efflux is the only mechanism by which macrophages can limit or reverse the cellular cholesterol accumulation. The importance of this pathway is highlighted by a broad spectrum of cholesterol efflux pathways. Two of them are independent of extracellular cholesterol acceptors, namely the secretion of lipid-rich apoE-containing particles and the oxidation of cholesterol into 27-hydroxycholesterol together with the subsequent secretion of this oxysterol. The appearance of foam cells in genetically modified mice lacking macrophage apoE as well as in cholesterol-27-hydroxylase (CYP27) deficient patients with cerebrotendinous xanthomatosis highlight the relevance of these pathways for the regulation of macrophage cholesterol homeostasis (Bjorkhem and Diczfalusy 2002).

However, the HDL-dependent cholesterol efflux pathways are generally considered as more important. HDL and lipid-free apolipoproteins induce at least four kinds of cholesterol efflux, two of which are independent of cellular proteins and are slow, and two of which depend on cellular proteins and are fast (Rothblat et al. 1999).

3.1
Receptor-Independent Cholesterol Efflux Pathways: Aqueous Diffusion and Microsolubilization

Unesterified cholesterol desorbs from the plasma membrane and diffuses across a concentration gradient to extracellular lipoproteins including HDL. This passive process of diffusional efflux is enhanced by esterification of cholesterol by LCAT that functions to maintain the gradient of cholesterol between the cell surface and the HDL particle (Rothblat et al. 1999). This passive process is not very efficient in mediating cholesterol removal from macrophages (Rothblat et al. 1999).

By the abundance of amphipathic helices rather than a specific domain, lipid-free apolipoproteins A-I, A-II, A-IV, Cs, and E but also amphipathic synthetic peptides can associate spontaneously with phospholipids of the cell membrane and sequester them into the extracellular compartment (Rothblat et al. 1999). This so-called microsolubilization is followed or paralleled by some cholesterol efflux but does not lead to the formation of distinct HDL precursors which mature to HDL. This efflux is mediated by amino terminal domains and by the interaction of amino terminal and carboxy terminal domains of apoA-I (Chroni et al. 2003).

3.2
Scavenger Receptor B1

Expression of SR-BI in macrophages enhances HDL-mediated cholesterol efflux. (Llera-Moya et al. 1999; Liu et al. 2002). This is in contrast to the effect of SR-BI in liver or steroidogenic cells, where SR-BI mediates influx of cholesterol (Silver and Tall 2001). The cellular and extracellular metabolism of cholesterol may dictate the inward or outward direction of cholesterol flux. According to this model, the synthesis of bile acids, lipoproteins or steroid hormones favours influx of cholesterol into liver and steroidogenic organs, respectively, whereas cellular cholesterol ester hydrolysis and extracellular LCAT-mediated cholesterol esterification favours cholesterol efflux from macrophages.

Another open question relates to the mechanism by which SR-BI facilitates cholesterol efflux. Since another HDL binding protein of the scavenger receptor B family, i.e. CD36, does not mediate cholesterol efflux, it has been suggested that binding of HDL to SR-BI facilitates cholesterol efflux by reorganization of lipids within the plasma membrane (Llera-Moya et al. 1999). Both SR-BI mediated cholesterol efflux and SR-BI mediated HDL lipid uptake into the liver are potentially anti-atherogenic pathways. In agreement with this, inactivation of SR-BI increases atherosclerosis in mice despite increasing HDL-C (Braun et al. 2002) and over-expression of SR-BI decreases atherosclerosis in mice despite decreasing HDL-C (Arai et al. 1999).

3.3
ATP Binding Cassette Transporter A1

Lipid-free apoA-I induces phospholipid and cholesterol efflux from various cells including macrophages by the interaction with ABCA1 (Oram 2002). This pathway depends on a distinct domain within the carboxy terminus of apoA-I whereas 'microsolubization' is also mediated by amino terminal domains and by the interaction of amino terminal and carboxy terminal domains of apoA-I (Chroni et al. 2003). Moreover, ABCA1-mediated lipid efflux but not microsolubilization results in the formation of HDL precursors which subsequently mature to HDL (Chroni et al. 2003).

The mechanism by which ABCA1 mediates lipid efflux is not resolved. Originally it was suggested that the transmembrane domains of ABCA1 form a pore within the plasma membrane into which lipids are translocated ('flopped') from the inner leaflet of the plasma membrane. From there they are then picked up by lipid-free apolipoproteins which may even bind to ABCA1. More recent data do not support this model but rather suggest that ABCA1 organizes the intracellular trafficking of lipids and proteins (Neufeld et al. 2001; Chen et al. 2001). HDL and apoA-I were previously found to be internalized by macrophages into an endosomal compartment from where they are resecreted together with lipids (Takahashi and Smith 1999). Tangier macrophages appear to have a defect in resecretion and aberrantly target internalized HDL to lysosomes for degradation. For this reason and because of the presence of hyperplastic Golgi structures within lipid laden macrophages of Tangier patients or ABCA1 deficient mice, it has been suggested that ABCA1 serves as a protein component of vesicles which shuttles lipids (and proteins including interleukin 1β and apoE) between lipid-rich intracellular organelles such as the trans-Golgi network, lysosomes, and the plasma membrane (von Eckardstein et al. 2001a; Zhou et al. 2002). Actually, the transfection of cells with fluorescent ABCA1 showed intensive cycling of fluorescent vesicles between the trans-Golgi network and the plasma membrane (Neufeld et al. 2001).

Whatever the mechanism, HDL deficiency and the abundance of macrophage foam cells in patients with Tangier disease highlight the importance of ABCA1 for the regulation of both HDL-C plasma concentration and the regulation of cellular cholesterol homeostasis. However, the site of foam cell formation is variable and involves arteries, liver, spleen, tonsils, and peripheral nerves. Some but not all Tangier disease patients have premature atherosclerosis, others have hepatosplenomegaly and peripheral neuropathy.

These biochemical, pathological and clinical findings make ABCA1 an interesting target for anti-atherosclerotic drug therapy. To reach this aim it is important to understand the regulation of ABCA1. The promoter of the ABCA1 gene contains binding motifs for several transcription factors including the sterol regulatory binding protein (SREBP) and the liver-X-receptor/retinoid-X-receptor (LXRα/RXRα) (Santamarina-Fojo et al. 2001). In agreement with a regulatory role of these transcription factors, ABCA1 expression and lipid efflux are up-regulated by cholesterol, oxysterols, retinoids and cAMP analogues (Santamarina-Fojo et al. 2001).

On the other hand, ABCA1 expression is downregulated in mice with diabetes mellitus, possibly as a result of the inhibitory effects of free unsaturated fatty acids on oxysterol- and retinoid-induced ABCA1 expression (von Eckardstein et al. 2003). This observation and the stimulatory effect of unsaturated fatty acids on ABCA1 degradation (Wang and Oram 2002) provide a direct link between defective cholesterol efflux and the accelerated development of atherosclerosis in patients with diabetes mellitus. ABCA1 expression is also repressed by the inflammatory cytokine interferon γ and by lipopolysaccharides, but up-regulated by transforming growth factor (TGF) β (Santamarina-Fojo et al. 2001). Inflammation may hence represent another pathologic state in which disturbed cholesterol efflux favours the development of atherosclerosis.

4
Effect of Drug-Mediated Increase in HDL on Atherosclerosis

Outcomes of several prospective intervention studies have been interpreted as proofs for the beneficial effect of increasing HDL-C on CHD prevention. However, it is important to emphasize that these studies used fibrates and statins which exert a broad spectrum of metabolic effects (see chapters by Paoletti et al. and Staels et al. in this volume), only one of which is the moderate increase in HDL-C. Moreover, the conclusions on the beneficial effects of increased HDL-C were drawn from results of post hoc analyses of some big trials but not confirmed in post hoc analyses of others.

In the Helsinki Heart (HHS) and VA-HIT studies (both gemfibrozil) increases in HDL-C and HDL_3-C, respectively, were significantly associated with reduction in event rates (Manninen et al. 1992; Robins et al. 2001). No such associations, however, were seen in the BIP trial (bezafibrate) or the AFCAPS (lovastatin), 4S (simvastatin), WOCSCOPS, CARE and LIPID trials (pravastatin) (BIP 2000; Sacks et al. 2000; WOSCOPS 1998; Ballantyne et al. 2001; Gotto, Jr. et al. 2000). Likewise post hoc and meta analyses of some (e.g. BECAIT, bezafibrate, LCAS, fluvastatin) (Ruotolo et al. 1998; Ballantyne et al. 1999) but not all (e.g. LOCAT, gemfibrozil) (Frick et al. 1997) angiographic trials provided evidence for a moderate but significant association between changes in HDL-C and regression of atherosclerotic lesions.

In view of the strong LDL-C lowering effects of statins and the strong triglyceride lowering effects of fibrates together with the pleiotropic effects of both drug groups on vascular inflammation and insulin sensitivity, it is not justified to take these studies as proof for a general atheroprotective effect of increased HDL-C. These studies only show that patients with low HDL-C and additional risk factors benefit from treatment with fibrates or statins. In this context it is also important to reconcile that in the two controlled intervention studies on cardiovascular effects of hormone replacement therapy (HRT) in postmenopausal women, a combination of conjugated equine estrogens and medroxyprogesterone did not reduce (Heart Estrogen/Progestin Replacement Study; HERS) but even increased coronary event rates (Women's Health Initiative) despite increased HDL-C (Hulley et al. 1998; Grady et al. WHI 2002; Manson et al. 2003).

5
Drug Effects on HDL Metabolism

5.1
Statins

In addition to decreasing LDL-C concentrations in a dose-dependent manner (Gotto 2002) statins also increase HDL-C by about 4%–10% with no general dose-response and independent of the HDL-C baseline level (4S 1994). Most of these studies have systematically excluded patients with low HDL-C levels, except for the AFCAPS/TexCAPS primary prevention study which specifically included participants with an average normal total cholesterol of 5.7 mmol/l and LDL-C of 3.9 mmol/l but low HDL-C of 0.94 mmol/l for men and 1.03 mmol/l for women (Downs et al. 1998). In this study lovastatin treatment increased HDL-C by 6% while the beneficial effect of this increase on coronary outcomes did not reach significance. Only the increase in apoA-I in the lovastatin treated group had a significant association with the decrease of CHD events (Gotto et al. 2000).

HDL-C elevation was also not significantly associated with the reduction of CHD events in any of the other large scale primary or secondary prevention studies with the exception of the recent post hoc subgroup analysis of the 4S trial. There patients with the lipid triad of elevated LDL-C (5.1 mmol/l), low HDL-C (0.86 mmol/l) and elevated triglycerides (2.17 mmol/l) were shown to receive a greater benefit from statin treatment than patients with isolated LDL-C elevation and high HDL-C (Ballantyne et al. 2001).

In a small turnover study using stable isotopes, pravastatin was found to increase the production and catabolism of apoA-I (Schaefer et al. 1999). This was corroborated by in vitro experiments where statins directly up-regulate apoA-I gene transcription through peroxisome proliferator activator receptor alpha (PPARα) (Martin et al. 2001). And it seems that statin dependent activation of PPARα is independent of activation by fibrates because simultaneous treatment of statins and fibrates resulted in synergistic effects on PPARα transactivation (Martin et al. 2001).

The hypercatabolic effect of statins on HDL metabolism appears to be mediated by up-regulation of SR-BI and down-regulation of ABCA1 (Trigatti et al. 2000; Krieger 1999). Statin-mediated down-regulation of cholesterol synthesis may enhance selective uptake of HDL-C in the liver through up-regulation of SR-BI which is expected to increase HDL catabolism and lower plasma HDL-C (Trigatti et al. 2000; Krieger 1999). Furthermore, down-regulation of ABCA1 by inhibition of cholesterol synthesis would reduce HDL maturation and as a secondary effect enhance the catabolism of apoA-I. SR-BI up-regulation and ABCA1 down-regulation are expected to lower HDL-C in plasma and cannot explain the statin induced elevation of HDL-C. However, statin treated patients also have reduced CETP activity in plasma, which impairs cholesterol-ester transfer from HDL to apoB containing lipoproteins and thereby increases HDL-C.

Taken together the in vitro data suggest that statins increase HDL-C via enhanced apoA-I production which appears to override the HDL-C lowering effect of increased HDL catabolism. However for some statins or at high dosages these relative effects may vary so that the HDL-C increase is reduced. Because of the divergent effects of statins on the expression of ABCA1 (down) and SR-BI (up) and because of their inhibition of CETP, the effects of statins on RCT from peripheral cells to the liver are difficult to predict.

5.2
Fibrates

Fibrates were found to regulate the expression of several genes involved in lipoprotein metabolism and inflammation by activation of the nuclear receptor PPARα. Activated PPARα binds to PPAR-response elements and increases the transcription of downstream genes. Several pivotal genes of HDL metabolism including apoA-I, apoA-II, SR-BI and ABCA1 harbour such PPAR response elements and are up-regulated in the presence of PPARα agonists (Fruchart 2001).

Enhanced hepatic secretion of apoA-I and apoA-II increase HDL production whereas up-regulation of ABCA1 helps to supply HDL precursors with phospholipid and cholesterol from peripheral cells. Furthermore, LPL is up-regulated and apoC-III, an inhibitor of LPL, is suppressed by PPARα activation. Hence, fibrate treatment enhances lipolysis of triglyceride-rich lipoproteins and thereby increases the production of surface remnants and finally the formation of HDL. The combination of these processes is thought to increase HDL-C levels and to enhance RCT.

Fibrates primarily lower triglyceride levels and were shown to increase HDL-C between 6% and 18% in three large clinical trials for primary prevention and secondary prevention of CHD (Robins et al. 2001, BIP 2000). Effects of fibrates on serum levels of lipids and lipoproteins differ widely depending on the baseline lipoprotein profile in treated patients. For fenofibrate, the increase in HDL-C has been shown to be related to baseline HDL-C. Individuals with low baseline levels of HDL-C experience the strongest increase in HDL-C (Despres 2001). In two large open-label trials, fenofibrate increased HDL-C by 41% and 44% when baseline levels were lower than 0.9 mmol/l (Despres 2001).

In a subgroup analysis of the HHS primary prevention trial, individuals with low HDL-C were also found to benefit most effectively from gemfibrozil treatment (Manninen et al. 1988). The HHS trial showed that in middle aged men with an average total cholesterol level of 7 mmol/l and an average HDL-C of 1.22 mmol treatment with gemfibrozil increased HDL-C by 11% which was significantly associated with a reduction in fatal and non-fatal coronary event rates. Gemfibrozil also produced a significant increase in HDL_3-C in the secondary prevention trial VA-HIT which was related to a reduction of CHD events (Robins et al. 2001). VA-HIT selected men with low HDL-C levels (average 0.82 mmol/l) and low LDL-C (average 2.9 mmol/l) (Robins et al. 2001). Multivariate analysis calculated that CHD events were reduced by 11% for every 0.13 mmol/l increase in HDL-C, however, mean HDL-C increased in average by only 0.05 mmol/l (Robins et al. 2001).

Furthermore, men with low HDL-C (average 0.9 mmol/l) and moderately elevated cholesterol (LDL-C average 3.8 mmol/l) did not benefit from bezafibrate treatment in the BIP secondary prevention trial (BIP 2000). This lack of reduction in CHD events was observed despite a 18% increase of HDL-C and a 21% decrease in triglycerides (BIP 2000). The difference between the outcomes of the VA-HIT and the BIP trial may have resulted from differences in study design and populations examined. The BIP trial recruited a smaller proportion of hypertriglyceridaemic individuals than the VA-HIT trial. Interestingly, a subgroup of the BIP trial with triglycerides greater than 2.3 mmol/l benefited from bezafibrate treatment. Moreover, a post hoc analysis of the VA-HIT trial revealed that men with diabetes mellitus or increased fasting glucose benefited more from gemfibrozil treatment than euglycaemic men. Hence, it may well be that several metabolic mechanisms which differ in their response to fibrates lead to low HDL-C .

5.3
Nicotinic Acid (Niacin)

Treatment with nicotinic acid leads to favourable changes of all major lipid fractions and exerts the strongest HDL increasing effect of all commercially available drugs with increments of up to 30% (Vega and Grundy 1994; Tavintharan and Kashyap 2001).

In vivo kinetic studies attributed the increase of HDL-C by nicotinic acid to a decreased fractional catabolic rate of apoA-I (Shepherd et al. 1979). This conclusion was corroborated by cell culture experiments, showing that nicotinic acid did not increase apoA-I expression but inhibited the uptake of HDL-apoA-I without blocking the uptake of HDL-C esters. Such a mechanism would improve RCT possibly through SR-BI mediated cholesterolester uptake (Kamanna and Kashyap 2000).

Two randomized double-blind studies revealed that 2–3 g nicotinic acid increases HDL-C by 25%–29% in individuals with low baseline HDL-C (Elam et al. 2000; Sakai et al. 2001). There is only one controlled secondary prevention trial which assessed the effect of nicotinic acid on clinical end-points, the Coronary Drug Project. During the first 6 years of follow-up, treatment with nicotinic acid had no effect on coronary and total morbidity. However, after an additional follow-up of 9 years, death rates were lower among individuals who received nicotinic acid than among those who received placebo (Canner et al. 1986).

5.4
Sex Steroids

5.4.1
Oestrogens

Oestrogens increase HDL-C by increasing apoA-I production and by decreasing HDL catabolism through inhibition of HL and SR-BI. Intriguingly, oestrogen treatment decreased SR-BI expression in hepatic tissue but increased SR-BI expression in steroidogenic tissue of rats (Graf et al. 2001). Oral HRT with oestrogens increases HDL-C in postmenopausal women and hypogonadal men by about 8% (Binder et al. 2001). In non-hysterectomized women, oestrogens must be combined with progestins to reduce the risk of endometrial cancer. The 17-hydroxyprogesterone derivatives like medroxyprogesterone acetate possess no or only little androgen activity and partly anti-androgenic activities, whereas the nortestosterone derivatives have an androgenic potency.

Androgenic progestins were shown to diminish the HDL-raising effect of oestrogens in combined oestrogen/progestin HRT. However, low dose progestin and novel progestins with primarily anti-androgenic activity such as medroxyprogesterone acetate do not offset the HDL-increasing effect of oestrogens (Manson et al. 2003).

Meta analyses of observational studies suggested that HRT lowers risk for CHD in post-menopausal women. However, two recent controlled intervention studies revealed that a combination of unconjugated oestrogen and medroxyprogesterone acetate did not reduce or even increased coronary event rates in post-menopausal women despite their beneficial effects on lipoprotein levels which included a 14% decrease in LDL-C, a 10% increase in triglycerides and an 8% elevation of HDL-C (Hulley et al. 1998; Fletcher and Colditz 2002; WHI 2002). The HERS was a controlled 4.1-year trial with an unblinded follow up of 2.7 years in 2763 postmenopausal women with CHD (Grady et al. 2002), while the Women's Health Initiative (WHI) was a controlled trial in 16,608 healthy post-menopausal women with a follow up of 5.2 years (WHI 2002). The WHI trial was stopped early because health risks exceeded health benefits in women using the combined oestrogen/progestin treatment. Women receiving oestrogen plus progestin experienced increased incidences of coronary events, venous thromboembolism and breast cancer (WHI 2002; Manson et al. 2003).

These data motivated the search for alternative HRT regimens. Selective oestrogen receptor modulators act as oestrogen agonists or antagonists depending on the target tissue. This may explain why their influence on lipid metabolism diverges significantly. Raloxifene has been shown to competitively inhibit oestrogen action in the breast and the endometrium and to act as an agonist on bone and lipid metabolism. Three years of follow-up data from two controlled trials in 1,145 post-menopausal women showed decreased LDL levels with unaltered HDL levels (Johnston et al. 2000). The MORE trial showed raloxifene's benefit for breast cancer in a large 3-year controlled study with no difference in overall mortality, however, there was an increase in venous thromboembolism (Cummings et al. 1999).

Tibolone is a synthetic steroid which is used for treatment of post-menopausal complaints and bone loss and of which three major metabolites exert oestrogenic, gestagenic and androgenic effects. While tibolone exerts beneficial effects on triglycerides and lipoprotein(a) levels, it also decreases HDL-C by 20%, probably by increasing HL activity (Nofer et al. 2002). The clinical consequences of these changes in lipoprotein metabolism are not yet known. But it is interesting to note that treatment with this drug does not cause significant changes in the cholesterol efflux capacity of plasma (von Eckardstein et al. 2001c; von Eckardstein and Assmann 2000).

5.4.2
Testosterone

There is an increasing interest in testosterone for treatment of male hypogo-
nadism especially in the elderly. Testosterone was shown to lower HDL-C dose-
and concentration-dependently (Bhasin et al. 2001), probably by increasing the
expression of HL and SR-BI (Langer et al. 2002). In the physiological range,
testosterone treatment decreases HDL-C by about 0.05–0.13 mmol/l whereas
supraphysiologcal doses cause a pronounced decrease in HDL-C by more than
20%. How these changes in HDL-C translate into coronary risk is not known because testosterone was also shown to stimulate the efflux of cellular cholesterol
to HDL (Langer et al. 2002).

5.5
Fish Oil and Omega-3 Fatty Acids

Greenland Eskimos have a lower cardiovascular mortality than Danish co-
inhabitants. Comparison of the lifestyle of the two groups revealed that both
groups consumed a diet high in fat. However, Eskimos mainly ate fish and
marine mammals which are rich in the omega-3 fatty acids eicosapentaenoic
acid (EPA) and docosahexaenoic acid (DHA) whereas Danes ate a diet rich in
meat and dairy products which is high in saturated fat and cholesterol (Connor
2001). Several other population studies corroborated the initial finding that
fish consumption is associated with a reduced CHD incidence.

Combined EPA and DHA containing pharmacological supplementation was
consistently shown to reduce triglycerides. In normolipidaemic humans, fish
oil supplementation was shown to lower plasma triglycerides by 25% and
slightly increase LDL-C and HDL-C by 4% and 3%, respectively (Harris 1996).
A similar reduction in triglycerides and a similar increase in LDL-C was observed by fish oil supplementation in hypertriglyceridaemic diabetics but no
change in HDL-C was observed (Farmer et al. 2001).

Combined EPA and DHA supplementation was also investigated in a large
secondary prevention trial (GISSI) in patients surviving a recent myocardial
infarction. Treatment with n-3 fatty acids in addition to optimal pharmacological treatment and life-style advice led to a significant reduction in total
mortality mainly from a reduction in sudden death (Marchioli et al. 2002).
Intriguingly, this risk reduction was already significant after 3 months on n-3
fatty acid treatment. The conclusion from this study was that not the lipid
changes protected from sudden death but rather the anti-arrhythmic effect of
the n-3 fatty acids (Marchioli et al. 2002).

Fish oil also was shown to modulate the activity of several enzymes of lipid
metabolism that resulted in increased fatty acid mitochondrial β-oxidation and
in inhibition of de novo fatty acid synthesis (Schoonjans et al. 1996). Lipoprotein metabolism is further modified by an increase of the catabolic rate of HDL,

a decrease of apoC-III and an increase in LPL expression partially mediated by PPARα (Schoonjans et al. 1996). PPARα is not rate limiting for fish oil to exert its triglyceride lowering effect as the decrease in apoC-III production is affected in a PPARα independent manner (Dallongeville et al. 2001).

Recently, EPA and DHA were shown to inhibit the activation of the transcription factor LXRα by oxysterols (Yoshikawa et al. 2002). LXRs are key sensors of sterol metabolism and maintain normal cholesterol balance by promoting sterol efflux from peripheral cells, increasing circulating HDL-C, increasing hepatic sterol catabolism and excretion, and inhibiting further sterol absorption (Laffitte and Tontonoz 2002; Edwards et al. 2002). After activation through binding of oxysterols, LXRs bind as a heterodimer with the retinoic acid receptor to LXR-response elements in the promoter of genes such as SREBP-1c, LPL, CETP, ApoE, and ABCA1 and thereby activate transcription of these genes (Edwards et al. 2002; Yoshikawa et al. 2002). In line with this, fish oil inhibits LXR activation by oxysterols and as a consequence inhibits the binding to the LXR-responsive element which leads to down-regulation of SREBP-1c, to reduced de novo fatty acid synthesis and subsequently to reduced plasma triglyceride levels (Ou et al. 2001). In contrast, the net effect of fish oil on HDL-C is small, possibly through a counterbalance of PPAR activation and LXR inactivation. For example, LPL and ABCA1 are both up-regulated by PPARs and LXRs.

6
Drugs in Evaluation to Modify HDL Metabolism

6.1
CETP Inhibitors

Several CETP inhibitors were developed which form disulphide bonds with CETP and reduce its activity (Okamoto et al. 2000). At least two of them are currently being investigated in clinical trials (Brousseau et al. 2004; Clark et al. 2004; de Groot et al. 2004). The original rational of CETP inhibition was to mimic the anti-atherogenic lipoprotein profile of CETP deficiency where HDL-C is high and LDL-C low (Hirano et al. 2000). Additional arguments for the clinical use of CETP inhibitors was the previous finding that this group of drugs also inhibits PLTP and thereby the hepatic production of apoB-containing lipoproteins (Jiang et al. 2001).

In rabbits, the orally bioavailable CETP-inhibitor JTT-705 decreased CETP activity in a dose-dependent manner, decreased non-HDL-C and increased HDL-C. In addition, treatment of rabbits for 6 months led to a marked reduction of atherosclerotic lesions (Okamoto et al. 2000). In a recent randomized dose–response study, 4 weeks of treatment with JJT-705 resulted in a 37% reduction in CETP activity, a 34% increase in HDL-C and a 7% decrease in LDL-C with no change in the level of triglycerides (de Grooth et al. 2002).

The consequences of these lipoprotein changes are not clear and further research is necessary to investigate long-term benefits and adverse effects of this drug. Treatment with torcetrapib also caused dose-dependent decreases in CETP activity and increases in HDL cholesterol (Clark et al. 2004). Treatment with 120 mg torcetrapib per day increased HDL cholesterol by 46% if given alone and by 61% if given together with atorvastatin (Brousseau et al. 2004). If given twice daily, torcetrapib doubled HDL cholesterol. In addition, torcetrapib caused moderate decreases in LDL cholesterol and triglycerides (Brousseau et al. 2004; Clark et al. 2004). In rabbits, JTT-705 decreased CETP activity in a dose-dependent manner, decreased non-HDL cholesterol and increased HDL choesterol, and led to a significant reduction of atherosclerotic lesions in the presence of moderate but not severe hypercholesterolaemia (Huang et al. 2002; Okamoto et al. 2002). It may thus be that at least in hypercholesterolaemic subjects this class of drugs needs combination with statins. This may be important not only for the correction of hypercholesterolaemia but also for the efficient removal of apoE containing HDL which are formed in conditions of CETP deficiency and CETP inhibition. In this regard it is also important to recall possible risks of CETP inhibition. Subgroups of CETP deficient patients with low HL activity or hypertriglyceridaemia as well as carriers of certain genetic CETP variants were found to have an increased risk of CHD despite low CETP activity and elevated HDL-C. It may thus be that only subgroups of patients benefit from this class of drugs.

6.2
Exogenous ApoA-I or Reconstituted HDL

The beneficial effects of apoA-I and HDL on atherogenesis triggered the investigation of their potential therapeutic use to cure atherosclerosis. Intravenous infusion of apoA-I/lecithin discs (so-called reconstituted HDL) was shown to increase pre-β-HDL concentrations in lymph and to accelerate bile acid excretion in humans (Nanjee et al. 2001). Similar results were obtained following infusion of reconstituted HDL containing pro-apolipoprotein A-I where bile acid and cholesterol excretion were increased by about one-third without signs of increased cholesterol synthesis (Eriksson et al. 1999). Hence, metabolic studies in man support the view that precursors of HDL can stimulate RCT.

Further support for the use of apoA-I or reconstituted HDL therapy to stimulate RCT and to protect from atherosclerosis comes from animal studies. Infusion of a single high dose of recombinant apoA-I$_{milano}$ in rabbits was shown to decrease the lipid content and the number of macrophages in atherosclerotic lesions (Shah et al. 2001). Importantly, this effect was documented 48 h after apoA-I administration suggesting a very efficient way of mobilizing lipids from atherosclerotic plaques and eventually stabilizing them. In line with these findings, repetitive administration of apoA-I$_{milano}$ halted the progression of atherosclerosis in a hyperlipidaemic mouse model when mice were given recombinant apoA-I$_{milano}$ intravenously every second day for 5 weeks (Shah et al. 1998). In pigs apoA-I$_{milano}$ was recently shown to be inhibitory in stent restenosis (Kaul et al. 2003). In a recent double-blind, randomized intravascular ultrasound study, treatment of 123 patients with five weekly infusions containing either placebo or recombinant apoA-I$_{milano}$/phospholipid complexes at 15 mg/kg or 45 mg/kg dosages intravenously led to a 4% reduction in coronary atheroma load (Nissen et al. 2003). It is important to note that this intervention did not change HDL cholesterol. These data look encouraging and need to be confirmed in larger studies with clinical endpoints. In addition, the design of these studies does not allow the conclusion of whether the atheroprotective effects of the interventions are related to phospholipids, apoA-I or the specific apoA-I$_{milano}$ mutant.

Effects independent of RCT were also attributed to apoA-I infusion in humans. Infusion of apoA-I/phosphatidylcholine normalized the impaired endothelial function in hypercholesterolaemic patients. Endothelial dependent vasodilation upon acetylcholine stimulation was improved within minutes of apoA-I infusion reaching forearm blood flow levels similar to normolipidaemics (Spieker et al. 2002).

In all of the above studies apoA-I had to be given intravenously and this limits its use for long-term pharmacological therapy in humans. In contrast, an 18-amino acid long apoA-I mimetic peptide synthesized from D-amino acids which forms an amphipathic lipid binding class A alpha helix could be given to mice orally. The D-peptide was bioavailable and stable in circulation whereas the identical peptide from L-amino acids was rapidly degraded (Navab et al. 2002). Treatment with the apoA-I mimetic peptide did not affect lipoprotein levels but significantly inhibited the formation of atherosclerotic plaques in hyperlipidaemic mouse models (Navab et al. 2002, 2004). The same peptide was recently shown to increase plasma HDL-C activity when injected intraperitoneally (Van Lenten et al. 2002). Several apoA-I mimetic peptides have previously been synthesized and investigated for their atheroprotective potential. Many of these peptides strongly associated with phospholipids, promoted cholesterol efflux from lipid-laden cells and interacted with lipoproteins.

In addition to the atheroprotective mechanism, apoA-I mimetic peptides were shown to possess antiviral activity. An orally available apoA-I mimetic peptide protected mice from influenza infection and other apoA-I mimetic peptides inhibited HIV-induced syncytium formation and herpes simplex virus-induced cell fusion in cell cultures (Van Lenten et al. 2002).

7
Future Targets for Modulation of HDL Metabolism

From the current knowledge of HDL metabolism and RCT, three major targets for an anti-atherogenic strategy in HDL metabolism have emerged. Stimulation of apoA-I synthesis and secretion, stimulation of ABCA1 expression, and up-regulation of SR-BI are all expected to improve RCT (von Eckardstein 2004).

Stimulation of apoA-I synthesis and secretion is one key target for an anti-atherosclerotic therapy because of the pivotal role of apoA-I for the formation of HDL and because of the unequivocal finding of reduced atherosclerosis in transgenic animals over-expressing human apoA-I. Stimulation of ABCA1 expression and activity is also an attractive target because this transporter is essential for HDL formation and for the removal of cellular cholesterol from macrophages. Stimulation of both apoA-I and ABCA1 would increase HDL-C and would be easily accepted as preventive or curative treatment regimens. In contrast, up-regulation of SR-BI would cause a decrease rather than an increase of HDL-C and therefore create problems in clinical surveillance and acceptance of this therapy. Nevertheless, SR-BI has an important impact on cholesterol efflux from macrophages and on selective uptake of lipids from lipoproteins into the liver and up-regulation will improve RCT.

In many patients low HDL-C is not caused by dysregulation of a single pivotal gene but results from dysregulation of several genes. Moreover, low HDL-C is a prototype symptom of the metabolic syndrome which is frequently confounded with other risk factors. Even more so, low HDL-C frequently precedes the manifestation of other sequelae of the metabolic syndrome such as diabetes mellitus (von Eckardstein et al. 2000). Therefore, common regulatory pathways appear to be dysregulated in most individuals with low HDL-C which lead to increased coronary risk or even manifest atherosclerosis.

These common pathways may organize essential metabolic steps on the level of single cells, distinct organs, and the entire organism. The most likely candidate genes for these common denominators are transcription factors that regulate the transcription of several downstream genes and/or kinases or phosphatases which regulate signal transduction cascades involved in RCT. At present, the main targets for anti-atherosclerotic therapy are the transcription factors PPARα, PPARγ, PPARδ, LXRα, RXRα, and other orphan members of the nuclear receptor gene family.

Agonists of PPARα (fibrates) and PPARγ (glitazones) are already used as drugs for prevention of atherosclerosis and treatment of diabetes mellitus, respectively. More potent agonists of PPARα ('superfibrates') are sought and glitazones will have to be investigated for their capacity to prevent diabetes mellitus and CHD. The metabolic effects of PPARδ agonists have just started to be explored with the indication that selective PPARδ activation improves RCT (Oliver et al. 2001). Natural agonists of LXRα (oxysterols) and RXRα (retinoids) improve cholesterol efflux from macrophages but also induce hypertriglyceridaemia and are therefore not suitable for preventing atherosclerosis. However, one may consider synthetic agonists which only exert non-hepatic effects.

In addition to these transcription factors with known ligands, pivotal genes of HDL metabolism are also regulated by orphan receptors with unknown ligands, e.g. HNF1α and ZNF202 (Shih et al. 2001). For these orphan receptors it will be important to identify the physiological ligands. Because geographic differences in the prevalence of low HDL-C, diabetes mellitus type 2 and atherosclerotic vessel diseases are frequently paralleled with changes or differences in dietary habits, it is very likely that small molecules taken up with the diet are ligands of these nuclear receptors. Their elucidation may help to develop new compounds needed for the modulation of HDL metabolism. Likewise, several upstream effects of HDL on cell cycle and activation are mediated by its lipid components which can be exploited for drug development (von Eckardstein 2004).

References

4S (1994) Randomised trial of cholesterol lowering in 4444 patients with coronary heart disease: the Scandinavian Simvastatin Survival Study (4S). Lancet 344:1383–1389

WOSCOPS (1998) Influence of pravastatin and plasma lipids on clinical events in the West of Scotland Coronary Prevention Study (WOSCOPS). Circulation 97:1440–1445

BIP (2000) Secondary prevention by raising HDL cholesterol and reducing triglycerides in patients with coronary artery disease: the Bezafibrate Infarction Prevention (BIP) study. Circulation 102:21–27

WHI (2002) Risks and benefits of estrogen plus progestin in healthy postmenopausal women: principal results From the Women's Health Initiative randomized controlled trial. JAMA 288:321–333

Arai T, Wang N, Bezouevski M, Welch C, Tall AR (1999) Decreased atherosclerosis in heterozygous low density lipoprotein receptor-deficient mice expressing the scavenger receptor BI transgene. J Biol Chem 274:2366–2371

Ballantyne CM, Herd JA, Ferlic LL, Dunn JK, Farmer JA, Jones PH, Schein JR, Gotto AM, Jr. (1999) Influence of low HDL on progression of coronary artery disease and response to fluvastatin therapy. Circulation 99:736–743

Ballantyne CM, Olsson AG, Cook TJ, Mercuri MF, Pedersen TR, Kjekshus J (2001) Influence of low high-density lipoprotein cholesterol and elevated triglyceride on coronary heart disease events and response to simvastatin therapy in 4S. Circulation 104:3046–3051

Barter PJ (2002) Hugh sinclair lecture: the regulation and remodelling of HDL by plasma factors. Atheroscler Suppl 3:39–47

Bhasin S, Woodhouse L, Casaburi R, Singh AB, Bhasin D, Berman N, Chen X, Yarasheski KE, Magliano L, Dzekov C, Dzekov J, Bross R, Phillips J, Sinha-Hikim I, Shen R, Storer TW (2001) Testosterone dose-response relationships in healthy young men. Am J Physiol Endocrinol Metab 281:E1172–E1181

Binder EF, Williams DB, Schechtman KB, Jeffe DB, Kohrt WM (2001) Effects of hormone replacement therapy on serum lipids in elderly women. a randomized, placebo-controlled trial. Ann Intern Med 134:754–760

Bjorkhem I, Diczfalusy U (2002) Oxysterols: friends, foes, or just fellow passengers? Arterioscler Thromb Vasc Biol 22:734–742

Braun A, Trigatti BL, Post MJ, Sato K, Simons M, Edelberg JM, Rosenberg RD, Schrenzel M, Krieger M (2002) Loss of SR-BI expression leads to the early onset of occlusive atherosclerotic coronary artery disease, spontaneous myocardial infarctions, severe cardiac dysfunction, and premature death in apolipoprotein E-deficient mice. Circ Res 90:270–276

Brousseau ME, Schaefer EJ, Wolfe ML, Bloedon LT, Digenio AG, Clark RW, Mancuso JP, Rader DJ (2004) Effects of an inhibitor of cholesteryl ester transfer protein on HDL cholesterol. N Engl J Med 350:1505–1515

Canner PL, Berge KG, Wenger NK, Stamler J, Friedman L, Prineas RJ, Friedewald W (1986) Fifteen year mortality in Coronary Drug Project patients: long-term benefit with niacin. J Am Coll Cardiol 8:1245–1255

Chen W, Sun Y, Welch C, Gorelik A, Leventhal AR, Tabas I, Tall AR (2001) Preferential ATP-binding cassette transporter A1-mediated cholesterol efflux from late endosomes/lysosomes. J Biol Chem 276:43564–43569

Christensen EI, Birn H (2002) Megalin and cubilin: multifunctional endocytic receptors. Nat Rev Mol Cell Biol 3:256–266

Chroni A, Liu T, Gorshkova I, Kan HY, Uehara Y, von Eckardstein A, Zannis VI (2003) The central helices of APOA-I can promote ABCA1-mediated lipid efflux: amino acid residues 220–231 of the wild-type APOA-I are required for lipid efflux in vitro and HDL formation in vivo. J Biol Chem 278:6719–6730

Clark RW, Sutfin TA, Ruggeri RB, Willauer AT, Sugarman ED, Magnus-Aryitey G, Cosgrove PG, Sand TM, Wester RT, Williams JA, Perlman ME, Bamberger MJ (2004) Raising high-density lipoprotein in humans through inhibition of cholesteryl ester transfer protein: an initial multidose study of torcetrapib. Arterioscler Thromb Vasc Biol 24:490–497

Cohen JC, Vega GL, Grundy SM (1999) Hepatic lipase: new insights from genetic and metabolic studies. Curr Opin Lipidol 10:259–267

Connor WE (2001) n-3 Fatty acids from fish and fish oil: panacea or nostrum? Am J Clin Nutr 74:415–416

Cummings SR, Eckert S, Krueger KA, Grady D, Powles TJ, Cauley JA, Norton L, Nickelsen T, Bjarnason NH, Morrow M, Lippman ME, Black D, Glusman JE, Costa A, Jordan VC (1999) The effect of raloxifene on risk of breast cancer in postmenopausal women: results from the MORE randomized trial. Multiple Outcomes of Raloxifene Evaluation. JAMA 281:2189–2197

Curtiss LK, Boisvert WA (2000) Apolipoprotein E and atherosclerosis. Curr Opin Lipidol 11:243–251

Dallongeville J, Bauge E, Tailleux A, Peters JM, Gonzalez FJ, Fruchart JC, Staels B (2001) Peroxisome proliferator-activated receptor alpha is not rate-limiting for the lipoprotein-lowering action of fish oil. J Biol Chem 276:4634–4639

de Grooth GJ, Kuivenhoven JA, Stalenhoef AF, de Graaf J, Zwinderman AH, Posma JL, van Tol A, Kastelein JJ (2002) Efficacy and safety of a novel cholesteryl ester transfer protein inhibitor, JTT-705, in humans: a randomized phase II dose-response study. Circulation 105:2159–2165

Despres JP (2001) Increasing high-density lipoprotein cholesterol: an update on fenofibrate. Am J Cardiol 88:30N–36N

Downs JR, Clearfield M, Weis S, Whitney E, Shapiro DR, Beere PA, Langendorfer A, Stein EA, Kruyer W, Gotto AM, Jr. (1998) Primary prevention of acute coronary events with lovastatin in men and women with average cholesterol levels: results of AFCAPS/TexCAPS. Air Force/Texas Coronary Atherosclerosis Prevention Study. JAMA 279:1615–1622

Edwards PA, Kast HR, Anisfeld AM (2002) BAREing it all: the adoption of LXR and FXR and their roles in lipid homeostasis. J Lipid Res 43:2–12

Elam MB, Hunninghake DB, Davis KB, Garg R, Johnson C, Egan D, Kostis JB, Sheps DS, Brinton EA (2000) Effect of niacin on lipid and lipoprotein levels and glycemic control in patients with diabetes and peripheral arterial disease: the ADMIT study: A randomized trial. Arterial Disease Multiple Intervention Trial. JAMA 284:1263–1270

Eriksson M, Carlson LA, Miettinen TA, Angelin B (1999) Stimulation of fecal steroid excretion after infusion of recombinant proapolipoprotein A-I. Potential reverse cholesterol transport in humans. Circulation 100:594–598

Farmer A, Montori V, Dinneen S, Clar C (2001) Fish oil in people with type 2 diabetes mellitus. Cochrane Database Syst Rev CD003205

Fletcher SW, Colditz GA (2002) Failure of estrogen plus progestin therapy for prevention. JAMA 288:366–368

Frick MH, Syvanne M, Nieminen MS, Kauma H, Majahalme S, Virtanen V, Kesaniemi YA, Pasternack A, Taskinen MR (1997) Prevention of the angiographic progression of coronary and vein-graft atherosclerosis by gemfibrozil after coronary bypass surgery in men with low levels of HDL cholesterol. Lopid Coronary Angiography Trial (LOCAT) Study Group. Circulation 96:2137–2143

Fruchart JC (2001) Peroxisome proliferator-activated receptor-alpha activation and high-density lipoprotein metabolism. Am J Cardiol 88:24N–29N

Glass CK, Witztum JL (2001) Atherosclerosis. the road ahead. Cell 104:503–516

Gotto AM, Jr. (2002) Management of dyslipidemia. Am J Med 112 Suppl 8A:10S–18S

Gotto AM, Jr., Whitney E, Stein EA, Shapiro DR, Clearfield M, Weis S, Jou JY, Langendorfer A, Beere PA, Watson DJ, Downs JR, de Cani JS (2000) Relation between baseline and on-treatment lipid parameters and first acute major coronary events in the Air Force/Texas Coronary Atherosclerosis Prevention Study (AFCAPS/TexCAPS). Circulation 101:477–484

Grady D, Herrington D, Bittner V, Blumenthal R, Davidson M, Hlatky M, Hsia J, Hulley S, Herd A, Khan S, Newby LK, Waters D, Vittinghoff E, Wenger N (2002) Cardiovascular disease outcomes during 6.8 years of hormone therapy: Heart and Estrogen/progestin Replacement Study follow-up (HERS II). JAMA 288:49–57

Graf GA, Roswell KL, Smart EJ (2001) 17beta-Estradiol promotes the up-regulation of SR-BII in HepG2 cells and in rat livers. J Lipid Res 42:1444–1449

Harris WS (1996) n-3 fatty acids and lipoproteins: comparison of results from human and animal studies. Lipids 31:243–252

Hersberger M, von Eckardstein A (2003) Low high-density lipoprotein cholesterol: physiological background, clinical importance and drug treatment. Drugs 63:1907–1945

Hirano K, Yamashita S, Matsuzawa Y (2000) Pros and cons of inhibiting cholesteryl ester transfer protein. Curr Opin Lipidol 11:589–596

Huang Z, Inazu A, Nohara A, Higashikata T, Mabuchi H (2002) Cholesteryl ester transfer protein inhibitor (JTT-705) and the development of atherosclerosis in rabbits with severe hypercholesterolaemia. Clin Sci (Lond) 103:587–594

Hulley S, Grady D, Bush T, Furberg C, Herrington D, Riggs B, Vittinghoff E (1998) Randomized trial of estrogen plus progestin for secondary prevention of coronary heart disease in postmenopausal women. Heart and Estrogen/progestin Replacement Study (HERS) Research Group. JAMA 280:605–613

Jiang XC, Qin S, Qiao C, Kawano K, Lin M, Skold A, Xiao X, Tall AR (2001) Apolipoprotein B secretion and atherosclerosis are decreased in mice with phospholipid-transfer protein deficiency. Nat Med 7:847–852

Johnston CC, Jr., Bjarnason NH, Cohen FJ, Shah A, Lindsay R, Mitlak BH, Huster W, Draper MW, Harper KD, Heath H, III, Gennari C, Christiansen C, Arnaud CD, Delmas PD (2000) Long-term effects of raloxifene on bone mineral density, bone turnover, and serum lipid levels in early postmenopausal women: three-year data from 2 double-blind, randomized, placebo-controlled trials. Arch Intern Med 160:3444–3450

Kamanna VS, Kashyap ML (2000) Mechanism of action of niacin on lipoprotein metabolism. Curr Atheroscler Rep 2:36–46

Kaul S, Rukshin V, Santos R, Azarbal B, Bisgaier CL, Johansson J, Tsang VT, Chyu KY, Cercek B, Mirocha J, Shah PK (2003) Intramural delivery of recombinant apolipoprotein A-IMilano/phospholipid complex (ETC-216) inhibits in-stent stenosis in porcine coronary arteries. Circulation 107:2551–2554

Krieger M (1999) Charting the fate of the "good cholesterol": identification and characterization of the high-density lipoprotein receptor SR-BI. Annu Rev Biochem 68:523–558

Laffitte BA, Tontonoz P (2002) Orphan nuclear receptors find a home in the arterial wall. Curr Atheroscler Rep 4:213–221

Langer C, Gansz B, Goepfert C, Engel T, Uehara Y, von Dehn G, Jansen H, Assmann G, von Eckardstein A (2002) Testosterone up-regulates scavenger receptor B1 and stimulates cholesterol efflux from macrophages. Biochem Biophys Res Commun 296:1051–1057

Liu T, Krieger M, Kan HY, Zannis VI (2002) The effects of mutations in helices 4 and 6 of ApoA-I on scavenger receptor class B type I (SR-BI)-mediated cholesterol efflux suggest that formation of a productive complex between reconstituted high density lipoprotein and SR-BI is required for efficient lipid transport. J Biol Chem 277:21576–21584

Llera-Moya M, Rothblat GH, Connelly MA, Kellner-Weibel G, Sakr SW, Phillips MC, Williams DL (1999) Scavenger receptor BI (SR-BI) mediates free cholesterol flux independently of HDL tethering to the cell surface. J Lipid Res 40:575–580

Manninen V, Elo MO, Frick MH, Haapa K, Heinonen OP, Heinsalmi P, Helo P, Huttunen JK, Kaitaniemi P, Koskinen P (1988) Lipid alterations and decline in the incidence of coronary heart disease in the Helsinki Heart Study. JAMA 260:641–651

Manninen V, Tenkanen L, Koskinen P, Huttunen JK, Manttari M, Heinonen OP, Frick MH (1992) Joint effects of serum triglyceride and LDL cholesterol and HDL cholesterol concentrations on coronary heart disease risk in the Helsinki Heart Study. Implications for treatment. Circulation 85:37–45

Manson JE, Hsia J, Johnson KC, Rossouw JE, Assaf AR, Lasser NL, Trevisan M, Black HR, Heckbert SR, Detrano R, Strickland OL, Wong ND, Crouse JR, Stein E, Cushman M (2003) Estrogen plus progestin and the risk of coronary heart disease. N Engl J Med 349:523–534

Marchioli R, Barzi F, Bomba E, Chieffo C, Di Gregorio D, Di Mascio R, Franzosi MG, Geraci E, Levantesi G, Maggioni AP, Mantini L, Marfisi RM, Mastrogiuseppe G, Mininni N, Nicolosi GL, Santini M, Schweiger C, Tavazzi L, Tognoni G, Tucci C, Valagussa F (2002) Early protection against sudden death by n-3 polyunsaturated fatty acids after myocardial infarction: time-course analysis of the results of the Gruppo Italiano per lo Studio della Sopravvivenza nell'Infarto Miocardico (GISSI)-Prevenzione. Circulation 105:1897–1903

Martin G, Duez H, Blanquart C, Berezowski V, Poulain P, Fruchart JC, Najib-Fruchart J, Glineur C, Staels B (2001) Statin-induced inhibition of the Rho-signaling pathway activates PPARalpha and induces HDL apoA-I. J Clin Invest 107:1423–1432

Martinez LO, Jacquet S, Esteve JP, Rolland C, Cabezon E, Champagne E, Pineau T, Georgeaud V, Walker JE, Terce F, Collet X, Perret B, Barbaras R (2003) Ectopic beta-chain of ATP synthase is an apolipoprotein A-I receptor in hepatic HDL endocytosis. Nature 421:75–79

Nanjee MN, Cooke CJ, Garvin R, Semeria F, Lewis G, Olszewski WL, Miller NE (2001) Intravenous apoA-I/lecithin discs increase pre-beta-HDL concentration in tissue fluid and stimulate reverse cholesterol transport in humans. J Lipid Res 42:1586–1593

Navab M, Anantharamaiah GM, Hama S, Garber DW, Chaddha M, Hough G, Lallone R, Fogelman AM (2002) Oral administration of an Apo A-I mimetic Peptide synthesized from D- amino acids dramatically reduces atherosclerosis in mice independent of plasma cholesterol. Circulation 105:290–292

Navab M, Anantharamaiah GM, Reddy ST, Hama S, Hough G, Grijalva VR, Wagner AC, Frank JS, Datta G, Garber D, Fogelman AM (2004) Oral D-4F causes formation of pre-beta high-density lipoprotein and improves high-density lipoprotein-mediated cholesterol efflux and reverse cholesterol transport from macrophages in apolipoprotein E-null mice. Circulation 109:3215–3220

Neufeld EB, Remaley AT, Demosky SJ, Stonik JA, Cooney AM, Comly M, Dwyer NK, Zhang M, Blanchette-Mackie J, Santamarina-Fojo S, Brewer HB, Jr. (2001) Cellular localization and trafficking of the human ABCA1 transporter. J Biol Chem 276:27584–27590

Nissen SE, Tsunoda T, Tuzcu EM, Schoenhagen P, Cooper CJ, Yasin M, Eaton GM, Lauer MA, Sheldon WS, Grines CL, Halpern S, Crowe T, Blankenship JC, Kerensky R (2004) Effect of recombinant ApoA-I Milano on coronary atherosclerosis in patients with acute coronary syndromes: a randomized controlled trial. JAMA 290:2292–2300

Nofer JR, Kehrel B, Fobker M, Levkau B, Assmann G, von Eckardstein A (2002) HDL and arteriosclerosis: beyond reverse cholesterol transport. Atherosclerosis 161:1–16

Okamoto H, Yonemori F, Wakitani K, Minowa T, Maeda K, Shinkai H (2000) A cholesteryl ester transfer protein inhibitor attenuates atherosclerosis in rabbits. Nature 406:203–207

Oliver WR, Jr., Shenk JL, Snaith MR, Russell CS, Plunket KD, Bodkin NL, Lewis MC, Winegar DA, Sznaidman ML, Lambert MH, Xu HE, Sternbach DD, Kliewer SA, Hansen BC, Willson TM (2001) A selective peroxisome proliferator-activated receptor delta agonist promotes reverse cholesterol transport. Proc Natl Acad Sci USA 98:5306–5311

Oram JF (2002) ATP-binding cassette transporter A1 and cholesterol trafficking. Curr Opin Lipidol 13:373–381

Ou J, Tu H, Shan B, Luk A, DeBose-Boyd RA, Bashmakov Y, Goldstein JL, Brown MS (2001) Unsaturated fatty acids inhibit transcription of the sterol regulatory element-binding protein-1c (SREBP-1c) gene by antagonizing ligand-dependent activation of the LXR. Proc Natl Acad Sci USA 98:6027–6032

Rader DJ, Jaye M (2000) Endothelial lipase: a new member of the triglyceride lipase gene family. Curr Opin Lipidol 11:141–147

Robins SJ, Collins D, Wittes JT, Papademetriou V, Deedwania PC, Schaefer EJ, McNamara JR, Kashyap ML, Hershman JM, Wexler LF, Rubins HB (2001) Relation of gemfibrozil treatment and lipid levels with major coronary events: VA-HIT: a randomized controlled trial. JAMA 285:1585–1591

Rothblat GH, Llera-Moya M, Atger V, Kellner-Weibel G, Williams DL, Phillips MC (1999) Cell cholesterol efflux: integration of old and new observations provides new insights. J Lipid Res 40:781–796

Ruotolo G, Ericsson CG, Tettamanti C, Karpe F, Grip L, Svane B, Nilsson J, de Faire U, Hamsten A (1998) Treatment effects on serum lipoprotein lipids, apolipoproteins and low density lipoprotein particle size and relationships of lipoprotein variables to progression of coronary artery disease in the Bezafibrate Coronary Atherosclerosis Intervention Trial (BECAIT). J Am Coll Cardiol 32:1648–1656

Rye KA, Clay MA, Barter PJ (1999) Remodelling of high density lipoproteins by plasma factors. Atherosclerosis 145:227–238

Sacks FM, Tonkin AM, Shepherd J, Braunwald E, Cobbe S, Hawkins CM, Keech A, Packard C, Simes J, Byington R, Furberg CD (2000) Effect of pravastatin on coronary disease events in subgroups defined by coronary risk factors: the Prospective Pravastatin Pooling Project. Circulation 102:1893–1900

Sakai T, Kamanna VS, Kashyap ML (2001) Niacin, but not gemfibrozil, selectively increases LP-AI, a cardioprotective subfraction of HDL, in patients with low HDL cholesterol. Arterioscler Thromb Vasc Biol 21:1783–1789

Santamarina-Fojo S, Remaley AT, Neufeld EB, Brewer HB, Jr. (2001) Regulation and intracellular trafficking of the ABCA1 transporter. J Lipid Res 42:1339–1345

Schaefer JR, Schweer H, Ikewaki K, Stracke H, Seyberth HJ, Kaffarnik H, Maisch B, Steinmetz A (1999) Metabolic basis of high density lipoproteins and apolipoprotein A-I increase by HMG-CoA reductase inhibition in healthy subjects and a patient with coronary artery disease. Atherosclerosis 144:177–184

Schoonjans K, Staels B, Auwerx J (1996) Role of the peroxisome proliferator-activated receptor (PPAR) in mediating the effects of fibrates and fatty acids on gene expression. J Lipid Res 37:907–925

Shah PK, Nilsson J, Kaul S, Fishbein MC, Ageland H, Hamsten A, Johansson J, Karpe F, Cercek B (1998) Effects of recombinant apolipoprotein A-I(Milano) on aortic atherosclerosis in apolipoprotein E-deficient mice. Circulation 97:780–785

Shah PK, Yano J, Reyes O, Chyu KY, Kaul S, Bisgaier CL, Drake S, Cercek B (2001) High-dose recombinant apolipoprotein A-I(milano) mobilizes tissue cholesterol and rapidly reduces plaque lipid and macrophage content in apolipoprotein e-deficient mice. Potential implications for acute plaque stabilization. Circulation 103:3047–3050

Shepherd J, Packard CJ, Patsch JR, Gotto AM, Jr., Taunton OD (1979) Effects of nicotinic acid therapy on plasma high density lipoprotein subfraction distribution and composition and on apolipoprotein A metabolism. J Clin Invest 63:858–867

Shih DQ, Bussen M, Sehayek E, Ananthanarayanan M, Shneider BL, Suchy FJ, Shefer S, Bollileni JS, Gonzalez FJ, Breslow JL, Stoffel M (2001) Hepatocyte nuclear factor-1alpha is an essential regulator of bile acid and plasma cholesterol metabolism. Nat Genet 27:375–382

Silver DL, Tall AR (2001) The cellular biology of scavenger receptor class B type I. Curr Opin Lipidol 12:497–504

Silver DL, Wang N, Xiao X, Tall AR (2001) High density lipoprotein (HDL) particle uptake mediated by scavenger receptor class B type 1 results in selective sorting of HDL cholesterol from protein and polarized cholesterol secretion. J Biol Chem 276:25287–25293

Spieker LE, Sudano I, Hurlimann D, Lerch PG, Lang MG, Binggeli C, Corti R, Ruschitzka F, Luscher TF, Noll G (2002) High-density lipoprotein restores endothelial function in hypercholesterolemic men. Circulation 105:1399–1402

Takahashi Y, Smith JD (1999) Cholesterol efflux to apolipoprotein AI involves endocytosis and resecretion in a calcium-dependent pathway. Proc Natl Acad Sci USA 96:11358–11363

Tall AR, Jiang X, Luo Y, Silver D (2000) 1999 George Lyman Duff memorial lecture: lipid transfer proteins, HDL metabolism, and atherogenesis. Arterioscler Thromb Vasc Biol 20:1185–1188

Tavintharan S, Kashyap ML (2001) The benefits of niacin in atherosclerosis. Curr Atheroscler Rep 3:74–82

Thuren T (2000) Hepatic lipase and HDL metabolism. Curr Opin Lipidol 11:277–283

Trigatti B, Rigotti A, Krieger M (2000) The role of the high-density lipoprotein receptor SR-BI in cholesterol metabolism. Curr Opin Lipidol 11:123–131

Van Lenten BJ, Wagner AC, Anantharamaiah GM, Garber DW, Fishbein MC, Adhikary L, Nayak DP, Hama S, Navab M, Fogelman AM (2002) Influenza infection promotes macrophage traffic into arteries of mice that is prevented by D-4F, an apolipoprotein A-I mimetic peptide. Circulation 106:1127–1132

Vega GL, Grundy SM (1994) Lipoprotein responses to treatment with lovastatin, gemfibrozil, and nicotinic acid in normolipidemic patients with hypoalphalipoproteinemia. Arch Intern Med 154:73–82

von Eckardstein A, Crook D, Elbers J, Ragoobir J, Ezeh B, Helmond F, Miller N, Dieplinger H, Coelingh Bennink H, Assmann G (2003) Tibolone lowers HDL cholesterol by increasing hepatic lipase activity but does not impair cholesterol efflux. Clin Endocrinol (Oxford) 58:49–58

von Eckardstein A (2004) Therapeutic approaches for the modification of high-density lipoproteins. Drug Discovery Today: Therapeutic Strategies 1:177–187

von Eckardstein A, Assmann G (2000) Prevention of coronary heart disease by raising high-density lipoprotein cholesterol? Curr Opin Lipidol 11:627–637

von Eckardstein A, Langer C, Engel T, Schaukal I, Cignarella A, Reinhardt J, Lorkowski S, Li Z, Zhou X, Cullen P, Assmann G (2001a) ATP binding cassette transporter ABCA1 modulates the secretion of apolipoprotein E from human monocyte-derived macrophages. FASEB J 15:1555–1561

von Eckardstein A, Nofer JR, Assmann G (2001b) High density lipoproteins and arteriosclerosis. Role of cholesterol efflux and reverse cholesterol transport. Arterioscler Thromb Vasc Biol 21:13–27

von Eckardstein A, Schmiddem K, Hovels A, Gulbahce E, Schuler-Luttmann S, Elbers J, Helmond F, Bennink HJ, Assmann G (2001c) Lowering of HDL cholesterol in post-menopausal women by tibolone is not associated with changes in cholesterol efflux capacity or paraoxonase activity. Atherosclerosis 159:433–439

von Eckardstein A, Schulte H, Assmann G (2000) Risk for diabetes mellitus in middle-aged Caucasian male participants of the PROCAM study: implications for the definition of impaired fasting glucose by the American Diabetes Association. Prospective Cardiovascular Munster. J Clin Endocrinol Metab 85:3101–3108

Wang Y, Oram JF (2002) Unsaturated fatty acids inhibit cholesterol efflux from macrophages by increasing degradation of ATP-binding cassette transporter A1. J Biol Chem 277:5692–5697

Yoshikawa T, Shimano H, Yahagi N, Ide T, Amemiya-Kudo M, Matsuzaka T, Nakakuki M, Tomita S, Okazaki H, Tamura Y, Iizuka Y, Ohashi K, Takahashi A, Sone H, Osuga JJ, Gotoda T, Ishibashi S, Yamada N (2002) Polyunsaturated fatty acids suppress sterol regulatory element-binding protein 1c promoter activity by inhibition of liver X receptor (LXR) binding to LXR response elements. J Biol Chem 277:1705–1711

Zhou X, Engel T, Goepfert C, Erren M, Assmann G, von Eckardstein A (2002) The ATP binding cassette transporter A1 contributes to the secretion of interleukin 1beta from macrophages but not from monocytes. Biochem Biophys Res Commun 291:598–604

HEP (2005) 170:563–590

Inhibition of Lipoprotein Lipid Oxidation

O. Cynshi[1] · R. Stocker[2] (✉)

[1] Fuji-Gotemba Research Laboratories, Chugai Pharmaceutical Co. Ltd, 1-135 Komakado, 412-8513 Gotemba, Shizuoka, Japan

[2] Centre for Vascular Research, School of Medical Sciences, Faculty of Medicine, University of New South Wales, 2052 Sydney, NSW, Australia
r.stocker@unsw.au

Abstract According to the oxidative modification hypothesis, antioxidants that inhibit the oxidation of low-density lipoprotein (LDL) are expected to attenuate atherosclerosis, yet not all antioxidants that inhibit LDL oxidation in vitro inhibit disease in animal models of atherosclerosis. As with animal studies, a benefit with dietary supplements of antioxidants in general and vitamin E in particular was anticipated in humans, yet the overall outcome of large, randomized controlled studies has been disappointing. However, in recent years it has become clear that the role of vitamin E in LDL oxidation and the relationship between in vitro and in vivo inhibition of LDL oxidation are more complex than previously appreciated, and that oxidative events in addition to LDL oxidation in the extracellular space need to be considered in the context of an antioxidant as a therapeutic drug against atherosclerosis. This review focuses on some of these complexities, proposes a novel method to assess in vitro 'oxidizability' of lipoprotein lipids, and summarizes the present situation of development of antioxidant compounds as drugs against atherosclerosis and related cardiovascular disorders.

Keywords AGI-1067 · Antioxidants · Atherosclerosis · BO-653 · Lipid oxidation · Oxidation · Oxidized LDL · Restenosis

1
Introduction

1.1
Oxidative Modification Hypothesis

There have been numerous efforts to explain the complex events associated with the development of atherosclerosis. As a result three distinct hypotheses, the response-to-injury, the response-to-retention, and the oxidative modification hypothesis, have emerged and are currently under investigation. These hypotheses are not mutually exclusive but rather emphasize different concepts as the necessary and sufficient events to support the development of atherosclerosis. For the purposes of this review, we will focus on the oxidative modification hypothesis.

The oxidative modification hypothesis focuses on the concept that low-density lipoprotein (LDL) in its native state is not atherogenic. However, LDL modified chemically is readily internalized by macrophages through a so-called 'scavenger receptor' pathway (Goldstein et al. 1979). The scavenger receptor was identified by Kodama et al. (Kodama et al. 1990) and its targeted disruption was shown to lead to a reduction in atherosclerosis in hypercholesterolemic apolipoprotain E-deficient mice (Suzuki et al. 1997). Exposure to vascular cells in medium that contains transition metals also results in modification of LDL such that it serves as a ligand for the scavenger receptor pathway (Henriksen et al. 1981). It is now clear that one mechanism whereby cells in vitro render LDL a substrate for the scavenger receptor pathway is via oxidation of LDL lipids and the resulting modification of apolipoprotein B-00 (Steinbrecher et al. 1984).

According to the oxidative modification hypothesis of atherosclerosis (Steinberg et al. 1989), LDL traverses the subendothelial space of lesion-prone arterial sites. During this process, LDL lipids are subject to oxidation and, as a consequence, apolipoprotein B-100 lysine groups are modified so that the net negative charge of the lipoprotein particle increases (Haberland et al. 1982). This modification renders LDL susceptible to macrophage uptake via a number of scavenger receptor pathways, producing cholesterol ester-laden foam cells (Haberland et al. 1984). It is this accumulation of foam cells that forms the nidus of a developing atherosclerotic lesion. In addition, oxidized LDL contributes to atherogenesis by aiding the recruitment of circulating monocytes into the intimal space, inhibiting the ability of resident macrophages to leave the intima, and being cytotoxic, leading to loss of endothelial integrity (Quinn et al. 1985). The latter property was proposed to provide the link between fatty streak formation due to lipid infiltration and the progression of the fatty streak to more advanced lesions according to the response-to-injury hypothesis of atherogenesis (Steinberg et al. 1989).

The process of LDL oxidation is associated with a number of other potentially pro-atherogenic events. For example, during the initial stages of in vitro LDL oxidation, modification of LDL lipids can occur in the absence of any changes to apolipoprotein B-100. Such modified LDL has been termed 'minimally modified LDL' and shown in vitro to induce the synthesis of monocyte chemotactic protein-1 in both smooth muscle and endothelial cells (Cushing et al. 1990; Rajavashisth et al. 1990) resulting in the recruitment of inflammatory cells (Navab et al. 1991). This particular step appears critical as mice lacking the receptor for monocyte chemotactic protein-1 are resistant to atherosclerosis (Boring et al. 1998; Gosling et al. 1999). More heavily in vitro oxidized LDL, commonly termed 'ox-LDL', is chemotactic for monocytes (Quinn et al. 1987) and T lymphocytes (McMurray et al. 1993), perhaps as the result of lysophosphatidylcholine formed during oxidation (Steinbrecher et al. 1984). Oxidized LDL has also been shown to stimulate the proliferation of smooth muscle cells, and to be immunogenic by eliciting the production of autoantibodies (Parums et al. 1990; Salonen et al. 1992) and the formation of immune complexes that can also facilitate macrophage internalization of LDL (Klimov et al. 1985; Griffith et al. 1988). The recruitment of inflammatory cells may result in the continued oxidation of LDL, setting the stage for catalytic expansion of the atherosclerotic lesion and the full-blown spectrum of atherosclerosis.

1.2
Inhibition of Atherosclerosis by Antioxidants

There are several lines of evidence that support the oxidative modification hypothesis. For example, oxidized LDL can support foam cell formation in vitro, the lipid in human lesions is substantially oxidized, there is evidence for the presence of oxidized LDL in vivo, and in vitro oxidized LDL has a number of potentially pro-atherogenic activities (reviewed in Stocker and Keaney 2004). In addition, support for the hypothesis comes from studies showing that several structurally unrelated anti-oxidants inhibit atherosclerosis in animals.

Arguably the strongest evidence in support of anti-oxidant compounds providing protection against atherosclerosis comes from studies with probucol (Mashima et al. 2001). Probucol is a synthetic cholesterol-lowering drug that also possesses anti-oxidant activity (Marshall 1982; Parthasarathy et al. 1986). The lipophilic drug associates with and effectively protects LDL against in vitro oxidation induced by copper ions (Parthasarathy et al. 1986; Kita et al. 1987), although it is a sterically hindered phenol, and its peroxyl radical scavenging activity is only about 16% of that of α-tocopherol (Pryor et al. 1993).

Early studies with probucol demonstrated inhibition of atherosclerosis in rabbits (Kritchevsky et al. 1971; Tawara et al. 1986) and monkeys (Wissler and Vesselinovitch 1983). Kita and colleagues (Kita et al. 1987) treated Watanabe heritable hyperlipidemic (WHHL) rabbits with probucol and observed an 87% reduction in lesion area and LDL resistance to oxidation compared to those animals not treated with probucol. These findings prompted the authors to conclude that the reduction of atherosclerosis was due to the anti-oxidant effect of probucol; however, probucol also produced a 17% reduction in serum cholesterol. Carew and colleagues (Carew et al. 1987) controlled for the cholesterol-lowering effect of probucol with lovastatin. Similar reductions in total cholesterol were observed with lovastatin and probucol; however, the latter provided an additional 48% reduction in atherosclerosis (Carew et al. 1987), suggesting that probucol inhibited atherosclerosis due to its anti-oxidant activity. This contention was supported in a study with WHHL rabbits treated with a structural analog of probucol devoid of cholesterol-lowering properties (Mao et al. 1991). Both probucol and the analog inhibited LDL oxidation and reduced atherosclerosis, suggesting an anti-oxidant-mediated mechanism for lesion reduction. Subsequent studies in primates (Sasahara et al. 1994), cholesterol-fed rabbits (Shaish et al. 1995), and hamsters (Parker et al. 1995) also demonstrated a reduction in atherosclerosis with probucol. The situation appears more complex in mouse models of atherosclerosis, where probucol promotes atherosclerosis in the aortic root (Zhang et al. 1997, Bird et al. 1998, Moghadasian et al. 1999) but inhibits disease formation at more distal sites (Witting et al. 2000).

There have been two studies testing the antiatherosclerotic activity of probucol in humans. The Probucol Quantitative Regression Study reported probucol to be ineffective in attenuating lumen loss in the femoral arteries in hypercholesterolemic subjects over 3 years, as assessed by quantitative angiography (Walldius et al. 1994). Importantly however, this method does not directly assess disease burden. In contrast, the Fukoaka Atherosclerosis Trial observed probucol to significantly decrease atherosclerosis progression in the carotid artery of hypercholesterolemic patients, as assessed by the intima-to-media thickness determined by B-mode ultrasound (Sawayama et al. 2002). In addition, probucol (Tardif et al. 1997, 2003), and a probucol analog with one of its two phenol moieties present as succinate ester (Tardif et al. 2003), also protect against restenosis after percutaneous coronary intervention (see Sect. 3.2).

A number of other anti-oxidants have also been tested for their ability to inhibit atherosclerosis in animal models of the disease. N,N'-diphenyl-phenylenediamine is an aniline compound that attenuates atherosclerosis in the aorta of cholesterol-fed rabbits (Sparrow et al. 1992), and similar findings have been reported in a murine model of atherosclerosis (Tangirala et al. 1995). In addition, 2,3-dihydro-5-hydroxy-2,2-dipentyl-4,6-di-*tert*-butylbenzofuran (BO-653), a synthetic anti-oxidant with structural components of vitamin E (Noguchi et al. 1997), inhibits atherosclerosis in both rabbit and murine models (Cynshi et al. 1998) (see Sect. 3.3). Similarly, 3,3',5,5'-tetrabutyl 1,1'-biphenyl 4,4'diol, a lipophilic bisphenol, inhibits atherosclerosis in mice deficient in apolipoprotein E and the LDL receptor (Witting et al. 1999). Furthermore, supplementation of the diet with butylated hydroxytoluene reduces atherosclerotic lesions in cholesterol-fed rabbits (Bjorkhem et al. 1991; Freyschuss et al. 1993), and another recent study showed that boldine, an alkaloid anti-oxidant, inhibits atherosclerosis in LDL receptor-deficient mice (Santanam et al. 2004).

A common feature of all of these compounds is that they inhibit LDL oxidation in vitro. Thus, a number of lipid-soluble, synthetic anti-oxidants have been used to demonstrate an association between a reduction in atherosclerosis and ex vivo inhibition of LDL oxidation.

1.3
Insights from Overall Lack of Beneficial Effect of Antioxidants on Cardiovascular Diseases

It is important to point out, however, that not all synthetic anti-oxidants offer protection against atherosclerosis in animals (reviewed by Stocker 1999). This is particularly intriguing in situations where the anti-oxidants have been shown to decrease the extent of lipid oxidation. For example, supplementation of a butter-based atherogenic diet with butylated hydroxytoluene and butylated hydroxyanisole (both phenolic lipid-soluble anti-oxidants that effectively inhibit LDL oxidation in vitro) does not prevent atherosclerosis in rabbits (Wilson et al. 1978). Also, compared with probucol, its structural analog *bis*(3,5-di-*tert*-butyl-4-hydroxy-phenylether)propane offers superior protection to LDL against in vitro oxidation, yet the analog is ineffective in inhibiting atherosclerosis in LDL receptor-deficient rabbits (Fruebis et al. 1994). Perhaps even more striking, another structural analog of probucol, 3,3'-5,5'-tetra-*tert*-butyl-4,4'-bisphenol, prevents lipoprotein lipid oxidation in the vessel wall of LDL receptor-deficient rabbits as effectively as probucol, yet the analog, unlike probucol, does not protect against atherosclerosis (Witting et al. 1999). Conversely, probucol inhibits atherosclerosis in the aortic arch and thoracic and abdominal aorta of apolipoprotein E-deficient mice without inhibiting aortic lipoprotein oxidation (Witting et al. 2000). These latter studies establish that at least in some animal models, the process of lipoprotein oxidation can be dissociated from atherosclerosis.

In addition to the synthetic lipid-soluble anti-oxidants referred to above, vitamin E has been used repeatedly for intervention studies in a variety of experimental models. This is not surprising, considering it is the most abundant endogenous anti-oxidant associated with LDL extracts (Esterbauer et al. 1992). A majority of studies report a null effect of vitamin E supplements on lesion formation in animals on a normal diet (Stocker and Keaney 2004). Only 11 of the 44 studies carried out over the last 50 years show vitamin E to attenuate disease. In 4 of these 11 studies vitamin E supplements lowered plasma lipids (Brattsand 1975; Wilson et al. 1978; Westrope et al. 1982; Prasad and Kalra 1993) so that this hypolipidemic rather than the anti-oxidant function may have been responsible for the outcome. Thus, an anti-atherogenic effect independent of lipid lowering has been observed in only seven studies (Prasad and Kalra 1993; Qiao et al. 1993; Sun et al. 1997; Böger et al. 1998; Pratico et al. 1998; Thomas et al. 2001; Cyrus et al. 2003). Notably, a similar number of investigations (n=5) have shown increased lesion formation with vitamin E supplements, particularly when given at high concentration (Bruger 1945; Moses et al. 1952; Godfried et al. 1989; Keaney et al. 1994; Upston et al. 2001).

As with the animal studies, a benefit with dietary supplements of antioxidants in general and vitamin E in particular was also anticipated in humans. However, the overall outcome, particularly the results of the large, randomized controlled studies, has been disappointing (reviewed by Kritharides and Stocker 2002). In primary prevention studies, low dose α-tocopherol does not reduce the incidence of coronary events (ATBC study), and β-carotene either has no effect or increases the incidence of coronary events and cancer death (ATBC, CARET, Physician's Health studies). Secondary preventions, those with small populations and short duration of follow up have shown some benefit (CHAOS, SPACE), but larger randomized studies indicate no benefit from α-tocopherol supplements (HOPE, GISSI, PPP). Recent studies with anti-oxidant combinations also show no benefit (HATS, MPS).

Importantly however, these studies do not rule out that oxidative modification plays an important role in atherogenesis and that other anti-oxidants may not provide protection against atherosclerosis and related cardiovascular disease. In fact, recent basic research can help explain why α-tocopherol and other anti-oxidants may have failed to inhibit atherosclerosis. For example, contrary to expectations, α-tocopherol does not become depleted as atherosclerotic lesions develop (Terentis et al. 2002). Also, it has become clear that the role of α-tocopherol in LDL oxidation is more complex than previously assumed, that the efficacy of different anti-oxidants varies depending on the nature of the oxidants involved, and that oxidative events taking place within vascular cells also need to be considered in addition to, or separate from LDL oxidation in the extracellular space.

Discerning the role of α-tocopherol in LDL oxidation, each lipoprotein particle contains 6–12 vitamin molecules (Stocker et al. 1991; Esterbauer et al. 1992) as its major redox-active constituent. If LDL particles are exposed to a strong oxidant or encounter radicals with high frequency, α-tocopherol is consumed rapidly and there is little concomitant formation of lipid hydroperoxides (Esterbauer et al. 1989, 1992; Bowry et al. 1992; Bowry and Stocker 1993; Ingold et al. 1993). Under these conditions, α-tocopherol ostensibly performs an anti-oxidant role. However, there is little evidence that strongly oxidizing conditions persist in vivo. In atherosclerotic vessels LDL is surrounded by a myriad of other molecules, some of which will react with the oxidants present, thereby essentially decreasing the frequency with which the lipoprotein particles themselves encounter radicals. Therefore, conditions of mild oxidants and low 'fluxes' of radical oxidants appear more likely to be relevant in vivo.

If LDL particles encounter mild oxidants or radicals with low frequency, α-tocopherol is consumed much slower and large amounts of lipid hydroperoxides accumulate simultaneously, in accordance with the model of tocopherol-mediated peroxidation (Stocker et al. 1991; Bowry and Stocker 1993; Ingold et al. 1993; Iwatsuki et al. 1995; Kontush et al. 1996; Witting et al. 1997, 1998; Bowry and Ingold 1999; Stocker 1999; Upston et al. 1999; Culbertson et al. 2001). In tocopherol-mediated peroxidation, α-tocopherol does not act as a classic chain-breaking anti-oxidant. Rather the fate of α-tocopheroxyl radical determines whether vitamin E exhibits pro- or anti-oxidant activity. A number of endogenous reducing agents, termed 'co-anti-oxidants', can impede the pro-oxidant activity of α-tocopherol (Bowry et al. 1995; Thomas et al. 1996; Witting et al. 1996; Neuzil et al. 1997). These co-anti-oxidants reduce the α-tocopheroxyl radical and eliminate the radical character from the LDL particle thereby inhibiting tocopherol-mediated peroxidation. Thus, this line of experimentation suggests that vitamin E requires co-anti-oxidants to inhibit LDL lipid oxidation in vivo, a notion that has been verified experimentally (Witting et al. 1999, 2000; Choy et al. 2003).

It is also important to consider that depletion of LDL's α-tocopherol is required for accumulation of secondary lipid oxidation products such as aldehydes (Esterbauer et al. 1987) and F_2-isoprostanes (Lynch et al. 1994) that are responsible for the atherogenic properties of in vitro oxidized LDL (Steinbrecher et al. 1989, Hörkkö et al. 1999, Podrez et al. 2002). However, as pointed out earlier, α-tocopherol does not become depleted in atherosclerotic lesions or lipoproteins isolated from such lesions (Suarna et al. 1995; Niu et al. 1999; Terentis et al. 2002). Thus, modifications other than those induced by radical oxidants need to be considered as important in the conversion of LDL into particles recognized by scavenger receptors. Indeed, 2e-oxidants such as hypochlorite and peroxynitrite are implicated in oxidative processes in atherosclerosis (Carr et al. 2000). Of potential importance, α-tocopherol does not protect LDL against oxidative modification by these 2e-oxidants (Hazell and Stocker 1997; Thomas et al. 1998). It is difficult to predict the overall contribution of α-TOH to LDL oxidation in atherosclerosis.

It follows from the above discussion that inhibition of tocopherol-mediated peroxidation is a useful strategy to inhibit lipoprotein lipid oxidation in the vessel wall, and that in addition to radical oxidants 2e-oxidants also need to be considered as potentially relevant when designing anti-oxidant-based drug therapies. In addition, it is increasingly clear that oxidative events in a developing atherosclerotic lesion are not limited to LDL oxidation in the extracellular space, but also include a variety of cellular events and functions (Griendling and FitzGerald 2003; Stocker and Keaney 2004). The latter include cell signaling, the regulation of nitric oxide bioactivity, cell growth and apoptosis, as well as necrosis and platelet aggregation. Therefore, in the context of a therapeutic drug against atherosclerosis and related vascular disease, it is important to also consider potential protective cellular activities by the anti-oxidant.

2
Methods to Assess Lipid and Lipoprotein Oxidizability in Humans

2.1
Conventional Methods

If oxidative modification of lipid and lipoprotein contributes to atherogenesis, the accumulation of oxidation products may be expected to reflect the disease process. Furthermore, oxidation products formed in diseased arteries and released into the circulation may provide the basis for a diagnostic of atherosclerosis, particularly if the concentration of the oxidation products in the blood increases with increasing severity of the disease. However, many of the oxidation products formed are chemically reactive and undergo further reactions including the formation of covalent bonds with other molecules, so that oxidation products 'disappear' rather than accumulate. In addition, metabolism and excretion of oxidation products complicates the assessment of the extent of oxidation in the body by determining the concentration of oxidation products in blood. This is compounded further by a varying dilution effect, given that oxidation likely happens locally, for example in a coronary artery, while assessment of a blood borne oxidation parameter provides systemic information. Nevertheless, the measurement of oxidation products has the potential to provide direct evidence for oxidation processes occurring and contributing to atherosclerosis, and hence to serve as a clinical marker of the disease.

2.1.1
Oxidation Products

Given the central role proposed for lipoprotein oxidation in atherogenesis, much emphasis has been placed on markers of lipid oxidation. The evaluation of thiobarbituric acid-reactive substances (TBARS) in plasma has been proposed as a convenient method to assess lipid peroxidation (Yagi 1984). The method requires no expensive equipment and is feasible for common laboratories. It comprises heating the plasma with thiobarbituric acid under acidic conditions followed by measuring its fluorescence as an index of the amount of lipid hydroperoxides present. During the heating, lipid hydroperoxides are converted to malondialdehyde (MDA) that reacts with thiobarbituric acid to form a fluorescent adduct. While simple, the assay has, however, several major drawbacks:

1. MDA can be generated by molecules other than lipid hydroperoxides, and several biological molecules interfere with the fluorescence assay.
2. Lipid hydroperoxides (and hence MDA) can be formed ex vivo during the heating process.
3. The yield of MDA formed varies for different types of lipid hydroperoxides.

Therefore, the TBARS assay generally lacks specificity and it is a measure of endogenous lipid hydroperoxides and lability of plasma lipids to oxidation.

To improve specificity, MDA can be determined by gas chromatography-mass spectrometry (GC-MS). This method can also be applied to biological samples (Yeo et al. 1994), by first releasing MDA trapped in proteins as a Schiff base, derivatizing it to a stable adduct, N-pentafluorophenylpyrazole, and detecting this adduct by negative chemical ionization. An advantage of this method is that compared to the commonly used TBARS assay, all steps are performed at room temperature thereby suppressing artifactual oxidation of the sample.

As an alternative to the detection of MDA, plasma lipid hydroperoxides can be determined by high performance liquid chromatography (HPLC) with post-column chemiluminescence detection (Yamamoto and Ames 1987). In this method, plasma lipids are carefully extracted using methanol and hexane, and the different classes of lipids are then separated from each other and endogenous lipid-soluble anti-oxidants by HPLC. Separation of anti-oxidants from lipid hydroperoxides is important as the former interfere with the detection of the latter. The lipid hydroperoxides are then detected by chemiluminescence based on the degradation of the hydroperoxide moiety by microperoxidase and the oxidation of isoluminol. This method has been successfully applied to determine the concentration of cholesterylester hydroperoxides (CE–OOH), a predominant species of lipid hydroperoxides, in plasma of healthy subjects. The value obtained of 3.4 ± 2.0 nM (Yamamoto and Niki 1989) is about 10^3-fold lower than commonly reported plasma TBARS levels of 2.7 ± 1.2 μM (Efe et al. 1999). This discrepancy between plasma concentrations of CE–OOH and TBARS may reflect the difference in specificity and ex vivo oxidation. It has also been argued that the extraction of lipids and subsequent chromatography results in loss of endogenous lipids hydroperoxides, based on a method where plasma is added to a reaction mixture containing luminol, hemin, and Triton X-100, and single photon emission recorded as a measure of lipid hydroperoxides (Zamburlini et al. 1995). A problem with this single photon counting technology is, however, that lipid-soluble anti-oxidants present in plasma lipoproteins inhibit the chemiluminescence, yet are not separated from lipid hydroperoxides. Thus, this method probably underestimates the concentration of lipid hydroperoxides. The application of the HPLC post-column chemiluminescence method to human plasma indicates that the concentration of circulating lipid hydroperoxides in healthy subjects is close to the lower detection limit of the assay. This may simply reflect the low concentration of these types of oxidized lipids in human plasma or, alternatively, it may mirror active metabolism lipid hydroperoxides, such as their chemical reduction to the corresponding hydroxides by methionine residues of lipoprotein-associated proteins (Garner et al. 1998; Mashima et al. 1999).

Oxidation products of arachidonic acid are additional candidates for serving as markers of lipid oxidation. Arachidonic acid is oxidized by free radical reactions into up to 64 species of F_2-isoprostanes that can be divided into four structural classes of regioisomers (Morrow et al. 1994). These F_2-isoprostanes are thought to be relatively stable and specific products of lipid peroxidation, much superior to TBARS. They can be detected in measurable quantities using reasonable amounts of plasma, and are now commonly used markers for lipid peroxidation. 8-iso-Prostaglandin $F_{2\alpha}$ (also referred to as 8-epiPGF$_{2\alpha}$ or iPF$_{2\alpha}$-III), representative of one of the four classes of regioisomers, is relatively abundant in vivo in humans and was the first isoprostane proposed as a new oxidation marker for lipid peroxidation (Patrono and FitzGerald 1997). The most reliable method to determine F_2-isoprostanes is to use GC-MS (Morrow et al. 1990). An immunoassay for F_2-isoprostanes is also available (Wang et al. 1995), although its specificity for different biological samples remains to be established. 8-iso-Prostaglandin $F_{2\alpha}$ is of interest due to its ability to induce vasoconstriction. A corollary of this is, however, that if such activity were important, the stability of 8-iso-prostaglandin $F_{2\alpha}$ and hence its utility as a marker of oxidative stress may be limited.

The levels of this oxidation marker increase dramatically in animal models of oxidant injury (Morrow et al. 1992) as well as in hypercholesterolemia (Davi et al. 1997), diabetes mellitus (Davi et al. 1999) and in cigarette smokers (Morrow et al. 1995). On the other hand, no significant change in urinary 8-iso-PGF$_2$ was observed following 8 weeks of supplementation of healthy subjects with vitamin E (200–2000 IU/day) (Meagher et al. 2001), or with ascorbate (500 mg/day) or vitamin E (400 IU/day) or a combination of the two anti-oxidants (Huang et al. 2002). Similarly, vitamin E (100 or 800 IU/day) supplementation for 5 days did not decrease urinary 8-iso-PGF$_2$ in smokers (Reilly et al. 1996). As discussed earlier, it is increasingly appreciated that vitamin E has both anti- and pro-oxidant activity toward lipid peroxidation, and therefore vitamin E supplements may not be appropriate to reduce in vivo lipid peroxidation in humans.

2.1.2
Oxidizability

Assessing lipid and lipoprotein oxidizability may provide valuable information, particularly if an increased atherosclerotic burden is associated with increased oxidizability. The term oxidizability implies the involvement of both oxidative stress and endogenous anti-oxidant activity, and therefore has the potential to provide direct information on the protecting power of the body against lipid peroxidation. A typical method is based on subjecting a sample containing endogenous anti-oxidants to ex vivo oxidation and assessing the protecting power of the sample against this oxidation. Samples of plasma, serum or lipoprotein fractions are commonly used to evaluate oxidizability.

The oxidant chosen should be such that the results obtained are unambiguous and applicable to the type of sample used, although it is important to keep in mind that the results may be representative only of the specific condition applied in the assay. To achieve a short assay time, high reproducibility and low costs, most assays apply severe oxidizing conditions in which endogenous anti-oxidants are consumed completely by the oxidant used. This contrasts the in vivo situation, where anti-oxidant components are replenished constantly and initiation of oxidation my not be a frequent event. Furthermore, we still have only limited knowledge of how oxidation occurs at different sites in human tissue, so that at present it is not clear which oxidizing conditions best reflect the in vivo situation in a particular disease state, and therefore should be used for in vitro oxidizability assessment. Keeping these limitations in mind, three methods to assess oxidizability are introduced in the following.

TAS (Total Antioxidant Status) Test   This assay (Rice-Evans and Miller 1994) was proposed as a rapid, clinical test to assess the total anti-oxidant status of plasma or tissue homogenate. The test assesses the total anti-oxidant power within a short reacting time (typically 6 min) using small amounts of a sample, thereby allowing the assay to be automated. In the assay, 75 µM hydrogen peroxides and 7.5 µM metmyoglobin are reacted to induce oxidation of 150 µM 2,2'-azinobis(3-ethylbenzothiazoline 6-sulfonate) (ABTS) as the indicator of oxidation, with different compounds present in the biological sample competing with ABTS for the oxidants produced by hydrogen peroxide and methemoglobin. The biological samples are tested in a highly diluted form and TAS-values represented as a Trolox equivalent anti-oxidant capacity (mM). Under standard conditions, 2.5 mM of Trolox are completely consumed in 6 min, implying the presence of highly oxidizing conditions. Lipid peroxidation does not appear to contribute greatly to the TAS-value determined, whereas anti-oxidant components suppress the formation of the ABTS radical cation in a concentration- and time-dependent manner.

Total Radical-Trapping Antioxidant Potential (TRAP)   In this assay oxidation is mediated by peroxyl radicals generated by the thermal decomposition of water-soluble azo-initiator, 2,2'-azobis (2-amidinopropane) hydrochloride (AAPH) at a known constant rate (Wayner et al. 1985). A problem with the original method is that the oxygen electrode used to measure the endpoint is hard to maintain at a stable performance, thereby limiting reproducibility and sensitivity of this assay. As an alternative, a chemiluminescence-based detection method has been proposed (Alho and Leinonen 1999), in which luminol is used as a chemiluminescent substrate instead of the electrode. AAPH (40 mM) and luminol (1 mM) are incubated under aerobic conditions and at 37°C to generate chemiluminescence at a constant rate. The biological sample is then added (at 5% of the reaction mixture) and chemiluminescence is measured for 90 min. The TRAP value of the biological sample is calculated as the total concentration (µM) of peroxyl radicals trapped. From this it is possible to calculate the theoretical TRAP value for individual anti-oxidants, knowing their individual concentrations present in the sample and using the respective stoichiometric peroxyl radical-scavenging factors, i.e., the number of peroxyl radicals scavenged by one molecule of the anti-oxidant. Among endogenous anti-oxidants in human plasma, the most efficient components are uric acid, ascorbic acid, α-tocopherol and proteins. As in plasma the concentration of uric acid is much higher than that of other anti-oxidants, it contributes most prominently to TRAP. It should be noted that in this assay, the aqueous peroxyl radicals generated react with luminol mainly in the aqueous solution, so that TRAP values are poor indicators of the lipid oxidizability of a sample.

LDL Oxidation A popular method to assess LDL oxidizability is the so-called lag-time assay proposed by Esterbauer (Esterbauer et al. 1989). This assay uses isolated LDL that should be freshly prepared using ultracentrifugation and from which chelating reagent such as EDTA should be removed. The oxidation comprises adding copper ions to the LDL sample at a molar copper/LDL ratio of 16:1, and maintaining the mixture at 37°C to induce oxidation, monitored as an increase in the absorbance at 234 nm. In this assay, the absorbance initially remains largely unchanged (for a period of time referred to as the 'lag phase'), and then increases rapidly (propagation phase) before reaching a plateau (termination phase). These different phases of LDL oxidation are considered relevant indicators of the initiation, propagation and termination of LDL lipid peroxidation, respectively. Different to TAS and TRAP, this method is thought to assess the chain reaction of lipid peroxidation. Although several analytical endpoints related to oxidizability can be measured in the assay, lag time is the most commonly used parameter. The lag time, defined as the period from the start of the incubation until the beginning of the rapid increase in absorbance, provides direct information on the amount of anti-oxidants present in LDL as all anti-oxidants are essentially depleted during the lag time, although the precise relationship between LDL's endogenous anti-oxidants and the duration of the lag phase remains obscure (Esterbauer et al. 1991). In clinical trials, administration of α-tocopherol to healthy subjects results in an extension of the time lag (Dieber-Rotheneder et al. 1991) and similar results have been reported in patients with coronary artery diseases (Mosca et al. 1997). Importantly, however, to date there has been no report demonstrating a correlation between lag time and risk of coronary heart disease.

2.2
Relationship Between Oxidizability and Cardiovascular Disease

Upon oxidation by a radical oxidant, the anti-oxidant molecule itself becomes a radical that has the potential to initiate further biological damage. A common feature of the in vitro tests described above is that they all generate oxidants at very high rates, much higher than can be reasonably expected to occur in vivo. A consequence of such high radical flux conditions is that the anti-oxidant-derived radical most likely reacts with another initiating radicals (e.g., a peroxyl radical derived from AAPH), as reflected in the stoichiometric factor that is commonly two (or higher) for most anti-oxidants in the tests used. However, if the flux of initiating radicals is low, the likelihood increases for the anti-oxidant-derived radical to participate in radical-transfer reactions involving biological targets, such as lipids containing a pair of bisallylic hydrogen atoms. In this scenario, the anti-oxidant becomes a prooxidant. In fact, all anti-oxidants that scavenge radicals are Janus faced, i.e., they have the potential to act as anti-oxidant or prooxidant. The model of tocopherol-mediated peroxidation discussed earlier, represents a good example of a Janus-faced anti-oxidant for the case of α-tocopherol. By contrast, conventional in vitro oxidizability assays artificially generate conditions that selectively probe for only one of the two Janus faces, i.e., the anti-oxidant face of anti-oxidants. This may explain why there is no apparent correlation between in vitro 'LDL oxidizability' and the extent of coronary artery disease (Karmansky et al. 1996), and why vitamin E supplements can improve in vitro LDL oxidizability (Dieber-Rotheneder et al. 1991) but not in vivo lipid peroxidation (Meagher et al. 2001).

Concerning atherosclerosis, α-tocopherol remains essentially intact even in the most advanced stages of atherosclerosis, yet the lipid present in these lesions is substantially oxidized (Terentis et al. 2002; Upston et al. 2002). Furthermore, there is evidence that the oxidized lipoprotein-derived lipids detected in human lesions are mostly generated in the presence of α-tocopherol (Upston et al. 2002). Therefore, we must consider the possibility that lipoprotein lipid oxidation in atherosclerotic lesions proceeds in the presence of anti-oxidants. If so, it would be desirable to establish an in vitro test that mimics this situation, i.e., where oxidation takes place in the presence of endogenous anti-oxidants. This can be achieved using conditions of low radical flux. Ideally, this should also involve a biological sample of complex composition rather than an isolated component such as LDL, thereby providing the possibility of interaction between water- and lipid-soluble anti-oxidants.

2.3
New Concept for Oxidizability Assessment

It follows from the above discussion that to assess oxidizability in vitro such that it more closely reflects in vivo conditions, an oxidizability assay should have the following features (Cynshi and Stocker 2003):

1. Use the biological sample as intact as possible and without dilution.
2. Expose the biological sample to a low flux of oxidizing radicals.
3. Select an endpoint where at least some of the endogenous anti-oxidants remain present.

The first feature allows synergistic interaction between endogenous anti-oxidants in the sample, whereas the second feature allows for the potential prooxidant action of endogenous anti-oxidants, and the third feature mimics the situation occurring in atherosclerotic lesions. The two major challenges here are to: (a) obtain the required high degree of sensitivity (to detect a small amount of oxidation products) and selectivity (to distinguish these oxidation products from potentially interfering substances); and (b) establish an assay relevant to human diseases. Progress in technology has helped to master the first challenge, however, the second challenge continues to be unresolved.

As a first step towards achieving an improved in vitro oxidizability assay based on the above concepts, we have developed the Plasma Lipid Oxidizability (PLOX) assay in which a small volume of whole plasma is oxidized with 10 mM AAPH at 37°C for 8 h, before the oxidized lipid are extracted and analyzed by HPLC. In the assay, AAPH derived-peroxyl radicals promote lipid oxidation similarly to the situation in the TRAP assay. However, the rate at which these peroxyl radicals are generated relative to the concentration of available biological targets including lipoproteins is substantially lower in the PLOX than the TRAP assay. Furthermore, the PLOX assay measures the products of lipid peroxidation that occurs in a chain reaction via tocopherol-mediated peroxidation, whereas the TRAP assay predominantly measures oxidation reactions taking place in the aqueous phase and that are independent on lipid peroxidation. Compared to Esterbauer's LDL oxidation method, the PLOX assay assesses a complex biological sample, in which endogenous anti-oxidants interact with each other and prooxidant activities significantly contribute to the endpoint measured; the Esterbauer LDL assay uses isolated and diluted LDL under conditions that are restricted to radical scavenging activities of anti-oxidants. Although both assays measure lipid peroxidation products, the PLOX assay utilizes oxidative processes taking place during the early stage of what corresponds to the lag phase in the Esterbauer LDL assay, and the latter does not provide information on the comparable phase of oxidation. The measurement of lipid peroxidation in the PLOX assay is based on an established method for the detection of the primary oxidation products of a cholesterylesters, i.e., cholesterylester hydroperoxides (CE–OOH) and cholesterylester hydroxides (CE–OH) by HPLC (Kritharides et al. 1993). Reproducibility is improved by measuring both CE–OOH and CE–OH as the former can be converted to the latter.

To illustrate some of the novel features of the PLOX assay, the effect of different lipophilic anti-oxidants was tested using pooled human plasma. As shown in Fig. 1, addition of α-tocopherol showed a prooxidant activity, as predicted by the model of tocopherol-mediated peroxidation. On the other hand, probucol had no effect on the PLOX value, indicating that under the conditions used this drug fails to inhibit lipoprotein lipid oxidation in the presence of endogenous anti-oxidants including α-tocopherol. This is not surprising given that the reactivity of probucol is 40 times lower than that of α-tocopherol (Cynshi et al. 1998). Among the lipid-soluble anti-oxidants, the PLOX value was inhibited by BO-653, a newly designed anti-oxidant discussed in the following section. Figure 1 illustrates that lipid oxidation in the presence of endogenous anti-oxidants and induced by a low rate of peroxyl radicals has features vastly different to those seen in the conventional in vitro oxidizability assays.

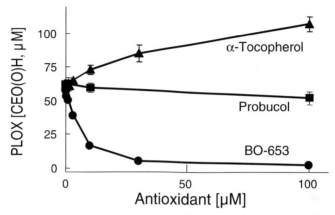

Fig. 1 Effect of lipid-soluble anti-oxidants on PLOX, a new in vitro oxidizability assay. The PLOX assay was performed by ex vivo oxidation induced by aerobic incubation of human plasma in the presence of 10 mM AAPH and at 37°C for 8 h. α-Tocopherol (*triangles*), probucol (*squares*) or BO-653 (*circles*) was added to pooled plasma from healthy subjects prior to the start of the oxidation. Data are expressed as mean±SD from three separate experiments. Where an SD cannot be seen, it is smaller than the symbol. The PLOX value is the total concentration of CE–OOH and CE–OH accumulated after oxidation. In the absence of added anti-oxidants, the PLOX-value was 61.7±2.9 μM

In conclusion, the PLOX assay is based on novel concepts that appear to reasonably reflect the situation of lipoprotein lipid oxidation taking place in human atherosclerotic lesions, and hence may be useful to further our understanding of the relevance of lipid oxidation in the pathogenesis of this and possibly other diseases. Therefore, we propose to test the suitability of this assay as a tool to investigate the relationship between the lipid oxidation and atherosclerosis in humans.

3
Antioxidants in Commercial Development as Drugs Against Cardiovascular Diseases

Antioxidants have potential as therapeutic drugs against various diseases, in particular atherosclerosis, as they can inhibit lipid peroxidation involved in LDL oxidation and reduce detrimental biological consequences caused by oxidative stress. Currently, two anti-oxidants are under commercial development as drugs to combat cardiovascular diseases. One is AGI-1067, the mono-succinate ester of probucol that is being developed as a vascular (v)-protectant (Hatch 2002). The other is BO-653 that shares structural features with probucol and α-tocopherol and is under development as an LDL anti-oxidant (Meng 2003).

3.1
AGI-1067

AGI-1067 is an orally active anti-oxidant v-protectant under development by AtheroGenics for the potential prevention of atherosclerosis and restenosis. Accumulation of leukocytes into the vessel wall is one of the earliest detectable events in the development of atherosclerosis. Leukocyte adhesion to the endothelium and their recruitment into the subendothelial space are regulated by adhesion molecules, such as vascular cell adhesion protein-1 (VCAM-1), and by monocyte chemoatractant protein-1 (MCP-1), the expression of which is thought to be under redox control (Marui et al. 1993). AGI-1067 has been synthesized as an anti-oxidant v-protectant that reduces the expression of VCAM-1 and MCP-1 (Medford 1997a, 1997b). Indeed, AGI-1067 reduces the expression of VCAM-1 and MCP-1 induced by tumor necrosis factor-α in vitro and lipopolysaccharide in vivo, and it significantly reduces atherosclerosis in LDL receptor-deficient and in apolipoprotein E-deficient mice (Sundell et al. 2003). The same authors reported that probucol failed to inhibit both the expression of VCAM-1 and MCP-1, as well as atherosclerosis, although the two compounds structurally differ only in one of two phenol groups being substituted with a succinate ester in AGI-1067 (Fig. 2). It is interesting to note in this context, that the succinate ester of α-tocopherol has also been reported to have a biological action distinct from that α-tocopherol, including inhibition of cell adhesion by suppressing NF-κB mobilization (Erl et al. 1997). Whereas in vivo α-tocopheryl succinate is metabolized readily to α-tocopherol, the ester bond in AGI-1067 is metabolically more stable due to the presence of bulky *tert*-butyl groups. Furthermore, AGI-1067 does not appear to reduce HDL-cholesterol or to prolong the QTc interval (Wasserman et al. 2003), i.e., side effects of probucol of potential concern that have resulted in the withdrawal of the drug by the Food and Drugs Administration.

Probucol has previously been shown to prevent coronary restenosis after balloon angioplasty (Tardif et al. 1997). In that study, probucol was administered for 4 weeks before angioplasty due to the limited bioavailability and accumulation of probucol in tissues (Reaven et al. 1992). Based on the same rationale, the Canadian Antioxidant Restenosis Trial (CART-1) was designed to investigate the efficacy of AGI-1067 against restenosis following stent placement or balloon angioplasty (Tardif et al. 2003). As the plasma levels of AGI-1067 appeared to reach steady state within 2 weeks, patients were treated for 2 weeks before and 4 weeks after percutaneous coronary intervention (PCI).

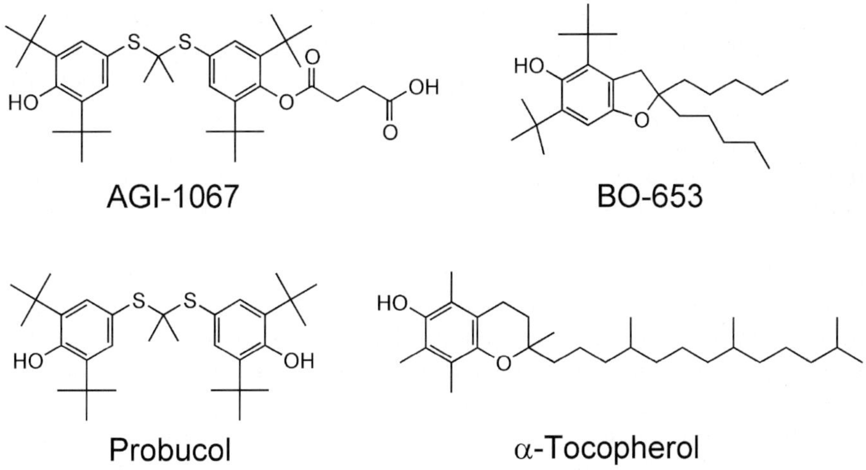

Fig. 2 Chemical structures of AGI-1067, BO-653, probucol and α-tocopherol

Three hundred and five patients were randomly assigned to one of five treatments: placebo, 500 mg probucol twice daily, or 70, 140 or 280 mg of AGI-1067 once daily; 85% of the patients received stents. Intravascular ultrasound evaluation was carried out at baseline and 6-months follow up by a blinded core laboratory. The luminal area at follow-up was 2.66 ± 1.58 mm^2 for placebo, 3.36 ± 2.69 mm^2 for probucol, 3.36 ± 2.12 mm^2 for AGI-1067 280 mg and this reduction was significant for probucol and significantly related to the AGI-1067 dose (Tardif et al. 2003). In addition, there was a trend for AGI-1067 to decrease the loss in lumen volume of a reference segment between baseline and follow up ($P = 0.077$ for dose–response). Prolongation of QTc interval occurred in 17.4% of probucol-treated patients, whereas its frequency was the same in AGI-1067- and placebo-treated patients. In summary, the CART-1 trial revealed that AGI-1067, like probucol, reduces restenosis after PCI, but, unlike probucol, does not cause QTc prolongation. The fact that AGI–067 also slowed lumen loss in a nonstented reference segment, in addition suggests for the first time that AGI-1067 may also protect against atherosclerosis. It will be interesting to investigate in future clinical trials whether the protection observed with AGI-1067 in humans is indeed due to an anti-oxidant action of the drug. Such information is presently not available although it is important to provide evidence in support of the oxidative modification hypothesis of atherosclerosis.

Considering that oxidative stress and inflammation may persist for the entire period of risk after PCI, treatment with AGI-1067 for periods of time exceeding 4 weeks post-PCI may further enhance the protection against luminal narrowing. An important practical consideration is that repeated administration of drugs before PCI, as done in the MVP (Tardif et al. 1997) and CART-1 trial (Tardif et al. 2003) cannot be applied to patients undergoing non-elective PCI. Therefore, the next trial, i.e., CART-2, determines the anti-restenotic effect of AGI-1067 when given for 12 months after PCI without pre-treatment, or with pre-treatment as a single dose on the day of PCI. CART-2 is a 12-month, 500-patient, double-blind, placebo-controlled trial with 280 mg AGI-1067, administered orally once daily; the trial was initiated in 2001. Enrolment has been completed and the results will provide important practical information on the efficacy of the drug to reduce restenosis after PCI and to reduce plaque growth in coronary arteries.

As the results of CART-1 were suggestive of AGI-1067 decreasing the rate of coronary artery lumen loss due to progression of atherosclerosis, another objective is to demonstrate a direct anti-atherosclerotic effect of AGI-1067 on coronary blood vessels in humans. For this purpose, AtheroGenics has initiated the Aggressive Reduction of Inflammation Stops Events (ARISE) trial. ARISE is a large, double-blind, placebo-controlled Phase III trial to be conducted in over 180 cardiac centers, and involving 4,000 patients who will be followed for an average of 18 months or until a minimum of 1,160 primary cardiovascular events have occurred. Clearly, the results from CART-2 and ARISE will provide important information about whether synthetic anti-oxidants may be beneficial in reducing atherosclerosis in humans.

3.2
BO-653

BO-653 (2,3-dihydro-5-hydroxy-2,2-dipentyl-4,6-di-*tert*-butylbenzofuran) is an orally active LDL anti-oxidant under development by Chugai for the potential prevention of atherosclerosis and restenosis, similar to AGI-1067. BO-653 was designed and synthesized in an attempt to overcome the limitations of probucol and α-tocopherol as inhibitors of LDL oxidation, and to test the oxidative modification theory (Cynshi 1997). As indicated earlier, BO-653 is able to inhibit tocopherol-mediated peroxidation and thus can inhibit plasma lipoprotein lipid oxidation in the presence of endogenous anti-oxidants, whereas probucol and α-tocopherol fail to do so (Fig. 1). This superior anti-oxidant action is encouraging, and BO-653 may provide useful support for the oxidative modification hypothesis in atherosclerosis. In fact, BO-653 has been shown to reduce atherosclerosis in three different animal models, i.e., mice fed a high fat diet fed, LDL receptor-deficient mice, and WHHL rabbits (Cynshi et al. 1998). Similar to the situation with AGI-1067, however, a direct link between this protective activity and in vivo inhibition of lipid oxidation has not been established, although BO-653 effectively protects LDL from in vitro oxidation (Noguchi et al. 1997).

In addition to inhibition of LDL oxidation, BO-653 has been reported to inhibit the expression of three α-type proteasome subunits (Takabe et al. 2001) that might limit the increase in NF-κB activity seen in atherosclerotic lesions. NF-κB is thought to be an important pro-inflammatory player in early stages of atherosclerosis. In the rabbit balloon injury model, BO-653 also inhibits induction of c-*MYC*, resulting in a reduction in neointimal thickening 4 weeks after the injury (Inoue et al. 2002). c-*MYC* is one of the early response genes in proliferating cells following NF-κB activation, and inhibition of c-*MYC* expression may be one of the mechanisms by which BO-653 suppresses the proliferation of vascular smooth muscle cells. Treatment of pigs with 500 mg of BO-653 daily starting 1 week before stent deployment reduces both coronary in-stent narrowing and collagen deposition (Miyauchi et al. 2000). Furthermore, BO-653 was similarly effective without pre-treatment before stent deployment. Thus, BO-653 not only has an anti-oxidant action different from probucol and α-tocopherol, but it also has anti-proliferative activity that may contribute to its ability to inhibit intimal thickening in animals and restenosis in humans.

A phase I trial was conducted as a double-blind, placebo-controlled study with healthy subjects (to be published). BO-653 was administered twice daily in dosages ranging from 200 to 800 mg/day and for up to 4 weeks. Adequate safety and tolerance profiles were established for BO-653. Antioxidant efficacy was assessed by the TBARS (using butylated hydroxy toluene to avoid ex vivo oxidation), LDL oxidation as lag-time and plasma oxidizability as a prototype assay of PLOX, using plasma samples from subjects participating in the repeated administration studies. Plasma TBARS were unchanged by all doses of BO-653, whereas the lag time was prolonged dose-dependently and in a treatment period-dependent manner. Plasma oxidizability (ex vivo oxidized by AAPH and determined by HPLC with post-column chemiluminescence) was dramatically decreased in plasma from BO-653 treated subjects even at the lowest dose of BO-653, 200 mg/day, at the first evaluation, 1 week after drug administration started. No dose–response relationship was observed as the lowest dose of BO-653, 100 mg twice daily, already completely suppressed plasma oxidation. Administration of BO-653 up to 800 mg/day did not alter the plasma concentrations of the endogenous anti-oxidants, ascorbate, α-tocopherol and coenzyme Q_{10}.

The results of the Phase I trial indicate that BO-653 acts as an anti-oxidant in healthy subjects as intended by the drug design. Therefore, in 2001 Chugai initiated the PREVention of post-Angioplasty restenosis In stented Lesions (PREVAIL) trial to assess the efficacy of BO-653 to inhibit in-stent restenosis in humans (http://www.chugaibio.com; November 2003). PREVAIL is a multicenter, double-blind, placebo-controlled, dose-ranging Phase II study to evaluate the safety and efficacy of BO-653. Patients are given placebo, 25, 50 or 100 mg of BO-653 twice daily for 6 months after the stent procedure. Enrolment was completed in 2003 and the results will provide the first clinical data on the efficacy of

BO-653 to reduce restenosis after PCI. In addition, as a secondary endpoint the lumen of a nonstented reference artery will be assessed to provide information on the potential anti-atherosclerotic activity of BO-653, although treatment for 6 months may be too short for the detection of regression of atherosclerotic lesions. PLOX assays are being conducted with the plasma samples of the subjects enrolled, in an attempt to establish a link between the clinical outcome and the anti-oxidant activities of BO-653. PREVAIL should provide useful information on whether BO-653, an efficient synthetic LDL anti-oxidant that also possesses protective cellular activities, improves clinical outcome in in-stent restenosis. If successful, a large scale follow-up study will be needed to establish whether BO-653 is able to inhibit atherosclerosis, and whether this is indeed due to inhibition of LDL oxidation and/or other oxidative events in the wall of affected vessels.

Acknowledgements R.S. is supported by a Senior Principal Research Fellowship from the National Health and Medical Research Council of Australia.

References

Alho H, Leinonen J (1999) Total anti-oxidant activity measured by chemiluminescence methods. Methods Enzymol 299:3–15

Bird DA, Tangirala RK, Fruebis J, Steinberg D, Witztum JL, Palinski W (1998) Effect of probucol on LDL oxidation and atherosclerosis in LDL receptor deficient mice. J Lipid Res 39:1079–1090

Bjorkhem I, Henriksson-Freyschuss A, Breuer O, Diczfalusy U, Berglund L, Henriksson P (1991) The anti-oxidant butylated hydroxytoluene protects against atherosclerosis. Arterioscler Thromb 11:15–22

Böger, RH, Bode-Böger SM, Phivthong-ngam L, Brandes RP, Schwedhelm E, Mügge A, Böhme M, Tsikas D, Frölich JC (1998) Dietary L-arginine and α-tocopherol reduce vascular oxidative stress and preserve endothelial function in hypercholesterolemic rabbits via different mechanisms. Atherosclerosis 141:31–43

Boring, L, Gosling J, Cleary M, Charo IF (1998) Decreased lesion formation in CCR2-/- mice reveals a role for chemokines in the initiation of atherosclerosis. Nature 394:894–897

Bowry VW, Ingold KU (1999) The unexpected role of vitamin E (α-tocopherol) in the peroxidation of human low-density lipoprotein. Acc Chem Res 32:27–34

Bowry VW, Ingold KU, Stocker R (1992) Vitamin E in human low-density lipoprotein. When and how this anti-oxidant becomes a pro-oxidant. Biochem J 288:341–344

Bowry VW, Mohr D, Cleary J, Stocker R (1995) Prevention of tocopherol-mediated peroxidation of ubiquinol-10-free human low density lipoprotein. J Biol Chem 270:5756–5763

Bowry VW, Stocker R (1993) Tocopherol-mediated peroxidation. The pro-oxidant effect of vitamin E on the radical-initiated oxidation of human low-density lipoprotein. J Am Chem Soc 115:6029–6044

Brattsand R (1975) Actions of vitamins A and E and some nicotinic acid derivatives on plasma lipids and on lipid infiltration of aorta in cholesterol-fed rabbits. Atherosclerosis 22:47–61

Bruger M (1945) Experimental Atherosclerosis. VII. Effect of vitamin E. Proc Soc Exp Biol Med 59:56–57

Carew TE, Schwenke DC, Steinberg D (1987) Antiatherogenic effect of probucol unrelated to its hypocholesterolemic effect: evidence that anti-oxidants in vivo can selectively inhibit low density lipoprotein degradation in macrophage-rich fatty streaks and slow the progression of atherosclerosis in the Watanabe heritable hyperlipidemic rabbit. Proc Natl Acad Sci USA 84:7725–7729

Carr AC, McCall MR, Frei B (2000). Oxidation of LDL by myeloperoxidase and reactive nitrogen species: reaction pathways and anti-oxidant protection. Arterioscler Thromb Vasc Biol 20:1716–1723

Choy KJ, Deng YM, Hou JY, Wu B, Lau AK, Witting PK, Stocker R (2003) Coenzyme Q10 supplementation inhibits aortic lipid oxidation but fails to attenuate intimal thickening in balloon-injured New Zealand White rabbits. Free Radic Biol Med 35:300–309

Culbertson SM, Vinqvist MR, Barclay LR, Porter NA (2001) Minimizing tocopherol-mediated radical phase transfer in low-density lipoprotein oxidation with an amphiphilic unsymmetrical azo initiator. J Am Chem Soc 123:8951–8960

Cushing SD, Berliner JA, Valente AJ, Territo MC, Navab M, Parhami F, Gerrity R, Schwartz CJ, Fogelman AM (1990) Minimally modified low density lipoprotein induces monocyte chemotactic protein (MCP-1) in human endothelial and smooth muscle cells. Proc Natl Acad Sci USA 87:5134–5138

Cynshi O (1997) Preventives/remedies for arteriosclerosis. Patent WO9850025

Cynshi O, Kawabe Y, Suzuki T, Takashima Y, Kaise H, Nakamura M, Ohba Y, Kato Y, Tamura K, Hayasaka A, Higashida A, Sakaguchi H, Takeya M, Takahashi K, Inoue K, Noguchi N, Niki E, Kodama T (1998) Antiatherogenic effects of the anti-oxidant BO-653 in three different animal models. Proc Natl Acad Sci USA 95:10123–10128

Cynshi O, Stocker R (2003) Methods for evaluating anti-oxidant potency of biological samples. WO2004083869

Cyrus T, Yao Y, Rokach J, Tang LX, Pratico D (2003) Vitamin E reduces progression of atherosclerosis in low-density lipoprotein receptor-deficient mice with established vascular lesions. Circulation 107:521–523

Davi G, Alessandrini P, Mezzetti A, Minotti G, Bucciarelli T, Costantini F, Cipollone F, Bon GB, Ciabattoni G, Patrono C (1997) In vivo formation of 8-Epi-prostaglandin F2 alpha is increased in hypercholesterolemia. Arterioscler Thromb Vasc Biol 17:3230–3235

Davi G, Ciabattoni G, Consoli A, Mezzetti A, Falco A, Santarone S, Pennese E, Vitacolonna E, Bucciarelli T, Costantini F, Capani F, Patrono C (1999) In vivo formation of 8-iso-prostaglandin $F_{2\alpha}$ and platelet activation in diabetes mellitus: effects of improved metabolic control and vitamin E supplementation. Circulation 99:224–229

Dieber-Rotheneder M, Puhl H, Waeg G, Striegl G, Esterbauer H (1991) Effect of oral supplementation with D-alpha-tocopherol on the vitamin E content of human low density lipoproteins and resistance to oxidation. J Lipid Res 32:1325–1332

Efe H, Deger O, Kirci D, Karahan SC, Orem A, Calapoglu M (1999) Decreased neutrophil antioxidative enzyme activities and increased lipid peroxidation in hyperlipoproteinemic human subjects. Clin Chim Acta 279:155–165

Erl W, Weber C, Wardemann C, Weber PC (1997) α-Tocopheryl succinate inhibits monocytic cell adhesion to endothelial cells by suppressing NF-kappa B mobilization. Am J Physiol 273: H634–H640

Esterbauer H, Dieber-Rotheneder M, Striegl G, Waeg G (1991) Role of vitamin E in preventing the oxidation of low-density lipoprotein. Am J Clin Nutr 53:314S–321S

Esterbauer H, Gebicki J, Puhl H, Jürgens G (1992) The role of lipid peroxidation and anti-oxidants in oxidative modification of LDL. Free Radic Biol Med 13:341–390

Esterbauer H, Jürgens G, Quehenberger O, Koller E (1987) Autoxidation of human low density lipoprotein: loss of polyunsaturated fatty acids and vitamin E and generation of aldehydes. J Lipid Res 28:495–509

Esterbauer H, Striegl G, Puhl H, Rotheneder M (1989) Continuous monitoring of in vitro oxidation of human low density lipoprotein. Free Rad Res Comms 6:67–75

Freyschuss A, Stiko-Rahm A, Swedenborg J, Henriksson P, Bjorkhem I, Berglund L, Nilsson J (1993) Antioxidant treatment inhibits the development of intimal thickening after balloon injury of the aorta in hypercholesterolemic rabbits. J Clin Invest 91:1282–1288

Fruebis J, Steinberg D, Dresel HA, Carew TA (1994) A comparison of the antiatherogenic effects of probucol and a structural analogue of probucol in low density lipoprotein receptor-deficient rabbits. J Clin Invest 94:392–398

Garner B, Waldeck AR, Witting PK, Rye K-A, Stocker R (1998) Oxidation of high density lipoproteins. II. Evidence for direct reduction of HDL lipid hydroperoxides by methionine residues of apolipoproteins AI and AII. J Biol Chem 273:6088–6095

Godfried SL, Combs GF, Saroka JM, Dillingham LA (1989) Potentiation of atherosclerotic lesions in rabbits by high dietary level of vitamin E. Br J Nutr 61:607–617

Goldstein JL, Ho YK, Basu SK, Brown MS (1979) Binding site on macrophages that mediates uptake and degradation of acetylated low density lipoprotein, producing massive cholesterol deposition. Proc Natl Acad Sci USA 76:333–337

Gosling J, Slaymaker S, Gu L, Tseng S, Zlot CH, Young SG, Rollins BJ, Charo IF (1999) MCP-1 deficiency reduces susceptibility to atherosclerosis in mice that overexpress human apolipoprotein B. J Clin Invest 103:773–778

Griendling KK, FitzGerald GA (2003) Oxidative stress and cardiovascular injury: Part I: basic mechanisms and in vivo monitoring of ROS. Circulation 108:1912–1916

Griffith RL, Virella GT, Stevenson HC, Lopes-Virella MF (1988) Low density lipoprotein metabolism by human macrophages activated with low density lipoprotein immune complexes. A possible mechanism of foam cell formation. J Exp Med 168:1041–1059

Haberland ME, Fogelman AM, Edwards PA (1982). Specificity of receptor-mediated recognition of malonydialdehyde-modified low density lipoproteins. Proc Natl Acad Sci USA 79:1712–1716

Haberland ME, Olch CL, Fogelman AM (1984) Role of lysines in mediating interaction of modified low density lipoproteins with the scavenger receptor of human monocyte macrophages. J Biol Chem 259:11305–11311

Hatch GM (2002) AGI-1067. AtheroGenics. Curr Opin Investig Drugs 3:433–436

Hazell LJ, Stocker R (1997) α-Tocopherol does not inhibit hypochlorite-induced oxidation of apolipoprotein B-100 of low-density lipoprotein. FEBS Lett 414:541–544

Henriksen T, Mahoney EM, Steinberg D (1981) Enhanced macrophage degradation of low density lipoprotein previously incubated with cultured endothelial cells: recognition by receptors for acetylated low density lipoproteins. Proc Natl Acad Sci USA 78:6499–6503

Hörkkö S, Bird DA, Miller E, Itabe H, Leitinger N, Subbanagounder G, Berliner JA, Friedman P, Dennis EA, Curtiss LK, Palinski W, Witztum JL (1999) Monoclonal autoantibodies specific for oxidized phospholipids or oxidized phospholipid-protein adducts inhibit macrophage uptake of oxidized low-density lipoproteins. J Clin Invest 103:117–128

Huang HY, Appel LJ, Croft KD, Miller ER, 3rd, Mori TA, Puddey IB (2002) Effects of vitamin C and vitamin E on in vivo lipid peroxidation: results of a randomized controlled trial. Am J Clin Nutr 76:549–555

Ingold KU, Bowry VW, Stocker R, Walling C (1993) Autoxidation of lipids and antioxidation by α-tocopherol and ubiquinol in homogeneous solution and in aqueous dispersions of lipids. The unrecognized consequences of lipid particle size as exemplified by the oxidation of human low density lipoprotein. Proc Natl Acad Sci USA 90:45–49

Inoue K, Cynshi O, Kawabe Y, Nakamura M, Miyauchi K, Kimura T, Daida H, Hamakubo T, Yamaguchi H, Kodama T (2002) Effect of BO-653 and probucol on c-MYC and PDGF-A messenger RNA of the iliac artery after balloon denudation in cholesterol-fed rabbits. Atherosclerosis 161:353–363

Iwatsuki M, Niki E, Stone D, Darley-Usmar VM (1995) α-Tocopherol mediated peroxidation in the copper (II) and met myoglobin induced oxidation of human low density lipoprotein: the influence of lipid hydroperoxides. FEBS Lett 360:271–276

Karmansky I, Shnaider H, Palant A, Gruener N (1996) Plasma lipid oxidation and susceptibility of low-density lipoproteins to oxidation in male patients with stable coronary artery disease. Clin Biochem 29:573–579

Keaney JF, Jr, Gaziano JM, Xu A, Frei B, Curran-Celentano J, Shwaery GT, Loscalzo J, Vita JA (1994) Low-dose α-tocopherol improves and high-dose α-tocopherol worsens endothelial vasodilator function in cholesterol-fed rabbits. J Clin Invest 93:844–851

Kita T, Nagano Y, Yokode M, Ishii K, Kume N, Ooshima A, Yoshida H, Kawai C (1987) Probucol prevents the progression of atherosclerosis in Watanabe heritable hyperlipidemic rabbit, an animal model for familial hypercholesterolemia. Proc Natl Acad Sci USA 84:5928–5931

Klimov AN, Denisenko AD, Popov AV, Nagornev VA, Pleskov VM, Vinogradov AG, Denisenko TV, Magracheva E, Kheifes GM, Kuznetzov AS (1985) Lipoprotein-antibody immune complexes. Their catabolism and role in foam cell formation. Atherosclerosis 58:1–15

Kodama T, Freeman M, Rohrer L, Zabrecky J, Matsudaira P, Krieger M (1990) Type I macrophage scavenger receptor contains alpha-helical and collagen-like coiled coils. Nature 343:531–535

Kontush A, Finckh B, Karten B, Kohlschütter A, Beisiegel U (1996) Antioxidant and prooxidant activity of α-tocopherol in human plasma and low density lipoprotein. J Lipid Res 37:1436–1448

Kritchevsky D, Kim HK, Tepper SA (1971) Influence of 4,4'-(isopropylidenedithio)bis(2,6-di-t-butylphenol) (DH-581) on experimental atherosclerosis in rabbits. Proc Soc Exp Biol Med 136:1216–1221

Kritharides L, Jessup W, Gifford J, Dean RT (1993) A method for defining the stages of LDL oxidation by the separation of cholesterol and cholesteryl ester- oxidation products by HPLC. Anal Biochem 213:79–89

Kritharides L, Stocker R (2002) The use of anti-oxidant supplements in coronary heart disease. Atherosclerosis 164:211–219

Lynch SM, Morrow JD, Roberts LJ, II, Frei B (1994) Formation of noncyclooxygenase-derived prostanoids (F_2-isoprostanes) in plasma and low-density lipoprotein exposed to oxidative stress in vitro. J Clin Invest 93:998–1004

Mao SJ, Yates MT, Parker RA, Chi EM, Jackson RL (1991) Attenuation of atherosclerosis in a modified strain of hypercholesterolemic Watanabe rabbits with use of a probucol analogue (MDL 29,311) that does not lower serum cholesterol. Arterioscler Thromb 11:1266–1275

Marshall FN (1982) Pharmacology and toxicology of probucol. Artery 10:7–21

Marui N, Offermann MK, Swerlick R, Kunsch C, Rosen CA, Ahmad M, Alexander RW, Medford RM (1993) Vascular cell adhesion molecule-1 (VCAM-1) gene transcription and expression are regulated through an anti-oxidant-sensitive mechanism in human vascular endothelial cells. J Clin Invest 92:1866–1874

Mashima R, Witting PK, Stocker R (2001) Oxidants and anti-oxidants in atherosclerosis. Curr Opin Lipidol 12:411–418

Mashima R, Yoshimura S, Yamamoto Y (1999) Reduction of lipid hydroperoxides by apolipoprotein B-100. Biochem Biophys Res Commun 259:185–189

McMurray HF, Parthasarathy S, Steinberg D (1993) Oxidatively modified low density lipoprotein is a chemoattractant for human T lymphocytes. J Clin Invest 92:1004–1008

Meagher EA, Barry OP, Lawson JA, Rokach J, FitzGerald G (2001) Effects of vitamin E on lipid peroxidation in healthy persons. JAMA 285:1178–1182

Medford RM, Somers P (1997) Monoesters of probucol for the treatment of cardiovascular and inflammatory disease. WO9851289

Medford RM, Somers PK, Hoong LK, Meng CQ (1997) Compounds and methods for the inhibition of the expression of VCAM-1. Patent WO9851662

Meng CQ (2003) BO-653. Chugai. Curr Opin Investig Drugs 4:342–346

Miyauchi K, Schwartz RS, Aihara K, Kurata T, Sato H, Yamaguchi H, Daida H (2000) Efficacy of a novel anti-oxidant on vascular remodelling after coronary angioplasty: Possible role of endothelial function and collagen accumulation. Circulation 102:915 (Abstract)

Moghadasian MH, McManus BM, Godin DV, Rodrigues B, Frohlich JJ (1999) Proatherogenic and antiatherogenic effects of probucol and phytosterols in apolipoprotein E–deficient mice: possible mechanisms of action. Circulation 99:1733–1739

Morrow JD, Awad JA, Kato T, Takahashi K, Badr KF, Roberts LJ, 2nd, Burk RF (1992) Formation of novel non-cyclooxygenase-derived prostanoids (F2-isoprostanes) in carbon tetrachloride hepatotoxicity. An animal model of lipid peroxidation. J Clin Invest 90:2502–2507

Morrow JD, Frei B, Longmire AW, Gaziano JM, Lynch SM, Shyr Y, Strauss WE, Oates JA, Roberts LJ, 2nd. (1995) Increase in circulating products of lipid peroxidation (F2-isoprostanes) in smokers. Smoking as a cause of oxidative damage. N Engl J Med 332:1198–1203

Morrow JD, Hill KE, Burk RF, Nammour TM, Badr KF, Roberts LJ, 2nd (1990) A series of prostaglandin F_2-like compounds are produced in vivo in humans by a non-cyclooxygenase, free radical-catalyzed mechanism. Proc Natl Acad Sci USA 87:9383–9387

Morrow JD, Minton TA, Badr KF, Roberts LJ, 2nd (1994) Evidence that the F2-isoprostane, 8-epi-prostaglandin F2 alpha, is formed in vivo. Biochim Biophys Acta 1210:244–248

Mosca L, Rubenfire M, Mandel C, Rock C, Tarshis T, Tsai A, Pearson T (1997) Antioxidant nutrient supplementation reduces the susceptibility of low density lipoprotein to oxidation in patients with coronary artery disease. J Am Coll Cardiol 30:392–399

Moses C, Rhodes GL, Levinson JP (1952) The effect of alpha-tocopherol on experimental aptherosclerosis. Angiology 3:397–407

Navab M, Imes SS, Hama SY, Hough GP, Ross LA, Bork RW, Valente AJ, Berliner JA, Drinkwater DC, Laks H, Fogelman AM (1991) Monocyte transmigration induced by modification of low density lipoprotein in cocultures of human aortic wall cells is due to induction of monocyte chemotactic protein 1 synthesis and is abolished by high density lipoprotein. J Clin Invest 88:2039–2046

Neuzil J, Witting PK, Stocker R (1997) α-Tocopheryl hydroquinone is an efficient multifunctional inhibitor of radical-initiated oxidation of low-density lipoprotein lipids. Proc Natl Acad Sci USA 94:7885–7890

Niu X, Zammit V, Upston JM, Dean RT, Stocker R (1999) Co-existence of oxidized lipids and α-tocopherol in all lipoprotein fractions isolated from advanced human atherosclerotic plaques. Arterioscler Thromb Vasc Biol 19:1708–1718

Noguchi N, Okimoto Y, Tsuchiya J, Cynshi O, Kodama T, Niki E (1997) Inhibition of oxidation of low-density lipoprotein by a novel anti-oxidant, BO-653, prepared by theoretical design. Arch Biochem Biophys 347:141–147

Parker RA, Sabrah T, Cap M, Gill BT (1995) Relation of vascular oxidative stress, α-tocopherol, and hypercholesterolemia to early atherosclerosis in hamsters. Arterioscler Thromb Vasc Biol 15:349–358

Parthasarathy S, Young SG, Witztum JL, Pittman RC, Steinberg D (1986). Probucol inhibits oxidative modification of low density lipoprotein. J Clin Invest 77:641–644

Parums DV, Brown DL, Mitchinson MJ (1990) Serum antibodies to oxidized low-density lipoprotein and ceroid in chronic periaortitis. Arch Pathol Lab Med 114:383–387

Patrono C, FitzGerald GA (1997) Isoprostanes: potential markers of oxidant stress in atherothrombotic disease. Arterioscler Thromb Vasc Biol 17:2309–2315

Podrez EA, Poliakov E, Shen Z, Zhang R, Deng Y, Sun M, Finton PJ, Shan L, Febbraio M, Hajjar DP, Silverstein RL, Hoff HF, Salomon RG, Hazen SL (2002) A novel family of atherogenic oxidized phospholipids promotes macrophage foam cell formation via the scavenger receptor CD36 and is enriched in atherosclerotic lesions. J Biol Chem 277:38517–38523

Podrez EA, Poliakov E, Shen Z, Zhang R, Deng Y, Sun M, Finton PJ, Shan L, Gugiu B, Fox PL, Hoff HF, Salomon RG, Hazen SL (2002) Identification of a novel family of oxidized phospholipids that serve as ligands for the macrophage scavenger receptor CD36. J Biol Chem 277:38503–38516

Prasad K, Kalra J (1993) Oxygen free radicals and hypercholesterolemic atherosclerosis: effect of vitamin E. Am Heart J 125:958–973

Pratico D, Tangirala RK, Radar D, Rokach J, FitzGerald GA (1998) Vitamin E suppresses isoprostane generation *in vivo* and reduces atherosclerosis in apoE-deficient mice. Nat Med 4:1189–1192

Pryor WA, Cornicelli JA, Devall LJ, Tait B, Trivedi BK, Witiak DT, Wu M (1993) A rapid screening test to determine the anti-oxidant potencies of natural and synthetic anti-oxidants. J Org Chem 58:3521–3532

Qiao Y, Yokoyama M, Kameyama K, Asano G (1993) Effect of vitamin E on vascular integrity in cholesterol-fed guinea pigs. Arterioscl Thromb 13:1885–1892

Quinn MT, Parthasarathy S, Fong LG, Steinberg D (1987) Oxidatively modified low density lipoproteins: a potential role in recruitment and retention of monocyte/macrophages during atherogenesis. Proc Natl Acad Sci USA 84:2995–2998

Quinn MT, Parthasarathy S, Steinberg D (1985) Endothelial cell-derived chemotactic activity for mouse peritoneal macrophages and the effects of modified forms of low density lipoprotein. Proc Natl Acad Sci USA 82:5949–5953

Rajavashisth TB, Andalibi A, Territo MC, Berliner JA, Navab M, Fogelman AM, Lusis AJ (1990) Induction of endothelial cell expression of granulocyte and macrophage colony-stimulating factors by modified low-density lipoproteins. Nature 344:254–257

Reaven PD, Parthasarathy S, Beltz WF, Witztum JL (1992) Effect of probucol dosage on plasma lipid and lipoprotein levels and on protection of low density lipoprotein against in vitro oxidation in humans. Arterioscler Thromb 12:318–324

Reilly M, Delanty N, Lawson JA, FitzGerald GA (1996) Modulation of oxidant stress in vivo in chronic cigarette smokers. Circulation 94:19–25

Rice-Evans C, Miller NJ (1994) Total anti-oxidant status in plasma and body fluids. Methods Enzymol 234:279–293

Salonen JT, Ylä-Herttuala S, Yamamoto R, Butler S, Korpela H, Salonen R, Nyyssönen K, Palinski W, Witztum JL (1992) Autoantibody against oxidised LDL and progression of carotid atherosclerosis. Lancet 339:883–887

Santanam N, Penumetcha M, Speisky H, Parthasarathy S (2004) A novel alkaloid anti-oxidant, Boldine and synthetic anti-oxidant, reduced form of RU486, inhibit the oxidation of LDL in-vitro and atherosclerosis in vivo in LDLR(-/-) mice. Atherosclerosis 173:203–210

Sasahara M, Raines EW, Chait A, Carew TE, Steinberg D, Wahl PW, Ross R (1994) Inhibition of hypercholesterolemia-induced atherosclerosis in the nonhuman primate by probucol. I. Is the extent of atherosclerosis related to resistance of LDL to oxidation? J Clin Invest 94:155–164

Sawayama Y, Shimizu C, Maeda N, Tatsukawa M, Kinukawa N, Koyanagi S, Kashiwagi S, Hayashi J (2002) Effects of probucol and pravastatin on common carotid atherosclerosis in patients with asymptomatic hypercholesterolemia. Fukuoka Atherosclerosis Trial (FAST). J Am Coll Cardiol 39:610–616

Shaish A, Daugherty A, O'Sullivan F, Schonfeld G, Heinecke JW (1995) Beta-carotene inhibits atherosclerosis in hypercholesterolemic rabbits. J Clin Invest 96:2075–2082

Sparrow CP, Doebber TW, Olszewski J, Wu MS, Ventre J, Stevens KA, Chao YS (1992) Low density lipoprotein is protected from oxidation and the progression of atherosclerosis is slowed in cholesterol-fed rabbits by the anti-oxidant N,N'-diphenyl-phenylenediamine. J Clin Invest 89:1885–1891

Steinberg D, Parthasarathy S, Carew TE, Khoo JC, Witztum JL (1989) Beyond cholesterol: Modifications of low-density lipoprotein that increase its atherogenicity. N Engl J Med 320:915–924

Steinbrecher UP, Lougheed M, Kwan W-C, Dirks M (1989) Recognition of oxidized low density lipoprotein by the scavenger receptor of macrophages results from derivatization of apolipoprotein B by products of fatty acid peroxidation. J Biol Chem 264:15216–15223

Steinbrecher UP, Parthasarathy S, Leake DS, Witztum JL, Steinberg D (1984) Modification of low density lipoprotein by endothelial cells involves lipid peroxidation and degradation of low density lipoprotein phospholipids. Proc Natl Acad Sci USA 81:3883–3887

Stocker R (1999) The ambivalence of vitamin E in atherogenesis. TiBS 24:219–223

Stocker R (1999) Dietary and pharmacological anti-oxidants in atherosclerosis. Curr Opin Lipidol 10:589–597

Stocker R, Bowry VW, Frei B (1991) Ubiquinol-10 protects human low density lipoprotein more efficiently against lipid peroxidation than does α-tocopherol. Proc Natl Acad Sci USA 88:1646–1650

Stocker R, Keaney JF, Jr (2004) The role of oxidative modifications in atherosclerosis. Physiol Rev 84:1381–1478

Suarna C, Dean RT, May J, Stocker R (1995) Human atherosclerotic plaque contains both oxidized lipids and relatively large amounts of α-tocopherol and ascorbate. Arterioscler Thromb Vasc Biol 15:1616–1624

Sun J, Giraud DW, Moxley RA, Driskell JA (1997) β-Carotene and α-tocopherol inhibit the development of atherosclerotic lesions in hypercholesterolemic rabbits. Int J Vitam Nutr Res 67:155–163

Sundell CL, Somers PK, Meng CQ, Hoong LK, Suen KL, Hill RR, Landers LK, Chapman A, Butteiger D, Jones M, Edwards D, Daugherty A, Wasserman MA, Alexander RW, Medford RM, Saxena U (2003) AGI-1067: a multifunctional phenolic anti-oxidant, lipid modulator, anti-inflammatory and antiatherosclerotic agent. J Pharmacol Exp Ther 305:1116–1123

Suzuki H, Kurihara Y, Takeya M, Kamada N, Kataoka M, Jishage K, Ueda O, Sakaguchi H, Higashi T, Suzuki T, Takashima Y, Kawabe Y, Cynshi O, Wada Y, Honda M, Kurihara H, Aburatani H, Doi T, Matsumoto A, Azuma S, Noda T, Toyoda Y, Itakura H, Yazaki Y, Horiuchi S, Takahashi K, Kruijt JK, van Berkel TJC, Steinbrecher UP, Ishibashi S, Maeda N, Gordon S, Kodama T (1997) A role for macrophage scavenger receptors in atherosclerosis and susceptibility to infection. Nature 386:292–296

Takabe W, Kodama T, Hamakubo T, Tanaka K, Suzuki T, Aburatani H, Matsukawa N, Noguchi N (2001) Anti-atherogenic anti-oxidants regulate the expression and function of proteasome alpha-type subunits in human endothelial cells. J Biol Chem 276:40497–40501

Tangirala RK, Casanada F, Miller E, Witztum JL, Steinberg D, Palinski W (1995) Effect of the anti-oxidant N,N'-diphenyl 1,4-phenylenediamine (DPPD) on atherosclerosis in apoE-deficient mice. J Lipid Res 15:1625–1630

Tardif J-C, Côté G, Lespérance J, Bourassa M, Lambert J, Doucet S, Bilodeau L, Nattel S, de Guise P (1997) Probucol and multivitamins in the prevention of restenosis after coronary angioplasty. N Engl J Med 337:365–372

Tardif JC, Gregoire J, Schwartz L, Title L, Laramee L, Reeves F, Lesperance J, Bourassa MG, L'Allier PL, Glass M, Lambert J, Guertin MC (2003) Effects of AGI-1067 and probucol after percutaneous coronary interventions. Circulation 107:552–558

Tawara K, Ishihara M, Ogawa H, Tomikawa M (1986) Effect of probucol, pantethine and their combinations on serum lipoprotein metabolism and on the incidence of atheromatous lesions in the rabbit. Jpn J Pharmacol 41:211–222

Terentis AC, Thomas SR, Burr JA, Liebler DC, Stocker R (2002) Vitamin E oxidation in human atherosclerotic lesions. Circ Res 90:333–339

Thomas SR, Davies MJ, Stocker R (1998) Oxidation and antioxidation of human low-density lipoprotein and plasma exposed to 3-morpholinosydnonimine and reagent peroxynitrite. Chem Res Toxicol 11:484–494

Thomas SR, Leichtweis SB, Pettersson K, Croft KD, Mori TA, Brown AJ, Stocker R (2001) Dietary co-supplementation with vitamin E and coenzyme Q_{10} inhibits atherosclerosis in apolipoprotein E gene knockout mice. Arterioscler Thromb Vasc Biol 21:585–593

Thomas SR, Witting PK, Stocker R (1996) 3-Hydroxyanthranilic acid is an efficient, cell-derived co-anti-oxidant for α-tocopherol, inhibiting human low density lipoprotein and plasma lipid peroxidation. J Biol Chem 271:32714–32721

Upston JM, Niu X, Brown AJ, Mashima R, Wang H, Senthilmohan R, Kettle AJ, Dean RT, Stocker R (2002) Disease stage-dependent accumulation of lipid and protein oxidation products in human atherosclerosis. Am J Pathol 160:701–710

Upston JM, Terentis AC, Morris K, Keaney JF, Jr., Stocker R (2002) Oxidized lipid accumulates in the presence of a-tocopherol in atherosclerosis. Biochem J 363:753–760

Upston JM, Terentis AC, Stocker R (1999) Tocopherol-mediated peroxidation (TMP) of lipoproteins: implications for vitamin E as a potential antiatherogenic supplement. FASEB J 13:977–994

Upston JM, Witting PK, Brown AJ, Stocker R, Keaney JF, Jr. (2001) Effect of vitamin E on aortic lipid oxidation and intimal proliferation after vascular injury in cholesterol-fed rabbits. Free Radic Biol Med 31:1245–1253

Walldius G, Olsson AG, Bergstrand L, Hadell K, Johansson J, Kaijser L, Lassvik C, Molgaard J, Nilsson S, et al. (1994) The effect of probucol on femoral atherosclerosis: the Probucol Quantitative Regression Swedish Trial (PQRST). Am J Cardiol 74:875–883

Wang Z, Ciabattoni G, Créminon C, Lawson J, FitzGerald GA, Patrono C, Maclouf J (1995) Immumological characterization of urinary 8-epi-prostaglandin $F_{2\alpha}$ excretion in man. J Pharmacol Exp Therapeutics 275:94–100

Wasserman MA, Sundell CL, Kunsch C, Edwards D, Meng CQ, Medford RM (2003) Chemistry and pharmacology of vascular protectants: a novel approach to the treatment of atherosclerosis and coronary artery disease. Am J Cardiol 91:34A–40A

Wayner DDM, Burton GM, Ingold KU, Locke S (1985) Quantitative measurement of the total, peroxyl radical-trapping anti-oxidant capability of human blood plasma by controlled peroxidation. FEBS Lett 187:33–37

Westrope KL, Miller RA, Wilson RB (1982) Vitamin E in a rabbit model of endogenous hypercholesterolemia and atherosclerosis. Nutr Rep Int 25:83–88

Wissler RW, Vesselinovitch D (1983) Combined effects of cholestyramine and probucol on regression of atherosclerosis in rhesus monkey aortas. Appl Pathol 1:89–96

Witting PK, Pettersson K, Letters J, Stocker R (2000) Anti-atherogenic effect of coenzyme Q_{10} in apolipoprotein E gene knockout mice. Free Radic Biol Med 29:295–305

Witting PK, Pettersson K, Letters J, Stocker R (2000) Site-specific anti-atherogenic effect of probucol in apolipoprotein E deficient mice. Arterioscler Thromb Vasc Biol 20: e26–e33

Witting PK, Pettersson K, Östlund-Lindqvist A-M, Westerlund C, Wågberg M, Stocker R (1999) Dissociation of atherogenesis from aortic accumulation of lipid hydro(pero)xides in Watanabe heritable hyperlipidemic rabbits. J Clin Invest 104:213–220

Witting PK, Pettersson K, Östlund-Lindqvist A-M, Westerlund C, Westin Eriksson A, Stocker R (1999) Inhibition by a co-anti-oxidant of aortic lipoprotein lipid peroxidation and atherosclerosis in apolipoprotein E and low density lipoprotein receptor gene double knockout mice. FASEB J 13:667–675

Witting PK, Upston JM, Stocker R (1997) The role of α-tocopheroxyl radical in the initiation of lipid peroxidation in human low density lipoprotein exposed to horse radish peroxidase. Biochemistry 36:1251–1258

Witting PK, Upston JM, Stocker R (1998) The molecular action of α-tocopherol in lipoprotein lipid peroxidation: pro- and anti-oxidant activity of vitamin E in complex heterogeneous lipid emulsions. In: Quinn PJ, Kagan VE (eds) Subcellular biochemistry: fat-soluble vitamins. Plenum Press, London, pp 345–390

Witting PK, Westerlund C, Stocker R (1996) A rapid and simple screening test for potential inhibitors of tocopherol-mediated peroxidation of LDL lipids. J Lipid Res 37:853–867

Yagi K (1984) Assay for blood plasma or serum. Methods Enzymol 105:328–331

Yamamoto Y, Ames BN (1987) Detection of lipid hydroperoxides and hydrogen peroxide at picomole levels by an HPLC and isoluminol chemiluminescence assay. Free Rad Biol Med 3:359–361

Yamamoto Y, Niki E (1989) Presence of cholesteryl ester hydroperoxide in human blood plasma. Biochem Biophys Res Comm 165:988–993

Yeo HC, Helbock HJ, Chyu DW, Ames BN (1994) Assay of malondialdehyde in biological fluids by gas chromatography- mass spectrometry. Anal Biochem 220:391–396

Zamburlini A, Maiorino M, Barbera P, Roveri A, Ursini F (1995) Direct measurement by single photon counting of lipid hydroperoxides in human plasma and lipoproteins. Anal Biochem 232:107–113

Zhang SH, Reddick RL, Avdievich E, Surles LK, Jones RG, Reynolds JB, Quarfordt SH, Maeda N (1997) Paradoxical enhancement of atherosclerosis by probucol treatment in apolipoprotein E-deficient mice. J Clin Invest 99:2858–2866

HEP (2005) 170:591–617
© Springer-Verlag Berlin Heidelberg 2005

Correction of Insulin Resistance and the Metabolic Syndrome

D. Müller-Wieland (✉) · J. Kotzka

Deutsches Diabetes-Zentrum, Institut für Klinische Biochemie und Pathobiochemie,
Auf'm Hennekamp 65, 40225 Düsseldorf, Germany
mueller-wieland@ddfi.uni-duesseldorf.de

Abstract Insulin resistance is a common phenomenon of the metabolic syndrome, which is clinically characterized by a clustering of various cardiovascular risk factors in a single individual and a higher prevalence of respective complications, such as coronary heart disease and stroke. At the cellular level, insulin resistance is defined as a reduced insulin action, which can affect not only glucose uptake, but also gene regulation. Elucidation of novel signaling networks within the cell which are mediating and affecting insulin action will reveal many new genes and drug targets that are potentially of clinical relevance in the future. In this chapter, we propose that the metabolic syndrome might be a clinical consequence of altered gene regulation. This is illuminated in the context of transcription factors, e.g., sterol regulatory element binding proteins (SREBPs), coupling signals from nutrients, metabolites, and hormones at the gene regulatory level with pathobiochemical features of increased lipid accumulation in lean nonadipose tissues. The phenomenon of ectopic lipid accumulation (lipotoxicity) appears to be a novel link between insulin resistance, obesity, and possibly other features of the metabolic syndrome. Therefore, the investigation of specific gene regulatory networks and their alterations might be a clue to understanding the development and clustering of different cardiovascular risk factors in different individuals. As cellular sensors transcription factors—as common denominators of gene regulatory networks—might thereby also determine the susceptibility of individuals to cardiovascular risk factors and their complications.

Keywords Insulin resistance · Metabolic syndrome · Signaling networks · Lipotoxicity

1
Introduction

Insulin resistance is a common phenomenon in the pathogenesis of frequent endocrine metabolic diseases such as type 2 diabetes, obesity, disorders of lipid metabolism, and hypertension. These cardiovascular risk factors often appear together in a single individual, and this clustering is also called 'insulin resistance syndrome' or 'metabolic syndrome'. There are several classification criteria for the definition of individuals with metabolic syndrome (Tables 1, 2 and 3) (Grundy et al. 2004; Reaven 2003). The National Cholesterol Education Program's Adult Treatment Panel III report identified the metabolic syndrome as a multiplex risk factor for cardiovascular disease. Using these criteria, several epidemiological data have recently been reported indicating a higher prevalence of coronary complications and stroke in individuals with metabolic syndrome. In the Prospective Cardiovascular Münster study 4,818 men aged of 35–65 years were investigated over a 10-year period. The acute coronary event rate was twofold higher in individuals with the metabolic syndrome compared to probands without (Assmann et al. 2003). In accordance with that, data of the National Health and Nutrition Examination Survey (NHANES) III show that the prevalence of coronary heart disease (CHD) in the US population aged 50 years and older is also almost twofold higher in individuals with metabolic syndrome compared to controls (Alexander et al. 2003). In this study, the highest prevalence of CHD was seen in patients with metabolic syndrome and clinically overt type 2 diabetes. Interestingly, the prevalence of CHD in patients with type 2 diabetes but without any other feature of the metabolic syndrome did not exceed the prevalence in control individuals. Considering the metabolic syndrome as a multiplex syndrome which deserves more clinical attention, it should also be noted that it affects almost half of the older population. For example, the overall prevalence of the metabolic syndrome in the NHANES population of 3,510 individuals aged 50 years and older was 44% (Alexander et al. 2003). Patients with type 2 diabetes had an even higher prevalence of the metabolic syndrome, i.e., 86%. In patients with impaired fasting glucose, the prevalence was 71.3% and in patients with impaired glucose tolerance, it was 33.1%. Attention should be paid to the investigated individuals with normal plasma glucose levels; even in this group, the prevalence was 25.8% (Alexander et al. 2003).

Table 1 ATP III clinical identification of the metabolic syndrome (modified from Grundy et al. 2004a, b)

Risk factor	Defining level
Abdominal obesity, given as waist circumference[a,b]	
Men	>102 cm (>40 in)
Women	>88 cm (>35 in)
Triglycerides	≥ 150 mg/dl
High-density lipoprotein cholesterol	
Men	<40 mg/dl
Women	<50 mg/dl
Blood pressure	$\geq 130/\geq 85$ mmHg
Fasting glucose	≥ 110 mg/dl[c]

[a] Overweight and obesity are associated with insulin resistance and the metabolic syndrome. However, the presence of abdominal obesity is more highly correlated with the metabolic risk factors than is an elevated BMI. Therefore, the simple measure of waist circumference is recommended to identify the body weight component of the metabolic syndrome.

[b] Some male patients can develop multiple metabolic risk factors when the waist circumference is only marginally increased, e.g., from 94 to 102 cm (from 37 to 39 inches). Such patients may have a strong genetic contribution to insulin resistance. They should benefit from changes in life habits, similarly to men with categorical increases in waist circumference.

[c] The American Diabetes Association has recently established a cut-off point of ≥ 100 mg/dl, above which persons have either prediabetes (impaired fasting glucose) or diabetes. This new cut-off point should be applicable to identification of the lower boundary to define an elevated glucose level as one criterion for the metabolic syndrome.

Table 2 WHO clinical criteria for metabolic syndrome (modified from Grundy et al. 2004a, b)

Insulin resistance, identified by one of the following:
Type 2 diabetes
Impaired fasting glucose
Impaired glucose tolerance
Or for those with normal fasting glucose levels (<110 mg/dl), glucose uptake below the lowest quartile for background population under investigation under hyperinsulinemic, euglycemic conditions

Plus any two of the following:
Antihypertensive medication and/or high blood pressure (≥ 140 mmHg systolic or ≥ 90 mmHg diastolic)
Plasma triglycerides ≥ 150 mg/dl (≥ 1.7 mmol/l)
High-density lipoprotein cholesterol <35 mg/dl (<0.9 mmol/l) in men or <39 mg/dl (1.0 mmol/l) in women
BMI >30 kg/m2 and/or waist:hip ratio >0.9 in men, >0.85 in women
Urinary albumin excretion rate ≥ 20 µg/min or albumin:creatinine ratio ≥ 30 mg/g

Table 3 AACE clinical criteria for diagnosis of the insulin resistance syndrome[a] (modified from Grundy et al. 2004a, b)

Risk factor components	Cutpoints for abnormality
Overweight/obesity	BMI ≥ 25 kg/m2
Elevated triglycerides	≥ 150 mg/dl (1.69 mmol/l)
Low high-density lipoprotein cholesterol	
Men	< 40 mg/dl (1.04 mmol/l)
Women	< 50 mg/dl (1.29 mmol/l)
Elevated blood pressure	≥ 130/85 mmHg
2-h postglucose challenge	> 140 mg/dl
Fasting glucose	Between 110 and 126 mg/dl
Other risk factors	Family history of type 2 diabetes, hypertension, or CVD
	Polycystic ovary syndrome
	Sedentary lifestyle
	Advancing age
	Ethnic groups having high risk for type 2 diabetes or CVD

[a] Diagnosis depends on clinical judgment based on risk factors.

This clinical observation in the latter group corresponds to the pathophysiological concept that in the metabolic syndrome, insulin resistance does not necessarily begin with glucose intolerance. Accordingly, at the cellular level, it makes sense to define insulin resistance as a reduced insulin action, which can affect not only glucose uptake, but also other cellular responses to insulin. Multiple defects and disorders in various signaling pathways of different cells and tissues can develop in diverse combinations over time, each contributing to the heterogeneous clinical phenotype of patients with metabolic syndrome. Several features associated with the metabolic syndrome are summarized in Table 4 (Reaven 2003). Furthermore, in the clinical manifestation of the metabolic syndrome, primary and secondary alterations add to the biochemical and clinical mixture linked to insulin resistance. Therefore, careful clinical characterization of different symptoms and signs of the metabolic syndrome and their association with genetic and cellular alterations will lead to new subclassifications and, consequently, to new diagnostic and therapeutic approaches. In addition, this knowledge will be a key step in the development of novel individually based preventive strategies.

In this article, we will summarize principle mechanisms of insulin action and insulin resistance at the cellular level, because each step might be a future target for therapy. This is followed by two paragraphs on gene regulatory control via transcription factors integrating signals of nutrients, metabolites, and hormones at the gene regulatory level. Transcription factors are sensors for cell responses to metabolic, endocrine, and inflammatory signals, thereby possibly

Table 4 Abnormalities associated with insulin resistance or metabolic syndrome (modified from Reaven 2003)

Clinical features

Cardiovascular disease

Type 2 diabetes

Essential hypertension

Polycystic ovary syndrome

Non-alcoholic fatty liver disease

Certain forms of cancer

'Occult' features

Some degree of glucose intolerance

Impaired fasting glucose

Impaired glucose tolerance

Dyslipidemia

↑ Triglycerides

↓ High-density lipoprotein cholesterol

↓ Low-density lipoprotein particle diameter (small, dense particles)

↑ Postprandial accumulation of triglyceride-rich lipoproteins

Endothelial dysfunction

↑ Mononuclear cell adhesion

↑ Plasma concentration of cellular adhesion molecules

↑ Plasma concentration of asymmetric dimethylarginine

↓ Endothelial-dependent vasodilatation

Procoagulant factors

↑ Plasminogen activator inhibitor-I

↑ Fibrinogen

Hemodynamic changes

↑ Sympathetic nervous system activity

↑ Renal sodium retention

Markers of inflammation

↑ C-reactive protein, leukocyte count

Abnormal uric acid metabolism

↑ Plasma uric acid concentration

---

determining individual susceptibilities to the development of cardiovascular complications. This concept of altered control of gene expression as a major player in the pathogenesis of metabolic syndrome has also shed new light on the link between body fat and insulin resistance, i.e., not the amount, but rather the localization or ectopic accumulation of fat appears to be a critical issue. Finally, the chapter looks at the pharmacological basis of old and new drugs and ends with a concluding perspective.

2
Cellular Mechanisms of Insulin Action and Insulin Resistance

One approach to understand the relation between insulin resistance and other features of the metabolic syndrome is the elucidation of complex cellular signaling mechanisms mediating not only insulin-stimulated glucose uptake but also many other cellular effects, including gene regulatory networks affecting cell growth and differentiation. Principle mechanisms of the cellular network of insulin signaling appear to be similar to the growing family of growth factors, because most of them act via receptor-associated tyrosine kinases (RTKs) at the cell surface (Saltiel and Kahn 2001; Avruch 1998; Ullrich and Schlessinger 1990; Pawson 2004). Activation of these receptors by ligand binding, for example the insulin receptor by insulin, leads to autophosphorylation of an intracellular receptor domain at tyrosine residues, thereby activating the intrinsic kinase activity of the receptor. The activated RTK phosphorylates substrates within the cell at tyrosine residues. The tyrosine phosphorylated substrates act as so-called docking or adapter proteins by binding other signaling molecules. There are many different substrates interacting directly with the insulin receptor in a tyrosine-dependent manner, e.g., various insulin receptor substrates (IRS), shc, Gab1–2, etc. Again, each of these receptor substrates affect the activity of different downstream signaling proteins, thereby generating signaling complexes inducing diverse cell responses to insulin. Therefore, insulin action of cells depends on the cell-specific sets of signaling complexes. Furthermore, in terms of signaling pathways and control, these cellular signaling complexes are not only points of signal diversification, but also crosspoints for integration into and adjustment to the activity of other pathways. For example, a single insulin receptor substrate can bind various other signaling proteins, but can also be used by different RTKs and modulated by different regulatory processes. As for the substrate Gab-1, we have shown that it is tyrosine-phosphorylated by different RTKs (Lehr et al. 2000). In this case, it is interesting that the RTKs phosphorylated the same tyrosine residues, but in a differential quantitative manner. Taken together, signaling complexes regulate the activity of different signaling cascades playing a role in diverse cellular functions, including glucose uptake and gene regulation. Each signaling step or protein appears to be a potential candidate for genetic as well as regulatory defects of insulin action and is therefore a potential drug target for various forms of insulin resistance including the metabolic syndrome.

2.1
Phosphorylation of Proteins Involved in Insulin Action

Signaling networks (Fig. 1) are generated by protein–protein interactions which are regulated by subcellular localization, phosphorylation, and abundance of each signaling molecule. Insulin action can be modulated by affecting

Principals of signaling cascades and networks

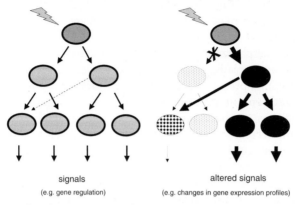

signals
(e.g. gene regulation)

altered signals
(e.g. changes in gene expression profiles)

Fig. 1 Insulin signaling by protein complexes or signalosomes. Representation of intracellular signaling networks regulated by their abundance, activity, and posttranslational modification coupling receptors at the cell surface to cellular responses including gene regulation. It is obvious that postreceptor defects can affect each signaling step alone or in combination. The pattern of disturbances of signal transduction pathways will lead to different clinical phenotypes or manifestations of the different components of the metabolic syndrome. Furthermore, the insulin resistant states are even more complex as the patterns of signaling proteins differ between cells and tissues. Furthermore, signaling defects in one tissue can affect insulin sensitivity in others. For further details, see text. (Modified from Kotzka and Müller-Wieland 2004)

the sites and amount of tyrosine as well as serine/threonine phosphorylation of signaling proteins.

Phosphorylation of proteins at tyrosine residues can stimulate the activity of enzymes and serve as recognition sites for downstream signaling proteins. Selective generation of signaling complexes by site-specific tyrosine phosphorylation is not only a cellular tool to control selectivity, endurance, and strength of signaling pathways towards different extracellular stimuli, but is also a key step of regulation and possibly drug treatment. Many peptides are being developed to simulate or inhibit tyrosine-mediated protein interactions or to mimic insulin action at the receptor level (Qureshi et al. 2000; Moller 2001; Zhang et al. 1999). In this context, it has become interesting to pharmacologically affect the counter-players of tyrosine kinases, i.e., the tyrosine phosphatases. Cell and animal studies have shown, for example, that the insulin signal can be inhibited at the receptor level by specific tyrosine phosphatases (Goldstein 2002a). Protein-tyrosine phosphatases (PT-Pases) that function as negative regulators of the insulin signaling cascade have been identified as novel targets for the therapeutic enhancement of insulin action in insulin-resistant disease states. Recent studies have provided compelling evidence that one of the main functions of the intracellular enzyme PTPase1B (PTP1B), and perhaps to a lesser extent of the transmembrane

PTPase leukocyte antigen-related, is to suppress insulin action (Zabolotny et al. 2004). Reducing PTP1B abundance not only enhances insulin sensitivity and improves glucose metabolism, but also protects against obesity induced by high-fat feeding.

Besides tyrosine phosphatases, another principle mechanism of downregulating insulin action is increased phosphorylation at serine and threonine residues of proximal proteins involved in the signal transduction pathways of insulin. Serine/threonine phosphorylation of the insulin receptor or insulin receptor substrates has been investigated in greater detail and shown to be associated with decreased insulin signaling (Lee and White 2004; Pirola et al. 2004; Werner et al. 2004; Aguirre et al. 2002; Al-Hasani et al. 1997). The detailed mechanisms are still unclear, but serine phosphorylation might impair the transferase activity of protein tyrosine kinases, affect phospho-tyrosine dependent protein–protein interactions, or accelerate the dissociation of signaling complexes. Insulin resistant states induced by inflammatory signals, hyperglycemia, free fatty acids, catecholamines, angiotensin II, and cytokines including tumor necrosis factor (TNF)α have been related to molecular mechanisms associated with increased serine phosphorylation of proximal signaling proteins involved in insulin action, like the insulin receptor or insulin receptor substrates. These effects are mediated by different serine/threonine kinases within cells of different insulin-sensitive tissues, like protein kinase A, protein kinase B, different members of the protein kinases C family, different MAP kinase families (Erk, JNK, p38), and JAK. We have recently shown that Erk-MAP kinases phosphorylate Gab-1 at serine residues, which are in proximity to the tyrosine phosphorylation sites binding the downstream signaling protein p85-PI 3 kinase (Lehr et al. 2004b). In accordance with that, Erk phosphorylation of Gab-1 at these sites abolishes the insulin-induced generation and activation of this specific signaling complex.

In respect of potential molecular mechanisms for the clinically observed association between inflammation and insulin resistance, it is worth mentioning that activation of the inhibitor kappa B kinase (IKK) has been brought into context with insulin resistance. This hypothesis was supported by the observation that heterogeneous gene deletion or high doses of salicylate, which then can inhibit IKK, increase insulin sensitivity in some circumstances (Hundal et al. 2002; Yuan et al. 2001; Shoelson et al. 2003). IKK phosphorylates a protein called IκB, which is an inhibitor for the gene regulatory nuclear factor (NF)-κB proteins playing a central role in most inflammatory responses. Phosphorylation of IκB leads to a release of NF-κB, which then can move into the nucleus and stimulate the transcription of specific genes. One additional essential feature of cellular inflammatory reactions is the induction of immediate-early genes, e.g., SOCS (suppressor of cytokine signaling) proteins in response to cytokine treatment. SOCS proteins, which also contain a central phospho-tyrosine interacting SH2-domain, can modulate insulin signaling by competing with other substrates and channeling IRS proteins to the proteosome for degradation (Rui et al. 2002). Accordingly, inhibition of SOCS proteins in mice improves insulin sensitivity and other features of the metabolic syndrome (Ueki et al. 2004).

2.2
Role of Abundance of Insulin Signaling Molecules

The pivotal role of insulin as well as the fact that absolute insulin deficiency leads to the development of ketoacidosis were proven in transgenic mice lacking insulin receptor (IR) (Accili et al. 1996; Joshi et al. 1996). These mice die shortly after birth due to severe ketoacidosis, but most of the heterozygous animals are clinically inapparent. This corresponds to the clinical observation of patients with genetic syndromes of severe insulin resistance. In these patients, two defective alleles of the IR can be identified, and the patients die soon after birth. The parents, however, which apparently have heterozygous alterations of the IR gene, are clinically silent or show only mild glucose intolerance. Adding a defective allele of the insulin receptor substrate (IRS) 1 to these heterozygous IR knockout mice, which increases the state of insulin resistance by adding a postreceptor defect, leads to clinical manifestation of diabetes (Bruning et al. 1997). This is a transgenic mice model for the development of polygenic disease states associated with insulin resistance, such as the metabolic syndrome.

Interestingly, mice deficient for IRS-1 alone exhibit the classical metabolic syndrome, i.e., insulin resistance with glucose intolerance, hypertriglyceridemia, and low high-density lipoprotein-cholesterol levels as well as elevated blood pressure (Abe et al. 1998; Araki et al. 1994; Kulkarni et al. 1999a; Tamemoto et al. 1994). The insulin resistance is compensated by an increased insulin production of the β-cells. Furthermore, these animals show a reduced embryonal and postnatal growth rate and a body weight in adulthood reduced by 40%–50%. IRS-2-deficient mice have a severe insulin resistance in liver and muscle (Kubota et al. 2000; Suzuki et al. 2004; Withers et al. 1998). However, in these animals, insulin resistance cannot be compensated by increased insulin production, because β-cell neogenesis is decreased.

Further transgenic mice studies have shown that decreased insulin action in one tissue can induce alterations and insulin resistance in others (Accili 2004). Therefore, metabolic and endocrine signals of different tissues communicate by regulating insulin sensitivity and glycemic state as well as lipid homeostasis. In the following, we will give examples of mice in which insulin action has been transgenically ablated in selective classical tissues such as skeletal muscle, liver, fat, and central nervous system.

It has been clinically observed that skeletal muscle is responsible for a major part of postprandial insulin-stimulated glucose uptake. Therefore, the hypothesis that insulin resistance in skeletal muscle plays an essential role in the development of clinically overt type 2 diabetes has always remained current. Surprisingly, transgenic mice in which the insulin receptor was deleted specifically in skeletal muscle had no clinically overt diabetes, no growth alteration or glucose intolerance, but showed features of the metabolic syndrome, i.e., mild insulin resistance with slightly elevated levels of insulin and triglycerides in plasma (Bruning et al. 1998b). Further studies showed that glucose was redistributed to adipose tissue. Mice being insulin receptor deficient in liver developed overt diabetes due to increased hepatic gluconeogenesis. Mice with an insulin receptor knockout in β-cells of the pancreas exhibited defects in insulin secretion similar to early stages of type 2 diabetes (Kulkarni et al. 1999b). For the first time, these data provided evidence that insulin resistance of β-cells can be associated with reduced glucose-stimulated insulin secretion. Therefore, insulin resistance can lead not only to reduced insulin-stimulated uptake of glucose and increased glucose production, but also to impaired insulin secretion, i.e., to all biochemical features of type 2 diabetes. Mice with fat-specific disruption of the insulin receptor gene are protected against age-related and hypothalamic lesion-induced obesity and obesity-related glucose intolerance (Bluher et al. 2002). In this context, it is interesting to note that insulin receptor deficiency in the central nervous system leads to hyperphagia with consecutive features of the metabolic syndrome, i.e., obesity, insulin resistance, and elevated triglyceride levels (Bruning et al. 1998a). The potential clinical relevance and role of cellular signaling proteins in the pathophysiology of insulin resistance can be tested best in transgenic mice models (Accili 2004; Kadowaki 2000; Mauvais-Jarvis et al. 2002; Nandi et al. 2004; Terauchi and Kadowaki 2002). Although it is still unclear whether the physiology of mice and its alterations induced by transgenic technology is applicable to human beings, these models can help to test and generate clinical hypotheses delineating different components in complex systems.

3
Metabolic Syndrome: Clinical Manifestation of Dysregulated Metabolic and Endocrine Control of Gene Expression?

Insulin action is not only related to the uptake of glucose, but also to the regulation of many different genes, including gene regulatory networks affecting cell growth and differentiation. Alterations in gene expression might play a central role in cellular insulin resistance and in the pathogenesis of associated clinical features. Therefore, proteins involved in gene regulatory pathways, such as transcription factors, might be a relevant pathogenic link in the clinical clustering of cardiovascular risk factors.

Transcription factors might be altered in their abundance and activity primarily, or secondarily as a consequence of altered insulin action and/or other metabolic features. One of the best examples of transcription factors integrating cellular information induced by nutrients, metabolites, hormones, growth factors, inflammatory signals, and drugs on insulin sensitivity as well as on intracellular lipid metabolism are peroxisomal proliferator activator receptors (PPARs) and SREBPs (Auwerx and Mangelsdorf 2000; Horton et al. 2002; Hyoun-Ju et al. 2002; Ziouzenkova et al. 2002).

PPARs are ligand-activated transcription factors and belong to the nuclear receptor family without well-known intrinsic ligands, also called orphan receptors. Three different PPARs have been characterized: PPARα, PPAR β/δ, and PPARγ. PPARα, which is a target of fibrates, is expressed mainly in liver and plays a central role in fatty acid metabolism. PPAR β/δ appears to be regulated by some fatty acids and is expressed in many different tissues. In contrast, PPARγ is a key player in the control of adipogenesis and insulin sensitivity (Rosen et al. 2000; Samuel et al. 2004; Vergès 2004). PPARγ is also a target for the class of insulin sensitizers called glitazones. The precise mechanisms by which glitazones or PPARγ-activity affect insulin sensitivity are still unclear. Several mechanisms have been discussed, for example redistributing visceral to subcutaneous fat, increasing lipid catabolism and thereby reducing lipotoxicity, affecting fat cell size, and secreting adipokines. PPARγ is controlled by coactivators. Most recently, the PPARγ coactivator (PGC)-1 has drawn increasing attention. Spiegelman's group showed that PGC-1α plays a central role in controlling PPARγ activity and thereby adipogenesis, but that it can also interact with other transcription factors controlling muscle differentiation and hepatic gluconeogenesis (Herzig et al. 2001; Lin et al. 2002; Michael et al. 2001; Puigserver et al. 2001, 2003; Yoon et al. 2001). Therefore, PGC-1α is an example of how a single signaling step controlling gene expression and cellular differentiation networks affects such diverse cellular phenomena, i.e., fat cell differentiation, muscle cell differentiation, hepatic gluconeogenesis, energy expenditure, etc. However, all these features and their alterations might play a role in the clinical manifestation and future drug therapy of metabolic syndrome. Another important family playing a role in this metabolism-related gene regulatory network is the SREBPs.

4
SREBP-1: A Novel Drug Target for Metabolic Syndrome?

SREBPs have been identified as transcription factors that are regulated by nutrients, metabolites, hormones, and drugs. These features of transcription factors seem to be key for bringing together open strings of gene regulation, cellular signaling networks, and the development of nutrition-related polygenic diseases like obesity and type 2 diabetes. About 10 years ago, SREBPs were independently identified by two different research groups working on cholesterol metabolism and the mechanisms of fat cell differentiation, respectively. The group of Goldstein and Brown isolated two SREBPs, SREBP-1 and SREBP-2, from human HeLa cell extracts because of their binding property to the cholesterol-regulated element [sterol regulatory element (sre)-1] in the promoter of the low-density lipoprotein (LDL) receptor (Briggs et al. 1993; Hua et al. 1993; Wang et al. 1993; Yokoyama et al. 1993). The group of Spiegelman isolated SREBP-1c by screening a rat adipocyte cDNA library using an E-box motive as probe. Since the isolated protein plays an important role in adipogenesis, it was called adipocyte-determination-and-differentiation-factor-1 (Tontonoz et al. 1993).

Until today, the family of SREBPs has essentially encompassed two isoforms, SREBP-1 and SREBP-2, which are encoded by two different genes called *SREBF-1* and *SREBF-2*. In contrast to *SREBF-2*, *SREBF-1* is transcribed into two major splice variants called SREBP-1a and SREBP-1c (Yokoyama et al. 1993; Hua et al. 1995; Shimomura et al. 1997). One essential feature of SREBPs is that they are embedded as transcriptional inactive precursor proteins in the membrane of the endoplasmatic reticulum and the nuclear envelope. Lowering of the intracellular sterol content leads to the release of the transcriptional active N-terminal domain by activation of a proteolytic cascade attacking the membrane-inserted portion of the SREBPs (Brown and Goldstein 1997, 1999).

An additional principle mechanism of regulation besides cleavage is the control of SREBP gene expression. It has been shown that the transcription of SREBPs can be regulated by hormones, e.g., insulin stimulates the transcriptional rate of SREBP-1c by phosphatidylinositol 3-kinase activated PKCλ (Foretz et al. 1999a, 1999b; Matsumoto et al. 2002, 2003). However, one has to consider that an increase in gene transcription does not necessarily correlate with an increased amount of transactive protein domains within the nucleus, as also increased amounts of precursor proteins underlie the sterol-dependent proteolytic processing described above. Therefore, the observation that insulin can stimulate the expression of the LDL-receptor gene to a similar degree in cholesterol-rich as well as lipid-depleted serum indicates that this phenomenon cannot be explained conclusively by increased insulin-induced expression of the *SREBP-1* gene alone (Streicher et al. 1996). Rather, a mechanism might be postulated by which the activity of the transactive SREBP domain may also be modulated directly. We have recently shown that SREBPs are substrates of mitogen-activated protein kinases (Kotzka et al. 2000). For example, hormonal effects on the LDL-receptor gene promoter are completely abolished in stable cell lines lacking either SREBP-1 or SREBP-2 and can be reconstituted by ectopic expression of the corresponding constitutively active N-terminal domains of SREBPs (Kotzka et al. 1998, 2000). Furthermore, hormonal regulation of the LDL-receptor promoter can be blocked by incubation of cells with inhibitors of mitogen activated protein (MAP) kinase cascades. Wortmannin, however, as an inhibitor of the PI-3 kinase pathway, had no effect. These data support the evidence that SREBPs and their corresponding *cis*-element are integral members of the MAP kinase signaling cascades linking effects of insulin and growth factors from the cell surface to gene regulatory networks. Additional analyses identified SREBPs as substrates of the Erk-MAP kinase family. Using a protein chemistry approach, e.g., the anion exchange chromatography, reversed phase HPLC, mass spectrometry, and Edman degradation, serine 117 has been identified as the major phosphorylation site within SREBP-1a for Erk-MAP kinases (Roth et al. 2000). Functional investigations show that transactivity of the N-terminal domain of SREBP-1a is stimulated by insulin and platelet-derived growth factor (PDGF) in a synergistic fashion. Mutation of the major phosphorylation site serine 117 to alanine completely abolishes this synergistic effect of insulin and PDGF on transactivity. Taken together, besides proteolytic cleavage, the mechanism of phosphorylation is a functional modification leading to an increased transactivity of SREBPs. From the cellular point of view, this is an additional possibility to react to environmental changes, indicating that the SREBPs are a gene regulatory point of convergence for diverse extracellular signals including hormones, nutrients, and even drugs.

There are several transgenic mice models of SREBPs which show that they are major players in the control of cellular lipid metabolism. In respect to the metabolic syndrome, SREBP-1 isoforms appear to have a predominant role. Therefore, we focus on the two mice models in which either SREBP-1a or SREBP-1c were overexpressed under the same promoter in fat cells. Transgenic mice overexpressing SREBP-1a under control of the PEPCK promoter, which is active not only in liver, but also in kidney and adipose tissue, do not only show steatosis hepatis, but also a reduced amount of white fat (Shimano et al. 1996). In contrast, mice overexpressing SREBP-1c under control of the PEPCK promoter do not show any gross change in white adipose tissue (Shimano et al. 1997). However, mice overexpressing SREBP-1c under control of the fat cell-specific aP2 promoter lack fat tissue due to an inhibited adipocyte differentiation (Shimomura et al. 1998). The mice that lack adipose tissue are insulin resistant, have hyperglycemia, and a massive steatosis hepatis including elevated plasma triglyceride levels. This phenotype resembles the clinical picture of congenital generalized lipodystrophy (Lawrence 1946; Seip 1996). Furthermore, the level of serum leptin was greatly reduced in these mice, and the application of leptin reconstituted insulin sensitivity (Shimomura et al. 1999). In contrast, mice overexpressing SREBP-1a under control of the aP2 promoter show a great increase in white and brown adipose tissue, which is most likely the consequence of a massively increased rate of cholesterol and fatty acid synthesis (Horton et al. 2003). Overexpression of SREBP-1a increased the number of differentiated hypertrophic adipocytes and induced only a mild hepatic steatosis, but no diabetic phenotype. In conclusion, these transgenic animal models show that SREBP-1a is a potent activator of all known SREBP-regulated gene targets. The splice variant SREBP-1c predominantly activates genes affecting fatty acid metabolism and is a major regulator of de novo lipid synthesis. In contrast, SREBP-2 is mainly a regulator of genes predominantly affecting cholesterol homeostasis. Based on this relative selectivity of different SREBP isoforms, one might speculate that SREBPs are an important link between metabolism, insulin sensitivity, and in the development of other cardiovascular risk factors at the gene regulatory level.

Apparently, SREBPs are key players in the control of intracellular lipid accumulation. One interesting aspect is that increased intracellular lipid accumulation might impair the function of the corresponding cell, e.g., insulin secretion in the case of pancreatic β-cells, or insulin-stimulated glucose uptake or insulin sensitivity in the case of adipose tissue, skeletal muscle, and liver. In this respect, intracellular lipid accumulation, called lipotoxicity, might be a link between insulin resistance, visceral obesity, and increased lipid deposition in nonadipose tissue, perhaps even including cells of the arterial vessel wall, being a feature of atherosclerosis. Accordingly, it is interesting to note that recently Mingrone et al. (2003) have shown that massive weight loss after biliopancreatic diversion is associated with reversion of insulin resistance, lowering of intra-myocytic triglyceride depots, reduction of SREBP-1c mRNA expression in skeletal muscle, and reduction of cardiovascular risk over 24 months. Furthermore, SREBP-1c appears to play a role in the development of the HIV treatment associated insulin resistance syndrome (Caron et al. 2003; Hadri et al. 2004; Kannisto et al. 2003; Williams et al. 2004). Therefore, SREBP-1a/c not only seem to regulate lipid metabolism, but also appear to be a target of insulin action and may therefore be a key link for different features of the metabolic syndrome (see Fig. 2; Müller-Wieland and Kotzka 2002). Furthermore, overexpression of SREBP-1a/c in liver can lead to IRS-2-related insulin resistance (Ide et al. 2004).

5
Lipotoxicity: A Novel Link Between Insulin Resistance and Fat

Several cell biological studies, animal studies, and an increasing number of clinical studies support the hypothesis of Unger (2002 and 2003) and McGarry (2002) that an increased intracellular lipid accumulation in nonfat cells is associated with a disturbance of the respective functions, i.e., insulin resistance in case of insulin action.

Studies in different groups of individuals, i.e., individuals with a normal glucose tolerance, impaired glucose tolerance, and clinically overt type 2 diabetes show that lipid accumulation within skeletal muscle (lipotoxicity) is a very early phenomenon. Jacob et al. (1999) have shown that the intracellular lipid content of skeletal muscle cells has a very strong correlation to the insulin sensitivity already in nondiabetic relatives of patients with type 2 diabetes. Accordingly, obese individuals who are not insulin resistant appear to have a relatively low intramyocellular lipid content, whereas insulin-resistant individuals with a lack or reduced white adipose tissue (lipodystrophy) have a relatively high intramyocellular lipid content. This is in accordance with the

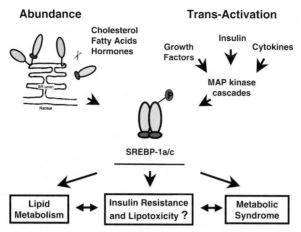

Fig. 2 Role of SREBP-1 as a link between lipid metabolism, insulin action, and clinical features of the metabolic syndrome or syndrome X. Abundance of SREBP-1a/c is regulated by intracellular cholesterol levels, nutrients (such as fatty acids), and hormones. The latter also appear to stimulate transactivity of these transcription factors by phosphorylation via MAP kinase cascades. SREBPs, in concert with other transcription factors, affect the expression of many genes controlling lipid metabolism, insulin sensitivity, and possibly genes involved in the development of visceral obesity, blood pressure control, inflammation, and other features of the metabolic syndrome. For further details, see text. (Modified from Kotzka and Müller-Wieland 2004)

hypothesis that insulin-stimulated glucose uptake or insulin sensitivity correlate much more strongly with the intramuscular cellular lipid content than with body mass index (BMI). Therefore, lipotoxicity might be a mechanism shedding new light on the intricate relationship between body weight and insulin sensitivity.

Based on the accumulating evidence that not the amount of subcutaneous fat but rather the amount of ectopic fat accumulation is the determinant of insulin resistance, one would predict that isolated removal of subcutaneous fat will have no effect on insulin sensitivity. This question was recently answered in an elegant clinical study of Klein et al. (2004), in which the effect of liposuction in eight women with normal glucose tolerance and a mean BMI of 35.1 kg/m^2 and in seven women with a BMI of 39.9 kg/m^2 and type 2 diabetes was investigated. The volume of subcutaneous fat was decreased by 44% in normal glucose tolerant individuals and by 28% in patients with type 2 diabetes, corresponding to a mean absolute loss of fat of 9.1 kg and 10.5 kg, respectively. Insulin sensitivity of liver, skeletal muscle, and adipose tissue was evaluated by assessing the stimulation of glucose disposal, suppression of glucose production, and inhibition of lipolysis before and 10–12 weeks after abdominal liposuction. This surgical procedure had no significant effect on insulin sensitivity of liver, muscle, adipose tissue, or other features of the metabolic syndrome, like blood pressure or plasma lipids. Furthermore, inflammatory markers in plasma, like C-reactive protein, interleukin-6, and TNFα were not altered. Plasma levels of adiponectin were not altered either, indicating that liposuction reduced the amount of subcutaneous tissue, but obviously not its endocrine activity. Furthermore, subcutaneous obesity appears to be associated with increased sympathetic activity, an essential feature of metabolic syndrome (Alvarez et al. 2004).

Also, Kim et al. (2000a, 2000b, 2002) have generated a transgenic mice model in which transcription factors involved in the development of white fat tissue were inhibited. These mice have a clinical phenotype resembling the one of congenital lipoatrophy. The lipoatrophic mice had an ectopic accumulation of fat in liver and skeletal muscle. Interestingly, insulin-stimulated PI3 kinase activation was greatly reduced in liver as well as in skeletal muscle. This cellular insulin resistance was almost restored by transplantation of small amounts of fat. The effect was associated with the reduction of lipid content in liver and skeletal muscle. Unlike in wild-type mice, blocking the uptake of fatty acids in muscle by knocking out the fatty acid transporter protein prevents metabolic induction of insulin resistance. These and other studies support not only the concept of ectopic fat accumulation, but also the increasing evidence that white adipose tissue is not only a passive reservoir for lipids, but also a very active endocrine organ (Guerre-Millo 2004). Several factors with endocrine activity (adipokines) are listed in Table 5. Some of them affect both insulin sensitivity and cellular lipid metabolism, e.g., by stimulating the rate of β-oxidation and reducing fatty acid synthesis. The cellular basis of the homeostasis is a potential treasure of drug targets (Orci et al. 2004).

Table 5 Adipocyte-secreted proteins as modulators of the metabolic syndrome

Nutrient intake	Leptin
Insulin sensitivity	Resistin
	Adiponectin
	TNFα
Ectopic lipid accumulation	Leptin
	Adiponectin
	FGFs?
Inflammation	Cytokines
	Acute phase response proteins
Prothrombotic state	Complement factors
	PAI 1
	Prostacyclin
Dyslipidemia	LPL
	CETP
Blood pressure	Angiotensinogen
	Adrenotopic substances

Malonyl-CoA is an intracellular link between β-oxidation and fatty acid synthesis. Malonyl-CoA inhibits the carnitine palmitoyltransferase system, which is required for long-chain fatty acetyl-CoA molecules to transverse the inner mitochondrial membrane. Acetyl-CoA carboxylase (ACC) is the enzyme that converts acetyl-CoA to malonyl-CoA. In mice lacking ACC2, fat storage is reduced due to continuous fatty acid oxidation. Novel issues for the metabolic syndrome appeared when it was reported that a previously metabolically unrelated growth factor, the fibroblast growth factor (FGF) 19, overexpressed in transgenic mice, induces resistance to diet-induced obesity and insulin desensitization (Fu et al. 2004; Strack and Myers 2004). Therefore, it is a sparkling observation that FGF19 inhibits ACC2, thus increasing fatty acid oxidation. This further supports the emerging concept that fatty acid oxidation may have beneficial effects on obesity, type 2 diabetes, and the metabolic syndrome. Accordingly, genetic reduction of malonyl-CoA in liver reduces lipotoxicity too (An et al. 2004).

Since the mitochondrion in eukaryotic cells is the place for oxidation of fatty acids, there is increasing interest in the role of this compartment in ectopic lipid accumulation and the metabolic syndrome. Recently, an excellent clinical study by Gerald Shulman's group has investigated this issue specifically in insulin-resistant offspring of patients with type 2 diabetes (Petersen et al. 2004). Compared to insulin-sensitive controls, the insulin-stimulated rate of glucose uptake by muscle was approximately 60% lower in the insulin-resistant group and associated with an increase of 80% in intramyocellular lipid content. Further investigations showed that this increase in intramyocellular lipids was most likely attributable to a reduction in mitochondrial phosphorylation. Therefore, this report provides direct evidence for impaired mitochondrial activity in individuals with features of lipotoxicity and insulin resistance.

To further elucidate the relationship between lipid accumulation and mitochondra at the cellular level, we generated cell lines overexpressing constitutively active SREBP-1a in human liver cells. These cells show massive intracellular lipid accumulation. We have further analyzed the protein pattern of mitochondria using the novel technique of two-dimensional difference gel electrophoresis (Lehr et al. 2004a). Mitochondria were enriched by subcellular fractionation using differential and isopyknic centrifugation. Proteins of isolated organelles were labeled with Cy-dyes and separated on 2D gels. These gels revealed more than 100 protein spots, which were significantly different in their abundance between wild-type and SREBP-1a (+) cells. MALDI MS showed that 68% of the identified proteins belonged to mitochondria. In SREBP-1a (+) cells, several enzymes involved in β-oxidation were notably reduced. Accordingly, GC-analyses of the intracellular fatty acid pattern revealed a significant increase in long-chain unsaturated fatty acids. Therefore, the detected protein differences might be an explanation for the observed intracellular lipid accumulation and again link SREBP-1a to mitochondria, lipotoxicity, and insulin resistance.

What exactly the role of subcutaneous and visceral fat is for the excessive lipid accumulation in other organs such as liver, skeletal muscle, and possibly heart is still a matter of discussion (Wu et al. 2001; Cancello et al. 2004; Giusti et al. 2004). Current research intends to delineate differences in endocrine and metabolic activity in fat of different body regions. One recent example of a potentially interesting target for the metabolic syndrome in fat tissue per se is the enzyme 11β-hydroxysteroid dehydrogenase type 1 (11β-HSD-1) (Duplomb et al. 2004; Masuzaki et al. 2003; Morton et al. 2004a, 2004b, Paterson et al. 2004; Walker and Seckl 2003). This enzyme increases intracellular glucocorticoid action and is elevated in adipose tissue of obese humans and animals. Fat-specific overexpression of 11β-HSD-1 produces a metabolic syndrome in mice, whereas mice lacking this enzyme are resistant to high-fat diet-induced visceral obesity and metabolic features.

The concept of ectopic lipid accumulation might be an explanation for many basic unresolved clinical observations, e.g., that insulin sensitivity does not correlate with the amount of subcutaneous fat, that insulin sensitivity is greatly increased by a modest body weight reduction of only 5%–10%, and that not all obese individuals are insulin-resistant. Several animal and human studies have provided evidence that intramyocellular lipid accumulation correlates best with a degree of insulin-stimulated glucose uptake of the body. In accordance with that, inactivation of fatty acid uptake prevents fat-induced insulin resistance (Kim et al. 2004). Mobilization or decrease in intramyocellular lipid appears to be more sensitive to weight reduction than fat of subcutaneous tissue (Houmard et al. 2002; Kelley and Goodpaster 2001). Similar observations have been made for the amount of visceral fat. In the context of these mechanisms, the amount of visceral fat might be as well a marker of the amount of lipid accumulation outside of white subcutaneous fat tissue. Accordingly, there are animal models with visceral obesity, but without insulin resistance (Brains et al. 2004). In addition, recent clinical studies have shown that intracellular lipid content of liver (steatosis hepatis) is associated with insulin resistance, too (Gupte et al. 2004; Hui et al. 2004; Marchesini et al. 2001; Michael et al. 2000; Samuel et al. 2004; Song 2002). Interestingly, there is increasing experimental evidence that intracellular lipid metabolism of pancreatic beta cells appears to play a pivotal role in the regulation of insulin secretion. Lipotoxicity therefore seems to be a novel mechanism (one of many that are still unknown) for the key phenomena of the pathogenesis of type 2 diabetes or metabolic syndrome, insulin resistance in skeletal muscle, disturbance of insulin secretion of the pancreatic beta cell, and increased hepatic glucose production as the consequence of hepatic insulin resistance (Boden and Shulman 2002; Shafrir and Raz 2003). Taken together, the metabolic syndrome represents a group of clinical disorders related to insulin resistance and altered liporegulation.

6
How Will Old and New Drugs Work in the Future?

The metabolic or insulin resistance syndrome is a clinical conglomerate of different symptoms and signs, which is also partially covered by other chapters in this book. Therefore, we will not address drug developments in the fields of dyslipoproteinemia, control of arterial blood pressure, and drugs affecting coagulation or obesity. Rather, we focus on the general mechanism of drugs possibly increasing insulin sensitivity and decreasing ectopic fat accumulation. Among the classical blood sugar-lowering drugs, there are several drugs which have been shown to reduce the development of clinically overt type 2 diabetes in a state of impaired glucose tolerance, e.g., metformine, troglitazone, and acarbose (Knowler et al. 2002; Chiasson et al. 2002; Buchanan et al. 2002; Xiang et al. 2004). Furthermore, it is interesting to note that the concept of multiple mechanisms leading to different states of insulin resistance is strengthened by the observation that large clinical studies using lipid-lowering drugs such as statins, or blood pressure-lowering drugs such as angiotensin converting enzyme inhibitors or angiotensin receptor blockers, also reduce the incidence of type 2 diabetes (Prisant 2004; Lithell et al. 2003; Julius et al. 2004). This indicates that there are several mechanisms causing the metabolic syndrome and that drugs which have been given due to an indication like hypertension might also reduce other components of the metabolic syndrome. In accordance with that, blood sugar-lowering drugs, e.g., metformine, acarbose, or glitazones also affect blood pressure, plasma lipids, and possibly fat distribution. For acarbose, it has been shown that treatment is associated with the lowering of cardiovascular risk and incidence of arterial hypertension (Chiasson et al. 2003). Interestingly, the increase in insulin sensitivity of glitazones appears to be associated with a redistribution from ectopic lipids to a subcutaneous fat tissue (Mudaliar and Henry 2004). This corresponds to the concept of lipotoxicity or ectopic lipid accumulation mentioned above. In this context, glitazones can also be understood not only as blood sugar-lowering agents or insulin sensitizers, but rather as 'anti-lipotoxica'. The role of glitazone as potential 'anti-lipotoxica' (Mayerson et al. 2002) on vascular cells and atherosclerosis is under investigation (Goldstein 2002b).

Based on the different mechanisms mentioned in this review, it is conceivable that each of these mechanisms could be a potential drug target (Bailey 2004; Goldstein 2002b; Moller 2001). A combination of clinical and molecular studies will have to show which different symptoms of the metabolic syndrome develop first, e.g., dyslipidemia first and then hypertension, or vice versa. The understanding of the major players and the background orchestra might lead to new indications for 'old drugs', the identification of novel drug targets and the development of new agents. Furthermore, the role of combinations in therapy and prevention will have to be investigated. One key issue in clinical medicine would be when and how to treat individuals with different features of the metabolic syndrome to prevent cardiovascular complications. At the moment, clinical medicine focuses on the treatment of clinically overt diseases or complications with drugs in rather high doses. The question will be whether, from a preventive point of view, it is more effective to treat early but perhaps with a low dose. Therefore, there might be a paradigm shift from 'late and high' treatment to prevention, i.e., 'early and low' drug taking.

7
Conclusions and Perspectives

Testing different hypotheses and candidate pathways in transgenic mice have identified complex communication pathways between different tissues controlling insulin sensitivity and the state of glucose as well as lipid homeostasis. The elucidation of novel signaling networks within the cell that are mediating and affecting insulin action will reveal many novel genes and drug targets which, in the future, might be of clinical relevance. Therefore, many different clinical subtypes of the metabolic syndrome will have to be investigated, which will enable us not only to perform effective prevention, but also to treat and care for our patients individually according to the best clinical practice.

Insulin resistance-related metabolic syndrome is associated with an increased cardiovascular risk. In this chapter, we proposed that these clinical states are not only a consequence of altered blood glucose, but rather of genetic dysregulation. Specific gene regulatory networks and their alterations might be the key to understanding the development and clustering of different cardiovascular risk factors in different individuals. The common denominators of gene regulatory networks are transcription factors which are cellular sensors and thereby determine the susceptibility of individuals to cardiovascular risk factors, including the metabolic syndrome.

References

Abe H, Yamada N, Kamata K, et al. (1998) Hypertension, hypertriglyceridemia and impaired endothelium-dependent vascular relaxation in mice lacking insulin receptor substrate-1. J Clin Invest 101:1784–1788

Accili D (2004) The struggle for mastery in insulin action: from triumvirate to republic. Diabetes 53:1633–1642

Accili D, Drago J, Lee EJ, Johnson MD, et al. (1996) Early neonatal death in mice homozygous for a null allele of the insulin receptor gene. Nature Genet 12:106–109

Aguirre V, Werner ED, Giraud J, et al. (2002) Phosphorylation of Ser307 in insulin receptor substrate-1 blocks interactions with the insulin receptor and inhibits insulin action. J Biol Chem 277:1531–1537

Alexander CM, Landsman PB, Teutsch SM, et al. (2003) NCEP-defined metabolic syndrome, diabetes, and prevalence coronary heart disease among NHANES III participants age 50 years and older. Diabetes 52:1210–1214

Al-Hasani H, Eisermann B, Tennagels N, et al. (1997) Identification of Ser-1275 and Ser-1309 as autophosphorylation sites of the insulin receptor. FEBS 400:65–70

Alvarez GE, Ballard TP, Beske SD, Davy KP (2004) Subcutaneous obesity is not associated with sympathetic neural activation. Am J Physiol Heart Circ Physiol 287:H414–H418

An J, Muoio DM, Shiota M, et al. (2004) Hepatic expression of malonyl-CoA decarboxylase reverses muscle, liver and whole-animal insulin resistance. Nature Med 10:268–274

Araki E, Lipes MA, Patti ME, et al. (1994) Alternative pathway of insulin signalling in mice with targeted disruption of the IRS-1 gene. Nature 372:186–190

Assmann G, Buyken A, Cullen P, et al. (2003) Prävention der koronaren Herzkrankheit. 1st Edn. Bruckmeier Verlag GmbH, Grünwald

Auwerx J, Mangelsdorf D (2000) X-ceptors, nuclear receptors for metabolism. In: Stemme S, Olsson AG (eds) Atherosclerosis XII. Elsevier Science BV, Amsterdam, pp 21–39

Avruch J (1998) Insulin signal transduction through protein kinase cascades. Mol Cell Biochem 182:31–48

Bailey CJ (2004) New Drugs for the Treatment of Diabetes Mellitus. In: DeFronzo RA, Ferrannini E, Keen H, Zimmet P (eds) International textbook of diabetes mellitus, 3rd Edn. John Wiley & Sons Ltd, Chichester pp 953–979

Bains RS, Wells SE, Flavell DM, et al. (2004) Visceral obesity without insulin resistance in late-onset obesity rats. Endocrinology 145:2666–2679

Bluher M, Michael MD, Perone OD, et al. (2002) Adipose tissue selective insulin receptor knockout protects against obesity and obesity-related glucose intolerance. Dev Cell 3:25–38

Boden G, Shulman GI (2002) Free fatty acids in obesity and type 2 diabetes: defining their role in the development of insulin resistance and beta-cell dysfunction. Eur J Clin Invest 32(Suppl. 3):14–23

Briggs MR, Yokoyama C, Wang X, Brown MS, Goldstein JL (1993) Nuclear protein that binds sterol regulatory element of low density lipoprotein receptor promoter. I. Identification of the protein and delineation of its target nucleotide sequence. J Biol Chem 268:14490–14496

Brown MS, Goldstein JL (1997) The SREBP pathway: regulation of cholesterol metabolism by proteolysis of a membrane-bound transcription factor. Cell 89:331–320

Brown MS, Goldstein JL (1999) A proteolytic pathway that controls the cholesterol content of membranes, cells, and blood. Proc Natl Acad Sci USA 96:11041–11048

Bruning JC, Winnay J, Bonner-Weir S, et al. (1997) Development of a novel polygenic model of NIDDM in mice heterozygous for IR and IRS-1 null alleles. Cell 88:561–572

Bruning JC, Gautam D, Burks DJ, et al. (1998a) Role of the brain insulin receptor in control of body weight and reproduction. Science 299:2122–2125

Bruning JC, Michael MD, Winnay JN, et al. (1998b) A muscle-specific insulin receptor knockout exhibits features of the metabolic syndrome of NIDDM without altering glucose tolerance. Mol Cell 2:559–569

Buchanan TA, Xiang AH, Peters RK, et al. (2002) Preservation of pancreatic beta-cell function and prevention of type 2 diabetes by pharmacological treatment of insulin resistance in high-risk hispanic women. Diabetes 51:2796–2803

Cancello R, Tounian A, Poitou Ch, Clément K (2004) Adiposity signals, genetic and body weight regulation in humans. Diabetes Metab 30:215–227

Caron M, Auclair M, Sterlingot H, et al. (2003) Some HIV protease inhibitors alter lamin A/C maturation and stability, SREBP-1 nuclear localization and adipocyte differentiation. AIDS 17:2437–2444

Chiasson JL, Josse RG, Gomis R, et al. (2002) Acarbose for prevention of type 2 diabetes mellitus : the STOPP-NIDDM randomized trial. Lancet 359:2072–2077

Chiasson JL, Josse RG, Gomis R, et al. (2003) Acarbose treatment and the risk of cardiovascular disease and hypertension in patients with impaired glucose tolerance: the STOPP-NIDDM trial. JAMA 290:486–494

Duplomb L, Lee Y, Wang MY, et al. (2004) Increased expression and activity of 11beta-HSD-1 in diabetic islets and prevention with troglitazone. Biochem Biophys Res Commun 313:594–599

Foretz M, Pacot C, Dugail I, et al. (1999a) ADD1/SREBP-1c is required in the activation of hepatic lipogenic gene expression by glucose. Mol Cell Biol 19:3760–3768

Foretz M, Guichard C, Ferre P, Foufelle F (1999b) Sterol regulatory element binding protein-1c is a major mediator of insulin action on the hepatic expression of glucokinase and lipogenesis-related genes. Proc Natl Acad Sci USA 96:12737–12742

Fu L, John ML, Adams SH, et al. (2004) Fibroblast growth factor 19 increases metabolic rate and reverses dietary and leptin-deficient diabetes. Endocrinology 145:2594–2603

Giusti V, Suter M, Verdumo C, et al. (2004) Molecular determinants of human adipose tissue: differences between visceral and subcutaneous compartments in obese women. J Clin Endocrinol Metab 89:1379–1384

Goldstein BJ (2002a) Protein-tyrosine phosphatases: emerging targets for therapeutic intervention in type 2 diabetes and related states of insulin resistance. J Clin Endocrinol Metab 87:2472–2480

Goldstein BJ (2002b) Possible vascular-protective effects of antidiabetic agents such as the thiazolidinediones (TZDs). Clin Ther 24:1358–1360

Grundy SM, Brewer HG, Cleeman JI, et al. for the conference participants (2004a) Definition of metabolic syndrome. Report of the National Heart, Lung, and Blood Institute/American Heart Association Conference on Scientific Issues Related to Definition. Circulation 109:433–438

Grundy SM, Hansen B, Smith SC, et al. for the conference participants (2004b) Clinical management of metabolic syndrome. Report of the American Heart Association/National Heart, Lung, and Blood Institute/American Diabetes Association Conference on Scientific Issues Related to Management. Circulation 209:551–556

Guerre-Millo M (2004) Adipose tissue and adipokines: for better or worse. Diabetes Metab 30:13–19

Gupte P, Amarapurkar D, Agal S, et al. (2004) Non-alcoholic steatohepatitis in type 2 diabetes mellitus. J Gastroenterol Hepatol 19:854–858

Hadri KE, Glorian M, Monsempes C, et al. (2004) In vitro suppression of the lipogenic pathway by the nonnucleoside reverse transcriptase inhibitor efavirenz in 3T and human preadipocytes or adipocytes. J Biol Chem 279:15130–15141

Herzig S, Long F, Jhala US, et al. (2001) CREB regulates hepatic gluconeogenesis through the coactivator PGC-1. Nature 413:179–183

Horton JD, Goldstein JL, Brown MS (2002) SREBPs: activators of the complete program of cholesterol and fatty acid synthesis in the liver. J Clin Invest 109:1125–1131

Horton JD, Shimomura I, Ikemoto S, et al. (2003) Overexpression of SREBP-1a in mouse adipose tissue produces adipocyte hypertrophy, increased fatty acid secretion, and fatty liver. J Biol Chem 278:36652–36660

Houmard JA, Tanner CJ, Yu C, et al. (2002) Effect of weight loss on insulin sensitivity and intramuscular long-chain fatty acyl-CoAs in morbidly obese subjects. Diabetes 51:2959–2963

Hua X, Yokoyama C, Wu J, et al. (1993) SREBP-2, a second basic-helix-loop-helix-leucine zipper protein that stimulates transcription by binding to a sterol regulatory element. Proc Natl Acad Sci USA 90:11603–11607

Hua X, Wu J, Goldstein JL, Brown MS, Hobbs HH (1995) Structure of the human gene encoding sterol regulatory element binding protein-1 (SREBF1) and localization of SREBF1 and SREBF2 to chromosomes 17p11.2 and 22q13. Genomics 10:667–673

Hui JM, Hodge A, Farrell GC, et al. (2004) Beyond insulin resistance in NASH: TNF-alpha or adiponectin. Hepatology 40:46–54

Hundal RS, Petersen KF, Mayerson AB, et al. (2002) Mechanism by which high-dose aspirin improves glucose metabolism in type 2 diabetes. J Clin Invest 109:1321–1326

Hyoun-Ju K, Miyazaki M, Man WC, et al. (2002) Sterol regulatory element-binding proteins (SREBPs) as regulators of lipid metabolism. Polyunsaturated fatty acids oppose cholesterols-mediated induction of SREBP-1 maturation. Ann NY Acad Sci 967:34–42

Ide T, Shimano H, Yahagi N, et al. (2004) SREBPs suppress IRS-2-mediated insulin signaling in the liver. Nat Cell Biol 6:351–357

Jacob S, Machann J, Rett K, et al. (1999) Association of increased intramyocellular lipid content with insulin resistance in lean nondiabetic offspring of type 2 diabetic subjects. Diabetes 48:1113–1119

Joshi RL, Lamothe B, Cordonnier N, et al. (1996) Targeted disruption of the insulin receptor gene in the mouse results in neonatal lethality. EMBO J 15:1542–1547

Julius S, Kjeldsen SE, Weber M (2004) Outcomes in hypertensive patients at high cardiovascular risk treated with regimes based on valsartan or amlodipine: the VALUE randomised trial. Lancet 363:2022–2031

Kadowaki T (2000) Insights into insulin resistance and type 2 diabetes from knockout mouse models. J Clin Invest 106:459–465

Kannisto K, Sutinen J, Korsheninnikova E, et al. (2003) Expression of adipogenic transcription factors, peroxisome proliferation-activated receptor gamma co-activator 1, IL-6 and CD45 in subcutaneous adipose tissue in lipodystrophy association with highly active antiretroviral therapy. AIDS 17:1753–1762

Kelley DE, Goodpaster BH (2001) Skeletal muscle triglyceride. an aspect of regional adiposity and insulin resistance. Diabetes 24:933–941

Kim JK, Gavrilova O, Chen Y, et al. (2000) Mechanisms of insulin resistance in A-ZIP/17-1 fatless mice. Biol Chem 276:8456–8460

Kim JK, Michael MD, Previs SF, et al. (2000a) Redistribution of substrates to adipose tissue promotes obesity in mice with selective insulin resistance in muscle. J Clin Invest 105:1791–1797

Kim YB, Shulman GI, Kahn BB (2002b) Fatty acid infusion selectively impairs insulin action on Akt1 and protein kinase C lambda/zeta but not on glycogen synthase kinase-3. J Biol Chem 277:32915–32922

Kim JK, Gimeno RE, Higashimori, et al. (2004) Inactivation of fatty acid transport protein 1 prevents fat-induaced insulin resistance in skeletal muscle. J Clin Invest 113:756–763

Klein S, Fontana L, Young L, et al. (2004) Absence of an effect of liposuction on insulin action and risk factors for coronary heart disease. N Engl J Med 350:2549–2557

Knowler WC, Barrett-Connor E, Fowler SE, et al. (2002) Reduction in the incidence of type 2 diabetes with lifestyle intervention or metformin. N Engl J Med 346:393–403

Kotzka J, Muller-Wieland D, Koponen A, et al. (1998) ADD1/SREBP-1c mediates insulin-induced gene expression linked to the MAP kinase pathway. Biochem Biophys Res Commun 249:375–379

Kotzka J, Muller-Wieland D, Roth G, et al. (2000) Sterol regulatory element binding proteins SREBP-1a and SREBP-2 are linked to the map kinase cascade. J Lipid Res 41:99–108

Kotzka J, Müller-Wieland D (2004) Sterol regulatory element-binding protein (SREBP)-1: gene regulatory target for insulin resistance? Expert Opin Ther Targets 8:141–149

Kubota N, Tobe K, Terauchi Y, et al. (2000) Disruption of insulin receptor substrate 2 causes type 2 diabetes because of liver insulin resistance and lack of compensatory ß-cell hyperplasia. Diabetes 49:1880–1889

Kulkarni RN, Winnay JN, Daniels M, et al. (1999a) Altered function of insulin receptor substrate 1-deficient mouse islets and cultured beta-cell lines. J Clin Invest 104:R67–R75

Kulkarni RN, Bruning JC, Winnay JN, et al. (1999b) Tissue-specific knockout of the insulin receptor in pancreatic beta cells creates an insulin secretory defect similar to that in type 2 diabetes. Cell 96:329–339

Lawrence RD (1946) Lypodystrophy and hepatomegaly with diabetes, lipaemia and other metabolic disturbances. A case throwing new light on the action of insulin. Lancet 1:724–731

Lee YH, White MF (2004) Insulin receptor substrate proteins and diabetes. Arch Pharm Res 27:361–370

Lehr S, Kotzka J, Herkner A, et al. (2000) Identification of major tyrosine phosphorylation sites in the human insulin receptor substrate Gab-1 by insulin receptor kinase in vitro. Biochemistry 49:10898–10907

Lehr S, Kotzka J, Avci H, et al. (2004a) Effect of SREBP-1a on intracellular lipids and mitochondrial protein pattern in human liver cells detected by 2D-DIGE. Biochemistry (in press)

Lehr S, Kotzka J, Avci H, et al. (2004b) Identification of Major ERK-Related Phosphorylation Sites in Gab1. Biochemistry 43:12133–12140

Lin J, Wu H, Tarr PT, et al. (2002) Transcriptional co-activator PGC-1α drives the formation of slow-twitch muscle fibres. Nature 418:797–801

Lithell H, Hansson L, Skoog I, et al. (2003) The Study on Cognition and Prognosis in the Elderly (SCOPE): principal results of a randomized double-blind intervention trial. J Hypertens 21:875–886

Marchesini G, Brizi M, Bianchi G, et al. (2001) Nonalcoholic fatty liver disease. A feature of the metabolic syndrome. Diabetes 50:1844–1850

Masuzaki H, Yamamoto H, Kenyon CJ, et al. (2003) Transgenic amplification of glucocorticoid action in adipose tissue causes high blood pressure in mice. J Clin Invest 112:83–90

Matsumoto M, Ogawa W, Teshigawara K, et al. (2002) Role of the insulin receptor substrate 1 and phosphatidylinositol 3-kinase signaling pathway in insulin-induced expression of sterol regulatory element binding protein 1c and glucokinase genes in rat hepatocytes. Diabetes 51:1672–1680

Matsumoto M, Ogawa W, Akimoto K, et al. (2003) PKClambda in liver mediates insulin-induced SREBP-1c expression and determines both hepatic lipid content and overall insulin sensitivity. J Clin Invest 112:935–944

Mauvais-Jarvis F, Kulkarni RN, Kahn CR (2002) Knockout models are useful tools to dissect the pathophysiology and genetics of insulin resistance. Clin Endocrinol 57:1–7

Mayerson AB, Hundal RS, Dufour S, et al. (2002) The effects of rosiglitazone on insulin sensitivity, lipolysis, and hepatic and skeletal muscle triglyceride content in patients with type 2 diabetes. Diabetes 51:797–802

McGarry JD (2002) Dysregulation of fatty acid metabolism in the etiology of type 2 diabetes. Diabetes 51:7–18

Michael LF, Wu Z, Cheatham RB, et al. (2001) Restoration of insulin-sensitive glucose transporter (GLUT4) gene expression in muscle cells by the transcriptional coactivator PGC-1. Proc Natl Acad Sci USA 98:3820–3825

Michael MD, Kulkarni RN, Postic C, et al. (2000) Loss of insulin signaling in hepatocytes leads to severe insulin resistance and progressive hepatic dysfunction. Mol Cell 6:87–97

Mingrone G, Rosa G, Greco AV, et al. (2003) Intramyocitic lipid accumulation and SREBP-1c expression related to insulin resistance and cardiovascular risk in morbid obesity. Atherosclerosis 170:155–161

Moller DE (2001) New drug targets for type 2 diabetes and the metabolic syndrome. Nature 414:821–827

Morton NM, Ramage L, Seckl JR (2004a) Down-regulation of adipose 11β-hydroxysteroid dehydrogenase type 1 by High-fat feeding in mice: a potential adaptive mechanism counteracting metabolic disease. Endocrinology 145:2707–2712

Morton NM, Paterson JM, Mauzaki H, et al. (2004b) Novel adipose tissue-mediated resistance to diet-induced visceral obesity in 11 beta-hydroxysteroid dehydrogenase type 1-deficient mice. Diabetes 53:931–938

Mudaliar S, Henry RR (2004) Thiazolidiones as PPAR Agonists. In: DeFronzo RA, Ferrannini E, Keen H, Zimmet P (eds) International textbook of diabetes mellitus, 3rd Edn. John Wiley & Sons Ltd, Chichester, pp 871–899

Müller-Wieland D, Kotzka J (2002) SREBP-1: gene regulatory key to Syndrome X? Ann NY Acad Sci 967:19–27

Nandi A, Kitamura Y, Kahn CR, et al. (2004) Mouse models of insulin resistance. Physiol Rev 84:623–647

Orci L, Cook WS, Ravazzola M (2004) Rapid transformation of white adipocyte into fat-oxidizing machines. Proc Natl Acad Sci USA 101:2058–2063

Paterson JM, Morteon NM, Fievet C, et al. (2004) Metabolic syndrome without obesity: Hepatic overexpression 11beta-hydroxysteroid dehydrogenase type 1 in transgenic mice. Proc Natl Acad Sci USA 101:7088–7093

Pawson R (2004) Specificity in signal transduction: from phosphotyrosine-SH2 domain interactions to complex cellular systems. Cell 116:191–203

Petersen KF, Dufour S, Befrey D, et al. (2004) Impaired mitochondrial activity in the insulin-resistant offspring of patients with type 2 diabetes. N Engl J Med 350:664–671

Pirola L, Johnston AM, Van Obberghen E (2004) Modulation of insulin action. Diabetologia 47:170–184

Prisant LM (2004) Preventing type II diabetes mellitus. J Clin Pharmacol 44:406–413

Puigserver P, Rhee J, Lin J, et al. (2001) Cytokine stimulation of energy expenditure through p38 MAP Ki activation of PPARγ Coactivator-1. Mol Cell 8:971–982

Puigserver P, Rhee J, Donovan J, et al. (2003) Insulin-regulated hepatic gluconeogenesis through FOXO1-PGC-1alpha interaction. Nature 423:550–555

Qureshi SA, Ding V, Li Z (2000) Activation of insulin signal transduction pathway and antidiabetic activity of small molecule insulin receptor activators. J Biol Chem 275:36590–36595

Reaven GM (2003) The insulin resistance syndrome. Curr Atherosclerosis Rep 5:365–371

Rosen ED, Walkey CJ, Puigserver P, Spiegelman BM (2000) Transcriptional regulation of adipogenesis. Genes Dev 14:1293–1307

Rosen ED, Hsu CH, Wang X, et al. (2002) C/EBPa induces adipogenesis through PPARγ: a unified pathway. Genes Dev 16:22–26

Roth G, Kotzka J, Kremer L, et al. (2000) MAP kinases Erk1/2 phosphorylate sterol regulatory element-binding protein (SREBP)-1a at serine 117 in vitro. J Biol Chem 275:33302–33307

Rui L, Yuan M, Frantz D, et al. (2002) SOCS-1 and SOCS-3 block insulin signalling by ubiquitin-mediated degradation of IRS1 and IRS2. J Biol Chem 277:42394–42398

Saltiel AR, Kahn CR (2001) Insulin signalling and the regulation of glucose and lipid metabolism. Nature 414:799–806

Samuel VT, Liu ZX, Qu X, et al. (2004) Mechanism of Hepatic Insulin Resistance in Non-alcoholic Fat Liver Disease. J Biol Chem 279:32345–32353

Seip M, Trygstad O (1996) Generalized lipodystrophy, congenital and acquired (lipoatrophy). Acta Paediatr Suppl 413:2–28

Shafrir E, Raz I (2003) For Debate. Diabetes: mellitus or lipidus? Diabetologia 46:433–440

Shimano H, Horton JD, Hammer RE, et al. (1996) Overproduction of cholesterol and fatty acids causes massive liver enlargement in transgenic mice expressing truncated SREBP-1a. J Clin Invest 98:1575–1584

Shimano H, Horton JD, Shimomura I, et al. (1997) Isoform 1c of sterol regulatory element binding protein is less active than isoform 1a in livers of transgenic mice and in cultured cells. J Clin Invest 99:846–854

Shimizu S, Ugi S, Maegawa H, et al. (2003) Protein-tyrosine phosphatase 1 as new activator for hepatic lipogenesis via sterol regulatory element-binding protein-1 gene expression. J Biol Chem 278:43095–43101

Shimomura I, Shimano H, Horton JD, et al. (1997) Differential expression of exons 1a and 1c in mRNAs for sterol regulatory element binding protein-1 in human and mouse organs and cultured cells. J Clin Invest 99:838–845

Shimomura I, Hammer RE, Richardson JA, et al. (1998) Insulin resistance and diabetes mellitus in transgenic mice expressing nuclear SREBP-1c in adipose tissue: model for congenital generalized lipodystrophy. Genes Dev 12:2182–3194

Shimomura I, Hammer RE, Ikemoto S, et al. (1999) Leptin reverses insulin resistance and diabetes mellitus in mice with congenital lipodystrophy. Nature 401:73–76

Shoelson SE, Lee J, Yuan M (2003) Inflammation and the IKKß/IκB/NF-κB axis in obesity- and diet-induced insulin resistance. Int J Obesity 27:S49–S52

Song S (2002) The role of increased liver triglyceride content: a culprit of diabetic hyperglycaemia? Diabetes Metab Res Rev 18:5–12

Strack AM, Myers RW (2004) Modulation of metabolic syndrome by fibroblast growth factor 19 (FGF19)? Endocrinology 145:2591–2593

Streicher R, Kotzka J, Muller-Wieland D, et al. (1996) SREBP-1 mediates activation of the low density lipoprotein receptor promoter by insulin and insulin-like growth factor-I. J Biol Chem 271:7128–7133

Suzuki R, Tobe K, Aoyama M, et al. (2004) Both insulin signaling defects in the liver and obesity contribute to insulin resistance and cause diabetes in Irs2(-/-) mice. J Biol Chem 279:25039–25049

Tamemoto H, Kadowaki T, Tobe K, et al. (1994) Insulin resistance and growth retardation in mice lacking insulin receptor substrate-1. Nature 372:182–186

Terauchi Y, Kadowaki T (2002) Insights into molecular pathogenesis of type 2 diabetes from knockout mouse models. Endocr J 49:247–263

Tontonoz P, Kim JB, Graves RA, Spiegelman BM (1993) ADD1: a novel helix-loop-helix transcription factor associated with adipocyte determination and differentiation. Mol Cell Biol 13:4753–4759

Ueki K, Kondo T, Kahn CR (2004) Suppressor of cytokine signalling 1 (SOCS-1) and SOCS-3 causes insulin resistance through inhibition of tyrosine phosphorylation of insulin receptor substrate proteins by discrete mechanisms. Mol Cell Biol 24:5434–5446

Ullrich A, Schlessinger J (1990) Signal transduction by receptors with tyrosine kinase activity. Cell 20:203–212

Unger RH (2002) Lipotoxic diseases. Ann Rev Med 53:319–336

Unger RH (2003) Minireview: weapons of lean body mass destruction: the role of ectopic lipids in the metabolic syndrome. Endocrinology 144:5159–5165

Vergès B (2004) Clinical interest of PPARs ligands. Particular benefit in type 2 diabetes and metabolic syndrome. Diabetes Metab 30:7–12

Walker BR, Seckl RJ (2003) 11beta-hydroxysteroid dehydrogenase type 1 as a novel therapeutic target in metabolic and neurodegenerative diseases. Expert Opin Ther Targets 7:771–783

Wang X, Briggs MR, Hua X, Yokoyama C, Goldstein JL, Brown MS (1993) Nuclear protein that binds sterol regulatory element of low density lipoprotein receptor promoter. II. Purification and characterization. J Biol Chem 268:14497–14504

Weiss R, Dufour S, Taksali SE, et al. (2003) Prediabetes in obese youth: a syndrome of impaired glucose tolerance, severe insulin resistance, and altered myocellular and abdominal fat partitioning. Lancet 362:1857–1858

Werner ED, Lee J, Hansen L, et al. (2004) Insulin resistance due to phosphorylation of insulin receptor substrate-1 at serine 302. J Biol Chem 279:35298–35305

Williams K, Rao YP, Natarajan R, et al. (2004) Indinavir alters sterol and fatty acid homeostatic mechanisms in primary rat hepatocytes by increasing levels of activated sterol regulatory element-binding proteins and decreasing cholesterol 7alpha-hydroxylase mRNA levels. Biochem Pharmacol 67:255–267

Withers DJ, Gutierrez JS, Towery H, et al. (1998) Disruption of IRS-2 causes type 2 diabetes in mice. Nature 391:900–904

Wu X, Hoffstedt J, Deeb W, et al. (2001) Depot-specific variation in protein-tyrosine phosphatase activities in human omental and subcutaneous adipose tissue: a potential contribution to differential insulin sensitivity. J Clin Endocrinol Metab 86:5973–5980

Xiang AH, Peters RK, Kjos SL, et al. (2004) Pharmacological treatment of insulin resistance at two different stages in the evolution of type 2 diabetes: impact of glucose tolerance and beta-cell function. J Clin Endocrinol Metab 89:2846–2851

Yokoyama C, Wang X, Briggs MR, et al. (1993) SREBP-1, a basic-helix-loop-helix-leucine zipper protein that controls transcription of the low density lipoprotein receptor gene. Cell 75:187–197

Yoon JC, Puigserver P, Chen G, et al. (2001) Control of hepatic gluconeogenesis through the transcriptional coactivator PGC-1. Nature 413:131–138

Yuan M, Konstantopoulos N, Lee J, Hansen L, Li ZW, Karin M, Shoelson SE (2001) Reversal of obesity- and diet-induced insulin resistance with salicylates or targeted disruption of Ikkbeta. Science 293:1673–1677

Zabolotny JM, Haj FG, Kim YB, et al. (2004) Transgenic overexpression of protein-tyrosine phosphatase 1B in muscle causes insulin resistance, but overexpression with leukocyte antigen-related phosphatase does not additively impair insulin action. J Biol Chem 279:24844–24851

Zhang B, Salituro G, Szalkowski D (1999) Discovery of a small molecule insulin mimetic with antidiabetic activity in mice. Science 284:974–977

Ziouzenkova O, Perrey S, Marx N, et al. (2002) Peroxisome Proliferator-activated Receptors. Curr Atheroscler Rep 4:59–64

HEP (2005) 170:619–644

Protection of Endothelial Function

L.E. Spieker · T.F. Lüscher (✉)

Cardiology, University Hospital, 8091 Zürich, Switzerland
cardiotfl@gmx.ch

Abstract The vascular endothelium synthesizes and releases a spectrum of vasoactive substances and therefore plays a fundamental role in the basal and dynamic regulation of the circulation. Nitric oxide (NO)—originally described as endothelium-derived relaxing factor—is released from endothelial cells in response to shear stress produced by blood flow, and in response to activation of a variety of receptors. After diffusion from endothelial to vascular smooth muscle cells, NO increases intracellular cyclic guanosine-monophosphat concentrations by activation of the enzyme guanylate cyclase leading to relaxation of the smooth muscle cells. NO has also antithrombogenic, antiproliferative, leukocyte-adhesion inhibiting effects, and influences myocardial contractility. Endothelium-derived NO-mediated vascular relaxation is impaired in spontaneously hypertensive animals. NO decomposition by free oxygen radicals is a major mechanism of impaired NO bioavailability. The resulting imbalance of endothelium-derived relaxing and contracting substances disturbs the normal function of the vascular endothelium. Endothelin acts as the natural counterpart to endothelium-derived NO. In man, besides its effect of increasing arterial blood pressure , ET-1 induces vascular and myocardial hypertrophy, which are independent risk factors for cardiovascular morbidity and mortality. Current therapeutic strategies concentrate mainly on lowering of low-density lipoprotein cholesterol and an impressive reduction in the risk for cardiovascular morbidity and mortality has been achieved. Inflammatory mechanisms play an important role in vascular disease and inflammatory plasma markers correlate with prognosis. Novel therapeutic strategies specifically targeting inflammation thus bear great potential for the prevention and treatment of atherosclerotic vascular disease.

Keywords Nitric oxide · Endothelin · Atherosclerosis · Free radicals · Inflammation · Cholesterol

1
Introduction

Atherosclerotic vascular disease is among the most frequent causes of death worldwide (Murray and Lopez 1997). Elevated cholesterol levels constitute a major risk factor for the development of atherosclerotic vascular disease. Focusing on lowering of low-density lipoprotein (LDL) cholesterol, an impressive reduction in cardiovascular morbidity and mortality has been achieved even in patients with normal cholesterol levels.

In contrast, high-density lipoprotein (HDL) exerts protective effects. The underlying mechanisms are pleiotropic as HDL mediates reverse cholesterol transport and has additional anti-inflammatory, pro-fibrinolytic, and anti-oxidative properties (Nofer et al. 2002). This review will focus on the role of HDL as a novel pharmacological target for the prevention of atherosclerotic vascular disease.

2
Endothelial Dysfunction

The endothelium—probably the largest and most extensive tissue in the body—forms a highly selective permeability barrier and is a continuous, uninterrupted, smooth, and nonthrombogenic surface. The endothelium synthesizes and releases a broad spectrum of vasoactive substances (Fig. 1). Functional impairment of the vascular endothelium in response to injury occurs long before the development of visible atherosclerotic changes of the artery (Fig. 2).

Nitric oxide (NO) prevents leukocyte adhesion and migration into the arterial wall, smooth muscle cell proliferation, and platelet adhesion and aggregation, i.e., key events in the development of atherosclerosis (Boulanger

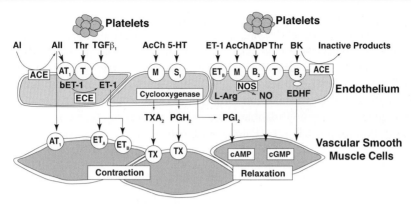

Fig. 1 Endothelium-derived vasoactive substances. Nitric oxide (*NO*) is released from endothelial cells in response to shear-stress and to activation of a variety of receptors. NO exerts vasodilating and antiproliferative effects on smooth muscle cells and inhibits thrombocyte-aggregation and leukocyte-adhesion. Endothelin-1 (*ET-1*) exerts its major vascular effects—vasoconstriction and cell proliferation—through activation of specific ETA receptors on vascular smooth muscle cells. In contrast, endothelial ETB receptors mediate vasodilation via release of NO and prostacyclin. Additionally, ETB receptors in the lung were shown to be a major pathway for the clearance of ET-1 from plasma. *ACE*, Angiotensin-converting enzyme; *ACh*, acetylcholine; *AII*, angiotensin II; *AT1*, angiotensin 1 recetor; *BK*, bradykinine; *COX*, cyclooxygenase; *ECE*, endothelin-converting enzyme; *EDHF*, endothelium-derived hyperpolarizing factor; *ETA* and *ETB*, endothelin A and B receptor; *ET-1*, endothelin-1; *L-Arg*, L-arginine; *PGH2*, prostaglandin H2; *PGI2*, prostacyclin; *S*, serotoninergic receptor; *Thr*, thrombine; *T*, thromboxane receptor; *TXA2*, thromboxane; *5-HT*, 5-hydroxytryptamine (serotonine). (Modified from Lüscher and Noll 1998)

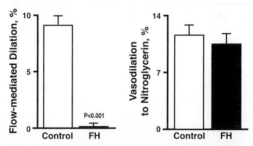

Fig. 2 Flow-mediated dilation of the brachial artery in children with familial hypercholesterolemia (*FH*). Flow-mediated dilatation is much reduced in comparison with the normocholesterolemic control group, whereas dilation in response to nitroglycerin, an endothelium-independent vasodilator, was equal in both groups. (Modified from Celermajer et al. 1992)

and Lüscher 1990; Bhagat et al. 1996; Bhagat and Vallance 1997; Ross 1999; Fichtlscherer et al. 2000; Hingorani et al. 2000). NO—synthesized by NO synthase (NOS) from L-arginine in presence of the cofactor tetrahydrobiopterin (BH_4)—is released from endothelial cells mainly in response to shear stress produced by blood flow or pharmacological stimulants such as acetylcholine

(Fig. 3) (Furchgott and Zawadzki 1980; Rubanyi et al. 1986; Palmer et al. 1988a, 1988b; Anderson and Mark 1989; Vallance et al. 1989; Stamler et al. 1994; Joannides et al. 1995a, 1995b). NO is a free radical gas with an in vivo half-life of a few seconds, and is able to cross biological membranes readily (Furchgott and Zawadzki 1980; Palmer et al. 1987; Stamler et al. 1992). After diffusion from endothelial to vascular smooth muscle cells, NO increases intracellular cyclic guanosine-monophosphate concentrations leading to relaxation of the smooth muscle cells (Fig. 1) (Palmer et al. 1988).

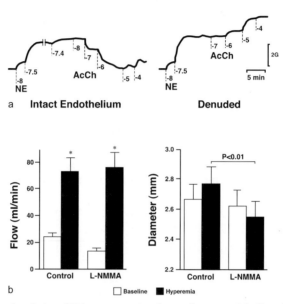

Fig. 3A In norepinephrine (*NE*)-preconstricted arteries, acetylcholine (*AcCh*) induces concentration-dependent relaxation in the presence of an intact endothelium. In endothelium-denuded arteries however, relaxation is abolished and converted to vasoconstriction. (Modified from Furchgott 1983). **B** Nitric oxide (*NO*) is essential for flow-mediated dilatation of large human arteries. Under control conditions, release of the occlusion induced a marked increase in radial blood flow followed by a delayed increase in radial diameter. L-NMMA, an inhibitor of NO synthesis, decreased basal forearm blood flow without affecting basal radial artery diameter. In the presence of L-NMMA, the flow-mediated dilatation of the radial artery was abolished and converted to vasoconstriction. (Modified from Joannides et al. 1995)

Oxidatively modified LDL (oxLDL) decreases the bioavailability of endothelium-derived NO. In patients with atherosclerotic vascular disease, endothelial NOS (eNOS) protein expression and NO release are markedly reduced (Oemar et al. 1998). Indeed, carotid wall thickening correlates with reduced NO-mediated vasodilation (Ghiadoni et al. 1998; Perticone et al. 1999). Impaired endothelium-dependent vasodilation is an adverse prognostic parameter in patients with atherosclerotic vascular disease.

In contrast to NO, circulating endothelin (ET)-1 levels are increased in patients with atherosclerotic vascular lesions and correlate with the severity of the disease (Lerman et al. 1991). The amount of ET-1 in the vascular wall corresponds to blood pressure, total serum cholesterol, and number of atherosclerotic sites (Rossi et al. 1999). ET-1 acts as the natural counterpart to endothelium-derived NO (Fig. 1) (Lüscher et al. 1990). Besides of its arterial blood pressure rising effect in man (Vierhapper et al. 1990; Kiely et al. 1997), ET-1 induces vascular and myocardial hypertrophy (Ito et al. 1991; Barton et al. 1998; Yang et al. 1999), which are independent risk factors for cardiovascular morbidity and mortality (Kannel et al. 1969; Bots et al. 1997; O'Leary et al. 1999).

ET-1 stimulates the release of inflammatory mediators such as interleukin (IL)-1, IL-6, and IL-8 (Fig. 1). Thereby, the anti-inflammatory effects of NO are antagonized. NO itself plays an important role in clinical systemic inflammatory syndromes when the inducible isoform of the NO generating enzyme, iNOS, is activated in sepsis.

3
Dyslipidemia and the Development of Atherosclerotic Plaques

Elevated LDL cholesterol is a risk factor for the development of atherosclerotic vascular disease and causes endothelial dysfunction (Fig. 2) (Anonymous 1982; Cohen et al. 1988) LDL gets trapped in the vascular wall and undergoes oxidative modification. Monocytes attach to the endothelial surface and migrate subendothelially where they accumulate LDL and take the appearance of foam cells (Fig. 4). The accumulation of these subendothelial macrophages, which have receptors for native and oxLDL, get visible as fatty streaks—the earliest manifestation of atherosclerosis—and later become fibrofatty lesions and fibrous plaques (Fig. 5).

3.1
HDL and Endothelial Function

In patients with endothelial dysfunction due to hypercholesterolemia (Fig. 2), intravenous infusion of HDL rapidly restores impaired endothelium-dependent vasodilation (Fig. 6). The underlying mechanism is an improvement in NO bioavailability (Zeiher et al. 1994; Spieker et al. 2002), which is of major importance for the prevention of thrombosis as the endothelium continuously releases NO, an inhibitor of platelet aggregation (Fig. 7). Indeed, HDL levels determine thrombus formation (Li et al. 1999; Naqvi et al. 1999). The anticoagulant activities of protein S and activated protein C are enhanced (Griffin et al. 1999). Furthermore, HDL has pro-fibrinolytic properties (Saku et al. 1985).

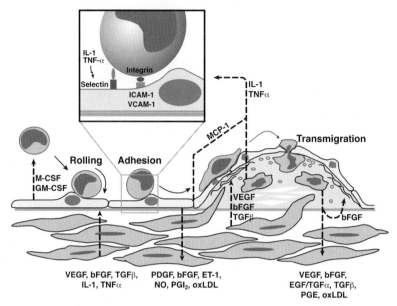

Fig. 4 Leukocyte adhesion and migration in atherosclerosis. Leukocytes adhering to the vascular endothelium migrate through the vascular wall to the subendothelium and secrete vasoactive and inflammatory substances. *bFGF*, Basic fibroblast growth factor; *EGF*, epidermal growth factor; *ET-1*, endothelin-1; *GM-CSF*, granulocyte-macrophage colony stimulating factor; *ICAM-1*, intercellular adhesion molecule; *IL-1*, interleukin-1; *MCP-1*, monocyte chemotactic protein; *M-CSF*, macrophage colony stimulating factor; *NO*, nitric oxide; *oxLDL*, oxidatively modified LDL; *PGE*, prostaglandin E; *PDGF*, platelet-derived growth factor; *PGI*$_2$, prostacyclin; *TNFα*, tumor necrosis factor alpha; *TGFβ*, transforming growth factor beta; *VCAM-1*, vascular cell adhesion molecule; *VEGF*, vascular endothelial growth factor

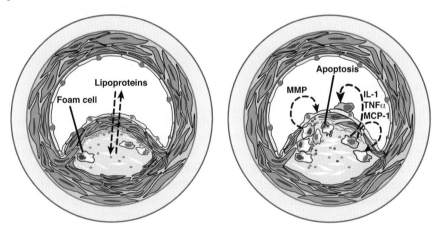

Fig. 5 Plaque rupture in unstable angina. Macrophage-rich areas of the plaque with only a thin fibrous cap are prone to rupture, whereas plaques with a thick fibrous cap remain clinically stable

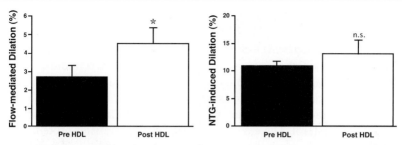

Fig. 6 Intravenous infusion of reconstituted high-density lipoprotein (rDHL, 80 mg/kg over 4 h) leads to improved flow-mediated dilation of the brachial artery in hypercholesterolemic patients. (Modified from Spieker et al. 2002)

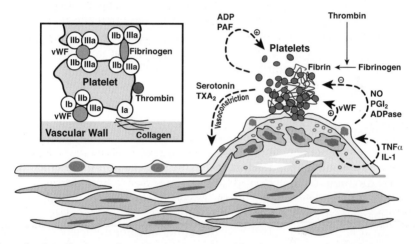

Fig. 7 Platelet adhesion and aggregation is mediated by glycoproteins Ib, IIb, and IIIa. *ADP*, adenosine diphosphate; *ADPase*, adenosine diphosphatase; *Ia*, *Ib*, *IIb*, and *IIIa*, glycoproteins; *IL-1*, interleukin-1; *NO*, nitric oxide; *PAF*, platelet aggregating factor; *PGI$_2$*, prostacyclin; *TNFα*, tumor necrosis factor alpha; *TXA$_2$*, thromboxane; *vWF*, von Willebrand factor

3.2
Reverse Cholesterol Transport

Reverse cholesterol transport is a pathway transporting cholesterol from peripheral cells and tissues to the liver for biliary excretion into the intestine. The process is mediated by HDL and its major carrier protein apolipoprotein (apo) A-I. Infusion of apoA-I in volunteers intensifies reverse cholesterol transport with subsequent fecal cholesterol excretion (Eriksson et al. 1999). Experimentally, elevating HDL or its main carrier protein, apoA-I even reduces atherosclerotic lesions (Badimon et al. 1990; Mach et al. 1998; Schieffer et al. 2000; Ridker et al. 2001).

Cholesterol is taken up by nascent HDL particles (preβ_1-HDL) produced by hepatocytes and in the intestine. Alternatively, these small discoid lipid-poor particles dissociate from chylomicrons and very-low-density lipoprotein during lipoprotein lipase-mediated hydrolysis of triglycerides. Cellular cholesterol efflux is mediated by ATP-binding cassette transporter protein 1 (ABCA1), the expression of which is regulated by sterol and liver-X/retinoid-X receptor (LXR/RXR). The accumulation of cholesterol transforms $pre\beta_1$-HDL particles into bigger particles, HDL_2. Cholesterol esterification by lecithin:cholesterol acyltransferase leads to the formation of spherical β_3-HDL particles which acquire more cholesterol. The enzyme cholesteryl ester transfer protein (CETP) exchanges accumulated cholesteryl esters for triglycerides and particles are remodeled into smaller HDL_3 particles and lipid-free apoA-I. The latter are re-lipidated by cellular phospholipid and cholesterol to form $pre\beta_1$-HDL particles. HDL-derived cholesteryl esters are removed from the circulation via the LDL receptor pathway. The uptake of HDL cholesterol to the liver is mediated by scavenger receptor (SR)-BI (respectively its human homologue, CLA-1).

The expression of the SR-BI, ABCA1, and CETP, but not apoA-I, genes is regulated by sterols. In addition, SR-BI is regulated by peroxisome-proliferator activated receptor-α, as is apoA-I and apoA-II expression.

3.3
HDL as an Antioxidant

Oxidative stress plays an important role in the pathogenesis of Atherosclerosis. Superoxide anion (O_2^-), an oxygen radical, can scavenge NO to form peroxynitrite ($ONOO^-$) effectively reducing the bioavailability of endothelium-derived NO (Rubanyi and Vanhoutte 1986). In addition, O_2^- can act as a vasoconstrictor (Katusic and Vanhoutte 1989). Nicotinamide adenine dinucleotide (NADH) dehydrogenase, a mitochondrial enzyme of the respiratory chain, seems to be a major source of O_2^-. Expression of NAD(P)H oxidase in human coronary artery smooth muscle cells is upregulated by pulsatile stretch, generating increased oxidative stress. Other sources of O_2^- are cyclooxygenase (COX), and xanthine oxidase.

HDL, due to its paraoxonase content is an important antioxidant. Several polymorphisms of the paraoxonase enzyme have been described. Indeed, paraoxonase enzymatic polymorphisms with different antioxidant capacity may influence the susceptibility to oxidative stress and thus the pathogenesis of atherosclerosis.

4
Endothelins

Over a decade ago, a novel vasoconstrictor peptide synthesized by vascular endothelial cells was identified (Hickey et al. 1985; Yanagisawa et al. 1988). The family of endothelins (ET) consists of three closely related peptides–ET-

1, ET-2, and ET-3–which are converted by endothelin-converting enzymes (ECE) from 'big endothelins' originating from large preproendothelin peptides cleaved by endopeptidases. The ET peptides are not only synthesized in vascular endothelial and smooth muscle cells (Fig. 1), but also in neural, renal, pulmonal, and some circulatory cells holding the genes for endothelins. The chemical structure of the endothelins is closely related to neurotoxins (sarafotoxins) produced by scorpions and snakes. Factors modulating the expression of ET-1 are shear-stress, epinephrine, angiotensin II, thrombin, inflammatory cytokines [tumor necrosis factor (TNF) α, IL-1 and -2], transforming growth factor β and hypoxia. ET-1 is metabolized by a neutral endopeptidase, which also cleaves natriuretic peptides.

Imbalance of endothelium-derived relaxing and contracting substances disturbs the normal function of the vascular endothelium. ET acts as the natural counterpart to endothelium-derived NO (Fig. 1), which exerts vasodilating, antithrombotic, and antiproliferative effects, and inhibits leukocyte adhesion to the vascular wall. Besides its effect of increasing arterial blood pressure in man (Vierhapper et al. 1990), ET-1 induces vascular and myocardial hypertrophy (Ito et al. 1991), which are independent risk factors for cardiovascular morbidity and mortality. Indeed, in patients with essential hypertension, carotid wall thickening and left ventricular mass correlate with reduced endothelium-dependent vasodilation.

ET-1 rather acts in a paracrine than an endocrine mode of action, which is reflected by plasma levels of ET-1 in the picomolar range. Infusion of an ET receptor antagonist into the brachial artery or systemically in healthy humans leads to vasodilation indicating a role of ET-1 in the maintenance of basal vascular tone. When ET-1 itself is infused, vasoconstriction follows a brief phase of vasodilation, which may be explained by relaxation of smooth muscle cells caused by ET_B receptor-mediated release of the vasodilators nitric oxide and prostacyclin (Fig. 1). Additionally, ET-1 may also exert effects on the central and autonomic nervous system and alter baroreflex function. In the kidney, sodium reabsorption is modulated.

Significant correlations between the amount of immunoreactive ET-1 in the tunica media and blood pressure, total serum cholesterol, and number of atherosclerotic sites were found (Rossi et al. 1999). However, because most ET-1 synthesized in endothelial cells is secreted abluminally, it might attain a higher concentration in the vessel wall than in plasma. In blood vessels of healthy controls, ET-1 was detectable almost exclusively in endothelial cells, whereas in patients with coronary artery disease and/or arterial hypertension, sizable amounts of ET-1 were detectable in the tunica media of different types of arteries (Rossi et al. 1999).

The ET system is activated in several but not all animal models of arterial hypertension. Correspondingly, ET plasma levels have been reported to be elevated in certain patients with essential hypertension (Saito et al. 1990), but this is a subject to controversy. Furthermore, there is evidence that certain gene polymorphisms of ET-1 and ET receptors could be associated with blood pressure levels. Moreover, in hypertensive patients, infusion of an $ET_{A/B}$ receptor antagonist causes significantly greater vasodilation than in normotensive subjects. Since in this study plasma levels of ET-1 were similar in normo- and hypertensive patients, increased sensitivity to endogenous ET-1 has to be postulated. As in certain patients with arterial hypertension, endogenous catecholamine production is increased, and catecholamines potentiate ET-1 induced vasoconstriction, these interactions with the ET-1 pathway is likely to be involved in the pathogenesis of hypertension. Decreased bioavailability of NO is also involved in this phenomenon, since NO antagonizes some of the effects of ET-1.

5
Inflammatory Pathways in Atherosclerosis

Circulating levels of apparently normal-range C-reactive protein (CRP)—an acute phase protein measurable by a high-sensitivity assay—correlates with prognosis of patients with an acute coronary syndrome (Liuzzo et al. 1994; Ridker et al. 1998). Moreover, CRP is a prognostic marker in stable coronary artery disease, and more surprising, even in apparently healthy subjects (Ridker et al. 1998a, 1998b). Inflammatory cytokines such as IL-6 and IL-18, and serum amyloid A are further prognostic markers in patients with coronary artery disease.

Indeed, the inflammatory activity of an atherosclerotic plaque determines the risk for rupture with following coronary thrombosis and vessel occlusion (Fuster et al. 1999; Libby 2001). A thin cap—due to high inflammatory activity of metalloproteinases—is prone to rupture, which may trigger platelet aggregation and thrombosis leading to the clinical spectrum of the acute coronary syndrome (Fig. 5). In contrast, a thick fibrous cap—formed by smooth muscle cells and connective-tissue matrix—covering these plaques with few inflammatory cells stabilizes the lipid core against exposition to the blood (Fig. 5).

Cholesterol triggers the release of inflammatory mediators such as CRP. Together with other inflammatory mediators such IL-1, IL-6, IL-8, and TNF-α, CRP activates the expression of adhesion molecules such as intercellular adhesion molecule (ICAM)-1 and E-selectin on endothelial cells and decreases NO bioavailabilty (Fig. 4). Adhesion molecules are essential for the transmigration of monocytes through the vascular wall into the intima where they take up oxidized cholesterol and accumulate as foam cells (Fig. 4). As CRP increases the expression of tissue factor in monocytes and thus activates the clotting system, it is not surprising that elevated CRP levels are associated with adverse outcome in patients with acute or chronic coronary artery disease (Liuzzo et al. 1994; Ridker et al. 1998).

Another important pathway is CD40L, a member of the TNF family and ligand for CD40, a receptor widely expressed in vascular cells. CD40L is released by $CD4^+$ T lymphocytes and activated platelets. The CD40L pathway increases endothelial adhesiveness for monocytes by stimulation of adhesion molecule and IL-6 and IL-8 expression (Henn et al. 1998). Furthermore, it induces monocyte chemoattractant protein-1 expression, which is a key mediator in chemotaxis of further monocytes to migrate into the subendothelial space (Fig. 4). Accumulation of macrophages with subsequent apoptosis and further stimulation of inflammation leads to plaque formation. In addition, a prothrombotic state arises, as CD40L induces tissue factor expression by monocytes and promotes platelet aggregation (Fig. 7) (Lindmark et al. 2000; Andre et al. 2002). In turn, CD40L is upregulated upon GpIIb/IIIa engagement (May et al. 2002). Patients with hypercholesterolemia show elevated soluble CD40L levels (Garlichs et al. 2001; Cipollone et al. 2002), as do patients with acute coronary syndrome (Aukrust et al. 1999). Blocking the CD40 pathway experimentally halts the progression of atherosclerosis (Mach et al. 1998).

HDL levels are inversely correlated with coronary endothelium-dependent vasodilation mediated by NO (Zeiher et al. 1994). Patients with elevated inflammatory markers unopposed by high HDL levels show much more pronounced endothelial dysfunction of the coronary arteries and higher levels of adhesion molecules. Circulating levels of adhesion molecules correlate with cardiovascular mortality in patients with coronary artery disease (Ridker et al. 1998; Blankenberg et al. 2001). The prevention of cytokine and adhesion molecule expression–in part mediated by NO–is an important anti-atherosclerotic feature of HDL (De Caterina et al. 1995; Ridker et al. 1998; Blankenberg et al. 2001; Cockerill et al. 2001).

Interestingly, inflammation in turn induces endothelial dysfunction with decreased NO bioavailability (Fichtlscherer et al. 2000; Hingorani et al. 2000). Acute-phase HDL is relatively poor in apoA-I and paraoxonase and becomes pro-inflammatory and pro-oxidant (Van Lenten et al. 2001). HDL may thus loose part of its beneficial effects under inflammatory conditions.

6
Impact of Drug Therapy on Vascular Function

6.1
Statins

Statins play an important part in the secondary prevention of cardiovascular disease in patients at risk from atherosclerosis. Statin therapy improves the prognosis of patients at risk from atherosclerotic vascular disease even in presence of normal cholesterol plasma levels (Anonymous 1994, 1995, 1998).

Moreover, it reduces transient myocardial ischemia and improves endothelial function by upregulation of eNOS expression leading to improved NO bioavailability (Leung et al. 1993; Egashira et al. 1994; Stroes et al. 1995; Treasure et al. 1995; van Boven et al. 1996; O'Driscoll et al. 1997; John et al. 1998; Laufs et al. 1998; Dupuis et al. 1999).

Influence of statin therapy on HDL cholesterol levels is modest (Table 1). As low HDL is a principal risk factor for the development of premature coronary artery disease (Genest et al. 1992), it will become a major target for the prevention of vascular disease.

Table 1 Large clinical trials with lipid-lowering drugs for cardiovascular prevention

Drug	Increase in HDL	Clinical endpoint trial
I° Prevention		
Gemfibrozil	11%	Helsinki Heart Study (Frick et al. 1987)
Lovastatin	6%	AFCAPS/TexCAPS (Downs et al. 1998)
Pravastatin	5%	WOSCOP (1995)
II° Prevention		
Gemfibrozil	6%	VA-HIT (Rubins et al. 1999)
Bezafibrate	18%	Bezafibrate Infarction Prevention Study (2000)
Nicotinic acid+simvastatin	26%	HATS (Brown et al. 2001)
Simvastatin	8%	4S (1994)
Simvastatin	n.a.	HPS (2002)
Pravastatin	5%	CARE (Sacks et al. 1996)
Pravastatin	5%	LIPID (1998)
Fluvastatin	22%	LIPS (Serruys et al. 2002)
Atorvastatin	1.6%	MIRACL (Schwartz et al. 2001)
Atorvastatin	8%	AVERT (Pitt et al. 1999)

4S denotes Scandinavian Simvastatin Survival Study; AFCAPS/TexCAPS, Air Force Texas Coronary Atherosclerosis Prevention Study; CARE, Cholesterol and Recurrent Events; HATS, HDL-Atherosclerosis Treatment Study; HPS, Heart Protection Study; LIPID, Long-term Intervention with Pravastatin in Ischemic Disease; LIPS, Lescol Intervention Prevention Study; MIRACL, Myocardial Ischemia Reduction with Aggressive Cholesterol Lowering; n.a., not available; VA-HIT, Veterans Affairs High-density Lipoprotein Cholesterol Intervention Trial; and WOSCOP, West of Scotland Coronary Prevention Study.

6.2
ACE Inhibitors

In the TREND study, ACE inhibition with quinapril improved endothelial dysfunction in patients with coronary artery disease who were normotensive and who did not have severe hyperlipidemia or evidence of heart failure

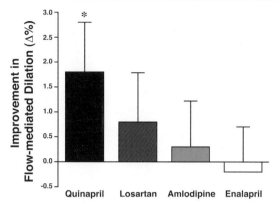

Fig. 8 Effects of quinapril, losartan, amlodipine, and enalapril on endothelial function in patients with coronary artery disease. Only quinapril was associated with a significant improvement in flow-mediated dilation of the brachial artery. (Modified from Anderson et al. 2000) (BANFF study)

(Mancini et al. 1996). However, the specific pharmacological features of an ACE inhibitor may be important for its effects on endothelial function, e.g., high tissue permeability. ACE inhibitors inhibit the breakdown of bradykinin, a stimulator of NO release, and antioxidant properties further improve NO bioavailability. They inhibit the endothelial production of angiotensin II and ET-1. Indeed, in a comparative study in patients with coronary artery disease, only quinapril but not enalapril was associated with a significant improvement in flow-mediated dilation of the brachial artery (Fig. 8) (Anderson et al. 2000). Improved NO bioavailability also affects platelet function. Indeed, inhibitors of the renin–angiotensin–aldosterone system inhibit platelet aggregation in vitro. The favorable effects of ACE inhibitors on endothelial function with antithrombotic, antiproliferative, and antimigratory actions may explain how they can prevent cardiovascular events in patients with atherosclerosis even in the absence of hypertension.

6.3
Angiotensin II Receptor Antagonists

Treatment with candesartan, an AT_1 receptor antagonist, reduced the vasodilator response to the mixed $ET_{A/B}$ receptor antagonist TAK-044 that was initially more pronounced in hypertensive patients than in normotensive controls (Ghiadoni et al. 2000). This was paralleled by a reduction in circulating plasma ET-1 levels. Furthermore, the impaired vasoconstrictor response to L-NMMA, an inhibitor of NO synthesis, was augmented by antihypertensive treatment in hypertensives. Thus, the angiotensin II receptor blocker candesartan improves tonic NO release and reduces vasoconstriction to endogenous ET-1 in the forearm of hypertensive patients. The reduction of oxidative stress by blockade

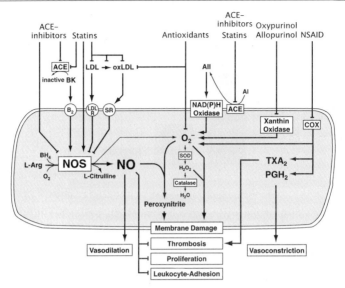

Fig. 9 Mechanisms of action of cardiovascular drugs on the endothelial L-arginine/nitric oxide pathway. Statins as well as ACE inhibitors increase endothelial nitric oxide synthase (*eNOS*) expression. In addition, ACE inhibitors inhibit the breakdown of bradykinin (*BK*), which in turn increases the release of nitric oxide (*NO*) via B$_2$-bradykinergic receptors. Furthermore, they inhibit the formation of angiotensin II (*AII*), which activates NAD(P)H oxidase to synthesize superoxide anions (*O$_2^-$*). Antioxidants prevent scavenging of NO by superoxide anions. Exogenous supply of L-arginine (*L-Arg*) and tetrahydrobiopterin (*BH$_4$*) increases their bioavailability in endothelial cells, which may be diminished in certain disease states. *ACE*, angiotensin-converting enzyme; *B$_2$*, bradykinin receptor; *BK*, bradykinin; *COX*, cyclooxygenase; *LDL-R*, low-density lipoprotein receptor; *oxLDL*, oxidatively modified LDL; *PGH$_2$*, prostaglandin H$_2$; *PGI$_2$*, prostacyclin; *SR*, scavenger receptor

of the angiotensin II-pathway is an important feature of this class of drugs (Fig. 9). Irbesartan, another AT$_1$ receptor antagonist, has also been investigated in hypertensive patients. Long-term irbesartan treatment enhanced both endothelium-dependent and -independent vascular vasodilation responses. In addition, irbesartan restored the vasoconstrictor capacity of the NO synthase inhibitor L-NMMA, suggesting a direct effect on tonic NO release, and decreased ET-1 production. Other AT$_1$ receptor antagonists such as telmisartan and losartan did not improve endothelium-dependent vasodilation in hypertensive patients. The potency of angiotensin II receptor blockers to increase NO bioavailability may be even greater in platelets than in endothelial cells. Indeed, angiotensin II receptor antagonists show antiaggregatory effects on platelets.

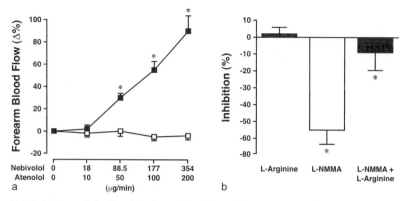

Fig. 10A, B Effects of the betablocker nebivolol on forearm blood flow in healthy human subjects. A Nebivolol, but not the betablocker atenolol, increases forearm blood flow. B This effect is prevented by co-infusion of the inhibitor of nitric oxide L-NMMA. (Modified from Cockcroft et al. 1995)

6.4
Betablockers

Interestingly, infusion of nebivolol, but not other betablockers, intra-arterially in the forearm of healthy subjects is associated with an increase in forearm blood flow (Fig. 10). The increase in forearm blood flow achieved by nebivolol can be prevented by co-infusion of the NO synthesis inhibitor L-NMMA. Similar results have been obtained in the human venous circulation. This strongly suggests that nebivolol stimulates the formation of NO in the vasculature and may therefore have an interesting hemodynamic profile which leads—unlike other betablockers—to peripheral vasodilation in addition to the classical betablocking effects on the sympathetic nervous system, heart rate and cardiac contractility. Indeed, nebivolol also causes NO-dependent vasodilation in hypertensive patients. However, this favorable effect did not last during chronic treatment (6 months) with this new type of β_1-blocker. Nebivolol also inhibits platelet aggregation by its NO-dependent mechanism. Traditional betablockers have little effect on platelet aggregation.

6.5
Calcium Channel Blockers

Besides certain ACE inhibitors, several calcium channel blocking agents were successful in improving endothelial function in human hypertension (Fig. 11). Antioxidative properties of an antihypertensive drug are important, since oxidative stress plays a central role in the pathophysiology of human hypertension. Endothelial function of patients with hypertension is improved by ascorbic acid, an antioxidant vitamin, which restores the imbalance of

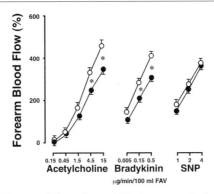

Fig. 11 Effects of lacidipine, a calcium channel blocker, on endothelial function in hypertensive patients. After chronic treatment with lacidipine, the vasodilation in response to the endothelium-dependent vasodilators acetylcholine and bradykinin, but not to sodium nitroprusside (*SNP*), an endothelium-independent vasodilator, was significantly increased. *FAV* denotes forearm volume. (Modified from Taddei et al. 1997)

increased NO decomposition by superoxide. Scavenging of reactive oxygen species by antioxidants may become an important therapeutic strategy (Fig. 9), since chronic treatment with vitamin C is in fact able to lower blood pressure in patients with hypertension (Duffy et al. 1999). The beneficial effects of calcium antagonists on endothelial function may not be confined to hypertension. Nifedipine, a dihydropyridine calcium channel blocker, also improves endothelium-dependent vasodilation to acetylcholine in hypercholesterolemics (Verhaar et al. 1999). Also in the coronary circulation, calcium antagonists reverse abnormal vasomotion in hypercholesterolemia. Indeed, in the INTACT study, angiographic progression of coronary artery disease was retarded by nifedipine (Lichtlen et al. 1990). However, in patients with coronary artery disease, the calcium antagonist amlodipine did not improve endothelial function.

An increase in intracellular platelet calcium concentration mediated by calcium channels is the main signal event in platelet activation. Unsurprisingly therefore, calcium channel blockers have been shown to inhibit platelet activation.

6.6
Endothelin Antagonists and Vasopeptidase Inhibitors

In rats with angiotensin II-induced and chronic NO-deficient hypertension, endothelial dysfunction is ameliorated by treatment with an ET receptor antagonist. Furthermore, ET receptor antagonism prevents vascular hypertrophy in a variety of other experimental models of hypertension. Similarly, treatment with a selective ET_A receptor antagonist attenuates the development of left ventricular hypertrophy in renovascular hypertensive rats. In hypertension and

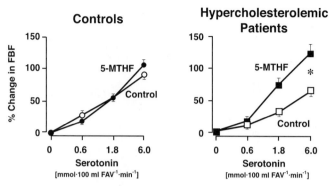

Fig. 12 Effects of 5-methyltetrahydrofolate (*5-MTHF*) on serotonin-induced endothelium-dependent vasodilation in the forearm circulation of patients with hypercholesterolemia and normocholesterolemic controls. These results show that the active form of folic acid restores endothelial function in hypercholesterolemia due to reduced catabolism of nitric oxide (*NO*). *FAV* denotes forearm volume. (Modified from Verhaar et al. 1998)

hypercholesterolemia, ET antagonism may be superior to ECE inhibition since vascular ECE activity is inversely correlated to serum LDL levels and blood pressure.

In hypertensive patients, bosentan, a mixed $ET_{A/B}$ receptor antagonist, effectively decreases arterial blood pressure in patients with essential hypertension. This effect is not accompanied by neurohormonal activation, as reflected by a lack of increase in heart rate, plasma catecholamines, plasma renin activity, and plasma angiotensin II levels. Further trials are needed to clarify if ET receptor antagonists offer additional benefits over conventional antihypertensive drugs.

6.7
COX Inhibitors

There are important interactions between NO and COX products. COX-dependent substances (e.g., thromboxane A_2 and prostaglandin H_2) impair NO bioavailability. Indeed, COX is a source of the NO-scavenger O_2^-. Aspirin improves the abnormal vasomotion in the forearm of hypertensive and hypercholesterolemic patients. Most likely, aspirin restores the altered balance between vasoconstrictor and dilator prostanoids, which favors vasoconstriction and thrombosis. These findings may partly explain the favorable effects of aspirin in patients with cardiovascular disease. A novel interesting concept in atherosclerosis is selective inhibition of COX-2, which lowers CRP levels and improves endothelial function (Fig. 12) (Chenevard et al. 2003). The improvement of endothelial function by selective COX-2 inhibition illustrates the potential of antiinflammatory drugs in atherosclerosis.

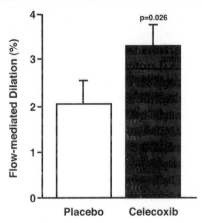

Fig. 13 Inhibition of the inducible isoform of cyclooxygenase (COX-2) leads to an improvement of endothelial function in patients with coronary artery disease. Flow-mediated dilation of the brachial artery was significantly improved after 2 weeks of therapy. C-reactive protein levels (CRP) decreased significantly. Endothelium-independent vasodilation to nitroglycerine was not affected, indicating a specific effect on the endothelium. (Modified from Chenevard et al. 2003)

6.8
Antioxidative Vitamins

Antioxidants scavenge reactive oxygen species and thereby reduce NO breakdown. In patients with familial hypercholesterolemia, 5-methyltetrahydrofolate, the active form of folic acid, improves endothelial function both when given acutely and chronically (Fig. 13). The effects of folic acid supplementation on morbidity and mortality in patients with coronary artery disease are currently tested in large clinical studies.

Vitamin C (ascorbic acid), an antioxidant vitamin, restores endothelial function in patients with hypercholesterolemia, diabetes mellitus, and patients who smoke. Also in patients with hypertension, endothelial dysfunction is improved by ascorbic acid, both in the coronary and the peripheral circulation. Scavenging of reactive oxygen species by antioxidants may become an interesting therapeutic strategy, since chronic treatment with vitamin C lowers blood pressure in patients with hypertension. In patients with coronary artery disease, long-term ascorbic acid supplementation also improves endothelial function.

The effects of vitamin E supplementation on endothelial function in patients at risk from or with established atherosclerotic vascular disease are less consistent. The beneficial effects of vitamin E may be confined to subjects with increased exposure to oxLDL, as is the case for hypercholesterolemics who smoke. Combined vitamin E and simvastatin therapy leads to an improvement in flow-mediated vasodilation of the brachial artery of hypercholesterolemic men, which is more pronounced than with lipid-lowering therapy alone. The results of clinical trials studying the clinical outcome of patients with coronary artery disease under vitamin E supplementation have been disappointing. Indeed, vitamin E supplementation had no effect on cardiovascular endpoints in the Heart Outcomes Prevention Evaluation Study (HOPE).

6.9
Tetrahydrobiopterin and L-Arginine

Tetrahydrobiopterin (BH_4), a cofactor for NO synthesis by eNOS, ameliorates endothelial dysfunction in hypercholesterolemic patients and smokers. In patients with coronary artery disease, BH_4 restores endothelium-dependent vasodilation to acetylcholine. Experimentally, BH_4 also improves endothelial function in arterial hypertension. In human studies, BH_4 improves endothelium-dependent vasodilation to acetylcholine in patients with arterial hypertension.

L-Arginine, the substrate for NO synthesis, improves endothelium-dependent vasodilation both in the coronary and peripheral circulation of patients with hypercholesterolemia. However, L-arginine does not improve endothelial function in diabetic subjects, indicating that the underlying pathophysiologies in subjects with different risk factors call for differential treatment strategies.

7
Conclusions

The vascular endothelium, synthesizing and releasing vasoactive substances, plays a crucial role in the pathogenesis of atherosclerosis. Due to its position between blood and vascular wall, the endothelium is thought to be both victim and offender in atherosclerosis. A clinically important consequence of endothelial dysfunction in patients with atherosclerosis is the generation of a prothrombotic situation. The delicate balance of endothelium-derived factors, which is disturbed in atherosclerosis, can be restored by specific treatment.

Elevated LDL cholesterol is the current therapeutic target in patients at risk from atherosclerosis. Inflammatory mechanisms play an important role in vascular disease and inflammatory plasma markers correlate with prognosis. Novel therapeutic strategies specifically targeting inflammation bear great potential for the prevention and treatment of atherosclerotic vascular disease.

Acknowledgements Original research of the authors reported in this article was supported by the Swiss National Research Foundation (Nos. 32–51069.97/1 and 32–52690.97), the Stanley Thomas Johnson Foundation, and the Swiss Heart Foundation.

References

Anderson EA, Mark AL (1989) Flow-mediated and reflex changes in large peripheral artery tone in humans. Circulation 79:93–100

Anderson TJ, Elstein E, Haber H, Charbonneau F (2000) Comparative study of ACE-inhibition, angiotensin II antagonism, and calcium channel blockade on flow-mediated vasodilation in patients with coronary disease (BANFF study). J Am Coll Cardiol 35:60–66

Andre P, Nannizzi-Alaimo L, Prasad SK, Phillips DR (2002) Platelet-derived CD40L: the switch-hitting player of cardiovascular disease. Circulation 106:896–899

Anonymous (1982) The MRFIT research group. Multiple Risk Factor Intervention Trial. Risk factor changes and mortality results. JAMA 248:1465–1477

Anonymous (1994) The Scandinavian Simvastatin Survival Study group. Randomised trial of cholesterol lowering in 4444 patients with coronary heart disease: the Scandinavian Simvastatin Survival Study (4S). Lancet 344:1383–1389

Anonymous (1995) The West of Scotland Coronary Prevention Study group. Prevention of coronary heart disease with pravastatin in men with hypercholesterolemia. N Engl J Med 333:1301–1307

Anonymous (1998) The Long-Term Intervention with Pravastatin in Ischaemic Disease (LIPID) Study Group. Prevention of cardiovascular events and death with pravastatin in patients with coronary heart disease and a broad range of initial cholesterol levels. N Engl J Med 339:1349–1355

Anonymous (2000) Secondary prevention by raising HDL cholesterol and reducing triglycerides in patients with coronary artery disease: the Bezafibrate Infarction Prevention (BIP) study. Circulation 102:21–27

Anonymous (2002) MRC/BHF Heart Protection Study of cholesterol lowering with simvastatin in 20,536 high-risk individuals: a randomised placebo-controlled trial. Lancet 360:7–22

Aukrust P, Muller F, Ueland T, Berget T, Aaser E, Brunsvig A, Solum NO, Forfang K, Froland SS, Gullestad L (1999) Enhanced levels of soluble and membrane-bound CD40 ligand in patients with unstable angina. Possible reflection of T lymphocyte and platelet involvement in the pathogenesis of acute coronary syndromes. Circulation 100:614–620

Badimon JJ, Badimon L, Fuster V (1990) Regression of atherosclerotic lesions by high density lipoprotein plasma fraction in the cholesterol-fed rabbit. J Clin Invest 85:1234–1241

Barton M, d'Uscio LV, Shaw S, Meyer P, Moreau P, Luscher TF (1998) ET(A) receptor blockade prevents increased tissue endothelin-1, vascular hypertrophy, and endothelial dysfunction in salt-sensitive hypertension. Hypertension 31:499–504

Bhagat K, Moss R, Collier J, Vallance P (1996) Endothelial 'stunning' following a brief exposure to endotoxin: a mechanism to link infection and infarction? Cardiovasc Res 32:822–829

Bhagat K, Vallance P (1997) Inflammatory cytokines impair endothelium-dependent dilatation in human veins in vivo. Circulation 96:3042–3047

Blankenberg S, Rupprecht HJ, Bickel C, Peetz D, Hafner G, Tiret L, Meyer J, et al. (2001) Circulating cell adhesion molecules and death in patients with coronary artery disease. Circulation 104:1336–1342

Bots ML, Hoes AW, Koudstaal PJ, Hofman A, Grobbee DE et al. (1997) Common carotid intima-media thickness and risk of stroke and myocardial infarction: the Rotterdam Study. Circulation 96:1432–1437

Boulanger C, Lüscher TF (1990) Release of endothelin from the porcine aorta. Inhibition of endothelium-derived nitric oxide. J Clin Invest 85:587–590

Brown BG, Zhao XQ, Chait A, Fisher LD, Cheung MC, Morse JS, Dowdy AA, Marino EK, Bolson EL, Alaupovic P, Frohlich J, Albers JJ (2001) Simvastatin and niacin, antioxidant vitamins, or the combination for the prevention of coronary disease. N Engl J Med 345:1583–1592

Celermajer DS, Sorensen KE, Gooch VM, Spiegelhalter DJ, Miller OI, Sullivan ID, Lloyd JK, Deanfield JE (1992) Non-invasive detection of endothelial dysfunction in children and adults at risk of atherosclerosis. Lancet 340:1111–1115

Chenevard R, Hurlimann D, Bechir M, Enseleit F, Spieker L, Hermann M, Riesen W, Gay S, Gay RE, Neidhart M, Michel B, Luscher TF, Noll G, Ruschitzka F (2003) Selective COX-2 inhibition improves endothelial function in coronary artery disease. Circulation 107:405–409

Cipollone F, Mezzetti A, Porreca E, Di Febbo C, Nutini M, Fazia M, Falco A, Cuccurullo F, Davi G (2002) Association between enhanced soluble CD40L and prothrombotic state in hypercholesterolemia: effects of statin therapy. Circulation 106:399–402

Cockcroft JR, Chowienczyk PJ, Brett SE, Chen CP, Dupont AG, Van Nueten L, Wooding SJ, Ritter JM (1995) Nebivolol vasodilates human forearm vasculature: evidence for an L-arginine/NO-dependent mechanism. J Pharmacol Exp Ther 274:1067–1071

Cockerill GW, Huehns TY, Weerasinghe A, Stocker C, Lerch PG, Miller NE, Haskard DO (2001) Elevation of plasma high-density lipoprotein concentration reduces interleukin-1-induced expression of E-selectin in an in vivo model of acute inflammation. Circulation 103:108–112

Cohen RA, Zitnay KM, Haudenschild CC, Cunningham LD (1988) Loss of selective endothelial cell vasoactive functions caused by hypercholesterolemia in pig coronary arteries. Circ Res 63:903–910

De Caterina R, Libby P, Peng HB, Thannickal VJ, Rajavashisth TB, Gimbrone Jr MA, Shin WS, Liao JK (1995) Nitric oxide decreases cytokine induced endothelial activation: nitric oxide selectively reduces endothelial expression of adhesion molecules and proinflammatory cytokines. J Clin Invest 96:60–68

Downs JR, Clearfield M, Weis S, Whitney E, Shapiro DR, Beere PA, Langendorfer A, Stein EA, Kruyer W, Gotto AM, Jr. (1998) Primary prevention of acute coronary events with lovastatin in men and women with average cholesterol levels: results of AFCAPS/TexCAPS. Air Force/Texas Coronary Atherosclerosis Prevention Study. JAMA 279:1615–1622

Duffy SJ, Gokce N, Holbrook M, Huang A, Frei B, Keaney JFJ, Vita JA (1999) Treatment of hypertension with ascorbic acid. Lancet 354

Dupuis J, Tardif JC, Cernacek P, Theroux P (1999) Cholesterol reduction rapidly improves endothelial function after acute coronary syndromes. The RECIFE (Reduction of cholesterol in ischemia and function of the endothelium) trial. Circulation 99:3227–3233

Egashira K, Hirooka Y, Kai H, Sugimachi M, Suzuki S, Inou T, Takeshita A (1994) Reduction in serum cholesterol with pravastatin improves endothelium-dependent coronary vasomotion in patients with hypercholesterolemia. Circulation 89:2519–2524

Eriksson M, Carlson LA, Miettinen TA, Angelin B (1999) Stimulation of fecal steroid excretion after infusion of recombinant proapolipoprotein A-I. Potential reverse cholesterol transport in humans. Circulation 100:594–598

Fichtlscherer S, Rosenberger G, Walter G, Breuer S, Dimmeler S, Zeiher AM (2000) Elevated C-reactive protein levels and impaired endothelial vasoreactivity in patients with coronary artery disease. Circulation 102:1000–1006

Frick MH, Elo O, Haapa K, Heinonen OP, Heinsalmi P, Helo P, Huttunen JK, Kaitaniemi P, Koskinen P, Manninen V, et al. (1987) Helsinki Heart Study: primary-prevention trial with gemfibrozil in middle-aged men with dyslipidemia. Safety of treatment, changes in risk factors, and incidence of coronary heart disease. N Engl J Med 317:1237–1245

Furchgott RF (1983) Role of endothelium in responses of vascular smooth muscle. Circ Res 53:557–573

Furchgott RF, Zawadzki JV (1980) The obligatory role of endothelial cells in the relaxation of arterial smooth muscle by acetylcholine. Nature 288:373–376

Fuster V, Fayad ZA, Badimon JJ (1999) Acute coronary syndromes: biology. Lancet 353 (suppl II):5–9

Garlichs CD, John S, Schmeisser A, Eskafi S, Stumpf C, Karl M, Goppelt-Struebe M, Schmieder R, Daniel WG (2001) Upregulation of CD40 and CD40 ligand (CD154) in patients with moderate hypercholesterolemia. Circulation 104:2395–2400

Genest J, Jr., McNamara JR, Ordovas JM, Jenner JL, Silberman SR, Anderson KM, Wilson PW, Salem DN, Schaefer EJ (1992) Lipoprotein cholesterol, apolipoprotein A-I and B and lipoprotein (a) abnormalities in men with premature coronary artery disease. J Am Coll Cardiol 19:792–802

Ghiadoni, L, S Taddei, Virdis A, Sudano I, Di Legge V, Meola M, Di Venanzio L, Salvetti A (1998) Endothelial function and common carotid artery wall thickening in patients with essential hypertension. Hypertension 32:25–32

Ghiadoni L, Virdis A, Magagna A, Taddei S, Salvetti A (2000) Effect of the angiotensin II type 1 receptor blocker candesartan on endothelial function in patients with essential hypertension. Hypertension 35:501–506

Griffin JH, Kojima K, Banka CL, Curtiss LK, Fernandez JA (1999) High-density lipoprotein enhancement of anticoagulant activities of plasma protein S and activated protein C. J Clin Invest 103:219–227

Henn V, Slupsky JR, Grafe M, Anagnostopoulos I, Forster R, Muller-Berghaus G, Kroczek RA (1998) CD40 ligand on activated platelets triggers an inflammatory reaction of endothelial cells. Nature 391:591–594

Hickey KA, Rubanyi G, Paul RJ, Highsmith RF (1985) Characterization of a coronary vaso-constrictor produced by cultured endothelial cells. Am J Physiol 248: C550–C556

Hingorani AD, Cross J, Kharbanda RK, Mullen MJ, Bhagat K, Taylor M, Donald AE, Palacios M, Griffin GE, Deanfield JE, MacAllister RJ, Vallance P (2000) Acute systemic inflamma-tion impairs endothelium-dependent dilatation in humans. Circulation 102:994–999

Ito H, Hirata Y, Hiroe M, Tsujino M, Adachi S, Takamoto T, Nitta M, Taniguchi K, Marumo F (1991) ET-1 induces hypertrophy with enhanced expression of muscle specific genes in cultured neonatal rat cardiomyocytes. Circ Res 69:209–215

Joannides R, Haefeli WE, Linder L, Richard V, Bakkali EH, Thuillez C, Lüscher TF (1995a) Nitric oxide is responsible for flow-dependent dilatation of human peripheral conduit arteries in vivo. Circulation 91:1314–1319

Joannides R, Richard V, Haefeli WE, Linder L, Lüscher TF, Thuillez C (1995b) Role of basal and stimulated release of nitric oxide in the regulation of radial artery caliber in humans. Hypertension 26:327–331

John S, Schlaich M, Langenfeld M, Weihprecht H, Schmitz G, Weidinger G, Schmieder RE (1998) Increased bioavailability of nitric oxide after lipid-lowering therapy in hyperc-holesterolemic patients: a randomized, placebo-controlled, double-blind study. Circu-lation 98:211–216

Kannel WB, Gordon T, Offutt D (1969) Left ventricular hypertrophy by electrocardiogram. Prevalence, incidence, and mortality in the Framingham study. Ann Intern Med 71:89–105

Katusic ZS, Vanhoutte PM (1989) Superoxide anion is an endothelium-derived contracting factor. Am J Physiol 257:H33–H37

Kiely DG, Cargill RI, Struthers AD, Lipworth BJ (1997) Cardiopulmonary effects of endo-thelin-1 in man. Cardiovasc Res 33:378–386

Laufs U, La Fata V, Plutzky J, Liao JK (1998) Upregulation of endothelial nitric oxide synthase by HMG CoA reductase inhibitors. Circulation 97:1129–1135

Lerman A, Edwards BS, Hallett JW, Heublein DM, Sandberg SM, Burnett JJ (1991) Circulating and tissue endothelin immunoreactivity in advanced atherosclerosis. N Engl J Med 325:997–1001

Leung W-H, Lau C-P, Wong C-K (1993) Beneficial effect of cholesterol-lowering therapy on coronary endothelium-dependent relaxation in hypercholesterolemic patients. Lancet 341:1496–1500

Li D, Weng S, Yang B, Zander DS, Saldeen T, Nichols WW, Khan S, Mehta JL (1999) Inhibition of arterial thrombus formation by ApoA1 Milano. Arterioscler Thromb Vasc Biol 19:378–383

Libby P (2001) Current concepts of the pathogenesis of the acute coronary syndromes. Circulation 104:365–372

Lichtlen PR, Hugenholtz PG, Rafflenbeul W, Hecker H, Jost S, Deckers JW (1990) Retardation of angiographic progression of coronary artery disease by nifedipine. Results of the International Nifedipine Trial on Antiatherosclerotic Therapy (INTACT). INTACT Group Investigators. Lancet 335:1109–1113

Lindmark E, Tenno T, Siegbahn A (2000) Role of platelet P-selectin and CD40 ligand in the induction of monocytic tissue factor expression. Arterioscler Thromb Vasc Biol 20:2322–2328

Liuzzo G, Biasucci LM, Gallimore JR, Grillo RL, Rebuzzi AG, Pepys MB, Maseri A (1994) The prognostic value of C-reactive protein and serum amyloid a protein in severe unstable angina. N Engl J Med 331:417–424

Lüscher TF, Yang Z, Tschudi M, Von SL, Stulz P, Boulanger C, Siebenmann R, Turina M, Bühler FR (1990) Interaction between endothelin-1 and endothelium-derived relaxing factor in human arteries and veins. Circ Res 66:1088–1094

Mach F, Schonbeck U, Sukhova GK, Atkinson E, Libby P (1998) Reduction of atherosclerosis in mice by inhibition of CD40 signalling. Nature 394:200–203

Mancini GB, Henry GC, Macaya C, O'Neill BJ, Pucillo AL, Carere RG, Wargovich TJ, Mudra H, Luscher TF, Klibaner MI, Haber HE, Uprichard AC, Pepine CJ, Pitt B (1996) Angiotensin-converting enzyme inhibition with quinapril improves endothelial vasomotor dysfunction in patients with coronary artery disease. The TREND (Trial on Reversing ENdothelial Dysfunction) Study [published erratum appears in Circulation 1996; 94:1490]. Circulation 94:258–265

May AE, Kälsch T, Massberg S, Herouy Y, Schmidt R, Gawaz M (2002) Engagement of glycoprotein IIb/IIIa ($\alpha_{IIb}\beta_3$) on platelets upregulates CD40L and triggers CD40L-dependent matrix degradation by endothelial cells. Circulation 106:2111–2117

Murray CJ, Lopez AD (1997) Mortality by cause for eight regions of the world: Global Burden of Disease Study. Lancet 349:1269–1276

Naqvi TZ, Shah PK, Ivey PA, Molloy MD, Thomas AM, Panicker S, Ahmed A, Cercek B, Kaul S (1999) Evidence that high-density lipoprotein cholesterol is an independent predictor of acute platelet-dependent thrombus formation. Am J Cardiol 84:1011–1017

Nofer, JR, Kehrel B, Fobker M, Levkau B, Assmann G, von Eckardstein A (2002) HDL and arteriosclerosis: beyond reverse cholesterol transport. Atherosclerosis 161:1–16

O'Driscoll G, Green D, Taylor RR (1997) Simvastatin, an HMG-coenzyme A reductase inhibitor, improves endothelial function within 1 month. Circulation 95:1126–1131

O'Leary DH, Polak JF, Kronmal RA, Manolio TA, Burke GL, Wolfson SK, Jr. (1999) Carotid-artery intima and media thickness as a risk factor for myocardial infarction and stroke in older adults. Cardiovascular Health Study Collaborative Research Group. N Engl J Med 340:14–22

Oemar BS, Tschudi MR, Godoy N, Brovkovich V, Malinski T, Luscher TF (1998) Reduced endothelial nitric oxide synthase expression and production in human atherosclerosis. Circulation 97:2494–2498

Palmer RM, Ashton DS, Moncada S (1988a) Vascular endothelial cells synthesize nitric oxide from L-arginine. Nature 333:664–666

Palmer RM, Ferrige AG, Moncada S (1987) Nitric oxide release accounts for the biological activity of endothelium-derived relaxing factor. Nature 327:524–526

Palmer RMJ, Rees DD, Ashton DS, Moncada S (1988b) L-arginine is the physiological precursor for the formation of nitric oxide in endothelium-dependent relaxation. Biochem Biophys Res Commun 153:1251–1256

Perticone F, Maio R, Ceravolo R, Cosco C, Cloro C, Mattioli PL (1999) Relationship between left ventricular mass and endothelium-dependent vasodilation in never-treated hypertensive patients. Circulation 99:1991–1996

Pitt B, Waters D, Brown WV, van Boven AJ, Schwartz L, Title LM, Eisenberg D, Shurzinske L, McCormick LS (1999) Aggressive lipid-lowering therapy compared with angioplasty in stable coronary artery disease. Atorvastatin versus Revascularization Treatment Investigators. N Engl J Med 341:70–76

Ridker PM, Buring JE, Shih J, Matias M, Hennekens CH (1998a) Prospective study of C-reactive protein and the risk of future cardiovascular events among apparently healthy women. Circulation 98:731–733

Ridker PM, Glynn RJ, Hennekens CH (1998b) C-Reactive protein adds to the predictive value of total and HDL cholesterol in determining risk of first myocardial Infarction. Circulation 97:2007–2011

Ridker PM, Hennekens CH, Roitman-Johnson B, Stampfer MJ, Allen J (1998c) Plasma concentration of soluble intercellular adhesion molecule 1 and risks of future myocardial infarction in apparently healthy men. Lancet 351:88–92

Ridker PM, Rifai N, Clearfield M, Downs JR, Weis SE, Miles JS, Gotto AMJ (2001) Measurement of C-reactive protein for the targeting of statin therapy in the primary prevention of acute coronary events. N Engl J Med 344:1959–1965

Ridker PM, Rifai N, Pfeffer MA, Sacks FM, Moye LA, Goldman S, Flaker GC, Braunwald E (1998d) Inflammation, pravastatin, and the risk of coronary events after myocardial infarction in patients with average cholesterol levels. Cholesterol and Recurrent Events (CARE) Investigators. Circulation 98:839–844

Ross R (1999) Atherosclerosis—an inflammatory disease. N Engl J Med 340:115–126

Rossi GP, Colonna S, Pavan E, Albertin G, Della Rocca F, Gerosa G, Casarotto D, Sartore S, Pauletto P, Pessina AC (1999) Endothelin-1 and its mRNA in the wall layers of human arteries ex vivo. Circulation 99:1147–1155

Rubanyi GM, JC Romero, Vanhoutte PM (1986) Flow-induced release of endothelium-derived relaxing factor. Am J Physiol 250: H1145–H1149

Rubanyi GM, Vanhoutte PM (1986) Superoxide anions and hyperoxia inactivate endothelium-derived relaxing factor. Am J Physiol 250: H822–H827

Rubins, HB, SJ Robins, Collins D, Fye CL, Anderson JW, Elam MB, Faas FH, Linares E, Schaefer EJ, Schectman G, Wilt TJ, Wittes J (1999) Gemfibrozil for the secondary prevention of coronary heart disease in men with low levels of high-density lipoprotein cholesterol. Veterans Affairs High-Density Lipoprotein Cholesterol Intervention Trial Study Group. N Engl J Med 341:410–418

Sacks FM, Pfeffer MA, Moye LA, Rouleau JL, Rutherford JD, Cole TG, Brown L, Warnica JW, Arnold JMO, Wun C-C, Davis BR, Braunwald E (1996) The effects of pravastatin on coronary events after myocardial infarction in patients with average cholesterol levels. N Engl J Med 335:1001–1009

Saito Y, Nakao K, Mukoyama M, Imura H (1990) Increased plasma endothelin level in patients with essential hypertension [letter]. N Engl J Med 322:205

Saku K, Ahmad M, Glas-Greenwalt P, Kashyap ML (1985) Activation of fibrinolysis by apolipoproteins of high density lipoproteins in man. Thromb Res 39:1–8

Schieffer B, Schieffer E, Hilfiker-Kleiner D, Hilfiker A, Kovanen PT, Kaartinen M, Nussberger J, Harringer W, Drexler H (2000) Expression of angiotensin II and interleukin 6 in human coronary atherosclerotic plaques: potential implications for inflammation and plaque instability. Circulation 101:1372–1378

Schwartz GG, Olsson AG, Ezekowitz MD, Ganz P, Oliver MF, Waters D, Zeiher A, Chaitman BR, Leslie S, Stern T (2001) Effects of atorvastatin on early recurrent ischemic events in acute coronary syndromes: the MIRACL study: a randomized controlled trial. Jama 285:1711–1718

Serruys PW, de Feyter P, Macaya C, Kokott N, Puel J, Vrolix M, Branzi A, Bertolami MC, Jackson G, Strauss B, Meier B (2002) Fluvastatin for prevention of cardiac events following successful first percutaneous coronary intervention: a randomized controlled trial. JAMA 287:3215–3222

Spieker LE, Sudano I, Hurlimann D, Lerch PG, Lang MG, Binggeli C, Corti R, Ruschitzka F, Luscher TF, Noll G (2002) High-density lipoprotein restores endothelial function in hypercholesterolemic men. Circulation 105:1399–1402

Stamler JS, Loh E, Roddy MA, Currie KE, Creager MA (1994) Nitric oxide regulates basal systemic and pulmonary vascular resistance in healthy humans. Circulation 89:2035–2040

Stamler JS, Singel DJ, Loscalzo J (1992) Biochemistry of nitric oxide and its redox-activated forms. Science 258:1898–1902

Stroes ES, Koomans HA, de Bruin TW, Rabelink TJ (1995) Vascular function in the forearm of hypercholesterolaemic patients off and on lipid-lowering medication. Lancet 346:467–471

Taddei S, Virdis A, Ghiadoni L, Uleri S, Magagna A, Salvetti A (1997) Lacidipine restores endothelium-dependent vasodilation in essential hypertensive patients. Hypertension 30:1606–1612

Treasure CB, Klein JL, Weintraub WS, Talley JD, Stillabower ME, Kosinski AS, Zhang J, Boccuzzi SJ, Cedarholm JC, Alexander RW et al. (1995) Beneficial effects of cholesterol-lowering therapy on the coronary endothelium in patients with coronary artery disease. N Engl J Med 332:481–487

Vallance P, Collier J, Moncada S (1989) Effects of endothelium-derived nitric oxide on peripheral arteriolar tone in man. Lancet 2:997–1000

van Boven AJ, Jukema JW, Zwinderman AH, Crijns HJ, Lie KI, Bruschke AV (1996) Reduction of transient myocardial ischemia with pravastatin in addition to the conventional treatment in patients with angina pectoris. REGRESS Study Group [see comments]. Circulation 94:1503–1505

Van Lenten B, Wagner AC, Nayak DP, Hama S, Navab M, Fogelman A (2001) High-density lipoprotein loses its anti-inflammatory properties during acute influenza a infection. Circulation 103:2283–2288

Verhaar MC, Honing ML, van Dam T, Zwart M, Koomans HA, Kastelein JJ, Rabelink TJ (1999) Nifedipine improves endothelial function in hypercholesterolemia, independently of an effect on blood pressure or plasma lipids. Cardiovasc Res 42:752–760

Verhaar MC, Wever RM, Kastelein JJ, van Dam T, Koomans HA, Rabelink TJ (1998) 5-methyl-tetrahydrofolate, the active form of folic acid, restores endothelial function in familial hypercholesterolemia. Circulation 97:237–241

Vierhapper H, Wagner O, Nowotny P, Waldhausl W (1990) Effect of endothelin-1 in man. Circulation 81:1415–1418

Yanagisawa M, Kurihara H, Kimura S, Tomobe Y, Kobayashi M, Mitsui Y, Yazaki Y, Goto K, Masaki T (1988) A novel potent vasoconstrictor peptide produced by vascular endothelial cells. Nature 332:411–415

Yang Z, Krasnici N, Lüscher TF (1999) Endothelin-1 potentiates smooth muscle cell growth to PDGF: role of ETA and ETB receptor blockade. Circulation 100:5–8

Zeiher AM, SchachlingerV, Hohnloser SH, Saurbier B, Just H (1994) Coronary atherosclerotic wall thickening and vascular reactivity in humans. Elevated high-density lipoprotein levels ameliorate abnormal vasoconstriction in early atherosclerosis. Circulation 89:2525–2532

HEP (2005) 170:645–663

Modulation of Smooth Muscle Cell Proliferation and Migration: Role of Smooth Muscle Cell Heterogeneity

M.-L. Bochaton-Piallat (✉) · G. Gabbiani

Department of Pathology and Immunology, University of Geneva, CMU,
1 rue Michel-Servet, 1211 Geneva 4, Switzerland
marie-luce.piallat@medecine.unige.ch

Abstract Proliferation and migration of smooth muscle cells (SMCs) from the media towards the intima are key events in atherosclerosis and restenosis. During these processes, SMC undergo phenotypic modulations leading to SMC dedifferentiation. The identification and characterization of factors controlling these phenotypic changes are crucial in order to prevent the formation of intimal thickening. One of the questions which presently remains open, is to know whether any SMCs of the media are capable of accumulating into the intima or whether only a predisposed medial SMC subpopulation is involved in this process. The latter hypothesis implies that arterial SMCs are phenotypically heterogenous. In this chapter, we will describe the distinct SMC phenotypes identified in arteries of various species, including humans. Their role in the formation of intimal thickening will be discussed.

Keywords Atherosclerosis · Restenosis · Intimal thickening · Actin · Myosin

1
The Concept of SMC Heterogeneity

The accumulation of smooth muscle cells (SMCs) in the intima is a characteristic of atheromatosis and restenosis following angioplasty or stent implantation. It has been demonstrated that the combined action of growth factors, proteolytic agents and extracellular matrix proteins, produced by a dysfunctional endothelium and/or inflammatory cells, induce migration of SMCs from the media towards the intima where they proliferate (Ross 1999). During this process, SMCs undergo phenotypic changes, i.e. they switch from a contractile to a synthetic phenotype (Campbell and Campbell 1990; Thyberg et al. 1995). The contractile phenotype is typical of SMCs in healthy arteries i.e., differentiated arteries; these SMCs contain many microfilament bundles. The synthetic phenotype is typical of developing and pathological arteries, i.e. barely differentiated or dedifferentiated arteries and is characterized by a cytoplasm with a predominance of rough endoplasmic reticulum and containing a well-developed Golgi apparatus. One of the main interests in the field of atherosclerosis is the identification of factors which control the dedifferentiation process of SMCs. However, the question remains open as to whether any SMCs in the media can undergo phenotypic modulation or whether a pre-existing SMC subpopulation is prone to accumulate into the intimal thickening. In this respect, Benditt and Benditt (1973) have suggested that the origin of SMC accumulation in the atheromatous plaque is monoclonal or oligoclonal. More recently, microdissection of different portions of human plaques followed by polymerase chain reaction amplification of the DNA of an X-inactivated gene has confirmed that SMCs of the fibrous cap are monoclonal (Murry et al. 1997). All together, the SMC phenotypic changes and the monoclonal hypothesis support the concept of SMC heterogeneity. This notion has been reinforced by the description in vitro of morphologically distinct SMC populations in many species, including man (for review see Hao et al. 2003). The understanding of the biological features of different subtypes within the SMC population is crucial in the development of a strategy with which to control SMC accumulation into the intimal thickening.

2
SMC Phenotypes

2.1
Morphological Features

SMC heterogeneity has been established mainly in vitro by identifying SMC populations with two distinct morphologies: a spindle-shaped phenotype with the classical 'hills and valleys' growth pattern and an epithelioid phenotype in which cells grow as a monolayer and exhibit a cobblestone morphology at confluence. The spindle-shaped SMCs were isolated from the normal media of carotid artery and aorta whereas the epithelioid SMCs were obtained from the experimental intimal thickening induced 15 days after endothelial injury of these vessels (Walker et al. 1986; Orlandi et al. 1994a; Bochaton-Piallat et al. 1996; Yan and Hansson 1998). Several groups using different methods of cell isolation have demonstrated that epithelioid SMCs exist within the normal media supporting the hypothesis that this particular population is prone to accumulate within the intima. Villaschi et al. (1994) have shown that epithelioid SMCs are predominant in the luminal part of the rat aortic media. By producing clones from the normal media and intimal thickening, we have demonstrated that spindle-shaped and epithelioid clones can be recovered from both locations albeit in different proportions, the normal media predominantly yielding spindle-shaped clones and the intimal thickening yielding a majority of epithelioid clones (Bochaton-Piallat et al. 1996). Several groups have confirmed the production of distinct SMC clones from the normal media of rat (Yan and Hansson 1998; Lau 1999; Li et al. 2000) and mouse (Ehler et al. 1995). Taken together, these studies provide evidence that the normal media contains phenotypically heterogeneous SMCs and support the possibility that intimal thickening develops essentially from a distinct medial subpopulation exhibiting an epithelioid phenotype when placed into culture.

According to the age of the rat, spindle-shaped and epithelioid SMCs were recovered in variable proportions from the healthy aorta (Seifert et al. 1984; Gordon et al. 1986; McCaffrey et al. 1988; Hültgardh-Nilsson et al. 1991; Majesky et al. 1992; Bochaton-Piallat et al. 1993; Cook et al. 1994; Lemire et al. 1994). As shown in adult rats, spindle-shaped SMCs were predominant in fetuses at different developmental stages (Cook et al. 1994) as well as in newborn rats (4–5 days) (Hültgardh-Nilsson et al. 1991; Bochaton-Piallat et al. 1992, 1993) whereas epithelioid SMCs were prevalent in old rats (older than 18 months) (McCaffrey et al. 1988; Bochaton-Piallat et al. 1993). It is, however, noteworthy that a predominant population of epithelioid SMCs is recovered from the normal media of 12-day-old rats (Seifert et al. 1984; Gordon et al. 1986; Majesky et al. 1992; Lemire et al. 1994), an age when sexual maturation occurs. These results suggest that a variable proportion of SMCs exhibiting an epithelioid phenotype in vitro exists within the media throughout the whole life span and that this proportion increases with age. In this respect, several studies have shown that the intimal thickening in response to injury is more pronounced in old rats compared to adult rats (Stemerman et al. 1982; Hariri et al. 1986; Chen et al. 2000).

More recently, distinct phenotypes similar to those isolated from rat arteries have been recovered in arteries of larger animals, such as pig (Hao et al. 2002), dog (Holifield et al. 1996), and cow (Frid et al. 1997). Our group has identified two distinct SMC subpopulations from the porcine coronary artery (Hao et al. 2002). SMCs isolated by enzymatic digestion from the normal media exhibit a spindle-shaped phenotype and grow in a 'hills and valleys' configuration (Christen et al. 1999; Hao et al. 2002). In contrast, SMCs obtained by tissue explantation are either spindle-shaped or rhomboid (flat but more elongated than epithelioid rat SMCs): the luminal portion of the media yields equal proportions of spindle-shaped and rhomboid SMCs whereas the abluminal portion yields a high proportion of rhomboid SMCs (Hao et al. 2002). Using the same technique, intimal thickening induced 15 days after stent implantation gives rise to a high proportion of rhomboid SMCs. These cells, hence, represent good candidates for the formation of intimal thickening in the porcine coronary artery. In the canine carotid artery, spherical SMCs, similar to the rat epithelioid cells were isolated from the abluminal part of the normal media and were found to be predominant in the intimal thickening produced 14 days after endothelial injury (Holifield et al. 1996). SMC subpopulations exhibiting spindle-shaped, rhomboid and epithelioid morphologies were isolated from morphologically distinct compartments within the normal media of bovine pulmonary artery and aorta (Frid et al. 1997). Taken together, these studies further extend the notion of SMC heterogeneity to large animals.

Albeit sporadically, distinct SMC subpopulations have been isolated from healthy and atherosclerotic arteries (Benzakour et al. 1996; Bonin et al. 1999; Llorente-Cortes et al. 1999; Li et al. 2001; Martinez-Gonzalez et al. 2001) and displayed phenotypic features similar to those observed in rat and pig. In particular, the finding that epithelioid SMC can be cloned from the human arterial media (Li et al. 2001) supports the hypothesis that an SMC subset expands in atherosclerotic lesions. However, the relevance of SMC heterogeneity to human disease still remains to be demonstrated.

2.2
Proliferative Activity and Apoptosis

SMC proliferation is an essential process at the onset of intimal thickening formation (Clowes et al. 1983). Apoptosis has also been detected in SMCs of experimental intimal thickening, atherosclerotic and restenotic lesions (for a review see Kockx and Herman 2000; McCarthy and Bennett 2000; Geng and Libby 2002). Apoptosis could participate in the regulation of cellularity in restenosis and in the stability of the plaque. Hence it is of major importance to investigate whether the distinct SMC subpopulations display differences in proliferative activity and/or susceptibility to apoptosis. In all species studied, epithelioid and rhomboid SMCs show a higher proliferative activity than spindle-shaped SMCs; however, in contrast to spindle-shaped SMCs they stop growing at confluence because of cell contact inhibition (Walker et al. 1986; Bochaton-Piallat et al. 1996; Frid et al. 1997; Li et al. 2001; Hao et al. 2002). It is notable that epithelioid SMCs isolated from the rat are able to grow in the absence of serum (Grünwald and Haudenschild 1984; Seifert et al. 1984; McCaffrey et al. 1988; Schwartz et al. 1990; Majesky et al. 1992; McCaffrey and Falcone 1993; Lemire et al. 1994; Orlandi et al. 1994a; Bochaton-Piallat et al. 1996). Rat epithelioid SMCs produce platelet-derived growth factor (PDGF)-BB, which is a potent SMC mitogen (Seifert et al. 1984; Majesky et al. 1992; Lemire et al. 1994), and fail to respond to the growth inhibitory effect of transforming growth factor (TGF)-β (McCaffrey and Falcone 1993). However, the factor(s) responsible for serum independence have never been clearly identified. Autonomous growth of epithelioid and rhomboid SMCs has been observed in other species (Topouzis and Majesky 1996; Frid et al. 1997) with the exception of pig (Hao et al. 2002), which in this respect is similar to man (Li et al. 2001; Martinez-Gonzalez et al. 2001).

Much less information is available on the mechanisms of apoptosis in distinct SMC subpopulations. An enhanced susceptibility of rat epithelioid SMCs to apoptosis induced by reactive oxygen species (Li et al. 2000), retinoic acid (RA) and anti-mitotic drugs (Orlandi et al. 2001) has been recently described. Interestingly, SMCs isolated from healthy human coronary artery show marked heterogeneity to Fas-induced apoptosis (Chan et al. 2000).

All together, the studies demonstrating the enhanced proliferative as well as apopototic activities of epithelioid and rhomboid SMCs in various species fit well with the expected features of candidates for the intimal thickening formation.

2.3
Migratory Activity

Cell migration, a major event of the intimal thickening formation, is a complex process that includes the degradation of extracellular matrix components by enzymes belonging to two families: serine proteases, in particular the plasminogen activator (PA)/plasmin system, and matrix metalloproteinases. Both tissue-PA (tPA) and urokinase-type PA (uPA) have been detected in both experimental intimal thickening (Clowes et al. 1990; Reidy et al. 1996; Carmeliet et al. 1997) and human atherosclerotic lesions (Lupu et al. 1995; Noda-Heiny et al. 1995; Raghunath et al. 1995; Steins et al. 1999). It has been shown in rat (Bochaton-Piallat et al. 1996; Li et al. 1997) (Fig. 1A and B), pig (Hao et al. 2002) (Fig. 2A and B), and man (Li et al. 2001) that epithelioid or rhomboid SMCs exhibit a high migratory activity compared to spindle-shaped SMCs. It has been also demonstrated that rat epithelioid SMCs display high tPA activity (Bochaton-Piallat et al. 1998) (Fig. 1C) and pig rhomboid SMCs display high uPA activity (Hao et al. 2002) (Fig. 2C). Likewise, Lau (1999) has shown that rat epithelioid SMCs may produce tPA, uPA, and metalloproteinase-2 under particular growth conditions.

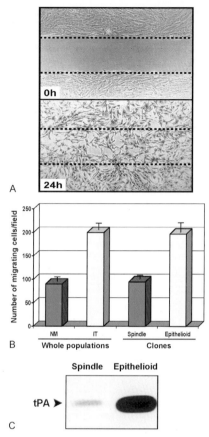

Fig. 1A–C Migratory and plasminogen activator (*PA*) activities of spindle-shaped and ep-ithelioid SMCs cultured as whole populations or clones isolated from rat aortic normal media (*NM*) and intimal thickening (*IT*) induced 15 days after endothelial injury. **A** 'In vitro wound' model: photomicrographs showing a confluent culture at 0 h scratched with a silicon rubber to obtain a 0.8-mm-wide 'in vitro wound'; after 24 h migrating cells invading the empty space are counted using an image analysis system. **B** Bar graph showing results of 'in vitro wound' model, calculated as the total number of migrated cells per field. Note that epithelioid SMCs cultured as whole populations or clones (*white bars*) exhibit a higher migratory activity than do spindle-shaped SMCs (*dark gray bars*) (*P*<0.05 in epithelioid vs. spindle-shaped SMCs). **C** Zymography of cell extracts showing that tissue-PA (*tPA*) activity is increased in IT-derived epithelioid SMCs compared to NM-derived spindle-shaped SMCs

2.4
Cytoskeletal Features

The contractile and synthetic SMC phenotypes have been characterized by their expression of cytoskeletal proteins, which are accepted as reliable differ-entiation markers (for a review see Schwartz et al. 1995; Owens 1998; Shana-han and Weissberg 1998; Sartore et al. 1999). Essentially, the main difference

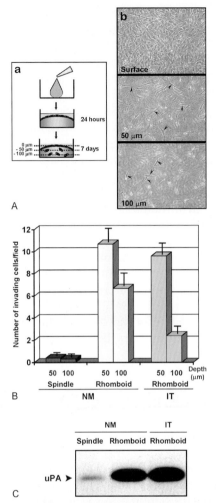

Fig. 2A–C Migratory and plasminogen activator (*PA*) activities of spindle-shaped and rhomboid SMCs isolated from porcine coronary artery normal media (*NM*) and intimal thickening (*IT*) induced 15 days after stent implantation. **A** Collagen gel invasion assay: (*a*) 24 h after collagen gel deposition, SMCs are seeded at the surface of the gel; at 7 days, cells are counted at focal levels of 50 and 100 μm beneath the surface of the gel; (*b*) photomicrographs showing SMCs at the surface of the gel, 50 μm and 100 μm beneath the surface of the gel after 7 days; invading cells are highlighted with *arrowheads*. **B** Bar graph showing results of collagen gel invasion assay, calculated as the total number of invading cells per field at 50 μm and 100 μm beneath the surface of the gel. Note that a high number of rhomboid SMCs isolated from NM (*white bars*) or IT (*light gray bars*) invade the collagen gel compared to spindle-shaped SMCs (*dark gray bars*) (*P*<0.01 in rhomboid vs. spindle-shaped SMCs). **C** Zymography of cell extracts showing that urokinase type-PA (*uPA*) activity is increased in rhomboid SMCs compared to spindle-shaped SMCs

between these two phenotypes appears to reside in their degree of differentiation. It should be noted that when placed into culture, all SMCs tend to show a dedifferentiated phenotype (Campbell and Campbell 1990; Thyberg et al. 1995). With this limitation, the phenotypic variations of cultured SMCs furnish important information concerning the influence of many factors on their biological features. The best studied markers are α-smooth muscle (SM) actin, the actin isoform typical of vascular SMCs, desmin, an intermediate filament protein, and SM myosin heavy chains (MHCs) isoforms SM1 and SM2. α-SM actin is expressed in vascular SMCs even at early stages of development, thus representing the most general marker of SMC lineage, whereas desmin and SMMHCs are markers of well differentiated SMCs (Owens 1995; Sartore et al. 1999). These three proteins are generally more abundant in spindle-shaped SMCs than in epithelioid or rhomboid SMCs in any species studied (Bochaton-Piallat et al. 1992, 1996; Lemire et al. 1994; Holifield et al. 1996; Frid et al. 1997; Li et al. 1997, 2001; Hao et al. 2002). Other cytoskeletal proteins have been less extensively studied. In particular, smoothelin, SM22α, calponin, h-caldesmon and meta-vinculin (Sartore et al. 1999) serve as late differentiation markers and are more abundant in spindle-shaped SMCs compared to epithelioid and rhomboid SMCs (Holifield et al. 1996; Topouzis and Majesky 1996; Frid et al. 1997; Hao et al. 2002). The level of expression of these proteins is much higher in larger animals such as pig and cow, than in rodents (Frid et al. 1997; Hao et al. 2002). For instance, in rat spindle-shaped SMCs, desmin is generally absent and SMMHCs are hardly detectable whereas they are maintained at a significant level of expression in porcine spindle-shaped SMCs (Hao et al. 2002). In this respect, SMCs isolated from large animals such as pig behave similarly to SMCs derived from human arteries (Li et al. 2001).

An interesting correlation has been demonstrated, albeit occasionally, between dedifferentiated and/or highly proliferating SMC phenotypes and increased low-density lipoprotein (LDL) uptake (Campbell et al. 1985; Parlavecchia et al. 1989; Llorente-Cortes et al. 1999; Thyberg 2002) or decreased high-density lipoprotein (HDL) binding sites (Dusserre et al. 1994). The role of LDL and HDL processes in atheromatous plaque formation with respect to SMC heterogeneity should be further investigated. Taken together, the data obtained in different species suggest that the degree of differentiation of SMCs changes with the phenotype; this integrates well in a view conciliating the heterogeneity with the modulation concepts.

2.5
Biochemical Markers

Once SMC populations have been defined, the ultimate aim is to identify genes and/or proteins that are differentially expressed among them and to test whether they are involved in the phenotypic changes that occur in vivo. By using 2D-PAGE followed by protein sequencing, we have identified three proteins specifically expressed in rat aortic epithelioid SMCs (Cremona et al. 1995; Neuville et al. 1997): cellular retinol binding protein-1 (CRBP-1), a protein involved in retinoid metabolism, and cytokeratins 8 and 18, intermediate filament proteins.

In vivo studies have demonstrated that CRBP-1 is constitutively expressed in very rarely occurring SMCs of the normal media of adult and old rats but not of newborn rats (Neuville et al. 1997). After endothelial injury, CRBP-1 is rapidly activated in a subset of medial SMCs located towards the lumen and is expressed in the large majority of SMCs present in the intimal thickening; it disappears when re-endothelialization is achieved. During these phases, CRBP-1 is present in replicative SMCs during the initial phase of intimal thickening formation and is detected in apoptotic cells during the late phase of intimal thickening remodeling (Neuville et al. 1997) known to be associated with SMC apoptosis (Bochaton-Piallat et al. 1995; Han et al. 1995; Perlman et al. 1997). In this respect, it has been shown that SMCs cultured from re-endothelialized intimal thickening (60 days after injury) are exclusively spindle-shaped (Orlandi et al. 1994a) suggesting that potentially epithelioid SMCs have disappeared. Moreover, cultured rat epithelioid SMCs are more sensitive to apoptosis than spindle-shaped SMCs (Li et al. 2000; Orlandi et al. 2001). These results suggest that a predisposed subset of medial SMCs becomes rapidly CRBP-1 positive after injury, undergoes replication during the early phase of intimal thickening development and then disappears, allegedly through apoptosis, when re-endothelialization takes place (Neuville et al. 1997). This also indicates that CRBP-1 is a marker of the epithelioid phenotype in vitro and SMC activation after endothelial injury in vivo. It is important to note that the in vitro and in vivo analysis of CRBP-1 expression in other animal models such as pig as well as in human specimens failed to confirm that this protein is a general marker of SMC activation in intimal thickening (M.-L. Bochaton-Piallat, P. Neuville, G. Gabbiani, unpublished observations). This further supports the assumption that rodent SMCs do not represent a reliable model for human SMCs.

Cytokeratin 8 and 18, intermediate filament proteins, as well as zonula occludens-2 protein and cingulin, two proteins of tight junctions, were thought to be exclusively expressed in epithelial or endothelial cells. They have since been identified as markers of rodent epithelioid SMCs (Ehler et al. 1995; Neuville et al. 1997; Adams et al. 1999) and are expressed in experimental intimal thickening (Adams et al. 1999) or human atheromatous plaque (Jahn et al. 1993). Studies of these proteins could give further insight into the mechanisms of SMC pathological modulation.

Several other genes have been discovered, mainly in rodents, as being specific or at least more abundant in one SMC population compared to the others. Epithelioid SMCs overexpress osteopontin (Giachelli et al. 1991a, 1993; Gadeau et al. 1993; Shanahan et al. 1993), tropoelastin (Majesky et al. 1992; Lemire et al. 1994; Adams et al. 1999), PDGF-BB (Majesky et al. 1992; Lemire et al. 1994), cytochrome P450 (Giachelli et al. 1991b), and peroxisome proliferator activated receptor-γ (Adams et al. 1999) whereas spindle-shaped SMCs overexpress procollagen type I and PDGF-α receptor (Majesky et al. 1992; Lemire et al. 1994; Adams et al. 1999). A study performed in the cow pulmonary artery model has shown that autonomously growing rhomboid SMCs exhibit constitutively activated extracellular signal-regulated kinase (ERK-1/2) and eicosanoid production (Frid et al. 1999). However, none of these genes has conclusively been proven to be relevant for the pathogenesis of human lesions.

3
Modulation of SMC Phenotype

Data suggesting SMC heterogeneity have been obtained essentially in vitro. It thus became important to study whether the distinct phenotypic features characterizing arterial SMC subpopulations are permanent or depend on the particular environment of cell culture. For this purpose, we have tested whether the features of spindle-shaped and epithelioid SMC subpopulations are retained when SMCs are implanted into rat carotid artery. We have observed that, after implantation, rat spindle-shaped and epithelioid SMCs keep their distinct differentiation features as defined, in addition to morphology, by the expression level of α-SM actin, SMMHCs and CRBP-1 (Bochaton-Piallat et al. 2001). This indicates that the phenotype of rat SMCs depends more on their intrinsic features rather than on their environment, thereby reinforcing the notion of SMC heterogeneity.

It is also important to evaluate whether microenvironmental factors influencing essential cellular processes such as proliferation, migration and differentiation modulate selectively the behavior of distinct SMC subpopulations. The factors tested up to now can be distributed into four categories: (1) those described as inhibitors of SMC proliferation and/or increasing SMC differentiation, e.g., heparin, TGF-β and RA; (2) those known to stimulate SMC proliferation and/or decrease SMC differentiation e.g., PDGF-BB, fibroblast-growth factor (FGF)-2, insulin-growth factor-I and II; (3) vasoactive substances such as endothelin-1, angiotensin II, histamine and norepinephrine; and finally (4) vasodilator factors such as nitric oxide (NO).

3.1
Factors Differentiating SMC

Heparin, which is the most powerful inhibitor of SMC growth in vitro and in vivo, at least in rat (Karnovsky et al. 1989; Au et al. 1993), acts similarly on rat (Orlandi et al. 1994b) and pig (Hao et al. 2002) SMC subpopulations. Contrasting with these results, heparin exerts a marked growth inhibition on rhomboid SMCs whereas it has almost no effect on spindle-shaped SMCs isolated from the cow pulmonary artery (Frid et al. 1997). These results indicate that the action of heparin on the diverse SMC subpopulation depends on the species studied.

TGF-β, which is a strong SMC growth inhibitor, increases the differentiation level of spindle-shaped and epithelioid SMCs of the rat model (Orlandi et al. 1994b); this is associated with a change in the epithelioid SMC morphology but which does not result in a typical spindle-shaped phenotype (Orlandi et al. 1994b). In pig coronary arterial SMCs, TGF-β does not influence SMC morphology although it decreases proliferation and increases differentiation of both SMC subtypes (Hao et al. 2002).

RA is considered to be a potent inducer of SMC differentiation (Blank et al. 1995; Colbert et al. 1996; Gollasch et al. 1998). In rat, RA slightly modifies cell morphology of epithelioid SMCs, similarly to TGF-β (Neuville et al. 1999). Interestingly RA increases the expression of α-SM actin only in epithelioid but not in spindle-shaped SMCs; however, in both cell types, it decreases proliferation and increases migration (Neuville et al. 1999). RA effects are mediated by the nuclear receptor RAR-α. These results indicate that rat epithelioid SMCs, i.e., CRBP-1-positive SMCs are more prone to respond to RA than spindle-shaped SMCs at least as far as their differentiation state is concerned. In vivo, feeding rats with RA or with a RAR-α agonist inhibits aortic or carotid artery intimal thickening formation (Miano et al. 1998; DeRose et al. 1999; Neuville et al. 1999), thus confirming functionally that CRBP-1 is a marker of SMC activation in the rat model.

3.2
Factors Dedifferentiating SMC

FGF-2 and PDGF-BB similarly increase the proliferation and migration of porcine SMC subpopulations (Hao et al. 2002). Human epithelioid SMC migrate more actively than spindle-shaped SMC in response to PFGF-BB (Li et al. 2001). We have shown that FGF-2 and PDGF-BB induce a switch from the spindle-shaped to the rhomboid phenotype in pig SMCs (Hao et al. 2002). This is associated with increased proliferation and decreased expression of differentiation markers. A similar effect has been obtained on spindle-shaped SMC clones. In both situations, this shape change is reversible when treatment is ceased. These results indicate that the switch depends on phenotypic modulation rather than on selection of a given population. Interestingly, endothelial cells isolated from the porcine coronary artery placed in co-culture with SMCs induce a switch from the spindle-shaped to the rhomboid phenotype (Hao et al. 2002). In these experiments, endothelial cells do not exhibit a quiescent state even after confluence, suggesting that they mimic an injured or dysfunctional endothelium. In other species, previous studies using endothelial cell/SMC co-culture have shown that endothelial cells stimulate SMC proliferation (Peiro et al. 1995; Nackman et al. 1996; Fillinger et al. 1997) and decrease the expression of α-SM actin and SMMHCs (Vernon et al. 1997), particularly when nonquiescent endothelial cells are used. It has been suggested that endothelial cells stimulate the proliferation of SMCs by producing plasminogen activator inhibitor-1 (PAI-1), which in turn inhibits TGF-β activation (Nackman et al. 1996; Petzelbauer et al. 1996; Powell et al. 1998). The mechanisms through which endothelial cells specifically act on porcine spindle-shaped SMCs remain to be clarified, but these results indicate that spindle-shaped SMCs can evolve, at least to some extent, into the rhomboid phenotype supporting the view that pig SMCs display an enhanced phenotypic plasticity compared to rat SMCs. It will be important to establish whether this plasticity is present in human SMCs.

3.3
Other Factors

It has been shown that spindle-shaped SMCs are more responsive than epithelioid SMCs to vasoactive factors such as endothelin-1 (Villaschi et al. 1994), angiotensin-2, histamine and norepinephrine (Li et al. 2001) either by measuring collagen gel contraction or by evaluating the intracellular calcium concentration. This is in accordance with the contractile feature of spindle-shaped SMCs. Conversely, epithelioid SMCs exhibit an increased expression of inducible NO synthase (Yan and Hansson 1998; Yan et al. 1999) that correlates with enhanced NF-κB expression when compared to spindle-shaped SMCs (Yan et al. 1999). Moreover, these cells fail to respond to NO (Yan and Hansson 1998; Chen et al. 2000) due to the lack of the β subunit of soluble guanylyl cyclase (Chen et al. 2000). This suggests that despite a large production of NO, epithelioid SMCs are less sensitive than spindle-shaped SMCs to NO action.

4
Conclusions and Perspectives

Taken together, the studies demonstrating the heterogeneity of SMCs in various species have led to the identification of particular SMC populations. These populations, which exhibit an epithelioid and/or rhomboid phenotype, possess features that explain their capacity of accumulating in the intimal thickening, thus representing an atheroma- or restenosis-prone phenotype. In particular they display: (1) enhanced capacity of proliferation and migration associated to a high proteolytic activity; (2) poorly differentiated state characteristic of intimal SMCs in vivo; and (3) they express proteins crucial for their behavior e.g. CRBP-1. It will be essential to identify molecules specific to the epithelioid/rhomboid phenotype in order to track in vivo atheroma- or restenosis-prone SMCs. Moreover, the finding of such molecules could lead to new strategies for the prevention of intimal SMC accumulation and/or to induce the differentiation of a potentially noxious cell into a more physiological phenotype, thus further stabilizing intimal thickening evolution. Using this approach we have identified CRBP-1 as a specific marker of intimal SMCs in the rat model (Cremona et al. 1995; Neuville et al. 1997). This observation has stimulated studies on RA that in turn has been shown to influence the biological behavior of epithelioid SMCs and inhibit intimal thickening formation. We are now analyzing porcine coronary artery SMCs using a proteomic strategy similar to that used in rats, with the hope of finding differentially expressed proteins that will be relevant for the human lesions.

It should be emphasized that the studies on the modulation of SMC phenotype have demonstrated diverging results in different species. Thus in rat, the best studied model, SMCs show two phenotypes that do not appear to be interchangeable, either in vitro or in vivo (Bochaton-Piallat et al. 1996, 2001). In contrast, in the porcine coronary model, spindle-shaped SMCs can change to rhomboid SMCs and, if the stimulus ceases, can return to the original phenotype, at least in vitro (Hao et al. 2002). This suggests that the evolution of in vivo lesions is more complex in pigs than in rats. In this respect, porcine SMCs appear to behave similarly to human SMCs.

In conclusion, studies on SMC heterogeneity are providing information useful for the precise characterization of the biological features of arterial SMCs and for a better understanding of the role of the different subpopulations in physiological and pathological situations. The discovery of new genes and/or proteins typical of the atheroma- or restenosis-prone phenotype in species other than the rat should give new insight into the understanding of human atherosclerosis and restenosis mechanisms.

Acknowledgements The authors acknowledge the support of the Swiss National Science Foundation (grant Nos. 31.061336.00 and 32-068034.02).

References

Adams LD, Lemire JM, Schwartz SM (1999) A systematic analysis of 40 random genes in cultured vascular smooth muscle subtypes reveals a heterogeneity of gene expression and identifies the tight junction gene zonula occludens 2 as a marker of epithelioid "pup" smooth muscle cells and a participant in carotid neointimal formation. Arterioscler Thromb Vasc Biol 19:2600–2608

Au YP, Kenagy RD, Clowes MM, Clowes AW (1993) Mechanisms of inhibition by heparin of vascular smooth muscle cell proliferation and migration. Haemostasis 23 Suppl 1:177–182

Benditt EP, Benditt JM (1973) Evidence for a monoclonal origin of human atherosclerotic plaques. Proc Natl Acad Sci USA 70:1753–1756

Benzakour O, Kanthou C, Kanse SM, Scully MF, Kakkar VV, Cooper DN (1996) Evidence for cultured human vascular smooth muscle cell heterogeneity: isolation of clonal cells and study of their growth characteristics. Thromb Haemost 75:854–858

Blank RS, Swartz EA, Thompson MM, Olson EN, Owens GK (1995) A retinoic acid-induced clonal cell line derived from multipotential P19 embryonal carcinoma cells expresses smooth muscle characteristics. Circ Res 76:742–749

Bochaton-Piallat ML, Gabbiani F, Ropraz P, Gabbiani G (1992) Cultured aortic smooth muscle cells from newborn and adult rats show distinct cytoskeletal features. Differentiation 49:175–185

Bochaton-Piallat ML, Gabbiani F, Ropraz P, Gabbiani G (1993) Age influences the replicative activity and the differentiation features of cultured rat aortic smooth muscle cell populations and clones. Arterioscler Thromb Vasc Biol 13:1449–1455

Bochaton-Piallat ML, Gabbiani F, Redard M, Desmouliere A, Gabbiani G (1995) Apoptosis participates in cellularity regulation during rat aortic intimal thickening. Am J Pathol 146:1059–1064

Bochaton-Piallat ML, Ropraz P, Gabbiani F, Gabbiani G (1996) Phenotypic heterogeneity of rat arterial smooth muscle cell clones. Implications for the development of experimental intimal thickening. Arterioscler Thromb Vasc Biol 16:815–820.

Bochaton-Piallat M-L, Gabbiani G, Pepper MS (1998) Plasminogen activator expression in rat arterial smooth muscle cells depends on their phenotype and is modulated by cytokines. Circ Res 82:1086–1093

Bochaton-Piallat ML, Clowes AW, Clowes MM, Fischer JW, Redard M, Gabbiani F, Gabbiani G (2001) Cultured arterial smooth muscle cells maintain distinct phenotypes when implanted into carotid artery. Arterioscler Thromb Vasc Biol 21:949–954

Bonin LR, Madden K, Shera K, Ihle J, Matthews C, Aziz S, Perez-Reyes N, McDougall JK, Conroy SC (1999) Generation and characterization of human smooth muscle cell lines derived from atherosclerotic plaque. Arterioscler Thromb Vasc Biol 19:575–587

Campbell G, Campbell J (1990) The phenotypes of smooth muscle expressed in human atheromaa. Ann NY Acad Sci 598:143–158

Campbell JH, Reardon MF, Campbell GR, Nestel PJ (1985) Metabolism of atherogenic lipoproteins by smooth muscle cells of different phenotype in culture. Arteriosclerosis 5:318–328

Carmeliet P, Moons L, Herbert JM, Crawley J, Lupu F, Lijnen R, Collen D (1997) Urokinase but not tissue plasminogen activator mediates arterial neointima formation in mice. Circ Res 81:829–839

Chan SW, Hegyi L, Scott S, Cary NR, Weissberg PL, Bennett MR (2000) Sensitivity to Fas-mediated apoptosis is determined below receptor level in human vascular smooth muscle cells. Circ Res 86:1038–1046

Chen L, Daum G, Fischer JW, Hawkins S, Bochaton-Piallat ML, Gabbiani G, Clowes AW (2000) Loss of expression of the β subunit of soluble guanylyl cyclase prevents nitric oxide-mediated inhibition of DNA synthesis in smooth muscle cells of old rats. Circ Res 86:520–525

Christen T, Bochaton-Piallat ML, Neuville P, Rensen S, Redard M, van Eys G, Gabbiani G (1999) Cultured porcine coronary artery smooth muscle cells. A new model with advanced differentiation. Circ Res 85:99–107

Clowes AW, Reidy MA, Clowes MM (1983) Kinetics of cellular proliferation after arterial injury. I. Smooth muscle growth in the absence of endothelium. Lab Invest 49:327–333

Clowes AW, Clowes MM, Au YP, Reidy MA, Belin D (1990) Smooth muscle cells express urokinase during mitogenesis and tissue-type plasminogen activator during migration in injured rat carotid artery. Circ Res 67:61–67

Colbert MC, Kirby ML, Robbins J (1996) Endogenous retinoic acid signaling colocalizes with advanced expression of the adult smooth muscle myosin heavy chain isoform during development of the ductus arteriosus. Circ Res 78:790–798

Cook CL, Weiser MC, Schwartz PE, Jones CL, Majack RA (1994) Developmentally timed expression of an embryonic growth phenotype in vascular smooth muscle cells. Circ Res 74:189–196

Cremona O, Muda M, Appel RD, Frutiger S, Hughes GJ, Hochstrasser DF, Geinoz A, Gabbiani G (1995) Differential protein expression in aortic smooth muscle cells cultured from newborn and aged rats. Exp Cell Res 217:280–287

DeRose JJ, Jr., Madigan J, Umana JP, Prystowsky JH, Nowygrod R, Oz MC, Todd GJ (1999) Retinoic acid suppresses intimal hyperplasia and prevents vessel remodeling following arterial injury. Cardiovasc Surg 7:633–639

Dusserre E, Bourdillon MC, Pulcini T, Berthezene F (1994) Decrease in high density lipoprotein binding sites is associated with decrease in intracellular cholesterol efflux in dedifferentiated aortic smooth muscle cells. Biochim Biophys Acta 1212:235–244

Ehler E, Jat PS, Noble MD, Citi S, Draeger A (1995) Vascular smooth muscle cells of H-2Kb-tsA58 transgenic mice. Characterization of cell lines with distinct properties. Circulation 92:3289–3296

Fillinger MF, Sampson LN, Cronenwett JL, Powell RJ, Wagner RJ (1997) Coculture of endothelial cells and smooth muscle cells in bilayer and conditioned media models. J Surg Res 67:169–178

Frid MG, Aldashev AA, Dempsey EC, Stenmark KR (1997) Smooth muscle cells isolated from discrete compartments of the mature vascular media exhibit unique phenotypes and distinct growth capabilities. Circ Res 81:940–952

Frid MG, Aldashev AA, Nemenoff RA, Higashito R, Westcott JY, Stenmark KR (1999) Subendothelial cells from normal bovine arteries exhibit autonomous growth and constitutively activated intracellular signaling. Arterioscler Thromb Vasc Biol 19:2884–2893

Gadeau AP, Campan M, Millet D, Candresse T, Desgranges C (1993) Osteopontin overexpression is associated with arterial smooth muscle cell proliferation in vitro. Arterioscler Thromb 13:120–125

Geng YJ, Libby P (2002) Progression of atheroma: a struggle between death and procreation. Arterioscler Thromb Vasc Biol 22:1370–1380

Giachelli C, Bae N, Lombardi D, Majesky M, Schwartz S (1991a) Molecular cloning and characterization of 2B7, a rat mRNA which distinguishes smooth muscle cell phenotypes in vitro and is identical to osteopontin (secreted phosphoprotein I, 2aR). Biochem Biophys Res Commun 177:867–873

Giachelli CM, Majesky MW, Schwartz SM (1991b) Developmentally regulated cytochrome P-450IA1 expression in cultured rat vascular smooth muscle cells. J Biol Chem 266:3981–3986

Giachelli CM, Bae N, Almeida M, Denhardt DT, Alpers CE, Schwartz SM (1993) Osteopontin is elevated during neointima formation in rat arteries and is a novel component of human atherosclerotic plaques. J Clin Invest 92:1686–1696

Gollasch M, Haase H, Ried C, Lindschau C, Morano I, Luft FC, Haller H (1998) L-type calcium channel expression depends on the differentiated state of vascular smooth muscle cells. Faseb J 12:593–601

Gordon D, Mohai LG, Schwartz SM (1986) Induction of polyploidy in cultures of neonatal rat aortic smooth muscle cells. Circ Res 59:633–644

Grünwald J, Haudenschild CC (1984) Intimal injury in vivo activates vascular smooth muscle cell migration and explant outgrowth in vitro. Arteriosclerosis 4:183–188

Han DK, Haudenschild CC, Hong MK, Tinkle BT, Leon MB, Liau G (1995) Evidence for apoptosis in human atherogenesis and in a rat vascular injury model. Am J Pathol 147:267–277

Hao H, Ropraz P, Verin V, Camenzind E, Geinoz A, Pepper MS, Gabbiani G, Bochaton-Piallat ML (2002) Heterogeneity of smooth muscle cell populations cultured from pig coronary artery. Arterioscler Thromb Vasc Biol 22:1093–1099

Hao H, Gabbiani G, Bochaton-Piallat ML (2003) Arterial smooth muscle cell heterogeneity. Implications for atherosclerosis and restenosis development. Arterioscler Thromb Vasc Biol (in press)

Hariri RJ, Alonso DR, Hajjar DP, Coletti D, Weksler ME (1986) Aging and arteriosclerosis. I. Development of myointimal hyperplasia after endothelial injury. J Exp Med 164:1171–1178

Holifield B, Helgason T, Jemelka S, Taylor A, Navran S, Allen J, Seidel C (1996) Differentiated vascular myocytes: are they involved in neointimal formation? J Clin Invest 97:814–825

Hültgardh-Nilsson A, Krondahl U, Querol-Ferrer V, Ringertz NR (1991) Differences in growth factor response in smooth muscle cells isolated from adult and neonatal rat arteries. Differentiation 47:99–105

Jahn L, Kreuzer J, von Hodenberg E, Kubler W, Franke WW, Allenberg J, Izumo S (1993) Cytokeratins 8 and 18 in smooth muscle cells. Detection in human coronary artery, peripheral vascular, and vein graft disease and in transplantation-associated arteriosclerosis. Arterioscler Thromb 13:1631–1639

Karnovsky MJ, Wright TC, Jr., Castellot JJ, Jr., Choay J, Lormeau JC, Petitou M (1989) Heparin, heparan sulfate, smooth muscle cells, and atherosclerosis. Ann NY Acad Sci 556:268–281

Kockx MM, Herman AG (2000) Apoptosis in atherosclerosis: beneficial or detrimental? Cardiovasc Res 45:736–746

Lau HK (1999) Regulation of proteolytic enzymes and inhibitors in two smooth muscle cell phenotypes. Cardiovasc Res 43:1049–1059

Lemire JM, Covin CW, White S, Giachelli CM, Schwartz SM (1994) Characterization of cloned aortic smooth muscle cells from young rats. Am J Pathol 144:1068–1081

Li S, Fan YS, Chow LH, Van Den Diepstraten C, van Der Veer E, Sims SM, Pickering JG (2001) Innate diversity of adult human arterial smooth muscle cells: cloning of distinct subtypes from the internal thoracic artery. Circ Res 89:517–525

Li WG, Miller FJ, Jr., Brown MR, Chatterjee P, Aylsworth GR, Shao J, Spector AA, Oberley LW, Weintraub NL (2000) Enhanced H_2O_2-induced cytotoxicity in "epithelioid" smooth muscle cells: implications for neointimal regression. Arterioscler Thromb Vasc Biol 20:1473–1479

Li Z, Cheng H, Lederer WJ, Froehlich J, Lakatta EG (1997) Enhanced proliferation and migration and altered cytoskeletal proteins in early passage smooth muscle cells from young and old rat aortic explants. Exp Mol Pathol 64:1–11

Llorente-Cortes V, Martinez-Gonzalez J, Badimon L (1999) Differential cholesteryl ester accumulation in two human vascular smooth muscle cell subpopulations exposed to aggregated LDL: effect of PDGF-stimulation and HMG-CoA reductase inhibition. Atherosclerosis 144:335–342

Lupu F, Heim DA, Bachmann F, Hurni M, Kakkar VV, Kruithof EK (1995) Plasminogen activator expression in human atherosclerotic lesions. Arterioscler Thromb Vasc Biol 15:1444–1455

Majesky MW, Giachelli CM, Reidy MA, Schwartz SM (1992) Rat carotid neointimal smooth muscle cells reexpress a developmentally regulated mRNA phenotype during repair of arterial injury. Circ Res 71:759–768

Martinez-Gonzalez J, Berrozpe M, Varela O, Badimon L (2001) Heterogeneity of smooth muscle cells in advanced human atherosclerotic plaques: intimal smooth muscle cells expressing a fibroblast surface protein are highly activated by platelet-released products. Eur J Clin Invest 31:939–949

McCaffrey TA, Nicholson AC, Szabo PE, Weksler ME, Weksler BB (1988) Aging and arteriosclerosis. The increased proliferation of arterial smooth muscle cells isolated from old rats is associated with increased platelet-derived growth factor-like activity. J Exp Med 167:163–174

McCaffrey TA, Falcone DJ (1993) Evidence for an age-related dysfunction in the antiproliferative response to transforming growth factor-β in vascular smooth muscle cells. Mol Biol Cell 4:315–322

McCarthy NJ, Bennett MR (2000) The regulation of vascular smooth muscle cell apoptosis. Cardiovasc Res 45:747–755

Miano JM, Kelly LA, Artacho CA, Nuckolls TA, Piantedosi R, Blaner WS (1998) all-trans-retinoic acid reduces neointimal formation and promotes favorable geometric remodeling of the rat carotid artery after balloon withdrawal injury. Circulation 98:1219–1227

Murry CE, Gipaya CT, Bartosek T, Benditt EP, Schwartz SM (1997) Monoclonality of smooth muscle cells in human atherosclerosis. Am J Pathol 151:697–705

Nackman GB, Bech FR, Fillinger MF, Wagner RJ, Cronenwett JL (1996) Endothelial cells modulate smooth muscle cell morphology by inhibition of transforming growth factor-β1 activation. Surgery 120:418–425

Neuville P, Geinoz A, Benzonana G, Redard M, Gabbiani F, Ropraz P, Gabbiani G (1997) Cellular retinol-binding protein-1 is expressed by distinct subsets of rat arterial smooth muscle cell in vitro and in vivo. Am J Pathol 150:509–521

Neuville P, Yan Z, Gidlof A, Pepper MS, Hansson GK, Gabbiani G, Sirsjo A (1999) Retinoic acid regulates arterial smooth muscle cell proliferation and phenotypic features in vivo and in vitro through an RARα-dependent signaling pathway. Arterioscler Thromb Vasc Biol 19:1430–1436

Noda-Heiny H, Daugherty A, Sobel BE (1995) Augmented urokinase receptor expression in atheroma. Arterioscler Thromb Vasc Biol 15:37–43

Orlandi A, Ehrlich HP, Ropraz P, Spagnoli LG, Gabbiani G (1994a) Rat aortic smooth muscle cells isolated from different layers and at different times after endothelial denudation show distinct biological features in vitro. Arterioscler Thromb 14:982–989

Orlandi A, Ropraz P, Gabbiani G (1994b) Proliferative activity and α-smooth muscle actin expression in cultured rat aortic smooth muscle cells are differently modulated by transforming growth factor-β1 and heparin. Exp Cell Res 214:528–536

Orlandi A, Francesconi A, Cocchia D, Corsini A, Spagnoli LG (2001) Phenotypic heterogeneity influences apoptotic susceptibility to retinoic acid and cis-platinum of rat arterial smooth muscle cells in vitro: Implications for the evolution of experimental intimal thickening. Arterioscler Thromb Vasc Biol 21:1118–1123

Owens GK (1995) Regulation of differentiation of vascular smooth muscle cells. Physiol Rev 75:487–517

Owens GK (1998) Molecular control of vascular smooth muscle cell differentiation. Acta Physiol Scand 164:623–635

Parlavecchia M, Skalli O, Gabbiani G (1989) LDL accumulation in cultured rat aortic smooth muscle cells with different cytoskeletal phenotypes. J Vasc Med Biol 1:308–313

Peiro C, Redondo J, Rodriguez-Martinez MA, Angulo J, Marin J, Sanchez-Ferrer CF (1995) Influence of endothelium on cultured vascular smooth muscle cell proliferation. Hypertension 25:748–751

Perlman H, Maillard L, Krasinski K, Walsh K (1997) Evidence for the rapid onset of apoptosis in medial smooth muscle cells after balloon injury. Circulation 95:981–987

Petzelbauer E, Springhorn JP, Tucker AM, Madri JA (1996) Role of plasminogen activator inhibitor in the reciprocal regulation of bovine aortic endothelial and smooth muscle cell migration by TGF-β1. Am J Pathol 149:923–931

Powell RJ, Bhargava J, Basson MD, Sumpio BE (1998) Coculture conditions alter endothelial modulation of TGF-β1 activation and smooth muscle growth morphology. Am J Physiol 274: H642–H649

Raghunath PN, Tomaszewski JE, Brady ST, Caron RJ, Okada SS, Barnathan ES (1995) Plasminogen activator system in human coronary atherosclerosis. Arterioscler Thromb Vasc Biol 15:1432–1443

Reidy MA, Irvin C, Lindner V (1996) Migration of arterial wall cells. Expression of plasminogen activators and inhibitors in injured rat arteries. Circ Res 78:405–414

Ross R (1999) Atherosclerosis: an inflammatory disease. N Engl J Med 340:115–126

Sartore S, Franch R, Roelofs M, Chiavegato A (1999) Molecular and cellular phenotypes and their regulation in smooth muscle. Rev Physiol Biochem Pharmacol 134:235–320

Schwartz SM, Foy L, Bowen-Pope DF, Ross R (1990) Derivation and properties of platelet-derived growth factor-independent rat smooth muscle cells. Am J Pathol 136:1417–1428

Schwartz SM, deBlois D, O'Brien ER (1995) The intima. Soil for atherosclerosis and restenosis. Circ Res 77:445–465

Seifert RA, Schwartz SM, Bowen-Pope DF (1984) Developmentally regulated production of platelet-derived growth factor- like molecules. Nature 311:669–671

Shanahan CM, Weissberg PL, Metcalfe JC (1993) Isolation of gene markers of differentiated and proliferating vascular smooth muscle cells. Circ Res 73:193–204

Shanahan CM, Weissberg PL (1998) Smooth muscle cell heterogeneity: patterns of gene expression in vascular smooth muscle cells in vitro and in vivo. Arterioscler Thromb Vasc Biol 18:333–338

Steins MB, Padro T, Li CX, Mesters RM, Ostermann H, Hammel D, Scheld HH, Berdel WE, Kienast J (1999) Overexpression of tissue-type plasminogen activator in atherosclerotic human coronary arteries. Atherosclerosis 145:173–180

Stemerman MB, Weinstein R, Rowe JW, Maciag T, Fuhro R, Gardner R (1982) Vascular smooth muscle cell growth kinetics in vivo in aged rats. Proc Natl Acad Sci USA 79:3863–3866

Thyberg J, Blomgren K, Hedin U, Dryjski M (1995) Phenotypic modulation of smooth muscle cells during the formation of neointimal thickenings in the rat carotid artery after balloon injury: an electron-microscopic and stereological study. Cell Tissue Res 281:421–433

Thyberg J (2002) Caveolae and cholesterol distribution in vascular smooth muscle cells of different phenotypes. J Histochem Cytochem 50:185–195

Topouzis S, Majesky MW (1996) Smooth muscle lineage diversity in the chick embryo. Two types of aortic smooth muscle cell differ in growth and receptor-mediated transcriptional responses to transforming growth factor-β. Dev Biol 178:430–445

Vernon SM, Campos MJ, Haystead T, Thompson MM, DiCorleto PE, Owens GK (1997) Endothelial cell-conditioned medium downregulates smooth muscle contractile protein expression. Am J Physiol 272: C582–C591

Villaschi S, Nicosia RF, Smith MR (1994) Isolation of a morphologically and functionally distinct smooth muscle cell type from the intimal aspect of the normal rat aorta. Evidence for smooth muscle cell heterogeneity. In Vitro Cell Dev Biol Anim 30A: 589–595

Walker LN, Bowen-Pope DF, Ross R, Reidy MA (1986) Production of platelet-derived growth factor-like molecules by cultured arterial smooth muscle cells accompanies proliferation after arterial injury. Proc Natl Acad Sci USA 83:7311–7315

Yan ZQ, Hansson GK (1998) Overexpression of inducible nitric oxide synthase by neointimal smooth muscle cells. Circ Res 82:21–29

Yan ZQ, Sirsjo A, Bochaton-Piallat ML, Gabbiani G, Hansson GK (1999) Augmented expression of inducible NO synthase in vascular smooth muscle cells during aging is associated with enhanced NF-κB activation. Arterioscler Thromb Vasc Biol 19:2854–2862

HEP (2005) 170:665–695
© Springer-Verlag Berlin Heidelberg 2005

Modulation of Macrophage Function and Metabolism

S. Bellosta[1] (✉) · F. Bernini[2]

[1] Department of Pharmacological Sciences, University of Milan, via Balzaretti 9,
20133 Milan, Italy
Stefano.Bellosta@unimi.it

[2] Department of Pharmacological and Biological Sciences and Applied Chemistry,
University of Parma, viale delle Scienze, 43100 Parma, Italy

Abstract Several drugs or pharmacologically active molecules such as statins, calcium antagonists, and PPAR agonists have been shown to affect macrophage functions that contribute to atherosclerosis and modulate plaque stability. For example, the modulation of matrix metalloproteinase secretion and cholesterol metabolism in macrophages may help to prevent cardiovascular disease independently of the correction of risk factors.

Keywords Atherosclerosis · Cholesterol metabolism · Drug treatment · Inflammation · Matrix metalloproteinase · Pleiotropic effects

1
Introduction

Atherosclerosis results from the interaction between blood elements and vessel wall abnormality that involves several pathological processes, namely increased endothelial permeability, blood cell adhesion, monocyte recruitment, smooth muscle cell (SMC) proliferation and migration, matrix synthesis, lipid accumulation, tissue degeneration, and cell necrosis (Ross 1999). Atherosclerotic plaque disruption with superimposed thrombosis is the main cause of the acute coronary syndrome of unstable angina, myocardial infarction, and sudden death. Most acute coronary events result from the disruption of mild-to-moderately stenosed atherosclerotic lesions, in which the degree of angiographic stenosis is less than 70%. Evidence is now accumulating that stabilizing atherosclerotic lesions prevents coronary events (Libby and Aikawa 2002). Indeed, atherosclerotic lesions, most often implicated in acute coronary events, have a soft, lipid-laden core and an excess of macrophages within the thin fibrous cap, which makes them prone to fissuring/rupture. The latter is the key primary event in the thrombotic process that ultimately leads to acute coronary events and sudden death (Brown et al. 1993). Plaque rupture usually occurs at the shoulder (Libby 1995), where macrophages accumulate and secrete matrix metalloproteinases (MMPs: collagenase, gelatinases, stromelysins) that weaken the thin fibrous cap (Libby 1995).

Besides lipid lowering therapy, which most probably affects the size and cholesterol content of the atheromatous core, plaque stabilization could be achieved by a direct inhibition of MMPs in the arterial wall. At least 23 different MMPs have been identified (Massova et al. 1998), and their number is still increasing. MMPs are a family of Zn^{2+}- and Ca^{2+}-dependent enzymes important in the resorption of extracellular matrixes in both physiological and pathological processes. MMPs act extracellularly at physiological pH and require activation by proenzyme precursors to attain enzymatic activity (Libby 1995) (Fig. 1). The regulation of these enzymes is very important and occurs at three levels: transcription, activation of latent proenzymes, and inhibition of proteolytic activity (Birkedal-Hansen et al. 1993; Matrisian 1994). The 92-kDa gelatinase B or metalloproteinase-9 (MMP-9) is expressed by virtually all activated macrophages and, through the degradation of the basement membrane, it facilitates the extravasation of macrophages. MMP-9 has been shown to be common in atherectomy materials from unstable angina (Brown et al. 1995) and abdominal aortic aneurysm (Newman et al. 1994).

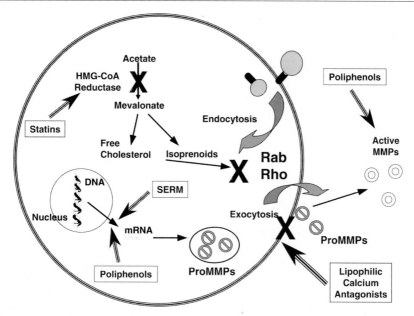

Fig. 1 Major mechanisms of pharmacological modulation of MMPs activity in macrophages

The expression of MMPs-1, -3, and -9 is up-regulated in cells present in atheromas, including endothelial cells, SMCs, and macrophages (Luan et al. 2003). Inflammatory mediators, including interleukin (IL)-1, CD-40 ligand, and tumour necrosis factor-α (TNF-α), up-regulate the MMP activity in vascular cells, especially in combination with platelet-derived growth factor (PDGF) or basic fibroblast growth factor (Luan et al. 2003). Ubiquitous inhibitors known as tissue inhibitors of metalloproteinases (TIMPs) control the activity of these enzymes under physiological conditions (Libby 1995). The activity of TIMPs in atherosclerotic plaques seems to correlate with a decreased MMP activity (Zaltsman et al. 1999) and hence with reduced matrix remodelling. MMPs can therefore perform their biological function only if a local excess prevails over endogenous inhibitors.

Macrophages of plasma monocyte origin also represent the majority of the cholesterol-loaded cells (foam cells) present in atherosclerotic lesions. This observation indicates that macrophages play a major role in atherogenesis (Ross 1999). Receptors (scavenger receptors) are present on the plasma membrane of these cells. The incubation of macrophages with modified LDL, obtained by modifications such as acetylation or oxidation, induces a massive accumulation of cholesterol esters with the in vitro formation of foam cells (Itabe 2003; Vainio and Ikonen 2003). The ability of macrophages to accumulate cholesterol from modified lipoproteins is due, at least in part, to the lack of a negative feedback regulation that down-regulates scavenger receptors even after a prolonged incubation with their ligands.

In mouse peritoneal macrophages it has been demonstrated that the accumulated cholesteryl esters undergo a constant turnover. Thus, the cholesterol esters are enzymatically hydrolysed and the released free cholesterol, if not removed from the cells by extracellular acceptors [i.e. high-density lipoprotein (HDL)], is re-esterified by the enzyme acyl CoA: cholesterol acyltransferase (ACAT) inducing a dynamic intracellular accumulation of this sterol. Interestingly, the plaques most susceptible to rupture have a high content of cholesterol (Vainio and Ikonen 2003). This chapter focuses on the effects of drugs or molecules that in macrophages modulate MMP secretion and cholesterol metabolism.

2
Pharmacological Control of MMPs

Proteases are particularly abundant in macrophages, where they are critical players in many key functions of the macrophage, such as the degradation of exogenous, potentially pathogenic proteins, the digestion of both foreign and self proteins into peptides for presentation by MHC class I and II, and the functional regulation of target proteins.

Increased activity of MMPs has been associated with a wide variety of pathological conditions, such as arthritis, cancer, multiple sclerosis, and atherosclerosis. The potential utility of MMP inhibitors in these diverse states of disease is evident, and several MMP inhibitors have entered clinical development (Whittaker et al. 2001). In addition, several other classes of drugs already in clinical use have been shown to modulate the activity of MMPs (Table 1, Fig. 1).

Table 1 Pharmacological modulation of MMPs in macrophages

Agents	Effect observed
Lipophilic statins	Inhibition of MMP-1, -3, -9 secretion
	No effect on TIMP-1, -2 expression
Calcium antagonists	
Lacidipine	Inhibition of MMP-9 and TIMP-1 secretion,
	reduced collagen degradation
Nifedipine	No effect
Polyphenols	Inhibition of MMP-9 secretion and activity
PPARα agonists	Inhibition of MMP-9 secretion
PPARγ agonists	Inihibition of MMP-9, ADAM, ADAMTS4 production
Raloxifene	Inhibition of MMP-1, -2, -3, -9 production

MMP, Matrix metalloproteinase; TIMP, tissue inhibitor of matrix metalloproteinase; ADAM, A disintegrin and metalloproteinase.

2.1
Statins

Statins are a structurally related group of 3-hydroxy-3-methylglutaryl coenzyme A (HMG-CoA) reductase inhibitors that are widely used to treat hyperlipidaemia. Their use is associated with a significant reduction of adverse coronary events, including myocardial infarction, and a marginal regression of plaque size (Libby and Aikawa 2002; Rabbani and Topol 1999). Furthermore, recent studies, both in vitro and in vivo, have suggested that the beneficial effects of statins may extend to mechanisms beyond cholesterol reduction (Luan et al. 2003). These pleiotropic effects of statins are mediated by their ability to block the synthesis of isoprenoid intermediates that serve as lipid attachments for a variety of intracellular signalling molecules whose proper membrane localization and function depend on isoprenylation (Bellosta et al. 2000).

We previously showed that statins inhibit the proteolytic activity of MMP-9 in macrophages in vitro (Bellosta et al. 1998). The inhibitory effect of fluvastatin on MMP-9 activity detected by zymography is not the consequence of a direct interference of the drug with the postsecretory activation of the MMPs, as the drug does not have any effect on the activity of MMP-9 already secreted into the growth media. In addition, fluvastatin reduces the amount of MMP-9 protein released by the cells, suggesting a direct effect on the secretion process. The reduced levels of MMP-9 detected in the media is not due to decreased MMP-9 gene expression either, because mRNA levels actually rise in fluvastatin-treated cells (Bellosta et al. 1998). The post-transcriptional inhibition of MMP-9 is reversible and appears to be mediated through a starvation of mevalonate and its derivatives, because the coincubation of the cells with statin and mevalonate completely overcomes the inhibitory effect of the drug. Recently, these results have been corroborated by new data showing that statins decrease the secretion of a broad spectrum of MMPs from both SMC and foamy macrophages, which implies a beneficial effect on plaque stability (Luan et al. 2003). Lovastatin decreases the collagenolytic, β-caseinolytic, and gelatinolytic activities that are predominantly associated with MMP-1, -3, and -9, respectively, and this effect is prevented by the addition of mevalonate or isoprenoid derivatives (Luan et al. 2003). By contrast, statins do not affect the production of TIMP-1 and -2, which potentially inhibits most MMPs and implies that statins shift the MMP/TIMP balance towards inactive enzymes.

The inhibition of HMG-CoA reductase by statins reduces intracellular levels of all intermediary products of cholesterol synthesis, including mevalonate, squalene, and isoprenoids needed for the prenylation of proteins. Prenylation is a type of stable lipid modification involving covalent addition of either farnesyl or geranylgeranyl isoprenoids (GGPP) to conserved cysteine residues at or near the C-terminus of proteins (Zhang and Casey 1996). Prenylated proteins include fungal mating factors, nuclear lamins, Ras and Ras-related GTP-binding proteins, protein kinases, and at least one viral protein. Prenylation promotes membrane interactions of most of these proteins and plays a major role in several protein–protein interactions and in signal transduction (Zhang and Casey 1996). Prenylated proteins, such as the Rab subgroup, i.e. small Ras-like GTPases in mammalian cells, play an important role in regulating membrane traffic and exocytic and endocytic transport processes (Zerial and Stenmark 1993). The inhibition of Rab prenylation blocks protein secretion (Seabra et al. 1993). For example, Rab3A is an important regulator of protein secretion by neuronal cells (Zhang and Casey 1996). Therefore, it has been postulated that the inhibition of isoprenoids formation by statins interferes with the MMP-9 secretion by macrophages (Bellosta et al. 1998).

Also, the translocation of Rho GTPase family members from the cytoplasm to the plasma membrane depends on geranylgeranylation (Takemoto and Liao 2001). Rescue of MMP secretion by GGPP confirms that the mechanism responsible for the inhibitory effect of statins on MMP secretion is the inhibition of prenylation. Previous studies demonstrated that the inhibition of geranylgeranyl transferase with L-839,867 and the inhibition of Rho by C3 exoenzyme significantly decreases the production of MMPs (Ikeda et al. 2000; Wong et al. 2001). Rho are small GTP-binding proteins that cycle between the inactive and the active GDP-bound state. They play crucial roles in diverse cellular events, such as cytoskeleton organization, membrane trafficking, secretion, transcriptional regulation, cell growth control, and development (Takemoto and Liao 2001).

As observed with fluvastatin, lovastatin had no significant effects on the mRNA levels of MMP-1, -3, and -9 (Luan et al. 2003). The previously reported inhibitory effect of fluvastatin on MMP-9 secretion from human macrophages was accompanied by a doubling of steady-state mRNA levels for MMP-9 (Bellosta et al. 1998). Thus, both studies agree that statins inhibit MMP secretion through a post-translational mechanism. Such a mechanism helps to explain the inhibition of MMPs secretion by statins with widely differing transcriptional regulation. For example, MMP-1, -3, and -9 secretion in SMC and MMP-1 and -3 secretion in foam cells are regulated and depend on the transcription factor nuclear factor-κB (NF-κB), but MMP-2 secretion in SMC and constitutive MMP-9 secretion in macrophages are independent of NF-κB (Chase et al. 2002). The secretion of TIMPs is unaffected by statins, which implies that the post-translational mechanism is selective for MMPs and not merely an overall inhibition of protein synthesis (Luan et al. 2003).

The extrapolation of the in vitro results to the in vivo condition is difficult, of course. The final net level of proteinase activity depends on several factors, such as the relative concentrations of active enzymes and specific inhibitors (i.e. TIMPs), and further studies are required to assess the in vivo relevance of these observations. Nevertheless, several clinical studies demonstrated the ability of statins to reduce the incidence of coronary heart disease (4S Investigators 1994; Shepherd et al. 1995), most probably by increasing the stability of the atherosclerotic plaque affecting macrophage functions rather than by reducing the stenotic occlusion (Falk et al. 1995).

2.2
Calcium Antagonists

It has been shown that various calcium-channel antagonists (blockers, CA) delay plaque formation in animal models (Bellosta and Bernini 2000). Although the mechanism of this beneficial effect is still not well understood, it appears to be unrelated to the anti-hypertensive properties of this class of drugs. They have been shown to modulate the low-density lipoprotein (LDL) metabolism in cell culture and to interfere directly with the major processes of atherogenesis in the arterial wall (Bellosta and Bernini 2000). These drugs inhibit SMC migration and proliferation as well as cholesterol accumulation in macrophages by inhibiting ACAT activity, both in vitro and in vivo. Studies have shown that the majority of CA of the 1,4-dihydropyridine type interact with calcium channels from a location near the surface of the cell membrane (Herbette et al. 1991). We have recently shown that the in vitro incubation of human macrophages with lacidipine reduces the secretion of MMP-9 by up to 50%, while nifedipine is ineffective (Bellosta et al. 2001). Lacidipine also reduces the secretion of TIMP-1, the endogenous inhibitor of MMP-9, and of other MMPs. This effect can counteract the inhibitory action of lacidipine on MMP-9 final activity. However, the drug effectively reduces the amount of free MMP-9 not complexed with TIMP-1, both in the active and in the latent form. Consistently, the treatment of the cells with lacidipine results in an overall reduction of the gelatinolytic activity of the cells, to an even higher degree than expected from the reduction of MMP-9 mass secretion (Bellosta et al. 2001). The fact that lacidipine inhibits the secretion of other MMPs with collagenolytic activity, such as MMP-2, MMP-8, and MMP-13, may be responsible for this high degree of reduction (Ikeda et al. 2000). The reduced levels of MMP-9 secreted into the medium by human macrophages is not caused by decreased MMP-9 gene expression, as the mRNA levels do not change appreciably after treatment of the cells with lacidipine. This suggests that the drug affects post-transcriptional processes of MMP-9 production and secretion, similar to the effect seen with statins. Alternatively, lacidipine treatment could cause a reduced translational efficiency combined with normal secretion of the translated product, but there is no evidence for such a mechanism. Therefore, the treatment with this CA interferes with the gelatinolytic capacity of human macrophages in culture. Data published on the involvement of intracellular calcium levels in the regulation of the activity of MMPs are quite controversial. Some reports demonstrated that low intracellular calcium levels decrease the gelatinolytic activity of MMP-2 (Kohn et al. 1994), whereas other authors have found that high intracellular calcium levels decrease the MMP-2 activity in human fibrosarcoma cells (Lohi and Keski-Oja 1995). Analogously, it has been reported that low intracellular calcium levels increase the proteolytic activity of MMP-2 and inhibit the TIMP-2 transcription and collagen deposition (Roth et al. 1996). Nifedipine, the prototype dihydropyridine with high affinity to calcium channel, has been shown to be completely inactive in MMP inhibition. In addition, the presence of lacidipine in the incubation medium does not affect intracellular Ca^{2+} levels, which indicates that the effect of the drug on the MMP-9 secretion process is independent of the variation in intracellular Ca^{2+} concentration (Bellosta et al. 2001).

The effect of lacidipine might be related to its physico-chemical properties. Unlike nifedipine, lacidipine is a highly lipophilic compound and binds to lipid membranes with a long half-life. This elevated lipophilicity raises its concentration in the cellular membrane by up to 800 times (Herbette et al. 1993). Therefore, the presence of lacidipine may alter the composition of the biophase, thus interfering with the MMP-9 secretion process. A similar hypothesis was proposed to explain its effect on cholesterol esterification (Bernini et al. 1997).

Galis and colleagues showed that MMPs are sensitive to antioxidant treatment (Galis et al. 1998). The possibility that macrophage gelatinolytic activity is redox dependent was suggested by previous studies showing activation of gelatinase zymogens by reactive oxygen species (ROS) known to be produced by macrophage foam cells (Rajagopalan et al. 1996). The macrophage-derived gelatinolytic activity was also inhibited by a treatment with N-acetyl-cysteine, a ROS scavenger. Activated macrophages, especially those of atherosclerotic lesions, are a major source of ROS. Thus, such an activation mechanism would result in the activation of MMP zymogens secreted by the macrophages themselves as well as by the neighbouring cells (Galis et al. 1998). Lacidipine has an antioxidant capacity similar to the one of vitamin E (Bellosta et al. 2001), and this chemical property could complete its inhibitory action on MMP-9 secretion through a mechanism still unknown, regardless of its CA activity.

The concentrations of lacidipine used in these studies on MMP secretion are higher than those reported in the plasma of treated patients. However, as mentioned before, lacidipine concentrates several fold in arterial cells, and its duration of action in vivo is unrelated to its plasma half-life (Herbette et al. 1993). In fact, peritoneal macrophages obtained from mice treated with lacidipine showed a reduced ex vivo ability to secrete MMP-9 (Bellosta et al. 2001). These results support the concept that therapeutic dosages of lacidipine can accumulate in macrophages of the vessel wall and hence modulate macrophage functions involved in atherogenesis.

2.3
Polyphenols

The modulation of the proteolytic activity of MMPs can also be achieved by affecting the MMP production on the gene level. We have recently shown that simple and natural molecules such as polyphenols, which are readily available from dietary sources, may exert an effect on the MMP-9 gelatinolytic potential by directly inhibiting enzyme activity and by modulating the MMP promotor activity and hence the release of MMP-9 from macrophages, (Bellosta et al. 2003) (Fig. 1). The results may represent a beneficial effect of this type of polyphenols on the therapeutic control of excessive extracellular matrix breakdown. These effects may be biologically relevant in that they interact at different steps (i.e. transcription, secretion, and activity) in the modulation of MMP-9. In particular, this was the first study reporting an inhibitory effect of the MMP-9 gene transcription with these compounds. These results provide new insights regarding the ability of polyphenols to act at the gene level in macrophages (Bellosta et al. 2003).

2.4
Selective Estrogen Receptor Modulators

Raloxifene, a selective estrogen receptor modulator (SERM), has been shown to affect the MMP-1, -2, -3, and -9 production and the macrophage accumulation in an animal model of atherosclerosis (Baetta et al. 2001). The decreased expression of MMPs in collar-induced carotid lesions may reflect diminished macrophage accumulation during raloxifene treatment. However, the in vitro data obtained from experiments with mouse macrophages suggest that raloxifene may also reduce the amount of MMPs released by the cells through a direct effect on the cell function. This effect is dose dependent and, at least for MMP-9, caused by reduced transcription. Thus, both of these mechanisms may contribute to the overall reduction of MMP expression observed in our in vivo model (Baetta et al. 2001). Interestingly, the in vitro effects of raloxifene on MMP-mediated proteolytic activity were evident at concentrations not too different from the average plasma levels of raloxifene reported for rabbits treated with an oral dose of raloxifene comparable with the one used in the present study (Bjarnason et al. 1997). No estrogen responsive element sequence can be found in the MMP-9 promoter. However, reports showed that the expression of different MMPs is inhibited by several ligands of the nuclear receptor superfamily (Schroen and Brinckerhoff 1996), although few consensus hormone responsive elements are present in their promoters. In addition, crosstalk among the endoplasmic reticulum and membrane-associated signalling pathways modify the promoter activity of different genes involved in monocyte–macrophage physiology. These interactions may underlie the mechanism responsible for the blockage of the MMP-9 promoter by raloxifene. Moreover, raloxifene reduces macrophage accumulation in the carotid lesions, and this effect may have several molecular bases. For example, raloxifene has been found to enhance vascular nitric oxide (NO) production in rabbit coronary arteries (Figtree et al. 1999) and in human endothelial cells (ECs) (Simoncini and Genazzani 2000), thereby potentially limiting endothelial activation in response to proinflammatory stimuli. In particular, it might be hypothesized that, similarly to natural estrogens (Nathan et al. 1999), SERMs affect the vascular expression of leukocyte adhesion receptors, as suggested by the observation that the raloxifene analogue LY117,018 is able to inhibit vascular cell adhesion molecule-1 (VCAM-1) expression in cultured human ECs (Mendelsohn and Karas 1999).

2.5
PPAR Agonists

Peroxisome proliferator-activated receptors (PPARs) also play an important role in the regulation of macrophage functions. PPARs are members of the nuclear receptor superfamily of ligand-dependent transcription factors and function as transcriptional regulators of gene expression. Upon ligand binding, nuclear receptors undergo a conformational change that mediates the exchange of corepressor and coactivator proteins to enable transcriptional activation or repression (Glass and Rosenfeld 2000). A rapidly evolving line of investigation has recently linked PPARs and liver X receptors (LXRs) to the regulation of both lipid homeostasis and inflammatory responses in macrophages. PPARs function as receptors for fatty acids and their metabolites, while LXRs are receptors for certain derivatives of cholesterol (Ricote et al. 2004). PPARs and LXRs activate gene expression by binding to specific DNA response elements in target genes as heterodimers with retinoid X receptors (RXR), which are themselves members of the nuclear receptor superfamily that can be regulated by 9-*cis* retinoic acid and long-chain polyunsaturated fatty acids (Ricote et al. 2004). PPARs and LXRs also negatively regulate gene expression in a ligand-dependent manner by antagonizing the activities of other signal-dependent transcription factors, such as NF-κB (Chinetti et al. 1998; Ricote et al. 1998b). The three known PPAR subtypes α, γ, and δ (β) show distinct tissue distribution and are associated with selective ligands (Ricote et al. 1999).

PPARα is strongly expressed in liver, kidney, heart, and muscle and regulates the production of enzymes involved in the β-oxidation of fatty acids and lipoprotein metabolism. PPARα is the molecular target of fibrates, such as gemfibrizol, that are clinically used to treat hypertriglyceridaemia (Fruchart et al. 1999, Staels et al. 1998).

PPARγ is most strongly expressed in adipose tissue and has been demonstrated to be essential for adipocyte differentiation and normal glucose metabolism (Ricote et al. 2004). PPARγ is expressed in numerous tissues and in cells of the monocyte/macrophage lineage (Ricote et al. 1998b), and it is involved in the development of monocytes along the macrophage lineage, in particular in the conversion of monocytes to foam cells (Tontonoz et al. 1998). Low levels of PPARγ are present in bone marrow-derived macrophages, whereas higher levels are present in activated peritoneal macrophages obtained after thioglycollate injection, which suggests that PPARγ is up-regulated during macrophage activation (Ricote et al. 1998a). Monocytes/macrophages in human atherosclerotic lesions express PPARγ, while normal arteries reveal minimal levels of PPARγ (Marx et al. 1998). PPARγ is activated by the thiazolidinedione drug class, exemplified by rosiglitazone, which acts as insulin sensitizer and is used in the treatment of type 2 diabetes mellitus (Willson et al. 1996; Worley et al. 2003).

PPARδ is ubiquitously expressed, it still lacks a clinical agonist, and its biological roles are less well established than those of PPARα and γ. However, recent studies suggest roles in skin homeostasis, lipid metabolism, and energy homeostasis (Ricote et al. 2004).

PPARα agonists (fibrates) cause a profound down-regulation of lipopolysaccharide (LPS)-induced secretion of MMP-9 by human monocytic THP-1 cells, although they fail to modulate LPS-induced secretion of IL-8 (Shu et al. 2000). These findings suggest that PPARs regulate only a subset of the proinflammatory genes controlled by AP-1, STAT, and NF-κB. Effects of PPARs on MMP-9 may account for the beneficial effect of PPAR agonists in animal models of atherosclerosis.

However, it has been postulated that the PPARα-mediated decrease in MMP-9 mRNA steady-state and zymogen levels is not attributable to an inhibition of MMP-9 gene expression. The inhibitory effects of PPARα agonists on cytokine-induced MMP-9 expression are indirect and primarily due to post-transcriptional regulatory events with a superinduction of inducible NO synthase (iNOS), leading to high levels of NO that subsequently reduce the half-life of MMP-9 mRNA (Eberhardt et al. 2002).

PPARγ may exert anti-inflammatory effects by negatively regulating the expression of pro-inflammatory genes that are induced during macrophage differentiation and activation, most probably by antagonizing the activity of different transcription factors (Ricote et al. 1998b). PPARγ agonists have been shown to suppress the inflammatory cytokines TNF-α, IL-1β, and IL-6 (Jiang et al. 1998), and iNOS (Ricote et al. 1998b) in monocytes and macrophages as well as MMP-9 (Marx et al. 1998; Patel et al. 2002; Ricote et al. 1998b; Shu et al. 2000). The actual mechanism of MMP-9 down-regulation has not yet been studied directly, although it is thought to involve transrepression of AP-1 and/or NF-κB sites in the MMP-9 promoter (Ricote et al. 1998b). No PPAR response element (PPRE) has been located in the human MMP-9 promoter yet, although two possible PPREs have recently been identified in 1.8 kb of the rat MMP-9 promoter (Eberhardt et al. 2002). It has recently been shown that PMA-stimulated THP-1 monocytic cells show altered MMP, ADAM (A Disintegrin And Metalloproteinase), and ADAMTS4 mRNA expression, which can be differentially regulated by the addition of PPARγ and RXR agonists (Worley et al. 2003). This has important implications for the use of PPARγ and RXR agonists in the treatment of diseases, especially type 2 diabetes and atherosclerosis.

3
Pharmacological Control of Cholesterol Metabolism in Macrophages

Accumulation of cholesterol in macrophages in the arterial wall is a major process in atheroma formation. These cells may accumulate an excess of cholesterol from acetylated LDL (AcLDL) and oxidized LDL (OxLDL) via scavenger receptors that mediate the internalization and degradation of modified lipoproteins (Itabe 2003). The cholesteryl esters transported by these lipoproteins are hydrolysed in lysosomes, and free cholesterol is released to a pool where it participates as a substrate for the esterification reaction catalysed by the microsomal enzyme ACAT (Brown et al. 1979). Several compounds have been reported to reduce cholesterol esterification. Some of them act indirectly by reducing intracellular cholesterol movement, impairing lysosomal lipoprotein degradation and cholesteryl ester hydrolysis (Bernini et al. 1989; Goldstein et al. 1980), or by inhibiting scavenger receptor expression and cellular influx of modified lipoproteins (Bottalico et al. 1991; Geng and Hansson 1992). Drugs may also act directly by inhibiting ACAT activity (Sliskovic and White 1991). Finally, some agents may act on the rate of cholesterol efflux from cells (Ricote et al. 2004). Depending on the mechanism involved, each agent may have different effects on the cellular cholesterol content and localization and on the ratio of esterified and unesterified cholesterol. ACAT inhibitors may increase the free cholesterol content of the plasma membrane, with a minor effect on total cellular cholesterol (Xu and Tabas 1991). Accumulation of cholesteryl esters in lysosomes is achieved with agents inhibiting the activity of lysosomal enzymes (Bernini et al. 1989; Goldstein et al. 1980). Free cholesterol accumulation in these organelles is observed with compounds active on intracellular cholesterol movement (Butler et al. 1992; Liscum and Faust 1989).

Cardiovascular drugs or potential antiatherosclerotic agents may affect lipid metabolism in macrophages (Table 2, Fig. 2).

3.1
Calcium Antagonists

CA interfere with cholesteryl ester hydrolysis and reesterification, thus affecting the intracellular deposition of cholesteryl esters. Nifedipine and verapamil analogues, but not diltiazem and flunarizine, inhibit the β-very-low-density lipoprotein (VLDL)-induced cholesterol esterification in rabbit macrophages. The same effect was achieved with the dihydropyridine calcium agonist BAY K 8644. The investigators concluded that these effects are independent from calcium entry blockade (Daugherty et al. 1987). Stein and Stein (1987) reported that verapamil has two major effects on cholesteryl ester metabolism in macrophages. First, verapamil inhibits LDL degradation and cholesteryl ester hydrolysis in lysosomes. This effect results in an accumulation

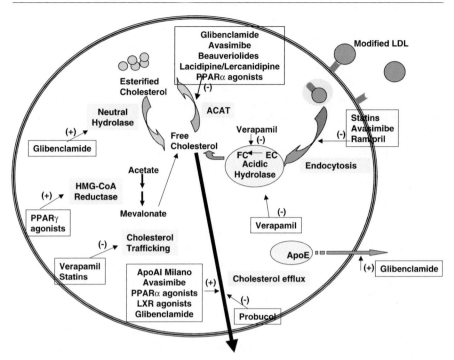

Fig. 2 Major mechanisms of pharmacological modulation of cholesterol metabolism in macrophages

of the esterified sterol. Second, verapamil reduces cholesterol esterification by inhibiting the delivery of cholesterol to the ACAT esterification site. This effect is independent of the inhibition of lysosomal cholesteryl ester hydrolysis. A reduction of ACAT activity reduces the cholesteryl ester content deposition. Therefore, the net effect of verapamil on cellular cholesteryl ester content will result from the balance of these two processes. Although the aforementioned activities have opposite consequences on the cellular cholesteryl ester content, both reduce the delivery of cholesterol to the cholesteryl ester cycle operating in the cytoplasm of macrophages, where esterified and free cholesterol are continuously hydrolysed and reesterified (Brown et al. 1980). Because verapamil reduces the delivery of the substrate (i.e. cholesterol), this 'futile' cycle will be reduced by the drug. Partial inhibition of lysosomal lipoprotein degradation and cholesteryl ester hydrolysis by basic CA, including amlodipine, may therefore be regarded as a beneficial effect rather than a possible proatherogenic side effect. In fact, these compounds may modulate the excessive release of free cholesterol not only to the cytoplasmic compartment (as previously discussed), but also to the plasma membrane (Tabas et al. 1988) where cholesterol may exert toxic effects (Kellner-Weibel et al. 1999; Spector et al. 1979). The non-hydrolysed cholesteryl ester, retained in the cells as a result of the lysoso-

Table 2 Pharmacological modulation of cholesterol metabolism in macrophages

Agents	Effect observed
ApoAI$_{Milano}$	Induction of cholesterol efflux
Avasimibe	Inhibition of: ACAT, modified LDL uptake
	Induction of cholesterol efflux
Beauveriolides I and III	Inhibition of ACAT
Glibenclamide	Inhibition of ACAT
	Induction of: cholesteryl ester hydrolysis cholesterol efflux,
	secretion of apolipoprotein E
Lacidipine, lercanidipine	Inhibition of cholesterol esterification
Lipophilic statins	Inhibition of: modified LDL endocytosis, cholesterol trafficking,
	LDL oxidation
PPARα agonists	Induction of cholesterol efflux
	Inhibition of ACAT1 and 2 activities
PPARγ agonists	Induction of HMG-CoA expression
Probucol	Inhibition of apoAI-mediated cholesterol efflux
Ramipril	Inhibition of CD36 expression and oxLDL uptake
Verapamil	Inhibition of: Beta VLDL-induced esterification, LDL degradation,
	acid cholesteryl ester hydrolysis, cholesterol trafficking
	Induction of cholesterol efflux

ACAT, Acyl CoA: cholesterol acyltransferase.

mal inhibition by CA, is eventually eliminated. This hypothesis is supported by data on smooth muscle cells where verapamil induces an initial increase (2–7 days) in cellular cholesteryl ester content that, at longer incubation times (18–35 days), is followed by a net decrease as compared with control cells (Stein and Stein 1987).

Lacidipine is a highly lipophilic third-generation CA whose pharmacokinetics are controlled by the tissue cell membrane compartment. Its duration of action classifies it as a once-a-day CA. Lercanidipine is a new third-generation CA with high lipophilicity and a chiral centre. Its pharmacokinetic and pharmacodynamic characteristics are similar to those of lacidipine, and it is also classified as a once-a-day CA. The long duration of action of lercanidipine and lacidipine is controlled by the tissue cell membrane compartment from which both drugs are slowly released once they have been distributed throughout the patient's body (Herbette et al. 1993). Therefore, these two lipophilic CA combine a relatively short plasma half-life, a gradual onset of action, and an intrinsically long duration of action.

Our group has shown that lacidipine affects intracellular cholesterol homeostasis in mouse peritoneal macrophages. Pre-treatment of macrophages with lacidipine reduces the formation of cholesteryl esters by up to 95%. Lacidipine inhibitory effect is observed at concentrations as low as 3 µM (Bernini et al.

1989, 1997), and we proposed that the drug directly inhibits ACAT that catalyses the esterification of cholesterol. Lacidipine consistently inhibits cholesterol esterification by more than 80% when added to cell-free homogenate (Bernini et al. 1997).

Lercanidipine is also able to inhibit cholesterol esterification by up to 70% in a concentration-dependent manner, both in whole cells and in cell-free homogenate. The mechanism by which lipophilic CA interferes with cholesterol esterification is still unknown. However, because the activity of ACAT is sensitive to variations in the lipophilicity and composition of the biophase (Suckling and Stange 1985), the presence of these drugs could alter the availability of the substrate (i.e. cholesterol) for the enzyme. This mechanism is consistent with the inhibitory activity observed in both living cells and cell-free homogenates. In our experience, nifedipine is ineffective under these experimental conditions. This observation suggests that lipophilic CA acts independently of voltage-operated calcium-channel blockade (Bernini et al. 1997). However, nifedipine may potentially exert antiatherosclerotic properties via a reduction of the oxidative modification of LDL, consequently reducing foam cell formation rather than inducing a direct reduction in cholesterol accumulation (Lesnik et al. 1997).

Recently, verapamil and other CA have been demonstrated to affect not only the intracellular processes involved in lipoprotein and cholesterol metabolism, but also to stimulate the pathways involved in cholesterol excretion from cells. This effect is achieved by inducing the expression of the cholesterol transporter ABCA1 (Tsujita and Yokoyama 1996). ABCA1 belongs to the ATP-binding cassette transporter family and promotes a unidirectional efflux of membrane cholesterol and phospholipid to lipid-poor apolipoproteins. ABCA1 expression can be stimulated in macrophages and other cells by the agonists of the nuclear receptor LXR, a potentially new class of drugs. Since cholesterol efflux is the first step of reverse cholesterol transport, molecules able to modulate this process may have an antiatherogenic activity by reducing lipid accumulation in cells and/or promoting cholesterol excretion from the body (Lund et al. 2003).

Even before the identification of ABCA1 as a mediator of cell cholesterol and phospholipid efflux to lipid-free apoproteins, it was demonstrated that probucol treatment of cells in culture produces a marked inhibition of apolipoprotein A-I-mediated lipid efflux from macrophages. Both cholesterol and phospholipid efflux to lipid-free apoA-I were greatly reduced if the cells were exposed to acetyl LDL containing probucol for 24 h (Tsujita and Yokoyama 1996). Sakr et al. (1999) were able to produce very rapid and extensive inhibition of lipid efflux from J774 macrophages incubated with probucol/albumin complexes.

3.2
ACE Inhibitors

The modulation of the cholesterol metabolism in macrophages has also been reported to occur in the presence of angiotensin converting enzyme (ACE) inhibitors. Treatment of mice with ramipril was found to significantly decrease the mRNA levels of OxLDL receptor CD36 in peritoneal macrophages and concomitantly inhibited the uptake of these modified lipoproteins (Hayek et al. 2002). This effect may provide ACE inhibitors with antiatherosclerotic properties.

3.3
Statins

Statins were found to decrease cholesterol esterification and deposition in macrophages (Bernini et al. 1993, Kempen et al. 1991). The inhibition of cholesterol esterification by statins is completely overcome by mevalonate and geranylgeraniol and takes place in the presence of an excess of exogenous cholesterol (Bernini et al. 1993; Kempen et al. 1991). These results indicate that statins do not affect esterification by preventing the intracellular formation of substrate for ACAT (i.e. cholesterol), but rather by inhibiting the formation of non-sterol mevalonate product(s).

The effect of statins on cholesterol esterification does not occur in cell-free homogenates (Kempen et al. 1991) and is observed only under conditions of simultaneous incubation of statins with AcLDL but not in cholesterol-preloaded cells (Bernini et al. 1993), thus indicating that these drugs are not direct ACAT inhibitors.

Our results indicate that fluvastatin and simvastatin reduce, depending on the concentration, more than 50% of the ^{125}I-AcLDL degradation by macrophages. This effect is not caused by a decrease in lysosomal enzyme activity and is paralleled by the retention of AcLDL-associated cholesteryl ester in the incubation medium. Also, the ability of fluvastatin to inhibit AcLDL degradation is completely overcome by mevalonate and its derivative geranylgeraniol. Binding experiments suggest that the inhibitory effect of fluvastatin on lipoprotein catabolism does not involve the decreased expression of scavenger receptors (Bernini et al. 1993).

Fluorescent microscope analysis of cellular internalization of AcLDL labelled with the fluorochrome 3,3'-dioctadecyl indocarbocyanine demonstrates that fluvastatin inhibits lipoprotein endocytosis.

In addition to simvastatin and fluvastatin, lovastatin has also been shown to reduce the cholesterol esterification in cholesterol-loaded human macrophages. This effect may be caused by the interference of the drug with the intracellular cholesterol delivery to the plasma membrane, resulting in increased free cholesterol and lower levels of cholesteryl ester. Lovastatin action may occur independently of the inhibition of the binding or uptake of AcLDL, ACAT activity, lysosomal hydrolysis of cholesteryl esters and the secretion of cholesterol into the medium (Cignarella et al. 1998). Lovastatin has also been reported to interfere with a modified lipoprotein uptake into macrophages by inhibiting the scavenger receptor expression or the oxidative modification of LDL (Aviram et al. 1992; Umetani et al. 1996).

It has recently been reported that pitavastatin, a new statin, inhibits CD36 expression, thus preventing OxLDL uptake by macrophages (Han et al. 2004).

A strong effect on cholesterol metabolism can also be obtained if the rate of cholesteryl ester synthesis is reduced by using ACAT inhibitors. However, studies conducted with the ACAT inhibitors avasimibe (CI-1011) indicate that the compound not only inhibits the rate of formation of cholesteryl esters, but also induces a reduction of the cellular cholesterol content. Similarly to statins, this effect appears to be mediated by a reduction of modified LDL uptake by the treated cells. Unlike with statins, with avasimibe the effect appears to involve a reduction in lipoprotein binding to cells. In addition, avasimibe appears to induce cellular cholesterol efflux (Rodriguez and Usher 2002).

It has been suggested that the inhibition of both ACAT and HMG-CoA reductase may exert a synergistic direct antiatherosclerotic effect on the vessel wall. In cultivated macrophages, atorvastatin approximately doubled the ability of avasimibe to reduce the mass of esterified cholesterol, and this was reversed by co-incubation with mevalonate or geranylgeraniol (Llaverias et al. 2002). As mentioned before, avasimibe and statins may reduce the cholesterol content in macrophages by different mechanisms, which may explain the synergistic effect reported in in vivo and in vitro models.

3.4
PPAR Agonists

PPARα activation may promote the cholesterol efflux from macrophages by inducing the ABCA1 pathway (Ricote et al. 2004). In human macrophages and foam cells, fibrates and synthetic PPARα activators reduce the ACAT1 activity and the cholesteryl ester to free cholesterol (FC) ratio. PPARα activation does not alter ACAT1 gene expression, but induces mRNA levels of carnitine palmitoyltransferase type 1, a key enzyme in mitochondrial fatty acid catabolism. PPARα activation also inhibits cholesteryl ester formation induced by TNF-α. This effect may involve the inhibition of neutral sphingomyelinase activation by TNF-α. The authors concluded that PPAR may control cholesterol esterification in macrophages and enhance the ABCAI mediated FC efflux.

In addition to PPARα, macrophages express PPARγ. In the THP-1 macrophages troglitazone or pioglitazone, two ligands of this receptor, increase the expression of HMG-CoA synthase and reductase through a PPRE. Treatment with troglitazone was found to significantly increase the activity of HMG-CoA reductase and the amount of intracellular cholesterol. Thus, opposite to

PPARα, PPARγ and its agonists increase the cholesterol content of macrophages by the increased expression of genes involved in cholesterol biosynthesis (Iida et al. 2002).

3.5
Other Compounds

The ATP-sensitive potassium channel inhibitor glibenclamide is used for treating diabetes mellitus. Cell culture studies in macrophages indicate that glibenclamide may inhibit the accumulation of cellular cholesteryl ester by increasing the hydrolysis of cholesteryl ester as well as cholesterol efflux, and possibly by increasing the secretion of apolipoprotein E (Nobusawa et al. 2000). In an ACAT assay using CHO cells that overexpress ACAT-1 or ACAT-2, it was reported that glibenclamide also inhibits the activity of the two isozymes (Ohgami et al. 2000).

It has recently been reported that the fungal derivative beauveriolides have the ability to reduce lipid droplet accumulation in macrophages (Namatame et al. 2004). Beauveriolides I and III, isolated from the *Beauveria* sp. FO-6979, specifically inhibit the macrophage ACAT activity, resulting in the blockage of cholestery ester synthesis and leading to the reduction of lipid droplets in macrophages. ACAT activity in the membrane fractions prepared from mouse liver and Caco-2 cells was also inhibited, indicating that beauveriolides block both ACAT-1 and -2.

Another approach to the prevention of cardiovascular disease is currently recommended by ATP III: the management of the HDL level. In this regard, recent work by Nissen et al. (2003) provided the first evidence of the clinical benefit of an HDL mimetic on coronary artery disease. In a multicentre pilot trial, they studied the effect of infusion of apoA-I$_{Milano}$/phospholipid complexes on the atheroma burden in patients with acute coronary syndrome and discovered a significant regression of coronary atherosclerosis as measured by intravascular ultrasound. This effect may, at least in part, involve the increased ability of apoA-I$_{Milano}$ in reconstituted HDL to promote cholesterol efflux and to inhibit cholesterol esterification in macrophages in culture (Calabresi et al. 1999).

4
Modulation of Other Macrophage Functions

Numerous other macrophages functions have been shown to be a possible target for a pharmacological intervention (Table 3).

Table 3 Pharmacological modulation of other macrophage functions

Agents	Effect observed
Lipophilic statins	Inhibition of macrophage proliferation, TF expression, LDL oxidation, CD36 and type I scavenger receptor expression, adhesion molecule expression, MCP-1 expression
	Immusoppressive effects
PPARγ agonists	Inhibition of inflammatory cytokine production
	Increased expression of CD36
PPARδ agonists	Inhibition of MCP-1 production
LXR agonists	Inhibition of pro-inflammatory gene expression
Raloxifene	Inhibition of macrophage accumulation
MIF antibody	Inhibition of macrophage recruitment, shift towards a plaque with a more stable phenotype

TF, tissue factor; MCP-1, monocyte chemoattractant protein 1; MIF, macrophage migration inhibitory factor.

4.1
PPAR Agonists

PPARγ activation has been shown to possibly exert pro-inflammatory effects by increasing the expression of the type 2 scavenger receptor CD36 (Nagy et al. 1998), which could promote differentiation and foam cell formation of macrophages in atherosclerotic plaques (Tontonoz et al. 1998). It has recently been shown that pitavastatin prevents the OxLDL uptake by macrophages through PPARγ-dependent inhibition of CD36 expression, thus suggesting that pitavastatin may be able to modulate CD36-mediated atherosclerotic foam cell formation (Han et al. 2004).

However, Patel et al. (2002) contested that PPARγ plays a role in monocyte differentiation, and the PPARγ antagonist GW9662 was unable to reverse 15d-PGJ2 and all-*trans*-retinoic acid-induced CD36 expression in THP-1 monocytes.

Chawla et al. (2003) demonstrated that in macrophages VLDL functions as a transcriptional regulator via the activation of the nuclear receptor PPARδ. The signalling components of native VLDL are its triglycerides, whose activity is enhanced by lipoprotein lipase. Thus, these data show a pathway through which dietary triglycerides and VLDL can directly regulate gene expression in atherosclerotic lesions.

Lee et al. (2003) proposed that PPAR-δ controls the inflammatory status of macrophages and thus may be a good target for treating atherosclerosis. Although the overexpression or deletion of PPAR-δ in macrophages suggested that PPAR-δ is proinflammatory, treating macrophages with a synthetic PPAR-δ ligand had the opposite effect, decreasing the production of inflammatory molecules such as monocyte chemoattractant protein 1 (MCP-1). Lee et al.

(2003) postulated that the effect of PPAR-δ depends on whether it is bound or unbound to a ligand. In the absence of a ligand, PPAR-δ sequesters a transcriptional repressor of inflammatory responses, which leads to inflammation. In the presence of a ligand, PPAR-δ releases the repressor and sets it free to exert its anti-inflammatory effects.

Tontonoz and colleagues have established a link between infection, foam cell formation, and nuclear receptor activity (Castrillo et al. 2003b). They showed that treating macrophages with model pathogens leads to the activation of Toll-like receptors and blocks the activation of LXR. As a result, expression of the LXR-regulated cholesterol transporter ABCA1 is reduced, which increases the foam cell formation. These findings establish a new connection between pathogens and the way in which macrophages handle cholesterol.

4.2
LXR Agonists

Interestingly, LXRs may have functions overlapping with the ones of PPARs in the negative control of the inflammatory response. LXR agonists have been shown to inhibit the macrophage response to bacterial pathogens and to antagonize a number of pro-inflammatory genes in macrophages. These include iNOS, COX-2, IL-1β and IL-6, MMP-9 and chemokines such as MCP-1 and -3, macrophage inflammatory protein-1β, and IP-10 (Castrillo et al. 2003a; Joseph et al. 2003). Similar to what has been described for PPARγ, LXR antagonizes the NF-κB pathway through a mechanism that is not completely understood. LXR-deficient mice exhibited enhanced responses to inflammatory stimuli, and LXR ligands reduced inflammation in murine models of atherosclerosis (Ricote et al. 2004). These observations lead to the idea that LXR and PPAR agonists may exert their antiatherogenic effect not only by promoting cholesterol efflux, but also by limiting the production of inflammatory mediators in the arterial wall. PPARs and LXRs have emerged as key regulators of macrophage biology controlling transcriptional programs involved in macrophage lipid homeostasis and inflammatory response.

Using DNA array-based global gene expression profiling experiments in human primary macrophages, Chinetti et al. (2004) found that AdipoR2, one of the two recently identified receptors for adiponectin, an adipocyte-specific secreted hormone with anti-diabetic and anti-atherogenic activities, is induced by both PPARα and PPARγ. AdipoR1 and AdipoR2 are both present in human atherosclerotic lesions. AdipoR1 is more abundant in monocytes than AdipoR2, and its expression decreases upon differentiation into macrophages, whereas AdipoR2 remains constant. Interestingly, treatment with a synthetic LXR agonist induced the expression of both AdipoR1 and AdipoR2. Furthermore, co-incubation with a PPARα ligand and adiponectin resulted in an additive effect on the reduction of the macrophage cholesteryl ester content. In conclusion, AdipoR1 and AdipoR2 are expressed in human atherosclerotic lesions and macrophages and can be modulated by PPAR and LXR ligands, thus identifying a mechanism of crosstalk between adiponectin and these nuclear receptor signalling pathways (Chinetti et al. 2004).

Asada et al. (2004) have recently demonstrated a strong expression of PPARs messenger RNA and protein in freshly isolated human alveolar macrophages (AMs). Ligands of PPARγ significantly decreased LPS-induced TNF-α production by AM. These ligands markedly up-regulated the expression of CD36, a scavenger receptor that mediates the phagocytosis of apoptotic neutrophils. Indeed, ligand-treated AM ingested a significantly higher number of apoptotic neutrophils than untreated AM. These data indicate that PPARγ expressed by AM play an anti-inflammatory role by inhibiting the cytokine production and increasing their CD36 expression together with the enhanced phagocytosis of apoptotic neutrophils, which is an essential process for the resolution of inflammation. This suggests a potential therapeutic application of PPARγ ligands in inflammatory disorders of the lung.

4.3
Statins

4.3.1
Macrophage Proliferation

Macrophages proliferate in atheroma, and this phenomenon most probably plays an important role in the formation of macrophage-rich vulnerable plaques. Thus, the inhibition of macrophage proliferation may promote the stabilization of atheroma. It has been shown that cerivastatin, in a concentration achievable in patients, suppresses the proliferation and activation of macrophages (Aikawa et al. 2001) and thereby reduces the expression of MMPs and tissue factor in atheroma of rabbits. Thus, statin can reduce the growth of macrophages expressing proteolytic enzymes and a thrombogenic factor in atheroma of animals with endogenous hypercholesterolaemia (Aikawa et al. 2001).

4.3.2
Modulation of LDL Oxidation

Oxidative modification of LDL is a key step in the atherogenic process (Ross 1999). The proatherogenic effects of OxLDL include impairment of endothelial-dependent vasodilation through the inhibition of NOS activity (Laufs et al. 1998), proliferation and apoptosis of SMC (Bjorkerud and Bjorkerud 1996), tissue factor expression by monocytes (Broze 1992) and generation of an inflammatory response (Rosenson and Tangney 1998; Ross 1999).

Statins have been shown to reduce the enhanced susceptibility of LDL to oxidation both in vitro and in vivo (Aviram et al. 1998b; Hussein et al. 1997). In vitro studies showed a consistent dose-dependent antioxidant effect of statins on LDL oxidation (Girona et al. 1999; Suzumura et al. 1999). Indeed, statins prolonged the lag time of oxidation in the initiation step and decreased the rate of oxidation in the propagation step depending on the concentration. Several mechanisms may explain their antioxidant properties. First, statins bind to the phospholipid fraction of LDL, thereby preventing the diffusion of free radicals generated under oxidative stress into the lipoprotein core (Aviram et al. 1998a). Second, statins decrease the cell oxygen production. In macrophages, a reduction of superoxide formation and LDL oxidation was shown after cell treatment with simvastatin. This effect was prevented by the addition of mevalonate (Giroux et al. 1993). These authors suggested the involvement of prenylated proteins, probably belonging to the Rac family, in mediating the generation of superoxide by macrophages.

4.3.3
Effects on Inflammation

Monocyte and T lymphocyte adhesion to the endothelium and their subsequent transendothelial migration is an early event in atherogenesis (Ross 1999). Molecules associated with the migration of leukocytes across the endothelium, such as platelet-endothelial-cell adhesion molecules, act in conjunction with chemoattractant molecules generated by the endothelium, SMC, and monocytes, such as MCP-1, osteopontin, and modified LDL, to attract monocytes and T cells into the artery (Ross 1999). Inflammatory cytokines secreted by macrophages and T lymphocytes can modify endothelial functions, SMC proliferation, collagen degradation and thrombosis (Ross 1999). Statins may have a direct anti-inflammatory effect on monocytes and macrophages through, for example, a decreased expression of intracellular adhesion molecule-1 by endothelial cells, an effect that was completely reversed by the addition of mevalonate (Niwa et al. 1996). This effect of statins may be mediated through a decrease in the expression of the OxLDL receptor on monocytes (Draude et al. 1999; Han et al. 2004). Moreover, statins suppress the LPS-induced secretion of IL-6 and IL-8, but not IL-1β, by activated monocytes in vitro (Comparato et al. 2001). The addition of mevalonate prevents the attenuation of IL-8 production by lovastatin.

More recently, Romano investigated the effect of different statins on the in vitro and in vivo production of MCP-1 (Romano et al. 2000). The in vitro findings showed that statins are able to induce a dose-dependent inhibition of MCP-1 production in peripheral blood mononuclear cells.

Finally, Mach demonstrated that statins inhibit the expression of major histocompatibility class II (MHC II) antigens by primary human macrophages and endothelial cells in response to interferon-γ (Kwak et al. 2000). This suggests that the immunosuppressive activity of statins may greatly contribute to the beneficial effect exerted by these drugs in cardiac transplant patients (Kwak et al. 2000, Palinski 2000).

Evidence has been provided that statins suppress the expression and function of leukocyte cell surface molecules, such as the integrin heterodimer CD11b/CD18, required for monocytes to adhere to endothelial monolayers. In fact, human blood monocytes isolated from statin-treated hypercholesterolaemic patients showed reduced CD11b surface expression and adhesion to the endothelium (Weber et al. 1997).

4.3.4
Macrophage Migration

Macrophage migration inhibitory factor (MIF) is a pleiotropic macrophage and T-cell cytokine, endocrine factor, and enzyme that controls cell-mediated inflammatory responses by affecting monocyte and T-cell recruitment (Schober et al. 2004). The inhibition of the random migration of macrophages has been described as one of the first activities of MIF. MIF enhances proinflammatory functions of macrophages when externally administered or endogenously expressed by macrophages. Up-regulation of MIF has been observed in endothelial cells, SMCs, and macrophages during the progression of atherosclerotic plaques in humans and in a hypercholesterolaemic rabbit model. Neutralizing MIF with a monoclonal antibody resulted in a marked reduction of neointimal macrophages and inhibited the transformation of macrophages into foam cells (Schober et al. 2004), although serum levels of the cytokines IL-2, IL-4, IL-6, IL-10, and TNF-α were increased in MIF monoclonal antibody-treated mice (Schober et al. 2004). Inhibition of MIF resulted in a shift in the cellular composition of neointimal plaques toward a stabilized phenotype with reduced macrophage/foam cell and increased SMC content. Total plaque size, however, was not significantly changed by the MIF blockade, probably as a result of the marked increase in neointimal SMC and collagen type I content (Schober et al. 2004).

4.3.5
Modulation of Tissue Factor Expression

Tissue factor (TF) plays a prominent role as the initiator of the extrinsic coagulation pathway and has been localized in lipid-enriched macrophages of human atherosclerotic plaque (Wilcox et al. 1989). It has been shown that lipophylic statins (simvastatin, fluvastatin) decreased the TF expression and activity in cultured human monocyte-derived macrophages (Colli et al. 1997). This effect was prevented by the addition of mevalonate and all-*trans*-geranylgeraniol, thus suggesting a role of the mevalonate pathway in regulating TF activity. Moreover, a recent study showed a dose-dependent inhibition of the rate of thrombin generation and of TF expression by simvastatin in LPS-stimulated monocytes, suggesting that simvastatin inhibits the rate of thrombin generation by directly interfering with the monocyte expression of TF (Ferro et al. 2000). It has recently been confirmed that cerivastatin treatment of Watanabe heritable hyperlipidaemic rabbits diminished the accumulation of macrophages in aortic atheroma and decreased the expression of MMPs and TF, prominent sources of molecules responsible for plaque instability and thrombogenicity (Aikawa et al. 2001).

5
Conclusion

Atherosclerotic lesions that are most often implicated in acute coronary events have a soft, lipid-laden core and an excess of macrophages within the thin fibrous cap, which makes them prone to fissuring/rupture. In the future, the prevention of cardiovascular disease will involve not only the correction of risk factors but also the direct pharmacological control of the processes occurring in the arterial wall. Agents able to modulate macrophage functions involved in plaque stability and atherothrombotic processes will be of particular importance.

Acknowledgements Supported partially by grant no. QLG1-1999-01007 from the European Commission to the consortium 'Macrophage Function and Stability of the Atherosclerotic Plaque (MAFAPS)' as part of the Fifth Framework Programme of the European Union.

References

4SInvestigators (1994) Randomised trial of cholesterol lowering in 4444 patients with coronary heart disease: the Scandinavian Simvastatin Survival Study (4S). Lancet 344:1383–1389

Aikawa M, Rabkin E, Sugiyama S, Voglic SJ, Fukumoto Y, Furukawa Y, Shiomi M, Schoen FJ, Libby P (2001) An HMG-CoA reductase inhibitor, cerivastatin, suppresses growth of macrophages expressing matrix metalloproteinases and tissue factor in vivo and in vitro. Circulation 103:276–283

Asada K, Sasaki S, Suda T, Chida K, Nakamura H (2004) Antiinflammatory roles of peroxisome proliferator-activated receptor gamma in human alveolar macrophages. Am J Respir Crit Care Med 169:195–200

Aviram M, Dankner G, Cogan U, Hochgraf E, Brook JG (1992) Lovastatin inhibits low-density lipoprotein oxidation and alters its fluidity and uptake by macrophages: in vitro and in vivo studies. Metabolism 41:229–235

Aviram M, Hussein O, Rosenblat M, Schlezinger S, Hayek T, Keidar S (1998a) Interactions of platelets, macrophages, and lipoproteins in hypercholesterolaemia: antiatherogenic effects of HMG-CoA reductase inhibitor therapy. J Cardiovasc Pharmacol 31:39–45

Aviram M, Rosenblat M, Bisgaier CL, Newton RS (1998b) Atorvastatin and gemfibrozil metabolites, but not the parent drugs, are potent antioxidants against lipoprotein oxidation. Atherosclerosis 138:271–280

Baetta R, Comparato C, Altana C, Canavesi M, Monetti M, Eberini I, Puglisi L, Corsini A, Bellosta S (2001) Raloxifene reduces macrophage accumulation and matrix metalloproteinase expression in carotid lesions of ovariectomized, cholesterol-fed rabbits. Abstract. Circulation (Suppl II) 104:11–67

Bellosta S, Bernini F (2000) Lipophilic calcium antagonists in antiatherosclerotic therapy. Curr Atheroscler Rep 2:76–81

Bellosta S, Via D, Canavesi M, Pfister P, Fumagalli R, Paoletti R, Bernini F (1998) HMG-CoA reductase inhibitors reduce MMP-9 secretion by macrophages. Arterioscler Thromb Vasc Biol 18:1671–1678

Bellosta S, Ferri N, Bernini F, Paoletti R, Corsini A (2000) Non-lipid-related effects of statins. Ann Med 32:164–176

Bellosta S, Canavesi M, Favari E, Cominacini L, Gaviraghi G, Fumagalli R, Paoletti R, Bernini F (2001) Lacidipine [correction of Lalsoacidipine] modulates the secretion of matrix metalloproteinase-9 by human macrophages. J Pharmacol Exp Ther 296:736–743

Bellosta S, Dell'Agli M, Canavesi M, Mitro N, Monetti M, Crestani M, Verotta L, Fuzzati N, Bernini F, Bosisio E (2003) Inhibition of metalloproteinase-9 activity and gene expression by polyphenolic compounds isolated from the bark of Tristaniopsis calobuxus (Myrtaceae). Cell Mol Life Sci 60:1440–1448

Bernini F, Catapano AL, Corsini A, Fumagalli R, Paoletti R (1989) Effects of calcium antagonists on lipids and atherosclerosis. Am J Cardiol 64:129I–133I; discussion 133I–134I

Bernini F, Didoni G, Bonfadini G, Bellosta S, Fumagalli R (1993) Requirement for mevalonate in acetylated LDL induction of cholesterol esterification in macrophages. Atherosclerosis 104:19–26

Bernini F, Canavesi M, Bernardini E, Scurati N, Bellosta S, Fumagalli R (1997) Effect of lacidipine on cholesterol esterification: in vivo and in vitro studies. Br J Pharmacol 122:1209–1215

Birkedal-Hansen H, Moore WG, Bodden MK, Windsor LJ, Birkedal-Hansen B, DeCarlo A, Engler JA (1993) Matrix metalloproteinases: a review. Crit Rev Oral Biol Med 4:197–250

Bjarnason NH, Haarbo J, Byrjalsen I, Kauffman RF, Christiansen C (1997) Raloxifene inhibits aortic accumulation of cholesterol in ovariectomized, cholesterol-fed rabbits. Circulation 96:1964–1969

Bjorkerud B, Bjorkerud S (1996) Contrary effects of lightly and strongly Oxidized LDL with potent promotion of growth versus apoptosis on arterial smooth muscle cells, macrophages, and fibroblasts. Arterioscler Thromb Vasc Biol 16:416–424

Bottalico LA, Wager RE, Agellon LB, Assoian RK, Tabas I (1991) Transforming growth factor-beta 1 inhibits scavenger receptor activity in THP-1 human macrophages. J Biol Chem 266:22866–22871

Brown MS, Goldstein JL, Krieger M, Ho YK, Anderson RG (1979) Reversible accumulation of cholesteryl esters in macrophages incubated with acetylated lipoproteins. J Cell Biol 82:597–613

Brown MS, Ho YK, Goldstein JL (1980) The cholesteryl ester cycle in macrophage foam cells. Continual hydrolysis and re-esterification of cytoplasmic cholesteryl esters. J Biol Chem 255:9344–9352

Brown BG, Zhao XQ, Sacco DE, Albers JJ (1993) Arteriographic view of treatment to achieve regression of coronary atherosclerosis and to prevent plaque disruption and clinical cardiovascular events. Br Heart J 69:S48–S53

Brown DL, Hibbs MS, Kearney M, Loushin C, Isner JM (1995) Identification of 92-kD gelatinase in human coronary atherosclerotic lesions. Association of active enzyme synthesis with unstable angina. Circulation 91:2125–31

Broze GJ, Jr. (1992) The role of tissue factor pathway inhibitor in a revised coagulation cascade. Semin Hematol 29:159–169

Butler JD, Blanchette-Mackie J, Goldin E, O'Neill RR, Carstea G, Roff CF, Patterson MC, Patel S, Comly ME, Cooney A, et al. (1992) Progesterone blocks cholesterol translocation from lysosomes. J Biol Chem 267:23797–23805

Calabresi L, Canavesi M, Bernini F, Franceschini G (1999) Cell cholesterol efflux to reconstituted high-density lipoproteins containing the apolipoprotein A-IMilano dimer. Biochemistry 38:16307–16314

Castrillo A, Joseph SB, Marathe C, Mangelsdorf DJ, Tontonoz P (2003a) Liver X receptor-dependent repression of matrix metalloproteinase-9 expression in macrophages. J Biol Chem 278:10443–10449

Castrillo A, Joseph SB, Vaidya SA, Haberland M, Fogelman AM, Cheng G, Tontonoz P (2003b) Crosstalk between LXR and toll-like receptor signaling mediates bacterial and viral antagonism of cholesterol metabolism. Mol Cell 12:805–816

Chase AJ, Bond M, Crook MF, Newby AC (2002) Role of nuclear factor-kappa B activation in metalloproteinase-1, -3, and -9 secretion by human macrophages in vitro and rabbit foam cells produced in vivo. Arterioscler Thromb Vasc Biol 22:765–771

Chawla A, Lee C-H, Barak Y, He W, Rosenfeld J, Liao D, Han J, Kang H, Evans RM (2003) PPARdelta is a very low-density lipoprotein sensor in macrophages. Proc Natl Acad Sci USA 100:1268–1273

Chinetti G, Griglio S, Antonucci M, Torra IP, Delerive P, Majd Z, Fruchart JC, Chapman J, Najib J, Staels B (1998) Activation of proliferator-activated receptors alpha and gamma induces apoptosis of human monocyte-derived macrophages. J Biol Chem 273:25573–25580

Chinetti G, Zawadski C, Fruchart JC, Staels B (2004) Expression of adiponectin receptors in human macrophages and regulation by agonists of the nuclear receptors PPARalpha, PPARgamma, and LXR. Biochem Biophys Res Commun 314:151–158

Cignarella A, Brennhausen B, von Eckardstein A, Assmann G, Cullen P (1998) Differential effects of lovastatin on the trafficking of endogenous and lipoprotein-derived cholesterol in human monocyte-derived macrophages. Arterioscler Thromb Vasc Biol 18:1322–1329

Colli S, Eligini S, Lalli M, Camera M, Paoletti R, Tremoli E (1997) Vastatins inhibit tissue factor in cultured human macrophages. A novel mechanism of protection against atherothrombosis. Arterioscler Thromb Vasc Biol 17:265–272

Comparato C, Altana C, Bellosta S, Baetta R, Paoletti R, Corsini A (2001) Clinically relevant pleiotropic effects of statins: drug properties or effects of profound cholesterol reduction? Nutr Metab Cardiovasc Dis 11:328–343

Daugherty A, Rateri DL, Schonfeld G, Sobel BE (1987) Inhibition of cholesteryl ester deposition in macrophages by calcium entry blockers: an effect dissociable from calcium entry blockade. Br J Pharmacol 91:113–118

Draude G, Hrboticky N, Lorenz RL (1999) The expression of the lectin-like oxidized low-density lipoprotein receptor (LOX-1) on human vascular smooth muscle cells and monocytes and its down-regulation by lovastatin. Biochem Pharmacol 57:383–386

Eberhardt W, Akool el S, Rebhan J, Frank S, Beck KF, Franzen R, Hamada FM, Pfeilschifter J (2002) Inhibition of cytokine-induced matrix metalloproteinase 9 expression by peroxisome proliferator-activated receptor alpha agonists is indirect and due to a NO-mediated reduction of mRNA stability. J Biol Chem 277:33518–33528

Falk E, Shah PK, Fuster V (1995) Coronary plaque disruption. Circulation 92:657–671

Ferro D, Basili S, Alessandri C, Cara D, Violi F (2000) Inhibition of tissue-factor-mediated thrombin generation by simvastatin. Atherosclerosis 149:111–116

Figtree GA, Lu Y, Webb CM, Collins P (1999) Raloxifene acutely relaxes rabbit coronary arteries in vitro by an estrogen receptor-dependent and nitric oxide-dependent mechanism. Circulation 100:1095–1101

Fruchart JC, Duriez P, Staels B (1999) Peroxisome proliferator-activated receptor-alpha activators regulate genes governing lipoprotein metabolism, vascular inflammation and atherosclerosis. Curr Opin Lipidol 10:245–257

Galis ZS, Asanuma K, Godin D, Meng X (1998) N-acetyl-cysteine decreases the matrix-degrading capacity of macrophage-derived foam cells: new target for antioxidant therapy? Circulation 97:2445–2453

Geng YJ, Hansson GK (1992) Interferon-gamma inhibits scavenger receptor expression and foam cell formation in human monocyte-derived macrophages. J Clin Invest 89:1322–1330

Girona J, La Ville AE, Sola R, Plana N, Masana L (1999) Simvastatin decreases aldehyde production derived from lipoprotein oxidation. Am J Cardiol 83:846–851

Giroux LM, Davignon J, Naruszewicz M (1993) Simvastatin inhibits the oxidation of low-density lipoproteins by activated human monocyte-derived macrophages. Biochim Biophys Acta 1165:335–338

Glass CK, Rosenfeld MG (2000) The coregulator exchange in transcriptional functions of nuclear receptors. Genes Dev 14:121–141

Goldstein JL, Ho YK, Brown MS, Innerarity TL, Mahley RW (1980) Cholesteryl ester accumulation in macrophages resulting from receptor-mediated uptake and degradation of hypercholesterolemic canine beta-very low density lipoproteins. J Biol Chem 255:1839–1848

Han J, Zhou X, Yokoyama T, Hajjar D, Gotto AMJ, Nicholson AC (2004) Pitavastatin down-regulates expression of the macrophage type B scavenger receptor, CD36. Circulation 109:790–796

Hayek T, Kaplan M, Raz A, Keidar S, Coleman R, Aviram M (2002) Ramipril administration to atherosclerotic mice reduces oxidized low-density lipoprotein uptake by their macrophages and blocks the progression of atherosclerosis. Atherosclerosis 161:65–74

Herbette LG, Rhodes DG, Mason RP (1991) New approaches to drug design and delivery based on drug-membrane interactions. Drug Des Deliv 7:75–118

Herbette LG, Gaviraghi G, Tulenko T, Mason RP (1993) Molecular interaction between lacidipine and biological membranes. J Hypertens Suppl 11:S13–S19

Hussein O, Schlezinger S, Rosenblat M, Keidar S, Aviram M (1997) Reduced susceptibility of low density lipoprotein (LDL) to lipid peroxidation after fluvastatin therapy is associated with the hypocholesterolemic effect of the drug and its binding to the LDL. Atherosclerosis 128:11–18

Iida KT, Kawakami Y, Suzuki H, Sone H, Shimano H, Toyoshima H, Okuda Y, Yamada N (2002) PPAR gamma ligands, troglitazone and pioglitazone, up-regulate expression of HMG-CoA synthase and HMG-CoA reductase gene in THP-1 macrophages. FEBS Lett 520:177–181

Ikeda U, Shimpo M, Ohki R, Inaba H, Takahashi M, Yamamoto K, Shimada K (2000) Fluvastatin inhibits matrix metalloproteinase-1 expression in human vascular endothelial cells. Hypertension 36:325–329

Itabe H (2003) Oxidized low-density lipoproteins: what is understood and what remains to be clarified. Biol Pharm Bull 26:1–9

Jiang C, Ting AT, Seed B (1998) PPAR-gamma agonists inhibit production of monocyte inflammatory cytokines. Nature 391:82–86

Joseph SB, Castrillo A, Laffitte BA, Mangelsdorf DJ, Tontonoz P (2003) Reciprocal regulation of inflammation and lipid metabolism by liver X receptors. Nat Med 9:213–219

Kellner-Weibel G, Geng YJ, Rothblat GH (1999) Cytotoxic cholesterol is generated by the hydrolysis of cytoplasmic cholesteryl ester and transported to the plasma membrane. Atherosclerosis 146:309–319

Kempen HJ, Vermeer M, de Wit E, Havekes LM (1991) Vastatins inhibit cholesterol ester accumulation in human monocyte-derived macrophages. Arterioscler Thromb 11:146–153

Kohn EC, Jacobs W, Kim YS, Alessandro R, Stetler-Stevenson WG, Liotta LA (1994) Calcium influx modulates expression of matrix metalloproteinase-2 (72-kDa type IV collagenase, gelatinase A). J Biol Chem 269:21505–21511

Kwak B, Mulhaupt F, Myit S, Mach F (2000) Statins as a newly recognized type of immunomodulator. Nat Med 6:1399–1402

Laufs U, La Fata V, Plutzky J, Liao JK (1998) Upregulation of endothelial nitric oxide synthase by HMG CoA reductase inhibitors. Circulation 97:1129–1135

Lee CH, Chawla A, Urbiztondo N, Liao D, Boisvert WA, Evans RM, Curtiss LK (2003) Transcriptional repression of atherogenic inflammation: modulation by PPARdelta. Science 302:453–457

Lesnik P, Dachet C, Petit L, Moreau M, Griglio S, Brudi P, Chapman MJ (1997) Impact of a combination of a calcium antagonist and a beta-blocker on cell- and copper-mediated oxidation of LDL and on the accumulation and efflux of cholesterol in human macrophages and murine J774 cells. Arterioscler Thromb Vasc Biol 17:979–988

Libby P (1995) Molecular bases of the acute coronary syndromes. Circulation 91:2844–2850

Libby P, Aikawa M (2002) Stabilization of atherosclerotic plaques: new mechanisms and clinical targets. Nat Med 8:1257–1262

Liscum L, Faust JR (1989) The intracellular transport of low density lipoprotein-derived cholesterol is inhibited in Chinese hamster ovary cells cultured with 3-beta-[2-(diethylamino)ethoxy]androst-5-en-17-one. J Biol Chem 264:11796–11806

Llaverias G, Jove M, Vazquez-Carrera M, Sanchez RM, Diaz C, Hernandez G, Laguna JC, Alegret M (2002) Avasimibe and atorvastatin synergistically reduce cholesteryl ester content in THP-1 macrophages. Eur J Pharmacol 451:11–17

Lohi J, Keski-Oja J (1995) Calcium ionophores decrease pericellular gelatinolytic activity via inhibition of 92-kDa gelatinase expression and decrease of 72-kDa gelatinase activation. J Biol Chem 270:17602–17609

Luan Z, Chase AJ, Newby AC (2003) Statins inhibit secretion of metalloproteinases-1, -2, -3, and −9 from vascular smooth muscle cells and macrophages. Arterioscler Thromb Vasc Biol 23:769–775

Lund EG, Menke JG, Sparrow CP (2003) Liver X receptor agonists as potential therapeutic agents for dyslipidaemia and atherosclerosis. Arterioscler Thromb Vasc Biol 23:1169–1177

Marx N, Sukhova G, Murphy C, Libby P, Plutzky J (1998) Macrophages in human atheroma contain PPARgamma: differentiation-dependent peroxisomal proliferator-activated receptor gamma(PPARgamma) expression and reduction of MMP-9 activity through PPARgamma activation in mononuclear phagocytes in vitro. Am J Pathol 153:17–23

Massova I, Kotra LP, Fridman R, Mobashery S (1998) Matrix metalloproteinases: structures, evolution, and diversification. Faseb J 12:1075–1095

Matrisian LM (1994) Matrix metalloproteinase gene expression. Ann N Y Acad Sci 732:42–50

Mendelsohn ME, Karas RH (1999) The protective effects of estrogen on the cardiovascular system. N Engl J Med 340:1801–1811

Nagy L, Tontonoz P, Alvarez JG, Chen H, Evans RM (1998) Oxidized LDL regulates macrophage gene expression through ligand activation of PPARgamma. Cell 93:229–240

Namatame I, Tomoda H, Ishibashi S, Omura S (2004) Antiatherogenic activity of fungal beauveriolides, inhibitors of lipid droplet accumulation in macrophages. Proc Natl Acad Sci USA 101:737–742

Nathan L, Pervin S, Singh R, Rosenfeld M, Chaudhuri G (1999) Estradiol inhibits leukocyte adhesion and transendothelial migration in rabbits in vivo: possible mechanisms for gender differences in atherosclerosis. Circ Res 85:377–385

Newman KM, Ogata Y, Malon AM, Irizarry E, Gandhi RH, Nagase H, Tilson MD (1994) Identification of matrix metalloproteinases 3 (stromelysin-1) and 9 (gelatinase B) in abdominal aortic aneurysm. Arterioscler Thromb 14:1315–1320

Nissen SE, Tsunoda T, Tuzcu EM, Schoenhagen P, Cooper CJ, Yasin M, Eaton GM, Lauer MA, Sheldon WS, Grines CL, Halpern S, Crowe T, Blankenship JC, Kerensky R (2003) Effect of recombinant ApoA-I Milano on coronary atherosclerosis in patients with acute coronary syndromes: a randomized controlled trial. JAMA 290:2292–2300

Niwa S, Totsuka T, Hayashi S (1996) Inhibitory effect of fluvastatin, an HMG-CoA reductase inhibitor, on the expression of adhesion molecules on human monocyte cell line. Int J Immunopharmacol 18:669–675

Nobusawa A, Taniguchi T, Fujioka Y, Inoue H, Shimizu H, Ishikawa Y, Yokoyama M (2000) Glibenclamide inhibits accumulation of cholesteryl ester in THP-1 human macrophages. J Cardiovasc Pharmacol 36:101–108

Ohgami N, Kuniyasu A, Furukawa K, Miyazaki A, Hakamata H, Horiuchi S, Nakayama H (2000) Glibenclamide acts as an inhibitor of acyl-CoA:cholesterol acyltransferase enzyme. Biochem Biophys Res Commun 277:417–422

Palinski W (2000) Immunomodulation: a new role for statins? Nat Med 6:1311–1312

Patel L, Charlton SJ, Marshall IC, Moore GB, Coxon P, Moores K, Clapham JC, Newman SJ, Smith SA, Macphee CH (2002) PPARgamma is not a critical mediator of primary monocyte differentiation or foam cell formation. Biochem Biophys Res Commun 290:707–712

Rabbani R, Topol EJ (1999) Strategies to achieve coronary arterial plaque stabilization. Cardiovasc Res 41:402–417

Rajagopalan S, Meng XP, Ramasamy S, Harrison DG, Galis ZS (1996) Reactive oxygen species produced by macrophage-derived foam cells regulate the activity of vascular matrix metalloproteinases in vitro. Implications for atherosclerotic plaque stability. J Clin Invest 98:2572–2579

Ricote M, Huang J, Fajas L, Li A, Welch J, Najib J, Witztum JL, Auwerx J, Palinski W, Glass CK (1998a) Expression of the peroxisome proliferator-activated receptor gamma (PPARgamma) in human atherosclerosis and regulation in macrophages by colony stimulating factors and oxidized low density lipoprotein. Proc Natl Acad Sci USA 95:7614–7619

Ricote M, Li AC, Willson TM, Kelly CJ, Glass CK (1998b) The peroxisome proliferator-activated receptor-gamma is a negative regulator of macrophage activation. Nature 391:79–82

Ricote M, Huang JT, Welch JS, Glass CK (1999) The peroxisome proliferator-activated receptor(PPARgamma) as a regulator of monocyte/macrophage function. J Leukoc Biol 66:733–739

Ricote M, Valledor AF, Glass CK (2004) Decoding transcriptional programs regulated by PPARs and LXRs in the macrophage: effects on lipid homeostasis, inflammation, and atherosclerosis. Arterioscler Thromb Vasc Biol 24:230–239

Rodriguez A, Usher DC (2002) Anti-atherogenic effects of the acyl-CoA:cholesterol acyltransferase inhibitor, avasimibe (CI-1011), in cultured primary human macrophages. Atherosclerosis 161:45–54

Romano M, Diomede L, Sironi M, Massimiliano L, Sottocorno M, Polentarutti N, Gugliel-
motti A, Albani D, Bruno A, Fruscella P, Salmona M, Vecchi A, Pinza M, Mantovani A
(2000) Inhibition of monocyte chemotactic protein-1 synthesis by statins. Lab Invest
80:1095–1100

Rosenson RS, Tangney CC (1998) Antiatherothrombotic properties of statins: implications
for cardiovascular event reduction. JAMA 279:1643–1650

Ross R (1999) Atherosclerosis–an inflammatory disease. N Engl J Med 340:115–126

Roth M, Eickelberg O, Kohler E, Erne P, Block LH (1996) Ca2+ channel blockers modulate
metabolism of collagens within the extracellular matrix. Proc Natl Acad Sci USA 93:5478–
5482

Sakr SW, Williams DL, Stoudt GW, Phillips MC, Rothblat GH (1999) Induction of cellular cholesterol efflux to lipid-free apolipoprotein A-I by cAMP. Biochim Biophys Acta
1438:85–98

Schober A, Bernhagen J, Thiele M, Zeiffer U, Knarren S, Roller M, Bucala R, Weber C (2004)
Stabilization of atherosclerotic plaques by blockade of macrophage migration inhibitory
factor after vascular injury in apolipoprotein E-deficient mice. Circulation 109:380–385

Schroen DJ, Brinckerhoff CE (1996) Nuclear hormone receptors inhibit matrix metalloproteinase (MMP) gene expression through diverse mechanisms. Gene Expr 6:197–207

Seabra MC, Brown MS, Goldstein JL (1993) Retinal degeneration in choroideraemia: deficiency of rab geranylgeranyl transferase. Science 259:377–381

Shepherd J, Cobbe SM, Ford I, Isles CG, Lorimer AR, MacFarlane PW, McKillop JH, Packard
CJ (1995) Prevention of coronary heart disease with pravastatin in men with hypercholesterolemia. West of Scotland Coronary Prevention Study Group. N Engl J Med
333:1301–1307

Shu H, Wong B, Zhou G, Li Y, Berger J, Woods JW, Wright SD, Cai TQ (2000) Activation of
PPARalpha or gamma reduces secretion of matrix metalloproteinase 9 but not interleukin
8 from human monocytic THP-1 cells. Biochem Biophys Res Commun 267:345–349

Simoncini T, Genazzani AR (2000) Raloxifene acutely stimulates nitric oxide release from
human endothelial cells via an activation of endothelial nitric oxide synthase. J Clin
Endocrinol Metab 85:2966–2969

Sliskovic DR, White AD (1991) Therapeutic potential of ACAT inhibitors as lipid lowering
and anti-atherosclerotic agents. Trends Pharmacol Sci 12:194–199

Spector AA, Mathur SN, Kaduce TL (1979) Role of acylcoenzyme A: cholesterol o-acyltransferase in cholesterol metabolism. Prog Lipid Res 18:31–53

Staels B, Dallongeville J, Auwerx J, Schoonjans K, Leitersdorf E, Fruchart JC (1998) Mechanism of action of fibrates on lipid and lipoprotein metabolism. Circulation 98:2088–2093

Stein O, Stein Y (1987) Effect of verapamil on cholesteryl ester hydrolysis and reesterification
in macrophages. Arteriosclerosis 7:578–584

Suckling KE, Stange EF (1985) Role of acyl-CoA: cholesterol acyltransferase in cellular
cholesterol metabolism. J Lipid Res 26:647–671

Suzumura K, Yasuhara M, Tanaka K, Suzuki T (1999) Protective effect of fluvastatin sodium
(XU-62-320), a 3-hydroxy-3-methylglutaryl coenzyme A (HMG-CoA) reductase in-
hibitor, on oxidative modification of human low-density lipoprotein in vitro. Biochem
Pharmacol 57:697–703

Tabas I, Rosoff WJ, Boykow GC (1988) Acyl coenzyme A:cholesterol acyl transferase in
macrophages utilizes a cellular pool of cholesterol oxidase-accessible cholesterol as
substrate. J Biol Chem 263:1266–1272

Takemoto M, Liao JK (2001) Pleiotropic effects of 3-hydroxy-3-methylglutaryl coenzyme
a reductase inhibitors. Arterioscler Thromb Vasc Biol 21:1712–1719

Tontonoz P, Nagy L, Alvarez JG, Thomazy VA, Evans RM (1998) PPARgamma promotes monocyte/macrophage differentiation and uptake of oxidized LDL. Cell 93:241–252

Tsujita M, Yokoyama S (1996) Selective inhibition of free apolipoprotein-mediated cellular lipid efflux by probucol. Biochemistry 35:13011–13020

Umetani N, Kanayama Y, Okamura M, Negoro N, Takeda T (1996) Lovastatin inhibits gene expression of type-I scavenger receptor in THP-1 human macrophages. Biochim Biophys Acta 1303:199–206

Vainio S, Ikonen E (2003) Macrophage cholesterol transport: a critical player in foam cell formation. Ann Med 35:146–155

Weber C, Erl W, Weber KS, Weber PC (1997) HMG-CoA reductase inhibitors decrease CD11b expression and CD11b-dependent adhesion of monocytes to endothelium and reduce increased adhesiveness of monocytes isolated from patients with hypercholesterolemia. J Am Coll Cardiol 30:1212–1217

Whittaker M, Floyd CD, Brown P, Gearing AJ (2001) Design and therapeutic application of matrix metalloproteinase inhibitors. Chem Rev 101:2205–2206

Wilcox JN, Smith KM, Schwartz SM, Gordon D (1989) Localization of tissue factor in the normal vessel wall and in the atherosclerotic plaque. Proc Natl Acad Sci USA 86:2839–2843

Willson TM, Cobb JE, Cowan DJ, Wiethe RW, Correa ID, Prakash SR, Beck KD, Moore LB, Kliewer SA, Lehmann JM (1996) The structure-activity relationship between peroxisome proliferator-activated receptor gamma agonism and the antihyperglycemic activity of thiazolidinediones. J Med Chem 39:665–668

Wong B, Lumma WC, Smith AM, Sisko JT, Wright SD, Cai TQ (2001) Statins suppress THP-1 cell migration and secretion of matrix metalloproteinase 9 by inhibiting geranylgeranylation. J Leukoc Biol 69:959–962

Worley JR, Baugh MD, Hughes DA, Edwards DR, Hogan A, Sampson MJ, Gavrilovic J (2003) Metalloproteinase expression in PMA-stimulated THP-1 cells. Effects of peroxisome proliferator-activated receptor-gamma (PPAR gamma) agonists and 9-cis-retinoic acid. J Biol Chem 278:51340–51346

Xu XX, Tabas I (1991) Lipoproteins activate acyl-coenzyme A:cholesterol acyltransferase in macrophages only after cellular cholesterol pools are expanded to a critical threshold level. J Biol Chem 266:17040–17048

Zaltsman AB, George SJ, Newby AC (1999) Increased secretion of tissue inhibitors of metalloproteinases 1 and 2 from the aortas of cholesterol fed rabbits partially counterbalances increased metalloproteinase activity. Arterioscler Thromb Vasc Biol 19:1700–1707

Zerial M, Stenmark H (1993) Rab GTPases in vesicular transport. Curr Opin Cell Biol 5:613–620

Zhang FL, Casey PJ (1996) Protein prenylation: molecular mechanisms and functional consequences. Annu Rev Biochem 65:241–269

HEP (2005) 170:697–722

Inflammation Is a Crucial Feature of Atherosclerosis and a Potential Target to Reduce Cardiovascular Events

F. Mach

Division of Cardiology, Department of Medicine, University Hospital Geneva,
24 Rue Micheli-du-Crest, 1211 Geneva 4, Switzerland
francois.mach@medecine.unige.ch

Abstract Contrary to popular opinion, atherosclerosis is not a disease unique to modern civilization. In fact, atherosclerotic lesions have been found in the arteries of mummies dating back to 1,500 B.C., and yet our understanding of this complex process is still evolving. A fusion of basic science advances and clinical research findings has radically altered our traditional concepts about the pathogenesis and treatment of the clinical complications of atherosclerosis. Most physicians previously regarded the artery as a being merely a blood conduit that became encrusted with lipid detritus as part of the aging process. Modern-day treatment of atherosclerosis has arisen primarily from an understanding of the epidemiology of the disease rather than its pathophysiology, in that risk factors have traditionally been targeted. Our concepts of atherogenesis have evolved from vague ideas of inevitable degeneration to a much better defined scenario of molecular and cellular events. As we enhance our understanding of its fundamental mechanism, we can begin to approach atherogenesis as a modifiable rather than ineluctable process. Indeed, as we recognize now that inflammation plays a pivotal role in the process of atherosclerosis, it is noteworthy to evaluate the effect of modern therapies on this facet of the disease.

Keywords Atherosclerosis · Inflammation · Treatment

1
Introduction

Health trends in the next 25 years will be determined by the aging of the world's population, the decline in age-specific mortality rates from communicable, maternal, perinatal, and nutritional disorders, the spread of HIV, and the increase in tobacco-related mortality and disability. Today, ischemic heart disease is the leading cause of death in developed countries with more than 3 million deaths per year, followed by stroke (1.6 million) and lung cancer (0.7 million) (Lopez and Murray 1998; Morrow et al. 1998). By 2020, based on current trends, ischemic disease will be the leading cause of disease burden worldwide, followed by unipolar major depression, road traffic accidents, stroke and chronic obstructive lung disease. For worldwide ischemic disease only, the number of disability-adjusted life years estimated for 2020 is about 82.3 million per year (Murray and Lopez 1996). Thus, despite changes in lifestyle and the use of new pharmacological approaches, atherosclerosis and its devastating clinical complications such as ischemia and infarction of the heart, the brain and other vital organs, ruptured aortic aneurysm and peripheral vascular insufficiency, continue to account for the majority of mortality and morbidity in the adult population of industrialized countries, and would be so worldwide by 2020 (Morrow et al. 1998).

Not long ago, most physicians envisaged atheroma as an inert collection of cholesterol, calcium, and fibrous tissue that grew steadily and ineluctably until it eventually obstructed an artery and impeded blood flow. When atherosclerosis was viewed as a 'plumbing' problem, mechanical means such as bypass surgery or percutaneous intervention seemed the most appropriate therapeutic approach. Atherosclerosis is a progressive disease process that generally begins in childhood and has clinical manifestations in middle to late adulthood (Stary 1990, 1994, 2000). Atherosclerosis is characterized by the accumulation of lipids, inflammatory cells and fibrous elements in the large arteries. The link between lipids and atherosclerosis dominated our thinking until the 1970s, based on strong experimental and clinical relationships between hypercholesterolemia and atheroma. The emerging knowledge of vascular biology led to a focus on growth factors and the proliferation of smooth muscle cells in the 1970s and 1980s.

Over the past few years the picture has evolved considerably, as clinical and pathological insights have pointed the way for rethinking atherogenesis at the level of a series of highly specific cellular and molecular biological responses that can best be described, in aggregate, as an inflammatory disease. Formerly focused on luminal narrowing due to the bulk of atheroma, our current concepts recognize the biological attributes of the atheroma as key determinants of its clinical significance. Thus, we have come to appreciate a prominent role for inflammation in atherosclerosis and its complications.

For example, lowering lipid levels with inhibitors of 3-hydroxy-3-methylglutaryl coenzyme A (HMG CoA) reductase, known as statins, substantially reduces acute adverse coronary events, but unexpectedly produces only slight reductions in arterial obstruction, as determined by angiography. This apparent paradox has shifted our focus from the degree of stenosis to the biology of the atherosclerotic plaque. A subset of atherosclerotic plaques described as 'vulnerable' seem particularly prone to physical disruption, producing thrombosis that triggers the acute coronary syndromes, including acute myocardial infarction (MI). This shift from 'hydraulics' to biology has identified new therapeutic goals. Clinical studies have indicated that statins can also diminish vascular inflammation and activation, independent of their lowering of lipid levels. However, the clinical relevance of such 'pleiotropic' effects of statins remains speculative. Beyond statins, other drugs may also stabilize plaques in unexpected ways. For example, fibric acid derivatives originally used to treat dyslipidemia have direct anti-inflammatory effects through activation of peroxisomal proliferation activating receptor-α (PPAR-α). Agents that interfere with signaling of angiotensin II, originally intended to lower blood pressure, also have anti-inflammatory effects relevant to atherosclerosis.

Molecular and cellular studies have also demonstrated that inflammatory leukocytes are central in atherogenesis because they produce many inflammatory mediators. In particular, macrophages and T lymphocytes may contribute to the disruption of vulnerable atheroma that trigger thrombosis and the onset of the acute coronary syndromes, including unstable angina, MI and cardiac sudden death. The atheroma itself, previously regarded as a bland collection of lipid waste, is now recognized as a dynamic lesion characterized by intricate exchanges of messages among these vascular and inflammatory cells. With this new understanding of the disease process comes an enormous opportunity to improve therapeutic and preventive approaches to atherosclerotic disease.

2
Changing Concepts of Atherogenesis

As we enhance our understanding of its fundamental mechanisms, we can begin to approach atherogenesis as a modifiable rather than ineluctable process. The clinically important complications of atheroma usually involve thrombosis. Arterial stenosis by themselves seldom cause acute unstable angina or acute MI. Indeed, sizeable atheroma may remain silent for decades or produce only stable symptoms such as angina pectoris precipitated by increased demand. Recent research has furnished new insight into the molecular mechanisms that cause transition from the chronic to the acute phase of atherosclerosis.

2.1
Lesion Initiation

Recruitment of mononuclear leucocytes (monocytes/macrophages and T lymphocytes) to the intima is one of the earliest events in the formation of an atherosclerotic lesion. We now appreciate that specific adhesion molecules expressed on the surface of vascular endothelial cells mediate leukocyte adhesion (Carlos and Harlan 1994; Frenette and Wagner 1996; Gimbrone et al. 1997). Once adherent, the leucocytes may enter the artery wall. Current evidence suggests that certain cytokines (e.g., interleukin-1, tumor necrosis α, interferon-γ) and chemokines (chemoattractant-cytokines), such as the macrophage chemoattractant protein-1 are highly expressed by vascular cells in response to different cardiovascular risk factors (e.g., hypertension, hypercholesterolemia). These pro-inflammatory molecules play an important role in the migration of inflammatory cells from the circulation to the vascular wall (Fig. 1). Within the lumen of the vessel, local shear stress alterations may also influence the expression of adhesion molecules, cytokines and chemokines either directly or indirectly (Gimbrone et al. 1997). In addition, it has been demonstrated that the well known endogenous mediator nitric oxide (NO), usually thought as a vasodilator, can reduce the adhesion and recruitment of leukocyte to the vessel wall of arteries (Lefer and Ma 1993). NO reduces the expression of many adhesion molecule, cytokines and chemokines (De Caterina et al. 1995). Thus, NO acts as an anti-inflammatory mediator as well as a vasodilator. In areas of normal arterial blood flow, laminar shear stress augments the activity of endothelial-NO synthase, the enzyme that produces endogenous NO. Thus, the endogenous anti-inflammatory action of NO should operate at sites of undisturbed arterial flow. Disturbed flow, with shear stress, at sites prone to early atheroma formation, such as branches and bifurcations, probably attenuate this endogenous anti-inflammatory pathway. Once inflammatory cells collect in the intima, they typically accumulate lipid and become foam cells.

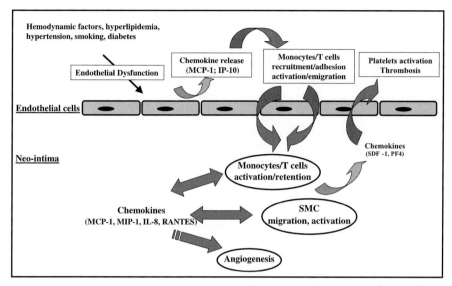

Fig. 1 Role of chemokins in atherogenesis. Various stimuli injure the vascular endothelium, inducing the release of several chemokines from the endothelial cells. These chemokines trigger chemokines receptors on circulating monocytes and T cells. Chemokine receptors/ligands interactions induce leukocyte activation, adhesion to the endothelium and subsequent migration into the underlying developing lesion. Once within the vascular wall, these mononuclear leukocytes release several chemokines and induce the release of chemokines by smooth muscle cells (*SMC*). This process implicates leukocyte retention, SMC migration and activation, angiogenesis, and may trigger platelet activation in atherosclerosis. (Adapted from Mach F. *Current Atherosclerosis Reports* 2001; 3:243–251)

2.2
Progression of Atheroma

Accumulation of macrophage foam cells, the hallmark of fatty streaks, may be reversible and does not itself cause clinical consequences. However, macrophage accumulation within the arterial intima sets the stage for progression of atheroma and evolution into more fibrous and eventually more complicated plaque that can indeed cause clinical disease.

Until recently, desquamation of the endothelium was previously considered responsible for causing adherence and degranulation of platelets with release of fibrogenic substances that could promote smooth muscle cell proliferation and extracellular matrix accumulation (Ross and Glomset 1976a, 1976b). Currently, we appreciate that atheroma can form in the absence of actual sloughing of endothelial cells. Mononuclear foam cells can insinuate themselves between intact endothelial cells and enter the intima by diapedesis. Migration and proliferation of smooth muscle cells that secret extracellular matrix macromolecules may contribute importantly to formation of fibrous lesions during this phase of atheroma progression. Pro-inflammatory cytokines regulate growth factor expression by vascular cells and leucocytes. For example, interleukin-1 increases production of platelet-derived-growth factor or basic fibroblast growth factor by human vascular smooth muscle cells and leukocytes (Raines et al. 1989). As in many biological control pathways, the balance of opposing forces determines the outcome. Growth factors can induce smooth muscle cell proliferation and stimulate their production of extracellular matrix. At the same time, interferon-γ, derived from activated T lymphocytes, can inhibit smooth muscle cell proliferation and matrix synthesis. Thus, smooth muscle cell accumulation depends on the equilibrium between growth-stimulatory and growth-inhibitory stimuli (Libby 2001).

2.3
The Molecular Mechanisms of the Thrombotic Complications of Atheroma

Arterial stenosis by themselves seldom cause acute unstable angina or acute MI. Indeed, sizeable atheroma may remain silent for decades or produce only stable symptoms such as angina pectoris precipitated by increased demand such as exertion. The majority of acute MIs result from atheroma that cause less than 50% stenosis of the artery, as assessed by arteriography (Smith 1996). Instead, thrombus formation usually occurs because of a physical disruption of atherosclerotic plaque (Falk et al. 1995). Because wall tension varies directly with radius (the Laplace relationship), the biomechanical stresses experienced by nonobstructing atheroma may be greater than that of stenosis, which yield a smaller residual lumen (Lee and Libby 1997). The physical disruption of the lesion that causes the thrombosis may be a superficial erosion that permits platelets to contact the pro-aggregatory collagen in the intima's basement membrane. However, the majority of coronary thrombosis result from a rupture of the plaque's protective fibrous cap, which permits contact between blood coagulation's factors and the highly thrombogenic material located in the lesion's lipid core (e.g., tissue factor). Because of the critical role of plaque rupture in coronary thrombosis, the biomechanical strength of the plaque's fibrous cap has considerable importance as a determinant of a particular lesion's stability. Approaching this issue in molecular terms, one must recognize that interstitial forms of collagen account for most of the tensile strength of the plaque's fibrous cap. The amount of collagen in the lesion's fibrous cap depends upon its rate of biosynthesis by the arterial smooth muscle cell, the main source of collagens in arteries. Certain growth factors stimulate collagen synthesis by vascular smooth muscle cells. In contrast, interferon-γ markedly inhibits interstitial gene expression and protein synthesis in these cells (Amento et al. 1991). This latter finding has particular bearing on the pathophysiology of plaque rupture because T lymphocytes accumulate at sites where plaques rupture and cause fatal thrombosis (van der Wal et al. 1994). Compared to regions lacking T lymphocyte infiltrates, pathological studies have shown low levels of interstitial collagen at sites of T lymphocyte accumulation (Rekhter et al. 1993). In addition to synthesis, degradation of the extracellular matrix can influence the level of collagen in the plaque's fibrous cap and thereby affect its tensile strength. Several specialized enzymes (e.g., matrix metal-loproteinases) can degrade the extracellular matrix, and thus participate in degradation of structurally important constituents of the arterial extracellular matrix. Activated macrophages within atheroma can elaborate a number of these matrix-degrading enzymes (Galis et al. 1994) (Fig. 2). Together, these findings suggest that release of inflammatory mediators by vascular leuco-cytes in particular places in atherosclerotic plaques may predispose them to rupture by impeding the ability of smooth muscle cells to maintain and re-pair the collagen crucial to the integrity of the plaque's fibrous cap (Libby 1995). Thus, far from being innocent bystanders, inflammatory leucocytes in the atherosclerotic plaque probably participate actively in the lesion initiation and progression as well as in the occurrence of acute coronary syndromes. These findings furnish additional connections between inflammation and the pathophysiology of atherosclerosis and its clinical complications.

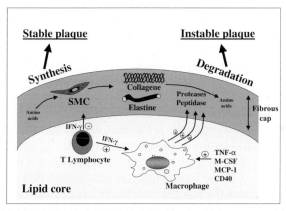

Fig. 2 Inflammatory processes in atheroma. The vascular smooth muscle cell (*SMC*) syn-thesizes the extracellular matrix protein, collagen, and elastin from amino acids. In the unstable plaque, interferon-γ (*IFN-γ*) secreted by activated T cells may inhibit collagen synthesis, interfering with the maintenance and repair of the collagenous framework of the plaque's fibrous cap. The activated macrophage secretes proteinases that can break down both collagen and elastin to peptides and eventually amino acids. Together, these processes can weaken the fibrous cap, rendering it particularly susceptible to rupture and precipitation of acute coronary syndromes. IFN-γ secreted by the T lymphocytes can in turn activate the macrophage. Plaques also contain other activators of macrophages, in-cluding tumor necrosis factor-α (*TNF-α*), macrophage colony-stimulating factor (*M-CSF*), and macrophage chemoattractant protein-1 (*MCP-1*), among others. (Adapted from Libby P. *Circulation* 1995; 91:2844–2850)

3
Role of Vascular Inflammation in Atherogenesis

3.1
Inflammation

Inflammation is a protective reaction against a variety of exogenous (micro-bial, chemical, physical) or endogenous (immunological, neurological) dis-turbances, which is characterized by the accumulation of specific subsets of leukocytes to sites of infection or tissue damage, and their subsequent ac-tivation (Sullivan et al. 2000). The attraction of leukocytes to tissues is es-sential for inflammation and the host response to infection (Springer 1996). This migration is a directional, nonrandom and selective process. The pro-cess of leukocyte trafficking manifests itself as inflammation with four classic cardinal signs: redness, swelling, heat and pain. In order to recruit leuko-cytes, the capillary blood flow and the vascular permeability are increased. This allows for enhanced migration of the leukocytes through the vascular endothelium, which is the boundary between the capillaries and the tissue, towards the site of inflammation. Depending on the cause, inflammation can resolve rapidly or develop into a complex process involving different leuko-cytes as well as endothelial and mesenchymal cells. When an infection or a lesion appears, the organism acts as quickly as possible in order to get rid of the injury. Among the first immune cells to arrive at the lesional site are neutrophils, which initiate a rapid, nonspecific phagocytic response (Picker 1992; Picker and Butcher 1992). These cells produce toxic substances includ-ing proteases and oxygenic radicals that suppress the pathogen quickly but nonspecifically. Whilst this process is efficient, a more specific antigenic recog-nition mechanism has evolved. In the specific antigen recognition process, antigen-presenting cells migrate to the site where antigen is present, followed by specific subsets of T and B lymphocytes (Baggiolini 1998). The activation of leukocytes generates the antigen-specific immune response, which results in the production of appropriate antibodies and activation of cytotoxic T lym-phocytes (Sullivan et al. 2000).

There are two classes of inflammation: acute inflammation, which is of short duration and is characteristically accompanied by plasma fluid exu-dates and neutrophil accumulation; and chronic inflammation which involves other leukocyte types such as monocytes/macrophages, T cells, eosinophils, basophils, mast cells and dendritic cells. This class of inflammation is of longer duration and is characterized by dense cellular infiltrates. Emerging ev-idence supports the implication of chronic inflammation as the crucial corner-stone of atherogenesis (Glass and Witztum 2001; Libby 2002; Libby et al. 2002; Lusis 2000; Ross 1999).

3.2
Atherosclerosis in Relation to Other Chronic Inflammatory Diseases

The cellular interactions in atherogenesis are fundamentally not different from those in chronic inflammatory-fibroproliferative disease such as cirrhosis, rheumatoid arthritis, glomerulosclerosis, pulmonary fibrosis, or chronic pancreatitis. The response of each particular tissue or organ depends on its characteristic cells and architecture, its blood and lymph supply, and the nature of offending agents. Thus, the cellular responses in the arteries (atherosclerosis), liver (cirrhosis), joints (rheumatoid arthritis), kidneys (glomerulosclerosis), lungs (pulmonary fibrosis), and pancreas (pancreatitis) are characteristic of each tissue or organ.

Rather then viewing atherosclerosis as progressive clogging of the pipes with nondescript, amorphous sludge, we now appreciate the dynamic and vital aspects of atheroma. The atherosclerotic lesions team with cells, particularly in early phases. The cellular residents of the atherosclerotic lesion include intrinsic vascular wall cells such as endothelial cells and smooth muscle cells (Glass and Witztum 2001; Libby 1995). In addition to these indigenous cells, the biological role of infiltrating leucocytes attracts ever-growing attention. Among these leukocytes, the principal (by number and functions) are monocyte-macrophages, usually named foam cells, and the T lymphocytes, mainly the T helper 1 subtype (Hansson 2001).

Does the inflammatory response in arteries differ from that in other tissues? Granulocytes are rare in atherosclerosis, and among the other diseases mentioned above, they are present only in rheumatoid arthritis and pulmonary fibrosis. In the case of arthritis, although the early response begins with granulocytes, they are found primarily within the joint cavity. Macrophages and lymphocytes predominate in the synovium, leading to erosion of cartilage and bone, which is replaced by fibrous tissue. In pulmonary fibrosis, granulocytes initially appear in the alveolar spaces; however, the lung parenchyma, where fibrosis ultimately occurs, is infiltrated by macrophages and lymphocytes. Thus, there are parallels between atherosclerosis and these other inflammatory disease (Ross 1999).

3.3
Atherosclerosis and Inflammation

A role for inflammation has become well established over the past decade or more in theories describing the atherosclerotic disease process. From a pathological viewpoint, all stages, i.e., initiation, growth, and complication of the atherosclerotic plaque, might be considered to be an inflammatory response to injury (Glass and Witztum 2001; Libby 2002; Libby et al. 2002; Lusis 2000; Ross 1999). In a variety of animal models of atherosclerosis, signs of inflammation occur hand-in-hand with incipient lipid accumulation in the artery wall. For example, blood leukocytes, mediators of host defenses and inflammation, localize in the earliest lesions of atherosclerosis, not only in experimental animals but in humans as well. The basic science of inflammation biology applied to atherosclerosis has afforded considerable new insight into the mechanisms underlying this recruitment of leukocytes. The normal endothelium does not in general support binding of white blood cells. However, early after initiation of an atherogenic diet, arterial endothelial cells begin to express on their surface selective adhesion molecules that bind to various classes of leukocytes. Interestingly, the foci of increased adhesion molecule expression overlap with sites in the arterial tree particularly prone to develop atheroma. Considerable evidence suggests that impaired endogenous atheroprotective mechanisms occur at branch points in arteries, where the endothelial cells experience disturbed flow. For example, absence of normal laminar shear stress may reduce local production of endothelium-derived NO. This endogenous vasodilator molecule also has anti-inflammatory properties (De Caterina et al. 1995). In addition to inhibiting natural protective mechanisms, disturbed flow can augment the production of certain leukocyte adhesion molecules (Nagel et al. 1994). Augmented wall stresses may also promote the production by arterial smooth muscle cells of proteoglycans that can bind and retain lipoprotein particles, facilitating their oxidative modification and thus promoting an inflammatory response at sites of lesion formation.

Once adherent to the endothelium, monocytes and T lymphocytes penetrate into the intima. Chemoattractant molecules appear to be responsible for the direct migration of monocytes and T lymphocytes into the intima at sites of lesion formation (Boring et al. 1998; Gu et al. 1998; Sheikine and Hansson 2004; Veillard et al. 2004). Once resident in the arterial wall, the blood-derived inflammatory cells participate in and perpetuate a local inflammatory response. The macrophages express scavenger receptors for modified lipoproteins, permitting them to ingest lipid and become foam cells. Several pro-inflammatory mediators, such as macrophage colony-stimulating factor contributes to the differentiation of the blood monocyte into the macrophage foam cell (Smith et al. 1995). T lymphocytes likewise encounter signals that cause them to elaborate inflammatory cytokines, such as interferon-γ, interleukins, or tumor necrosis factor-α, that in turn can stimulate macrophages as well as vascular endothelial cells and smooth muscle cells (SMCs) (Hansson and Libby 1996). Inflammatory processes not only promote initiation and evolution of atheroma, but also contribute decisively to precipitating acute thrombotic complications of atheroma. Most coronary arterial thrombi that cause fatal acute MI arise because of a physical disruption of the atherosclerotic plaque. The activated macrophage abundant in atheroma can produce proteolytic enzymes capable of degrading the collagen that lends strength to the plaque's protective fibrous cap, rendering that cap thin, weak, and susceptible to rupture. Interferon arising from the activated T lymphocytes in the plaque can halt collagen synthesis by SMCs, limiting the plaque's capacity to renew the collagen that reinforces it (Libby 1995). Macrophages also produce tissue factor, the major procoagulant and trigger to thrombosis found in plaques. Inflammatory mediators regulate tissue factor expression by plaque macrophages, demonstrating an essential link between arterial inflammation and thrombosis (Glass and Witztum 2001; Libby 2002; Lusis 2000).

3.4
Triggers for Inflammation in Atherogenesis

3.4.1
Oxidized Lipoproteins and Inflammation

According to the oxidation hypothesis, low-density lipoprotein (LDL) retained in the intima undergoes oxidative modification (Williams and Tabas 1998). These modified lipids can induce the expression of adhesion molecules, pro-inflammatory cytokines, chemokines and other mediators of inflammation from macrophages and vascular wall cells. Theses lipoprotein particles can also undergo modification within the artery wall, rendering them antigenic and capable of inciting T lymphocyte activation (Stemme et al. 1995; Witztum and Berliner 1998). Other lipoprotein particles such as very-low-density lipoprotein (VLDL) may activate inflammatory functions of vascular endothelial cells (Dichtl et al. 1999). On the other hand, high-density lipoprotein (HDL) protects against atherosclerosis. Reverse cholesterol transport effected by HDL likely accounts for some of its atheroprotective function (Asztalos 2004).

3.4.2
Hypertension and Inflammation

Increasing evidence supports the view that inflammation may participate in hypertension—providing a pathophysiological link between atherosclerosis and hypertension. Angiotensin II, in addition to its vasoconstrictor properties, can instigate intimal inflammation. For example, angiotensin II elicits the production of superoxide anion, a reactive oxygen species, from arterial endothelial cells and SMCs (Kon and Jabs 2004). Angiotensin II can also increase the expression by arterial SMCs of pro-inflammatory cytokines, chemokines or adhesion molecules from endothelial cells (Kranzhofer et al. 1999; Tummala et al. 1999). Some of the clinical benefits of angiotensin converting enzyme inhibitor therapy may derive from interrupting such pro-inflammatory pathways.

3.4.3
Diabetes and Inflammation

The hyperglycemia associated with diabetes can lead to modification of macro-molecules, for example, by forming advance glycation end products (AGE) (Schmidt et al. 1999). By binding surface receptors such as RAGE (recep-tor for AGE), these AGE-modified proteins can augment the production of pro-inflammatory cytokines and other inflammatory pathways in vascular en-dothelial cells. Beyond the hyperglycemia, the diabetic state promotes oxidative stress mediated by reactive oxygen species (Baynes and Thorpe 1999). Thus, as in the case of hypertension, inflammation links diabetes to atherosclerosis.

3.4.4
Obesity and Inflammation

Obesity not only predisposes to insulin resistance, diabetes and hyperten-sion, but also contributes to atherogenic dyslipidemia. High levels of free fatty acids originating from visceral fat reach the liver through the portal circu-lation and stimulate synthesis of the triglyceride-rich lipoprotein VLDL by hepatocytes. The resulting elevation in VLDL can lower HDL cholesterol by augmenting exchange from HDL to VLDL by cholesteryl ester transfer protein. Adipose tissue can also synthesize cytokines, such as tumor necrosis factor-α and interleukin-6 (Yudkin et al. 1999). In this way obesity itself promotes inflammation and potentiates atherogenesis independent of effects on insulin resistance or lipoproteins.

3.4.5
Infection

Infectious agents might also conceivably furnish inflammatory stimuli that accentuate atherogenesis (Libby et al. 1997). Acute infections can alter hemo-dynamics and the clotting and fibrinolytic systems in ways that can precipitate ischemic events. Chronic extravascular infections (e.g., gingivitis, prostatitis, bronchitis) can augment extravascular production of pro-inflammatory cy-tokines that may accelerate the evolution of remote atherosclerotic lesions. Intravascular infection might also provide a local inflammatory stimulus that could accelerate atherogenesis. Many human plaques show signs of infection by microbial agents such *Chlamydia pneumoniae*. When present in the arte-rial plaque, *Chlamydiae* may release lipopolysaccharide (endotoxin) and heat shock proteins that can stimulate the production of pro-inflammatory media-tors by vascular endothelial cells, SMCs and infiltrating leukocytes (Kol et al. 1999). Epidemiological studies of infection, however, have yielded mixed re-sults, with little prospective evidence that antibodies directed against *C. pneu-moniae, Helicobacter pylori*, herpes simplex virus, or cytomegalovirus predict vascular risk (Danesh et al. 1997).

4
Markers of Inflammation

The availability of effective therapies for preventing the occurrence of coronary disease renders imperative the need to identify individuals at risk for concerted intervention before problems become manifest. Based on the evidence supporting a role for inflammation in the pathogenesis of atherosclerosis, serum markers of inflammation have gained substantial interest as markers of atherosclerotic risk. In addition, many individuals develop coronary heart disease in the absence of abnormalities in the lipoprotein profile.

Potential targets for measurement include pro-inflammatory risk factors such as oxidized low-density lipoproteins, pro-inflammatory cytokines (e.g., interleukin-1, tumor necrosis factor-α), adhesion molecules (e.g., intercellular adhesion molecule-1, selectins), inflammatory stimuli with hepatic effects (e.g., interleukin-6) or the products of the hepatic stimulation, such as serum amyloid A or C-reactive protein (CRP) (Libby and Ridker 1999). Finally, other indicators of cellular responses to inflammation, such as elevated leukocyte count, might be evaluated. A sizable number of studies have examined the association between inflammation and cardiovascular disease (CVD) through measurement of a variety of analytes. Only some of assays are currently useable in clinical settings, after consideration of the stability of the analyte, the commercial availability of assays, the standardization of those assays to allow comparison of results, and the precision of the assays. Table 1 summarizes the currently available assays for inflammatory markers. These comparisons of the various inflammatory markers favor hs-CRP (high sensitive C-reactive protein) from the clinical chemistry perspective.

The coefficient of variation of hs-CRP assays is generally less than 10% from the 0.3- to 10-mg/l range (Roberts et al. 2001). Although CRP is an

Table 1 Available assays for inflammatory markers

Analyte	Stability	Assay availability	WHO Standards available	Interassay precision
Soluble adhesion molecules (e.g., VCAM-1)	Unstable (unless frozen)	Limited	No	CV < 15%
Cytokines (e.g., interleukin-6)	Unstable (unless frozen)	Few	Yes	CV < 15%
Fibrinogen	Unstable (unless frozen)	Many	Yes	CV < 8%
SAA	Stable	One	Yes	CV < 9%
hs-CRP	Stable	Many	Yes	CV < 10%
WBC count	Stable	Many	Yes	CV < 3%

acute-phase reactant and as such has higher within-subject variability than an established risk factor such as serum cholesterol, it also has a broader distribution in the population. Thus, in a manner similar to cholesterol, two separate measurements of hs-CRP are adequate to classify a person's risk level and to account for the increased within-individual variability (Ockene et al. 2001). The distribution of the logarithm of hs-CRP level is a normal distribution, and the non-transformed values are skewed toward the higher values, with most populations showing more than 95% of subjects with hs-CRP values of less than 10 mg/l. There seems to be little seasonal or diurnal variation with hs-CRP (Meier-Ewert et al. 2001). Several factors have been identified as being associated with increased or decreased levels of hs-CRP. For example, body weight and the metabolic syndrome are consistently associated with elevated hs-CRP, and weight loss is associated with reduction in hs-CRP levels, with some authors suggesting that hs-CRP is merely a marker for obesity and insulin resistance (McLaughlin et al. 2002; Visser et al. 1999; Ziccardi et al. 2002). Individuals with evidence of active infection, systemic inflammatory processes, or trauma should not be tested until these conditions disappear. An hs-CRP level of more than 10 mg/l, for example, should be discarded and repeated in 2 weeks to allow acute inflammations to subside before retesting. CRP is certainly a very good marker of inflammation that reflects the inflammatory load of the body. Alternatively, it has also been shown recently that CRP has more direct pro-inflammatory effects (Pasceri et al. 2000; Yeh 2004; Zwaka et al. 2001), observed at CRP levels frequently seen in patients.

4.1
CRP and Primary Prevention

A meta-analysis of prospective population-based studies has compared persons in the lower tertile of hs-CRP with those in the upper tertile. With a good consistency between studies, a relative odds of 2.0 (95% confidence interval, 1.6–2.5) for major coronary events was observed for the upper tertile with the lowest tertile used as a reference. These prospective studies include men, women, and the elderly (Kop et al. 2002; Ridker and Haughie 1998; Ridker et al. 2000). In general, most studies show a dose–response relationship between the level of hs-CRP and risk of incident coronary disease. Recent studies also suggest association with incidence of sudden death (Albert et al. 2002) and peripheral arterial disease (Ridker et al. 2001). It should be noted that studies of other, newer inflammatory markers such as interleukin-6 and serum amyloid A show similar results (Ridker et al. 2000).

The ability of hs-CRP to add to the predictive capacity of other, established risk factors has been examined in several studies. Through stratification or multivariable statistical adjustment, hs-CRP retains an independent association with incident coronary events after adjusting for age, total cholesterol,

HDL cholesterol, smoking, body mass index, diabetes, history of hypertension, exercise level, and family history of coronary disease (Ridker et al. 1998; Ridker 2001). Recent studies demonstrate the capability of elevated hs-CRP to predict coronary events in women after adjusting for risk factors used in the Framingham risk score (Ridker et al. 2002), and in the elderly with extensive adjustment for CVD risk factors and measures of sub-clinical atherosclerosis (Tracy et al. 1997).

4.2
CRP and Secondary Prevention

A growing number of studies has examined inflammatory markers as predictors of recurrent CVD and death in different settings, including the short-term risk, long-term risk, and risk after revascularization procedures such as percutaneous coronary intervention (PCI), including the risk of restenosis. CRP consistently predicts new coronary events in patients with unstable angina and acute MI (Bazzino et al. 2001; Bickel et al. 2002; Ridker et al. 1998; Ridker et al. 2005; Zebrack et al. 2002a, 2002b). For patients with acute coronary syndromes, cutpoints for elevated hs-CRP different than those for prediction in symptomatic patients may be useful. For example, a level of more than 10 mg/l in acute coronary syndromes may have better predictive qualities, whereas a level of more than 3 mg/l may be more useful in patients with stable coronary disease (Pearson et al. 2003).

Many analyses have adjusted for other prognostic factors, demonstrating continued predictive capacity with hs-CRP. In acute coronary syndromes, hs-CRP predicts recurrent MI independently of troponins, which suggests it is not merely a marker for the extent of myocardial damage (Morrow et al. 1998; Rebuzzi et al. 1998). Recent data also suggest that hs-CRP may be a marker for risk of restenosis after PCIs (Chew et al. 2001). Elevated hs-CRP levels also seem to predict prognosis and recurrent events in patients with stroke (Di Napoli et al. 2001a, 2001b) and peripheral arterial disease (Rossi et al. 2002). These data suggest that hs-CRP may have a role in risk stratification of patients with established CVD.

4.3
Recommendations for the Use of Inflammatory Markers in Clinical Practice

Current evidence supports the use of hs-CRP as the analyte of choice for the measure of vascular inflammation. The hs-CRP assay, to reduce within-individual variability, should be performed in a metabolically stable person without obvious inflammatory or infectious conditions. Results for hs-CRP should be expressed as mg/l only. The cutpoints of low risk (<1.0 mg/l), average risk (1.0 to 3.0 mg/l), and high risk (>3.0 mg/l) correspond to approximate tertiles of hs-CRP in the adult population. The high-risk tertile has a twofold increase in relative risk compared with the low-risk tertile (Pearson et al. 2003).

When and in whom should this inflammatory marker be measured? The optional use of hs-CRP is certainly to identify patients without known CVD who may be at higher absolute risk than estimated by major risk factors. Specifically, those patients at intermediate risk (e.g., 10%–20% risk of coronary heart disease over 10 years), in whom the physician may need additional information to guide considerations of further evaluation (e.g., imaging, exercise testing) or therapy (e.g., drug therapies with lipid-lowering, antiplatelet, or cardioprotective agents), may benefit from measurement of hs-CRP. Those who have a 10-year risk of more than 20% are designated as coronary heart disease equivalents and already qualify for intensive medical interventions. Current guidelines for secondary prevention generally recommend, without measuring hs-CRP, the aggressive application of secondary preventive interventions. Thus, secondary preventive care and acute coronary syndrome interventions should not depend on hs-CRP levels because the evidence for their effectiveness is already strong, so the utility of hs-CRP in secondary prevention seems to be more limited. Moreover, little evidence supports the use of serial testing for hs-CRP as a means to measure disease activity or to monitor therapy. Thus, the role of hs-CRP in secondary prevention is limited. Finally, the entire adult population should not be screened for hs-CRP for purposes of cardiovascular risk assessment. Little evidence supports a recommendation for widespread screening for hs-CRP as a public health measure. An interesting but untested use for hs-CRP is to motivate persons with moderate to high risk levels to improve their lifestyles (e.g., smoking cessation, dietary modification, exercise, weight loss) or to comply with drug therapies. Limited data support the effectiveness of this particular application at the present time, and it would require a randomized, controlled trial to prove efficacy.

5
Rationale for Reducing Vascular Inflammation in Atherosclerosis

Our new understanding of the pivotal position of inflammation in the pathogenesis of atherosclerosis raises questions and opens opportunities in prevention and therapy of this disease. A series of large, well-designed, randomized and controlled clinical trials have recently established the utility of several different pharmacological strategies for preventing recurrent MI or death beyond the recognized roles of aspirin and β-adrenergic blocking agents. Newer drug classes shown to be effective in this regard, including statins; angiotensin-converting enzyme inhibitors and angiotensin-receptor blockers; and fibric acid derivatives (activators of the nuclear receptor/transcription factor PPAR-α). The success of these categories of agents in the clinic has driven intense investigation, in the context of inflammation biology in atherosclerosis, to obtain a more complete picture of the mechanism of the clinical benefit observed.

For example, statins not only inhibit cholesterol synthesis, but also block the production of isoprenoid intermediates, which are important in many cellular biochemical effects. The possible nonlipid-lowering effects (pleiotropic) of statins include anti-inflammatory vascular properties (Veillard and Mach 2002). The degree to which certain clinical benefits of statins derive from such direct anti-inflammatory effects remains controversial. Statins certainly reduce inflammation in patients with atheroma, as reflected by the marker CRP (Ridker et al. 1998), and the degree of lowering of CRP correlates poorly with the reduction in lipids (either LDL or total cholesterol), demonstrating that some of the anti-inflammatory effect may not derive simply from a lipid-lowering action.

Just as reduced LDL may not account for all of the benefits of statins. Recent clinical trials suggest benefits of interrupting angiotensin II signaling that are not accounted for by the degree of blood pressure lowering (Yusuf 2000). Indeed, angiotensin II's actions extend far beyond vasoconstriction. Considerable evidence now supports a role for angiotensin II as a pro-inflammatory mediator (Kon and Jabs 2004).

The recent clinical success of fibric acid derivatives in certain patient populations, including those with diabetes or diabetic-like insulin-resistant states, has stimulated intense interest in the PPAR-α pathway. PPAR-α agonism increases the synthesis of apoA1, the main apoprotein of HDL, a particle that protects against lesion formation, probably owing to its role in reverse cholesterol transport (removing cholesterol from the artery wall and delivering it to peripheral tissues and the liver). PPAR-α agonists also possess anti-inflammatory properties of potential relevance to atherogenesis.

Looking at the way we have treated atherosclerosis over the years, we can see that inflammation has already been targeted, via aspirin, statin, fibrates and angiotensin converting enzyme inhibitors therapies. Furthermore, risk-factor modifications, such as body mass index reduction, smoking cessation and increase activity/endurance, may also reduce pro-inflammatory vascular processes through a decrease in circulating levels of CRP. These examples provide illustrations of unexpected anti-inflammatory effects of existing therapies for atherosclerosis.

6
Statins as Anti-inflammatory Agents

In the last decades, substantial progress has been made in understanding the relationship between lipid disorders and prevention of cardiac ischemic disease. The identification of new therapeutic targets and new lipid-modifying agents expend treatment options. HMG-CoA reductase inhibitors, the so-called statins, atorvastatin, fluvastatin, pravavstatin, lovastatin, simvastatin and rosu- vastatin can induce relatively large reductions in plasma cholesterol levels and are established drugs for the treatment of hypercholesterolemia (LaRosa 2000). Clinical trials have demonstrated that statins can induce regression of vascular atherosclerosis as well as reduction of cardiovascular-related morbidity and mortality in patients with and without coronary artery disease (Veillard and Mach 2002).

In most of these studies, statin-mediated lowering of cholesterol and triglyc- erides appeared to account for most but not all of the benefits, lending fur- ther support to the hypothesis that statins provide cardiovascular benefit be- yond lipid lowering (Sacks et al. 1998). Indeed, these findings suggested that treatment effects in certain subjects might not depend on LDL-cholesterol lowering alone and that the benefit conferred by statins is independent of baseline LDL-cholesterol levels. Similarly, statins reduce the risk of stroke and transplantation-associated coronary vasculopathy, complications incon- sistently associated with elevated lipid levels (Blauw et al. 1997; Hebert et al. 1997; Kobashigawa et al. 1995; Wenke et al. 1997). The observation that lipid lowering by means other than statins, such as ileal bypass surgery, re- quires markedly more time to manifest clinical benefits lent additional sup- port to the relevance of the potential 'pleiotropic' functions of this drug class (Buchwald et al. 1995).

Indeed, several in vitro studies have described the beneficial effects of statins by decreasing adhesion molecules, pro-inflammatory cytokine, chemokines as well as important immunological mediators (Fig. 3) (Schönbeck and Libby 2004; Veillard and Mach 2002). All these observations support recent human studies suggesting that statins reduce the number of inflammatory cells within atherosclerotic plaques (Crisby et al. 2001; Vaughan et al. 2000). Complemen- tary in vivo experiments have showed that many of these anti-inflammatory effects of statins might be related to the increased NO production induced by statins. Furthermore, as mentioned previously, the reduction of inflamma- tion by statin treatment in humans has been demonstrated by the decrease in circulating levels of hs-CRP (Ridker et al. 1998). Statin therapy lowers CRP levels, without correlation with lipid lowering (Musial et al. 2001; Ridker et al. 2001; Ridker et al. 2005). Indeed, almost all patients who clinically benefit from statin therapy had abnormal elevated CRP values. Although statins cer- tainly exert anti-inflammatory functions, both lipid-lowering-dependent and -independent functions of statins appear to be responsible. Such modulations in vascular inflammation might render atheroma less prone to rupture and thus may lower the risk of thromboembolic complications of atherosclero- sis, independently of alterations in luminal caliber (Libby and Aikawa 2002; Musial et al. 2001).

Further study of the pleiotropic functions of statins may provide insights into the biology of atherosclerosis that can yield benefits in terms of both

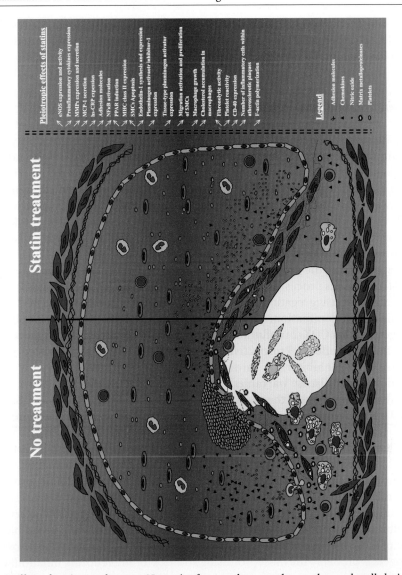

Fig. 3 Effect of statin on atheroma. Necrosis of macrophages and smooth muscle cell-derived foam cells leads to the formation of a necrotic core with accumulation of extracellular cholesterol. On the *left side* are represented the major pathophysiological features occurring within an arterial vessel wall of a patient not treated with statins. Numerous inflammatory cells, poor smooth muscle cells and collagen content of the fibrous cap, degraded principally by the matrix metalloproteinases often leads to plaque rupture followed by thrombus formation. On the *right side* are represented the main beneficial effects of statin therapy resulting in a more stable atherosclerotic plaque. (Reprinted from Veillard N. and Mach F. *Cellular and Molecular Life Sciences* 2002; 59: 1771–1786)

targeting therapy and developing novel strategies that will address the residual burden of atherosclerotic complications that occurs even those individuals who have achieved current lipid goals.

7
Future Potential Anti-inflammatory Agents

The discovery of new inflammatory pathways has raised the possibility that future treatments may target mediators of inflammation directly to add to the benefit of current treatments. Potential targets include proximal triggers such as cyclooxygenase (COX) enzyme or infectious agents, central signaling pathways in inflammation such as the transcription factor nuclear factor-κB (NF-κB), and distal effectors such as proteases, adhesion molecules, cytokines, chemokines, T lymphocytes, macrophages, SMC, and a variety of other inflammatory mediators.

By regulating the production of eicosanoids, COX (FitzGerald and Patrono 2001) modulates processes contributing to atherosclerosis and thrombosis, including platelet aggregation and the local inflammatory response. COX-2, a key mediator of inflammation, is upregulated in activated monocyte/macrophages, suggesting that COX-2 inhibition might reduce atherogenesis through its anti-inflammatory effects. Prospective randomized evaluation of the effects of selective COX-2 inhibitors on cardiovascular events in patients with or without cardiovascular disease warranted.

NF-κB is involved in the pathogenesis of atherosclerosis (Kutuk and Basaga 2003). NF-κB-induced target genes and signaling pathways mediating monocyte transmigration into the subendothelial space appears to be the point of intersection between inflammation and lipid peroxidation and is certainly a potential pharmaceutical target. Targeting NF-κB transcription pathways for a chronic disease such as atherosclerosis may well prove unrealistic given the key role of inflammation and innate immunity in normal host defenses. The redundancy of distal effectors of inflammation suggests that narrow-spectrum inhibition may not effectively modify the disease process, while broad blockade of these mediators will impair host defenses. Thus, targeting the proximal triggers is probably the most promising strategy for interrupting inflammation in atherogenesis.

8
Conclusions

Our concepts of atherogenesis have evolved from vague ideas of inevitable degeneration to a much better defined scenario of molecular and cellular events. As we enhance our understanding of its fundamental mechanism, we can begin to approach atherogenesis as a modifiable rather than ineluctable process.

Current evidence supports a central role for inflammation in all phases of the atherosclerotic process. Substantial biological data implicate inflammatory pathways in early atherogenesis, in the progression of lesions, and finally in the thrombotic complications of this disease. Many risk factors contribute as triggers of inflammatory reactions and injury to the endothelium. Growing evidence suggests that elevated plasma levels of vascular inflammation markers may help to predict future risk of cardiovascular events. Circulating acute-phase reactants elicited by inflammation may not only mark increased risk for vascular events, but in some cases may contribute to their pathogenesis. These new insights in the role of inflammation in atherosclerosis not only increase our understanding of this disease, but also have practical clinical applications in cardiovascular risk stratification and targeting of therapy. Prevention and current treatments for atherosclerosis are mainly based on drugs that lower plasma cholesterol concentration and high blood pressure. In particular, statins have proven to reduce the risk of cardiovascular events significantly, not only by their cholesterol-lowering properties, but also by their more recently identified anti-inflammatory effects. Nevertheless, atherosclerosis remains the primary cause for heart disease and stroke. Thus, a major challenge for future research would be the identification and development of promising novel anti-inflammatory therapies to reduce cardiovascular morbidity and mortality due to atherosclerosis.

References

Albert CM, Ma J, Rifai N, et al. (2002) Prospective study of C-reactive protein, homocysteine, and plasma lipid levels as predictors of sudden cardiac death. Circulation 105:2595–2599

Amento EP, Ehsani N, Palmer H, Libby P (1991) Cytokines positively and negatively regulate intersitial collagen gene expression in human vascular smooth muscle cells. Arteriosclerosis 11:1223–1230

Asztalos BF (2004) HDL Atherosclerosis Treatment Study. High-density lipoprotein metabolism and progression of atherosclerosis: new insights from the HDL Atherosclerosis Treatment Study. Curr Opin Cardiol 19:385–391

Baggiolini M (1998) Chemokines and leukocyte traffic. Nature 392:565–568

Baynes JW, Thorpe SR (1999) Role of oxidative stress in diabetic complications: a new perspective on an old paradigm. Diabetes 48:1–9

Bazzino O, Ferreiros ER, Pizarro R, et al. (2001) C-reactive protein and the stress tests for the risk stratification of patients recovering from unstable angina pectoris. Am J Cardiol 87:1235–1239

Bickel C, Rupprecht HJ, Blankenberg S, et al. (2002) Relation of markers of inflammation (C-reactive protein, fibrinogen, von Willebrand factor, and leukocyte count) and statin therapy to long-term mortality in patients with angiographically proven coronary artery disease. Am J Cardiol 89:901–908

Blauw GJ, Lagaay AM, Smelt AHM, et al. (1997) Stroke, statins, and cholesterol. A meta-analysis of randomized, placebo-controlled, double-blind trials with HMG-CoA reductase inhibitors. Stroke 28:946–950

Boring L, Gosling J, Cleary M, et al. (1998) Decreased lesion formation in CCR2-/- mice reveals a role for chemokines in the initiation of atherosclerosis. Nature 394:894–897

Buchwald H, Campos CT, Boen JR, et al. (1995) for the POSCH Group. Disease-free intervals after partial ileal bypass in patients with coronary heart disease and hypercholesterolemia: report from the Program on the Surgical Control of the Hyperlipidemias (POSCH). J Am Coll Cardiol 26:351–357

Carlos TM, Harlan JM (1994) Leukocyte-endothelial adhesion molecules. Blood 84:2068–2101

Chew DP, Bhatt DL, Robbins MA, et al. (2001) Incremental prognostic value of elevated baseline C-reactive protein among established markers of risk in percutaneous coronary intervention. Circulation104:992–997

Crisby M, Nordin-Fredriksson G, Shah PK, Yano J, Zhu J, Nilsson J (2001) Pravastatin treatment increases collagen content and decreases lipid content, inflammation, metalloproteinases, and cell death in human carotid plaques: implications for plaque stabilization. Circulation 103:926–933

Danesh J, Collins R, Peto R (1997) Chronic infections and coronary heart disease: is there a link? Lancet 350:430–436

De Caterina R, Libby P, Peng HB et al. (1995) Nitric oxide decreases cytokine-induced endothelial activation. Nitric oxide selectively reduces endothelial expression of adhesion molecules and proinflammatory cytokines. J Clin Invest 96:60–68

Di Napoli M, Papa F, Bocola V (2001a) C-reactive protein in ischemic stroke: an independent prognostic factor. Stroke 32:917–924

Di Napoli M, Papa F, Bocola V (2001b) Prognostic influence of increased C-reactive protein and fibrinogen levels in ischemic stroke. Stroke 32:133–138

Dichtl W, Nilsson L, Goncalves I, et al. (1999) Very low-density lipoprotein activates nuclear factor-κB in endothelial cells. Circ Res 84:1085–1094

Falk E, Shah P, Fuster V (1995) Coronary plaque disruption. Circulation 92:657–671

FitzGerald GA, Patrono C (2001). The coxibs, selective inhibitors of cyclooxygenase-2. N Engl J Med 345:433–442

Frenette P, Wagner D (1996) Adhesion molecules. New Engl J Med 334:1526–1529

Galis Z, Sukhova G, Lark M, Libby P (1994) Increased expression of matrix metalloproteinases and matrix degrading activity in vulnerable regions of human atherosclerotic plaques. J Clin Invest 94:2493–2503

Gimbrone MA Jr, Nagel T, Topper JN (1997) Biomechanical activation: an emerging paradigm in endothelial adhesion biology. J Clin Invest 100: S61

Glass CK, Witztum JL (2001) Atherosclerosis. the road ahead. Cell104:503–516

Gu L, Okada Y, Clinton S, et al. (1998) Absence of monocyte chemoattractant protein-1 reduces atherosclerosis in low-density lipoprotein-deficient mice. Mol Cell 2:275–281

Hansson G, Libby P (1996) The role of the lymphocyte. In: Fuster V, Ross R, Topol E (eds) Atherosclerosis and coronary artery disease. Lippincott-Raven: New York, pp 557–568

Hansson GK (2001) Immune mechanisms in atherosclerosis. Arterioscler Thromb Vasc Biol 21:1876–1890

Hebert PR, Gaziano JM, Chan KS, Hennekens CH (1997) Cholesterol lowering with statin drugs, risk of stroke, and total mortality. An overview of randomized trials. JAMA 278:313–321

Kobashigawa JA, Katznelson S, Laks H, et al. (1995) Effect of pravastatin on outcomes after cardiac transplantation. N Engl J Med 333:621–627

Kol A, Bourcier T, Lichtman AH, et al. (1999) Chlamydial and human heat shock protein 60 s activate human vascular endothelium, smooth muscle cells, and macrophages. J Clin Invest 103:571–577

Kon V, Jabs K (2004) Angiotensin in atherosclerosis. Curr Opin Nephrol Hypertens 13:291–297

Kop WJ, Gottdiener JS, Tangen CM, et al. (2002) Inflammation and coagulation factors in persons >65 years of age with symptoms of depression but without evidence of myocardial ischemia. Am J Cardiol 89:419–424

Kranzhofer R, Schmidt J, Pfeiffer CA, et al. (1999) Angiotensin induces inflammatory activation of human vascular smooth muscle cells. Arterioscler Thromb Vasc Biol 19:1623–1629

Kutuk O, Basaga H (2003) Inflammation meets oxidation: NF-kB as a mediator of initial lesion development in atheroscle. TRENDS in Mol Med 9:549–557

LaRosa JC (2000) Statins and risk of coronary heart disease. JAMA 283:2935–2936

Lee R, Libby P (1997) The unstable atheroma. Arterioscler Thromb Vasc Biol 17:1859–1867

Lefer AM, Ma XL (1993) Decreased basal nitric oxide release in hypercholesterolemia increases neutrophil adherence to rabbit coronary artery endothelium. Arterioscler Thromb 13:771–776

Libby P (1995) The molecular bases of the acute coronary syndromes. Circulation 91:2844–2850

Libby, P (2001) Current concepts of the pathogenesis of the acute coronary syndromes Circulation 104:365–372

Libby P (2002) Inflammation in atherosclerosis. Nature 420:868–874

Libby P, Aikawa M (2002) Stabilization of atherosclerotic plaques: New mechanisms and clinical targets. Nat Med 8:1257–1262

Libby P, Ridker PM (1999) Novel inflammatory markers of coronary risk theory versus practice Circulation 100:1148–1150

Libby P, Egan D, Skarlatos S (1997) Roles of infectious agents in atherosclerosis and restenosis: an assessment of the evidence and need for future research. Circulation 96:4095–4103

Libby P, Ridker PM, Maseri A (2002) Inflammation and atherosclerosis. Circulation 105:1135–1143

Lopez AD, Murray CC (1998) The global burden of disease, 1990–2020. Nat Med 4:1241–1243

Lusis AJ (2000) Atherosclerosis. Nature 407:233–241

McLaughlin T, Abbasi F, Lamendola C, et al. (2002) Differentiation between obesity and insulin resistance in the association with C-reactive protein. Circulation 106:2908–2912

Meier-Ewert HK, Ridker PM, Rifai N, et al. (2001) Absence of diurnal variation of C-reactive protein concentrations in healthy human subjects. Clin Chem 47:426–430

Morrow DA, Rifai N, Antman EM, et al. (1998) C-reactive protein is a potent predictor of mortality independently of and in combination with troponin T in acute coronary syndromes: a TIMI 11A substudy. Thrombolysis in Myocardial Infarction. J Am Coll Cardiol 31:1460–1465

Morrow RH, Hyder AA, Murray CJ, Lopez AD (1998) Measuring the burden of disease. Lancet 352:1859–1861

Murray CJ, Lopez AD (1996) The incremental effect of age-weighting on YLLs, YLDs, and DALYs: a response. Bull World Health Organ 74:445–446

Musial J, Undas A, Gajewski P, et al. (2001) Antiinflammatory effects of simvastatin in subjects with hypercholesterolemia. Int J Cardiol 77:247–253

Nagel T, Resnick N, Atkinson WJ, et al. (1994) Shear stress selectively upregulates intercellular adhesion molecule-1 expression in cultured human vascular endothelial cells. J Clin Invest 94:885–891

Ockene IS, Matthews CE, Rifai N, et al. (2001) Variability and classification accuracy of serial high-sensitivity C-reactive protein measurements in healthy adults. Clin Chem 47:444–450

Pasceri V, Willerson JT, Yeh ET (2000) Direct proinflammatory effect of C-reactive protein on human endothelial cells. Circulation 102:2165–2168

Pearson TA, Mensah GA, Alexander RW, Anderson JL, Cannon III RO, Criqui M, Fadl YY, Fortmann SP, Hong Y, Myers GL, Rifai N, Smith SC, Taubert K, Tracy RP, Vinicor F (2003) Markers of inflammation and cardiovascular disease application to clinical and public health practice. Circulation 107:499–511

Picker LJ (1992) Mechanisms of lymphocyte homing. Curr Opin Immunol 4:277–286

Picker LJ, Butcher EC (1992) Physiological and molecular mechanisms of lymphocyte homing. Annu Rev Immunol 10:561–591

Raines EW, Dower SK, Ross R (1989) Interleukin-1 mitogenic activity for fibroblasts and smooth muscle cells is due to PDGF-AA. Science 243:393–396

Rebuzzi AG, Quaranta G, Liuzzo G, et al. (1998) Incremental prognostic value of serum levels of troponin T and C-reactive protein on admission in patients with unstable angina pectoris. Am J Cardiol 82:715–719

Rekhter M, Zhang K, Narayanan A, Phan S, Schork M, Gordon D (1993) Type I collagen gene expression in human atherosclerosis. Localization to specific plaque regions. Am J Pathol 143:1634–1648

Ridker PM (2001) High-sensitivity C-reactive protein: potential adjunct for global risk assessment in the primary prevention of cardiovascular disease. Circulation 103:1813–1818

Ridker PM, Haughie P (1998) Prospective studies of C-reactive protein as a risk factor for cardiovascular disease. J Invest Med 46:391–395

Ridker PM, Glynn RJ, Hennekens CH (1998) C-reactive protein adds to the predictive value of total and HDL cholesterol in determining risk of first myocardial infarction. Circulation 97:2007–2011

Ridker PM, Rifai N, Pfeffer MA, et al. (1998) Inflammation, pravastatin, and the risk of coronary events after myocardial infarction in patients with average cholesterol levels. Cholesterol and Recurrent Events (CARE) Investigators. Circulation 98:839–844

Ridker PM, Hennekens CH, Buring JE, et al. (2000) C-reactive protein and other markers of inflammation in the prediction of cardiovascular disease in women. N Engl J Med 342:836–843

Ridker PM, Rifai N, Stampfer MJ, et al. (2000) Plasma concentration of interleukin-6 and the risk of future myocardial infarction among apparently healthy men. Circulation 101:1767–1772

Ridker PM, Rifai N, Clearfield M, et al. (2001) for the Air Force/Texas Coronary Atherosclerosis Prevention Study Investigators. Measurement of C-reactive protein for the targeting of statin therapy in the primary prevention of acute coronary events. N Engl J Med 344:1959–1965

Ridker PM, Stampfer MJ, Rifai N (2001) Novel risk factors for systemic atherosclerosis: a comparison of C-reactive protein, fibrinogen, homocysteine, lipoprotein(a), and standard cholesterol screening as predictors of peripheral arterial disease. JAMA 285:2481–2485

Ridker PM, Rifai N, Rose L, et al. (2002) Comparison of C-reactive protein and low-density lipoprotein cholesterol levels in the prediction of first cardiovascular events. N Engl J Med 347:1557–1565

Ridker PM, Cannon CP, Morrow D et al. (2005) C-reactive protein levels and outcomes after statin therapy. N Engl J Med 352:20–28

Roberts WL, Moulton L, Law TC, et al. (2001) Evaluation of nine automated high-sensitivity C-reactive protein methods: Implications for clinical and epidemiological applications: part 2. Clin Chem 47:418–425

Ross R (1999) Atherosclerosis: An inflammatory disease. N Engl J Med 340:115–126

Ross R, Glomset JA (1976a) The pathogenesis of atherosclerosis I. N Engl J Med 295:369–377

Ross R, Glomset JA (1976b) The pathogenesis of atherosclerosis II. N Engl J Med 295:420–425

Rossi E, Biasucci LM, Citterio F, et al. (2002) Risk of myocardial infarction and angina in patients with severe peripheral vascular disease: predictive role of C-reactive protein. Circulation 105:800–803

Sacks FM, Moye' LA, Davis BR, et al. (1998) Relationship between plasma LDL concentrations during treatment with pravastatin and recurrent coronary events in the Cholesterol and Recurrent Events trial. Circulation 97:1446–1452

Schmidt AM, Yan SD, Wautier JL, et al. (1999) Activation of receptor for advanced glycation end products: a mechanism for chronic vascular dysfunction in diabetic vasculopathy and atherosclerosis. Circ Res 84:489–497

Schönbeck U, Libby P (2004) Inflammation, Immunity, and HMG-CoA Reductase Inhibitors Statins as Antiinflammatory Agents? Circulation 109(suppl II):18–26

Sheikine Y, Hansson GK (2004) Chemokines and atherosclerosis. Ann Med 36:98–118

Smith S Jr (1996) Risk-reduction therapy: the challenge to change. Circulation 93:2205–2211

Smith JD, Trogan E, Ginsberg M, et al. (1995) Decreased atherosclerosis in mice deficient in both macrophage colony-stimulating factor (op) and apolipoprotein E. Proc Natl Acad Sci USA 92:8264–8268

Springer TA CM (1996) Traffic signals on endothelium for leukocytes in health, inflammation, and atherosclerosis. In: Fuster V, Ross R, Topol EJ (eds) Atherosclerosis and coronary artery disease. 1:595–606

Stary HC (1990) Atherosclerotic lesions in the young. G Ital Cardiol 20:1056–1058

Stary HC (1994) Changes in components and structure of atherosclerotic lesions developing from childhood to middle age in coronary arteries. Basic Res Cardiol 89:17–32

Stary HC (2000) Natural history and histological classification of atherosclerotic lesions: an update. Arterioscler Thromb Vasc Biol 20:1177–1178

Stemme S, Faber B, Holm J, et al. (1995) T lymphocytes from human atherosclerotic plaques recognize oxidized low density lipoprotein. Proc Natl Acad Sci USA 92:3893–3897

Sullivan GW, Sarembock IJ, Linden J (2000) The role of inflammation in vascular diseases. J Leukoc Biol 67:591–602

Tracy RP, Lemaitre RN, Psaty BM, et al. (1997) Relationship of C-reactive protein to risk of cardiovascular disease in the elderly: results from the Cardiovascular Health Study and the Rural Health Promotion Project. Arterioscler Thromb Vasc Biol 17:1121–1127

Tummala PE, Chen XL, Sundell CL, et al. (1999) Angiotensin II induces vascular cell adhesion molecule-1 expression in rat vasculature: a potential link between the renin-angiotensin system and atherosclerosis. Circulation 100:1223–1229

van der Wal AC, Becker AE, van der Loos CM (1994) Das PK. Site of intimal rupture or erosion of thrombosed coronary atherosclerotic plaques is characterized by an inflammatory process irrespective of the dominant plaque morphology. Circulation 89:36–44

Vaughan CJ, Gotto AM, Basson CT (2000) The evolving role of statins in the management of atherosclerosis. J Am Coll Cardiol 35:1–10

Veillard NR, Mach F (2002) Statins: the new aspirin? Cell Mol Life Sci 59:1771–1786

Veillard NR, Kwak B, Pelli G, Mulhaupt F, James RW, Proudfoot AEI, Mach F (2004) Antagonism of RANTES receptors reduces atherosclerotic plaque formation in mice. Circ Res 94: 253–261

Visser M, Bouter LM, McQuillan GM, et al. (1999) Elevated C-reactive protein levels in overweight and obese adults. JAMA 282:2131–2135

Wenke K, Meiser B, Thiery J, et al. (1997) Simvastatin reduces graft vessel disease and mortality after heart transplantation: a four-year randomized trial. Circulation 96:1398–1402

Williams KJ, Tabas I (1998) The response-to-retention hypothesis of atherogenesis reinforced. Curr Opin Lipidol 9:471–474

Witztum JL, Berliner JA (1998) Oxidized phospholipids and isoprostanes in atherosclerosis. Curr Opin Lipidol 9:441–448

Yeh ET (2004) CRP as a mediator of disease. Circulation 109 (suppl II):11–14

Yudkin JS, Stehouwer CD, Emeis JJ, et al. (1999) C-reactive protein in healthy subjects: associations with obesity, insulin resistance, and endothelial dysfunction: a potential role for cytokines originating from adipose tissue? Arterioscler Thromb Vasc Biol 19:972–978

Yusuf S. et al. (2000) Effects of an angiotensin-converting-enzyme inhibitor, ramipril, on cardiovascular events in high-risk patients. The Heart Outcomes Prevention Evaluation Study Investigators. N Engl J Med 342:145–153

Zebrack JS, Anderson JL, Maycock CA, et al. (2002a) Usefulness of highsensitivity C-reactive protein in predicting long-term risk of death or acute myocardial infarction in patients with unstable or stable angina pectoris or acute myocardial infarction. Am J Cardiol 89:145–149

Zebrack JS, Muhlestein JB, Horne BD, et al. (2002b) C-reactive protein and angiographic coronary artery disease: independent and additive predictors of risk in subjects with angina. J Am Coll Cardiol 39:632–637

Ziccardi P, Nappo F, Giugliano G, et al. (2002) Reduction of inflammatory cytokine concentrations and improvement of endothelial functions in obese women after weight loss over one year. Circulation 105:804–809

Zwaka TP, Hombach V, Torzewski J (2001) C-reactive protein-mediated low density lipoprotein uptake by macrophages: implications for atherosclerosis. Circulation 103:1194–1197

HEP (2005) 170:723–743

Autoimmune Mechanisms of Atherosclerosis

K. Mandal · M. Jahangiri · Q. Xu (✉)

Department of Cardiothoracic Surgery and Cardiological Sciences, St. George's Hospital
and Medical School, Cranmer Terrace, London SW17 0RE, UK
q.xu@sghms.ac.uk

Abstract Accumulating evidence supports an autoimmune mechanism as one of the prime
pathogenic processes involved in the development of atherosclerosis. So far, three proteins,
including heat shock proteins (HSPs), oxidized low-density lipoprotein (oxLDL), and β2
glycoprotein1 (β2GP1) have been recognized as autoantigens. It has been demonstrated
that risk factors for atherosclerosis, such as hypercholesterolemia, hypertension, infections,
and oxidative stress, evoke increased expression of HSPs in cells of atherosclerotic lesions.
Autoantibody levels against HSPs are significantly increased in patients with atherosclerosis
and T lymphocytes specifically responding to these autoantigens have been demonstrated
within atherosclerotic plaques. Subcutaneous immunization of animals with HSP65 induced
atheroma formation in the arterial wall. Furthermore, circulating immunoglobulin (Ig) G
and IgM oxidized low-density lipoprotein (oxLDL) antibodies are present in the plasma of
animals and humans and form immune complexes with oxLDL in atherosclerotic lesions.
These antibodies closely correlate with the progression and regression of atherosclerosis in
murine models. Interestingly, recent reports demonstrated that pneumococcal vaccination
to LDL receptor-deficient mice results in elevation of anti-oxLDL IgM Ab EO6, which is
inversely correlated with the development of atherosclerosis. Finally, it has been observed
that autoantigen β2GP1 localizes in the atheroma and that autoantibodies to β2GP1 are

correlated with the incidence of atherosclerosis in patients. Hence, these autoimmune reactions to HSPs, oxLDL and β2GP1 can contribute to the initiation and progression of atherosclerosis.

Keywords Heat shock protein (HSP) · Oxidised LDL (oxLDL) · Beta2 glycoprotein1 (β2GP1) · Autoimmunity · Atherosclerosis

1
Atherosclerosis: A Chronic Inflammatory Process

Atherosclerosis is a multifactorial process, characterized by the accumulation of lipid-laden macrophages and smooth muscle cell proliferation within the vessel wall (Ross 1993). However, its earliest lesions (fatty streaks) are characterized by a relative paucity of lipids and an abundance of inflammatory cells—such as activated T lymphocytes, mast cells, and macrophages—suggesting the involvement of inflammatory and immune processes in atherogenesis (Hansson 2001; Libby et al. 2002; Ross 1999; Wick and Xu 1999; Xu et al. 1990). In these early atherosclerotic lesions, the CD3$^+$ CD4$^+$ T cells bearing αβ T-cell receptor (TCR) predominate (Kleindienst et al. 1993; Xu et al. 1990). This suggests that the T cells recognize antigens that have been processed in macrophages via the endosomal pathway. The majority of T cells exhibit surface markers of memory cells in a state of chronic activation (Stemme et al. 1991). They are predominantly of T-helper (Th) 1 subtype, which secretes interferon-γ (IFN-γ), interleukin-2 (IL-2), and tumor necrosis factor (TNF) α and β, all of which cause macrophage stimulation and endothelial activation and induce an inflammatory state (Hansson 2001). In comparison to T cells, B cells are less frequently present in the atherosclerotic plaques, but occasionally, they can form prominent perivascular lymphoid aggregates (Wick et al. 1997). Immunoglobulin (Ig) G accumulation in human atheromas is a prominent feature (Vlaicu et al. 1985b). IgG co-localize with the terminal C5b-9 complement complex (Vlaicu et al. 1985a). Some of these immunoglobulins are likely to be specific for local antigens.

The antigens stimulating the recruitment of these T cells are increasingly believed to be microbial products such as heat shock proteins (HSPs), an evolutionarily conserved molecule. Proof in support of this notion comes from the findings of microbial antigens and DNA in atherosclerotic plaques (Curry et al. 2000; Wong et al. 1999) and from sero-epidemiological studies (Huittinen et al. 2002; Mayr et al. 2000). The recent finding of toll-like receptors (TLR) in atheromas (Edfeldt et al. 2002; Xu et al. 2001) provides a novel mechanism by which microbial and other local antigens could activate innate immunity and promote plaque growth. Evidence from in vitro studies and animal experiments also suggest an important role for oxidized low-density lipoprotein (oxLDL) in modulating immune mediators, both innate (Hajra et al. 2000; Walton et al. 2003; Xu et al. 2001) and adaptive (McMurray et al. 1993; Torzewski et al. 1998).

Endothelial cells, owing to their strategic location, also play a crucial role in these inflammatory responses (Bojakowski et al. 2000). Endothelial cells express TLRs (Edfeldt et al. 2002) and upon attachment of appropriate ligands, they express leukocyte adhesion molecules (Amberger et al. 1997), inducible nitric oxide (NO) synthase 2 (Akyurek et al. 1996), IL-1, and other inflammatory mediators. They can express scavenger receptors CD36 and LOX 1 (Li and Mehta 2000) and internalize modified low-density lipoprotein (LDL) particles. Their unique location renders them particularly important in recall responses to blood-borne antigens (Kol et al. 1999) and in the subsequent recruitment of leukocytes into atheromas.

2
Interplay Between the Innate and Adaptive Immunity in Atherosclerosis

Macrophages are of pivotal importance both in inflammation and innate immune responses. These attributes are largely due to their ability to produce proteases, free oxygen radicals, and cytokines and to activate complement. Their importance in atherogenesis is highlighted by the finding of reduced atherosclerosis in compound op/op/apoE-KO mice, a phenotype that is characterized by the lack of macrophages in tissues despite high blood cholesterol levels (Hansson 2001). They also serve as a crucial link between the innate and adaptive arms of the immune response by presenting foreign antigen to T cells.

T-cell activation leads to the secretion of IFN-γ, which in turn primes the macrophages to lower their threshold for TLR-dependent activation. T cells also produce TNF-α, another proatherogenic cytokine, which can activate nuclear factor kappaB (NF-κB) and link the adaptive arm back to innate immune pathways. Autoantigens like HSP60 can directly activate monocytes via the CD14-NFκB pathway (Kol et al. 2000). The activated T cells express CD40 ligand (Hansson et al. 2002; Henn et al. 1998), which binds with its receptors, CD40 on macrophages, B cells, platelets, and endothelial and smooth muscle cells. This interlinking and overlap of effector inflammatory pathways amplifies the downstream effect and is important in atherogenesis. In a recent epidemiological investigation, Kiechl et al. (2002) demonstrated that subjects carrying the rare allele of the Asp299Gly TLR4 polymorphism were more likely to have progressive carotid atherosclerosis, confirming the involvement of innate immunity in atherogenesis.

3
Autoantigens Initiate Adaptive Immunity in Atherosclerosis

The antigen specificity of T cells is determined by the unique conformation of the antigen-binding site in the CDR3 domain of the TCR protein, encoded in the sequence of their rearranged TCR gene. Upon activation, the stimulated T cell proliferates to give rise to a clone of cells with identical specificities. The presence in a tissue of a population of T cells with identical TCRs indicates clonal proliferation, arising as a result of stimulation by a specific local antigen.

The T cells within early atheromatous lesions of normocholesterolemic rabbits fed on a high cholesterol diet show evidence of such clonal proliferation (Curry et al. 2000). Evidence from studies on T cells isolated from human atherosclerotic plaques support the pathogenic role of autoantigens like HSPs (Xu et al. 1993a) and oxLDL (Caligiuri et al. 2000).

4
HSP60: Evidence Supporting Its Role as Autoantigen

Normocholesterolemic rabbits immunized with Freund's complete adjuvant, consisting of mineral oil and heat-killed mycobacteria, develop atherosclerotic lesions in the aorta at sites exposed to high hemodynamic stress. The same effect was observed when the experiments were repeated using recombinant mycobacterial HSP65 (mHSP65) as the immunogen (Xu et al. 1992), which forms a significant proportion of the whole protein content of mycobateria. The early atherosclerotic lesions, as induced in these experiments, are reversible and lack foam cells. However, in the presence of additional risk factors such as high blood cholesterol, the lesions became irreversible (Xu et al. 1996). Wild-type mice (C57BL/6J variety), which are normally very resistant to the induction of atherosclerosis by a high cholesterol diet alone, develop aggravated lesions when simultaneously immunized with mHSP65 (George et al. 1999).

4.1
Anti-HSP60 Antibodies

Our group (Xu et al. 1993c) was the first to report the association between anti-mHSP65 antibodies and atherosclerosis. Within the framework of the Brunneck study, a large prospective population-based survey on the pathogenesis of atherosclerosis, serum antibodies against mHSP65 were found to be significantly elevated in subjects aged 40–79 years with carotid atherosclerosis compared to those without lesions. This increased antibody titer was independent of age, sex, and other established risk factors. A subsequent follow-up study (Xu et al. 1999) confirmed that antibody levels for a given individual remained consistently elevated over a 5-year observation period and persisted at a higher level in subjects with progressive carotid atherosclerosis. This study also showed that mHSP65 antibody titers were significantly predictive of the 5-year mortality. Mayr et al. (2000) further demonstrated that anti mHSP65 antibody levels strongly correlated with human IgA to *Chlamydia pneumoniae* and with IgG to *Helicobacter pylori*, suggesting a role for infections as a stimulus for mHSP65 antibody production.

The association of anti HSP60 antibody levels and atherosclerosis has subsequently been confirmed by other groups (Table 1). The studies on patients with coronary atherosclerosis (Burian et al. 2001; Zhu et al. 2001) demonstrated that seropositive individuals not only had a higher prevalence of coronary artery disease but also that their disease severity correlated with the antibody titers, independently of traditional risk factors. A later study by Huittinen et al. (2002) demonstrated that patients with high human HSP60 IgA antibody titers in conjunction with elevated *C. pneumoniae* IgA antibody titers and an elevated C-reactive protein had a much higher risk (relative risk, 7.0) for adverse coronary events. These findings strongly suggest a pathogenic role for HSP60/65 autoantibodies in the progression of atherosclerosis.

Table 1 Summary of epidemiological studies on HSP antibodies

Reference	Cases/controls	Disease	HSPs	Odds ratio/P^*
Xu et al. 1993c	867	Carotid AS	HSP65	1.52 (1.09–2.02)
Gruber et al. 1996	107/90	Vasculitis	HSP65	$P < 0.001$
Hoppichler et al. 1996	203/76	CAD, MI	HSP65	$P < 0.05$
Mukherjee et al. 1996	28/12	CAD	HSP65	$P = 0.036$
Frostegard et al. 1997	66/67	Hypertension	HSP65	$P = 0.034$
Birnie et al. 1998	136	CAD	HSP65	$P = 0.012$
Prohaszka et al. 1999	74	CAD	HSP60	$P < 0.0001$
Xu et al. 1999	750	Carotid AS	HSP65	1.42 (1.02–1.98)
Chan et al. 1999	61/21	Peripheral AS	HSP70	$P = 0.0037$
Zhu et al. 2001	274/91	CAD	HSP60	1.86 (1.13–3.04)
Burian et al. 2001	276/129	CAD	HSP60	2.6 (1.3–5.0)
Gromadzka et al. 2001	180/64	Stroke	HSP65/70	$P < 0.0001$
Prohaszka et al. 2001	424/321	CAD	HSP60	$P < 0.007$
Ciervo et al. 2002	179/100	CAD	HSP60	$P < 0.05$
Huittinen et al. 2002	239/239	CAD	HSP60	2.0 (1.1–3.6)
Veres et al. 2002a	386/386	CV	HSP65	2.1 (1.2–3.9)
Biasucci et al. 2003	100/159	CAD	CHSP60	$P < 0.0001$
Huittinen et al. 2003	241/241	CAD	HSP60	2.1 (1.08–4.3)

$^*P$ values are shown when odds ratio was not documented in the paper. AS, Atherosclerosis; CAD, coronary artery disease; CV, cardiovascular events; MI, myocardial infarction.

The circulating anti-HSP antibodies mentioned above may be induced and maintained by different mechanisms. First, infection with microbes, containing homologous HSP60 proteins, could induce an anti-self response through molecular mimicry in susceptible individuals (Mollenhauer and Schulmeister 1992). Second, the protein itself could become immunogenic because of structural alteration resulting from oxidation or post-translational modification (Schattner and Rager-Zisman 1990). Third, other foreign or self-antigens could interact with HSP60 to form immunogenic complexes in which B cells recognize HSP60 and T cells direct their response at the associated antigen (Feige and van Eden 1996). Fourth, soluble HSP (Xu et al. 2000) might not be recognized as a self-protein by T and B cells because under physiological conditions, HSPs are located intracellularly (Multhoff and Botzler 1998). Finally, genetic variations, as suggested by strong association between the IL-6 promoter-174 polymorphism and anti-HSP60 antibody levels (Veres et al. 2002b), may yet be another way of maintaining high levels of anti-HSP antibodies in some individuals.

Because of high sequence homology between microbial and human HSPs (Morimoto 1993; Young and Elliott 1989), it is possible that such cross-reactive antibodies against HSPs of microbes and human beings can contribute to the development of atherosclerosis. Serum mHSP65 antibodies have been shown to react with the recombinant form of human HSP60 and homogenates from atherosclerotic plaques (Xu et al. 1993b). Human anti-mHSP65 antibodies react with HSP60 present on endothelial cells, macrophages, and smooth muscle cells within atheromas (Xu et al. 1993b). Schett et al. (1995) purified human anti-mHSP65 antibodies and demonstrated their cytotoxicity towards endothelial cells. The subsequent demonstration of specific reactivity of these antibodies with recombinant mycobacterial, human, chlamydial and *Escherichia coli* HSP60 (Mayr et al. 1999) strongly suggested their cross-reactive nature. In the presence of complement (complement-mediated cytotoxicity) or peripheral blood mononuclear cells (antibody-dependent cellular cytotoxicity), these antibodies induce lysis of stressed endothelial cells (Mayr et al. 1999). A population of autoreactive T cells, responding to HSP60, within the atherosclerotic lesions may play a similar proatherogenic role.

4.2
T Lymphocyte Response to HSP60/65

Studies have shown that T cells in human atheromas are mostly Th1 cells bearing the α/β receptor (Kleindienst et al. 1993). However, in the earliest stages of atherosclerosis, there is a relative abundance of T cells bearing the γ/δ receptor (Millonig et al. 2002). T cells bearing the γ/δ receptor have been proposed to constitute one of the first lines of defense and are known to participate in early stages of atherosclerosis (Millonig et al. 2002). The most probable antigens recognized by these T cells are HSPs, a hypothesis supported by the isolation of T cells from rabbit atheromas specifically responding to HSP65 in vitro (Xu et al. 1993a). IL-2 expanded T cell lines derived from atherosclerotic lesions showed a significantly higher HSP65 reactivity compared to the cells derived from peripheral blood of the same donor.

4.3
Soluble HSP60 as an Autoantigen

Chen et al. (1999) have shown that autologous HSP60 serves as a danger signal to the innate immune system, enhances the production of proinflammatory cytokines like TNFα, IL-12, and IL-15 and mediates monocyte adhesion to endothelial cells. In a large population-based study, Xu et al. (2000) showed the presence of high levels of serum soluble HSP60 (sHSP60) in subjects with carotid atherosclerosis and their correlation was found to be independent of age, sex, and other established risk factors. Furthermore, sHSP60 levels also correlated with anti HSP60, anti-LPS, anti-*Chlamydia* antibodies and a history of chronic infections. Elevated levels of sHSP60 have also been demonstrated in patients with borderline hypertension (Pockley et al. 2000) and have been correlated with a greater intima-media thickness. This provides further evidence to support the role of HSP60 in the progression of early atherosclerosis.

The likely source of these circulating sHSP60 are infectious agents such as *Chlamydia*, especially during the lytic phases of their life cycle (Beatty et al. 1994). The correlation of sHSP60 with anti-chlamydial antibodies (Xu et al. 2000) and their co-localization in human atheromas (Kol et al. 1998) provide evidence in support of this theory. Alternatively, surface expressed HSP60 (Gupta and Knowlton 2002; Kirchhoff et al. 2002) in stressed cells undergoing apoptosis may be released into the circulation as microparticles. This is corroborated by the finding of circulating microparticles in patients with acute coronary syndrome (Mallat et al. 1999), which also correlated with the degree of endothelial dysfunction in these patients (Boulanger et al. 2001).

Both chlamydial and human HSP60 can act as extracellular agonists, inducing macrophages to produce TNF-α and matrix metalloproteinase-9 (Kol et al. 1998) and causing endothelial cells to express adhesion molecules such as intracellular adhesion molecule-1 and E-selectin (Kol et al. 1999). Soluble HSP60 has also been shown to mediate the adhesion of monocytes to endothelial cells via CD14 receptor. These data, showing the ability of sHSP60 to activate the innate immunity (Srivastava 2002), not only support its proatherogenic role but also suggest that it might be a crucial link between infections and atherosclerosis (Fig. 1).

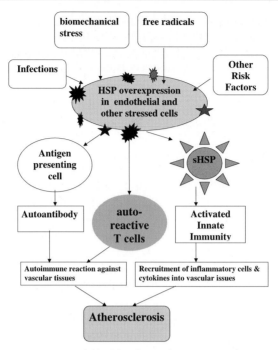

Fig. 1 Schematic representation of the role of autoimmunity in atherogenesis. Various endothelial stressors such as infections, hemodynamic stress (hypertension), oxidative stress (free radicals), and other vascular risk factors induce overexpression of HSPs in the vascular endothelial cells. HSPs, being highly immunogenic, can be processed by antigen presenting cells such as macrophages and presented to T and B lymphocytes. This can cause clonal expansion of auto-reactive T cells and B cells, producing autoimmunity. Alternatively, depending on the individual's genotype (polymorphism of receptors, such as MHC, toll-like receptors), the innate immune system can be directly activated by circulating sHSP, causing inflammation within the vascular tissues. Both of these mechanisms could contribute to atherogenesis

5
OxLDL: Evidence Supporting Its Role as Autoantigen

OxLDL is a commonly present neopitope detected in atherosclerotic lesions, both in animal models and in human specimens (Witztum and Steinberg 2001; Yla-Herttuala et al. 1994). When polyunsaturated fatty acids of LDL phospholipids undergo peroxidation/glycoxidation in the plaque microenvironment, a variety of highly reactive products such as malondialdehyde are formed, thus generating a variety of neo-self epitopes, which are recognized by the innate and adaptive immune system (Palinski et al. 1996). They can undergo further covalent bonding with apo-B with an intact phosphorylcholine moeity, forming adducts collectively termed as oxLDL. C-reactive protein, which has been suggested as a predictor of future cardiovascular events (Ridker et al. 2000), has been shown to co-localize (Chang et al. 2002) with oxLDL in atherosclerotic lesions, indicating that they both are involved in atherogenesis. The components of oxLDL are taken up by the macrophages through the scavenger receptor pathway and processed for presentation to T cells and B cells. Mice lacking scavenger receptor-A have a significant reduction of the extent of atherosclerosis (Binder et al. 2002). OxLDL contains platelet activating factor like lipids, which activate macrophages (Brand et al. 1994) and cause endothelial cell dysfunction (Dimmeler et al. 1997). Oxidised phospholipids also induce the secretion of chemotactic molecules like monocyte chemoattractant protein-1-1, facilitate the phenotypic transformation of monocytes into macrophages and stimulate smooth muscle cell proliferation (Witztum and Steinberg 2001). In addition, oxLDL can upregulate the proinflammatory and atherogenic activity of macrophages by directly modulating the expression of genes encoding for ATP-binding cassette transporter A1 and CD36 (Li and Glass 2002). Furthermore, oxLDL also leads to HSP overexpression in endothelial and smooth muscle cells (Amberger et al. 1997), thereby linking the two pathways involved in the autoimmune pathogenesis of atherosclerosis.

5.1
OxLDL Antibodies

Circulating IgG and IgM antibodies against malondialdehyde-LDL and CuOx-LDL have been identified in plasma (Holvoet et al. 2001, 1998, Meraviglia et al. 2002) and as immune complexes within atherosclerotic plaques (Craig et al. 1999; Tsimikas et al. 2001; Yla-Herttuala et al. 1994). This suggests that oxLDL is a locally formed autoantigen that elicits local cellular and humoral immune responses. These antibodies have been correlated with the progression of atherosclerosis in different vascular territories such as the carotid (Hulthe et al. 2001) and coronary artery (Lehtimaki et al. 1999). Some studies, however, document a negative correlation between the extent of atherosclerosis and levels of oxLDL antibodies, indicating a protective function for them (Fukumoto et al. 2000; Wu et al. 1999). Table 2 gives a brief overview of various epidemiological studies exploring the role of oxLDL antibodies and their influence on atherogenesis.

5.2
Cellular Immune Responses to oxLDL

A significant number of CD4$^+$ T cells, isolated and cloned from fresh human atheromas, recognized oxLDL in an HLA-DR/MHC class II restricted manner (Stemme et al. 1995; Zhou et al. 1996). Th1 cells are the dominant cell type in early atheromas with corresponding high expression of proinflammatory cytokines such as IFN-γ, IL-2, TNF-α and a predominance of IgG2a antibodies against oxLDL. In contrast, Th2 cells producing IL-4 and IL-10 which antag-

Table 2 Summary of epidemiological studies on oxLDL antibodies

Reference	Cases/ controls	Disease	IgG/IgM oxLDL antibody	Influence on atherogenesis
Lehtimaki et al. 1999	58/34	CAD	IgG	↑
Craig et al. 1999	66	CAD	IgM	↑
Bergmark et al. 1995	62/62	Peripheral AS	IgG	↑
Meraviglia et al. 2002	52	Carotid AS	IgG, IgM	↑
Hulthe et al. 2001	388	Carotid AS	IgG	↑
Hulthe et al. 2001	388	Peripheral AS	IgM	↓
Fukumoto et al. 2000	446	Carotid AS	IgG	↓
Wu et al. 1999	73/75	Hypertension	IgG, IgM	↓
Wu et al. 1999	73/75	Carotid AS	IgG, IgM	↔
Uusitupa et al. 1996	91/82	Carotid AS	IgG	↔
Hulthe et al. 1998	51/45	Carotid and peripheral AS	IgG, IgM	↔

↑, Progression of atherosclerosis; ↓, regression of atherosclerosis; ↔, no influence; AS, atherosclerosis; CAD, coronary artery disease.

onize proatherogenic effects of Th1 cells (Pinderski et al. 2002) and elicit the production of IgG1 antibodies, are detected only at very advanced stages of the disease and in extreme hypercholesterolemic situations (Hansson 2001). Exposure to oxLDL causes T cells to interact with macrophages (Hansson et al. 2002) and local dominance of T helper cell subsets determine the likely course of atherogenesis. OxLDL, on account of its closely spaced motif with multiple copies of oxidation specific epitopes, can also activate B cells via a T cell-independent pathway (Ochsenbein et al. 2000). These responses, however, are dominated by IgM antibodies. OxLDL can induce endothelial cell apoptosis (Dimmeler et al. 1997; Strachan et al. 1998), induce foam cell formation (Horvai et al. 1995), and cause various cells within the atheroma to express adhesion molecules (Palkama et al. 1993), all of which can contribute to the progression of atherosclerosis.

5.3
Autoimmunity Against OxLDL: Lessons from Animal Models

Autoimmunity modulates both the rate of atherogenesis and the composition of atheromas. When apoE-KO mice are crossed into a recombination activating gene (Rag)-deficient background, it generates hypercholesterolemic mice lacking both T and B cells. These mice, under conditions of extreme hypercholesterolemia (>1,300 mg/dl) for a sufficiently long duration (>16 weeks), do not show any alteration in the extent of atherosclerosis in comparison with controls (apoE-KO mice with normal immune function) (Dansky et al. 1997;

Daugherty et al. 1997). However, if the same immunodeficient mice are examined earlier (between 4–8 weeks) or even after an extended period but in the presence of much lower plasma cholesterol (600–800 mg/dl), the lack of T and B cells will result in significant reduction in atherosclerosis. These studies indicate that T and B cells are not obligatory, if there is sufficiently high atherogenic pressure such as extreme hypercholesterolemia for a prolonged duration. However, with less atherogenic pressure, autoimmunity could influence the course and extent of atherosclerosis.

Another interesting observation in such compound immunodeficient mice was that reduction in atherosclerosis was site-specific and dependent on the genetic background of the animals (Reardon et al. 2003). Hence, despite having a similar cardiovascular risk profile, the genetic background could selectively afford protection at certain sites while promoting atherosclerosis at others. Parenteral immunization of hypercholesterolemic mice with oxLDL (Ameli et al. 1996; Freigang et al. 1998; George et al. 1998) or infusion of polyclonal Ig into apoE-KO mice (Nicoletti et al. 1998) both lead to reduction of atherosclerosis, which highlights the fact that inhibition of cell-mediated immunity by removing the culprit autoantigens from circulation can be beneficial.

Active immunization of hypercholesterolemic (Apoe$^{-/-}$) mice with oxLDL has been shown to reduce the progression of atherosclerosis (Palinski et al. 1996). Monoclonal IgM autoantibodies, produced by splenic B-cells isolated from these mice, were shown to recognize oxidized phospholipids with a phosphorylcholine headgroup, especially those released from apoptotic cells (Shaw et al. 2000). The genes encoding the antigen binding site of these antibodies were found to be 100 % homologous with a natural murine IgA autoantibody (T15), which also recognizes phosphorylcholine and confers protection for mice against streptococcal infections. A positive selection of B1 cell lines secreting these autoantibodies occurs in Apoe$^{-/-}$ mice due to persistent stimulation by oxLDL, owing to their atherogenic burden (Binder et al. 2002). These antibodies also block the binding and degradation of oxLDL by macrophages in vitro (Shaw et al. 2001). These data suggest another possible way by which autoimmunity against an endogenous neo-epitope (oxLDL) may influence the progression of atherogenesis.

6
β2GP1: Evidence Supporting Its Role as Autoantigen

β2GP1 is implicated in several inflammatory disorders (Horkko et al. 2001), including atherosclerosis (Harats and George 2001). It causes platelet aggregation and endothelial dysfunction (Haviv 2000). Both hyperimmunization with β2GP1 and transfer of β2GP1 reactive T cells promote atherosclerosis in LDL receptor-deficient mice (George et al. 2000). The proatherogenic property of β2 GP1 is most probably related to its capacity to bind phospholipids.

Autoantibodies against β2GP1 share many of its pathological properties with antiphospholipid antibodies such as cardiolipin (Horkko et al. 2001) and lupus anticoagulant (Thiagarajan 2001). Furthermore, in patients with systemic lupus erythematosus, an autoimmune disorder with very high cardiovascular mortality, lupus anticoagulant levels strongly correlate with oxLDL antibody titers (Thiagarajan 2001) and predict progression of atherosclerosis. The cross-reactive nature of antiphospholipid and oxLDL antibodies (Horkko et al. 1996) suggests their likely involvement in the clearance of modified lipids from apoptotic cells, thereby influencing the course of atherogenesis.

7
Therapeutic Strategies: Based on an Autoimmune Model of Atherogenesis

From the discussion, it has so far become evident that CD4$^+$ T cells are the prime culprits in atherosclerosis. CD4$^+$ T cells can be broadly divided into two counterbalancing subgroups, i.e., Th 1 and Th 2 (Zhou et al. 1998). Th 1 cells are more abundant and proatherogenic, owing to their role as macrophage activator and IFN γ secretor. Counteracting them are the Th 2 cells, which suppress inflammation and decrease macrophage activity by acting through various effector cytokines i.e., IL-4, IL-10 and transforming growth factor (TGF)-β.

Developing tolerance towards HSP60/65 by mucosal administration of the autoantigen, resulting in a Th 2 bias, may help to reduce atherogenesis and could be a therapeutic strategy. Both nasal (Maron et al. 2002) and oral (Harats et al. 2002) administration of mHSP65 have been shown to decrease autoimmune responsiveness and are associated with a significant reduction of the number of infiltrating macrophages and the size of atherosclerotic plaques in LDL receptor-deficient mice. These animals, in comparison to controls, also had higher levels of IL-10, a potent anti-inflammatory cytokine, and a reduced number of CD4$^+$ T cells (Maron et al. 2002). All of these findings are compatible with the concept that a Th 1→Th 2 shift in the autoimmune reactivity could exert an athero-protective effect. These findings, however, were in complete contrast with the results obtained by parenteral immunization with mHSP65 (George et al. 2001).

Parenteral immunization using oxLDL as the immunogen, however, leads to a significant reduction of atherosclerosis (Freigang et al. 1998; George et al. 1998). It is hypothesized that the protective immunity works by inducing higher levels of oxLDL antibodies, which in turn increases the clearance of oxLDL from the extracellular space by way of scavenger receptors. Recently, Binder et al. (2003) immunized LDL receptor-deficient mice with *Streptococcus pneumoniae,* which induced high circulating levels of IgM-specific oxLDL antibodies and an accompanying expansion of oxLDL-specific T15 IgM secreting B cells in the spleen. These cross-reactive antibodies reduced the extent of atherosclerosis and were able to block the uptake of oxLDL by macrophages, thereby reducing foam cell formation. This suggests that molecular mimicry between oxLDL and microbial antigens elicit a beneficial, anti-atherogenic innate immune response.

In theory, immunomodulation towards an anti-inflammatory phenotype by enhancing Th 2/TGF β effector mechanisms or downregulating Th 1/proin-flammatory pathways are attractive treatment options. Broad spectrum im-munosuppressants such as cyclosporin and steroids have undesirable direct vascular effects that make them unsuitable as a treatment option. Some of the currently used drugs like statins (Horne et al. 2003) and glitazones, a per-oxisome proliferator activating receptor-γ agonist (Gralinski et al. 1998), are known to inhibit T cell activation and cytokine secretion. It is likely that some of their anti-atherogenic effects are due to the immunomodulatory properties. TNF-α antagonists are already being used for the treatment of rheumatoid arthritis and have undergone clinical trials investigating their use in heart failure. It will be important to see whether they are effective in ameliorating atherosclerosis as well. Experimental studies have also suggested a beneficial role for inhibitors of co-stimulatory molecules, CD40/CD40L, in halting the progression of atherosclerosis (Mach et al. 1998).

Time will be the final arbiter on whether these immune-based strategies get translated into active clinical use. The results presented above are certainly a reason for optimism in our ongoing search for the 'elixir of life' and the continuing battle against atherosclerosis.

References

Akyurek LM, Fellstrom BC, Yan ZQ, Hansson GK, Funa K, Larsson E (1996) Inducible and endothelial nitric oxide synthase expression during development of transplant arte-riosclerosis in rat aortic grafts. Am J Pathol 149:1981–1990

Amberger A, Maczek C, Jurgens G, Michaelis D, Schett G, Trieb K, Eberl T, Jindal S, Xu Q, Wick G (1997) Co-expression of ICAM-1, VCAM-1, ELAM-1 and Hsp60 in human arterial and venous endothelial cells in response to cytokines and oxidized low-density lipoproteins. Cell Stress Chaperones 2:94–103

Ameli S, Hultgardh-Nilsson A, Regnstrom J, Calara F, Yano J, Cercek B, Shah PK, Nilsson J (1996) Effect of immunization with homologous LDL and oxidized LDL on early atherosclerosis in hypercholesterolemic rabbits. Arterioscler Thromb Vasc Biol 16:1074–1079

Beatty WL, Morrison RP, Byrne GI (1994) Persistent chlamydiae: from cell culture to a paradigm for chlamydial pathogenesis. Microbiol Rev 58:686–699

Bergmark C, Wu R, de Faire U, Lefvert AK, Swedenborg J (1995) Patients with early-onset peripheral vascular disease have increased levels of autoantibodies against oxidized LDL. Arterioscler Thromb Vasc Biol 15:441–445

Biasucci LM, Liuzzo G, Ciervo A, Petrucca A, Piro M, Angiolillo DJ, Crea F, Cassone A, Maseri A (2003) Antibody response to chlamydial heat shock protein 60 is strongly associated with acute coronary syndromes. Circulation 107:3015–3017

Binder CJ, Chang MK, Shaw PX, Miller YI, Hartvigsen K, Dewan A, Witztum JL (2002) Innate and acquired immunity in atherogenesis. Nat Med 8:1218–1226

Binder CJ, Horkko S, Dewan A, Chang MK, Kieu EP, Goodyear CS, Shaw PX, Palinski W, Witztum JL, Silverman GJ (2003) Pneumococcal vaccination decreases atherosclerotic lesion formation: molecular mimicry between Streptococcus pneumoniae and oxidized LDL. Nat Med 9:736–743

Birnie DH, Holme ER, McKay IC, Hood S, McColl KE, Hillis WS (1998) Association between antibodies to heat shock protein 65 and coronary atherosclerosis. Possible mechanism of action of Helicobacter pylori and other bacterial infections in increasing cardiovascular risk. Eur Heart J 19:387–394

Bojakowski K, Religa P, Bojakowska M, Hedin U, Gaciong Z, Thyberg J (2000) Arteriosclerosis in rat aortic allografts: early changes in endothelial integrity and smooth muscle phenotype. Transplantation 70:65–72

Boulanger CM, Scoazec A, Ebrahimian T, Henry P, Mathieu E, Tedgui A, Mallat Z (2001) Circulating microparticles from patients with myocardial infarction cause endothelial dysfunction. Circulation 104:2649–2652

Brand K, Banka CL, Mackman N, Terkeltaub RA, Fan ST, Curtiss LK (1994) Oxidized LDL enhances lipopolysaccharide-induced tissue factor expression in human adherent monocytes. Arterioscler Thromb 14:790–797

Burian K, Kis Z, Virok D, Endresz V, Prohaszka Z, Duba J, Berencsi K, Boda K, Horvath L, Romics L, Fust G, Gonczol E (2001) Independent and joint effects of antibodies to human heat-shock protein 60 and Chlamydia pneumoniae infection in the development of coronary atherosclerosis. Circulation 103:1503–1508

Caligiuri G, Paulsson G, Nicoletti A, Maseri A, Hansson GK (2000) Evidence for antigen-driven T-cell response in unstable angina. Circulation 102:1114–1119

Chan YC, Shukla N, Abdus-Samee M, Berwanger CS, Stanford J, Singh M, Mansfield AO, Stansby G (1999) Anti-heat-shock protein 70 kDa antibodies in vascular patients. Eur J Vasc Endovasc Surg 18:381–385

Chang MK, Binder CJ, Torzewski M, Witztum JL (2002) C-reactive protein binds to both oxidized LDL and apoptotic cells through recognition of a common ligand: Phosphorylcholine of oxidized phospholipids. Proc Natl Acad Sci USA 99:13043–13048

Chen W, Syldath U, Bellmann K, Burkart V, Kolb H (1999) Human 60-kDa heat-shock protein: a danger signal to the innate immune system. J Immunol 162:3212–3219

Ciervo A, Visca P, Petrucca A, Biasucci LM, Maseri A, Cassone A (2002) Antibodies to 60-kilodalton heat shock protein and outer membrane protein 2 of Chlamydia pneumoniae in patients with coronary heart disease. Clin Diagn Lab Immunol 9:66–74

Craig WY, Rawstron MW, Rundell CA, Robinson E, Poulin SE, Neveux LM, Nishina PM, Keilson LM (1999) Relationship between lipoprotein- and oxidation-related variables and atheroma lipid composition in subjects undergoing coronary artery bypass graft surgery. Arterioscler Thromb Vasc Biol 19:1512–1517

Curry AJ, Portig I, Goodall JC, Kirkpatrick PJ, Gaston JS (2000) T lymphocyte lines isolated from atheromatous plaque contain cells capable of responding to Chlamydia antigens. Clin Exp Immunol 121:261–269

Dansky HM, Charlton SA, Harper MM, Smith JD (1997) T and B lymphocytes play a minor role in atherosclerotic plaque formation in the apolipoprotein E-deficient mouse. Proc Natl Acad Sci USA 94:4642–4646

Daugherty A, Pure E, Delfel-Butteiger D, Chen S, Leferovich J, Roselaar SE, Rader DJ (1997) The effects of total lymphocyte deficiency on the extent of atherosclerosis in apolipoprotein E-/- mice. J Clin Invest 100:1575–1580

Dimmeler S, Haendeler J, Galle J, Zeiher AM (1997) Oxidized low-density lipoprotein induces apoptosis of human endothelial cells by activation of CPP32-like proteases. A mechanistic clue to the 'response to injury' hypothesis. Circulation 95:1760–1763

Edfeldt K, Swedenborg J, Hansson GK, Yan ZQ (2002) Expression of toll-like receptors in human atherosclerotic lesions: a possible pathway for plaque activation. Circulation 105:1158–1161

Feige U, van Eden W (1996) Infection, autoimmunity and autoimmune disease. Exs 77:359–373

Freigang S, Horkko S, Miller E, Witztum JL, Palinski W (1998) Immunization of LDL receptor-deficient mice with homologous malondialdehyde-modified and native LDL reduces progression of atherosclerosis by mechanisms other than induction of high titers of antibodies to oxidative neoepitopes. Arterioscler Thromb Vasc Biol 18:1972–1982

Frostegard J, Lemne C, Andersson B, van der Zee R, Kiessling R, de Faire U (1997) Association of serum antibodies to heat-shock protein 65 with borderline hypertension. Hypertension 29:40–44

Fukumoto M, Shoji T, Emoto M, Kawagishi T, Okuno Y, Nishizawa Y (2000) Antibodies against oxidized LDL and carotid artery intima-media thickness in a healthy population. Arterioscler Thromb Vasc Biol 20:703–707

George J, Afek A, Gilburd B, Levkovitz H, Shaish A, Goldberg I, Kopolovic Y, Wick G, Shoenfeld Y, Harats D (1998) Hyperimmunization of apo-E-deficient mice with homologous malondialdehyde low-density lipoprotein suppresses early atherogenesis. Atherosclerosis 138:147–152

George J, Shoenfeld Y, Afek A, Gilburd B, Keren P, Shaish A, Kopolovic J, Wick G, Harats D (1999) Enhanced fatty streak formation in C57BL/6 J mice by immunization with heat shock protein-65. Arterioscler Thromb Vasc Biol 19:505–510

George J, Harats D, Shoenfeld Y (2000) Autoimmunity in atherosclerosis. The role of autoantigens. Clin Rev Allergy Immunol 18:73–86

George J, Afek A, Gilburd B, Shoenfeld Y, Harats D (2001) Cellular and humoral immune responses to heat shock protein 65 are both involved in promoting fatty-streak formation in LDL-receptor deficient mice. J Am Coll Cardiol 38:900–905

Gralinski MR, Rowse PE, Breider MA (1998) Effects of troglitazone and pioglitazone on cytokine-mediated endothelial cell proliferation in vitro. J Cardiovasc Pharmacol 31:909–913

Gromadzka G, Zielinska J, Ryglewicz D, Fiszer U, Czlonkowska A (2001) Elevated levels of anti-heat shock protein antibodies in patients with cerebral ischemia. Cerebrovasc Dis 12:235–239

Gruber R, Lederer S, Bechtel U, Lob S, Riethmuller G, Feucht HE (1996) Increased antibody titers against mycobacterial heat-shock protein 65 in patients with vasculitis and arteriosclerosis. Int Arch Allergy Immunol 110:95–98

Gupta S, Knowlton AA (2002) Cytosolic heat shock protein 60, hypoxia, and apoptosis. Circulation 106:2727–2733

Hajra L, Evans AI, Chen M, Hyduk SJ, Collins T, Cybulsky MI (2000) The NF-kappa B signal transduction pathway in aortic endothelial cells is primed for activation in regions predisposed to atherosclerotic lesion formation. Proc Natl Acad Sci USA 97:9052–9057

Hansson GK (2001) Immune mechanisms in atherosclerosis. Arterioscler Thromb Vasc Biol 21:1876–1890

Hansson GK, Libby P, Schonbeck U, Yan ZQ (2002) Innate and adaptive immunity in the pathogenesis of atherosclerosis. Circ Res 91:281–291

Harats D, George J (2001) Beta2-glycoprotein I and atherosclerosis. Curr Opin Lipidol 12:543–546

Harats D, Yacov N, Gilburd B, Shoenfeld Y, George J (2002) Oral tolerance with heat shock protein 65 attenuates Mycobacterium tuberculosis-induced and high-fat-diet-driven atherosclerotic lesions. J Am Coll Cardiol 40:1333–1338

Haviv YS (2000) Association of anticardiolipin antibodies with vascular injury: possible mechanisms. Postgrad Med J 76:625–628

Henn V, Slupsky JR, Grafe M, Anagnostopoulos I, Forster R, Muller-Berghaus G, Kroczek RA (1998) CD40 ligand on activated platelets triggers an inflammatory reaction of endothelial cells. Nature 391:591–594

Holvoet P, Theilmeier G, Shivalkar B, Flameng W, Collen D (1998) LDL hypercholesterolemia is associated with accumulation of oxidized LDL, atherosclerotic plaque growth, and compensatory vessel enlargement in coronary arteries of miniature pigs. Arterioscler Thromb Vasc Biol 18:415–422

Holvoet P, Mertens A, Verhamme P, Bogaerts K, Beyens G, Verhaeghe R, Collen D, Muls E, Van de Werf F (2001) Circulating oxidized LDL is a useful marker for identifying patients with coronary artery disease. Arterioscler Thromb Vasc Biol 21:844–848

Hoppichler F, Lechleitner M, Traweger C, Schett G, Dzien A, Sturm W, Xu Q (1996) Changes of serum antibodies to heat-shock protein 65 in coronary heart disease and acute myocardial infarction. Atherosclerosis 126:333–338

Horkko S, Miller E, Dudl E, Reaven P, Curtiss LK, Zvaifler NJ, Terkeltaub R, Pierangeli SS, Branch DW, Palinski W, Witztum JL (1996) Antiphospholipid antibodies are directed against epitopes of oxidized phospholipids. Recognition of cardiolipin by monoclonal antibodies to epitopes of oxidized low density lipoprotein. J Clin Invest 98:815–825

Horkko S, Olee T, Mo L, Branch DW, Woods VL, Jr., Palinski W, Chen PP, Witztum JL (2001) Anticardiolipin antibodies from patients with the antiphospholipid antibody syndrome recognize epitopes in both beta(2)-glycoprotein 1 and oxidized low-density lipoprotein. Circulation 103:941–946

Horne BD, Muhlestein JB, Carlquist JF, Bair TL, Madsen TE, Hart NI, Anderson JL (2003) Statin therapy interacts with cytomegalovirus seropositivity and high C-reactive protein in reducing mortality among patients with angiographically significant coronary disease. Circulation 107:258–263

Horvai A, Palinski W, Wu H, Moulton KS, Kalla K, Glass CK (1995) Scavenger receptor A gene regulatory elements target gene expression to macrophages and to foam cells of atherosclerotic lesions. Proc Natl Acad Sci USA 92:5391–5395

Huittinen T, Leinonen M, Tenkanen L, Manttari M, Virkkunen H, Pitkanen T, Wahlstrom E, Palosuo T, Manninen V, Saikku P (2002) Autoimmunity to human heat shock protein 60, Chlamydia pneumoniae infection, and inflammation in predicting coronary risk. Arterioscler Thromb Vasc Biol 22:431–437

Huittinen T, Leinonen M, Tenkanen L, Virkkunen H, Manttari M, Palosuo T, Manninen V, Saikku P (2003) Synergistic effect of persistent Chlamydia pneumoniae infection, autoimmunity, and inflammation on coronary risk. Circulation 107:2566–2570

Hulthe J, Wikstrand J, Lidell A, Wendelhag I, Hansson GK, Wiklund O (1998) Antibody titers against oxidized LDL are not elevated in patients with familial hypercholesterolemia. Arterioscler Thromb Vasc Biol 18:1203–1211

Hulthe J, Bokemark L, Fagerberg B (2001) Antibodies to oxidized LDL in relation to intima-media thickness in carotid and femoral arteries in 58-year-old subjectively clinically healthy men. Arterioscler Thromb Vasc Biol 21:101–107

Kiechl S, Lorenz E, Reindl M, Wiedermann CJ, Oberhollenzer F, Bonora E, Willeit J, Schwartz DA (2002) Toll-like receptor 4 polymorphisms and atherogenesis. N Engl J Med 347:185–192

Kirchhoff S, Gupta S, Knowlton AA (2002) Cytosolic HSP60, apoptosis, and myocardial injury. Circulation in press

Kleindienst R, Xu Q, Willeit J, Waldenberger FR, Weimann S, Wick G (1993) Immunology of atherosclerosis. Demonstration of heat shock protein 60 expression and T lymphocytes bearing alpha/beta or gamma/delta receptor in human atherosclerotic lesions. Am J Pathol 142:1927–1937

Kol A, Sukhova GK, Lichtman AH, Libby P (1998) Chlamydial heat shock protein 60 localizes in human atheroma and regulates macrophage tumor necrosis factor-alpha and matrix metalloproteinase expression. Circulation 98:300–307

Kol A, Bourcier T, Lichtman AH, Libby P (1999) Chlamydial and human heat shock protein 60 s activate human vascular endothelium, smooth muscle cells, and macrophages. J Clin Invest 103:571–577

Kol A, Lichtman AH, Finberg RW, Libby P, Kurt-Jones EA (2000) Cutting edge: heat shock protein (HSP) 60 activates the innate immune response: CD14 is an essential receptor for HSP60 activation of mononuclear cells. J Immunol 164:13–17

Lehtimaki T, Lehtinen S, Solakivi T, Nikkila M, Jaakkola O, Jokela H, Yla-Herttuala S, Luoma JS, Koivula T, Nikkari T (1999) Autoantibodies against oxidized low density lipoprotein in patients with angiographically verified coronary artery disease. Arterioscler Thromb Vasc Biol 19:23–27

Li AC, Glass CK (2002) The macrophage foam cell as a target for therapeutic intervention. Nat Med 8:1235–1242

Li D, Mehta JL (2000) Upregulation of endothelial receptor for oxidized LDL (LOX-1) by oxidized LDL and implications in apoptosis of human coronary artery endothelial cells: evidence from use of antisense LOX-1 mRNA and chemical inhibitors. Arterioscler Thromb Vasc Biol 20:1116–1122

Libby P, Ridker PM, Maseri A (2002) Inflammation and atherosclerosis. Circulation 105:1135–1143

Mach F, Schonbeck U, Sukhova GK, Atkinson E, Libby P (1998) Reduction of atherosclerosis in mice by inhibition of CD40 signalling. Nature 394:200–203

Mallat Z, Hugel B, Ohan J, Leseche G, Freyssinet JM, Tedgui A (1999) Shed membrane microparticles with procoagulant potential in human atherosclerotic plaques: a role for apoptosis in plaque thrombogenicity. Circulation 99:348–353

Maron R, Sukhova G, Faria AM, Hoffmann E, Mach F, Libby P, Weiner HL (2002) Mucosal administration of heat shock protein-65 decreases atherosclerosis and inflammation in aortic arch of low-density lipoprotein receptor-deficient mice. Circulation 106:1708–1715

Mayr M, Metzler B, Kiechl S, Willeit J, Schett G, Xu Q, Wick G (1999) Endothelial cytotoxicity mediated by serum antibodies to heat shock proteins of Escherichia coli and Chlamydia pneumoniae: immune reactions to heat shock proteins as a possible link between infection and atherosclerosis. Circulation 99:1560–1566

Mayr M, Kiechl S, Willeit J, Wick G, Xu Q (2000) Infections, immunity, and atherosclerosis: associations of antibodies to Chlamydia pneumoniae, Helicobacter pylori, and cytomegalovirus with immune reactions to heat-shock protein 60 and carotid or femoral atherosclerosis. Circulation 102:833–839

McMurray HF, Parthasarathy S, Steinberg D (1993) Oxidatively modified low density lipoprotein is a chemoattractant for human T lymphocytes. J Clin Invest 92:1004–1008

Meraviglia MV, Maggi E, Bellomo G, Cursi M, Fanelli G, Minicucci F (2002) Autoantibodies against oxidatively modified lipoproteins and progression of carotid restenosis after carotid endarterectomy. Stroke 33:1139–1141

Millonig G, Malcom GT, Wick G (2002) Early inflammatory-immunological lesions in juvenile atherosclerosis from the Pathobiological Determinants of Atherosclerosis in Youth (PDAY)-study. Atherosclerosis 160:441–448

Mollenhauer J, Schulmeister A (1992) The humoral immune response to heat shock proteins. Experientia 48:644–649

Morimoto RI (1993) Cells in stress: transcriptional activation of heat shock genes. Science 259:1409–1410

Mukherjee M, De Benedictis C, Jewitt D, Kakkar VV (1996) Association of antibodies to heat-shock protein-65 with percutaneous transluminal coronary angioplasty and subsequent restenosis. Thromb Haemost 75:258–260

Multhoff G, Botzler C (1998) Heat-shock proteins and the immune response. Ann N Y Acad Sci 851:86–93

Nicoletti A, Kaveri S, Caligiuri G, Bariety J, Hansson GK (1998) Immunoglobulin treatment reduces atherosclerosis in apo E knockout mice. J Clin Invest 102:910–918

Ochsenbein AF, Pinschewer DD, Odermatt B, Ciurea A, Hengartner H, Zinkernagel RM (2000) Correlation of T cell independence of antibody responses with antigen dose reaching secondary lymphoid organs: implications for splenectomized patients and vaccine design. J Immunol 164:6296–6302

Palinski W, Horkko S, Miller E, Steinbrecher UP, Powell HC, Curtiss LK, Witztum JL (1996) Cloning of monoclonal autoantibodies to epitopes of oxidized lipoproteins from apolipoprotein E-deficient mice. Demonstration of epitopes of oxidized low density lipoprotein in human plasma. J Clin Invest 98:800–814

Palkama T, Majuri ML, Mattila P, Hurme M, Renkonen R (1993) Regulation of endothelial adhesion molecules by ligands binding to the scavenger receptor. Clin Exp Immunol 92:353–360

Pinderski LJ, Fischbein MP, Subbanagounder G, Fishbein MC, Kubo N, Cheroutre H, Curtiss LK, Berliner JA, Boisvert WA (2002) Overexpression of interleukin-10 by activated T lymphocytes inhibits atherosclerosis in LDL receptor-deficient mice by altering lymphocyte and macrophage phenotypes. Circ Res 90:1064–1071

Pockley AG, Wu R, Lemne C, Kiessling R, de Faire U, Frostegard J (2000) Circulating heat shock protein 60 is associated with early cardiovascular disease. Hypertension 36:303–307

Prohaszka Z, Duba J, Lakos G, Kiss E, Varga L, Janoskuti L, Csaszar A, Karadi I, Nagy K, Singh M, Romics L, Fust G (1999) Antibodies against human heat-shock protein (hsp) 60 and mycobacterial hsp65 differ in their antigen specificity and complement-activating ability. Int Immunol 11:1363–1370

Prohaszka Z, Duba J, Horvath L, Csaszar A, Karadi I, Szebeni A, Singh M, Fekete B, Romics L, Fust G (2001) Comparative study on antibodies to human and bacterial 60 kDa heat shock proteins in a large cohort of patients with coronary heart disease and healthy subjects. Eur J Clin Invest 31:285–292

Reardon CA, Blachowicz L, Lukens J, Nissenbaum M, Getz GS (2003) Genetic background selectively influences innominate artery atherosclerosis: immune system deficiency as a probe. Arterioscler Thromb Vasc Biol 23:1449–1454

Ridker PM, Hennekens CH, Buring JE, Rifai N (2000) C-reactive protein and other markers of inflammation in the prediction of cardiovascular disease in women. N Engl J Med 342:836–843

Ross R (1993) The pathogenesis of atherosclerosis: a perspective for the 1990 s. Nature 362:801–809

Ross R (1999) Atherosclerosis–an inflammatory disease. N Engl J Med 340:115–126

Schattner A, Rager-Zisman B (1990) Virus-induced autoimmunity. Rev Infect Dis 12:204–222

Schett G, Xu Q, Amberger A, Van der Zee R, Recheis H, Willeit J, Wick G (1995) Autoantibodies against heat shock protein 60 mediate endothelial cytotoxicity. J Clin Invest 96:2569–2577

Shaw PX, Horkko S, Chang MK, Curtiss LK, Palinski W, Silverman GJ, Witztum JL (2000) Natural antibodies with the T15 idiotype may act in atherosclerosis, apoptotic clearance, and protective immunity. J Clin Invest 105:1731–1740

Shaw PX, Horkko S, Tsimikas S, Chang MK, Palinski W, Silverman GJ, Chen PP, Witztum JL (2001) Human-derived anti-oxidized LDL autoantibody blocks uptake of oxidized LDL by macrophages and localizes to atherosclerotic lesions in vivo. Arterioscler Thromb Vasc Biol 21:1333–1339

Srivastava P (2002) Roles of heat-shock proteins in innate and adaptive immunity. Nat Rev Immunol 2:185–194

Stemme S, Rymo L, Hansson GK (1991) Polyclonal origin of T lymphocytes in human atherosclerotic plaques. Lab Invest 65:654–660

Stemme S, Faber B, Holm J, Wiklund O, Witztum JL, Hansson GK (1995) T lymphocytes from human atherosclerotic plaques recognize oxidized low density lipoprotein. Proc Natl Acad Sci USA 92:3893–3897

Strachan DP, Mendall MA, Carrington D, Butland BK, Yarnell JW, Sweetnam PM, Elwood PC (1998) Relation of Helicobacter pylori infection to 13-year mortality and incident ischemic heart disease in the caerphilly prospective heart disease study. Circulation 98:1286–1290

Thiagarajan P (2001) Atherosclerosis, autoimmunity, and systemic lupus erythematosus. Circulation 104:1876–1877

Torzewski M, Klouche M, Hock J, Messner M, Dorweiler B, Torzewski J, Gabbert HE, Bhakdi S (1998) Immunohistochemical demonstration of enzymatically modified human LDL and its colocalization with the terminal complement complex in the early atherosclerotic lesion. Arterioscler Thromb Vasc Biol 18:369–378

Tsimikas S, Palinski W, Witztum JL (2001) Circulating autoantibodies to oxidized LDL correlate with arterial accumulation and depletion of oxidized LDL in LDL receptor-deficient mice. Arterioscler Thromb Vasc Biol 21:95–100

Uusitupa MI, Niskanen L, Luoma J, Vilja P, Mercuri M, Rauramaa R, Yla-Herttuala S (1996) Autoantibodies against oxidized LDL do not predict atherosclerotic vascular disease in non-insulin-dependent diabetes mellitus. Arterioscler Thromb Vasc Biol 16:1236–1242

Veres A, Fust G, Smieja M, McQueen M, Horvath A, Yi Q, Biro A, Pogue J, Romics L, Karadi I, Singh M, Gnarpe J, Prohaszka Z, Yusuf S (2002a) Relationship of anti-60 kDa heat shock protein and anti-cholesterol antibodies to cardiovascular events. Circulation 106:2775–2780

Veres A, Prohaszka Z, Kilpinen S, Singh M, Fust G, Hurme M (2002b) The promoter polymorphism of the IL-6 gene is associated with levels of antibodies to 60-kDa heat-shock proteins. Immunogenetics 53:851–856

Vlaicu R, Niculescu F, Rus HG, Cristea A (1985a) Immunohistochemical localization of the terminal C5b-9 complement complex in human aortic fibrous plaque. Atherosclerosis 57:163–177

Vlaicu R, Rus HG, Niculescu F, Cristea A (1985b) Immunoglobulins and complement components in human aortic atherosclerotic intima. Atherosclerosis 55:35–50

Walton KA, Cole AL, Yeh M, Subbanagounder G, Krutzik SR, Modlin RL, Lucas RM, Nakai J, Smart EJ, Vora DK, Berliner JA (2003) Specific phospholipid oxidation products inhibit ligand activation of toll-like receptors 4 and 2. Arterioscler Thromb Vasc Biol 23:1197–1203

Wick G, Xu Q (1999) Atherosclerosis–an autoimmune disease. Exp Gerontol 34:559–566

Wick G, Romen M, Amberger A, Metzler B, Mayr M, Falkensammer G, Xu Q (1997) Atherosclerosis, autoimmunity, and vascular-associated lymphoid tissue. Faseb J 11:1199–1207

Witztum JL, Steinberg D (2001) The oxidative modification hypothesis of atherosclerosis: does it hold for humans? Trends Cardiovasc Med 11:93–102

Wong Y, Thomas M, Tsang V, Gallagher PJ, Ward ME (1999) The prevalence of Chlamydia pneumoniae in atherosclerotic and nonatherosclerotic blood vessels of patients attending for redo and first time coronary artery bypass graft surgery. J Am Coll Cardiol 33:152–156

Wu R, de Faire U, Lemne C, Witztum JL, Frostegard J (1999) Autoantibodies to OxLDL are decreased in individuals with borderline hypertension. Hypertension 33:53–59

Xu Q, Dietrich H, Steiner HJ, Gown AM, Schoel B, Mikuz G, Kaufmann SH, Wick G (1992) Induction of arteriosclerosis in normocholesterolemic rabbits by immunization with heat shock protein 65. Arterioscler Thromb 12:789–799

Xu Q, Kleindienst R, Waitz W, Dietrich H, Wick G (1993a) Increased expression of heat shock protein 65 coincides with a population of infiltrating T lymphocytes in atherosclerotic lesions of rabbits specifically responding to heat shock protein 65. J Clin Invest 91:2693–2702

Xu Q, Luef G, Weimann S, Gupta RS, Wolf H, Wick G (1993b) Staining of endothelial cells and macrophages in atherosclerotic lesions with human heat-shock protein-reactive antisera. Arterioscler Thromb 13:1763–1769

Xu Q, Willeit J, Marosi M, Kleindienst R, Oberhollenzer F, Kiechl S, Stulnig T, Luef G, Wick G (1993c) Association of serum antibodies to heat-shock protein 65 with carotid atherosclerosis. Lancet 341:255–259

Xu Q, Kleindienst R, Schett G, Waitz W, Jindal S, Gupta RS, Dietrich H, Wick G (1996) Regression of arteriosclerotic lesions induced by immunization with heat shock protein 65-containing material in normocholesterolemic, but not hypercholesterolemic, rabbits. Atherosclerosis 123:145–155

Xu Q, Kiechl S, Mayr M, Metzler B, Egger G, Oberhollenzer F, Willeit J, Wick G (1999) Association of serum antibodies to heat-shock protein 65 with carotid atherosclerosis: clinical significance determined in a follow-up study. Circulation 100:1169–1174

Xu Q, Schett G, Perschinka H, Mayr M, Egger G, Oberhollenzer F, Willeit J, Kiechl S, Wick G (2000) Serum soluble heat shock protein 60 is elevated in subjects with atherosclerosis in a general population. Circulation 102:14–20

Xu QB, Oberhuber G, Gruschwitz M, Wick G (1990) Immunology of atherosclerosis: cellular composition and major histocompatibility complex class II antigen expression in aortic intima, fatty streaks, and atherosclerotic plaques in young and aged human specimens. Clin Immunol Immunopathol 56:344–359

Xu XH, Shah PK, Faure E, Equils O, Thomas L, Fishbein MC, Luthringer D, Xu XP, Rajavashisth TB, Yano J, Kaul S, Arditi M (2001) Toll-like receptor-4 is expressed by macrophages in murine and human lipid-rich atherosclerotic plaques and upregulated by oxidized LDL. Circulation 104:3103–3108

Yla-Herttuala S, Palinski W, Butler SW, Picard S, Steinberg D, Witztum JL (1994) Rabbit and human atherosclerotic lesions contain IgG that recognizes epitopes of oxidized LDL. Arterioscler Thromb 14:32–40

Young RA, Elliott TJ (1989) Stress proteins, infection, and immune surveillance. Cell 59:5–8

Zhou X, Stemme S, Hansson GK (1996) Evidence for a local immune response in atherosclerosis. CD4$^+$ T cells infiltrate lesions of apolipoprotein-E-deficient mice. Am J Pathol 149:359–366

Zhou X, Paulsson G, Stemme S, Hansson GK (1998) Hypercholesterolemia is associated with a T helper (Th) 1/Th2 switch of the autoimmune response in atherosclerotic apo E-knockout mice. J Clin Invest 101:1717–1725

Zhu J, Quyyumi AA, Rott D, Csako G, Wu H, Halcox J, Epstein SE (2001) Antibodies to human heat-shock protein 60 are associated with the presence and severity of coronary artery disease: evidence for an autoimmune component of atherogenesis. Circulation 103:1071–1075

HEP (2005) 170:745–776

Drug Therapies to Prevent Coronary Plaque Rupture and Erosion: Present and Future

P.T. Kovanen (✉) · M. Mäyränpää · K.A. Lindstedt

Wihuri Research Institute, Kalliolinnantie 4, 00140 Helsinki, Finland
petri.kovanen@wri.fi

Abstract Patients at high risk for coronary heart disease usually have a number of atherosclerotic plaques in their coronary arteries. Some plaques grow inward and, once they have caused a critical degree of luminal stenosis, lead to chronic anginal symptoms. Other plaques grow outward and remain silent unless they disrupt and trigger an acute coronary event. Either type of plaque may become vulnerable to rupture or erosion once they have reached an advanced stage. Typically, a highly stenotic fibrotic plaque is prone to erosion, whereas an advanced lipid-rich thin-cap fibroatheroma is prone to rupture. Because of the multitude and complex nature of the coronary lesions and our inability to detect silent rupture-prone plaques, the best practical approach to prevent acute coronary events is to treat the vulnerable patient, i.e., to eliminate the risk factors of coronary disease. Despite such preventive measures, a sizable number of patients still experience acute coronary events due to plaque erosion or rupture. Thus, there is room for new avenues to pharmacologically stabilize vulnerable plaques. The development of new noninvasive tools to detect the progression and regression of individual non-stenotic rupture-prone plaques will allow testing of such novel pharmacotherapies. Because no specific plaque-targeted therapies are available at present, we give an overview of the current pharmacotherapy to treat the vulnerable patient and also discuss potential novel therapies to prevent acute coronary events.

Keywords Coronary heart disease · Plaque rupture · Plaque erosion · Therapy

1
Introduction

Atherosclerosis of epicardial coronary arteries is the disease behind coronary artery disease (CAD). The growth and maturation of a coronary atherosclerotic plaque is a long-lasting process, whereas the conversion of a plaque into an atherothrombotic lesion takes place within a short time. The decade-long process of plaque evolution culminates when a voluminous stable plaque turns into an unstable plaque, also called vulnerable plaque, which is prone to thrombosis (Schaar et al. 2004a). It is the actual disruption of the vulnerable plaque that will expose a subendothelial prothrombotic surface, trigger local thrombus formation and cause an acute coronary syndrome. The challenge today is to stabilize the vulnerable plaques, to prevent the formation of new vulnerable plaques, and to prevent thrombosis on disrupted plaques (Schroeder and Falk 1995; Libby and Aikawa 2002). Here, we discuss the various drug therapies aimed at either preventing (a) the development of a vulnerable plaque, or (b) the actual event of plaque disruption. Because any pharmacological treatment aimed at averting acute coronary events may successfully prevent either of the two, it is often not possible to separate treatments by their mode of action. Accordingly, present clinical practice is to treat the high-risk, i.e., vulnerable patient instead of the vulnerable plaque (Naghavi et al. 2003a, 2003b).

The disruption of a vulnerable plaque may be superficial and is then called erosion, or it may be deep and is then called a rupture (Schaar et al. 2004a). The characteristics of vulnerable plaques that erode are different from those of plaques that rupture (Virmani et al. 2004). Thus, a plaque with a thick fibrous cap and a small lipid core is prone to erosion, whereas a plaque with a thin fibrous cap and a large lipid core is prone to rupture (Fig. 1). Essentially, in the former type, accumulation of fibrous tissue predominates, whereas in the latter type, accumulation of lipids predominates. Hence, both the composition

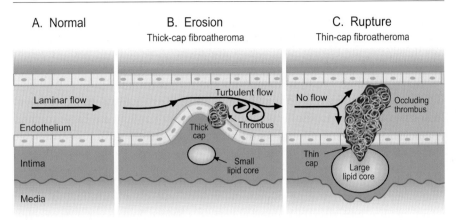

Fig. 1A–C Typical clinical course of the two types of vulnerable plaques in a coronary artery leading to an acute coronary syndrome. **A** Normal coronary artery with laminar flow of bypassing blood. **B** A highly stenotic thick-cap fibroatheroma has eroded, and a small nonoccluding thrombus has formed downstream in the area of turbulent flow. Thrombus formation and ensuing local spasm may lead to acute reduction in blood flow and trigger an episode of unstable angina. **C** A nonstenotic thin-cap fibroatheroma has ruptured and a large occluding thrombus has formed. Without thrombolysis, either spontaneous or therapeutic, acute myocardial infarction ensues

and the structure of a vulnerable plaque prone to erosion differ from those of a vulnerable plaque prone to rupture (Libby and Aikawa 2002). At present, we do not know why some plaques become fibrous and some lipid rich, although in severe dyslipidemia, coronary plaques in general tend to be lipid rich.

As the coronary plaques advance into late-stage lesions, they also grow in size. Fundamentally, there are two different types of growth: growth 'inwards' into the arterial lumen (Fig. 1B), and growth 'outwards' in the direction of the middle layer and the outer layer of the coronary wall (Fig. 1C). The former type leads to luminal stenosis, whereas the latter primarily does not (Naghavi et al. 2003a, 2003b). The inward growth or 'negative remodeling' is usually associated with stable coronary angina and decreases the tendency to develop acute coronary syndromes (Schoenhagen et al. 2000). The outward growth, referred to as 'compensatory enlargement' or 'positive remodeling', critically depends on the ability of the medial and adventitial layers of the arterial wall to yield to pressure, partly due to remodeling of the extracellular matrix and apoptotic cell death, which can be seen as thinning of the medial layer (Glagov et al. 1987). Of these two types of plaque, the nonobstructive type is prone to rupture. Indeed, 70% of acute coronary occlusions do not occur in the obstructive segments causing chronic anginal symptoms, but in the areas that have been angiographically normal (Little et al. 1988). Consequently, coronary atherosclerosis is a multifocal disease, and a multitude of plaques of different types and stages (ruptured and nonruptured) coexist in a single affected coronary artery (von Birgelen et al. 2001). This usually means that a stenotic plaque causing chronic angina pectoris is accompanied by a number of nonstenotic advanced, vulnerable plaques, which are silent. Any of these lesions might progress to the culprit lesion responsible for the fatal cardiovascular event.

As stated above, the most dangerous lesions are usually silent and hidden within the wall of the coronary artery and escape from early detection. Therefore, from a clinical point of view, there is an urgent need for a reliable method capable of identifying vulnerable patients (Naghavi et al. 2003a, 2003b). Currently the identification of vulnerable patients is based on the assessment of cumulative data provided by measurements of variables of blood vulnerability, myocardial vulnerability and plaque vulnerability. However, the sensitivity and specificity of currently used noninvasive risk stratification methods are unsatisfactory in recognizing the vulnerable plaques before they rupture. At present, there are several intracoronary technologies available for such detection, but these can be applied only to patients already undergoing an invasive diagnostic examination. This means that a silent rupture-prone vulnerable plaque can be detected before disruption only in patients with symptomatic coronary artery disease (Schaar et al. 2004b). Fortunately, the high-resolution noninvasive magnetic resonance imaging offers a promise of molecular imaging of coronary plaques and may, in the near future, allow to characterize plaque composition and microanatomy and identify lesions vulnerable to rupture or erosion already in asymptomatic vulnerable patients (Fayad 2003; Nikolaou et al. 2003).

The clinical consequences of plaque rupture and erosion tend to be different: a rupture is often followed by the formation of an occluding thrombus, and erosion by a non-occluding thrombus. However, erosion of a highly stenotic fibrotic plaque may cause the formation of an occluding thrombus (Falk 1983), and vice versa, rupture of a nonstenotic lipid-rich plaque may only induce a nonoccluding thrombus. Accordingly, it may sometimes be difficult to decide whether an acute coronary syndrome is caused by a ruptured or an eroded plaque. Inasmuch as the depth of the fissure distinguishes rupture from erosion, there must be many intermediate forms between the two extremes, which could also partly explain the overlapping clinical features between rupture and erosion. Based on the above plethora of arguments, it is currently not feasible to definitely separate the two forms of fissuring in the clinical setting when discussing the prevention of plaque fissuring as a target of drug therapy.

2
Rupture and Erosion of a Vulnerable Plaque: Potential Targets for Drug Therapy

Drug therapy for the vulnerable plaque has recently been reviewed in an elegant and comprehensive way by Forrester (2002), Libby and Aikawa (2002), as well as by Ambrose and D'Agate (2004).

2.1
Plaque Rupture

By definition, a plaque has ruptured when a breach in the fibrous cap allows the flowing blood to come in contact with the necrotic lipid core (Virmani et al. 2004) (Fig. 2A). Many cellular and molecular mechanisms within the plaque are amenable targets for drug treatment (Libby 1995; Forrester 2002; Libby and Aikawa 2002; Ambrose and D'Agate 2004). The multitude of such targets also reflects the complexity of the process of plaque rupture. Yet, at the level of the microanatomy of a rupture-prone plaque, we can define two elementary targets for drug therapy: the necrotic lipid core and the fibrous cap. Accordingly, to prevent the genesis of a rupture-prone plaque, we need to prevent the formation and expansion of a necrotic lipid core and inhibit the thinning of the fibrous cap.

The necrotic lipid core is formed when circulating low-density lipoprotein (LDL) particles enter the arterial intima, become modified, and form lipid droplets (Guyton and Klemp 1994; Öörni et al. 2000). Since the LDL-modifying processes are many, the best thinkable approach today is to slow

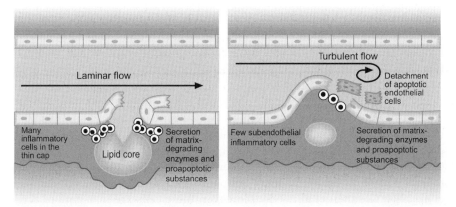

Fig. 2 Schematic presentation of the mechanisms of plaque rupture (**A**) and plaque erosion (**B**). **A** Thin-cap fibroatheromas are typically outward growing plaques with a large lipid core and many inflammatory cells. These lesions are commonly asymptomatic, as they do not interfere with blood flow until they rupture. The inflammatory cells (macrophages, lymphocytes and mast cells) secrete matrix degrading enzymes and proapoptotic substances and so predispose to plaque rupture. The mechanisms of the actual rupture include both intrinsic (plaque related) and extrinsic (hemodynamic) factors. **B** Thick-cap fibroatheromas are typically symptomatic inward growing plaques with a small lipid core and only few inflammatory cells. The inflammatory cells secrete matrix degrading enzymes and other proapoptotic factors. Together with turbulent blood flow, these mediators may induce apoptosis of endothelial cells and their detachment (i.e., erosion of the plaque)

down the influx of LDL particles into the coronary intima. This again should be achieved, at least theoretically, by lowering the plasma concentration of LDL particles. Also, maintenance of the endothelial barrier function by preventing endothelial dysfunction may be of value in the regulation of LDL influx into the intima (Sharma and Andrews 2000). The other component in the necrotic lipid core is dead macrophages. As at least part of the extracellular lipid in the core is derived from dead lipid-filled macrophage foam cells, their death should be prevented. At present, the mechanisms leading to macrophage death in vivo, either apoptotic or necrotic, are unknown and therefore not amenable to specific therapy. However, the influx of monocytes into the arterial intima should be reduced, which may be achieved by the use of a statin (Crisby et al. 2001).

The formation of a fibrous cap is intimately linked to the formation of a necrotic lipid core. Actually, a cap without a core does not exist. However, since we do not know whether a thin fibrous cap is the result of gradual thinning of a thick cap or results from a failure to thicken a thin cap, the therapeutic choices to prevent the formation of a thin cap are highly uncertain and remain theoretical as well. Interestingly, attenuation of apoptotic death of smooth muscle cells (SMCs) has been achieved by the use of a statin in human carotid plaques (Crisby et al. 2001).

2.2
Plaque Erosion

Erosion of a plaque denotes its de-endothelialization (Virmani et al. 2000) (Fig. 2B). As noted above, plaques with a thick fibrous cap and a small lipid pool typically erode rather than rupture (Libby and Aikawa 2002). Mechanistically, this is understandable, as a thick cap effectively prevents a superficial erosion from extending more deeply into the plaque core. In contrast, the molecular mechanisms leading to erosion are not well understood and are presently under intensive debate (Fuster 2002). It has been found that, similar to the actual site of rupture, the site of erosion is also infiltrated by inflammatory cells, such as macrophages, T lymphocytes, and mast cells (van der Wal et al. 1994; Kovanen et al. 1995). Moreover, these cells are in a state of activation and therefore secrete proteolytic enzymes and other pro-inflammatory mediators into their immediate surroundings (Libby 2002; Lindstedt et al. 2004; Lindstedt and Kovanen 2004). These findings provide a basis for designing pharmacological strategies to prevent erosion. These include targeted anti-inflammatory therapy aimed at regulating the number and activity of the subendothelial inflammatory cells as well as diminishing endothelial dysfunction. At present all these goals may be achieved by the use of statins (Crisby et al. 2001; Davignon 2004).

In sharp contrast to the above observations, another group of scientists has found no or only very few inflammatory cells in eroded areas (Virmani et al. 2004). Rather, they found an abundance of subendothelial SMCs, surrounded by extracellular matrix enriched with hyaluronic acid (Kolodgie et al. 2002). Possibly, the changes observed in the SMCs and the extracellular matrix were secondary rather than primary to erosion, when locally activated platelets had released growth factors and the growth-inhibitory effects of endothelial cells were lost. As growth and survival of the SMCs in the lesions (at least in the cap region) are considered to stabilize plaques and should therefore prevent them from rupturing, it is easy to understand that the experimentalists in the field and the pharmaceutical industry hesitate to plan new strategies for the prevention of plaque erosion by blocking SMC growth and matrix-producing activity. The likely presence of thin-cap atheromas in a diseased coronary artery with stenotic lesions actually precludes systemic administration of drugs with SMC-inhibiting actions in patients with angina pectoris.

Since a superficial erosion leading to endothelial denudation often occurs on the surface of a highly stenotic plaque, it is very likely that also the turbulent flow bypassing such a plaque contributes to the erosion. In summary, the functionality and well being of the endothelial cells at the interface between the external mechanical forces of blood flow and the subendothelial biochemical milieu is critical in determining whether erosion will take place or not.

The flow conditions can be improved by antihypertensive and heart rate reducing drugs. Therefore, irrespective of the denuding mechanism, any therapeutic intervention aimed at preventing endothelial dysfunction will also aid in the prevention of plaque erosion.

2.3
Repetitive Silent Ruptures and Erosions of a Plaque

The growth mechanisms of an obstructive plaque have remained enigmatic. As early as in the 1940s Duguid (1946) observed that stenotic lesions may show multiple layers of organized thrombi in their caps, suggesting repetitive disruptions and organization of mural thrombi as one mode of plaque growth. More recently, Virmani et al. (2004) confirmed in an elegant series of studies that plaques may become stenotic through thrombotic growth. Importantly, they suggest that at first, a nonstenotic vulnerable plaque, probably a thin cap fibroatheroma with a large lipid core, undergoes a subclinical small rupture. The luminal thrombus formed is nonocclusive and remains unnoticed by the patient. However, due to platelet-derived mediators and loss of the endothelium, the SMCs start dividing and secreting extracellular matrix rich in hyaluronic acid. In addition, the thrombus itself is overlaid by newly formed endothelium and becomes part of the cap. In essence, the clinically asymptomatic repetitive cycles of wounding and healing are the actual mechanisms of plaque progression leading to progressive luminal stenosis (Mann and Davies 1999).

Since after each small rupture the cap thickens, the likelihood of a large rupture, i.e., the formation of a fissure extending into the lipid core, becomes successively smaller. At the same time, as the degree of obstruction increases, the turbulence of flow also increases, and endothelial denudation becomes more likely. Thus, ultimately, a shift from small ruptures to erosions ensues. The growth of a plaque via repetitive silent ruptures resembles that of an active volcano and could be called 'eruption', a term that also emphasizes the existence of a continuum between erosion and rupture in specific types of vulnerable plaques.

To prevent a plaque from becoming highly stenotic by the above-described mechanism, the following therapeutic measures can be envisioned. In the first place, the formation of a rupture-prone plaque should be prevented (see above under 'plaque rupture'). Once the sequence of repetitive thrombotic events has begun (either due to rupture or erosion), the formation of an occluding thrombus by antiplatelet drugs is the primary goal of treatment. Finally, if a highly occlusive anginal symptom-causing plaque has evolved, vasodilators need to be added to the therapeutic armamentarium.

Our therapeutic options to prevent the actual event of rupture are modest. First of all, we are not able to specifically target the plaque cap-specific molecular mechanisms responsible for such an event. At best, we can attempt to eliminate the external triggers, known to increase the likelihood of a sudden plaque rupture. This includes lessening the hemodynamic stress acted upon a rupture-prone plaque (Bank et al. 2000; Finet et al. 2004) and preventing spasm of the coronary segment bearing a rupture-prone plaque (Bogaty et al. 1994).

3
Pharmacotherapy for the Vulnerable Plaque: Present and Future

3.1
Drugs Currently Used in Clinical Practice

We know now that the thrombosed plaques are responsible for the complications of coronary atherosclerosis, which include stable angina and the acute coronary syndromes, unstable angina, myocardial infarction, and sudden cardiac death. Thus, the cardiovascular drug trials in which such clinical events have been defined as endpoints can be considered as drug therapies for the vulnerable plaque (see Table 1). At the moment, the most convincing evidence in the prevention of acute coronary events has been obtained with studies using lipid-lowering, antithrombotic, antihypertensive, and antidiabetic drugs. They will be reviewed below. The reader is advised to learn more about the various therapies in other chapters of this book.

Table 1 Pharmacotherapy for vulnerable plaques: present and future

Anatomic target	Functional target	Current and future drugs
Endothelium	Maintaining vasorelaxation	Nitrates
	Maintaining the barrier function (to prevent LDL entry)	Antihistamines
	Prevention of endothelial denudation by prevention of endothelial dysfunction	Anti-inflammatory drugs (ASA, leukotriene receptor antagonists, mast cell stabilizers)
		Antihypertensive agents (ACE inhibitors, beta-blockers, calcium channel blockers)
		Antihyperlipidemic agents (e.g., statins, fibrates, niacin)
		Antihyperglycemic agents (glitazones)
		Antimicrobial agents
Fibrous cap	Prevention of cap thinning	Drugs also having anti-inflammatory effects (statins, leukotriene receptor antagonists, mast cell stabilizers)
		Antimicrobial agents
Lipid core	Prevention of lipid accumulation	All plasma lipid-regulating drugs (lowering plasma non-HDL lipoproteins and increasing HDL)
	Stimulation of lipid efflux	Statins
		Fibrates
		Niacin
		Resins
		Cholesterol absorption inhibitors
		ApoA-I Milano
		CETP inhibitors

3.1.1
Lipid-Regulating Drugs

3.1.1.1
HMG-CoA Reductase Inhibitors (Statins)

Various statins have been used in both primary prevention studies with asymptomatic patients and in secondary prevention studies with patients suffering from various symptoms of coronary artery disease. Thus, double-blind, placebo-controlled large long-term studies (at least 5 years) have been published using either lovastatin, simvastatin, or pravastatin. In these studies, the incidence of major adverse coronary events including coronary death decreased by 30%–40% (Grundy et al. 2004). The beneficial effect on hard coronary endpoints appears to be a common property of this class of drugs and includes the newer statins, such as fluvastatin and atorvastatin. The beneficial effects also include the diminution of ischemic stroke. This effect is probably due to the prevention of rupture and erosion of vulnerable carotid plaques.

It has been noted that the lipid-lowering therapy by statins decreases the number of acute coronary events earlier than a substantial regression of the coronary plaques is expected to take place (Brown et al. 1993). The likely explanation is that the plaques were stabilized, either directly by the action of statins (pleiotropic effects) (Davignon 2004) or indirectly through lowering of plasma LDL concentration (Law et al. 2003). Indeed, direct analysis of the sum volumes of all the plaques in an affected coronary artery, i.e., the plaque burden, has revealed the following intriguing results. A moderate dose of statin (40 mg pravastatin), which has been the average dose in many primary prevention care studies, only slows down the progression of atheroma burden, whereas the maximum dose of a statin (80 mg atorvastatin) halts progression of the atheroma burden (Nissen et al. 2004).

Recently, increasing evidence has been pointing towards a beneficial effect of statins when started already while the acute coronary syndrome is present. In the largest randomized study, patients suffering from unstable angina received high-dose atorvastatin (Schwartz et al. 2001). During the 16-week follow-up, ischemic events were significantly lower than in the placebo-treated group. This fast effect strongly supports the notion that statins may have rapid plaque-stabilizing effects, either preventing plaque rupture or erosion. It remains to be shown whether these effects are due to anti-inflammatory action on the plaque or to lowering of LDL-particle concentration in the circulation. Support for the latter possibility is obtained from the clinical observations showing that lowering of LDL-particle concentration by LDL apheresis in patients with very high levels improves the endothelial function, an effect which can be considered anti-inflammatory (Bosch and Wendler 2004).

Statins also increase the concentration of high-density lipoprotein (HDL). Since HDL has opposing effects to those of LDL, the HDL-increasing effects could potentially be plaque stabilizing. First, HDL initiates the so-called reverse cholesterol transport, i.e., induces removal of cholesterol from the macrophage foam cells rather than directly from the extracellular lipid pool. Second, HDL also has direct anti-inflammatory effects on endothelial cells which too could stabilize the plaques (Barter et al. 2004). Another chapter of this book discusses the effects of statins more thoroughly in an evidence-based manner (see the chapter by Paoletti et al., this volume).

3.1.1.2
Lipid Absorption Inhibitors

The two established bile acid sequestrants or resins (cholestyramine and colestipol) effectively lower plasma LDL-cholesterol, but their use is limited because of unacceptable gastrointestinal side effects. Cholestyramine was successfully used in the Coronary Primary Prevention Trial (Lipid Research Clinics Program 1984), one of the first studies to document that lowering of LDL-cholesterol prevents acute coronary events, such as myocardial infarction.

Ezetimibe is a new drug which specifically inhibits cholesterol absorption from the gut and effectively lowers plasma LDL-cholesterol (Bruckert et al. 2003). If equal lowering of LDL with ezetimibe, cholestyramine, and statins results in equipotent prevention of acute coronary events, the plaque-stabilizing effects of all these drugs are likely to be responsible for their LDL lowering rather than pleiotropic effects. The inhibition of cholesterol resorption is discussed more thoroughly in another chapter of this book (see the chapter by Plösch et al., this volume).

3.1.1.3
Fibrates

The effects of this class of drugs are discussed in Sect. 3.1.6.

3.1.2
Antiplatelet Drugs

All vulnerable patients should be treated with an antiplatelet drug both in the primary prevention of acute coronary events and in the prevention of recurrent ischemic events. Current evidence suggests that either aspirin or clopidogrel are appropriate first-line agents. The use of platelet activation and aggregation inhibitors as a part of anti-atherosclerotic drug regimen is discussed more thoroughly in an evidence-based manner in the chapter by Ahrens et al., this volume. A few highlights in terms of drug therapy of the vulnerable plaque are given below. The pharmaceutical treatment of acute coronary syndromes directed primarily at the dissolution of the developing intracoronary thrombosis is not part of the prevention of plaque rupture and erosion and is not discussed here.

3.1.2.1
Aspirin

Currently, the use of low-dose aspirin (75–100 mg/day) is recommended for the primary prevention of acute coronary events in vulnerable patients, and the same recommendation applies to the secondary prevention (patients with a prior coronary event) (Patrono et al. 2004; Hankey and Eikelboom 2003). It should be noted that the low dose used to block platelet activation is not likely to possess any direct anti-inflammatory effects on the plaque. Thus, aspirin cannot be considered as a plaque-stabilizing drug. It is now recognized that a patient with type 2 diabetes mellitus who has never had a myocardial infarction has the same high risk for a myocardial infarction as a nondiabetic individual who has already had a myocardial infarction (Haffner et al. 1998). Therefore, aspirin is an essential part of the primary prevention strategy in patients with diabetes mellitus (Colwell 2004).

3.1.2.2
Clopidogrel

Besides aspirin, clopidogrel is presently used as an antiplatelet drug in the treatment and prevention of ischemic cardiovascular disease (Patrono et al. 2004; Tendera and Wojakowski 2003). The availability of other antiplatelet drugs besides aspirin has been valuable, since cardiovascular events occur despite the administration of aspirin. This may be due to platelet activation by pathways not blocked by aspirin or to aspirin resistance. Indeed, since aspirin and clopidogrel exert complementary modes of inhibitory action on platelet activation, such synergistic action should result in a more effective prevention of cardiovascular events. In the CAPRIE (Clopidogrel versus Aspirin in Patients at Risk of Ischaemic Events) study, clopidogrel was more effective than aspirin in preventing the endpoint of myocardial infarction (CAPRIE Steering Committee 1996). In the CURE trial, it was found that the addition of clopidogrel to aspirin in patients with an acute coronary syndrome is superior to the administration of aspirin alone (The Clopidogrel in Unstable Angina to Prevent Recurrent Events Trial Investigators 2001). Thus, the addition of clopidogrel to aspirin was found to reduce, after a mean follow-up of 9 months, the relative risk for myocardial infarctions by 23%. The reduction of thrombotic complications of coronary atherosclerosis, reflect the prevention of future atherothrombosis, i.e., formation of a platelet-rich thrombus formation on a fissured plaque. Notably, it cannot be decided whether such inhibition targets the original destabilized culprit lesion or other rupture- or erosion-prone plaques in the affected coronary artery. It should be noted that adding aspirin to clopidogrel in high-risk patients with recent ischemic stroke or transient ischemic attack may increase the risk of hemorrhagic complications outweighing the benefit of clopidogrel alone in the prevention of vascular events (Diener et al. 2004).

3.1.3
Angiotensin-Converting Enzyme Inhibitors and Angiotensin Receptor Blockers

Clinical trials using angiotensin-converting enzyme (ACE) inhibitors have documented notable reductions in cardiovascular events despite only moderate effects on blood pressure (Yusuf et al. 2000). A reasonable explanation for the greater than expected beneficial effect of ACE inhibitors is their ability to inhibit the formation of angiotensin II, and thereby to inhibit its various effects on vascular biology. Locally produced angiotensin II may contribute to the instability of an atherosclerotic plaque by e.g., stimulating expression of endothelial adhesion molecules and of pro-inflammatory mediators and so increase the influx of inflammatory cells into the plaque (Schieffer et al. 2000). By inhibiting these pro-inflammatory processes, ACE inhibitors and also angiotensin II type 1 receptor blockers may directly contribute to plaque passivation in patients suffering from acute coronary syndromes (Monroe et al. 2003; Cipollone et al. 2004). Moreover, as discussed in this chapter, atherosclerotic plaque rupture is thought to occur because of changes in the plaque itself and systemic changes in the patient, such as hemodynamic alterations. The ACE inhibitor ideally acts at both levels—the plaque biology and the systemic biology of the patient (Lutgens et al. 2003). The use of ACE inhibitors as a part of an anti-atherosclerotic drug regimen is discussed by Schunkert and colleagues more thoroughly in an evidence-based manner in the chapter by Dendorfer et al., this volume.

3.1.4
Antihypertensive Agents, Beta-Blocking Agents and Nitrates

Antihypertensive agents other than ACE inhibitors have also been shown to affect the biology of atherosclerotic plaques (Chobanian et al. 1986). In contrast to the ACE inhibitors, neither specific mediator molecules nor specific target molecules in the plaques have been identified for these drugs. Rather, the effects seem to be mediated indirectly via the hemodynamic effects of the drugs. Oscillating shear stress may alter the endothelial function and promote atherogenesis below the intact endothelium, not only in stenotic inward growing, but also in nonstenotic outward growing areas in which large intramural plaques reside. In an outward growing eccentric plaque with a large lipid pool, the circumferential stress due to blood pressure is concentrated near the shoulder areas of the plaques, the common site of plaque rupture (Richardson et al. 1989). Indeed, of all the rupture-prone areas, the shoulder areas are most vulnerable, their rupture being the most common cause of myocardial infarction (Falk 1992).

Inward growth of the plaque with ensuing severe stenosis usually reflects the growth of the fibrotic component of the plaque. Such highly stenotic plaques are less prone to rupture but rather erode. The high velocity and turbulent flow of the blood passing such stenotic lesions may contribute to the denudation of the endothelium of the lesion (Gertz et al. 1981). It should be noted, however, that laminar flow seems to improve the endothelial cell function at least to a certain point (Berk et al. 2002). Endothelial denudation seems to be of importance especially at the downstream sides of the stenosed segments, in which the endothelial cells show morphological signs of senescence (Bürrig 1991). Moreover, endothelial apoptosis is most common at the downstream shoulders of human atherosclerotic plaques (Tricot et al. 2000).

Generally, lower blood pressure means less circumferential stress and less shear stress. Thus, lowering of blood pressure or the heart rate should lessen such untoward effects. Similarly, a low heart rate means low-cycle repetitive stress on the plaque. The use of beta blockers as a part of the anti-atherosclerotic drug regimen is discussed by Schmitz more thoroughly in an evidence-based manner.

An abnormal coronary vasospasm is important in the pathogenesis of plaque rupture and erosion (Kalsner 1995). Thus, pharmaceutical therapy aimed at treating the vasospasm is an essential part of the stabilization of a vulnerable plaque. Nitrates are safe and effective agents to relieve coronary vasoconstriction in patients with acute coronary syndromes (Hennekens et al. 1996).

3.1.5
Influenza Vaccinations

Influenza epidemics correlate with increased morbidity and mortality to acute coronary events (Gurfinkel et al. 2004). It appears that the latency period between acute infection and an atherothrombotic event is commonly about 2 weeks (Madjid et al. 2003). A number of potential mechanisms have been suggested to be responsible for the postinfluenzal triggering of coronary artery thrombosis (Madjid et al. 2003). In addition to the acute 'trigger effects', influenza has been attributed to also exert chronic pro-atherogenic actions (Madjid et al. 2003).

In several studies, influenza vaccinations have been associated with a reduced risk of acute coronary events in vulnerable patient groups (Naghavi et al. 2000; Nichol et al. 2003; Gurfinkel et al. 2004). Moreover, influenza vaccinations have proved to be safe and cost-effective (Madjid et al. 2003). Therefore, the recommendation of annual influenza vaccination to elderly and other vulnerable patient groups is reasonable (Nichol et al. 2003; Gurfinkel et al. 2004).

3.1.6
Peroxisome Proliferator-Activated Receptor Agonists

Peroxisome proliferator-activated receptors (PPARs) are nuclear receptors present in several organs and cell types, and notably also in atherosclerotic plaques. The PPAR family consists of three members: alpha, gamma, and beta/delta (Marx et al. 2004). All PPARs are activated by fatty acids, and importantly, PPAR alpha is activated by the lipid-regulating fibrates and PPAR gamma by the insulin-sensitizing glitazones, which have also beneficial effects on lipoprotein metabolism (Verges 2004).

3.1.6.1
PPAR Alpha Agonists (Fibrates)

Similar to statins, fibrates also regulate the concentration of plasma lipids. They are particularly well suited for the treatment of the 'deadly triad' of lipids, in which triglycerides are elevated, HDL-cholesterol is low, and the concentration of the especially atherogenic small-dense LDL particles is increased. Indeed, the best clinical benefits, in terms of reduction of coronary events, have been obtained in men having the above characterized dyslipidemia (Manninen et al. 1992). This applies to gemfibrozil in the setting of both primary and secondary prevention, and to bezafibrate when used for secondary prevention (Chapman 2003). No clinical endpoint studies are available yet for fenofibrate, although this drug clearly diminished the progression of coronary plaques in diabetic patients (Diabetes Atherosclerosis Intervention Study Group 2001). The use of fibrates as a part of anti-atherosclerotic drug regimen is discussed by Staels more thoroughly in an evidence-based manner in the chapter by Robillard et al., this volume.

3.1.6.2
PPAR Gamma Agonists (Glitazones)

The new group of clinically used antidiabetic thiazolidinediones (pio-, rosi-, and troglitazones) activate the ligand-activated nuclear transcription factor, PPAR gamma. This subtype of PPAR receptors controls a number of inflammatory processes in the atherosclerotic arterial wall and actually regulates gene expression in most of the cell types present in the vulnerable plaques: the endothelial cells, SMCs, macrophages, and T lymphocytes (Marx et al. 2004). Accordingly, the activators (agonists) of PPAR gamma have emerged as drugs with potential plaque-stabilizing effects. Among the cellular effects which can be regarded as plaque-stabilizing are the inhibition of the release of pro-inflammatory cytokines and matrix-degrading metalloproteinases by macrophages and SMCs, the modulation of the expression of chemokines and endothelin in endothelial cells, and the reduction of the secretion of interferon-gamma by T lymphocytes (Puddu et al. 2003; Marx et al. 2002). Thus, the drugs should reduce chemoattraction and adhesion of monocytes and T lymphocytes to endothelial cells by reducing the cytokine-induced expression of vascular cell adhesion molecule-1 and intercellular adhesion molecule-1. Indeed, studies with the atherosclerosis-prone apoE-null mice have provided in vivo evidence that troglitazone reduces monocyte/macrophage recruitment to atherosclerotic lesions (Pasceri et al. 2000). Moreover, glitazone treatment improves the coronary endothelial function in patients with diabetes mellitus (Murakami et al. 1999).

Although outcome data on the effects of glitazones on cardiovascular mortality are still lacking, beneficial effects on various surrogate markers of atherosclerosis have been reported, particularly in patients with metabolic syndrome and type 2 diabetes (Marx et al. 2004; Verges 2004). Thus, rosiglitazone treatment of patients with type 2 diabetes significantly reduces the plasma levels of interleukin-6 and C-reactive protein, the two pro-inflammatory components strongly related to inflammation in advanced atherosclerotic lesions (Libby and Aikawa 2002). In addition to the indirect markers of atherosclerosis, glitazones also reduce the progression of atherosclerosis, both in patients with type 2 diabetes (Satoh et al. 2003) and in patients without diabetes (Sidhu et al. 2004). Taken together, the experimental and human studies suggest that the glitazones may exert, in addition to systemic metabolic actions, direct anti-atherogenic actions at the level of the vascular wall (Barbier et al. 2002).

3.2
Drugs Currently in Experimental Use for the Prevention of Acute Coronary Events
3.2.1
Nonsteroidal Anti-inflammatory Drugs

As discussed in this chapter, there is substantial evidence supporting the notion that atherosclerosis in general, and rupture-prone plaques in particular, have a strong inflammatory component. Therefore, it is somewhat surprising that drugs developed to treat chronic inflammatory diseases, such as arthritis, have not been advocated to be used as first-line drugs to prevent atherosclerosis and its clinical complications.

Theoretically, the finding of increased expression of the pro-inflammatory cyclooxygenase isoform cyclooxygenase-2 (COX-2) in human atherosclerotic lesions (Schonbeck et al. 1999), and particularly in macrophages of the lesions (Baker et al. 1999), makes the use of selective COX-2 inhibitors a very attractive choice for the management of inflammation in the vulnerable plaque. However, endothelial cells too contain COX-2, which may be induced by the shear stress generated by blood flow. The elevated COX-2 in the endothelium generates the antithrombotic and vasodilatory eicosanoid prostacyclin, and inhibition of endothelial prostacyclin formation could potentially promote thrombosis. In addition, the COX-2 inhibitors let free the other cyclooxygenase isoform, COX-1, present in platelets, to synthesize thromboxane A_2, which promotes thrombosis. Thus, the net effect of COX-2 inhibitors on cardiovascular home-ostasis would be a prothrombotic shift in the dynamic balance between endothelial prostacyclin production and platelet thromboxane A_2 production. The above considerations may explain the occurrence of adverse cardiovascu-lar events in the COX-2 inhibitor rofecoxib trial (VIGOR). Indeed, in this trial a fivefold increase in atherothrombotic events was observed in comparison with naproxen, which inhibits not only COX-2 but also COX-1 (Bombardier et al. 2000; Pitt et al. 2002). Rofecoxib has now been withdrawn from the mar-ket, following the premature cessation of the Adenomatous Polyp Prevention on Vioxx (APPROVe) study, because of significant increase by a factor of 3.9 in the incidence of serious thromboembolic adverse events in the group receiving the drug, as compared with the placebo group (FitzGerald 2004).

The traditional NSAIDs such as aspirin inhibit both COX-1 and COX-2. As discussed previously, the small doses of aspirin used for platelet inhibition are likely to be without effect on the plaque itself. High doses of nonaspirin nonsteroidal anti-inflammatory drugs (NANSAIDs), with their potential abil-ity to maintain the platelet-endothelium balance and to inhibit macrophage COX-2, should theoretically be able to reduce the risk of acute coronary syndromes, even without the concurrent use of aspirin. A recent study by Kimmel et al. (2004) concludes that, in the absence of aspirin, NANSAIDs, particularly ibuprofen, are associated with a reduced risk of myocardial infarction. Some reports have suggested that a concurrent administration of aspirin and ibuprofen might be associated with lower cardioprotection than of aspirin alone due to pharmacodynamic interaction. A recent large study could not demonstrate any detectable risk reduction of myocardial infarction by NANSAIDs (ibuprofen and naproxen) (Garcia Rodriguez et al. 2004). Neither was there any noticeable clinical interaction that would affect the cardioprotection provided by aspirin when concurrently taking aspirin and NANSAID. The overall conclusion from the many studies is that NANSAIDs lack the protective effect against myocardial infarction afforded by aspirin. Hence, this class of drugs cannot be considered as a drug therapy for the vulnerable plaque.

3.2.2
Antibiotics

Besides lipid accumulation, also local and systemic inflammation has been shown to play a role in the generation of atherosclerosis and acute coronary events. In numerous serological and experimental studies, many microorganisms have been implicated as pathogenic components of atherosclerosis (see Table 2), although conflicting data has been reported for most, if not all microorganisms listed in Table 2. The most convincing evidence exists for the pro-atherogenic effects of chronic infections, such as chronic gingivitis and bronchitis. Acute infections seem to be associated with an increased risk of acute atherothrombotic events, suggesting a triggering role for acute infections (Madjid et al. 2003). At present, the total lifetime inflammatory burden seems to be associated more strongly with the increased risk of atherosclerosis than any of the single infections (Prasad et al. 2002).

Table 2 Microorganisms associated with increased risk of atherosclerosis and its complications

Bacteria	*Chlamydia pneumoniae* (Prasad et al. 2002)
	Helicobacter pylori (Prasad et al. 2002)
	Haemophilus influenzae (Espinola-Klein et al. 2002)
	Mycoplasma pneumoniae (Espinola-Klein et al. 2002)
Viruses	Cytomegalovirus (CMV) (Prasad et al. 2002)
	Herpes simplex virus (HSV-1 and HSV-2) (Prasad et al. 2002)
	Epstein-Barr Virus (EBV) (Espinola-Klein et al. 2002)
	Hepatitis viruses (Prasad et al. 2002)
	Influenza viruses (Gurfinkel et al. 2004)
	Human immunodeficiency virus (Neumann et al. 2004)

In order to affect atherogenesis in its various stages, the mechanisms by which the microorganisms operate must be different. One obvious problem in studying the effects of microorganisms on human coronary atherosclerosis and its complications is the lack of accurate measurements of development of atherosclerotic lesions in human coronary arteries. We are, therefore, left with studies on the possible relations between infections and the clinical complications of atherosclerosis.

To date, a few small secondary prevention studies have shown positive effects in the prevention of cardiac events with antibiotics (Sinisalo et al. 2002). However, a recent meta-analysis of randomized controlled trials on the secondary prevention of ischemic heart disease did not show beneficial effect of antibiotics on cardiovascular endpoints (Wells et al. 2004). In summary, due to the potential harmful effects of antibiotics, their use cannot be recommended for the treatment or prevention of atherosclerosis or acute coronary syndromes. However, further studies are warranted.

Promising results have been obtained in the prevention of acute coronary events in vulnerable patients with influenza vaccinations (Gurfinkel et al. 2004). Interestingly, there are no data on the anti-influenzaviral neuraminidase inhibitors (oseltamivir and zanamivir) in the prevention of acute coronary syndromes.

3.2.3
Antioxidants

As one of the main hypotheses of atherogenesis, the oxidation hypothesis has placed antioxidants in a prime position as potential inhibitors of atherogenesis and its clinical complications. Theoretically, by preventing the oxidation of LDL, antioxidants should have the ability to inhibit lesion progression via multiple mechanisms (Chisolm and Steinberg 2000; Carr et al. 2000). They include inhibition of recruitment of monocytes into the lesions and their activation and transformation into lipid-filled foam cells. Also, oxidized LDL can induce apoptotic death of monocytes, and the lipid-rich plaques contain increased numbers of macrophages with signs of apoptosis (Hutter et al. 2004). Thus, antioxidant therapies could prevent the formation of a necrotic lipid core. Finally, reactive oxygen species produced by macrophage foam cells activate vascular matrix metalloproteinases capable of degrading the extracellular matrix of plaque caps (Rajagopalan et al. 1996). Taken together, there is abundant data suggesting that oxidized LDL could contribute to the generation of both the necrotic lipid core and cap thinning, the two critical components of rupture-prone vulnerable plaques.

The numerous studies in experimental animals showing an inhibitory effect of antioxidants have served as a 'proof of principle' that antioxidants can halt the progression of atherosclerosis (Meagher and Rader 2001). Yet, several recent large-scale, double-blind, placebo-controlled trials have convincingly shown that neither beta-carotene nor vitamin E, alone or in combination with other antioxidant vitamins (vitamin C, beta-carotene and selenium), will reduce the risk of fatal or nonfatal infarction in an unselected population of people with established coronary artery disease or at high risk for it (Steinberg and Witztum 2002). A very recent small-scale, well-controlled clinical trial using doses of antioxidant vitamins similar to the ones used in the large-scale trials provided one plausible explanation for the negative outcomes of the large trials (Kinlay et al. 2004). In this study, long-term oral administration of vitamins C and E failed to improve the two key mechanisms in the biology of coronary atherosclerosis, i.e., coronary endothelial function or LDL oxidation. Even though the clinical trials with antioxidants present a negative picture in terms of prevention of coronary plaque rupture or erosion, they do not disprove the oxidant stress hypothesis. Rather, they call for more potent and effective, and perhaps entirely differently acting, antioxidants in this clinical setting.

3.3
Potential Future Drug Therapies for the Vulnerable Plaque

3.3.1
Vaccination Against Atherogenesis: Which Is the Correct Antigen?

Atherosclerosis has many similarities to inflammatory and autoimmune diseases such as rheumatoid arthritis and multiple sclerosis (Ross 1999; Hansson 2001). There is compelling evidence from experimental animal models that such autoimmune diseases may be treated by vaccination. There is also much evidence for the involvement of bacteria in the pathogenesis of atherosclerosis, which also opens up new avenues for the vaccination approach. Atherosclerosis is a complex disease with a myriad of molecules able to be modified to generate autoantigens (Nilsson and Kovanen 2004). Therefore, the key to designing successful vaccination is the choice of the correct target antigen (Hansson 2002). In atherosclerosis, two major autoantigens have so far been implicated: oxidized LDL and heat shock protein 60 (HSP60). Parenteral immunization with oxidized LDL was found to inhibit atherogenesis in experimental animals, suggesting that vaccination with this disease-associated autoantigen could be a possible strategy to treat atherosclerosis. The situation with heat shock proteins is more complex. Because heat shock proteins have been conserved in evolution, human HSP60 is highly homologous to and immunologically cross-reacts with mycobacterial HSP65 and chlamydial HSP60 (Wick et al. 2004). It is therefore possible that at least part of the immune responses to HSP60 is caused by microbial infections, and this cross-reactivity may explain why certain infections are associated with increased atherosclerosis.

Based on the above findings, there is potential for an antigen-specific therapy against atherosclerosis. The antigen-specific prophylaxis would not affect the resistance of the host against other pathogens or autoantigens. Actually, this is the only option, since generalized immunomodulation achieved with immunosuppressive drugs is unacceptable in the prevention of a common disease such as atherosclerosis. However, although immunization with the two different autoantigens, oxidized LDL and HSP65/60, can protect atherosclerosis-susceptible mice against advanced disease, the autoimmune reactions in the large portion of the human population affected by atherosclerosis are likely to involve many different antigens (Hansson 2002). It may, obviously, take a long time until vaccination trials against atherogenesis can begin. It will take even longer to obtain results, if young persons are to be vaccinated.

3.3.2
Proteinase Inhibitors

In the unstable plaque, a major component leading to cap thinning and weakening is the increased breakdown of the extracellular matrix of the fibrous cap. The activated macrophages and mast cells secrete proteases that can break down the framework consisting of collagen, elastin, and proteoglycans (Libby 1995; Lindstedt and Kovanen 2004). Breakdown of these structural molecules of the extracellular matrix can weaken the fibrous cap, rendering it more susceptible to rupture and precipitation of an acute coronary syndrome.

The proteases secreted by macrophages and SMCs include a variety of matrix metalloproteinases (MMPs) and cathepsins. Distinct approaches have been proposed for pharmacological inhibition of MMPs in atherosclerosis (Beaudeux et al. 2004). They include the decrease in cellular expression and activation of MMPs, the increase in cellular expression of TIMPs, the natural inhibitors of MMPs, and the direct inhibition of activated MMPs by pseudopeptide inhibitors, nonpeptide inhibitors, and tetracycline analogs. Of special practical importance is the fact that statins inhibit, at least in vitro, the secretion of certain MMPs by macrophages (Bellosta et al. 1998). Despite original enthusiasm for the novel idea of inhibiting plaque rupture by blocking MMPs, there is at present a lack of interest in planning new strategies for the prevention of acute coronary events by this principle. This is because, MMPs are also likely to have beneficial physiological effects in the arterial wall. In addition to being involved in clearance of debris, MMPs are involved in cell migration and proliferation needed for repair processes of injured arteries. Yet, in cancer and degenerative diseases such as arthritis, several MMP inhibitors are undergoing clinical trials (Brown 2000).

Atherosclerotic lesions in humans overexpress the elastolytic and collagenolytic cysteine proteases, the cathepsins S, K, and L, but show relatively reduced expression of cystatin C, their endogenous inhibitor (Liu et al. 2004). Extracts of human atheromatous tissue show greater elastolytic activity in vitro than the extracts from healthy donors. Moreover, the cysteinyl protease inhibitor E64d limits such an increase in elastolysis, indicating an involvement of cysteine proteases in elastin degradation during atherogenesis. Yet, as recently discussed by Liu et al. (2004), the cysteine proteases could play dual roles. Cathepsin-mediated fragmentation of the barrier between the medial and intimal layer of the atherosclerotic arterial wall would allow the migration of SMCs from the media into the intima, where they would produce collagen and reinforce the fibrous cap. On the other hand, the SMCs in the fibrous cap can also produce collagenolytic cathepsins, which would have the opposite effect. Accordingly, due to their important role in arterial remodeling, cysteine proteases are not at present a feasible target when planning strategies to prevent plaque rupture.

The two proteases secreted by mast cells are tryptase and chymase. Indeed, mast cells are filled with these neutral proteases, and the major secretory product of human mast cells is tryptase. Importantly, there is therapeutic potential of inhibition of either enzyme (He et al. 2001). Recently, APC2059, a highly specific and selective tryptase inhibitor, has been used to treat ulcerative colitis in humans (Tremaine et al. 2002). Similarly, tryptase inhibitors are also considered as potential therapeutic agents for asthma. Several orally active inhibitors of chymase are now available, but they have yet to be tested in humans (Doggrell and Wanstall 2004).

Since a multitude of proteases are acting in the inflamed cap of a vulnerable plaque, the key enzymes responsible for the pathological matrix degradation should be identified before specific drug therapy can be envisioned. For the time being, anti-inflammatory therapies aiming at lowering the numbers of the cells secreting such matrix-degrading enzymes, or their stabilization, may be the best way of lessening the proteolytic burden in the vulnerable cap.

3.3.3
Mast Cell Stabilizers, Antihistamines and Leukotriene Receptor Blockers: Agents Potentially Counteracting Atherosclerotic Vasoconstriction

Inflamed atherosclerotic coronary segments are known to constrict in response to various stimuli, especially in response to soluble mediators derived from inflammatory cells such as mast cells (Forman et al. 1985). In fact, such coronary segments paradoxically constrict in response to the very same stimuli known to exert a dilatatory effect on healthy coronary arteries. The key factor responsible for such an unfavorable effect is a dysfunctional or absent endothelium on the vulnerable plaques. Most importantly, the pathological vasoconstriction plays an important role in acute coronary syndromes and has also been suggested to predispose to plaque rupture and erosion (Hackett et al. 1987; Kalsner and Richards 1984; Kalsner 1995).

Mast cells are inflammatory cells capable of secreting a variety of preformed (histamine) and newly generated (leukotrienes) vasoactive mediators (Galli et al. 2002). As a sign of coronary mast cell activation in vivo, elevated levels of mast cell-derived histamine have been observed in the coronary circulation of patients with variant angina shortly before coronary spasm and the ensuing angina (Sakata et al. 1996). Also, the levels of histamine in the systemic circulation of patients with stable and unstable coronary heart disease may be elevated (Clejan et al. 2002). In variant angina, the numbers of coronary adventitial mast cells are highest in the spastic coronary segment (Forman et al. 1985). Finally, the number of activated histamine containing mast cells is increased in the intimal and adventitial layers of culprit lesions of patients with acute coronary syndromes as a reflection of an ongoing inflammation in the coronary plaques and also in the adventitia surrounding the plaque (Kovanen et al. 1995; Laine et al. 1999).

Also, leukotrienes have been shown to constrict atherosclerotic coronary arteries. This constriction was markedly attenuated by the leukotriene receptor antagonist ICI198.615 in an organ bath experiment (Allen et al. 1993). Although mast cells are a source of leukotrienes in atherosclerotic coronary arteries, there are also other likely sources such as macrophages.

Recently, mast cells have been shown to be structurally connected with sensory nerve fibers in the adventitia of atherosclerotic coronary arteries (Laine et al. 2000). This structural connection may be of pathological significance, since the identified sensory nerves contain peptide neurotransmitter substance P, vasoactive intestinal peptide, and calcitonin gene-related peptide, all capable of stimulating mast cells. Furthermore, the number of mast cells in contact with the sensory nerve fibers is significantly higher in the inflamed adventitia of atherosclerotic segments of coronary arteries than in the normal segments. Therefore, it is reasonable to hypothesize that neuroendocrine mechanisms of mast cell activation may also play a role in triggering acute coronary events (Huang et al. 2002; Kario et al. 2003).

The mast cell-derived histamine and leukotrienes also act as pro-inflammatory mediators and may thus aggravate coronary syndromes and lead to an increased risk of plaque rupture. Accordingly, blocking the local actions of these vasoactive and proinflammatory compounds is potentially beneficial in the treatment of the vulnerable plaques. Importantly, both antihistamines and leukotriene receptor antagonists are available for clinical use and have proved to be safe (Simons and Simons 2002; Drazen et al. 1999).

Taken together, the therapeutic targets of antihistamines and leukotriene receptor antagonists could possibly be widened to include also the prevention of coronary artery spasm in patients with stable or unstable angina, with an ultimate goal to reduce the risk of plaque rupture or erosion (De Caterina and Zampolli 2004).

3.3.4
Inductors of Cholesterol Efflux from Atherosclerotic Plaques

Very promising results have been obtained in a small, well-controlled clinical study with apoprotein (apo)A-I Milano intravenous infusions (Nissen et al. 2003). Notably, this was the first study to show a reduction of plaque size using an intravascular imaging method. This agent, the apoA-I Milano, is capable of removing cholesterol from the plaques, and, surprisingly, apparently also from the extracellular stores which have traditionally been considered to be very resistant to removal by HDL. This is the first 'drug' ever to directly and selectively affect the human plaque. Actually, by being injected into the systemic circulation, the apoA-I Milano is not 'plaque specific', as it can remove cholesterol from any tissue in the body. However, because in the common type of atherosclerosis cholesterol accumulates only in the arterial intima there is no excess to remove from other sites in extrahepatic tissues. Since accumulation of cholesterol is the very key element in the development of a rupture-prone plaque, its removal is the ultimate goal and the curative therapy of such a vulnerable plaque.

Finally, intravenous administration of apoA-I Milano, albeit theoretically attractive, will not be available for all patients at high risk for plaque rupture requiring stabilization and regression of the vulnerable plaques. Indeed, at present, such therapy is restricted to the patients with acute coronary syndromes (Nissen et al. 2003). However, with the advent of novel potent HDL-raising oral drugs, such as inhibitors of cholesteryl ester transfer protein, potentially plaque regression-inducing drug therapy will be available to a significantly larger group of vulnerable patients (Le Goff et al. 2004). The use of HDL metabolism-modulating agents as a potential anti-atherosclerotic drug therapy is discussed more thoroughly in the chapter by Hersberger and von Eckardstein, in this volume.

3.3.5
Progenitor Cells as Therapeutic Targets and Tools

Endothelial progenitor cells (EPCs) are bone marrow-derived cells, which are considered generally to be beneficial in the prevention of atherosclerosis and its complications (Szmitko et al. 2003; Urbich and Dimmeler 2004). The number of circulatory ECPs can be measured, and recent evidence suggests that the determination of their number in peripheral blood may provide a useful novel index of cumulative cardiovascular risk and also serve as a surrogate marker for vascular function (Hill et al. 2003). Interestingly, the number of circulatory EPCs appears to be regulated by factors which are also related to the risk of coronary artery disease (Vasa et al. 2001). Thus, nonpharmacological or pharmacological interventions aimed at reducing the risk factors of coronary artery disease seem to rapidly increase the number of EPCs (Assmus et al. 2003; Laufs et al. 2004; Kondo et al. 2004; Min et al. 2004). Taken together, ECPs seem to offer a novel diagnostic marker for the risk evaluation of coronary artery disease and hold considerable therapeutic potential for the treatment of coronary artery disease and its complications (Melo et al. 2004).

The hematopoietic stem cells can also differentiate into SMCs in various experimental models of vascular lesions. Indeed, it has been suggested that they participate in the pathogenesis of atherosclerosis (Sata et al. 2002). Therefore, it would be of great interest to know whether such SMC progenitors also contribute to the genesis of an obstructive coronary lesion in humans, too.

4
Summary

As discussed in this chapter, the current drug therapies for the vulnerable plaque aim mainly at inhibiting the development of vulnerable plaques, i.e., they are nonspecific systemic therapies which act at many levels of the long-lasting development of a vulnerable plaque (Fig. 3). Ideally, such preventive therapies could be optimal in that they halt or even reverse the progression of atherosclerosis at a clinically safe stage.

Even in the face of these visionary prospects, and the fact that coronary artery mortality rates have been dramatically declining (Tunstall-Pedoe et al. 1999), coronary artery disease has been predicted to be the killer number one worldwide also in the future (WHO 2002). The challenge to open up new fields for pharmacological rethinking in the prevention of plaque rupture remains (Rodgers 2003).

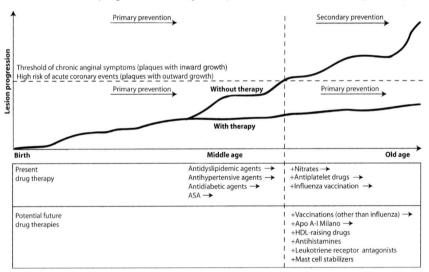

Fig. 3 Schematic representation of lesion progression in a vulnerable patient with and without therapy. One should note that, by definition, the secondary prevention in patients with outward-growing plaques begins after the first acute coronary event, provided that no symptoms causing inward-growing plaques are present. Current and potential future drug therapies are summarized in the *lower part* of the figure

References

Allen SP, Dashwood MR, Chester AH, et al. (1993) Influence of atherosclerosis on the vascular reactivity of isolated human epicardial coronary arteries to leukotriene C4. Cardioscience 4:4754

Ambrose JA, D'Agate DJ (2004) Drug therapy for the vulnerable plaque. In: Waksman R, Serruys PW (eds) Handbook of the vulnerable plaque. Taylor & Francis Group, London, pp 255–281

Assmus B, Urbich C, Aicher A, et al. (2003) HMG-CoA reductase inhibitors reduce senescence and increase proliferation of endothelial progenitor cells via regulation of cell cycle regulatory genes. Circ Res 92:1049–1055

Baker CS, Hall RJ, Evans TJ, et al. (1999) Cyclooxygenase-2 is widely expressed in atherosclerotic lesions affecting native and transplanted human coronary arteries and colocalizes with inducible nitric oxide synthase and nitrotyrosine particularly in macrophages. Arterioscler Thromb Vasc Biol 19:646–655

Bank AJ, Versluis A, Dodge SM, et al. (2000) Atherosclerotic plaque rupture: a fatigue process? Med Hypoteses 55:480–484

Barbier O, Torra IP, Duguay Y, et al. (2002) Pleiotropic actions of peroxisome proliferator-activated receptors in lipid metabolism and atherosclerosis. Arterioscler Thromb Vasc Biol 22:717–726

Barter PJ, Nicholls S, Rye KA, et al. (2004) Antiinflammatory properties of HDL. Circ Res 95:764–772

Beaudeux JL, Giral P, Bruckert E (2004) Matrix metalloproteinases, inflammation and atherosclerosis: therapeutic perspectives. Clin Chem Lab Med 42:121–131

Bellosta S, Via D, Canavesi M, et al. (1998) HMG-CoA reductase inhibitors reduce MMP-9 secretion by macrophages. Arterioscler Thromb Vasc Biol 18:1671–1678

Berk BC, Min W, Yan C, et al. (2002) Atheroprotective Mechanisms Activated by Fluid Shear Stress in Endothelial Cells. Drug News Perspect 15:133–139

Bogaty P, Hackett D, Davies G, et al. (1994) Vasoreactivity of the culprit lesion in unstable angina. Circulation 90:5–11

Bombardier C, Laine L, Reicin A, et al. (2000) Comparison of upper gastrointestinal toxicity of rofecoxib and naproxen in patients with rheumatoid arthritis. VIGOR Study Group. N Engl J Med 343:1520–1528

Bosch T, Wendler T (2004) State of the art of low-density lipoprotein apheresis in the year. Ther Apher Dial 8:76–79

Brown BG, Zhao XQ, Sacco DE, et al. (1993) Lipid lowering and plaque regression. New insights into prevention of plaque disruption and clinical events in coronary disease. Circulation 87:1781–1791

Brown PD (2000) Ongoing trials with matrix metalloproteinase inhibitors. Expert Opin Investig Drugs 9:2167–2177

Bruckert E, Giral P, Tellier P (2003) Perspectives in cholesterol-lowering therapy: the role of ezetimibe, a new selective inhibitor of intestinal cholesterol absorption. Circulation 107:3124–3128.

Bürrig KF (1991) The endothelium of advanced arteriosclerotic plaques in humans. Arterioscler Thromb 11:1678–1689

CAPRIE Steering Committee (1996) A randomised, blinded trial of clopidogrel versus aspirin in patients at risk of ischaemic events (CAPRIE). Lancet 348:1329–1339

Carr AC, Zhu BZ, Frei B (2000) Potential antiatherogenic mechanisms of ascorbate (vitamin C) and alpha-tocopherol (vitamin E). Circ Res 87:349–354

Chapman MJ (2003) Fibrates in 2003: therapeutic action in atherogenic dyslipidaemia and future perspectives. Atherosclerosis 171:1–13

Chisolm GM, Steinberg D (2000) The oxidative modification hypothesis of atherogenesis: an overview. Free Radic Biol Med 28:1815–1826

Chobanian AV, Brecher P, Haudenschild CC, et al. (1986) Effects of hypertension and of antihypertensive therapy on atherosclerosis. Hypertension 8(Suppl I):I-15–I-21

Cipollone F, Fazia M, Iezzi A, et al. (2004) Blockade of the angiotensin II type 1 receptor stabilizes atherosclerotic plaques in humans by inhibiting prostaglandin E2-dependent matrix metalloproteinase activity. Circulation 109:1482–1488

Clejan S, Japa S, Clemetson C, et al. (2002) Blood histamine is associated with coronary artery disease, cardiac events and severity of inflammation and atherosclerosis. J Cell Mol Med 6:583–592

Colwell JA (2004) Antiplatelet agents for the prevention of cardiovascular disease in diabetes mellitus. Am J Cardiovasc Drugs 4:87–106

Crisby M, Nordin-Fredriksson G, Shah PK, et al. (2001) Pravastatin treatment increases collagen content and decreases lipid content, inflammation, metalloproteinases, and cell death in human carotid plaques: implications for plaque stabilization. Circulation 103:926–933

Davignon J (2004) Beneficial cardiovascular pleiotropic effects of statins. Circulation 109(23 Suppl 1):III39–43.

De Caterina R, Zampolli A (2004) From asthma to atherosclerosis — 5-lipoxygenase, leukotrienes, and inflammation. N Engl J Med 350:4–7

Diabetes Atherosclerosis Intervention Study Group (2001) Effect of fenofibrate on progression of coronary-artery disease in type 2 diabetes: the Diabetes Atherosclerosis Intervention Study, a randomised study. Lancet 357:905–910

Diener HC, Bogousslavsky J, Brass LM, et al. (2004) Aspirin and clopidogrel compared with clopidogrel alone after recent ischaemic stroke or transient ischaemic attack in high-risk patients (MATCH): randomised, double-blind, placebo-controlled trial. Lancet 364:331–337

Doggrell SA, Wanstall JC (2004) Vascular chymase: pathophysiological role and therapeutic potential of inhibition. Cardiovasc Res 61:653–662

Drazen JM, Israel E, O'Byrne PM (1999) Drug therapy: Treatment of asthma with drugs modifying the leukotriene pathway. N Engl J Med 340:197–206

Duguid JB (1946) Thrombosis as a factor in the pathogenesis of coronary atherosclerosis. J Pathol Bacteriol 58:207–212

Espinola-Klein C, Rupprecht HJ, Blankenberg S, et al. (2002) Impact of infectious burden on progression of carotid atherosclerosis. Stroke 33:2581–2586

Falk E (1983) Plaque rupture with severe pre-existing stenosis precipitating coronary thrombosis. Characteristics of coronary atherosclerotic plaques underlying fatal occlusive thrombi. Br Heart J 50:127–134

Falk E (1992) Why do plaques rupture? Circulation 86(Suppl III):III30–42

Fayad ZA (2003) MR imaging for the noninvasive assessment of atherothrombotic plaques. Magn Reson Imaging Clin N Am 11:101–113

Finet G, Ohayon J, Rioufol G (2004) Biomechanical interaction between cap thickness, lipid core composition and blood pressure in vulnerable coronary plaque: impact on stability or instability. Coron Artery Dis 15:13–20

FitzGerald GA (2004) Coxibs and cardiovascular disease. N Engl J Med 351:1709–1711

Forman MB, Oates JA, Robertson D, et al. (1985) Increased adventitial mast cells in a patient with coronary spasm. N Engl J Med 313:1138–1141

Forrester JS (2002) Prevention of plaque rupture: a new paradigm of therapy. Ann Intern Med 137:823–833

Fuster V (2002) Assessing and modifying vulnerable atherosclerotic plaque. Futura Publishing Company, New York

Galli SJ, Wedemeyer J, Tsai M (2002) Analyzing the roles of mast cells and basophils in host defense and other biological responses. Int J Hematol 75:363–369

Garcia Rodriguez LA, Varas-Lorenzo C, Maguire A, et al. (2004) Nonsteroidal antiinflammatory drugs and the risk of myocardial infarction in the general population. Circulation 109:3000–3006

Gertz SD, Uretsky G, Wajnberg RS, et al. (1981) Endothelial cell damage and thrombus formation after partial arterial constriction: relevance to the role of coronary artery spasm in the pathogenesis of myocardial infarction. Circulation 63:476–486

Glagov S, Weisenberg E, Zarins CK, et al. (1987) Compensatory enlargement of human atherosclerotic coronary arteries. N Engl J Med 316:1371–1375

Grundy SM, Cleeman JI, Merz CN, et al. (2004) Implications of recent clinical trials for the National Cholesterol Education Program Adult Treatment Panel III Guidelines. J Am Coll Cardiol 44:720–732

Gurfinkel EP, Leon de la Fuente R, Mendiz O, et al. (2004) Flu vaccination in acute coronary syndromes and planned percutaneous coronary interventions (FLUVACS) Study. Eur Heart J 25:25–31

Guyton JR, Klemp KF (1994) Development of the atherosclerotic core region. Chemical and ultrastructural analysis of microdissected atherosclerotic lesions from human aorta. Arterioscler Thromb 14:1305–1314

Hackett D, Davies G, Chierchia S, et al. (1987) Intermittent coronary occlusion in acute myocardial infarction: Value of combined thrombolytic and vasodilator therapy. N Engl J Med 317:1055–1059

Haffner SM, Lehto S, Ronnemaa T, et al. (1998) Mortality from coronary heart disease in subjects with type 2 diabetes and in nondiabetic subjects with and without prior myocardial infarction. N Engl J Med 339:229–234

Hankey GJ, Eikelboom JW (2003) Antiplatelet drugs. Med J Aust 178:568–574

Hansson GK (2001) Immune mechanisms in atherosclerosis. Arterioscler Thromb Vasc Biol 21:1876–1890

Hansson GK (2002) Vaccination against atherosclerosis: science or fiction? Circulation 106:1599–1601

He S, Gaca MD, Walls AF (2001) The activation of synovial mast cells: modulation of histamine release by tryptase and chymase and their inhibitors. Eur J Pharmacol 412:223–229

Hennekens CH, Albert CM, Godfried SL, et al. (1996) Adjunctive drug therapy of acute myocardial infarction—evidence from clinical trials. N Engl J Med 335:1660–1667

Hill JM, Zalos G, Halcox JP, et al. (2003) Circulating endothelial progenitor cells, vascular function, and cardiovascular risk. N Engl J Med 348:593–600

Huang M, Pang X, Letourneau R, et al. (2002) Acute stress induces cardiac mast cell activation and histamine release, effects that are increased in apolipoprotein E knockout mice. Cardiovasc Res 55:150–160

Hutter R, Valdiviezo C, Sauter BV, et al. (2004) Caspase-3 and tissue factor expression in lipid-rich plaque macrophages: evidence for apoptosis as link between inflammation and atherothrombosis. Circulation 109:2001–2008

Kalsner S (1995) Coronary artery spasm. Multiple causes and multiple roles in heart disease. Biochem Pharmacol 49:859–871

Kalsner S, Richards R (1984) Coronary arteries of cardiac patients are hyperreactive and contain stores of amines: a mechanism for coronary spasm. Science 223:1435–1437

Kario K, McEwen BS, Pickering TG (2003) Disasters and the heart: a review of the effects of earthquake-induced stress on cardiovascular disease. Hypertens Res 26:355–367

Kimmel SE, Berlin JA, Reilly M, et al. (2004) The effects of nonselective non-aspirin non-steroidal anti-inflammatory medications on the risk of nonfatal myocardial infarction and their interaction with aspirin. J Am Coll Cardiol 43:985–990

Kinlay S, Behrendt D, Fang JC, et al. (2004) Long-term effect of combined vitamins E and C on coronary and peripheral endothelial function. J Am Coll Cardiol 43:629–634

Kolodgie FD, Burke AP, Farb A, et al. (2002) Differential accumulation of proteoglycans and hyaluronan in culprit lesions: insights into plaque erosion. Arterioscler Thromb Vasc Biol 22:1642–1648

Kondo T, Hayashi M, Takeshita K, et al. (2004) Smoking cessation rapidly increases circulating progenitor cells in peripheral blood in chronic smokers. Arterioscler Thromb Vasc Biol 24:1442–1447

Kovanen PT, Kaartinen M, Paavonen T (1995) Infiltrates of activated mast cells at the site of coronary atheromatous erosion or rupture in myocardial infarction. Circulation 92:1084–1088

Laine P, Kaartinen M, Penttilä A, et al. (1999) Association between myocardial infarction and the mast cells in the adventitia of the infarct-related coronary artery. Circulation 99:361–369

Laine P, Naukkarinen A, Heikkilä L, et al. (2000) Adventitial mast cells connect with sensory nerve fibers in atherosclerotic coronary arteries. Circulation 101:1665–1669

Laufs U, Werner N, Link A, et al. (2004) Physical training increases endothelial progenitor cells, inhibits neointima formation, and enhances angiogenesis. Circulation 109:220–226

Law MR, Wald NJ, Rudnincka R (2003) Quantifying effect of statins on low density lipoprotein cholesterol, ischaemic heart disease, and stroke: systematic review and meta-analysis. BMJ 326:1–7

Le Goff W, Guerin M, Chapman MJ (2004) Pharmacological modulation of cholesteryl ester transfer protein, a new therapeutic target in atherogenic dyslipidemia. Pharmacol Ther 101:17–38

Libby P (1995) Molecular bases of the acute coronary syndromes. Circulation 91:2844–2850

Libby P (2002) Inflammation in atherosclerosis. Nature 420:868–874

Libby P, Aikawa M (2002) Stabilization of atherosclerotic plaques: new mechanisms and clinical targets. Nat Med 8:1257–1262

Lindstedt KA, Kovanen PT (2004) Mast cells in vulnerable coronary plaques: potential mechanisms linking mast cell activation to plaque erosion and rupture. Curr Opin Lipidol 15:567–573

Lindstedt KA, Leskinen MJ, Kovanen PT (2004) Proteolysis of the pericellular matrix – a novel element determining cell survival and death in the pathogenesis of plaque erosion and rupture. Arterioscler Thromb Vasc Biol 24:1350–1358

Lipid Research Clinics Program (1984) The Lipid Research Clinics Coronary Primary Prevention Trial results II. The relationship of reduction in incidence of coronary heart disease to cholesterol lowering. JAMA 251:365–374

Little WC, Constantinescu M, Applegate RJ, et al. (1988) Can coronary angiography predict the site of a subsequent myocardial infarction in patients with mild-to-moderate coronary artery disease? Circulation 78:1157–1166

Liu J, Sukhova GK, Sun JS, et al. (2004) Lysosomal cysteine proteases in atherosclerosis. Arterioscler Thromb Vasc Biol 24:1359–1366

Lutgens E, van Suylen RJ, Faber BC, et al. (2003) Atherosclerotic plaque rupture: local or systemic process? Arterioscler Thromb Vasc Biol 23:2123–2130

Madjid M, Naghavi M, Litovsky S, et al. (2003) Influenza and cardiovascular disease: a new opportunity for prevention and the need for further studies. Circulation 108:2730–2736

Mann J, Davies MJ (1999) Mechanisms of progression in native coronary artery disease: role of healed plaque disruption. Heart 82:265–268

Manninen V, Tenkanen L, Koskinen P, et al. (1992) Joint effects of serum triglyceride and LDL cholesterol and HDL cholesterol concentrations on coronary heart disease risk in the Helsinki Heart Study. Implications for treatment. Circulation 85:37–45

Marx N, Kehrle B, Kohlhammer K, et al. (2002) PPAR activators as antiinflammatory mediators in human T lymphocytes: implications for atherosclerosis and transplantation-associated arteriosclerosis. Circ Res 90:703–710

Marx N, Duez H, Fruchart JC, et al. (2004) Peroxisome proliferator-activated receptors and atherogenesis: regulators of gene expression in vascular cells. Circ Res 94:1168–1178

Meagher E, Rader DJ (2001) Antioxidant therapy and atherosclerosis: animal and human studies. Trends Cardiovasc Med 11:162–165

Melo LG, Pachori AS, Kong D, et al. (2004) Gene and cell-based therapies for heart disease. FASEB J 18:648–663

Min TQ, Zhu CJ, Xiang WX, et al. (2004) Improvement in endothelial progenitor cells from peripheral blood by ramipril therapy in patients with stable coronary artery disease. Cardiovasc Drugs Ther 18:203–209

Monroe VS, Kerensky RA, Rivera E, et al. (2003) Pharmacologic plaque passivation for the reduction of recurrent cardiac events in acute coronary syndromes. J Am Coll Cardiol 41:23S–30S

Murakami T, Mizuno S, Ohsato K, et al. (1999) Effects of troglitazone on frequency of coronary vasospastic-induced angina pectoris in patients with diabetes mellitus. Am J Cardiol 84:92–94

Naghavi M, Barlas Z, Siadaty S, et al. (2000) Association of influenza vaccination and reduced risk of recurrent myocardial infarction. Circulation 102:3039–3045

Naghavi M, Libby P, Falk E, et al. (2003a) From vulnerable plaque to vulnerable patient: a call for new definitions and risk assessment strategies: Part I. Circulation 108:1664–1672

Naghavi M, Libby P, Falk E, et al. (2003b) From vulnerable plaque to vulnerable patient: a call for new definitions and risk assessment strategies: Part II. Circulation 108:1772–1778

Neumann T, Woiwod T, Neumann A, et al. (2004) Cardiovascular risk factors and probability for cardiovascular events in HIV-infected patients. Part II: gender differences. Eur J Med Res 9:55–60

Nichol KL, Nordin J, Mullooly J, et al. (2003) Influenza vaccination and reduction in hospitalizations for cardiac disease and stroke among the elderly. N Engl J Med 348:1322–1332

Nikolaou K, Poon M, Sirol M, et al. (2003) Complementary results of computed tomography and magnetic resonance imaging of the heart and coronary arteries: a review and future outlook. Cardiol Clin 21:639–655

Nilsson J, Kovanen PT (2004) Will autoantibodies help to determine severity and progression of atherosclerosis? Curr Opin Lipidol 15:499–503

Nissen SE, Tsunoda T, Tuzcu EM, et al. (2003) Effect of recombinant ApoA-I Milano on coronary atherosclerosis in patients with acute coronary syndromes: a randomized controlled trial. JAMA 290:2292–2300

Nissen SE, Tuzcu EM, Schoenhagen P, et al. (2004) For the REVERSAL Investigators. Effect of intensive compared with moderate lipid-lowering therapy on progression of coronary atherosclerosis: a randomized controlled trial. JAMA 291:1071–1080

Öörni K, Pentikäinen MO, Ala-Korpela M, Kovanen PT (2000) Aggregation, fusion, and vesicle formation of modified low density lipoprotein particles: molecular mechanisms and effects on matrix interactions. J Lipid Res 41:1703–1714

Pasceri V, Wu HD, Willerson JT, et al. (2000) Modulation of vascular inflammation in vitro and in vivo by peroxisome proliferator-activated receptor-gamma activators. Circulation 101:235–238

Pitt B, Pepine C, Willerson JT (2002) Cyclooxygenase-2 inhibition and cardiovascular events. Circulation 106:167–169

Prasad A, Zhu J, Halcox JP, et al. (2002) Predisposition to atherosclerosis by infections: role of endothelial dysfunction. Circulation 106:184–190

Puddu P, Puddu GM, Muscari A (2003) Peroxisome proliferator-activated receptors: are they involved in atherosclerosis progression? Int J Cardiol 90:133–140

Rajagopalan S, Meng XP, Ramasamy S (1996) Reactive oxygen species produced by macrophage-derived foam cells regulate the activity of vascular matrix metalloproteinases in vitro. Implications for atherosclerotic plaque stability. J Clin Invest 98:2572–2579

Richardson PD, Davies MJ, Born GV (1989) Influence of plaque configuration and stress distribution on fissuring of coronary atherosclerotic plaques. Lancet 2:941–944

Rodgers A (2003) A cure for cardiovascular disease? Combination treatment has enormous potential, especially in developing countries. BMJ 326:1407–1408

Ross R (1999) Atherosclerosis is an inflammatory disease. Am Heart J 138:S419–S420

Sakata Y, Komamura K, Hirayama A, et al. (1996) Elevation of the plasma histamine concentration in the coronary circulation in patients with variant angina. Am J Cardiol 77:1121–1126

Sata M, Saiura A, Kunisato A, et al. (2002) Hematopoietic stem cells differentiate into vascular cells that participate in the pathogenesis of atherosclerosis. Nat Med 8:403–409

Satoh N, Ogawa Y, Usui T, et al. (2003) Antiatherogenic effect of pioglitazone in type 2 diabetic patients irrespective of the responsiveness to its antidiabetic effect. Diabetes Care 26:2493–2499

Schaar JA, Muller JE, Falk E (2004a) Terminology for high-risk and vulnerable coronary artery plaques. Eur Heart J 25:1077–1082

Schaar JA, Regar E, Saia F, et al. (2004b) Diagnosing the vulnerable plaque in the cardiac catheterization laboratory. In: Waksman R, Serruys PW (eds) Handbook of the vulnerable plaque. Taylor & Francis Group, London, pp 81–95

Schieffer B, Schieffer E, Hilfiker-Kleiner D, et al. (2000) Expression of angiotensin II and interleukin 6 in human coronary atherosclerotic plaques: potential implications for inflammation and plaque instability. Circulation 101:1372–1378

Schoenhagen P, Ziada KM, Kapadia SR, et al. (2000) Extent and direction of arterial remodeling in stable versus unstable coronary syndromes: an intravascular ultrasound study. Circulation 101:598–603

Schonbeck U, Sukhova GK, Graber, et al. (1999) Augmented expression of cyclooxygenase-2 in human atherosclerotic lesions. Am J Pathol 155:1281–1291

Schroeder AP, Falk E (1995) Vulnerable and dangerous coronary plaques. Atherosclerosis 118 Suppl:S141–S149

Schwartz GG, Olsson AG, Ezekowitz MD, et al. (2001) Myocardial Ischemia Reduction with Aggressive Cholesterol Lowering (MIRACL) Study Investigators. Effects of atorvastatin on early recurrent ischemic events in acute coronary syndromes: the MIRACL study: a randomized controlled trial. JAMA 285:1711–1718

Sharma N, Andrews TC (2000) Endothelial function as a therapeutic target in coronary artery disease. Curr Atheroscler Rep 2:303–307

Sidhu JS, Kaposzta Z, Markus HS, et al. (2004) Effect of rosiglitazone on common carotid intima-media thickness progression in coronary artery disease patients without diabetes mellitus. Arterioscler Thromb Vasc Biol 24:930–934

Simons FE, Simons KJ (2002) Clinical pharmacology of H1-antihistamines. Clin Allergy Immunol 17:141–178

Sinisalo J, Mattila K, Valtonen V, et al. (2002) Clarithromycin in Acute Coronary Syndrome Patients in Finland (CLARIFY) Study Group. Effect of 3 months of antimicrobial treatment with clarithromycin in acute non-q-wave coronary syndrome. Circulation 105:1555–1560

Steinberg D, Witztum JL (2002) Is the oxidative modification hypothesis relevant to human atherosclerosis? Do the antioxidant trials conducted to date refute the hypothesis? Circulation 105:2107–2111

Szmitko PE, Fedak PW, Weisel RD, et al. (2003) Endothelial progenitor cells: new hope for a broken heart. Circulation 107:3093–3100

Tendera M, Wojakowski W (2003) Role of antiplatelet drugs in the prevention of cardiovascular events. Thromb Res 110:355–359

The Clopidogrel in Unstable Angina to Prevent Recurrent Events Trial Investigators (2001) Effects of clopidogrel in addition to aspirin in patients with acute coronary syndromes without ST-segment elevation. N Engl J Med 345:494–502

Tremaine WJ, Brzezinski A, Katz JA, et al. (2002) Treatment of mildly to moderately active ulcerative colitis with a tryptase inhibitor (APC 2059): an open-label pilot study. Aliment Pharmacol Ther 16:407–413

Tricot O, Mallat Z, Heymes C, et al. (2000) Relation between endothelial cell apoptosis and blood flow direction in human atherosclerotic plaques. Circulation 101:2450–2453

Tunstall-Pedoe H, Kuulasmaa K, Mähönen M, et al. (1999) Contribution of trends in survival and coronary-event rates to changes in coronary heart disease mortality: 10-year results from 37 WHO MONICA project populations. Monitoring trends and determinants in cardiovascular disease. Lancet 353:1547–1557

Urbich C, Dimmeler S (2004) Endothelial progenitor cells: characterization and role in vascular biology. Circ Res 95:343–353

van der Wal AC, Becker AE, van der Loos CM, et al. (1994) Site of intimal rupture or erosion of thrombosed coronary atherosclerotic plaques is characterized by an inflammatory process irrespective of the dominant plaque morphology. Circulation 89:36–44

Vasa M, Fichtlscherer S, Aicher A, et al. (2001) Number and migratory activity of circulating endothelial progenitor cells inversely correlate with risk factors for coronary artery disease. Circ Res 89:E1–E7

Verges B (2004) Clinical interest of PPARs ligands. Diabetes Metab 30:7–12

Virmani R, Kolodgie FD, Burke AP, et al. (2000) Lessons from sudden coronary death: a comprehensive morphological classification scheme for atherosclerotic lesions. Arterioscler Thromb Vasc Biol 20:1262–1275

Virmani R, Burke AP, Farb A, et al. (2004) Pathology of the vulnerable plaque. In: Waksman R, Serruys PW (eds) Handbook of the vulnerable plaque. Taylor & Francis Group, London, pp 33–48

von Birgelen C, Klinkhart W, Mintz GS, et al. (2001) Plaque distribution and vascular remodeling of ruptured and nonruptured coronary plaques in the same vessel: an intravascular ultrasound study in vivo. J Am Coll Cardiol 37:1864–1870

Wells BJ, Mainous AG 3rd, Dickerson LM (2004) Antibiotics for the secondary prevention of ischemic heart disease: a meta-analysis of randomized controlled trials. Arch Intern Med 164:2156–2161

Wick G, Knoflach M, Xu Q (2004) Autoimmune and inflammatory mechanisms in atheroscle-
    rosis. Annu Rev Immunol 22:361–403
World Health Organization (2002) Secondary prevention of non-communicable disease
    in low and middle income countries through community-based and health service
    interventions. Geneva: WHO
Yusuf S, Sleight P, Pogue J, et al. (2000) Effects of an angiotensin-converting-enzyme in-
    hibitor, ramipril, on cardiovascular events in high-risk patients. The Heart Outcomes
    Prevention Evaluation Study Investigators. N Engl J Med 342:145–153

HEP (2005) 170:777–783

Reciprocal Role of Vasculogenic Factors and Progenitor Cells in Atherogenesis

T. Murayama[1] · O.M. Tepper[2] · T. Asahara[3] (✉)

[1] Department of Clinical Innovative Medicine, Kyoto University Hospital, Kyoto, Japan

[2] Department of Surgery, Institute of Reconstructive Plastic Surgery, New York University Medical Center, New York , USA

[3] Institute of Biomedical Research and Innovation/RIKEN Center for Developmental Biology, 2-2 Minatojima-Minamimachi, 650-0047 Chuo-ku, Kobe, Japan
asa777@aol.com

Abstract While neovascularization plays an integral role in atherosclerosis, stimulation of angiogenesis does not appear to promote atherogenesis. This observation is important in view of recent advancements in angiogenic gene and cell therapy aimed at promoting new blood vessel growth in humans with vascular disease. Endothelial progenitor cells (EPCs) may actually prevent rather than provoke intimal thickening and vascular remodeling by promoting re-endothelialization in response to vascular trauma, as occurs with per-cutaneous transluminal vascular intervention for treating atherosclerotic vessels. Further support for the hypothesis that EPCs continuously repair vascular injury and contribute to the rejuvenation of vessels has been derived from animal studies demonstrating that serial injection of bone marrow-derived EPCs prevent atherogenesis, but that the quantity and quality of these cells deteriorate with aging. This chapter provides a summary of the influence of angiogenesis on atheromatous disease. Furthermore, the increasingly impor-tant relationship between atherosclerosis and newly emerging techniques in therapeutic angiogenesis (i.e., gene therapy and cell therapy with EPCs) is discussed.

Keywords Atherosclerosis · Endothelial progenitor cells · Neovascularization · Vascular injury

The involvement of the vasa vasorum in atherosclerotic disease has long been debated. Recently, this discussion has been re-ignited, following the work of Moulton and Folkman that demonstrated anti-angiogenic agents reduce plaque growth. They showed that systemic administration of endostatin or fumagillin-analog TP-470 to apolipoprotein E-deficient (apoE$^{-/-}$) mice for 16 weeks re-duced intimal neovascularization and subsequent plaque growth by 70%–85% (Fig. 1) (Moulton et al. 1999). Further experiments with angiostatin have high-lighted an important role of macrophages as well as neovascularization in plaque formation (Moulton et al. 2003).

The finding that neovascularization is a necessary condition for plaque growth thus raises the important question of whether increased angiogenesis

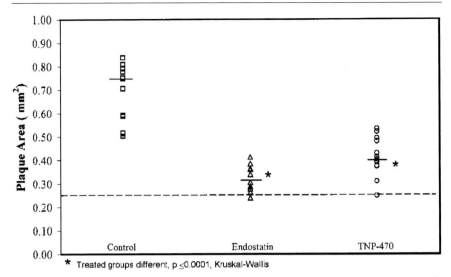

Fig. 1 Size of lesions at aortic origin after treatment with angiogenesis inhibitors in apoE$^{-/-}$ mice aged 20–36 weeks. Control (□), endostatin (▲), and TNP-470 (○) animals were treated for 16 weeks. *Dashed line* centered at 0.25 mm^2 represents median plaque area at aortic sinus lesions measured in a cohort (n=10) analyzed at 20 weeks. (From Moulton et al. 1999)

may lead to the progression of atherosclerosis. In this regard, the relationship between neovascularity and atherosclerosis is analogous to that of neovascularization and cancer. Folkman previously outlined "The hypothesis that tumor growth is angiogenesis-dependent is consistent with the observation that angiogenesis is necessary but not sufficient for continued tumor growth. While the absence of angiogenesis will severely limit tumor growth, the onset of angiogenic activity in a tumor permits, but does not guarantee, continued expansion of the tumor population." (Folkman 1993). The same is true for angiogenesis and atherosclerosis (Isner 1999).

The relationship between angiogenesis and atherosclerosis is particularly intriguing in light of recent advancements in angiogenic gene therapy. After all, therapeutic angiogenesis aims at promoting blood vessel growth in patients in whom atherosclerotic vascular disease is likely to be present. Of initial concern were the findings of Dake and colleagues from Stanford University claiming that vascular endothelial growth factor (VEGF) administration to apoE/apoB100 doubly deficient mice quadrupled the aortic plaque area after 3 weeks (Celletti et al. 2001b). The same group reported similar results from experiments performed in rabbits (Celletti et al. 2001a). However, VEGF pioneers, Losordo and Isner, took a very different stance on this issue (Isner 2001; Losordo and Isner 2001) and pointed out the following: (1) In a series of preclinical experiments, VEGF administration in vascular injury models demonstrated promotion of re-endothelialization, reduction of intimal thickening and mural thrombosis, and restoration of vasomotor function (Asahara et al. 1995, 1996; Van Belle et al. 1997a, 1997b, 1997c; Hiltunen et al. 2000); (2) the total of their 42 clinical cases of VEGF gene therapy of arteriosclerosis obliterans disclosed no evidence of new atherosclerotic lesion development (Baumgartner et al. 1998; Isner 1998).

Perhaps equally important is the question on the relationship between atheromatous disease and the recently identified endothelial progenitor cells (EPCs) (Asahara et al. 1997). First, it has been shown that bone marrow (BM)-derived EPCs are mobilized in the acute phase of acute myocardial infarction (Shintani et al. 2001; Vasa et al. 2001), and that their number in the circulation inversely correlates with the number and severity of risk factors for ischemic heart disease (Gill et al. 2001; Hill et al. 2003). While EPCs were initially shown to promote neovascularization at capillary levels in ischemic organs and tissues (Asahara et al. 1997, 1999), their role to atherosclerosis they may be repair of the intima in injured great vessels and the prevention of their remodeling. Indeed, EPCs were discovered for the first time in a vascular injury model to which VEGF was administered (Asahara et al. 1995, 1996, 1997). Our group (Walter et al. 2002) (Fig. 2) and others (Werner et al. 2002) recently reported similar results showing that administration of a 3-hydroxy-3-methylglutaryl coenzyme A (HMG-CoA) reductase inhibitor (statin) to vascular injury models in rats or mice mobilizes EPCs from the BM into the vascular lesion, promotes re-endothelialization, and prevents intimal thickening/vascular remodeling. Thus, it is reasonable to postulate that in humans EPCs actively participate in endothelial injury and vascular remodeling in response to percutaneous transluminal vascular intervention aimed at the treatment of atheromatous diseases.

Whether EPCs play a role in the natural course of atherosclerosis (i.e., without artificial/iatrogenic vascular injury) has remained unclear. However, Goldschmidt-Clermont and Taylor from Duke University (Rauscher et al. 2003) offer novel insight into this subject. In this study, the authors discovered that

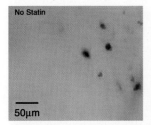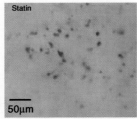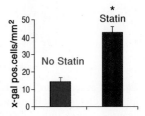

Fig. 2. Bone marrow-derived EPCs contribute to neoendothelium. Representative photomacrographs of luminal surface of X-gal-stained injured segments from control and simvastatin-treated animals at ×200 magnification. *Bar graph* (mean±SEM) depicts numbers of X-gal-positive cells/mm^2 expressing Tie-2, indicative of EPCs. *P <0.01 statin (n=5) vs. saline-injected (n=7). (Modified from Walter et al. 2002)

BM cells from young apoE$^{-/-}$ mice (4 weeks of age) prevent atherosclerosis progression in apoE$^{-/-}$ recipients when 10^6 cells were injected every 2 weeks beginning at 3 weeks of age. Several histological analyses disclosed that in this setting the atherosclerotic burden was reduced by 40% at 14 weeks of age. In contrast, treatment with BM cells from older apoE$^{-/-}$ mice (6 months of age) provided far less benefit (Fig. 3). Furthermore, the percentage of CD31$^+$CD45$^-$ cells from BM (defining vascular progenitor cells) decreased with the aging of apoE$^{-/-}$ mice. Taken together, they have postulated that vascular progenitor cells are continuously repairing vascular damage and contribute to the rejuvenation of vessels, but that the number of these cells decreases with aging, ultimately resulting in atherosclerosis. Although the character of the injected BM cells was not clarified, it is likely that they included EPCs. We also obtained evidence for the adverse effect of aging on EPCs: cultivated EPCs from patients with ischemic heart disease showed decreases in migratory activity in vitro and therapeutic efficacy in mouse model of hindlimb ischemia in vivo, depending on the age of the donors. In other words, EPCs from older patients (>75 years) show significantly less migratory activity and therapeutic effect than those from younger ones (<65 years) (Murayama et al. 2001). Hence, the quality and quantity of EPCs can deteriorate with aging, which may modify a variety of pathophysiological conditions in the elderly.

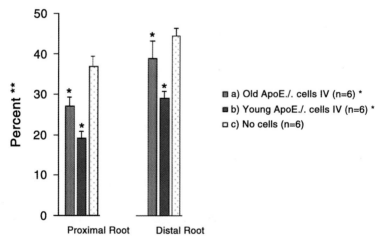

Fig. 3 All atherosclerosis data (mean±SEM) are for apoE$^{-/-}$ 'recipient' mice maintained on high-fat diet, sorted into one of three groups (a–c), at 14 weeks of age. Cell injections were given at 2-week intervals from 3 weeks until 13 weeks of age (10^6 cells/injection). Groups a and b received cells intravenously. Donor cells originated from severely atherosclerotic 6-month-old apoE$^{-/-}$ mice, maintained on high-fat diet (a), or preatherosclerotic 4-week-old apoE$^{-/-}$ mice (b). Group c indicates mice given no cells (negative control). Groups a and b differed from each other only in age of cell donor. Atherosclerotic burden differs significantly between groups a and b (P<0.05). (Modified from Rauscher et al. 2003)

Half a century ago, Rudolf Altschul exquisitely stated, "A person is as old as his endothelium." (Altschul 1954). Are there any strategies to overcome aging of an individual and his blood vessels, i.e., the most important risk factor for atheromatous disease? Unlike stem cells, EPCs cannot escape from cell senescence, and if EPC function deteriorates with aging, simple autologous cell therapy itself is insufficient to solve the paradigm. What about an EPC bank where EPCs are collected from young people, expanded, and stored for their future treatment? What happens if fortified autologous EPCs, obtained for example by overexpression of VEGF (Iwaguro et al. 2002), or the telomerase gene (Murasawa et al. 2002) are continuously administered to the patients in order to prevent vascular aging or atherosclerosis? We look forward to further advancements in this field and potential novel cell therapy techniques that translate into clinical practice.

This paper is supported in part by the Establishment of International COE for Integration of Transplantation Therapy and Regenerative Medicine (COE program of the Ministry of Education, Culture, Sports, Science and Technology, Japan).

References

Altschul R (1954) Endothelium, its development, morphology, function, and Pathology. Macmillan, New York

Asahara T, Bauters C, Pastore C, Kearney M, Rossow S, Bunting S, Ferrara N, Symes JF, Isner JM (1995) Local delivery of vascular endothelial growth factor accelerates reendothelialization and attenuates intimal hyperplasia in balloon-injured rat carotid artery. Circulation 91:2793–2801

Asahara T, Chen D, Tsurumi Y, Kearney M, Rossow S, Passeri J, Symes JF, Isner JM (1996) Accelerated restitution of endothelial integrity and endothelium-dependent function after phVEGF165 gene transfer. Circulation 94:3291–3302

Asahara T, Murohara T, Sullivan A, Silver M, van der Zee R, Li T, Witzenbichler B, Schatteman G, Isner JM (1997) Isolation of putative progenitor endothelial cells for angiogenesis. Science 275:964–967

Asahara T, Masuda H, Takahashi T, Kalka C, Pastore C, Silver M, Kearne M, Magner M, Isner JM (1999) Bone marrow origin of endothelial progenitor cells responsible for postnatal vasculogenesis in physiological and pathological neovascularization. Circ Res 85:221–228

Baumgartner I, Pieczek A, Manor O, Blair R, Kearney M, Walsh K, Isner JM (1998) Constitutive expression of phVEGF165 after intramuscular gene transfer promotes collateral vessel development in patients with critical limb ischemia. Circulation 97:1114–1123

Celletti FL, Hilfiker PR, Ghafouri P, Dake MD (2001a) Effect of human recombinant vascular endothelial growth factor165 on progression of atherosclerotic plaque. J Am Coll Cardiol 37:2126–2130

Celletti FL, Waugh JM, Amabile PG, Brendolan A, Hilfiker PR, Dake MD (2001b) Vascular endothelial growth factor enhances atherosclerotic plaque progression. Nat Med 7:425–429

Folkman J (1993) Tumor angiogenesis. In: Holland J, Frei EI, Bast RJ, Kute D, Morton D, Weichselbaum R (eds) Cancer medicine. Lea & Febiger, Philadelphia, pp 153–170

Gill M, Dias S, Hattori K, Rivera ML, Hicklin D, Witte L, Girardi L, Yurt R, Himel H, Rafii S (2001) Vascular trauma induces rapid but transient mobilization of VEGFR2(+)AC133(+) endothelial precursor cells. Circ Res 88:167–174

Hill JM, Zalos G, Halcox JP, Schenke WH, Waclawiw MA, Quyyumi AA, Finkel T (2003) Circulating endothelial progenitor cells, vascular function, and cardiovascular risk. N Engl J Med 348:593–600

Hiltunen MO, Laitinen M, Turunen MP, Jeltsch M, Hartikainen J, Rissanen TT, Laukkanen J, Niemi M, Kossila M, Hakkinen TP, Kivela A, Enholm B, Mansukoski H, Turunen AM, Alitalo K, Yla-Herttuala S (2000) Intravascular adenovirus-mediated VEGF-C gene transfer reduces neointima formation in balloon-denuded rabbit aorta. Circulation 102:2262–2268

Isner JM (1998) Arterial gene transfer of naked DNA for therapeutic angiogenesis: early clinical results. Adv Drug Deliv Rev 30:185–197

Isner JM (1999) Cancer and atherosclerosis: the broad mandate of angiogenesis. Circulation 99:1653–1655

Isner JM (2001) Still more debate over VEGF. Nat Med 7:639–641

Iwaguro H, Yamaguchi J, Kalka C, Murasawa S, Masuda H, Hayashi S, Silver M, Li T, Isner JM, Asahara T (2002) Endothelial progenitor cell vascular endothelial growth factor gene transfer for vascular regeneration. Circulation 105:732–738

Losordo DW, Isner JM (2001) Vascular endothelial growth factor-induced angiogenesis: crouching tiger or hidden dragon? J Am Coll Cardiol 37:2131–2135

Moulton KS, Heller E, Konerding MA, Flynn E, Palinski W, Folkman J (1999) Angiogenesis inhibitors endostatin or TNP-470 reduce intimal neovascularization and plaque growth in apolipoprotein E-deficient mice. Circulation 99:1726–1732

Moulton KS, Vakili K, Zurakowski D, Soliman M, Butterfield C, Sylvin E, Lo KM, Gillies S, Javaherian K, Folkman J (2003) Inhibition of plaque neovascularization reduces macrophage accumulation and progression of advanced atherosclerosis. Proc Natl Acad Sci USA 100:4736–4741

Murasawa S, Llevadot J, Silver M, Isner JM, Losordo DW, Asahara T (2002) Constitutive human telomerase reverse transcriptase expression enhances regenerative properties of endothelial progenitor cells. Circulation 106:1133–1139

Murayama T, Kalka C, Silver M, Ma H, Asahara T (2001) Aging impairs therapeutic contribution of human endothelial progenitor cells to postnatal neovascularization. Circulation 104:II-68–69

Rauscher FM, Goldschmidt-Clermont PJ, Davis BH, Wang T, Gregg D, Ramaswami P, Pippen AM, Annex BH, Dong C, Taylor DA (2003) Aging, progenitor cell exhaustion, and atherosclerosis. Circulation 108:457–463

Shintani S, Murohara T, Ikeda H, Ueno T, Honma T, Katoh A, Sasaki K, Shimada T, Oike Y, Imaizumi T (2001) Mobilization of endothelial progenitor cells in patients with acute myocardial infarction. Circulation 103:2776–2779

Van Belle E, Maillard L, Tio FO, Isner JM (1997a) Accelerated endothelialization by local delivery of recombinant human vascular endothelial growth factor reduces in-stent intimal formation. Biochem Biophys Res Commun 235:311–316

Van Belle E, Tio FO, Chen D, Maillard L, Kearney M, Isner JM (1997b) Passivation of metallic stents after arterial gene transfer of phVEGF165 inhibits thrombus formation and intimal thickening. J Am Coll Cardiol 29:1371–1379

Van Belle E, Tio FO, Couffinhal T, Maillard L, Passeri J, Isner JM (1997c) Stent endothelialization. Time course, impact of local catheter delivery, feasibility of recombinant protein administration, and response to cytokine expedition. Circulation 95:438–448

Vasa M, Fichtlscherer S, Aicher A, Adler K, Urbich C, Martin H, Zeiher AM, Dimmeler S (2001) Number and migratory activity of circulating endothelial progenitor cells inversely correlate with risk factors for coronary artery disease. Circ Res 89:E1–7

Walter DH, Rittig K, Bahlmann FH, Kirchmair R, Silver M, Murayama T, Nishimura H, Losordo DW, Asahara T, Isner JM (2002) Statin therapy accelerates reendothelialization: a novel effect involving mobilization and incorporation of bone marrow-derived endothelial progenitor cells. Circulation 105:3017–3024

Werner N, Priller J, Laufs U, Endres M, Bohm M, Dirnagl U, Nickenig G (2002) Bone marrow-derived progenitor cells modulate vascular reendothelialization and neointimal formation: effect of 3-hydroxy-3-methylglutaryl coenzyme a reductase inhibition. Arterioscler Thromb Vasc Biol 22:1567–1572

HEP (2005) 170:785–807

Gene Therapy of Atherosclerosis

E. Vähäkangas[1] · S. Ylä-Herttuala[1,2] (✉)

[1]Department of Biotechnology and Molecular Medicine, A.I. Virtanen Institute for Molecular Sciences, Kuopio, Finland

[2]Department of Medicine, University of Kuopio and Gene Therapy Unit, Kuopio University Hospital, 70210 Kuopio, Finland
Seppo.YlaHerttuala@uku.fi

Abstract Atherosclerosis and related diseases are the leading cause of death in Western world. The disease process begins with the formation of fatty streaks already during the first decade of life but does not manifest clinically until several decades later. Gene therapy is a potential new way to target multiple factors playing a role in the development and progression of atherosclerosis. A great number of genes involved in the development of atherosclerosis have been identified and have been tested both in vitro and in vivo as potential new targets for therapy. Pre-clinical experiments have shown the feasibility and safety of several gene therapy applications for the treatment of atherosclerosis and clinical trials have also provided evidence for the applicability of gene therapy for the treatment of cardiovascular diseases. In this review we discuss vectors and potential gene therapy approaches for intervention and therapy of atherosclerosis.

Keywords Atherosclerosis · Gene therapy · Viral vector

1
Introduction

Gene therapy aims to treat diseases by introducing therapeutic genes into the somatic cells of patients. Target diseases are by origin either multigenic or single gene defects. Atherosclerosis is a complex disease developing over a long period of time, affecting many cell types in the vessel wall and involving a multitude of different genes. Atherogenesis begins already during the first decade of life but is clinically manifested only decades later (Yla-Herttuala et al. 1986).

Foam cell formation is one of the early events of atherosclerosis. Increased expression of cytokines, chemokines and adhesion molecules leads to increased adhesion of monocyte-macrophages to endothelium and their transmigration into the subendothelial space. There macrophages and, to some extent smooth muscle cells (SMCs), accumulate lipid through scavenger receptors converting these cells into lipid-laden foam cells. Oxidation of low-density lipoprotein (LDL) by lipoxygenases and other mechanisms enables it to be recognized by scavenger receptors, which do not recognize native LDL and mediate unregulated uptake of cholesterol into the cells. SMCs, migrated from media into the intima, proliferate and produce extracellular matrix in the intima leading to the formation of atherosclerotic lesions with a necrotic core of lipid and a fibrous cap of SMCs and extracellular matrix. In the worst case, rupture of these lesions leads to thrombosis and infarction (Ross 1999).

Many risk factors contribute to the development of atherosclerosis and related complications (Lusis 2000). Among them, high plasma LDL and low high-density lipoprotein (HDL) levels are major contributing factors. There are also several inherited diseases such as familial hypercholesterolemia (FH) that lead to accelerated atherosclerosis. Current treatment strategies use drug treatment to affect cholesterol levels, hypertension and thrombosis. However, these approaches have not been effective in all patients.

Critical elements for successful gene therapy involve the identification of suitable target genes through which it is possible to influence disease development and progression, delivering the transgenes to the target tissue efficiently, achieving sufficient levels of gene expression for therapeutic effects and reaching these goals with minimal side effects. Additionally, regulated and tissue specific gene expression are goals for future gene therapy applications.

2
Vectors for Gene Therapy

The first critical point for successful gene therapy is the delivery and subsequent expression of the therapeutic gene in target cells. Delivery of therapeutic genes to cells ex vivo or tissues in vivo is possible by viral and nonviral vectors (Yla-Herttuala and Martin 2000). Different vector systems have inherent characteristics that make them suitable for specific applications (Table 1). Desired expression times and levels vary depending on the therapeutic aim (Kay et al. 2001). Some applications, such as vein-graft failure, may require only transient expression of a therapeutic gene whereas atherosclerosis requires long-lasting and sustained expression of gene(s). Several factors influence persistence of transgenes in target tissues, including the choice of promoter and enhancer elements, immune response to the vector and/or transgene product and turnover of the transduced cells (Ehrhardt et al. 2003; Stone et al. 2003; Yang et al. 1995).

Main target tissues for gene therapy of atherosclerosis include the liver due to its central role in lipoprotein metabolism, and the vessel wall. Both viral and nonviral vectors have demonstrated relatively low efficiency and lack of selectivity in vascular cells but recently vectors targeted into the vascular cells have emerged (Nicklin et al. 2001). Long-lasting expression is possible with lentiviral vectors or adeno-associated virus vectors. Persistent gene expression with both vectors has also been achieved in the liver (Follenzi et al. 2002; Snyder et al. 1997). Muscle-directed gene transfer could also be feasible for the production of secreted apolipoproteins (Harris et al. 2002).

2.1
Nonviral Vectors

Nonviral vectors include naked plasmid DNA, cationic liposomes and cationic polymers. Plasmids are safe, have high capacity to accommodate transgenes and large scale production and purification are relatively easy. The major drawback of naked plasmids is their low transfection efficiency and transient transgene expression. Transfection efficiency has been improved with the use plasmid:liposomes and plasmid:polymer complexes (Pakkanen et al. 2000) but has not yet reached the levels achieved with viral vectors (Turunen et al. 2002).

2.2
Viral Vectors

Viruses have evolved specific mechanisms for entering target cells and using cellular machinery to progress viral lifecycle. This interaction with specific cell surface receptors and subsequent entry into the cells has provided a good basis for the development of viral gene transfer vectors. Viral vectors are constructed by removing some or all of the viral coding sequences and providing *cis*-acting

Table 1 Vector systems for cardiovascular gene delivery

Vector	Advantages	Disadvantages
Adenovirus	Transduce dividing and nondividing cells	Short-lasting expression
	High-level expression	Host immune and inflammatory reactions
	Relatively easy to produce to high titer	
	Nonintegrating	
	Large transgene capacity	
Adeno-associated virus	Transduce dividing and nondividing cells	Limited transgene capacity ($\sim$4.7 kb)
	Nonpathogenic	Risk of insertional mutagenesis due to random integration
	Low immunogenicity	Laborous production procedure
	Integrating	
	Long-lasting and stable transgene expression	
Lentivirus	Transduce dividing and nondividing cells	Relatively low transfection efficiency
	Low immunogenicity	Risk of insertional mutagenesis due to random integration
	Integrating	Laborous production procedure
	Long-lasting and stable transgene expression	
Retroviruses	Low immunogenicity	Able to transduce only dividing cells
	Integrating	Low efficiency
	Long-lasting and stable transgene expression	Risk of insertional mutagenesis due to integration
Baculovirus	Transduces dividing and nondividing cells	Host immune and inflammatory reactions
	Large transgene capacity	Transient expression
	Nonreplicative in mammalian cells	
	Nonpathogenic	
Nonviral vectors: Naked plasmids plasmid/liposomes	Nonpathogenic	Poor efficiency
	Easy to produce	Transient expression

sequences required for packaging from helper plasmids or stable packaging cell lines. This eliminates the production of replication competent wild-type viruses during the vector production (Kay et al. 2001).

The main advantage of the viral vectors over the nonviral vectors is their high transduction efficiency as the desired therapeutic effect is usually proportional to the number of cells expressing the therapeutic gene. The main limitation of viral vectors is the potential of immune reactions. Immune responses can be directed either towards antigens of the viral backbone or specific antibodies can develop towards the transgene products. Recent development of vectors has aimed at removing as much of the viral genome as possible from the vector backbone, both to increase safety and to make space for larger transgene cassettes. Another important feature to increase safety of the viral vectors would be cell or tissue specific expression achieved by the use of tissue specific and inducible promoters (Koponen et al. 2003; Walther and Stein 1996).

2.2.1
Adenoviral Vectors

Adenoviruses are nonenveloped DNA viruses. There are over 50 adenovirus serotypes with serotypes 2 and 5 being the most commonly used in gene therapy. Other serotypes are, however, gaining more interest in order to avoid possible pre-existing immunity that can reduce efficiency of vector administration. Alternative serotypes may also be used to avoid neutralizing antibody responses if re-administration of the vector is required (Parks et al. 1999).

Adenoviruses provide strong expression in both dividing and nondividing cells but remain episomal leading to loss of gene expression within 2 weeks. Immune response elicited by the vector also contributes to the loss of transgene expression (Pastore et al. 1999).

Adenoviruses with a much higher capacity to accept foreign genetic material have been obtained with 'gutless' adenoviral vectors where the wild-type genome is replaced with a transgene cassette and regulatory elements. These vectors are also less immunogenic because no viral gene expression can result after removal of the entire adenovirus genome (Kochanek et al. 1996). Adenoviruses have been used for efficient gene delivery into many tissues including the vessel wall, liver and muscle (Gruchala et al. 2004; Jalkanen et al. 2003; Rissanen et al. 2003). However, adenoviruses are not the optimal vectors for treating atherosclerosis due to the short-term expression of the transgene but can instead be beneficial for the treatment of complications resulting from atherosclerosis, such as restenosis or bypass graft stenosis (Rutanen et al. 2002).

2.2.2
Retroviral Vectors

Retroviruses are lipid-enveloped particles with a diploid RNA genome. After entry into cells, the genome is reverse transcribed into double-stranded DNA and integrated into the host genome providing the ability to confer long-lasting transgene expression (Kay et al. 2001). Retroviral vectors can transduce only dividing cells limiting the range of target cells. Ex vivo approaches with retroviral vectors have been used to transduce lymphocytes and bone marrow stem cells among others (Engels et al. 2003; Hacein-Bey-Abina et al. 2002; Li et al. 2003; Muul et al. 2003). The retroviral envelope restricts its tropism to certain cell types expressing suitable receptors. Expanded host cell range has been achieved by pseudotyping the vectors with envelope proteins from other viruses e.g., the G protein of the vesicular stomatitis virus (VSV-G). Also, pseudotyping with VSV-G makes the envelope of the virus more stable allowing for concentration to high titers (Burns et al. 1993). Retroviruses are able to accommodate up to 8 kb of exogenous DNA in place of removed viral genes. The required *cis*-acting sequences are stably expressed from packaging cell lines (Ory et al. 1996). Retroviral vectors have been used for gene transfer in the cardiovascular system and liver, both in vivo and ex vivo (Grossman et al. 1995; Laitinen et al. 1997; Pakkanen et al. 1999a).

2.2.3
Lentiviral Vectors

Lentiviruses belong to the family of retroviruses. They are able to transduce nondividing, terminally differentiated cells and integrate into the host cell genome providing stable and long-lasting gene expression, a requirement in the treatment of atherosclerosis. Only a fraction of the parental genome of the lentivirus is required to produce a functional vector. The nonrequired genes are important for viral pathogenesis so packaging constructs with the minimal amount of helper genes have been developed (Dull et al. 1998). Biosafety of lentiviral vectors has been increased by the development of self-inactivating vectors (Miyoshi et al. 1998). Pseudotyping lentiviral vectors with VSV-G has led to increased stability of the viral particle and expanded tropism (Akkina et al. 1996; Naldini et al. 1996). VSV-G pseudotyped lentiviral vectors have been used to efficiently transduce liver (Follenzi et al. 2002; Kankkonen et al. 2004). They could prove beneficial in the treatment of FH or other diseases involving lipid homeostasis and requiring long-term expression of therapeutic genes in the liver. Lentiviruses are also being extensively studied for transduction of hematopoietic stem cells (Miyoshi et al. 1999).

2.2.4
Adeno-associated Virus-Vectors

Adeno-associated viruses (AAVs) are replication defective parvoviruses that require a helper virus to complete their productive life cycle. In the absence of a helper virus they establish a latent infection by integrating into the host genome in a site-specific manner. This ability of the wild-type AAV for site-specific integration has been one main property generating interest in developing gene transfer vectors based on AAVs. Eight serotypes of AAV have been identified with AAV2 being the most studied and used to date.

AAV vectors have many properties that make them ideal tools for gene transfer: they are nonpathogenic as they do not cause any known disease in humans, they mediate long-lasting transgene expression, transduce both dividing and nondividing cells, are nontoxic and exhibit low immunogenicity in vivo (Monahan and Samulski 2000). The major limitation is the low capacity of the vector backbone of only 4.7 kb. This is, however, being addressed by utilizing the property of the vectors to form heterodimers inside cells, so that either the therapeutic gene could be split in half and delivered by two separate vectors or the gene and regulatory elements could be split into two separate vectors (Sun et al. 2000; Yan et al. 2000). AAV-mediated long-term expression and the ability to transduce vascular SMCs makes it an attractive vector for treatment of atherosclerosis (Gruchala et al. 2004; Pajusola et al. 2002; Pruchnic et al. 2000).

2.2.5
Baculovirus Vectors

The baculovirus *Autographa californica* nuclear polyhedrosis virus (AcMNPV) is an enveloped virus with a double-stranded DNA genome. Baculoviruses are insect-specific and do not replicate in mammalian cells despite being able to enter certain vertebrate cells (Volkman et al. 1983). It has been shown, however, that when containing the appropriate eukaryotic promoter AcMNPV is able to transfer and express target genes in several mammalian cell types (Boyce and Bucher 1996). Baculoviruses can incorporate large amounts of foreign DNA into their nucleocapsid. Baculoviral vectors do not integrate into the host genome leading to transient transgene expression. The advantages of baculoviral vectors include transducing both dividing and nondividing cells, relatively easy preparation of high-titer virus stocks and very high capacity for foreign DNA (Pieroni and La Monica 2001). Their use in vivo has been hampered by inactivation by serum complement. Inactivation could be avoided by preventing contact with blood components (Airenne et al. 2000). The usefulness of baculoviral vectors in cardiovascular gene therapy remains to be elucidated.

3
Targets for Gene Therapy of Atherosclerosis

The most promising target diseases for gene therapy are monogenic diseases caused by a defect in one gene leading to the absence or dysfunction of the protein encoded by that gene. Atherosclerosis is a multifactorial disease developing over a long period of time with many environmental factors influencing its development and progression. This suggests that local gene therapy approaches might not be effective in primary prevention of atherosclerosis. There are, however, inherited disorders that can lead to atherosclerosis and where treatment by gene therapy may be feasible (Figs.1 and 2).

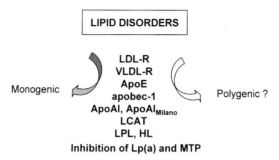

Fig. 1 Potential target genes for treatment of inherited lipid disorders

3.1
Genetic and Acquired Disorders of Lipid Metabolism

Increased plasma concentration of LDL is a major risk factor for the development of atherosclerosis. Numerous environmental factors and genetic loci contribute to increased plasma LDL levels but specific monogenic diseases leading to high plasma concentrations of LDL have also been identified (Rader et al. 2003).

FH is caused by mutations in the gene encoding the LDL receptor (LDL-R). This results in defective or total absence of hepatic uptake of LDL and increased plasma LDL concentrations. The disease is characterized by premature atherosclerosis and related complications (Rader et al. 2003). FH could be treated with liver-directed transfer of the LDL- or very-low-density lipoprotein (VLDL) receptor gene to restore, at least partially, liver uptake of LDL and to lower plasma cholesterol levels. This has been shown in animal models of FH with prolonged lowering of cholesterol after LDL-R gene transfer (Kankkonen et al. 2004; Pakkanen et al. 1999b) and protection from atherosclerosis after VLDL-R gene transfer (Oka et al. 2001). Transplantation of ex vivo transduced autologous hepatocytes expressing LDL-R also resulted in modestly lowered cholesterol levels in some patients (Grossman et al. 1995).

Dyslipoproteinemias such as hypoalphalipoproteinemia—low levels of HDL cholesterol—could be treated with gene transfer of the apoA-I or lecithin:cholesterol acyltransferase (LCAT) genes (Brousseau et al. 1998). In addition to affecting HDL concentrations LCAT also modulates LDL cholesterol concentrations by accelerating LDL catabolism. However, the LDL cholesterol lowering and anti-atherogenic properties of LCAT overexpression are dependent on at least one functional allele of the LDL-R gene (Brousseau et al. 2000). This makes LCAT an attractive target gene for treatment of heterozygous FH patients and dyslipoproteinemic patients with at least one functional allele of the LDL-R gene.

Apolipoprotein E (apoE) functions as a ligand for lipoprotein clearance and has an important role in the metabolism of triglyceride-rich VLDL and

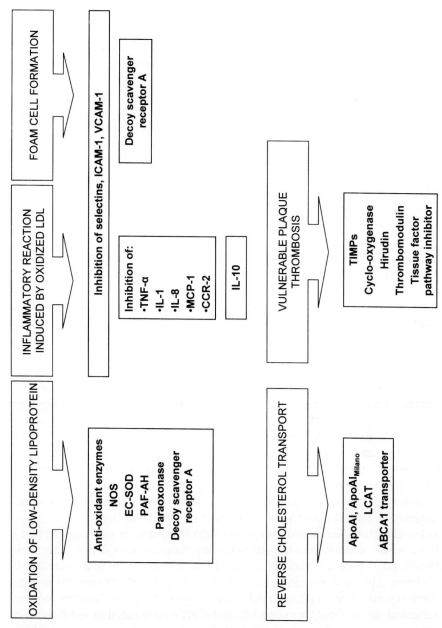

Fig. 2 Therapeutic targets and potential treatment genes

remnant metabolism. As such, apoE gene transfer could be used for the treatment of type III hyperlipoproteinemia which is due to the presence of specific apoE isoforms. Macrophage apoE expression has been shown to reduce lesion area in the early, but not in the later stages of atherogenesis without major changes in plasma cholesterol levels (Hasty et al. 1999). In contrast, hepatic expression of apoE lowers plasma cholesterol levels and induces regression of both fatty streak and more complex, advanced lesions (Tsukamoto et al. 1999).

ApoB100 is synthesized in the liver and is the major component of plasma LDL and also a component of other atherogenic lipoproteins such as lipoprotein (a) [Lp(a)] and VLDL. Transgenic mice with liver-specific expression of apobec-1 as well as adenoviral delivery to rabbit liver resulted in reduced LDL cholesterol levels (Kozarsky et al. 1996; Teng et al. 1997). High concentrations of apoB100 could be reduced with transfer of the catalytic subunit of the apoB mRNA editing enzyme. Hepatic overexpression of apobec-1 can also reduce atherogenic Lp(a) concentrations (Hughes et al. 1996). Lp(a) levels can also be targeted with ribozymes to inhibit the synthesis of this protein (Morishita et al. 1998).

Genetic deficiency of lipoprotein lipase (LPL), a critical enzyme for the catabolism of triglyceride-rich lipoproteins, leads to hyperlipidemia and may be a significant risk factor for the development of atherosclerosis (Benlian et al. 1996). Increased activity of LPL after liver-directed gene transfer has been shown to normalize lipoprotein profiles in LPL deficient animals and also to protect against atherosclerosis (Ashbourne Excoffon et al. 1997; Shimada et al. 1996). Hepatic lipase (HL) is an endothelial bound lipolytic enzyme which functions both as a phospholipase and triacylglycerol hydrolase, and is required for the metabolism of intermediate density lipoproteins and HDL. Patients with HL deficiency display a variable phenotype that may include hypertriglyceridemia with triglyceride enrichment of LDL and HDL particles, hypercholesterolemia, β-VLDL, and in some cases premature coronary artery disease (Connelly et al. 1990; Hegele et al. 1993). Gene transfer of HL to HL-deficient mice is able to correct the abnormal lipid profile (Applebaum-Bowden et al. 1996).

Plasma lipoprotein levels could also be reduced by inhibiting the microsomal triglyceride transfer protein (MTP) which catalyzes the transport of triglyceride, cholesteryl ester and phosphatidylcholine between membranes, and is required in the assembly of apoB containing lipoproteins (Gordon et al. 1995). Inhibition of MTP has been shown to inhibit apoB secretion from HepG2 cells and virtually eradicate atherosclerotic lesions in $LDLR^{-/-}/ApoB^{100/100}$ mice homozygous for a conditional allele for the gene for MTP (Jamil et al. 1996; Lieu et al. 2003). Specific inhibition of the MTP gene could be achieved with siRNA techniques (Scherer and Rossi 2003).

3.2
Oxidation of LDL

The accumulation of LDL in the intima of vessels where it is modified is one of the initial events in the development of atherosclerosis. These modifications contribute to both foam cell formation and inflammation in the vessel wall. The most important form of modification in humans is most likely oxidation of LDL. Oxidatively modified LDL has been detected in atherosclerotic lesions (Yla-Herttuala et al. 1989).

LDL can be oxidized by several mechanisms, such as by metal ions, lipoxygenases, myeloperoxidase and reactive nitrogen species. However, oxidation by metal ions probably does not play an important role in the in vivo oxidation of LDL (Leeuwenburgh et al. 1997). The presence of 15-lipoxygenase in macrophage-rich areas of human and rabbit atherosclerotic lesions has been shown by immunohistochemical studies (Yla-Herttuala et al. 1991b) as well as has the presence of HOCl-modified epitopes, i.e., markers of myeloperoxidase modified LDL (Malle et al. 2000). Nitric oxide (NO) is a free radical released by many vascular cells. NO itself causes little modification of LDL particles and it inhibits both cell-mediated and copper-mediated oxidation of LDL. Under aerobic conditions NO is converted into nitrite, and low concentrations of nitrite have been shown to inhibit myeloperoxidase-mediated oxidation of LDL (Carr and Frei 2001). However, when NO reacts with molecular oxygen or superoxide radicals it forms a multitude of reactive nitrogen species that are able to modify LDL in vitro. The presence of oxidized LDL leads to a proinflammatory reaction in the vessel wall that can accelerate atherosclerosis (Steinberg and Witztum 2002). Beneficial effects on endothelial dysfunction caused by oxidized LDL could be achieved by overexpression of antioxidant enzymes and nitric oxide synthase. Local catheter-mediated delivery, but not systemic delivery, of extracellular superoxide dismutase was able to reduce macrophage accumulation and restenosis in balloon-denuded rabbit aorta (Laukkanen et al. 2002). Reduction of macrophage accumulation could be advantageous for the treatment of atherosclerosis as macrophages secrete many cytokines and growth factors implicated in the pathogenesis of atherosclerosis.

Platelet-activating factor acetylhydrolase (PAF-AH), present in HDL particles, hydrolyzes and inactivates PAF and PAF-like oxidized or polar phospholipids thus having an anti-atherogenic role. It also has, however, atherogenic properties as it generates potent inflammatory lipid mediators after hydrolysis of oxidized lysophosphatidylcholines. PAF-AH has been detected in human and rabbit atherosclerotic lesions (Häkkinen et al. 1999). The role of PAF-AH as an anti-atherogenic molecule is supported by the fact that adenovirus-mediated gene transfer of PAF-AH led to a decrease in atherosclerosis. PAF-AH protected lipoproteins from oxidation and HDL particles with PAF-AH were able to reduce foam cell formation (Noto et al. 2003; Quarck et al. 2001; Turunen et al. 2004).

Serum paraoxonase 1 (PON1) is an HDL associated enzyme as well, and is expressed in the liver (Blatter et al. 1993). It inhibits LDL oxidation in vitro and PON1 transgenic mice are protected from atherosclerosis (Aviram et al. 1998; Tward et al. 2002).

Oxidized LDL is recognized by scavenger receptors that mediate its uptake into macrophages turning them into foam cells. Members of the scavenger receptor family include class A, class B, mucin-like and endothelial receptors (Terpstra et al. 2000). Scavenger receptor A and CD36 are considered the main receptors involved in foam cell formation, mediating the uptake of oxidized LDL into macrophages. Scavenger receptors also play a part in cell adhesion (Fraser et al. 1993), phagocytosis of apoptotic cells (Platt et al. 1999) and host immune functions (Dunne et al. 1994). Accumulation of lipid in macrophages and infiltration of monocytes into the vessel wall could be prevented by decoy scavenger receptors (Jalkanen et al. 2003).

3.3
Inflammation

Inflammation is mediated by several proinflammatory cytokines and plays an important role in the development and progression of atherosclerosis. Tumor necrosis factor-α (TNF-α) and interleukin (IL)-1 are potent pro-inflammatory cytokines that mediate some of their effects through up-regulation of other cytokines, chemokines and adhesion molecules (Laukkanen and Yla-Herttuala 2002). Circulating monocytes attach to endothelial cells by cell adhesion molecules such as selectins, vascular cell adhesion molecule and intercellular adhesion molecule-1 that are induced in response to inflammatory signals. Monocyte chemoattractant protein-1 (MCP-1) and IL-8 play crucial roles in the initiation of atherosclerosis by recruiting monocytes/macrophages into the vessel wall promoting lesion formation and plaque vulnerability. MCP-1 has been detected in macrophage-rich areas of human atherosclerotic lesions (Yla-Herttuala et al. 1991a). The effects of MCP-1 are mediated through the CC chemokine receptor 2 (CCR2) and modulation of MCP-1 levels or CCR2 activity lead to reduced atherosclerosis (Dawson et al. 1999; Gosling et al. 1999; Gu et al. 1998). Soluble adhesion molecules could be used to inhibit the migration of monocytes/macrophages into the vessel wall (Chen et al. 1994). Further, decoy scavenger receptors could be used to inhibit adhesion of monocytes to endothelium (Jalkanen et al. 2003).

The action of transcription factors involved in SMC proliferation, oxidative stress and inflammation, such as E2F and NFκB, could be inhibited by the use of decoy oligodeoxynucleotides (ODN) of these factors (Nakamura et al. 2002; Yoshimura et al. 2001). These ODNs have been shown to reduce neointimal formation but the inhibition of NFκB has also been shown to increase atherosclerosis in LDL-R-deficient mice, possibly by affecting the pro- and anti-inflammatory balance controlling the development of atherosclerosis (Kanters et al. 2003).

IL-10 is an anti-inflammatory cytokine produced by activated lympho-cytes and monocytes. Expression of IL-10 has been demonstrated in human atherosclerotic lesions and it also reduces atherosclerotic lesion formation in vivo in mouse models (Mallat et al. 1999; Pinderski Oslund et al. 1999). The reduction in lesion area is accompanied by a change in lesion composition into a more stable phenotype. Systemic expression of IL-10 has both metabolic and immunological effects (Von Der Thusen et al. 2001).

3.4
HDL and Reverse Cholesterol Transport

Reduced plasma HDL levels have been linked with increased risk of coronary heart disease in epidemiological studies (Gordon et al. 1977) and an increase of 1 mg/dl in HDL cholesterol has been shown to decrease CAD risk by ap-proximately 2.5% (Gordon et al. 1989). The atheroprotective role of HDL has been linked to its role in reverse cholesterol transport, inhibition of lipopro-tein oxidation and direct protection of the vessel wall (Assmann and Nofer 2003). Reverse cholesterol transport is the process whereby excess cholesterol in the peripheral tissues is transported to the liver for excretion. The process involves the efflux of cellular free cholesterol to HDL, esterification of free HDL cholesterol by LCAT, transport of HDL cholesterol to the liver and uptake of the cholesterol ester by the liver (Assmann and Nofer 2003).

ApoA-I is the major protein component of HDL and in addition to its structural role it also activates LCAT (Jonas 1991). Deficiency of apoA-I, which results in an increased risk of premature atherosclerosis, could be treated with transfer of apoA-I or apoA-I$_{Milano}$, a naturally occurring mutant of apoA-I, to the liver (Belalcazar et al. 2003; Benoit et al. 1999; Tangirala et al. 1999). ApoA-I$_{Milano}$ is associated with freedom from vascular disease despite reduced HDL and elevated triglyseride levels (Sirtori et al. 2001).

The ATP binding cassette transporter A1 (ABCA1) facilitates the efflux of cellular phospholipids and cholesterol to apolipoprotein acceptors, such as apoA-I, playing a key role in the initial step of reverse cholesterol transport (Wang et al. 2001). A defect in the gene encoding ABCAI has been identified as the cause of familial HDL-deficiency syndromes such as Tangiers disease (Brooks-Wilson et al. 1999). Increased expression of ABCA1 is atheroprotec-tive and leads to increased biliary cholesterol excretion in transgenic mice (Singaraja et al. 2002; Vaisman et al. 2001).

The scavenger receptor B type I (SR-BI) plays a major role in HDL metabo-lism. It functions as an HDL receptor (Acton et al. 1996) mediating the selective uptake of cholesterol esters from plasma HDL but binds also apoB containing lipoproteins, anionic phospholipids and apoptotic cells (Acton et al. 1996). It has also been shown to promote HDL-mediated cellular cholesterol efflux. SR-BI modulates plasma HDL cholesterol levels and affects HDL particle size and composition (Rigotti et al. 1997). Adenovirus-mediated overexpression of

SR-BI in the liver leads to a significant decrease in plasma HDL concentrations and an increase in cholesterol secretion to the bile (Kozarsky et al. 1997).

The human homolog of SR-BI is CLA-1 (Calvo and Vega 1993). The highest expression of CLA-1 is detected in the adrenal gland, and mRNA is also found in liver, testis and monocytes (Murao et al. 1997). It is also expressed in human atherosclerotic lesions and was found to colocalize with macrophages (Chinetti et al. 2000). The function of CLA-1 in lipoprotein metabolism is unknown but if it is shown to have a function similar to that of SR-BI it will provide a feasible target for interventions in the treatment of lipid disorders and/or atherosclerosis in humans.

3.5
Vulnerable Plaque

Primary prevention of atherosclerosis and plaque formation in the general population seems unlikely in light of the complex pathogenesis of the disease. This means that prevention of the complications of atherosclerosis, such as acute coronary events due to plaque rupture and thrombus formation, is an important goal. Vulnerable plaques are characterized by thin fibrous caps, increased numbers of inflammatory cells and reduced SMC and collagen content. Ruptures usually occur in the shoulder areas of the lipid-rich lesions containing macrophages. Therapeutic strategies include prevention of the degradation of the plaque cap, promotion of extracellular matrix formation and lowering of the lesion lipid and macrophage content.

Vulnerable plaques are characterized by reduced collagen content that can result from decreased synthesis of extracellular matrix by SMCs or increased breakdown by proteases resulting in thinning and weakening of the fibrous cap. Manipulation of cytokines and growth factors to inhibit SMC apoptosis or promote SMC proliferation and stimulation of matrix synthesis could lead to plaque stabilization. On the other hand, excess enhancement of matrix synthesis can lead to increased plaque growth, stenosis and arterial occlusion.

Matrix degradation is increased in unstable plaques and this can lead to thinning of the fibrous cap and result in plaque rupture. Matrix metalloproteinases (MMPs) have the major role in this degradation. Expression of MMPs from SMC and macrophages is increased in atherosclerotic lesions (Galis et al. 1994). MMP activity can be inhibited by increasing the natural inhibitors of matrix metalloproteinases (TIMPs) by gene transfer.

The CD40 receptor belongs to the TNF receptor family and is expressed on SMCs and macrophages. Activated T-lymphocytes can express CD40 ligand, a TNF-like molecule, on their cell surface. Interaction of CD40 ligand with its receptor promotes the expression of atherogenic molecules including MMPs, cytokines, adhesion molecules and tissue factor (Mach et al. 1998). Inhibition of CD40 signaling can modify plaques into a more stable phenotype and also inhibit lesion formation (Mach et al. 1998).

Thrombosis could be prevented with gene transfer of cyclo-oxygenase, hirudin, thrombomodulin or tissue factor pathway inhibitor (Rade et al. 1996; Zoldhelyi et al. 1996). IL-10 also inhibits tissue factor expression by activated monocytes.

4
Conclusion

Atherosclerosis is a complex disease influenced both by genes and environment. Characterization of the pathophysiology and identification of genes involved in atherogenesis has provided many therapeutic targets for intervention with gene therapy. More therapeutic targets will be identified with the use of DNA array technology and this may allow for 'gene cocktails' to be devised to allow better treatment of atherosclerosis (Yla-Herttuala and Alitalo 2003). At the moment, monogenic diseases leading to premature atherosclerosis provide the most attractive targets for gene therapy of atherosclerosis.

Currently the major limitation in gene therapy is the low transfection efficiency achieved in target tissues. Efficiency will be improved with the development of better vectors and gene delivery methods. Immunological tolerance of viral vectors has progressed with the development of new vectors with larger deletions or removal of the viral genes. As vector systems advance and become more efficient, development of targeted and regulated vectors for the treatment of atherosclerosis will become a major focus. Expression in specific target cells will decrease the risk of side effects due to reduced transduction of surrounding tissues, and could even lead to enhanced and prolonged gene expression. Targeted expression can be achieved with the use of tissue specific promoters, genetic modifications of viral capsid proteins or targeting peptides inserted in the viral envelope. Development of regulated expression systems will provide additional safety by allowing for activation of the transgene expression only by administration of pharmacological agents or by certain conditions in vivo like hypoxia or shear stress.

Acknowledgements This work was supported by grants from the Finnish Academy, the National Technology Agency of Finland, Sigrid Juselius foundation and Foundation for Cardiovascular Research.

References

Acton S, Rigotti A, Landschulz KT, Xu S, Hobbs HH, Krieger M (1996) Identification of scavenger receptor SR-BI as a high density lipoprotein receptor. Science 271:518–520

Airenne KJ, Hiltunen MO, Turunen MP, Turunen AM, Laitinen OH, Kulomaa MS, Yla-Herttuala S (2000) Baculovirus-mediated periadventitial gene transfer to rabbit carotid artery. Gene Ther 7:1499–1504

Akkina RK, Walton RM, Chen ML, Li QX, Planelles V, Chen IS (1996) High-efficiency gene transfer into CD34+ cells with a human immunodeficiency virus type 1-based retroviral vector pseudotyped with vesicular stomatitis virus envelope glycoprotein G. J Virol 70:2581–2585

Applebaum-Bowden D, Kobayashi J, Kashyap VS, Brown DR, Berard A, Meyn S, Parrott C, Maeda N, Shamburek R, Brewer HB Jr, Santamarina-Fojo S (1996) Hepatic lipase gene therapy in hepatic lipase-deficient mice. Adenovirus-mediated replacement of a lipolytic enzyme to the vascular endothelium. J Clin Invest 97:799–805

Ashbourne Excoffon KJ, Liu G, Miao L, Wilson JE, McManus BM, Semenkovich CF, Coleman T, Benoit P, Duverger N, Branellec D, Denefle P, Hayden MR, Lewis ME (1997) Correction of hypertriglyceridemia and impaired fat tolerance in lipoprotein lipase-deficient mice by adenovirus-mediated expression of human lipoprotein lipase. Arterioscler Thromb Vasc Biol 17:2532–2539

Assmann G, Nofer JR (2003) Atheroprotective effects of high-density lipoproteins. Annu Rev Med 54:321–341

Aviram M, Rosenblat M, Bisgaier CL, Newton RS, Primo-Parmo SL, La Du BN (1998) Paraoxonase inhibits high-density lipoprotein oxidation and preserves its functions. A possible peroxidative role for paraoxonase. J Clin Invest 101:1581–1590

Belalcazar LM, Merched A, Carr B, Oka K, Chen KH, Pastore L, Beaudet A, Chan L (2003) Long-term stable expression of human apolipoprotein A-I mediated by helper-dependent adenovirus gene transfer inhibits atherosclerosis progression and remodels atherosclerotic plaques in a mouse model of familial hypercholesterolemia. Circulation 107:2726–2732

Benlian P, Degennes JL, Foubert L, Zhang HF, Gagne SE, Hayden M (1996) Premature atherosclerosis in patients with familial chylomicronemia caused by mutations in the lipoprotein lipase gene. N Engl J Med 335:848–854

Benoit P, Emmanuel F, Caillaud JM, Bassinet L, Castro G, Gallix P, Fruchart JC, Branellec D, Denefle P, Duverger N (1999) Somatic gene transfer of human ApoA-I inhibits atherosclerosis progression in mouse models. Circulation 99:105–110

Blatter MC, James RW, Messmer S, Barja F, Pometta D (1993) Identification of a distinct human high-density lipoprotein subspecies defined by a lipoprotein-associated protein, K-45. Identity of K-45 with paraoxonase. Eur J Biochem 211:871–879

Boyce FM, Bucher NL (1996) Baculovirus-mediated gene transfer into mammalian cells. Proc Natl Acad Sci USA 93:2348–2352

Brooks-Wilson A, Marcil M, Clee SM, Zhang LH, Roomp K, van Dam M, Yu L, Brewer C, Collins JA, Molhuizen HO, Loubser O, Ouelette BF, Fichter K, Ashbourne-Excoffon KJ, Sensen CW, Scherer S, Mott S, Denis M, Martindale D, Frohlich J, Morgan K, Koop B, Pimstone S, Kastelein JJ, Hayden MR (1999) Mutations in ABC1 in Tangier disease and familial high-density lipoprotein deficiency. Nat Genet 22:336–345

Brousseau ME, Kauffman RD, Herderick EE, Demosky SJ, Jr., Evans W, Marcovina S, Santamarina-Fojo S, Brewer HB, Jr., Hoeg JM (2000) LCAT modulates atherogenic plasma lipoproteins and the extent of atherosclerosis only in the presence of normal LDL receptors in transgenic rabbits. Arterioscler Thromb Vasc Biol 20:450–458

Brousseau ME, Wang J, Demosky SJJ, Vaisman BL, Talley GD, Santamarina-Fojo S, Brewer HBJ, Hoeg JM (1998) Correction of hypoalphalipoproteinemia in LDL receptor-deficient rabbits by lecithin cholesterol acyltransferase. J Lipid Res 39:1558–1567

Burns JC, Friedmann T, Driever W, Burrascano M, Yee JK (1993) Vesicular stomatitis virus G glycoprotein pseudotyped retroviral vectors: concentration to very high titer and efficient gene transfer into mammalian and nonmammalian cells. Proc Natl Acad Sci USA 90:8033–8037

Calvo D, Vega MA (1993) Identification, primary structure, and distribution of CLA-1, a novel member of the CD36/LIMPII gene family. J Biol Chem 268:18929–18935

Carr AC, Frei B (2001) The nitric oxide congener nitrite inhibits myeloperoxidase/H2O2/ Cl- -mediated modification of low density lipoprotein. J Biol Chem 276:1822–1828

Chen SJ, Wilson JM, Muller DW (1994) Adenovirus-mediated gene transfer of soluble vascular cell adhesion molecule to porcine interposition vein grafts. Circulation 89:1922–1928

Chinetti G, Gbaguidi FG, Griglio S, Mallat Z, Antonucci M, Poulain P, Chapman J, Fruchart JC, Tedgui A, Najib-Fruchart J, Staels B (2000) CLA-1/SR-BI is expressed in atherosclerotic lesion macrophages and regulated by activators of peroxisome proliferator-activated receptors. Circulation 101:2411–2417

Connelly PW, Maguire GF, Lee M, Little JA (1990) Plasma lipoproteins in familial hepatic lipase deficiency. Arteriosclerosis 10:40–48

Dawson TC, Kuziel WA, Osahar TA, Maeda N (1999) Absence of CC chemokine receptor-2 reduces atherosclerosis in apolipoprotein E-deficient mice. Atherosclerosis 143:205–211

Dull T, Zufferey R, Kelly M, Mandel RJ, Nguyen M, Trono D, Naldini L (1998) A third-generation lentivirus vector with a conditional packaging system. J Virol 72:8463–8471

Dunne DW, Resnick D, Greenberg J, Krieger M, Joiner KA (1994) The type I macrophage scavenger receptor binds to gram-positive bacteria and recognizes lipoteichoic acid. Proc Natl Acad Sci USA 91:1863–1867

Ehrhardt A, Xu H, Kay MA (2003) Episomal persistence of recombinant adenoviral vector genomes during the cell cycle in vivo. J Virol 77:7689–7695

Engels B, Cam H, Schuler T, Indraccolo S, Gladow M, Baum C, Blankenstein T, Uckert W (2003) Retroviral vectors for high-level transgene expression in T lymphocytes. Hum Gene Ther 14:1155–1168

Follenzi A, Sabatino G, Lombardo A, Boccaccio C, Naldini L (2002) Efficient gene delivery and targeted expression to hepatocytes in vivo by improved lentiviral vectors. Hum Gene Ther 13:243–260

Fraser I, Hughes D, Gordon S (1993) Divalent cation-independent macrophage adhesion inhibited by monoclonal antibody to murine scavenger receptor. Nature 364:343–346

Galis ZS, Sukhova GK, Lark MW, Libby P (1994) Increased expression of matrix metallopro-teinases and matrix degrading activity in vulnerable regions of human atherosclerotic plaques. J Clin Invest 94:2493–2503

Gordon DA, Wetterau JR, Gregg RE (1995) Microsomal triglyceride transfer protein: a pro-tein complex required for the assembly of lipoprotein particles. Trends Cell Biol 5:317–321

Gordon DJ, Probstfield JL, Garrison RJ, Neaton JD, Castelli WP, Knoke JD, Jacobs DR, Jr., Bangdiwala S, Tyroler HA (1989) High-density lipoprotein cholesterol and cardiovascu-lar disease. Four prospective American studies. Circulation 79:8–15

Gordon T, Castelli WP, Hjortland MC, Kannel WB, Dawber TR (1977) High density lipopro-tein as a protective factor against coronary heart disease. The Framingham Study. Am J Med 62:707–714

Gosling J, Slaymaker S, Gu L, Tseng S, Zlot CH, Young SG, Rollins BJ, Charo IF (1999) MCP-1 deficiency reduces susceptibility to atherosclerosis in mice that overexpress human apolipoprotein B. J Clin Invest 103:773–778

Grossman M, Rader DJ, Muller DW, Kolansky DM, Kozarsky K, Clark BJI, Stein EA, Lupien PJ, Brewer HB, Jr., Raper SE, Wilson JM (1995) A pilot study of ex vivo gene therapy for homozygous familial hypercholesterolaemia. Nat Med 1:1148–114

Gruchala M, Bhardwaj S, Pajusola K, Roy H, Rissanen T, Kokina I, Kholova I, Markkanen J, Rutanen J, Heikura T, Alitalo K, Büeler H, Yla-Herttuala S (2004) Gene transfer into rabbit arteries with adeno-associated virus and adenovirus vectors. J Gene Med 6:545–554

Gu L, Okada Y, Clinton SK, Gerard C, Sukhova GK, Libby P, Rollins BJ (1998) Absence of monocyte chemoattractant protein-1 reduces atherosclerosis in low density lipoprotein receptor-deficient mice. Mol Cell 2:275–281

Hacein-Bey-Abina S, Le Deist F, Carlier F, Bouneaud C, Hue C, De Villartay JP, Thrasher AJ, Wulffraat N, Sorensen R, Dupuis-Girod S, Fischer A, Davies EG, Kuis W, Leiva L, Cavazzana-Calvo M (2002) Sustained correction of X-linked severe combined immun-odeficiency by ex vivo gene therapy. N Engl J Med 346:1185–1193

Häkkinen T, Luoma JS, Hiltunen MO, Macphee CH, Milliner KJ, Patel L, Rice SQ, Tew DG, Karkola K, Ylä-Herttuala S (1999) Lipoprotein-associated phospholipase A(2), platelet-activating factor acetylhydrolase, is expressed by macrophages in human and rabbit atherosclerotic lesions. Arterioscler Thromb Vasc Biol 19:2909–2917

Harris JD, Schepelmann S, Athanasopoulos T, Graham IR, Stannard AK, Mohri Z, Hill V, Hassall DG, Owen JS, Dickson G (2002) Inhibition of atherosclerosis in apolipoprotein-E-deficient mice following muscle transduction with adeno-associated virus vectors encoding human apolipoprotein-E. Gene Ther 9:21–29

Hasty AH, Linton MF, Brandt SJ, Babaev VR, Gleaves LA, Fazio S (1999) Retroviral gene therapy in ApoE-deficient mice: ApoE expression in the artery wall reduces early foam cell lesion formation. Circulation 99:2571–2576

Hegele RA, Little JA, Vezina C, Maguire GF, Tu L, Wolever TS, Jenkins DJ, Connelly PW (1993) Hepatic lipase deficiency. Clinical, biochemical, and molecular genetic characteristics. Arterioscler Thromb 13:720–728

Hughes SD, Rouy D, Navaratnam N, Scott J, Rubin EM (1996) Gene transfer of cytidine deam-inase apoBEC-1 lowers lipoprotein(a) in transgenic mice and induces apolipoprotein B editing in rabbits. Hum Gene Ther 7:39–49

Jalkanen J, Leppanen P, Narvanen O, Greaves DR, Yla-Herttuala S (2003) Adenovirus-mediated gene transfer of a secreted decoy human macrophage scavenger receptor (SR-AI) in LDL receptor knock-out mice. Atherosclerosis 169:95–103

Jamil H, Gordon DA, Eustice DC, Brooks CM, Dickson JK, Jr., Chen Y, Ricci B, Chu CH, Harrity TW, Ciosek CP, Jr., Biller SA, Gregg RE, Wetterau JR (1996) An inhibitor of the microsomal triglyceride transfer protein inhibits apoB secretion from HepG2 cells. Proc Natl Acad Sci USA 93:11991–11995

Jonas A (1991) Lecithin-cholesterol acyltransferase in the metabolism of high-density lipoproteins. Biochim Biophys Acta 1084:205–220

Kankkonen H, Vähäkangas E, Marr R, Pakkanen T, Laurema A, Leppänen P, Jalkanen J, Verma I, Ylä-Herttuala S (2004) Long-term lowering of serum cholesterol levels in LDL-receptor deficient WHHL rabbits by gene therapy. Mol Ther 9:548–556

Kanters E, Pasparakis M, Gijbels MJ, Vergouwe MN, Partouns-Hendriks I, Fijneman RJ, Clausen BE, Forster I, Kockx MM, Rajewsky K, Kraal G, Hofker MH, de Winther MP (2003) Inhibition of NF-kappaB activation in macrophages increases atherosclerosis in LDL receptor-deficient mice. J Clin Invest 112:1176–1185

Kay MA, Glorioso JC, Naldini L (2001) Viral vectors for gene therapy: the art of turning infectious agents into vehicles of therapeutics. Nat Med 7:33–40

Kochanek S, Clemens PR, Mitani K, Chen HH, Chan S, Caskey CT (1996) A new adenoviral vector: Replacement of all viral coding sequences with 28 kb of DNA independently expressing both full-length dystrophin and beta-galactosidase. Proc Natl Acad Sci USA 93:5731–5736

Koponen JK, Kankkonen H, Kannasto J, Wirth T, Hillen W, Bujard H, Yla-Herttuala S (2003) Doxycycline-regulated lentiviral vector system with a novel reverse transactivator rtTA2S-M2 shows a tight control of gene expression in vitro and in vivo. Gene Ther 10:459–466

Kozarsky KF, Bonen DK, Giannoni F, Funahashi T, Wilson JM, Davidson NO (1996) Hepatic expression of the catalytic subunit of the apolipoprotein B mRNA editing enzyme (apobec-1) ameliorates hypercholesterolemia in LDL receptor-deficient rabbits. Hum Gene Ther 7:943–957

Kozarsky KF, Donahee MH, Rigotti A, Iqbal SN, Edelman ER, Krieger M (1997) Overexpression of the HDL receptor SR-BI alters plasma HDL and bile cholesterol levels. Nature 387:414–417

Laitinen M, Pakkanen T, Donetti E, Baetta R, Luoma J, Lehtolainen P, Viita H, Agrawal R, Miyanohara A, Friedmann T, Risau W, Martin JF, Soma M, Ylä-Herttuala S (1997) Gene transfer into the carotid artery using an adventitial collar: comparison of the effectiveness of the plasmid- liposome complexes, retroviruses, pseudotyped retroviruses, and adenoviruses. Hum Gene Ther 8:1645–1650

Laukkanen J, Yla-Herttuala S (2002) Genes involved in atherosclerosis. Exp Nephrol 10:150–163

Laukkanen MO, Kivelä A, Rissanen TT, Rutanen J, Kärkkäinen MK, Leppänen O, Brasen JH, Ylä-Herttuala S (2002) Adenovirus-mediated extracellular superoxide dismutase gene therapy reduces neointima formation in balloon denuded rabbit aorta. Circulation 106:1999–2003

Leeuwenburgh C, Rasmussen JE, Hsu FF, Mueller DM, Pennathur S, Heinecke JW (1997) Mass spectrometric quantification of markers for protein oxidation by tyrosyl radical, copper, and hydroxyl radical in low density lipoprotein isolated from human atherosclerotic plaques. J Biol Chem 272:3520–3526

Li Z, Schwieger M, Lange C, Kraunus J, Sun H, van den AE, Modlich U, Serinsoz E, Will E, von Laer D, Stocking C, Fehse B, Schiedlmeier B, Baum C (2003) Predictable and efficient retroviral gene transfer into murine bone marrow repopulating cells using a defined vector dose. Exp Hematol 31:1206–1214

Lieu HD, Withycombe SK, Walker Q, Rong JX, Walzem RL, Wong JS, Hamilton RL, Fisher EA, Young SG (2003) Eliminating atherogenesis in mice by switching off hepatic lipoprotein secretion. Circulation 107:1315–1321

Lusis AJ (2000) Atherosclerosis. Nature 407:233–241

Mach F, Schonbeck U, Sukhova GK, Atkinson E, Libby P (1998) Reduction of atherosclerosis in mice by inhibition of CD40 signalling. Nature 394:200–203

Mallat Z, Heymes C, Ohan J, Faggin E, Leseche G, Tedgui A (1999) Expression of interleukin-10 in advanced human atherosclerotic plaques: relation to inducible nitric oxide synthase expression and cell death. Arterioscler Thromb Vasc Biol 19:611–616

Malle E, Waeg G, Schreiber R, Grone EF, Sattler W, Grone HJ (2000) Immunohistochemical evidence for the myeloperoxidase/H2O2/halide system in human atherosclerotic lesions: colocalization of myeloperoxidase and hypochlorite-modified proteins. Eur J Biochem 267:4495–4503

Miyoshi H, Blömer U, Takahashi M, Gage FH, Verma IM (1998) Development of a self-inactivating lentivirus vector. J Virol 72:8150–8157

Miyoshi H, Smith KA, Mosier DE, Verma IM, Torbett BE (1999) Transduction of human CD34+ cells that mediate long-term engraftment of NOD/SCID mice by HIV vectors. Science 283:682–686

Monahan PE, Samulski RJ (2000) AAV vectors: is clinical success on the horizon? Gene Ther 2000 7:24–30

Morishita R, Yamada S, Yamamoto K, Tomita N, Kida I, Sakurabayashi I, Kikuchi A, Kaneda Y, Lawn R, Higaki J, Ogihara T (1998) Novel therapeutic strategy for atherosclerosis: ribozyme oligonucleotides against apolipoprotein(a) selectively inhibit apolipoprotein(a) but not plasminogen gene expression. Circulation 98:1898–1904

Murao K, Terpstra V, Green SR, Kondratenko N, Steinberg D, Quehenberger O (1997) Characterization of CLA-1, a human homologue of rodent scavenger receptor BI, as a receptor for high density lipoprotein and apoptotic thymocytes. J Biol Chem 272:17551–17557

Muul LM, Tuschong LM, Soenen SL, Jagadeesh GJ, Ramsey WJ, Long Z, Carter CS, Garabedian EK, Alleyne M, Brown M, Bernstein W, Schurman SH, Fleisher TA, Leitman SF, Dunbar CE, Blaese RM, Candotti F (2003) Persistence and expression of the adenosine deaminase gene for 12 years and immune reaction to gene transfer components: long-term results of the first clinical gene therapy trial. Blood 101:2563–2569

Nakamura T, Morishita R, Asai T, Tsuboniwa N, Aoki M, Sakonjo H, Yamasaki K, Hashiya N, Kaneda Y, Ogihara T (2002) Molecular strategy using cis-element 'decoy' of E2F binding site inhibits neointimal formation in porcine balloon-injured coronary artery model. Gene Ther 9:488–494

Naldini L, Blömer U, Gallay P, Ory D, Mulligan R, Gage FH, Verma IM, Trono D (1996) In vivo gene delivery and stable transduction of nondividing cells by a lentiviral vector. Science 272:263–267

Nicklin SA, Buening H, Dishart KL, de Alwis M, Girod A, Hacker U, Thrasher AJ, Ali RR, Hallek M, Baker AH (2001) Efficient and selective AAV2-mediated gene transfer directed to human vascular endothelial cells. Mol Ther 4:174–181

Noto H, Hara M, Karasawa K, Iso O, Satoh H, Togo M, Hashimoto Y, Yamada Y, Kosaka T, Kawamura M, Kimura S, Tsukamoto K (2003) Human plasma platelet-activating factor acetylhydrolase binds to all the murine lipoproteins, conferring protection against oxidative stress. Arterioscler Thromb Vasc Biol 23:829–835

Oka K, Pastore L, Kim IH, Merched A, Nomura S, Lee HJ, Merched-Sauvage M, Arden-Riley C, Lee B, Finegold M, Beaudet A, Chan L (2001) Long-term stable correction of low-density lipoprotein receptor-deficient mice with a helper-dependent adenoviral vector expressing the very low-density lipoprotein receptor. Circulation 103:1274–1281

Ory DS, Neugeboren BA, Mulligan RC (1996) A stable human-derived packaging cell line for production of high titer retrovirus/vesicular stomatitis virus g pseudotypes. Proc Natl Acad Sci USA 93:11400–11406

Pajusola K, Gruchala M, Joch H, Luscher TF, Yla-Herttuala S, Bueler H (2002) Cell-type-specific characteristics modulate the transduction efficiency of adeno-associated virus type 2 and restrain infection of endothelial cells. J Virol 76:11530–11540

Pakkanen TM, Laitinen M, Hippeläinen M, Hiltunen MO, Alhava E, Ylä-Herttuala S (2000) Periadventitial lacZ gene transfer to pig carotid arteries using a biodegradable collagen collar or a wrap of collagen sheet with adenoviruses and plasmid-liposome complexes. J Gene Med 2:52–60

Pakkanen TM, Laitinen M, Hippeläinen M, Hiltunen MO, Lehtolainen P, Leppänen P, Luoma JS, Alhava E, Ylä-Herttuala S (1999a) Improved gene transfer efficiency in liver with vesicular stomatitis virus G-protein pseudotyped retrovirus after partial liver resection and thymidine kinase-ganciclovir pre-treatment. Pharmacol Res 40:451–457

Pakkanen TM, Laitinen M, Hippeläinen M, Kallionpää H, Lehtolainen P, Leppänen P, Luoma JS, Tarvainen R, Alhava E, Ylä-Herttuala S (1999b) Enhanced plasma cholesterol lowering effect of retrovirus- mediated LDL receptor gene transfer to WHHL rabbit liver after improved surgical technique and stimulation of hepatocyte proliferation by combined partial liver resection and thymidine kinase ganciclovir treatment. Gene Ther 6:34–41

Parks R, Evelegh C, Graham F (1999) Use of helper-dependent adenoviral vectors of alternative serotypes permits repeat vector administration. Gene Ther 6:1565–1573

Pastore L, Morral N, Zhou H, Garcia R, Parks RJ, Kochanek S, Graham FL, Lee B, Beaudet AL (1999) Use of a liver-specific promoter reduces immune response to the transgene in adenoviral vectors. Hum Gene Ther 10:1773–1781

Pieroni L, La Monica N (2001) Towards the use of baculovirus as a gene therapy vector. Curr Opin Mol Ther 3:464–467

Pinderski Oslund LJ, Hedrick CC, Olvera T, Hagenbaugh A, Territo M, Berliner JA, Fyfe AI (1999) Interleukin-10 blocks atherosclerotic events in vitro and in vivo. Arterioscler Thromb Vasc Biol 19:2847–2853

Platt N, da Silva RP, Gordon S (1999) Class A scavenger receptors and the phagocytosis of apoptotic cells. Immunol Lett 65:15–19

Pruchnic R, Cao B, Peterson ZQ, Xiao X, Li J, Samulski RJ, Epperly M, Huard J (2000) The use of adeno-associated virus to circumvent the maturation-dependent viral transduction of muscle fibers. Hum Gene Ther 11:521–536

Quarck R, De Geest B, Stengel D, Mertens A, Lox M, Theilmeier G, Michiels C, Raes M, Bult H, Collen D, Van Veldhoven P, Ninio E, Holvoet P (2001) Adenovirus-mediated gene transfer of human platelet-activating factor-acetylhydrolase prevents injury-induced neointima formation and reduces spontaneous atherosclerosis in apolipoprotein E-deficient mice. Circulation 103:2495–2500

Rade JJ, Schulick AH, Virmani R, Dichek DA (1996) Local adenoviral-mediated expression of recombinant hirudin reduces neointima formation after arterial injury. Nat Med 2:293–298

Rader DJ, Cohen J, Hobbs HH (2003) Monogenic hypercholesterolemia: new insights in pathogenesis and treatment. J Clin Invest 111:1795–1803

Rigotti A, Trigatti BL, Penman M, Rayburn H, Herz J, Krieger M (1997) A targeted mutation in the murine gene encoding the high density lipoprotein (HDL) receptor scavenger receptor class B type I reveals its key role in HDL metabolism. Proc Natl Acad Sci USA 94:12610–12615

Rissanen TT, Markkanen JE, Gruchala M, Heikura T, Puranen A, Kettunen MI, Kholova I, Kauppinen RA, Achen MG, Stacker SA, Alitalo K, Yla-Herttuala S (2003) VEGF-D is the strongest angiogenic and lymphangiogenic effector among VEGFs delivered into skeletal muscle via adenoviruses. Circ Res 92:1098–1106

Ross R (1999) Mechanisms of disease—Atherosclerosis—An inflammatory disease. N Engl J Med 340:115–126

Rutanen J, Markkanen J, Yla-Herttuala S (2002) Gene therapy for restenosis: current status. Drugs 62:1575–1585

Scherer LJ, Rossi JJ (2003) Approaches for the sequence-specific knockdown of mRNA. Nat Biotechnol 21:1457–1465

Shimada M, Ishibashi S, Inaba T, Yagyu H, Harada K, Osuga JI, Ohashi K, Yazaki Y, Yamada N (1996) Suppression of diet-induced atherosclerosis in low density lipoprotein receptor knockout mice overexpressing lipoprotein lipase. Proc Natl Acad Sci USA 93:7242–7246

Singaraja RR, Fievet C, Castro G, James ER, Hennuyer N, Clee SM, Bissada N, Choy JC, Fruchart JC, McManus BM, Staels B, Hayden MR (2002) Increased ABCA1 activity protects against atherosclerosis. J Clin Invest 110:35–42

Sirtori CR, Calabresi L, Franceschini G, Baldassarre D, Amato M, Johansson J, Salvetti M, Monteduro C, Zulli R, Muiesan ML, Agabiti-Rosei E (2001) Cardiovascular status of carriers of the apolipoprotein A-I (Milano) mutant: the Limone sul Garda study. Circulation 103:1949–1954

Snyder RO, Miao CH, Patijn GA, Spratt SK, Danos O, Nagy D, Gown AM, Winther B, Meuse L, Cohen LK, Thompson AR, Kay MA (1997) Persistent and therapeutic concentrations of human factor IX in mice after hepatic gene transfer of recombinant AAV vectors. Nat Genet 16:270–276

Steinberg D, Witztum JL (2002) Is the oxidative modification hypothesis relevant to human atherosclerosis? Do the antioxidant trials conducted to date refute the hypothesis? Circulation 105:2107–2111

Stone D, Xiong W, Williams JC, David A, Lowenstein PR, Castro MG (2003) Adenovirus expression of IL-1 and NF-kappaB inhibitors does not inhibit acute adenoviral-induced brain inflammation, but delays immune system-mediated elimination of transgene expression. Mol Ther 8:400–411

Sun L, Li J, Xiao X (2000) Overcoming adeno-associated virus vector size limitation through viral DNA heterodimerization. Nat Med 6:599–602

Tangirala RK, Tsukamoto K, Chun SH, Usher D, Pure E, Rader DJ (1999) Regression of atherosclerosis induced by liver-directed gene transfer of apolipoprotein A-I in mice. Circulation 100:1816–1822

Teng B, Ishida B, Forte TM, Blumenthal S, Song LZ, Gotto AMJ, Chan L (1997) Effective lowering of plasma, LDL, and esterified cholesterol in LDL receptor-knockout mice by adenovirus-mediated gene delivery of ApoB mRNA editing enzyme (Apobec1). Arterioscler Thromb Vasc Biol 17:889–897

Terpstra V, van Amersfoort ES, van Velzen AG, Kuiper J, Van Berkel TJ (2000) Hepatic and extrahepatic scavenger receptors: function in relation to disease. Arterioscler Thromb Vasc Biol 20:1860–1872

Tsukamoto K, Tangirala R, Chun SH, Pure E, Rader DJ (1999) Rapid regression of atherosclerosis induced by liver-directed gene transfer of ApoE in ApoE-deficient mice. Arterioscler Thromb Vasc Biol 19:2162–2170

Turunen MP, Puhakka HL, Koponen JK, Hiltunen MO, Rutanen J, Leppanen O, Turunen AM, Narvanen A, Newby AC, Baker AH, Yla-Herttuala S (2002) Peptide-retargeted adenovirus encoding a tissue inhibitor of metalloproteinase-1 decreases restenosis after intravascular gene transfer. Mol Ther 6:306–312

Turunen P, Jalkanen J, Heikura P, Puhakka H, Karppi J, Nyyssönen K, Ylä-Herttuala S (2004) Adenivirus-mediated gene transfer of Lp-PLA2 reduces LDL degradation and foam cell formationin vitro. J Lipid Res 45:1633–1639

Tward A, Xia YR, Wang XP, Shi YS, Park C, Castellani LW, Lusis AJ, Shih DM (2002) Decreased atherosclerotic lesion formation in human serum paraoxonase transgenic mice. Circulation 106:484–490

Vaisman BL, Lambert G, Amar M, Joyce C, Ito T, Shamburek RD, Cain WJ, Fruchart-Najib J, Neufeld ED, Remaley AT, Brewer HB, Jr., Santamarina-Fojo S (2001) ABCA1 overexpression leads to hyperalphalipoproteinemia and increased biliary cholesterol excretion in transgenic mice. J Clin Invest 108:303–309

Von Der Thusen JH, Kuiper J, Fekkes ML, De Vos P, Van Berkel TJ, Biessen EA (2001) Attenuation of atherogenesis by systemic and local adenovirus-mediated gene transfer of interleukin-10 in LDLr-/- mice. FASEB J 15:2730–2732

Walther W, Stein U (1996) Cell type specific and inducible promoters for vectors in gene therapy as an approach for cell targeting. J Molecular Med 74:379–392

Wang N, Silver DL, Thiele C, Tall AR (2001) ATP-binding cassette transporter A1 (ABCA1) functions as a cholesterol efflux regulatory protein. J Biol Chem 276:23742–23747

Yan Z, Zhang Y, Duan D, Engelhardt JF (2000) From the cover: trans-splicing vectors expand the utility of adeno-associated virus for gene therapy. Proc Natl Acad Sci USA 97:6716–6721

Yang Y, Li Q, Ertl HC, Wilson JM (1995) Cellular and humoral immune responses to viral antigens create barriers to lung-directed gene therapy with recombinant adenoviruses. J Virol 69:2004–2015

Yla-Herttuala S, Alitalo K (2003) Gene transfer as a tool to induce therapeutic vascular growth. Nat. Med. 9:694–701

Yla-Herttuala S, Lipton BA, Rosenfeld ME, Sarkioja T, Yoshimura T, Leonard EJ, Witztum JL, Steinberg D (1991a) Expression of monocyte chemoattractant protein 1 in macrophage-rich areas of human and rabbit atherosclerotic lesions. Proc Natl Acad Sci USA 88:5252–5256

Yla-Herttuala S, Martin JF (2000) Cardiovascular gene therapy. Lancet 355:213–222

Yla-Herttuala S, Nikkari T, Hirvonen J, Laaksonen H, Mottonen M, Pesonen E, Raekallio J, Akerblom HK (1986) Biochemical composition of coronary arteries in Finnish children. Arteriosclerosis 6:230–236

Yla-Herttuala S, Palinski W, Rosenfeld ME, Parthasarathy S, Carew TE, Butler S, Witztum JL, Steinberg D (1989) Evidence for the presence of oxidatively modified low density lipoprotein in atherosclerotic lesions of rabbit and man. J Clin Invest 84:1086–1095

Yla-Herttuala S, Rosenfeld ME, Parthasarathy S, Sigal E, Sarkioja T, Witztum JL, Steinberg D (1991b) Gene expression in macrophage-rich human atherosclerotic lesions. 15-lipoxygenase and acetyl low density lipoprotein receptor messenger RNA colocalize with oxidation specific lipid-protein adducts. J Clin Invest 87:1146–1152

Yoshimura S, Morishita R, Hayashi K, Yamamoto K, Nakagami H, Kaneda Y, Sakai N, Ogihara T (2001) Inhibition of intimal hyperplasia after balloon injury in rat carotid artery model using cis-element 'decoy' of nuclear factor-kappaB binding site as a novel molecular strategy. Gene Ther 8:1635–1642

Zoldhelyi P, McNatt J, Xu XM, Loose-Mitchell D, Meidell RS, Clubb FJJ, Buja LM, Willerson JT, Wu KK (1996) Prevention of arterial thrombosis by adenovirus-mediated transfer of cyclooxygenase gene. Circulation 93:10–17

Subject Index

Printing: Krips bv, Meppel
Binding: Litges & Dopf, Heppenheim